Robert J. Townley

Immunopharmacology of
Allergic Diseases

CLINICAL ALLERGY AND IMMUNOLOGY

Series Editor

MICHAEL A. KALINER, M.D.

Medical Director
Institute for Asthma and Allergy
Washington, D.C.

1. Sinusitis: Pathophysiology and Treatment, *edited by Howard M. Druce*
2. Eosinophils in Allergy and Inflammation, *edited by Gerald J. Gleich and A. Barry Kay*
3. Molecular and Cellular Biology of the Allergic Response, *edited by Arnold I. Levinson and Yvonne Paterson*
4. Neuropeptides in Respiratory Medicine, *edited by Michael A. Kaliner, Peter J. Barnes, Gert H. H. Kunkel, and James N. Baraniuk*
5. Provocation Testing in Clinical Practice, *edited by Sheldon L. Spector*
6. Mast Cell Proteases in Immunology and Biology, *edited by George H. Caughey*
7. Histamine and H_1-Receptor Antagonists in Allergic Disease, *edited by F. Estelle R. Simons*
8. Immunopharmacology of Allergic Diseases, *edited by Robert G. Townley and Devendra K. Agrawal*

ADDITIONAL VOLUMES IN PREPARATION

Indoor Air Pollution and Health, *edited by Emil J. Bardana, Jr., and Anthony Montanaro*

Genetics of Allergy and Asthma: Methods for Investigative Studies, *edited by Malcolm Blumenthal and Bengt Björkstén*

Immunopharmacology of Allergic Diseases

edited by
Robert G. Townley
Devendra K. Agrawal

Creighton University School of Medicine
Omaha, Nebraska

Marcel Dekker, Inc.

New York•Basel•Hong Kong

Library of Congress Cataloging-in-Publication Data

Immunopharmacology of allergic diseases / edited by Robert G. Townley, Devendra K. Agrawal.
  p. cm. — (Clinical allergy and immunology ; 8)
  Includes index.
  ISBN 0-8247-9513-X (hardcover : alk. paper)
  1. Allergy—Pathophysiology. 2. Allergy—Chemotherapy. 3. Immunopharma-cology. I. Townley, Robert G. II. Agrawal, Devendra K. III. Series.
  [DNLM: 1. Hypersensitivity—drug therapy. 2. Hypersensitivity—immunology. 3. Anti-Allergic Agents—therapeutic use. 4. Anti-Allergic Agents—immunology. 5. Immunotherapy.   W1 CL652 v. 8 1996 / WD 300 I336 1996]
  RC585.I446 1996
  616.97'079—dc20
  DNLM/DLC
  for Library of Congress   96-20570
                                                                        CIP

The publisher offers discounts on this book when ordered in bulk quantities. For more information, write to Special Sales/Professional Marketing at the address below.

This book is printed on acid-free paper.

Marcel Dekker, Inc.
270 Madison Avenue, New York, New York 10016

Current printing (last digit):
10 9 8 7 6 5 4 3 2 1

PRINTED IN THE UNITED STATES OF AMERICA

Series Introduction

I well remember when *Immunopharmacology of the Lung* was published because it represented the beginning of an era where immunology, pharmacology, and allergy-asthma were combined. That book brought a lot of attention to the mechanisms involved in both the pathogenesis and treatment of asthma, and helped define the course that research in asthma was to follow. Thus, when we were considering which direction to take the "Clinical Allergy and Immunology" series, it seemed timely and appropriate to develop a new book on the immunopharmacology of allergic diseases. The opportunity to recruit Robert Townley to be the senior editor occurred in Paris while he and I were attending an international meeting on asthma. Dr. Townley has devoted himself to this topic throughout his career and was the perfect choice. When presented with the chance to create this book, he did not hesitate to accept. In fact, the only problem we encountered with this book was in limiting the topics to a single text rather than two!

Dr. Townley and his colleagues have assembled an international team of experts to construct an exciting book that combines basic science with clinical needs. The contributors have produced first-rate chapters on a wide range of topics and have created a book that will be of use to both investigators and clinicians.

Clinicians are faced with the dilemma of an ever-increasing body of clinical science to follow and an ever-changing science base to understand. Many clinicians complain that they do not know where to turn in their attempts to keep up. Let me suggest that books like this one allow clinicians to overview those areas of science that apply to their needs. In this text, Drs. Townley and Agrawal have brought together eloquent reviews of the most current processes involved in cell activation, the cells involved in the allergic response, the mediators of allergy, and how these advances apply to the allergic diseases. I for one have found this book essential for keeping abreast of the field as we move to the next century and recommend it to all clinicians in this field.

Michael A. Kaliner

iii

Preface

In 1937, when Bauer and Staub began using antihistaminic drugs for the symptomatic treatment of allergic manifestations, a new area of immunopharmacology emerged. Shortly thereafter, immunosuppressive drugs for use in transplantation immunity were developed, and Benacerraf discovered genetic control of the immune response. In the last decade, with the development of genetic engineering technology, there has been an exponential growth in our understanding of the complex network of hematopoietic growth factors, interleukins, and cell adhesion molecules.

Some 13 years have passed since the publication of *Immunopharmacology of the Lung* by H. H. Newball. At that time, the major focus was on histamine as the mediator of immediate hypersensitivity. The development of molecular biology techniques and our understanding of novel allergic mediators have made rapid strides recently and we have attempted to place the role of these mediators in perspective and to point out some of the complexities and questions that remain to be resolved.

This book provides clinicians and scientists with a comprehensive review of the ever-changing field of immunopharmacology of allergic diseases, and we hope that it will provide an important link between a number of other volumes in this series. We have divided this book into four major sections. Part I, Basic Aspects of Immunopharmacology, addresses receptor-response coupling and lymphokine-induced transmembrane signaling, as well as structure and involvement of the IgE receptors. The role of cell adhesion molecules in allergic diseases, the mechanisms underlying the release of chemical mediators, and the immunological basis for the action of immune substances are presented. Part II, Inflammatory Cells in Allergic Diseases, includes a discussion on the differentiation and maturation of these cells along with their innervation, subtypes, and function. Part III, Inflammatory Mediators in Allergic Diseases, presents state-of-the-art reviews on neuropeptides, histamine releasing factors and their inhibitors, cytokines, nitric oxide, leukotrienes, and platelet-activating factors, as well as on the role of these cells and mediators, in particular, in allergic airway diseases. Finally, Part IV focuses on the clinical aspect of immunopharmacology and allergy, and includes adrenergic agents, phosphodiesterase inhibitors, potential agents that affect ion channels in the airways, neuropeptides, antihistamines, agents that affect mast cells and their degranulation, and corticosteroids.

The contributors to this book are internationally recognized authorities in their fields. Their contributions to this volume are truly at the cutting edge of research and we wish to express our sincerest thanks to all of them for their efforts and patience during the preparation of this book.

The editors wish to give special mention to Julie Boilesen, Dori Kojima, Susan Donahoe, and Cristine Mito for their many hours of untiring work with typing, correspondence, filing, proofreading, and indexing.

Robert G. Townley
Devendra K. Agrawal

Contents

Contributors

Devendra K. Agrawal, Ph.D.   Associate Professor, Departments of Internal Medicine and Medical Microbiology and Immunology, Creighton University School of Medicine, Omaha, Nebraska

Rafeul Alam, M.D., Ph.D.   Director, Division of Allergy and Immunology, Department of Internal Medicine, The University of Texas Medical Branch, Galveston, Texas

Bernard Arnoux, Ph.D.   Clinique des Maladies Respiratoires and INSERM, Hopital Arnaud de Villeneuve, Montpellier, France

James N. Baraniuk, M.D.   Assistant Professor, Department of Medicine, Georgetown University, Washington, D.C.

Peter J. Barnes, M.D.   Professor, Department of Thoracic Medicine, National Heart and Lung Institute, London, England

Jean Bousquet, M.D., Ph.D.   Professor, Clinique des Maladies Respiratoires and INSERM, Hopital Arnaud de Villeneuve, Montpellier, France

Joshua A. Boyce, M.D.   Harvard Medical School and Department of Rheumatology and Immunology, Brigham and Women's Hospital, Boston, Massachusetts

Pierre G. Braquet, Ph.D., D.Sc.   President, Bio-Inova, Plaisir, France

William W. Busse, M.D.   Professor, Department of Medicine, University of Wisconsin, Madison, Wisconsin

Pascal Chanez, M.D., Ph.D.   Clinique des Maladies Respiratoires and INSERM, Hopital Arnaud de Villeneuve, Montpellier, France

Anoop J. Chauhan, M.R.C.P.   MRC Training Fellow, University Medicine, University of Southampton, Southampton, England

Daniel H. Conrad   Professor, Department of Microbiology and Immunology, Virginia Commonwealth University, Richmond, Virginia

John J. Costa, M.D.   Instructor and Clinical Associate, Departments of Pathology and Medicine, Beth Israel Hospital and Harvard Medical School, Boston, Massachusetts

I. Caroline Crocker, M.Sc.   Creighton University School of Medicine, Omaha, Nebraska

Marcelle Damon, M.D.*   INSERM, Montpellier, France.

Judah A. Denburg, M.D., F.R.C.P.   Professor, Department of Medicine, McMaster University, Hamilton, Ontario, Canada

Charles A. Dinarello, M.D.   Professor, Department of Medicine, Tufts University School of Medicine and New England Medical Center, Boston, Massachusetts

Roy J. Duhe, Ph.D.   Biological Carcinogenesis and Development Program, Program Resources, Inc./Dyn Corp., National Cancer Institute, Frederick Cancer Research and Development Center, Frederick, Maryland

Gerald A. Evans, Ph.D.   Biological Carcinogenesis and Development Program, Program Resources, Inc./Dyn Corp., National Cancer Institute, Frederick Cancer Research and Development Center, Frederick, Maryland

William L. Farrar, Ph.D.   Cytokine Molecular Mechanisms Section, Laboratory of Immunoregulation, Biological Response Modifiers Program, National Cancer Institute, Frederick Cancer Research and Development Center, Frederick, Maryland

Stephen J. Galli, M.D.   Director, Division of Experimental Pathology, Department of Pathology, Beth Israel Hospital, and Professor of Pathology, Harvard Medical School, Boston, Massachusetts

Mark A. Giembycz, B.Sc., Ph.D.   Department of Thoracic Medicine, Royal Brompton National Heart and Lung Institute, London, England

Philippe Godard, M.D.   Professor, Clinique de Maladies Respiratoires and INSERM, Hopital Arnaud de Villeneuve, Montpellier, France

Edward J. Goetzl, M.D.   Professor of Medicine and Microbiology, Director of Allergy/ Immunology, University of California, San Francisco, California

J. Andrew Grant, M.D.   Professor, Department of Medicine, Microbiology, and Immunology, The University of Texas Medical Branch, Galveston, Texas

Stephen T. Holgate, M.D., D.Sc. F.R.C.P.   MRC Clinical Professor of Immunopharmacology, Honorary Consultant Physician, University Medicine, University of Southampton, Southampton, England

Russell J. Hopp, D.O.   Professor, Department of Pediatrics, Creighton University School of Medicine, Omaha, Nebraska

David Hosford, Ph.D.   Director of Research and Development Coordination, Institut Henri Beaufour, Le Plessis Robinson, France

---

*Deceased.

O. M. Zack Howard, Ph.D.   Biological Carcinogenesis and Development Program, Program Resources, Inc./Dyn Corp., National Cancer Institute, Frederick Cancer Research and Development Center, Frederick, Maryland

David A. Ingram, M.D.   Department of Pediatrics, University of California, San Francisco, California

Yoshinori Katada, M.D.   Department of Internal Medicine III, Osaka University Medical School, Osaka, Japan

Arthur F. Kavanaugh, M.D.   Assistant Professor, Department of Internal Medicine, University of Texas Southwestern Medical Center, Dallas, Texas

Robert A. Kirken, Ph.D.   Laboratory of Molecular Immunoregulation, Cytokine Mechanism Section, Biological Response Modifiers Program, National Cancer Institute, Frederick Cancer Research and Development Center, Frederick, Maryland

Tadamitsu Kishimoto, M.D., Ph.D.   Professor and Chairman, Department of Medicine III, Osaka University Medical School, Osaka, Japan

Jeffrey L. Kishiyama, M.D.   Assistant Clinical Professor, Department of Medicine and Laboratory Medicine, University of California, San Francisco, California

Matyas Koltai, M.D., Ph.D.   Cardiology Consultant, Institut Henri Beaufour, Le Plessis Robinson, France

Brian F. Leber, M.D.   Assistant Professor, Department of Medicine, McMaster University, Hamilton, Ontario, Canada

E. Maggi   Clinical Immunology Department, Institute of Clinica Medica III, University of Florence, Florence, Italy

François-Bernard Michel, M.D.   Professor and Director, Clinique de Maladies Respiratoires and INSERM, Hopital Arnaud de Villeneuve, Montpellier, France

Hiroshi Ochi, Ph.D.   Department of Medicine III, Osaka University Medical School, Osaka, Japan

William F. Owen, Jr., M.D.   Harvard Medical School and Department of Rheumatology and Immunology, Brigham and Women's Hospital, Boston, Massachusetts

Mary E. Paul, M.D.   Assistant Professor of Pediatrics, Department of Allergy and Immunology, Baylor College of Medicine, Houston, Texas

Frederick L. Pearce, B.Sc., Ph.D.   Professor, Department of Chemistry, University College London, London, England

Stephen I. Rennard, M.D.   Chief, Pulmonary and Critical Care Medicine, Department of Internal Medicine, University of Nebraska Medical Center, Omaha, Nebraska

Richard A. Robbins, M.D.   Associate Professor, Department of Internal Medicine, University of Nebraska Medical Center, Omaha, Nebraska

S. Romagnani, M.D.   Clinical Immunology Department, Institute of Clinica Medica III, University of Florence, Florence, Italy

Debra J. Romberger, M.D.   Assistant Professor, Department of Pulmonary and Critical Care Medicine, University of Nebraska Medical Center, Omaha, Nebraska

Hallgeir Rui, M.D., Ph.D.   Laboratory of Molecular Immunoregulation, Cytokine Mechanism Section, Biological Response Modifiers Program, National Cancer Institute, Frederick Cancer Research and Development Center, Frederick, Maryland

Eric T. Sandberg, M.D.   Assistant Professor, Department of Pediatrics, Baylor College of Medicine, Houston, Texas

Julie B. Sedgwick, Ph.D.   Associate Scientist, Allergy and Clinical Immunology Unit, Department of Medicine, University of Wisconsin, Madison, Wisconsin

William T. Shearer, M.D., Ph.D.   Professor, Pediatrics, Microbiology, and Immunology, Baylor College of Medicine, and Chief, Allergy and Immunology Service, Texas Children's Hospital, Houston, Texas

Joseph H. Sisson   Associate Professor, Department of Internal Medicine, Pulmonary and Critical Care Medicine Section, University of Nebraska Medical Center, Omaha, Nebraska

John E. Souness, B.Sc., Ph.D.   Discovery Biology, Dagenham Research Centre, Rhône-Poulenc Rorer, Ltd., Essex, England

John R. Spurzem, M.D., M.S.P.H.   Associate Professor, Department of Internal Medicine, University of Nebraska Medical Center, Omaha, Nebraska

Sunil P. Sreedharan, Ph.D.   Assistant Professor, Department of Medicine, University of California, San Francisco, California

Andrzej M. Stanisz   Associate Professor, Department of Pathology and Intestinal Disease Research Program, McMaster University, Hamilton, Ontario, Canada

Ron H. Stead   Associate Professor, Department of Pathology and Intestinal Disease Research Program, McMaster University, Hamilton, Ontario, Canada

Masaki Suemura, M.D., Ph.D.   Associate Professor, Department of Medicine III, Osaka University Medical School, Osaka, Japan

Toshio Tanaka, M.D., Ph.D.   Assistant Professor, Department of Medicine III, Osaka University Medical School, Osaka, Japan

John H. Toogood, M.D., F.R.C.P.(C.)   Professor of Medicine, Division of Clinical Immunology and Allergy, University of Western Ontario, London, Ontario, Canada

Robert G. Townley, M.D.   Professor of Medicine, Microbiology, and Immunology, and Director of Allergy/Immunology, Creighton University School of Medicine, Omaha, Nebraska

Edouard Vannier, Ph.D.   Assistant Professor, Department of Medicine, Tufts University School of Medicine and New England Medical Center, Boston, Massachusetts

A. Maurizio Vignola, M.D.   Instituto di Fisiopatologia Respiratoria, Palermo, Italy

Frederick A. White, M.D., F.R.C.P. (C)   Division of Clinical Immunology and Allergy, Department of Medicine, University of Western Ontario, London, Ontario, Canada

Ruth M. Williams, Ph.D.   Klinische und Experimentelle Immunologie, Eberhard-Karls-Universitat, Tubingen, Germany

Immunopharmacology of
Allergic Diseases

1

Biochemical and Pharmacological Basis of Receptor–Response Coupling and the Role of G-Proteins in the Action of Immune-Reacting Substances

Devendra K. Agrawal
Creighton University School of Medicine, Omaha, Nebraska

INTRODUCTION

Signals, in the form of chemicals carried by endogenous mediators, such as neurotransmitters, antigens, growth hormones, cytokines, and other humoral factors, are selectively recognized by highly specific receptors present on cell surface or in the cytoplasm or nucleoplasm. In general, water-soluble ligands bind to cell surface receptors, whereas lipid-soluble molecules, such as steroids and thyroid hormones, cross the bilipid membrane layer and bind to receptors present in the cytosol or in the nucleoplasm. In cell surface receptors, biological signals are converted into an internal cell language through a cascade of intracellular reactions. This involves the generation or release of several second messengers, including cyclic nucleotides (cAMP, cGMP), inositol triphosphate (IP_3), diacylglycerol (DAG), and an increase in cytosolic free Ca^{2+}. The signal carried by the second messengers is then amplified, transmitted, and propagated within the internal plasma membrane and cell cytosol where phosphorylation and dephosphorylation of several proteins takes place to regulate a cellular response.

In this chapter I will discuss general concepts of drug–receptor interaction, various signal transduction mechanisms, mechanisms underlying mediator release, and a brief overview of the intracellular pathways involved in the receptor–response coupling of growth factor receptors, cytokine receptors, immunoglobulin receptors, and corticosteroid receptors. A detailed discussion of various mediators and cytokines and their individual receptors follows in the subsequent chapters.

MEMBRANE RECEPTOR CLASSES

With the advent of molecular biology techniques, it has become easier to deduce the amino acid sequences of many of the subunits of signal-transducing membrane receptors. A receptor is defined on the basis of the secondary structure of its subunits, rather than its primary structure. The amino acid sequence of the hydrophobic transmembrane domain determines the type of receptor. Although a receptor may be monomeric or polymeric, most receptors contain at least one transmembrane domain.

In general, there are three major classes of cell surface receptor proteins (Fig. 1):

Ion Channel-Linked Receptors

The ion channel-linked receptors transduce the chemical signal by opening a cation or anion channel, thereby increasing the permeability of the plasma membrane for certain ions that, in turn, initiate electrical excitation of the cell leading to depolarization. Most of these receptor subunits have structure that can assemble in an oligomer surrounding a membrane pore. A well-studied example of such a phenomenon is the γ-aminobutyric acid (GABA) receptor present in the brain. Other examples include receptors for glycine, glutamate, ATP, and nicotinic acetylcholine. Interestingly, the extracellularly activated ATP receptor transduces a signal by opening Ca^{2+}, Na^+, or Mg^{2+} channels, whereas the intracellularly activated ATP receptors elicit a signal by closing K^+ channel (1).

Single-Hydrophobic Domain or Catalytic Receptors

The catalytic receptors contain one transmembrane domain sequence, the subunit of the receptor being monomers or homodimers. The binding subunit itself is a ligand-stimulated tyrosine kinase or a ligand-stimulated guanylate cyclase. However, the involvement of some unknown novel enzymes or pathways cannot be ruled out. The intrinsic tyrosine kinase activity is usually present at the COOH-terminal site of the receptor (see Fig. 1). A

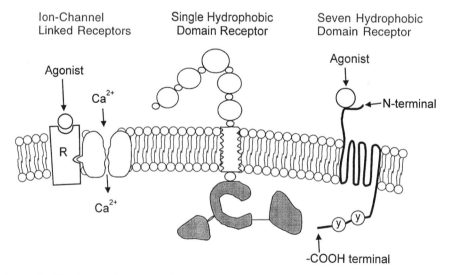

Figure 1 The three major classes of cell surface receptor proteins: in the ion channel-linked receptor, receptor coupling with Ca^{2+} channels has been shown. However, a receptor may be coupled to any other ion including Na^+ or Cl^-. The single-hydrophobic–domain receptors usually contain an intrinsic tyrosine kinase moiety. Seven-hydrophobic–domain receptors may contain tyrosine residues (as shown by Y residues) and thus can activate tyrosine kinases.

specific signal is translated into tyrosine kinase activity. Characteristic examples of this class of receptors include receptors for mitogenic growth factors, insulin, natriuretic peptides, and many cytokines. Phosphorylation (or dephosphorylation) of tyrosine residues triggers conformational changes in regulatory intracellular proteins that alter their properties. This leads to the physiological responses to an agonist.

Two mechanisms by which activated receptor tyrosine kinases transmit information are by protein phosphorylation and by protein–protein interactions. Autophosphorylation is an extremely rapid response of growth factor receptors to ligand binding that allows phosphorylation of exogenous substrates. Tyrosine phosphorylation creates high-affinity sites for binding of proteins that contain the SH2 domain, a motif comprising approximately 100 amino acids (2). Some proteins that contain SH2 domains bind to autophosphorylated growth factor receptors.

Seven-Hydrophobic Domain Receptors

The seven-hydrophobic domain receptors span the bilipid membrane seven times, the subunit mass of the receptor being packed within the membrane. The NH_2-terminal ligand-binding site of the receptor is present extracellularly, whereas the COOH-terminal is intracellular (see Fig. 1). Each subunit carries a G-protein recognition sequence. A large number of receptor-mediated generation of second messengers and activation of ion channels involve GTP-binding regulatory proteins (G-proteins). G-proteins are linked to many cell surface receptors and appear to regulate a variety of effector systems located in the plasma membrane, in the secretory granules of the cells, and in other cellular organelles. In general, in seven-transmembrane domain receptor activation two major pathways for signal transduction have been proposed: (1) activation or inhibition of the adenylate cyclase pathway and (2) stimulation of the turnover of phosphatidylinositol. Both of these pathways involve G-proteins.

Adenylate Cyclase Pathway and Nuclear Transcription Factors

Agonist–receptor interactions converge on the amplifier system, adenylate cyclase, which converts ATP into cAMP (Fig. 2). An agonist may be either stimulatory, such as β-adrenoceptors, or inhibitory such as α_2-adrenoceptors. Such an excitatory or inhibitory effect on adenylate cyclase is regulated by stimulatory G-proteins (G_s) or inhibitory G-proteins (G_i) (These are discussed in a subsequent section in this chapter.) Cyclic-AMP exerts most of its effect by activating cAMP-dependent protein kinase (protein kinase A; PKA). Both cAMP and PKA are ubiquitous in all animal cells. The cAMP binds cooperatively to two sites on the regulatory subunit of PKA, releasing the active catalytic subunit. The active catalytic subunit is translocated from its cytoplasmic and Golgi complex-anchoring sites and phosphorylates serine or threonine residues in cytoplasmic and nuclear proteins or in enzymes leading to cellular response.

Activated PKA modulates the function of nuclear transcriptional factors, such as cAMP-response element (CRE)-binding protein (CREB) that bind to DNA sequences in the 5′ upstream promoter regions of cAMP-inducible genes that contain CRE (see Fig. 2). Several CRE-binding factors have been recognized that function either as activators, such as CREB and activating transcription factors (ATFs), or as repressors, such as the CRE modulators, $CREM_\alpha$, $CREM_\beta$, $CREM_\gamma$, and the CREM-generated products: *i*nducible *c*AMP *e*arly *r*epressor (ICER), together with E4BP4 (3) and CREB-2 (4). The activation of CREB in response to increased levels of cAMP or Ca^{2+} appears to be regulated by the inducible phosphorylation of a specific amino acid, Ser-133, which acts as a critical positive regula-

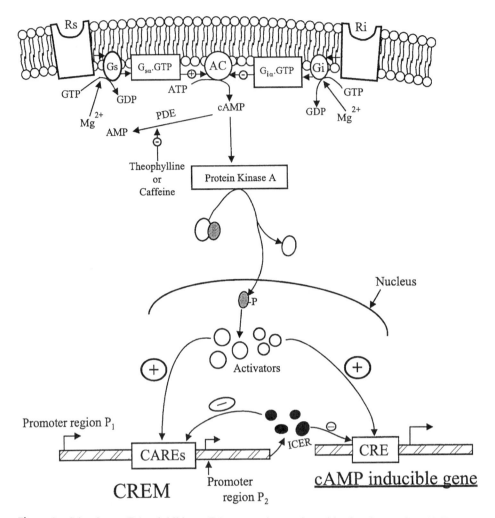

Figure 2 Stimulatory (R_s) or inhibitory (R_i) receptor interaction with adenylate cyclase (AC) system by guanine nucleotide-binding regulatory proteins (G_s or G_i). Increase in intracellular cAMP concentration activates protein kinase A (PKA). The catalytic subunit of protein kinase A translocates into the nucleus and phosphorylates activators, which act by binding to the cAMP-responsive elements (CRE) that are present in the promoter region of cAMP-inducible genes. Activators also bind to the cAMP-autoregulatory elements that are present in the promoter region of the cAMP-responsive element modulator (CREM). Inducible cAMP early repressor (ICER) proteins repress transcription by binding to the CRE and from the CREM promoter region P_2 that contains four DNA elements capable of binding ICER. (Adapted from Ref. 5.)

tory site. Induction of cAMP-responsive transcription by PKA function is regulated by the combined activation of the activators and down-regulation of ICERs which are CREM isoforms and function as transcriptional antagonists in several tissues and cells. Both activators and repressors can bind CREs or cAMP autoregulatory elements (CAREs; see Fig. 2). In response to cAMP stimulation, CREM transcripts increase rapidly with a peak at 2–4 h, followed by a rapid down-regulation.

A role for CRE-binding factors has been proposed in several neuroendocrine processes (5). Since cAMP is important in various receptor–response-coupling pathways (6,7), it is reasonable to speculate that CRE-binding proteins play an important role in allergic diseases, especially in bronchial asthma. The cAMP activators and receptor proteins may also be involved in desensitization of β-adrenoceptors following a long-term administration of β-agonist therapy (see Chap. 22).

Phosphatidylinositol Turnover Pathway and Nuclear Transcription Factors

Breakdown of cellular phosphoinositides occurs in response to a calcium-mobilizing stimulus (Fig. 3). Phosphoinositides are ubiquitous components of eukaryotic cell membranes and include phosphatidylinositol (PI), phosphatidylinositol-4-phosphate (PIP) and phosphatidylinositol 4,5-diphosphate (PIP_2) (8). Various kinases and phosphatases maintain an equilibrium among the phosphoinositides (9). Hydrolysis of these membrane-bound inositol lipids occurs following the interaction of an external signal with its specific receptor on the cell surface. This hydrolysis is catalyzed by phospholipase C (PLC). Activation of PLC by an agonist–receptor complex is governed by G-proteins (G_p or G_q) (10). Recently, tyrosine-phosphorylated proteins have been shown to activate an isoenzyme of PLC, PLCγ1, either directly or by a G-protein (see Fig. 3). Hydrolysis of phosphoinositides is then followed by the production of at least two second messengers, diacylglycerol (DAG) and inositol triphosphate (IP_3). Diacylglycerol remains in the membrane and, in conjunction with a small amount of Ca^{2+}, it translocates the inactive protein kinase C (PKC) to active C-kinase at the inner plasma membrane. In this process, the membrane phospholipid phosphatidylserine may act as a cofactor activating PKC. Phosphokinase C has a broad spectrum specificity, phosphorylating serine and threonine residues of many intracellular proteins, thereby producing a cellular response. It can also activate the enzyme NADPH oxidase to generate superoxide radicals (Fig. 4). In addition to its activation of PKC, DAG can also be converted into arachidonic acid, either by DAG kinase or by DAG lipase (see Fig. 4). An increase in $[Ca^{2+}]_i$ can also activate phospholipase A_2 (PLA_2), which can degrade membrane phospholipids into arachidonic acid. Thus, arachidonic acid could be formed either by the activation of PLA_2 or through DAG formation. In either event, the arachidonic acid thus formed can generate prostaglandins, thromboxanes, or leukotrienes by the action of cyclooxygenase or lipoxygenase.

Inositol triphosphate is water-soluble, and so diffuses into the cytoplasm, where it can mobilize Ca^{2+} from an intracellular pool, resulting in increased cytoplasmic concentrations of Ca^{2+} (9). It releases calcium from a nonmitochondrial pool, mainly endoplasmic reticulum. However, the existence of an IP_3-insensitive intracellular Ca^{2+} pool has also been suggested (9,11).

In addition to the release of Ca^{2+} from intracellular stores, an increase in cytosolic free calcium in response to a stimulus can occur by the influx of extracellular calcium through voltage-operated calcium channels, or through second–messenger-operated calcium channels (see Fig. 4). Voltage-operated calcium channels are usually present only in excitable cells, including airway smooth muscle. The presence of such channels in nonexcitable cells, such as lymphocytes or eosinophils, is highly unlikely.

There is a considerable uncertainty concerning the mechanism and control of second–messenger-operated channels. Both IP_3 and IP_4 have been implicated in controlling the entry of extracellular Ca^{2+} through slow calcium channels (9,11). It has been suggested that IP_3, together with IP_4, causes a second mobilization of intracellular Ca^{2+}, probably by activation of Ca^{2+} entry (see Fig. 3).

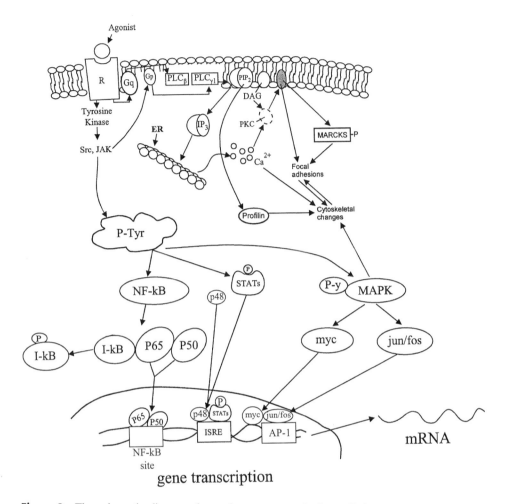

Figure 3 The schematic diagram shows the most extensively studied components involved in receptor–response coupling by phosphatidylinositol (PI) hydrolysis and the activation of tyrosine kinase. An agonist–receptor complex activates phospholipase C (PLC) either directly by G_q-protein or by tyrosine protein phosphorylation and G_p-protein. The PI hydrolysis generates inositol triphosphate (IP$_3$), which releases Ca^{2+} from endoplasmic reticulum (ER), and diacylglycerol (DAG). The Ca^{2+} and DAG translocate protein kinase C (PKC) from the cytosol to associate with the inner plasma membrane. Activated PKC enhances cell adhesion through the formation of focal contacts and also through phosphorylation of the PKC-specific substrate MARCKS (myristoylated alanine-rich C kinase substrate), a phosphoprotein that localizes to focal contact-like sites. Phosphatidylinositol diphosphate (PIP$_2$) can regulate actin-binding proteins, such as profilin to regulate cytoskeletal changes. Tyrosine kinases, such as Src and JAK family kinases, can phosphorylate various transcription factors that then migrate to the nucleus, bind to their respective sites, and regulate gene transcription. The *myc* and *jun/fos* transcription factors bind to the active AP-1 transcription factor complexes site in the nucleus. NF-κB, nuclear factor κB; I-κB, inhibitor of κ-B; STAT, signal transducers and activators of transcription; MAPK, mitogen-activated protein kinase; ISRE, interferon-stimulated response element.

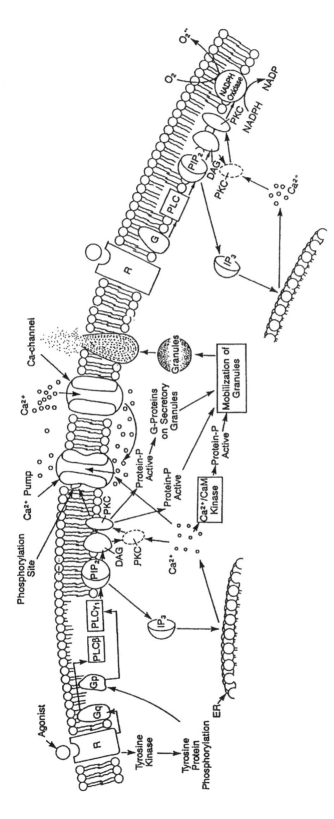

Figure 4 A model for mediator release by PI metabolism. The phosphorylated proteins in response to protein kinase C (PKC) or Ca^{2+}–calmodulin (CAM) kinase in conjunction with increase in intracellular free Ca^{2+} may mobilize secretory granules for exocytosis either directly or by the activation of a distinct G-protein in the granules. On the right hand side, a model for the synthesis and release of superoxide radicals is shown. Phosphorylation of a set of proteins by PKC can stimulate NADPH oxidase to generate and release superoxide anions (O_2^-). For other abbreviations, see Figs. 2 and 3.

Activation of tyrosine kinases has also been reported in receptor–response coupling of seven-transmembrane domain receptors. In this pathway, the phosphorylation of proteins on tyrosine residues by tyrosine kinases has been suggested to contribute to signaling processes that lead to cellular responses, such as muscle contraction (12,13). After activation of tyrosine kinases, signal is transduced by the phosphorylation of a family of transcriptional factors in the cytosol. The active domain of the transcriptional factor translocates to the nucleus to elicit a response that includes gene transcription. Several transcription factors have been recognized (14). These include nuclear factor κB (NF-κB), *myc, jun/fos*, and signal transducers and activators of transcription (STATS). NF-κB in its inactive state exists as a tetramer consisting of three proteins, p65, p50, and inhibitory-κB (I-κB). Tyrosine kinase activation phosphorylates the I-κB, which then dissociates, and the dimer of p65 and p50 translocates to the nucleus and binds to the NF-κB-binding site to induce gene transcription (see Fig. 3). The STATs, which were originally identified as signal transducers involved in activation of interferon (IFN)-α receptors, after phosphorylation migrate to the nucleus and bind to the interferon-stimulated response element (ISRE) sequence upstream from their promoter regions (see Fig. 3; 15,16). The ISREs placed upstream or downstream from reporter genes activate transcription in an IFN-α-dependent manner. Interferon-γ stimulates transcription of genes that function in the immune response, and it causes immediate transcriptional activation of the gene encoding guanylate-binding protein and several other genes. The consensus immediate-response element involved in IFN-γ-stimulated cells has been characterized and is termed the IFN-γ activation site (GAS; 17). Phosphorylation of the mitogen-activated protein kinases activates *myc* and *jun/fos* transcription factors that bind to the AP-1 site in the nucleus to induce gene transcription.

Assessment of the correlation between biochemical and functional events has been made primarily by use of compounds that inhibit tyrosine kinases. For example, we have recently reported that genistein and tyrphostin-sensitive tyrosine kinases are involved in norepinephrine-induced contraction of rat aortic smooth muscle (18). Similar observations have also been made in methacholine-induced contraction of guinea pig tracheal smooth muscle (our unpublished observations). These studies suggest that the activation of seven-transmembrane domain receptors can trigger a series of reactions involving not only the adenylate cyclase and phosphatidylinositol turnover pathways, but also the tyrosine kinase pathways. There are some indications that all these pathways are interconnected and talk to each other to elicit a final response. This will be discussed in the next section.

GUANINE NUCLEOTIDE-BINDING REGULATORY PROTEINS (G-PROTEINS)

There is increasing evidence that receptor-mediated generation of second messengers by both the aforementioned pathways involves G-proteins. These proteins are believed to couple extracellular signals generated by activated membrane receptors to intracellular effector molecules. A wide variety of G-proteins have been identified in many cell types, subserving specific functions. However, the mechanism of the multitude of functions regulated by G-proteins is not yet fully understood.

Classification and Characteristics of G-Proteins

Two major classes of G-proteins have been described in the literature: (1) Heterotrimeric G-proteins that consist of α-, β-, and γ-subunits. G-proteins appear to be built to a common design. However, the α-subunit of every heterotrimeric G-protein differs and characterizes an individual G-protein (19,20). The relative molecular mass of the α-subunit ranges from M_r 39 to 52 kDa, that of the β-subunit is 35–36 kDa, and of the γ-subunit approximately 7–10 kDa. The α-subunit has high-affinity Mg^{2+}-modulated guanine nucleotide-binding site. (2) Low molecular mass monomeric G-proteins (or small G-proteins) with M_r ranging from 18 to 32 kDa. These include *ras*-related proteins and many other oncogene products (21). Both major classes of G-proteins are rapidly expanding. Therefore, these are categorized into subclasses that, in turn, may contain more than one individual member.

The G-proteins share the following properties: (1) They require GTP for their action. (2) G-proteins possess slowly hydrolyzing intrinsic guanosine triphosphatase (GTPase) activity. In response to agonist occupation of receptors, G-protein interacts with GTP to give a free α-subunit bound to GTP and βγ-dimers (22). It is the GTP-bound state of the α-subunit that is active and interacts with effector enzyme (e.g., adenylate cyclase; see Fig. 2). On hydrolysis of GTP to GDP, the α-subunit is inactivated and recycled back to associate with β- and γ-subunits. (3) The α-subunits of heterotrimeric G-proteins serve as substrates for ADP-ribosylation by bacterial toxin and can also be modified covalently by *N*-myristylation. Toxins (pertussis and cholera) covalently modify the α-subunits by catalyzing the transfer of ADP-ribose from NAD^+ to specific amino acid residues (23). Botulinum toxin ADP-ribosylates some of the low molecular mass G-proteins.

Molecular biology has revealed that many G-proteins, such as G_s, G_i, G_o, G_t, G_q, $G_{p/PLC}$, G_{PLA2}, G_{K^+}, $G_{Ca^{2+}}$, and so on, are derived from a large gene family (24). The family is now known to contain at least 16 different genes that encode the α-subunit, 4 that encode the β-subunit, and multiple genes encoding the γ-subunits (25). G_s and G_i, the stimulatory and inhibitory G-proteins of adenylate cyclase, were among the first G-proteins to be identified and characterized. Pharmacologically, G_s and G_i can be distinguished on the basis of their ability to be ADP-ribosylated by cholera and pertussis toxins, respectively (26).

The subtypes of α-subunits are produced by alternative splicing of mRNA, probably from a single gene (27,28) and are classified on the basis of similarity in their amino acid sequence. A given subtype may have more than one isotype. Thus G_s comprises four isotypes including $G_{\alpha olf}$, G_i consists of $G_{\alpha i-1}$, $G_{\alpha i-2}$, $G_{\alpha i-3}$; G_q includes $G_{\alpha 15}$, $G_{\alpha 16}$, $G_{\alpha 14}$, $G_{\alpha 11}$, $G_{\alpha q}$; and G_{12} consists of G_{12} and G_{13} (29).

Small G-proteins (18–32 kDa), which currently include more than 40 individual members, are categorized into several subfamilies. These include those encoded by *ras*, *ral*, *rab*, *rho*, *rac*, *YPT*, *SEC4*, and many other genes (30–32). They possess sequence homology with the proteins encoded by these oncogenes. The *ras*-related proteins are proto-oncogenes and generally are involved in cellular differentiation and transformation and with vesicular trafficking in the cell (33). Low molecular mass G-proteins are involved in the regulation of fusion events along the secretory pathway (21,34,35). They lack a site for ADP-ribosylation with either pertussis or cholera toxin, although some of them can be ADP-ribosylated with botulinum toxin.

More recently, relatively high molecular mass GTP-binding proteins (e.g., 100 kDa implicated in receptor recycling during endocytosis) have been detected in liver (36,37), parotid gland (38), eosinophils and neutrophils (39,40), blood vessels (41), and tracheal smooth muscle (42,43). The functions of these proteins are not yet clear, but their locations at secretory granules suggest possible involvement in secretory functions.

Cellular Functions of G-Proteins

An immense amount of research has been conducted investigating G-proteins in various cell systems, including smooth muscles, such as vascular smooth muscle (44–48). These studies focused on the involvement of G-proteins in signal transduction mechanisms. The functional role of G-proteins was elucidated using various parameters, including the measurement of second messengers (Ca^{2+}, cAMP, IP_3) and muscle contraction, in response to various agonists (norepinephrine, acetylcholine, endothelin, GTPγS) in the presence and absence of different G-protein-interacting probes. However, the role of G-proteins in airway smooth muscle has not been extensively studied. In the following section, G-protein involvement in various cell systems will be discussed.

G-Proteins in Smooth-Muscle Function

The involvement of G-proteins in signal transduction, in relation to contraction of smooth muscle is supported by the observation that in permeabilized aortic cells, GTPγS (a nonhydrolyzable GTP analogue) increases IP_3 formation (49). GTPγS has also been reported to induce a Ca^{2+} influx in vascular smooth-muscle cells and contraction of permeabilized aortic strips (50).

Fluorides have long been known to influence the activity of hormone-sensitive adenylate cyclase systems (51). Fluoride exhibits a wide variety of pharmacological actions in vitro, including contraction of blood vessels (48). Therefore, sodium fluoride is used as a G-protein activator in adenylate cyclase research on smooth-muscle activity of guinea pig airways. Fluoride complexes with Al^{+3}, and the resulting fluoroaluminate (AlF_4^-) complex is an activator of G-proteins. This AlF_4^- species is able to mimic the action of GTP and, thereby, cause dissociation of the α-subunit of G-proteins and subsequent modulation of the target enzyme (adenylate cyclase) (52). The AlF_4^- can stimulate adenylate cyclase by direct action on the G_s protein. A recent report (53) indicated that AlF_4^- stimulates a small increase in cAMP levels in slices of bovine tracheal smooth muscle. The fluoride ion is able to modulate G-protein-mediated activation of PLC activity in various tissues (54–56). Moreover, Hall and colleagues (53) also reported that NaF stimulates the PI turnover in bovine tracheal smooth muscle. In guinea pig visceral smooth muscle addition of PLC to lung strips caused a rapidly developing contraction that was followed by a slow phase of contraction (57). These studies confirmed that activated PLC indeed causes contraction of guinea pig airway smooth muscle and strengthened the hypothesis that sodium fluoride-induced responses are mediated by a G-protein involved in the activation of PLC. Other studies have also demonstrated that NaF, in a concentration-dependent manner, stimulates PI hydrolysis in rat aorta and caudal artery (45). Although fluoride stimulates G-proteins in many tissues (58,59), the results imply that the fluoride evoked effects were not mediated by a pertussis toxin-sensitive G-protein (60).

Recently, our laboratory has identified various types of heterotrimeric (G_s and G_i), low molecular mass and high molecular mass G-proteins in the purified membranes of rat aorta and mesenteric artery (41). Interestingly, certain differences in G-proteins were observed between the aorta and mesenteric artery (41). These studies were supported by the contractile studies in the isolated ring segments of rat aorta and mesenteric artery. In guinea pig and bovine trachea, Joshi and colleagues (42,43) have identified several types of G-proteins. Functional studies in tracheal smooth muscle suggested the involvement of G_s- and G_i-like proteins, which are substrates for cholera toxin and pertussis toxin.

These data support the existence of multiple types of G-proteins in various smooth-muscle cells. The role of heterotrimeric G-proteins can be supported by the studies with cholera toxin, pertussis toxin, NaF, and N-ethylmaleimide (NEM). However, the functional significance of other proteins, such as high molecular mass and monomeric G-proteins, remains to be elucidated.

G-Proteins in Cells Other Than Smooth Muscles

Pertussis toxin has been used to identify the G-proteins controlling activation of PI turnover (20,61,62). Pretreatment of guinea pig neutrophils (63), human neutrophil membranes (64), human leukemic (HL-60) cells (65), rat renal mesangial cells (66), and rat mast cells (67) with pertussis toxin inhibited hormone-stimulated PIP_2 hydrolysis (68). Similar results were obtained for muscarinic stimulation in cultured chick heart cells (69) and α_1-adrenergic agonist stimulation in brown adipocytes (70). These results indicate that pertussis toxin inhibits receptor-mediated PI hydrolysis in some, but not all, cellular systems (71–73). Although pertussis toxin markedly attenuates muscarinic receptor-induced inhibition of cAMP in dog tracheal smooth muscle and in a variety of other cell systems (74), presumably by uncoupling the muscarinic receptor from the G-protein, there is no information on the effects of GTP or its analogues, or the bacterial toxins, on agonist-induced PI turnover and contraction in airway smooth muscle.

In addition to pertussis toxin, NEM (a sulfhydryl G-protein inhibitory agent) has been used for selective inhibition of adenylate cyclase inhibitors. It acts by alkylating SH-groups on proteins. Pertussis toxin-sensitive G-proteins are the most sensitive targets for the alkylating effects of NEM (75).

Despite heterotrimeric G-proteins being central to the signal transduction process and acting as switches that regulate information flow, there is evidence that, in certain systems, such as vascular smooth muscle, signal transduction processes and muscle contraction may occur without the involvement of G-proteins. It has been reported that treatment of vascular preparations with pertussis toxin failed to prevent PI metabolism, Ca^{2+} mobilization, and muscle responsiveness (45). Similarly, another group was not able to inhibit agonist-induced stimulation of Ca^{2+} channels in vascular smooth muscle pretreated with pertussis and cholera toxin. Although G-protein research in airway smooth muscle has not been vigorously pursued, the apparent role of the PI turnover in this tissue suggests that GTP-binding proteins might play a pivotal role as signal transducers in receptor–effector coupling.

CROSS-TALK AMONG INTRACELLULAR SIGNAL TRANSDUCTION PATHWAYS

With the advent of new molecular biology techniques and the cloning of various receptors, it has now become clear that there is enormous heterogeneity and differential cell expression with specific intracellular localization of various signaling proteins. Various intracellular signal-transducing proteins may interact with each other and, consequently, are capable of exerting either a synergistic or antagonistic effect. To regulate a cellular function, a positive signal is often followed by immediate negative-feedback control. These methods include the activation of Na^+–K^+ pump to decrease intracellular Na^+ concentration, sequestration of intracellular free Ca^{2+} after muscle contraction, and receptor down-regulation and internalization. All these interactions are important for our understanding of the dynamic aspects of cellular regulation.

Phospholipases play an important role in the signal transduction process inside the cell. Signal-activated phospholipases have been reported to modulate and regulate the information transmitted by two distinct channels. The major phospholipases that play an integral role in transmembrane signaling include phospholipase C (PLC), phospholipase D (PLD), and phospholipase A_2 (PLA_2). Phospholipase C stimulates the second messengers of the PI cascade that elevate intracellular Ca^{2+} and activate protein kinase C. Phospholipase A_2 is also activated, resulting in release of arachidonic acid. Phospholipase D has been reported to regulate phosphatidylinositol–PLC activity by altering the formation of its product, phosphatidic acid (76). Several lipid-derived messengers regulate the GTPase activity of small G-proteins of the *ras* superfamily. The lipid-derived mediators 1-stearoyl-2-arachidonoyl-phosphatidic acid and arachidonic acid inhibit the p21^{ras} GTPase-activating protein (77). In mitogen-stimulated cells, phospholipases regulate the activation of p21^{ras}. Thus, proteins that regulate the GTPase activity of low molecular size G-proteins could represent convergence points at which signals carried by lipid mediators are integrated.

Cross-talk between tyrosine kinases and the classic PI turnover pathway has also been reported (see Fig. 3). Receptor-stimulated tyrosine kinase may, in turn, activate phosphatidylinositol–PLC, PLD, or PLA$_2$ enzymes either directly or by a G-protein. Protein kinase C isoenzymes play an important role in coordinating the activation of these phospholipases. We have recently reported the activation of p60^{src} tyrosine kinase and JAK1-like kinases by endothelin-1 (ET-1) receptor activation in human umbilical vein endothelial cells (78). In several cell systems, endothelin-1 has been reported to activate PLC by a pertussis toxin-sensitive G-protein. In intact blood vessels ET-1 stimulation increases PLD activity (79). Endothelin-1 also alters the cell membrane potential, probably by a mechanism involving both ligand and voltage-gated calcium channels. All these data suggest that the ET-1 receptor, which belongs to the family of receptors with seven-transmembrane domains, is coupled to multiple signaling pathways. However, it is not clear whether these pathways are activated independently or in parallel. In view of the examples known in other cell systems, such as T-cell receptor stimulation, it is reasonable to speculate that the activation of tyrosine kinases and the resulting tyrosine phosphorylated proteins can activate a G-protein, which then activates PLC.

In conclusion, it appears that intracellular-signaling pathways are not independent. Rather, signaling pathways converge and coordinate with each other to regulate a cell function. Any disturbance in these pathways may result in a pathological phenomenon.

MECHANISMS UNDERLYING MEDIATOR RELEASE

Chemical mediators are released from various cells. These mediators may be preformed or newly synthesized. Preformed mediators are present in the form of granules-stored vesicles; for example, mast cells and basophils contain histamine; eosinophils contain major basic protein (MBP), eosinophil cationic protein (ECP), eosinophil-derived neurotoxin (EDN), and eosinophil peroxidase (EPO); and platelets contain serotonin. Newly synthesized mediators are synthesized and released in response to a stimulus; for example, leukotrienes, platelet-activating factor, and superoxide radicals, released from cells such as eosinophils and monocytes–macrophages.

The release of mediators appears to be stimulus-specific and involves different pathways in transmembrane signaling. In general, mediators that are present in granules are released by an exocytotic mechanism whereby the granules fuse with the membrane (see Fig. 4). Spry (80) has suggested that the exocytosis of eosinophil granules takes place through the solubilization of the granular material within the granule, with subsequent transport of the molecules through the cytoplasm individually, or by the endoplasmic reticulum. It is now clear from most of the studies that an increase in intracellular free Ca^{2+} is the key step in the mobilization of granular vesicles to the membrane (see Fig. 4). In guinea pig eosinophils, Nuesse and colleagues (81) observed that eosinophil degranulation occurred without any parallel increase in electrical conductivity and, therefore, by a conventional exocytotic membrane fusion mechanism. Cromwell et al. (82) reported that eosinophil degranulation was dependent on Ca^{2+} and GTPγS, but did not require ATP, although ATP enhanced the magnitude of the secretory response. In addition, ATP increased the affinity of Ca^{2+} and GTPγS for their degranulating activity. Furthermore, activation of PKC enhances the eosinophil responsiveness.

Phospholipid hydrolysis and protein phosphorylation may also be involved in the release of mediators. Holgate and colleagues (83) have reported that phorbol esters release the granule core protein MBP, without any effect on the release of matrix protein EPO or the small-granule protein arylsulfatase. This suggests the existence of a selective degranulation mechanism for MBP. Furthermore, agents such as calcium ionophore, phorbol esters, platelet-activating factor (PAF), and sodium fluoride, produced superoxide radicals from eosinophils. However, these stimuli had no effect on the release of EPO and arlysulfatase. Capron and colleagues (84) observed the release of EPO and MBP from anti-IgE-activated eosinophils, whereas anti-IgG antibodies released only ECP. These results clearly suggest that cellular degranulation and the release of mediators may be stimulus-specific, and that the exocytosis of small and large granules could be differentially regulated.

In newly synthesized mediators, there is also an involvement of inositol phosphates and protein kinases. For example, synthesis of PAF and leukotriene-C_4 (LTC$_4$) from various cells, including eosinophils, takes place by the degradation of membrane phospholipids by the action of Ca^{2+}-dependent PLA$_2$ or by the formation of DAG (Fig. 5). Any stimulus that is capable of activating the phosphatidylinositol pathway or activating PLA$_2$ theoretically should be able to generate these mediators from mast cells, eosinophils, or other cells that are capable of releasing these mediators. The activation of 5′-lipoxygenase requires its translocation from the cytosol fraction to the membrane in response to an increase in intracellular free Ca^{2+} (85). The translocated 5′-lipoxygenase interacts with a membrane-anchored protein (5′-lipoxygenase-activating protein) (86). Thus, a transient increase in intracellular free Ca^{2+} could activate not only PLA$_2$ to form arachidonic acid, but may also be involved in regulating the 5′-lipoxygenase activity (for further information on leukotrienes, see Chap. 20).

All these data suggest an involvement of the phosphatidylinositol metabolism and an increase in intracellular free Ca^{2+} in various cells in response to a stimulus which, in turn, may generate and release newly formed mediators. Similar to the granular proteins, the

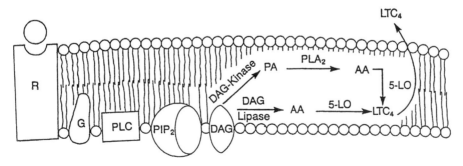

Figure 5 A schematic diagram showing the release of leukotriene C_4 (LTC$_4$). Arachidonic acid (AA) could be synthesized from phospholipids, such as phosphatidylinositol or phosphatidylcholine by the activation of phospholipase A$_2$ (PLA$_2$). In addition, diacylglycerol (DAG), generated during PI hydrolysis, can be converted to AA, either by the action of DAG kinase or DAG lipase.

newly formed mediators may also be stimulus-specific. Furthermore, if there is cross-talk between various signal transduction pathways, the role of tyrosine kinases and their interaction with phospholipid metabolism requires further attention to their effect on mediator release.

GROWTH FACTOR AND CYTOKINE RECEPTORS

Most growth factors stimulate a group of intracellular protein kinases that includes Raf1 kinase, MAP kinase, and protein kinase C (87,88). Activation of Raf1 kinase appears to be essential for serum-induced proliferation of fibroblasts. The Raf1 kinase may also be involved in activating specific genes, such as c-*fos* (89,90). Although Raf1 kinase can be directly activated by receptor tyrosine kinases in vitro, it is likely that in vivo there are intermediate molecules that mediate its activation.

Platelet-derived growth factor β-receptor (PDGFβR) and fibroblast growth factor receptor (FGFR) have been studied in detail (91). The activation of the PDGFβR involves a chain of reactions, including activation of phosphatidylinositol 3-kinase, GTPase-activating factor (GAP), PLCγ, and a variety of tyrosine kinases including the Src family of kinases (Fig. 6). In addition, several other signal transduction molecules interact with PDGFβR. These molecules include growth factor receptor-bound 2 (Grb2); small adaptor proteins, such as the SH2 domain and collagen-like (Shc); Nck, Shb, and GTPase-activating protein (GAP) or *ras*. Activation of tyrosine kinases regulates growth and differentiation of cells. Activation of PLC in human B cells is dependent on tyrosine phosphorylation (92).

Mitogen-activated protein kinase (MAPK) plays a critical role in a variety of signal transduction pathways (93–95). The MAPK activity peaks and declines following mitogen stimulation with kinetics reminiscent of immediate early-gene mRNA accumulation. Activation of MAPK is dependent on phosphorylation of a neighboring tyrosine and threonine residue. Evidence suggests that multiple isoforms of MAPK are expressed within a single cell type, each of which serves a particular cellular function (96). Recently, new classes of MAPK-related kinases have been reported (97,98). These Jun kinases and stress-activated protein kinases are phosphorylated on nearly juxtaposed threonine and tyrosine residues, similarly to MAPK. Furthermore, these phosphorylation events are important for kinase activity.

Cytokines, a large family of protein mediators, regulate proliferation, differentiation, and function of various lineages of cells. Each cytokine interacts with different types of cells and exhibits pleiotropic functions, depending on the target cell. Most of the cytokine receptors that constitute distinct superfamilies do not possess intrinsic protein tyrosine kinase domains, yet receptor stimulation usually invokes rapid tyrosine phosphorylation of intracellular proteins, including the receptors themselves. However, cytokine receptors are also capable of recruiting or activating a variety of nonreceptor protein tyrosine kinases to induce downstream-signaling pathways. The specificity of the later effect is governed by the intracytoplasmic structure of cytokine receptors (99). Individual cytokines will be discussed in the following chapters. In this section, I would like to briefly point out the synergistic interactions between various inflammatory mediators and a possible role of cytokines.

Recently, we reported that neuropeptides alone have no eosinophil chemotactic activity on human peripheral blood eosinophils in vitro (100). The peptides, however, potentiated the PAF- and LTB$_4$-induced eosinophil chemotaxis in allergic, but not in normal, subjects. These effects were considered specific for the neuropeptides that exist in the respiratory

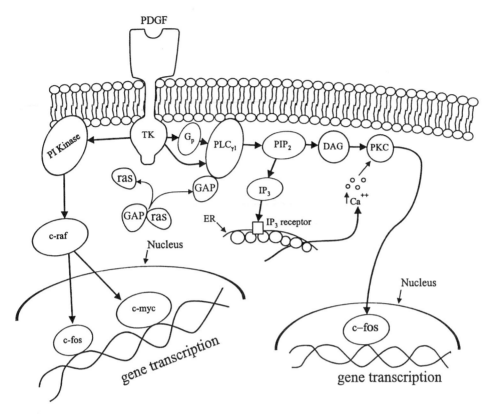

Figure 6 A schematic diagram showing the receptor–response coupling in platelet-derived growth factor (PDGF) receptor, which contains intrinsic tyrosine kinase moiety. The PDGF receptor binds PI3-kinase by the kinase insert region PLC$_{\gamma l}$ and *ras*-GAP are bound by the COOH-terminus. PI kinase activates c-*raf* transcription factor to induce gene transcription. Activated protein kinase C (PKC) can also regulate gene transcription through the c-*fos* transcription factor.

tract because pancreastatin, an unrelated polypeptide irrelevant to allergic airway inflammation, had no effect. These results support the hypothesis that neuropeptides play a significant role in eosinophil infiltration by priming cells in allergic inflammation.

The mechanism by which neuropeptides prime eosinophil chemotactic activity remains obscure. It is possible that peptides trigger a signal transduction sequence in human eosinophils. Activation by substance P (SP) of the respiratory burst and exocytosis in human neutrophils were associated with phosphoinositide turnover and with an increase in $[Ca^{2+}]_i$, which was mostly due to release from intracellular stores (101). Furthermore, PKC, which is activated by DAG formed by the hydrolysis of phosphatidylinositol diphosphates, not involved in the activation of the NADPH oxidase in the presence of substance P. The respiratory burst induced by *N*-formyl-methionyl-leucyl-phenylalanine (FMLP) was completely inhibited by pertussis toxin, which is known to catalyze the ADP-ribosylation of the α-subunit of a G-protein. Exocytosis, measured as the cytochalasin B-dependent secretion of specific and azurophilic granules of human neutrophils, was induced by both SP and FMLP. Collectively, these observations support the possibility that neuropeptides prime eosinophil chemotactic activity by activation of a signal transduction sequence. Alternatively or in addition, it is possible that neuropeptides trigger the synthesis and release of cytokines such as interleukin (IL)-3, IL-5, or granulocyte—macrophage colony-stimulating factor (GMCSF). These cytokines increase viability, degranulation, superoxide and leukotriene generation, and proteoglycan synthesis. Interleukin-5 and GM-CSF by themselves possess little degranulating effect, but IL-3, IL-5, and GM-CSF enhance the immunoglobulin-induced eosinophil-derived neurotoxin release. Interleukin-5 is the most potent and selective enhancer. Buckley and colleagues (102) recently reported synergistic interactions between IL-1 and calcitonin gene-related peptide (CGRP) in eliciting an increase in microvascular leakage. This suggests that classic mediators of inflammation and neuropeptides could interact synergistically at the inflammatory sites.

LEUKOCYTE ADHESION RECEPTORS

The leukocyte adhesion receptors belong to three families of cell adhesion molecules. These include (1) the immunoglobulin family, such as intercellular adhesion molecules (ICAM-1) and vascular cell adhesion molecules (VCAM1); (2) integrins, which include counterreceptors for ICAM or VCAM; and (3) selectins, which include E-selectin (ELAM-1), P-selectin (GMP-140), and L-selectin (lymphocyte-homing receptor, or LAM-1) (103–105). Among these receptors, integrins behave as classic receptors, capable of transducing external signal into a cell language by the generation of second messengers within the cell. Integrin receptors activate the $Na^+–H^+$ antiporter and, thereby, elevate intracellular pH (106,107). Integrins also increase intracellular free Ca^{2+} concentration. Cross-linking of LFA-1 on lymphocytes with antibodies against the α-chain resulted in phosphatidylinositol hydrolysis and a rise in intracellular $[Ca^{2+}]$ (108). In addition to the activation of these classic transmembrane-signaling pathways, integrins also induce tyrosine phosphorylation. Cross-linking of integrins on the surface of carcinoma cells induced tyrosine phosphorylation of a complex of 120-kDa proteins (109). A similar phenomenon has also been observed in the interaction of fibroblasts plated on fibronectin, with the involvement of 125-kDa focal adhesion kinase (110,111). Whether there is an interaction between various intracellular transmembrane-signaling pathways in integrin receptor activation remains unclear. There is cross-talk between integrins and other receptors in signal transduction, such as those found in stimulation of the T-cell receptor-induced proliferation of lymphocytes that occurs only when coreceptors such as LFA-1 are also involved (112). In another example, maximal synthesis of PAF in monocytes by serum opsonized zymosan requires both β_2-integrin and β-glucan receptors (113). Thus, integrins are capable of collaborating with other receptors. This permits the transduction of information both ways across the cell membrane (for a detailed description on cell adhesion molecules, see Chap. 4).

IMMUNOGLOBULIN RECEPTORS

Studies have investigated the activation of various immunoglobulin receptors (114). For example, the aggregation of the high-affinity IgE receptors (FcϵRI) on mast cells and basophils results in degranulation and the release of inflammatory mediators. The IgE receptor activation and aggregation in mast cells was initially shown to activate phospholipid methylation and the activation of PLA_2 and PLD, and to increase Ca^{2+} influx. Recent studies report the involvement of tyrosine kinase activation after IgE receptor activation in mast cells. The aggregation of the FcϵRI has induced tyrosine phosphorylation of several proteins, including the β- and γ-subunits of FcϵRI, p72^{syk}, PLCγ1, pp53/p56^{lyn}, pp60^{c-src}, pp95^{vav}, and pp125^{FAK}, and several other proteins (115–118). Recently, Hamaway and colleagues (119) reported that FcεRI aggregation induced tyrosine phosphorylation of paxillin, a 68-kDa cytoskeletal protein that accumulates at focal adhesion sites. Interestingly, the tyrosine phosphorylation of paxillin was induced by the direct increase in intracellular Ca^{2+} and the direct activation of PKC. A detailed discussion on these receptors is given in the chapter of IgE receptors in mast cells.

CORTICOSTEROID RECEPTORS

Steroid hormones are lipophilic. Therefore, they can enter the target cell and bind to an intracellular receptor protein. The hormone–receptor complex mobilizes to the nucleus, where it selectively regulates transcription by binding to specific DNA sequences, termed glucocorticoid-responsive elements (GREs), and activates transcription of downstream coding sequences. Thus, the DNA-binding species regulates the rate of gene expression. Steroid receptors can both stimulate and inhibit gene transcription, either by negative GREs, or indirectly, by protein–protein interaction.

Glucocorticoids are very potent anti-inflammatory agents. Dexamethasone, a synthetic glucocorticoid, is a potent inhibitor of gene transcription of many proinflammatory cytokines, including IL-1, tissue necrosis factor-α (TNF-α), IL-2, IL-3, GM-CSF, and others. Glucocorticoids down-regulate IL-2 receptors (120) and also inhibit the expression of cell adhesion molecules (121). Initially, it was thought that most of the effects of corticosteroids take place by the formation of lipocortins, which act on the cell membranes and inhibit PLA$_2$. However, recent studies clearly suggest that the anti-inflammatory effect of glucocorticoids is primarily through the interaction between glucocorticoid receptors and transcriptional factors at the nuclear level. Several cytokines and growth factors may interact with the effect of corticosteroids. Inflammatory agents, in general, up-regulate the relevant genes during inflammation. Up-regulation of inflammatory genes takes place by the action of transcriptional factors. Among various transcriptional factors, nuclear factor κB (NF-κB)/Rel proteins function as important positive regulators of inflammatory genes. Functional NF-κB/Rel-binding sites are increased in the nucleus in response to several cytokines and tumor-promoting agents (Fig. 7). Corticosteroid receptors and the RelA-mediated activation of NF-κB site interact with each other and regulate gene transcription (122); the corticosteroid receptor suppresses the NF-κB/RelA-binding site, and RelA physically interacts with the corticosteroid receptor and represses the transcriptional activation of corticosteroid receptors by a glucocorticosteroid response element (see Fig. 7). This could be a possible molecular mechanism underlying the anti-inflammatory effect of corticosteroids during inflammation.

Vig and colleagues (123) recently reported the evidence that glucocorticoid receptors and c-*jun* expression are functionally linked. In the inactive, untransformed state, a glucocorticoid receptor is present in the cytosol as hetero-oligomeric receptor, containing one subunit of receptor protein, two molecules of heat-shock protein, hsp90, and one molecule of the immunophilin, p59. A modulator or a metal ion stabilizes the untransformed receptor state. The binding of glucocorticosteroid with its receptor in the cytosol and the activation of kinases phosphorylate the receptor; heat-shock proteins, modulator, and p59 dissociate, leading to the transformed monomeric state of glucocorticosteroid receptor. This monomeric state combines with the Jun transcriptional factor to form a heteromeric complex, resulting in the inactivation of Jun and a decrease in c-*jun* mRNA levels (see Fig. 7).

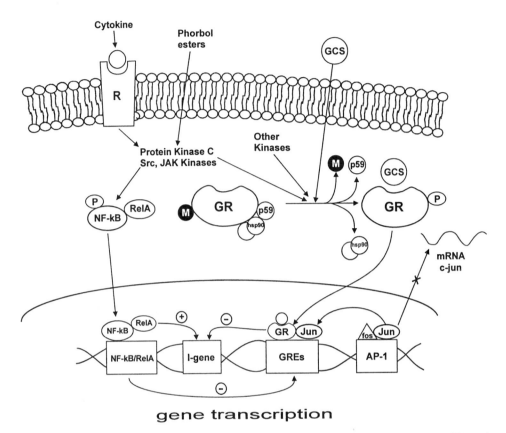

gene transcription

Figure 7 A proposed scheme for the mechanism of action of glucocorticosteroid (GCS) and regulation by various kinases. In an untreated cell, GCS receptors (GR) are present in the cytosol in an untransformed state, containing one subunit of GR protein; two molecules of the heat-shock protein, hsp90; one molecule of the immunophilin, p59; and a modulator or a metal of low molecular weight. After binding to GCS, the hormone–receptor complex migrates to the nucleus, binds to the GR elements (GREs). The *jun* or the *fos* factors migrate from the Ap-1 site to regulate the GREs. Overexpression of *jun* blunts GR-mediated gene expression, and overexpression of the GR can block AP-1 gene activation. NF-κB, especially the RelA can stimulate the I gene (gene for inflammatory mediators), whereas the activated GREs suppress the I gene. Increased activity of NF-κB/RelA has a negative effect on the gene transcription of the GR.

Interaction between the glucocorticoid receptor and the AP-1 transcription factor could also be mediated by glucocorticoid receptor–*fos* interactions (124,125). In general, overexpression of Jun in cells blunts cellular responsiveness to corticosteroids, and overexpression of glucocorticoid receptor in cells that respond to activators—such as phorbol esters—of the AP-1 transcription factor (*fos*/Jun) blunts AP-1 transactivation of responsive genes (126–128).

Thus, the anti-inflammatory effect of glucocorticoids involves a multitude of intracellular proteins that regulate the gene expression of glucocorticoid-responsive elements and cAMP-responsive elements. A detailed analysis of promoter function of various genes and studies on the interaction of glucocorticoid receptors and various transcription factors are required for a better understanding of the molecular mechanisms of action of glucocorticoids in various allergic diseases.

DRUG–RECEPTOR INTERACTIONS: AGONISM AND ANTAGONISM

The effect of endogenous mediators in a given organ determines the overall metabolic state of that organ. Endogenous mediators, as well as exogenously administered drugs, interact with their specific receptors to elicit a response. These mediators or drugs may act either as agonists or antagonists. *Agonists* are molecules that bind to a specific site, activate receptors, and elicit a response. Thus, agonists possess intrinsic activities and efficacies of varying magnitude. Compounds with a low-intrinsic activity can induce only a relatively small maximum effect. These are called partial agonists. *Antagonists*, on the other hand, bind, but do not activate, receptors. Antagonists have zero intrinsic activity. If an antagonist rapidly dissociates from the receptor site, it produces reversible antagonism. If the antagonist forms a chemical bond with, and alkylates the receptor, it produces irreversible antagonism. A drug or molecule may bind to the receptor site with a very high-energy covalent bond, producing a noncompetitive interaction. Phenoxybenzamine is a typical example of noncompetitive antagonist.

REGULATION OF RECEPTOR–RESPONSE COUPLING

In general, receptors can be regulated by an alteration in a receptor's density, its affinity, or its location. In addition, the response to receptor activation may also be regulated at several steps in the chain of events involved in the signal transduction pathways. The following discussion focuses on general pathways and mechanisms by which receptors can be regulated, including antagonism, desensitization, and supersensitivity phenomena. Detailed information about a specific receptor or mediator follows in subsequent sections of this book.

Desensitization (Refractoriness or Tachyphylaxis, "Fade Phenomenon")

Continuous stimulation of cells with agonists generally results in a state of desensitization, such that the effect that follows subsequent exposure to the same concentration of drug is diminished. This may lead to *tolerance*, which may be either slowly or rapidly developing. This phenomenon can become very important in therapeutic situations, such as opium alkaloids, β-agonist therapy in asthma, and so forth. The following mechanisms have been proposed to explain this: (1) slow regeneration from an inactive receptor form, (2) formation of an endogenous inhibitor, (3) agonist-mediated decrease in receptor number, and (4) depletion of second messenger or endogenously released factor.

Receptor number appears to be regulated by several general mechanisms. The first mechanism involves down-regulation or loss of receptors from the cell surface after receptor occupancy by the ligand. This phenomenon can involve internalization, deregulation, or altered recycling of the receptor and, in some cases, shedding of the receptor. This phenomenon has also been referred to as "homologous desensitization." In contrast, "heterologous desensitization" occurs when receptors for different hormones or neurotransmitters become less effective because of a defect at a postreceptor site. Down-regulation occurs on a number of cell types, with a variety of hormones. A well-established example is the down-regulation of β-adrenoceptors in lymphocytes and airway smooth muscles in asthmatic subjects (6). We have previously reported that PAF decreased the density of β-adrenoceptors in human lung parenchymal tissue (129,130). In functional studies in the isolated trachea and lung parenchyma of guinea pig or human, PAF significantly reduced the potency of isoproterenol to reverse methacholine or histamine-induced contraction (131). Such an effect of PAF on the down-regulation of β-adrenoceptor responses in the airways could be either direct or indirect by the release of other mediators, such as IL-1 or TNF-α. In this phenomenon, it is possible that the translocation of adenylate cyclase-coupled receptor kinase from the cytosol to the plasma membrane phosphorylates adenylate cyclase-coupled receptors (132).

A second mechanism is receptor desensitization, which indicates that the receptor is still present on the surface membrane, but is not in an accessible or active form for the ligand. Again, this process has been studied extensively for β-adrenoceptors and insulin receptors. In the β-adrenoceptors, the receptor undergoes phosphorylation and desensitization. Phosphorylation of the agonist-occupied receptor, which turns this signaling pathway off, is mediated by serine–threonine kinases, termed βARK for β-adrenoceptor kinase, or GRK2 for G-protein-coupled receptor kinase. Receptor activation triggers translocation of βARK from the cytosol to the plasma membrane, where it phosphorylates agonist-occupied receptors. More than 70% of the βARK is translocated within a few minutes of receptor activation, leading to an increased activity of membrane-associated kinases. However, within 20 min of receptor activation, βARK activity returns to normal in the cytosol. The βARK appears to bind to βγ-subunits of G-proteins after the α-subunit is dissociated from the αβγ-complex in response to receptor stimulation. The binding of the βARK to the βγ-subunit inhibits the response of the receptor to further stimulation, leading to desensitization: βARK-phosphorylated receptors are only minimally desensitized. An additional cytosolic protein, β-arrestin, is required to induce maximal homologous desensitization (133). A recent study by Sallese and colleagues (134) suggests that the NH_2-terminal of βARK contains some sites crucial for the normal processing of receptor proteins. For further discussion on β-adrenoceptors, please see Chapter 22.

In contrast with down-regulation, up-regulation, or increase of receptors after occupancy by their ligands, occurs with IL-2 receptors and prolactin receptors (see further discussion). The number of receptors can be altered by changes in the rate of synthesis of receptor.

Receptor affinity can be regulated by receptor-specific ligands, other ligands, and various chemical agents. Occasionally, occupancy of a receptor by its ligand results in either positive or negative cooperative effects, which change the affinity of the receptor. Several intracellular membrane proteins may alter receptor affinity.

Receptor organization and distribution can be regulated by at least three general mechanisms. The first mechanism involves the actual cross-linking of receptors by multivalent receptor-specific or other ligands, such as immunoglobulins or lectins. The second mechanism involves induction of biochemical membrane or cellular responses by occupancy of the receptor with monovalent ligands, such as insulin. Induced responses could regulate such processes as receptor migration, aggregation, internalization, and recycling. Finally, various agents that alter membrane or cellular constituents, such as disulfide bonds, phospholipids, and cytoskeletal elements, can alter receptor organization and distribution.

There are several classes of biochemical membrane reactions that could be involved in receptor regulation. One of these processes is phosphorylation, as several different receptors have tyrosine kinases that are capable of autophosphorylation. Another hormone-sensitive membrane process that could be involved in receptor regulation is phospholipid methylation (135). Finally, oxidation–reduction changes of membrane components containing disulfide bonds and sulfhydryl group result in receptor regulation (136).

Supersensitivity and Up-Regulation of Receptors

Up-regulation of receptors may lead to hypersensitivity or supersensitivity to receptor agonists. This may be due to long-term administration of antagonists, or to synthesis of additional receptors. Up-regulation of receptors can also be homologous or heterologous. The administration of prolactin in vivo, as well as angiotensin II and pentagastrin, up-regulates their respective receptors (137). Exposure of lymphocytes to IL-2 increases the number of functional IL-2 receptors on $CD4^+$ cells. A similar phenomenon has also been reported for IgE receptors. In heterologous up-regulation of receptors, steroid hormones acting through their specific receptors can increase the density of cell surface receptors for polypeptides. For instance, estrogen can increase the number of oxytocin receptors in rat uterus. Corticosteroids have been observed to elevate the density of β-adrenoceptors in animal lung tissue (138) and human lymphocytes and granulocytes (139). In addition, glucocorticoids can also cause a switch in subtype from β_1 to β_2 (140).

Thus, cellular desensitization following the repeated administration of a drug can be manifest by receptor down-regulation and also by attenuation of maximum response. The latter effect is mainly due to a defect at a postreceptor site. On the other hand, continuous blockade of a receptor by antagonist may result in receptor recruitment and hypersensitization of cells. These mechanisms have important implications for understanding the pathophysiology of various disease states, and thus help in the development of new therapeutic and curative approaches.

CONCLUDING REMARKS

The biological signals carried by an immune-reacting substance activate a receptor, which sends the message through the membrane, and initiates a cascade of enzymatic steps to amplify the signal. This process ultimately leads to an output response that may include contraction or relaxation of a muscle, release of a mediator, or turning on a gene. This process is very complex and diversified. Several protein kinases are activated and bind to specific anchoring proteins at their site of action. We are beginning to understand how these pathways transmit an external signal into the cell language to elicit the appropriate response. Cross-talk between the pathways allows integration of the multiple signals that a cell receives at any one time. The multiplicity of the incoming signals and the myriad of biological processes that are regulated suggest that there are more signal pathways than those already uncovered. Transcription factors regulate the expression of genes and appear to play a pivotal role in genetic differences in phenotypes. Elucidation of various pathways and the identification and isolation of the involved proteins hopefully will provide an important means of cell regulation in various pathological conditions, and thus will be helpful in the development of better therapeutic and curative approaches.

REFERENCES

1. Benham CD. ATP-activated channels gate calcium entry in single smooth muscle cells dissociated from rabbit ear artery. J Physiol Lond 1989; 419:689–701.

2. Koch CA, Anderson D, Moran MF, Ellis C, Pawson T. SH2 and SH3 domains: elements that control interactions of cytoplasmic signaling proteins. Science 1991; 252:668–674.

3. Cowell IG, Skinner A, Hurst HC. Transcriptional repression by a novel member of the bZIP family of transcription factors. Mol Cell Biol 1992; 12:3070–3077.

4. Karpinski BA, Morle GD, Huggenvik J, Uhler MD, Leiden JM. Molecular cloning of CREB-2: an ATF/CREB transcription factor that can negatively regulate transcription from the cAMP response element. Proc Natl Acad Sci USA 1992; 89:4820–4824.

5. Lalli E, Sassone-Corsi P. Signal transduction and gene regulation: the nuclear response to cAMP. J Biol Chem 1994; 269:17359–17362.

6. Agrawal DK. Adrenoceptors in the airways: their characteristics and clinical implications. In: Hollinger MA ed. Focus on Pulmonary Pharmacology and Toxicology. Boca Raton, FL: CRC Press, 1990:85–104.

7. Agrawal DK, Numao T. Transmembrane signaling in eosinophils. In: Makino S, Fukuda T, eds. Eosinophils: Biological and Clinical Aspects. Boca Raton, FL: CRC Press, 1993:171–192.

8. Nishizuka Y. Turnover of inositol phospholipids and signal transduction. Science 1984; 225:1365–1369.

9. Berridge MJ, Irvine RF. Inositol phosphates and cell signaling. Nature 1989; 341:197–201.

10. Smrcka AV, Hepler JR, Brown KO, Strenweis PC. Regulation of polyphosphoinositide-specific phospholipase C activity by purified G_q. Science 1991; 251:804–809.

11. Putney JW. Receptor-regulated calcium entry. Pharmacol Ther 1990; 48:427–435.

12. Cadena DL, Gill GN. Receptor tyrosine kinases. FASEB J 1992; 6:2332–2337.

13. Cooper JA, Howell B. The when and how of Src regulation. Cell 1993; 73:1051–1054.

14. Hunter T, Karin M. The regulation of transcription by phosphorylation. Cell 1992; 70:375–387.

15. Heim MH, Kerr IM, Stark GR, Darnell JE Jr. Contribution of STAT SH2 groups to specific interferon signaling by the Jak–STAT pathway. Science 1995; 267:1347–1349.

16. Ihle JN, Witthuhn BA, Quelle FW, Yamamoto K, Thierfelder WE, Kreider B, Silvennoinen O. Signaling by the cytokine receptor superfamily: JAKs and STATs. Trends Biochem Sci 1994; 19:222–227.

17. Darnell JE Jr, Kerr IM, Stark GR. Jak-STAT pathways and transcriptional activation in response to IFNs and other extracellular signaling proteins. Science 1994; 264:1421.

18. Abebe W, Agrawal DK. Role of tyrosine kinases in norepinephrine-induced contraction of vascular smooth muscle. J Cardiovasc Pharamcol 1995; 26:153–159.

19. Northup JK, Sternweis PC, Smigel MD, Schlifer LS, Ross EM, Gilman AG. Purification of the regulatory component of adenylate cyclase. Proc Natl Acad Sci USA 1980; 77:6516–6520.

20. Gilman AG. G-proteins: transducers of receptor generated signals. Annu Rev Biochem 1987; 56:615–649.

21. Burgoyne RD, Morgan A. Low molecular mass GTP-binding proteins of adrenal chromaffin secretory granules. FEBS Lett 1989; 245:122–126.

22. Northup JK, Sternweis PC, Gilman AG. The subunits of the stimulatory regulatory component of adenylate cyclase. Resolution, activity, and properties of the 35,000-dalton (beta) subunit. J Biochem 1983; 258:11361–11368.

23. Moss J, Vaughan M. ADP ribosylation of guanyl nucleotide-binding regulatory proteins by bacterial toxins. Adv Enzymol 1988; 61:303–379.

24. Gilman AT. Regulation of adenylate cyclase by G-proteins. Adv Second Messenger Phospho-protein Res 1990; 24:51–57.

25. Birnbaumer L. Transduction of receptor signal into modulation of effector activity by G-proteins: the first 20 years or so. FASEB J 1990; 4:3068–3078.

26. Gierschik P, Codina J, Simons C, Birnbaumer L, Spiegel A. Antisera against a guanine nucleotide binding protein from retina cross-react with the beta-subunit of adenylate cyclase-associated guanine nucleotide binding proteins N_s and N_i. Proc Natl Acad Sci USA 1985; 82:727–731.

27. Robishaw JD, Russell DW, Harris BA, Smigel MD, Gilman AG. Deduced primary structure

of the alpha-subunit of GTP-binding stimulatory protein of adenylate cyclase. Proc Natl Acad Sci USA 1986; 83:1251–1255.

28. Bray P, Carter A, Simons C, Guo V, Puckett C, Kamholz J, Spiegel A, Niremberg M. Human cDNA clones for four species of $G_{\alpha s}$ signal transduction protein. Proc Natl Acad Sci USA 1986; 83: 8893–8897.

29. Simon M, Michael P, Strathmann P, Narasimhan G. Diversity of G-proteins in signal transduction. Science 1991; 252:802–808.

30. Capon DJ, Chen EY, Levinson AD, Seeburg PH, Goeddel DV. Complete nucleotide sequence of the T24 human bladder carcinoma oncogene and its normal homologue. Nature 1983; 302: 33–37.

31. Schmidtt HD, Wagner P, Pfaff E, Gallwitz D. The *ras* related *YPT1* gene product in yeast: a GTP-binding protein that might be involved in microtubule organization. Cell 1986; 47: 401–412.

32. Yamamoto K, Kondo J, Hishida T, Teranishi Y, Takai Y. Purification and characterization of a GTP-binding protein with a molecular weight of 20,000 dalton in bovine membrane. Identification of the *rho* gene product. J Biol Chem 1988; 263:9926–9932.

33. Segev N, Mulholland J, Botstein D. The yeast GTP binding YPT1 protein and a mammalian counterpart are associated with the secretion machinery. Cell 1988; 52:915–924.

34. Mayorga LS, Diaz R, Colombo ML, Stahl PD. GTPγS stimulation of endosome fusion suggests a role for a GTP-binding protein in the priming of vesicles before fusion. Cell Regul 1989; 1:113–124.

35. Gomperts BD. A GTP-binding protein mediating exocytosis. Annu Rev Physiol 1990; 52: 591–606.

36. Traub LM, Evans WH, Sagieisenberg R. A novel 100 kDa protein, localized to receptor enriched endosomes, is immunologically related to the signal transducing G-proteins G_t and G_i. Biochem J 1990; 272:453–458.

37. Udrisar D, Rodbell M. Microsome and cytosolic fractions of guinea pig hepatocytes contain 100 kDa GTP-binding proteins reactive with antisera against α-subunits of stimulatory and inhibitory heterotrimeric GTP-binding proteins. Proc Natl Acad Sci USA 1990; 87:6321–6325.

38. Ali N, Agrawal D K, Cheung P. Identification of G-proteins in rat parotid gland plasma membrane and granule membranes: presence of distinct components in granule membrane. Mol Cell Biochem 1992; 115:155–162.

39. Numao T, Ali N, Agrawal DK. High molecular weight GTP-binding proteins in human blood eosinophils: modulation by platelet-activating factor. J Allergy Clin Immunol 1992; 89:294.

40. Agrawal DK, Ali N, Numao T. PAF receptors and G-proteins in human blood eosinophils and neutrophils. J Lipid Mediat 1992; 5:101–104.

41. Abebe W, Edwards JD, Agrawal DK. G-proteins in rat blood vessels -I. Identification. Gen Pharmacol 1995; 26:65–73.

42. Joshi S, Abebe W, Agrawal DK. Identification of guanine nucleotide binding regulatory proteins in bovine tracheal smooth muscle. Mol Cell Biochem 1995; 153 (in press).

43. Joshi S, Abebe W, Agrawal DK. G-proteins in guinea pig airway smooth muscle: identification and functional involvement. Pharmacol Res 1995 (in press).

44. Asano M, Masuzawa K, Matsuda T. Role of stimulation GTP-binding protein (G_s) in reduced beta-adrenoceptor coupling in the femoral arteries isolated from spontaneously hypertensive rats. J Pharmacol Exp Ther 1988; 246:709–714.

45. Cheung YD, Feltham I, Thompson P, Triggle CR. α-Adrenoceptor activation of polyphosphoinositide hydrolysis in the rat tail artery. Biochem Pharmacol 1990; 40:2425–2432.

46. Dortal DE, Murahazhi T, Peach M. Regulation of cytosolic calcium by angiotensins in vascular smooth muscle. Hypertension 1990; 15:815–822.

47. Kitazawa T, Kobayashi S, Homiuti K, Somlyo AV, Somlyo AP. Receptor-coupled permeabilized smooth muscle. J Biol Chem 1989; 264:5339–5342.

48. Zeng YY, Benisthin CG, Pang PKT. Guanine nucleotide binding protein may modulate gating of

calcium channels in vascular smooth muscle. I. Studies with fluoride. J Pharmacol Exp Ther 1989; 250:343–351.

49. Somlyo AP, Walker JW, Goldman YE, Trentham P, Kobayashi DR, Kitazawa S, Somlyo AV. Inositol trisphosphate, calcium and muscle contraction. Philos Trans R Soc Lond Biol Sci 1988; 320:399–414.

50. Abebe W, Edwards JD, Agrawal DK. G-protein in rat blood vessels—II. Assessment of functional involvement. Gen Pharmacol 1995; 26:75–83.

51. Rall TW, Sutherland EW. Formation of a cyclic adenine ribonucleotide by tissue particles. J Biochem 1958; 232:1065–1067.

52. Taylor CW, Merrit JE. Receptor coupling to polyphosphoinositide turnover: a parallel with the adenylate cyclase system. Trends Pharmacol Sci 1986; 7:238–242.

53. Hall IP, Donaldson J, Hill SJ. Modulation of fluoroaluminate-induced inositol phosphate formation by increase in tissue cyclic AMP content in bovine tracheal smooth muscle. Br J Pharmacol 1990; 100:646–650.

54. Godfrey PP, Watson SP. Fluoride inhibits agonist-induced formation of inositol phosphates in rat cortex. Biochem Biophys Res Commun 1988; 155:664–669.

55. Marc S, Leifer D, Harbon S. Fluoroaluminates muscarinic and oxytocin-receptor mediated generation of inositolphosphates and contraction in the intact guinea pig myometrium. Biochem J 1988; 255:705–713.

56. Watson SP, Stanley AF, Sasaguri T. Does the hydrolysis of inositol phospholipids lead to the opening of voltage operated Ca^{2+} channels in guinea pig ileum. Studies with fluoride ions and caffeine. Biochem Biophys Res Commun 1988; 153:14–20.

57. Popescu LM, Hinescu ME, Musat S, Ionescu M, Pistritzu F. Inositol trisphosphate and the contraction of vascular smooth muscle cells. Eur J Pharmacol 1986; 123:167–169.

58. Jope RS, Lally KM. Synaptosomal calcium influx is activated by sodium fluoride. Biochem Biophys Res Commun 1988; 151:774–780.

59. Hughes BP, Barritt GJ. The stimulation of sodium fluoride of plasma-membrane Ca^{2+} inflow in isolated hepatocytes. Evidence that a GTP-binding regulatory protein is involved in hormonal stimulation of Ca^{2+} inflow. Biochem J 1987; 245:41–47.

60. Ui M. G-proteins identified as pertussis toxin substrates. In: Naccache PH, ed. G-Protein and Calcium Signalling. Boca Raton, FL: CRC Press, 1990:3–27.

61. Iyengar R, Birnbaumer L. Signal transduction by G-proteins. ISI Atlas Sci Pharmacol 1987; 1:213–222.

62. Stryer L, Bourne HR. G-proteins: a family of signal transducers. Annu Rev Cell Biol 1986; 2: 391–419.

63. Ohta H, Okajima F, Ui M. Inhibition of islet-activating protein of a peptide-induced early breakdown of inositol phospholipids and Ca^{2+} mobilization in guinea pig neutrophils. J Biol Chem 1985; 260:15771–15780.

64. Smith JB, Smith L, Higgins BL. Temperature and nucleotide dependence of calcium release by *myo*-inositol 1, 4, 5-trisphosphate in cultured vascular smooth muscle cells. J Biol Chem 1985; 260:14413–14416.

65. Brandt SJ, Dougherty RW, Lapetina EG, Niedel JG. Pertussis toxin inhibits chemotactic peptide-stimulated generation of inositol phosphates and lysosomal enzyme secretion in human leukemic (HL) cells. Proc Natl Acad Sci USA 1985; 82:3277–3280.

66. Pfeilschifter J, Bauer C. Pertussis toxin abolishes angiotensin II-induced phosphoinositide hydrolysis and prostaglandin synthesis in rat renal mesengial cells. Biochem J 1986; 236:289–294.

67. Nakamura T, Ui M. Simultaneous inhibition of inositol phospholipid breakdown, arachidonic acid release and histamine secretion in mast cells by islet-activating protein, pertussis toxin. J Biol Chem 1985; 260:3584–3593.

68. Lynch CJ, Pepic V, Blackmore F, Exton JH. Effect of islet-activating pertussis toxin on the binding characteristics of Ca^{2+} mobilizing hormones and on agonist activation of phosphorylase in hepatocytes. Mol Pharmacol 1986; 29:196–203.

69. Masters SB, Martin MW, Harden TK, Brown JH. Pertussis toxin does not inhibit muscarinic-receptor-mediated PI hydrolysis or calcium mobilization. Biochem J 1985; 227:933–937.
70. Schimmel RJ, Elliott ME. Pertussis toxin does not prevent alpha-adrenergic stimulated breakdown of phosphoinositides in brown adipocytes. Biochem Biophys Res Commun 1986; 135: 823–829.
71. Cockcroft S. Polyphosphoinositide phosphodiesterase: regulation by a novel guanine nucleotide binding protein, G_p. Trends Biochem Sci 1987; 12:75–78.
72. Cockcroft S, Gomperts BD. Role of guanine nucleotide binding protein in the activation of polyphosphoinositide phosphodiesterase. Nature 1985; 314:534–536.
73. Abdel-Latif AA. Calcium-mobilizing receptors, polyphosphoinositide and the generation of second messengers. Pharmacol Rev 1986; 38:227–272.
74. Sankary RM, Jones CA, Madison JM, Brown JK. Muscarinic cholinergic inhibition of cAMP accumulation in airway smooth muscle. Role of a pertussis toxin-sensitive protein. Am Rev Respir Dis 1988; 138:145–150.
75. Jakobs KH, Lasch P, Minuth M, Aktories K, Schultz G. Uncoupling of α-adrenoceptor mediated inhibition of human platelet adenylate cyclase by NEM. J Biol Chem 1982; 257:2829–2833.
76. Qian Z, Drewes LR. Cross-talk between receptor-regulated phospholipase D and phospholipase C in brain. FASEB J 1991; 5:315–319.
77. Liscovitch M. Crosstalk among multiple signal-activated phospholipases. Trends Biochem Sci 1992; 17:393–399.
78. Chisholm L, Dovgan PS, Agrawal DK, McGregor PE, Edwards JD. Modulation of monocyte adherence to endothelial cells by endothelin-1: involvement of *src* (p60*src*) and JAK1-like kinases. J Vasc Surg 1996; 23 (in press).
79. Liu Y, Geisbuhler B, Jones AW. Activation of multiple mechanisms including phospholipase D by endothelin-1 in rat aorta. Am J Physiol 1992; 262:C941–C949.
80. Spry CJF. Eosinophils: A comprehensive Review and Guide to the Scientific and Medical Literature. Oxford: Oxford University Press, 1988:43–52.
81. Nuesse O, Lindau M, Cromwell O, Kay AB, Gomperts BD. Intracellular application of guanosine-5'-O-(3-thiotriphosphate) induces exocytotic granule fusion in guinea pig eosinophils. J Exp Med 1990; 171:775–782.
82. Cromwell O, Bennett JP, Hide I, Kay AB, Gomperts BD. Mechanism of granule enzyme secretion from permeabilized guinea pig eosinophils: dependence on Ca^{2+} and guanine nucleotides. J Immunol 1991; 147:1905–1910.
83. Holgate ST, Hutson PA, Shute JK, Rimmer SJ, Akkerman CL, Church MK. The role of neutrophils and eosinophils in a model of asthma in the guinea pig. In: Kay AB, ed. Eosinophils. London: Blackwell Scientific, 1990:83–92.
84. Capron M, Prin L, Ameisen J-C, Capron A. Immunoglobulin receptors on eosinophil leucocytes. In: Kay AB, ed. Eosinophils. London: Blackwell Scientific, 1990:11–18.
85. Puustinen T, Sheffer MM, Samuelsson B. Regulation of the human 5'-lipoxygenase: stimulation by micromolar Ca^{2+} levels and phosphatidylcholine vesicles. Biochim Biophys Acta 1988; 960:261–272.
86. Dixon RAF, Diehl RE, Opas E, Rands E, Vickers PJ, Evans JF, Gillard JW, Miller DK. Requirement of a 5-lipoxygenase-activating protein for leukotriene synthesis. Nature 1990; 343:282–288.
87. Anderson NG, Li P, Marsden LA, William N, Roberts TM, Sturgill TW. Raf-1 is a potential substrate for mitogen-activated protein kinase in vivo. Biochem J 1991; 277:573–576.
88. Karin M, Smeal T. Control of transcription factors by signal transduction pathways: the beginning of the end. Trends Biochem Sci 1992; 17:418–422.
89. Rapp UR. Role of Raf-1 serine/threonine protein kinase in growth factor signal transduction. Oncogene 1991; 6:495–500.
90. Howe LR, Leevers SJ, Gomez N, Nakielny S, Cohen P, Marshall CJ. Activation of the MAP kinase pathway by the protein kinase raf. Cell 1992; 71:335–342.

91. Claesson-Welsh L. platelet-derived growth factor receptor signals. J Biol Chem 1994; 269: 32023–32026.

92. Padeh S, Levitzki A, Gazit A, Mills GB, Roifman CM. Activation of phospholipase C in human B cells is dependent on tyrosine phosphorylation. J Clin Invest 1991; 87:1114–1118.

93. Pelech SL, Charest DL, Mordret GP, Siow YL, Palaty C, Campbell D, Charlton L, Samiei M, Sanghera JS. Networking with mitogen-activated protein kinases. Mol Cell Biochem 1993; 127/128:157–169.

94. Anderson N. MAP kinases—ubiquitous signal transducers and potentially important components of the cell cycling machinery in eukaryotes. Cell Signal 1992; 4:239–246.

95. Ahn NG. The MAP kinase cascade: discovery of a new signal transduction pathway. Mol Cell Biochem 1993; 127/128:201–209.

96. Whitmarsh AJ, Shore P, Sharrocks AD, Davis RJ. Integration of MAP kinase signal transduction pathways at the serum response element. Science 1995; 269:403–407.

97. Kyriakis JM, App H, Zhang X-F, Banerjee P, Brautigan DL, Rapp UR, Avruch J. Raf-1 activates MAP kinase-kinase. Nature 1992; 358:417–421.

98. Galcheva-Gargova Z. An osmosensing signal transduction pathway in mammalian cells. Science 1994; 265:806–808.

99. Taniguchi T. Cytokine signaling through nonreceptor protein tyrosine kinases. Science 1995; 268:251–255.

100. Numao T, Agrawal DK. Neuropeptides modulate human eosinophil chemotaxis. J Immunol 1992; 149:3309–3315.

101. Sera MCF, Bazzoni F, Bianca VD, Greskowiak M, Rossi F. Activation of human neutrophils by substance P: effect on oxidative metabolism, exocytosis, cytosolic Ca^{2+} concentration and inositol phosphate formation. J Immunol 1988; 141:2118–2125.

102. Buckley TL, Brain SD, Collins S, William TJ. Inflammatory edema induced by interactions between IL-1 and the neuropeptide calcitonin gene-related peptide. J Immunol 1991; 146:3424–3430.

103. Bevilacqua MP, Nelson RM. Selectins. J Clin Invest 1993; 91:379–387.

104. Clark EA, Brugge JS. Integrins and signal transduction pathways: the road taken. Science 1995; 268:233–239.

105. Abelda SM, Buck CA. Integrins and other cell adhesion molecules. FASEB J 1990; 4:2868–2880.

106. Hynes RO. Integrins: versatility, modulation, and signaling in cell adhesion. Cell 1992; 69: 11–25.

107. Schwartz M, Denninghoff K. alpha-V integrins mediate the rise in intracellular calcium in endothelial cells on fibronectin even though they play a minor role in adhesion. J Biol Chem 1994; 269:11133–11137.

108. Pardi R, Bender JR, Dettori C, Giannazza E, Engleman EG. Heterogeneous distribution and transmembrane signaling properties of lymphocyte function-associated antigen (LFA-1) in human lymphocyte subsets. J Immunol 1989; 143:3157–3166.

109. Kornberg LJ, Earp HS, Turner CE, Prockop C, Juliano RL. Signal transduction by integrins: increased protein tyrosine phosphorylation caused by clustering of beta-1 integrins. Proc Natl Acad Sci USA 1991; 88:8392–8396.

110. Hanks SK, Calalb MB, Harper MC, Patel SK. Focal adhesion protein-tyrosine kinase phosphorylated in response to cell attachment to fibronectin. Proc Natl Acad Sci USA 1992; 89:8487–8491.

111. Hildebrand JD, Schaller MD, Parsons JT. Identification of sequences required for the efficient localization of the focal adhesion kinase, pp125FAK, to cellular focal adhesions. J Cell Biol 1993; 123:993–1005.

112. van Noesel C, Miedema F, Brouwer M, de Rie MA, Aarden LA, van Lier RA. Regulatory properties of LFA-1 alpha and beta chains in human T-lymphocyte activation. Nature 1988; 333:850–852.

113. Elstad MR, Parker CJ, Cowley FS, Wilcox LA, McIntyre TM, Prescott SM, Zimmerman GA. CD11b/CD18 integrin and a beta-glucan receptor act in concert to induce the synthesis of platelet-activating factor by monocytes. J Immunol 1994; 152:220–230.

114. Ravetch JV, Kinet J-P. Fc receptors. Annu Rev Immunol 1991; 9:457–492.

115. Paolini R, Jouvin MH, Kinet JP. Phosphorylation and dephosphorylation of the high-affinity receptor for immunoglobulin E immediately after receptor engagement and disengagement. Nature 1991; 353:855–858.

116. Eiseman E, Bolen JB. Engagement of the high-affinity IgE receptor activates *src* protein-related tyrosine kinases. Nature 1992; 355:78–83.

117. Benhamou M, Siraganian RP. Protein–tyrosine phosphorylation: an essential component of FcεRI signaling. Immunol Today 1992; 13:195–199.

118. Hamawy MM, Mergenhagen S, Siraganian RP. Tyrosine phosphorylation of pp125^{FAK} by the aggregation of high-affinity immunoglobulin E receptors requires cell adherence. J Biol Chem 1993; 268:6851–6856.

119. Hamawy MM, Swaim WD, Minoguchi K, de Feijter AW, Mergenhagen SE, Siraganian RP. The aggregation of the high affinity IgE receptor induces tyrosine phosphorylation of paxillin, a focal adhesion protein. J Immunol 1994; 153:4655–4662.

120. Paliogianni F, Ahuja SS, Balow JP, Balow JE, Boumpas DT. Novel mechanism for inhibition of human T cells by glucocorticoids. Glucocorticoids inhibit signal transduction through IL-2 receptor. J Immunol 1993; 151:4081–4089.

121. Springer TA. Traffic signals for lymphocyte recirculation and leukocyte emigration: the multi-step paradigm. Cell 1994; 76:301–314.

122. Caldenhoven E, Liden J, Wissink S, Van de Stolpe A, Raaijmakers J, Koenderman L, Okret S, Gustafsson J-A, Van der Saag T. Negative cross-talk between RelA and the glucocorticoid receptor: a possible mechanism for the antiinflammatory action of glucocorticoids. Mol Endocrinol 1995; 9:401–412.

123. Vig E, Barrett TJ, Vedeckis WV. Coordinate regulation of glucocorticoid receptor and c-*jun* mRNA levels: evidence for cross-talk between two signaling pathways at the transcriptional level. Mol Endocrinol 1994; 8:1336–1346.

124. Lucibello FC, Slater EP, Jooss KU, Beato M, Mueller R. Mutual transrepression of Fos and the glucocorticoid receptor: involvement of a functional domain in Fos which is absent in FosB. EMBO J 1990; 9:2827–2834.

125. Kerppola TK, Luk D, Curran T. Fos is a preferential target of glucocorticoid receptor inhibition of AP-1 activity in vitro. Mol Cell Biol 1993; 13:3782–3791.

126. Jonat C, Rahmsdorf HJ, Park K-K, Cato ACB, Gebel S, Ponta H, Herrlich P. Antitumor promotion and antiinflammation: down-modulation of AP-1 (*fos/jun*) activity by glucocorticoid hormone. Cell 1990; 62:1189–1204.

127. Yang-Yen HF, Chambard JC, Sun Y-L, Smeal T, Schmidt TJ, Drouin J, Karin M. Transcriptional interference between c-*jun* and the glucocorticoid receptor: mutual inhibition of DNA binding due to direct protein–protein interaction. Cell 1990; 62:1205–1215.

128. Schuele R, Rangarajan P, Kliewer S, Ransone LJ, Bolado J, Yang N, Verma IM, Evans RM. Functional antagonism between the oncoprotein c-*jun* and the glucocorticoid receptor. Cell 1990; 62:1217–1226.

129. Agrawal DK, Townley RG. Effect of platelet-activating factor on beta adrenoceptors in human lung. Biochem Biophys Res Commun 1987; 143:1–6.

130. Agrawal DK. Platelet-activating factor in the airways. In: Agrawal DK, Townley RG, eds. Inflammatory Cells and Mediators in Bronchial Asthma. Boca Raton, FL: CRC Press, 1991:171–206.

131. Agrawal DK, Bergren DR, Byorth PJ, Townley RG. Platelet-activating factor induces non-specific desensitization to bronchodilators in guinea pigs. J Pharmacol Exp Ther 1991; 259:1–7.

132. Benovic JL, Strasser RH, Caron MJ, Lefkowitz RJ. beta-Adrenergic receptor-kinase: identifica-

tion of a novel protein kinase that phosphorylates the agonist-occupied form of the receptor. Proc Natl Acad Sci USA 1986; 83:2797–2802.

133. Wilson CJ, Applebury ML. Arresting G-protein coupled receptor activity. Curr Biol 1993; 3: 683–686.

134. Sallese M, Lombardi MS, Haske TN, Levine H III, De Blasi A. Molecular analysis of the functional role of β-adrenergic receptor kinase-1 amino-terminal. J Recept Signal Transd Res 1995; 15:81–90.

135. Hirata F, Axelrod J. Phospholipid methylation and biological signal transduction. Science 1980; 209:1082–1090.

136. Jacobs S, Cuatrecasas P. Disulfide reduction converts the insulin receptor of human placenta to a low affinity form. J Clin Invest 1980; 66;1424–1427.

137. Takeuchi K, Speir GR, Johnson LR. Mucosal gastrin receptor. III. Regulation by gastrin. Am J Physiol 1980; 238:G135–G140.

138. Mano K, Akbarzadeh A, Townley RG. Effect of hydrocortisone on beta-adrenergic receptors in lung membranes. Life Sci 1979; 25:195–201.

139. Davis AW, Lefkowitz RJ. Steroid-induced regulation of human leukocyte beta-adrenergic receptors. J Clin Endocrinol Metab 1980; 51:599–606.

140. Lai E, Rosen OM, Rubin CS. Dexamethasone regulates the β-adrenergic receptor subtype expressed by 3T3-L1 preadipocytes and adipocytes. J Biol Chem 1982; 257:6691–6696.

2

Lymphokine-Induced Signal Transduction

Hallgeir Rui, Robert A. Kirken, Roy J. Duhe, O. M. Zack Howard, Gerald A. Evans, and William L. Farrar*
National Cancer Institute, Frederick Cancer Research and Development Center, Frederick, Maryland

INTRODUCTION

Lymphokines constitute a diverse set of signaling proteins released from cells of the immune system, and they are intimately involved in the coordination of immune responses. These factors exert a wide range of influences, and regulate cellular growth, differentiation, activation state, and chemotaxis. Selective cell surface receptors bind and mediate the effects of lymphokines by initiating specific biochemical signaling cascades.

Insight into the molecular mechanisms of lymphokine-induced signal transduction is critical for our comprehension of the immune system and a variety of immunological diseases. Knowledge of function is essential for the understanding of malfunction, whether it be of genetic or environmental origin. Furthermore, information about receptor action is necessary for a directed development of receptor-specific drugs, which generally promise fewer side effects than pharmacological agents acting on downstream effector molecules shared by converging signaling pathways. Classification of receptors into related families based on primary sequence homologies, has greatly facilitated a concerted effort to elucidate their activation mechanisms. Conserved sequences typically indicate important domains of shared function, and results obtained from studies of one receptor family member can be rapidly applied to related receptors, thereby stimulating a synergistic disclosure of the common mechanisms of action for receptor relatives.

In most respects, there are no clear distinctions between lymphokines and other arbitrarily designated groups of extracellular signal proteins, including cytokines, hormones, and growth factors. Indeed several classic hormones and growth factors may also be lymphokines (e.g., prolactin and platelet-derived growth factor). Similarly, lymphokine receptors belong structurally and functionally to a number of different classes of receptors that are not restricted to lymphokine ligands. Hence, probably no unique signaling pathway has evolved exclusively for lymphokines and, consequently, this review of lymphokine-induced signal transduction will include information relating to transmembrane signal transduction in general.

The major families of lymphokine–cytokine receptors are the hematopoietin receptors, interferon receptors, tumor necrosis factor receptors, immunoglobulin-domain receptors, and chemokine receptors (1). Among these, hematopoietin receptors and interferon receptors are structurally and functionally related. This review will emphasize signal transduction by the hematopoietin receptors, the largest of these receptor families, but the function of the other classes of lymphokine receptors will also be discussed.

THE HEMATOPOIETIN RECEPTOR SUPERFAMILY

Researchers have interchangeably referred to this superfamily of receptors as the cytokine, hematopoietin, or the PRL/GH/IL receptor family (2–8). Although their respective ligands may not all have hematopoietic effects, the term hematopoietin receptor family will be used throughout this review.

The diverse group of ligands that bind to hematopoietin receptors includes most of the 13 currently known interleukins (except IL-1, IL-8, and IL-10), granulocyte–macrophage colony-stimulating factor (GM-CSF), granulocyte colony-stimulating factor (G-CSF), oncostatin M (OSM), leukemia inhibitory factor (LIF), and ciliary neurotrophic factor (CNTF), erythropoietin (EPO), growth hormone (GH), and prolactin (PRL) (2–8). Furthermore, the oncogene v-*mpl* has been shown to encode part of a recently cloned orphan receptor, MPL, which also belongs to this receptor family (9). A majority of the ligands binding to hematopoietin receptors constitute growth factors for many of their target cells, and at least two receptors, EPOR and MPL, have demonstrated oncogenic potential (9,10). However, most of these signaling proteins also seem capable of inducing differentiation as well as specific functional activities of their target cells.

Receptor Structure

Hematopoietin receptors share several conserved structural features, mainly in their extracellular domains (2–8). These include a double β-barrel organization, with four conserved cysteine residues and a characteristic Trp-Ser-X-Trp-Ser motif (WS-box). The paired cysteines are important for ligand binding, but no definite role beyond a possible involvement in protein–protein interaction has yet been established for the WS-box (11–13). Interestingly, in several receptors thus far cloned, this extracellular hematopoietin domain has been serially duplicated, providing chicken PRLR, murine IL-3Rα, and human MPL with a "double-antenna structure" (9,14,15). The resulting conceptual bivalency of these receptor forms may represent an evolutionary advantage that could shed light on the mechanism of activation for these receptors.

Hematopoietin receptors have a single transmembrane segment of approximately 25 amino acids, with a predicted α-helical structure. The cytoplasmic domains of the various family members show substantial diversity in size and structure, implying unique interaction capacities with primary and secondary effector proteins. However, a conserved membrane-proximal motif has been identified, denoted homology box 1 (16,17) or proline-rich motif (PRM) (18). A second, less conserved cytoplasmic region, box 2, is found in PRL receptors and several other hematopoietin receptors (16,17). Recent studies on the effect of systematic deletion of cytoplasmic segments from various hematopoietin receptors, including EPOR, gp130, GHR, PRLR, IL-2Rβ, and G-CSFR, have demonstrated that the capacity to generate mitogenic signal resides within these juxtamembrane regions (16,17,19–34). However, the removal of "dispensable" receptor regions may be compensated for by activating mutations in the transfected cell lines (35), and the mitogenic contribution of these segments may be underestimated.

Ligand-Specific Subunits and Shared Signal Transducers

The assembly of subunits for the various hematopoietin receptor complexes has proved surprisingly diverse and complex (6,36,37). Figure 1 represents a systematization of subgroups of hematopoietin receptors according to their ligands and receptor components. Some ligands appear to employ only one receptor protein, including PRL, GH, EPO, and G-CSF, whereas other ligands use unique, specificity-conferring subunits to facilitate binding and subsequent activation of a second signal-transducing subunit which, by itself, has only low affinity of the cytokine (6,36,37). In these latter cases, both receptor components are needed for high-affinity binding and signal transduction, but the signal-transducing subunit might be shared by several ligands. For instance, receptor complexes for human IL-3, IL-5, and GM-CSF comprise specific α-subunits in combination with the

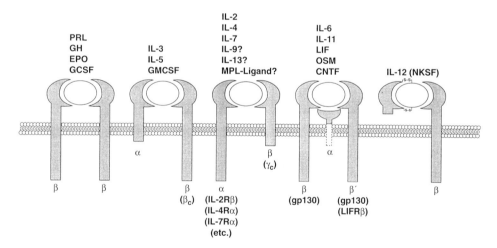

Figure 1 Systematization of hematopoietin receptors into subgroups based on common signal-transducing β-subunits: PRL, GH, EPO, and GCSF each activate a single form of signal-transducing proteins that also bind the ligand with high affinity. IL-3, IL-5, and GMCSF bind primarily to ligand-specific α-subunits and share the signal-transducing β-subunit, KH97 or β_c. IL-2, IL-4, IL-7, and IL-9 (and possibly IL-13 and the MPL-ligand, see text), share the IL-2 receptor γ-chain (γ_c), and have unique ligand-specific α-subunits. Note that the IL-2R β-chain (IL-2Rβ) is categorized as an α-subunit. It remains to be established if both IL-2Rγ and its associated α-subunits are signal transducers. The IL-6/LIF/OSM/CNTF/IL-11 subfamily of ligands utilize signal-transducing components gp130 or LIFRβ, or both, in addition to optional α-subunits. No transmembrane receptor has been identified for IL-12, which is a unique disulfide-linked hybrid of a ligand-like protein and an α-subunit-like receptor protein. See text for details.

common signal-transducing β-subunit, KH97 or β_c (6,38). The IL-2 receptors present another variant of complexity, since IL-2 interacts not only with two essential hematopoietin receptor subunits, IL-2Rβ and IL-2Rγ, but also with a third, nonconforming protein with a short cytoplasmic domain, IL-2Rα (39). This accessory receptor subunit serves as a positive affinity modulator through its regulated expression (40,41). Furthermore, IL-2Rγ was recently shown to be shared by several lymphoid growth factors, including IL-2, IL-4, and IL-7 (42–44), and an involvement in IL-9 and IL-13 signaling was postulated, based on sequence homologies and functional data (45,46). In Figure 1, we have also tentatively placed the unknown MPL-ligand in this subgroup, since hybrids comprising the extracellular MPL-domain and the cytoplasmic IL-4Rα-domain, function in a fashion analogous to that of wild-type IL-4Rα (47).

It was recently demonstrated that the X-linked, severe combined immunodeficiency syndrome (XSCID) is the clinical manifestation of a genetic inactivation of IL-2Rγ (48,49). This syndrome is substantially more serious than the relatively mild immunosuppression associated with isolated IL-2-deficiency, an observation that can now be explained by the synchronous abrogation of signal transduction by multiple cytokines (42–44,48,49).

Distinctive receptor subunit complexity is also seen with the IL-6/OSM/LIF/CNTF/ IL-11 subfamily of cytokines, which utilize either gp130, LIFRβ, or both, as signal-transducing components (36–38), in addition to optional, ligand-specific α-subunits. The CNTFRα has no transmembrane segment, but is anchored to the outer leaflet of the plasma membrane by a glycophosphatidylinositol linkage (50), whereas IL-6Rα has a short, but dispensable, cytoplasmic domain. In fact, soluble extracellular IL-6Rα is active in conjunction with IL-6, and this complex of ligand and soluble receptor transmits a signal into the cell by interacting with the extracellular domain of the signal transducer gp130 (51,52). Whether this represents a physiological endocrine mechanism remains to be established, but the majority of hematopoietin receptors exist also as soluble binding proteins, including IL-6Rα (53–57). Interleukin-12 represents an interesting conceptual variant of a complex between a ligand and its soluble receptor, since this lymphokine is a circulating, disulfide-liked heterodimer of a 35-kDa ligand-like protein and a 42-kDa WS–box-containing member of the hematopoietin receptor family (58,59). Its transmembrane, signal-transducing receptor protein has not yet been identified, but it could conceivably be, or be related to, gp130/LIFRβ. In Figure 1, we have provisionally placed this receptor–ligand hybrid in a group by itself.

Ligand–Induced Receptor Subunit Dimerization

Major progress has recently been made in the understanding of the molecular events that occur when ligand binds to hematopoietin receptors. Receptor dimerization or oligomerization appears to be the initial result of ligand binding, a phenomenon that is rapidly replacing the previously favored conformational change as a general mechanism of transmembrane signaling by growth factor receptors (37,38,60,61). Single-subunit receptors, including G-CSFR, PRLR, GHR, and EPOR, may undergo homodimerization, whereas multicomponent receptor complexes may aggregate by heterodimerization.

Several lines of evidence support such ligand-induced receptor aggregation. Direct structural confirmation of receptor homodimerization was obtained by high-resolution x-ray crystallography of GH–GHR complexes (62,63). The data showed that one molecule of GH simultaneously bound two molecules of soluble GHR. The binding interfaces were mapped, and a mutant GH, with affinity for only one receptor site, acted as a potent antagonist of GH-induced proliferation (64). This monovalent GHR antagonist also served as a PRLR antagonist, which can be explained by the fact that human GH cross-reacts with PRLR, implying a similar activation mechanism for PRLR (65). Additional evidence for dimerization being the inductive element of hematopoietin receptor activation came with the observation that a point mutation in EPOR resulted in a constitutively active, disulfide-linked dimer with oncogenic potential (10). Furthermore, recent evidence has been presented that gp130 and LIF, the signal-transducing components of IL-6/LIF/OSM/CNTF/IL-11 receptor complexes, undergo homo- or heterodimerization following ligand binding (36,37,66–68).

Further functional data in support of homodimerization of receptor components include the ability of bivalent monoclonal antireceptor antibodies to mimic the effect of several cognate ligands. This has been shown for PRLR (69, and references therein) and GHR (64,70,71), and indirectly for G-CSFR, using anti-GHR monoclonal antibodies (MAbs) to activate hybrid receptors consisting of extracellular GHR domains and cytoplasmic G-CSFR domains (64). Monovalent Fab-fragments of these agonistic antibodies remain inactive, unless religated with bivalent anti-Fab antibodies.

Involvement of JAK Tyrosine Kinases

The demonstration of a key role for cytoplasmic JAK tyrosine kinases in hematopoietin receptor signaling, ended several years of searching for the primary, hematopoietin receptor-associated tyrosine kinase(s) (72,73). Until recently, three known JAK kinases had been isolated from mammalian cells: JAK1, JAK2, and TYK2 (74–81). The JAK kinases are characterized by tandem phosphotransfer–kinase domains comprising the COOH-terminal third of the molecules, and an absence of typical src-homology domains and transmembrane segments. These enzymes are ubiquitously expressed in a variety of tissues and cells. Ihle and collaborators were the first to demonstrate that EPO, GH, and IL-3 rapidly activated and tyrosine phosphorylated JAK2 (72,73,82). Using similar methods, we have extended these findings to include JAK2 activation by PRL (83). Furthermore, the IL-6/LIF/OSM/CNTF/IL-11 subfamily of ligands appears to recruit JAK1, JAK2, and TYK2, depending on cell type (84). In contrast, a distinct JAK kinase migrating at 116 kDa is used by IL-2 (85,86). This conclusion was based on comparison of net charge and phosphopeptide maps between p116 and JAK2, as well as homologous functional characteristics. A polyclonal antibody raised against a peptide corresponding to the COOH-terminal region of a recently cloned, novel form of JAK kinase, L-JAK (87), identified p116 both in immunoblotting and immunoprecipitation experiments (88,89). Other laboratories have also obtained complete or partial sequence of this novel JAK kinase, tentatively designated JAK3 (90), TK5 (91), or ptk2 (92). In addition to regulating p116/L-JAK/JAK3, IL-2 also induced tyrosine phosphorylation of JAK1 in human YT cells, but this response was modest compared with the degree of p116/L-JAK/JAK3 phosphorylation (93).

Moreover, using rat Nb2 cells, which are responsive to multiple cytokines, we found that IL-2, IL-4, IL-7, and IL-9 selectively tyrosine phosphorylated p116/L-JAK/JAK3 (88,93), thereby providing a possible link between this JAK kinase and the common IL-2Rγ. Table 1 is a summary of the currently known ligand–JAK kinase partners. Work is in progress addressing the mode of interaction between JAK enzymes and individual receptor complexes. Although JAK kinases probably constitute the primary effector molecules triggered by hematopoietin receptor aggregation, many unanswered questions remain before a full understanding of the mechanisms and significance of JAK activation is achieved.

Table 1 Review of Lymphokine Activation of JAK Enzymes. Hematopoietin and Interferon Receptor Ligands and Their Reported JAK Kinase Partners. Only Positive Observations Are Indicated.

	JAK1	JAK2	TYK2	JAK3 (L-JAK/p116)	Ref.
PRL		+			83
GH		+			73
EPO		+			72
G-CSF					
IL-3		+			82
Il-5					
GM-CSF					
IL-2	+			+	86, 88, 89
IL-4				+	88, 89
IL-7				+	88
IL-9				+	93
IL-13					
Il-6	+		+		84
LIF					
OSM					
CNTF	+	+	+		84
IL-11					
IL-12					
IFNα/β	+		+		80, 151, 152, 153
IFNγ	+	+			152, 153

Are JAK Kinases Associated with Receptors Before Ligand Binding?

The absence of tyrosine kinase activity in PRL and GH receptor immune complexes from unstimulated cells (73,83,94–96) does not support the notion of preassociation of JAK enzymes with hematopoietin receptors. However, analysis of anti-PRL receptor immunoprecipitates by anti-JAK2 immunoblotting revealed that JAK2 was associated with PRLR both before and after ligand binding (83). The fact that JAK2 can be purified using immobilized EPOR fusion proteins as an affinity matrix also supports a direct interaction between the unactivated receptor and the kinase (72). A lesser degree of association might be expected if an adaptor protein was required to bridge the receptor and kinase. Similarly, the unexpectedly high efficiency of indirect affinity purification of GHR- and PRLR-associated JAK2 by antiligand antibodies (73, 94–96) further supports the notion of a direct interaction between receptor and kinase. Association of JAK kinases with the unactivated signal-transducing receptor components, gp130–LIFRβ, was also reported (84). Finally, in IL-2 receptor immune complexes from YT cells grown in the absence of IL-2, tyrosine kinase activity and phosphorylation of p116/L-JAK/JAK3 were observed in both stimulated and unstimulated receptor complexes (85,86). Taken together, these observations strongly suggest an association of JAK enzymes with the cytoplasmic segments of unactivated hematopoietin receptors. The absence of catalytic activity of immune complexes from unstimulated GH and PRL receptors may have technical reasons, such as disruption of key receptor components caused by detergent sensitivity.

Further work is needed to determine the site of interaction between receptor components and JAK kinases. The ability of EPO and PRL receptors with cytoplasmic deletions to mediate ligand-induced tyrosine phosphorylation of JAK2, correlated with the presence of intact homology boxes 1 and 2 (72,97). This is in agreement with the observation that these cytoplasmic homology regions are critical to the mitogenic activity of several hematopoietin receptors tested, including GHR, EPOR, PRLR, IL-2Rβ, and GM-CSFR (16,17,19–34).

How Do JAK Enzymes Become Activated?

The data reviewed in the foregoing indicate that the cytoplasmic domain of the unstimulated signal-transducing subunits of hematopoietin receptors are associated with JAK enzymes, and that the ligand induces receptor dimerization. In light of these observations, a simple model of activation, analogous to that of receptor tyrosine kinases, such as epidermal growth factor (EGF) and platelet-derived growth factor (PDGF) receptors, has been proposed (36,86). These growth factor receptors are stimulated by ligand-induced dimerization, which allows activation of the intrinsic kinase through intermolecular transphosphorylation (60). By using a series of bivalent monoclonal anti-PRL receptor antibodies, we have recently shown that receptor-associated JAK2 is tyrosine phosphorylated in response to antibody-induced receptor aggregation of PRL receptors in a transient manner similar to that induced by PRL (98). Monovalent antireceptor Fab-fragments required religation with bivalent anti-Fab antibodies to be active. Furthermore, the mitogenic potency of the five MAbs correlated with their ability to induce tyrosine phosphorylation of JAK2 (98).

It is expected that bivalent, monospecific antibodies toward other homodimerizing, signal-transducing receptor subunits, will also activate associated cytoplasmic JAK kinases. When heterodimerization of distinct receptor chains is the activating event, antibodies recognizing only one receptor component will probably be inactive. However, only three of the five anti-PRLR receptor antibodies acted as good receptor agonists, indicating that the resulting relative orientation and intermolecular distances of the dimerized receptors may also be important for receptor triggering, and that dimerization per se is not sufficient (98).

Specificity and Promiscuity of Receptor–JAK Interactions

Table 1 summarizes the involvement of JAK1, JAK2, TYK2, and the novel JAK kinase p116/L-JAK/JAK3, with various hematopoietin receptors. Further investigations of receptor and JAK kinase associations are needed to clarify to what extent there is promiscuity in their relationships. Does the relative expression levels of different JAK kinases in a cell influence the selection of kinase by receptor? The IL-6/LIF/OSM/CNTF/IL-11 subgroup of cytokines, which use at least two distinct signal transducers, gp130 and LIFRβ, has been reported to stimulate JAK1, JAK2, TYK2, or a combination thereof, depending on the cell type (84). It remains to be established to what extent this is due to the employment of distinct signal transducers, or is the result of molecular promiscuity and cellular variations in JAK expression levels. As noted earlier, this specific subgroup of ligands interact with a particularly challenging set of hematopoietin receptors. We have tested the activation of JAK2 by PRL in several cell lines, including rat Nb2 lymphoma cells, human T47D breast cancer cells, and mouse 32D myloid cells transfected with PRL receptors. Thus far, the PRL R has remained faithful to JAK2 (99).

Substrates of JAK Kinases: Involvement of SH2 Domain Proteins

With use of in vitro tyrosine kinase assays, the JAK enzymes have been shown to autophosphorylate. Furthermore, most hematopoietin receptors undergo tyrosine phosphorylation following activation, and at least some of this phosphorylation is probably the result of JAK activity. Receptor-associated proteins, either preassociated or associated following initial phosphorylation of critical tyrosine residues, constitute likely substrates for JAKs. Such substrates are most likely found among *src* homology domain 2 (SH2) proteins, which are known to associate specifically with tyrosine-phosphorylated protein motifs (for reviews, see 100, 101). Whether JAK2 substrates are confined to proteins permanently or transiently anchored to the receptor complex has not yet been determined.

Several SH2 domain proteins have been identified since the cloning of *src*. One group of SH2 domain proteins are enzymes, such as tyrosine kinases Abl, Syk, Csk, and the Src-family (Src, Lck, Hck, Fyn, Fgr, etc.), as well as other enzymes including phosphatidyl-inositol-3-kinase (PI3-K), phospholipase Cγ, Ras–GAP, tyrosine phosphatases, and Vav, a factor with G-nucleotide exchange activity. A second group of SH2-domain proteins do not have intrinsic enzymatic activity, but function as molecular linkers or adaptors by connecting components of signaling cascades (100). These include Crk, Shc, Nck, Grb2, and the p85 subunit of PI3K. Many of these SH2 domain proteins have been implicated in hematopoietin receptor signaling (102–109), and are also used by several additional growth factor receptors, including interferon (IFN) receptors, receptor tyrosine kinases, and probably other tyrosine kinase pathways. The selective recruitment of a given SH2 domain protein is determined by the phosphorylation of specific recognition sites on the docking protein. Differences in expression levels of SH2 domain proteins may give rise to some of the variation observed in response to the same lymphokine between different cell types. Thus, a given receptor may adopt different SH2 domain proteins in different cells, depending on availability, and distinct hematopoietin receptor subunits probably have unique selectivity for SH2 domain proteins owing to differences in their cytoplasmic structures.

Circuits from Membrane to Nucleus

The Ras–Raf–MAP Kinase Pathway

The Ras-signaling pathway is activated by many growth factor receptors, and its molecular details have recently been clarified to a large extent (for reviews, see 110,111). Phosphorylation of specific cytoplasmic receptor tyrosine residues in the cytoplasmic receptor tails allows the SH2 domain adaptor protein Grb2 to translocate from the cytoplasm to the membrane-associated receptor complex (Fig. 2). Alternatively, hematopoietin receptors may recruit Grb2 by first capturing another SH2 adaptor protein, Shc (112,113). Affiliated with Grb2 is the guanine nucleotide exchange protein, Sos, which on cotranslocation from the cytoplasm is brought in proximity of membrane-associated p21Ras. Nucleotide exchange occurs, and inactive Ras is converted into the active, GTP-bound form. Activated Ras interacts physically with the serine–threonine kinase Raf, and initiates a kinase cascade that involves phosphorylation and activation of MAP kinase kinase (MAPKK or MEK) and

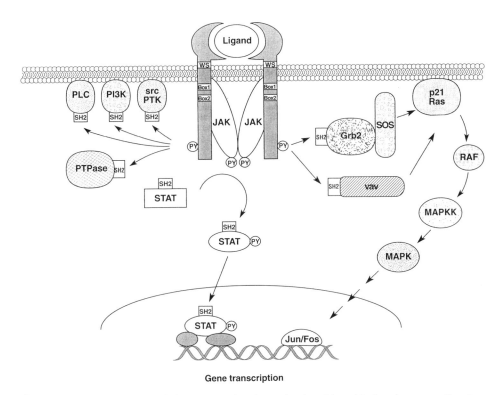

Figure 2 Model of hematopoietin receptor signal transduction. Ligand-induced receptor dimerization, activation of associated JAK tyrosine kinases, and subsequent recruitment of specific SH2 domain effector proteins represent the general signaling paradigm. WS (WSXWS motif), box 1 and box 2 denote the characteristic conserved motifs of hematopoietin receptors. See text for details.

MAP kinase (MAPK, including ERK1 and ERK2) (112). This signal is mediated into the nucleus. The MAPK activation correlates with activation–transcription of the AP1-transcription factors, *jun* and *fos*, thereby completing one circuit from the membrane to the nucleus (110,111).

The STAT Pathway

An alternative, more direct signaling route from membrane receptors to the nucleus was recently identified. STAT proteins have been named for their function as *s*ignal *t*ransducers and *a*ctivators of *t*ranscription, and are also SH2 domain proteins (see Fig. 2). Members of this growing class of proteins were first found to be activated by interferon receptors (115,116), but recent observations have disclosed an involvement of these factors also with hematopoietin receptors and receptor tyrosine kinases (107–109). The STAT proteins undergo rapid tyrosine phosphorylation after receptor activation, and may be directly phosphorylated by JAK enzymes. Activated STAT proteins migrate to the nucleus and interact with specific DNA response elements. A more detailed discussion on the function of STAT proteins is provided under interferon receptor signaling. Ongoing work is mapping the activation of individual STAT proteins by the various hematopoietin receptors.

Role of Tyrosine Phosphatases

The tyrosine phosphorylation kinetics of JAK enzymes, receptors, and SH2 domain proteins following hematopoietin receptor activation are normally transient, indicating an activation of tyrosine phosphatases. Recent work has identified two SH2 domain-containing tyrosine phosphatases, Syp (phosphotyrosine phosphatase; PTP1D) and hematopoietic cell phosphatase (HCP; PTP1C) (117–122). HCP has been shown to bind to activated, tyrosine phosphorylated IL-3 receptor β-chain, and constitutes a candidate off-switch (123). If the role of such tyrosine phosphatases in hematopoietin receptor signal transduction indeed is to neutralize the kinase effect, these proteins are potential antioncogenes (117,123). Interestingly, the COOH-terminal portion of the cytoplasmic domain of the EPO receptor has been demonstrated to be a negative regulatory region for receptor-mediated proliferation (26). The presence of a binding site for HCP or a related PTPase would provide a possible explanation for this observation. However, tyrosine phosphatases may have more complex regulatory roles in hematopoietin receptor signaling than simply counteracting JAK activity.

Preservation of Lymphokine-Specific Signals Across the Membrane

One intriguing element of hematopoietin receptor function is the ability of these receptors to induce overlapping, but distinct effects, despite their shared use of relatively few JAK kinases, as well as signal-transducing β-components (72). This is directly reflected in observed overlapping, but distinct protein phosphorylation patterns (124). For example, IL-2 and IL-4 share one receptor component, the IL-2Rγ (42,44) and activate the same JAK kinase, p116/L-JAK/JAK3 (88,89). However, in spite of these commonalities, the two lymphokines, in many instances, exert opposing effects (125). The simplest explanation for this phenomenon is the recruitment of distinct effector proteins by the cytoplasmic domain of their respective ligand-specific receptor subunits. Support for this notion was recently provided by the demonstration of the ability of IL-2, but not IL-4, to activate the Shc/Grb2/Sos/Ras pathway (102,112,113,126). Indeed, the IL-4Rα chain appears to couple the IL-4 receptor to a protein related to the insulin receptor substrate, IRS-1, which serves as a docking protein for multiple SH2 effector proteins (127). Hence, by the use of a single unique receptor subunit, and an economical sharing of signal transducing β-subunits and common JAK kinases, multicomponent hematopoietin receptors retain the ability to communicate lymphokine-specific messages across the cell membrane. Receptor-specific–signaling determinants in the cytoplasmic domains of hematopoietin receptors, as well as in other growth factor receptors, represent intriguing future targets for novel, ligand-independent receptor antagonists.

THE INTERFERON RECEPTOR SUPERFAMILY

Lymphokines that signal through members of the interferon (IFN) receptor superfamily, include IFN-α, IFN-β, IFN-γ, and IL-10 (3,7,128–130). The α-interferons are a group of more than 20 related signal proteins produced by virus-infected macrophages, whereas IFN-β is a single protein secreted by fibroblasts during viral infection (131,132). Interferons-α and IFN-β have approximately 25% amino acid identity and bind to the same receptors (132,133). Interferon-γ is secreted primarily by IL-2-stimulated T and NK cells, whereas IL-10 is produced by B cells, activated T cells, keratinocytes, as well as macrophages (130,132). Interferons and IL-10 have a broad range of activities, including regulation of target cell lymphokine production and general immunomodulatory influences, such as costimulation or inhibition of proliferation and differentiation induced by other lymphokines (for reviews, see Refs. 131,132,134).

Receptor Structure

Receptors for IFN-α and β, IFN-γ, and IL-10 have been cloned (135–140), and they are structurally and functionally related to hematopoietin receptors. Although IFN receptors lack the WS-box, the hallmark of hematopoietin receptors, and differ in the organization of their extracellular cysteine residues, overall sequence homologies of the extracellular domains indicate a common genetic origin (3,7,128–130). Accumulating evidence has suggested the presence of an additional receptor chain in IFN receptor complexes (138,140,141), analogous to oligoheteromeric hematopoietin receptors. The recent cloning of a second INF-γ receptor subunit verified this notion (142,143). This IFNγR β-chain does not bind IFN-γ by itself, but has structural features similar to previously cloned IFN receptor proteins. Although the cytoplasmic domains of currently known IFN receptors do not exhibit any distinct homologies, the IFNγR β-chain contains a region related to the homology box 2 of the hematopoietin receptors. This observation provides the first genetic link between the cytoplasmic domains of members of the two receptor families (142).

Mechanism of Transmembrane Signaling

Structural homologies and experimental data indicate that IFN receptors signal in a manner similar to that of hematopoietin receptors. Ligand-induced receptor aggregation is probably the initiating molecular event, as discussed earlier for hematopoietin receptors. Interestingly, IFN-γ exist as an active dimer (144–147), and cross-linking studies have demonstrated the formation of IFNγRα-dimers (148). It is still unclear whether parallel aggregation of β-chains is also essential. More knowledge is needed on the assembly and molecular stoichiometry of activated IFN receptor complexes. However, a common activation paradigm for IFN and hematopoietin receptors seems likely, since IFN receptor aggregation is also rapidly followed by activation of receptor-associated JAK kinases (133,149–151).

The critical role of JAK kinases in IFN receptor signaling was established by a series of remarkable genetic complementation studies, using a set of mutant HT1080 fibrosarcoma cells, which by random mutagenesis and systematic selection had been rendered unresponsive to either IFN-α/β, IFN-γ, or both types of IFNs. These studies revealed that IFN-α/β receptor signaling required coexpression of JAK1 and TYK2, whereas JAK1 and JAK2 were essential for IFN-γ receptor signaling (80,152,153).

Activation of JAK Tyrosine Kinases

A general activation mechanism of JAK tyrosine kinases has not yet crystallized, but evidence indicates a direct association between IFN receptors and JAK kinases (151), similar to what has been reported for hematopoietin receptors (72,73,83,84). Since one may assume that hematopoietin and IFN receptors share the same mechanism of JAK activation, the previously reviewed scheme of initial hematopoietin receptor activation also applied to IFN receptors (see earlier). In its simplest form, this model involves ligand-induced aggregation of preformed receptor–JAK complexes, with possible transphosphorylation and activation of the kinase molecules (36,60). It is conceivable that the corequirement for two distinct JAK enzymes for signaling by receptors for both IFN-α/β and IFN-γ (152,153), reflects an interdependent cross-activation of the two JAK enzymes, which are associated with their respective receptor subunit. This would be analogous to the demonstrated use of more than one JAK kinase by some of the multichain hematopoietin receptors (i.e., the IL-6 and IL-2 receptor systems; 36,37,89,93). However, considerable work is needed to thoroughly test this model of receptor-mediated JAK activation. Identification of additional IFN receptor components in particular, as well as their interaction sites with JAK kinases, will greatly facilitate our understanding of the immediate events of IFN receptor activation. The presence of a homology box 2-like region in the cytoplasmic domain of the IFN-γ receptor β-chain, offers a possible interaction site for JAK2, which is one of the JAK enzymes recruited by IFN-γ, since this homology motif is most well-defined in hematopoietin receptors known to activate JAK2 (97).

SH2 Domain Effector Proteins

Direct evidence for tyrosine phosphorylation of IFN receptors has been reported (154,155). Again, similar to the model of hematopoietin receptor signaling, docking of SH2 domain proteins onto cytoplasmic phosphotyrosyl residues of activated receptor components represents the most straightforward paradigm (36,86). One group of SH2 domain proteins that plays a major role in IFN receptor signaling, is the STAT family of transcription factors (150). Indeed, most of the pioneering work on these proteins has been carried out in the IFN system, although STAT proteins are also used by hematopoietin receptors, receptor tyrosine kinases, and possibly other tyrosine kinase pathways (107–109,115,116,156). Analysis of IFN-responsive genes and cloning of proteins binding to their regulatory domains led to the identification and cloning of the STAT molecules (115,133,150,156). There are now four members of this expanding protein family, STAT1α/β (the alternatively spliced p91 and p84 proteins of the ISGF-3α complex), STAT2 (p113 of ISGF-3α), STAT3, and STAT4 (150,157). These cytoplasmic transcription factors associate with specific phosphotyrosyl residues of the activated receptor complex, on JAK enzymes, cytoplasmic receptor domains, or additional receptor-associated proteins (151), and undergo tyrosine phosphorylation, possibly directly by JAK kinases (158–161). Specifically, IFN-induced receptor-docking of STAT1α/β (p91/p84) leads to phosphorylation of tyrosine residue Y701 which, in turn, causes the protein to oligomerize and translocate to the nucleus and interact with specific DNA response elements (162–164). Other STAT proteins also become activated by tyrosine phosphorylation on analogous tyrosine residues (150). Interferon-α/β induces tyrosine phosphorylation, activation, and heterooligomerization of STAT1α/β, STAT2, and a third 48-kDa component. This heteromeric complex then binds to the interferon-stimulated response element (ISRE; 131,150). In contrast, IFN-γ causes phosphorylation and homodimerization of STAT1α/β, without involvement of STAT2 and p48, and dimerized STAT1α/β then interacts with the IFN-γ-activated site (GAS; 131,150). Specific palindromic DNA interaction sequences have been identified in a number of IFN-responsive genes (131). As mentioned earlier, the STAT pathway is used by IFN receptors, hematopoietin receptors, as well as growth factor receptor tyrosine kinases, such as the EGF receptor, and constitutes a fundamental signaling circuit from the membrane to nucleus. Understanding the molecular details of activation of STAT proteins as well as their assembly into functional complexes with specific DNA recognition are some of the many challenging problems awaiting solution by future research efforts.

THE TUMOR NECROSIS FACTOR RECEPTOR FAMILY

A third class of lymphokine receptors is the tumor necrosis factor (TNF) receptor super-family. The knowledge of the signal transduction mechanisms of this receptor family is still scarce, with key elements of receptor activation unsettled. In addition, several receptors as well as ligands have not yet been matched with their cognate partner, and exist solely as unwed family members with genetic ties. One interesting feature of many, if not all, of the TNF-related ligands, is their dual existence as active membrane-bound and secreted forms. Whereas the secreted proteins operate as traditional lymphokines by activating cell surface receptors on target cells, the membrane-anchored forms of these ligands require cell-to-cell contact to interact with the same receptors. Under these latter circumstances there is a distinct possibility of bilateral signal transduction by the cytoplasmic domains of the interacting transmembrane proteins, thereby obscuring the traditional concepts of receptors and ligands (165). Furthermore, the extracellular domains of many of these transmembrane receptors can be proteolytically released and can conceivably interact with surface-bound ligands on separate cells, possibly acting as neutralizing antagonists or functional agonists. These observations set the stage for a remarkably intricate signaling network by this ligand–receptor system.

Cloned ligands for this receptor family include TNF-α, lymphotoxin-α (LT-α or TNF-β), lymphotoxin-β (LT-β), CD27 ligand, CD30 ligand, CD40 ligand, and 4-1BB ligand (166–173). Nerve growth factor (NGF) and related neurotropins have limited homology to these ligands, but interact nonetheless with a receptor which belongs to the TNF receptor family, the low-affinity p75 NGF receptor (165,174). The sequence homology of the TNF ligands is restricted to approximately 150 COOH-terminal amino acids, which in soluble TNF-α and LT-α form β-pleated sheet sandwiches that facilitate homotrimerization (165,175–177). The two homologues of tumor necrosis factor, TNF-α and LT-α, share approximately 30% amino acid identity (168). Sequence alignment indicates that the remaining members of this ligand family have a similar tertiary structure and form oligomers (165). In addition to structural similarities, several of these lymphokines can act both as growth factors and propagators of apoptotic cell death, largely depending on the target cell. Moreover, the multivalency of these ligands, owing to their oligomeric state, explains their ability to aggregate receptors. Determination of the crystal structure of LT-α complexed to soluble p55 TNFR1 (178), revealed that three molecules of soluble, extra-cellular domains of p55 TNFR1 bound to one LT-α homotrimer, thereby providing direct structural evidence for the mechanism of ligand-induced receptor clustering. This ligand-induced receptor aggregation is probably the initial molecular event causing receptor activation.

The currently known members of the TNF receptor family include the 55- to 60-kDa TNF-R1 (CD120a) (179,180), the 70- to 80-kDa TNF-R2 (CD120b) (181), the low-affinity p75 NGFR (182), CD27 (183), CD30 (184), CD40 (185), Fas (186), OX-40 (187), 4-1BB (188), LT-β receptor (189), SFV-T2 (PV-T2) (190), and VACC (PV-A53R) (191). Figure 3 presents an alignment of their extracellular amino acid sequences. The main common structural element of the extracellular domains of these receptors is a series of four cysteine-rich pseudorepeats consisting of approximately 40 amino acids, each containing five or six cysteines. CD30 contains an additional pseudorepeat (184), whereas FAS and CD27 have only three of these cysteine-rich regions (165). These segments appear to be important for ligand interaction (192,193). SFV-T2 (PV-T2) and VACC (PV-A53R) are

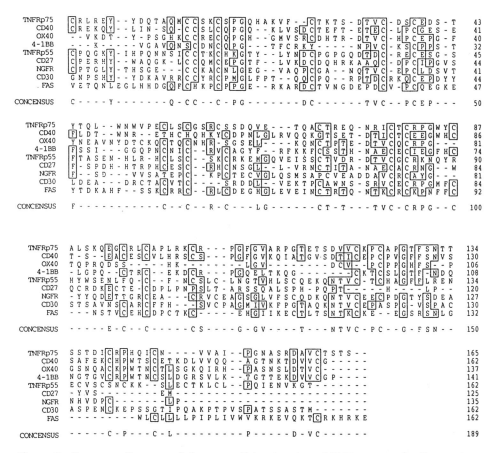

Figure 3 Sequence alignment of the extracellular domains of TNF receptor family members. Human Tnfrp80 ("p75 TNFR2" in text), human CD40, rat OX40, human 4-1BB, human Tnfrp60 ("p55 TNFR1" in text), human CD27, human low-affinity nerve growth factor receptor (p75 NGFR), human CD30, and human FAS are presented. Amino acids are numbered from the predicted initiation methionine, and identical residues are boxed. Amino acids that are conserved in four or more of the family members are indicated as consensus below the alignment. The analysis was performed using the PILEUP algorithm of the Sequence Analysis Software Package, ver. 7.0, by Genetics Computer, Inc., Madison, Wisconsin.

virally encoded, soluble proteins corresponding to extracellular receptor domains. The cytoplasmic domains of the transmembrane receptor family members share very limited homology, which implies distinct interaction capacities with effector proteins, and possibly different signaling mechanisms (165). However, most hematopoietin and interferon receptors also differ widely in their cytoplasmic domains, yet they share cytoplasmic tyrosine kinases of the JAK family as their primary effector proteins (see foregoing; 36,37,86).

TNF and TNF Receptors

The TNF-α and LT-α have been studied extensively and there are several reviews on their structure and function (166–168). These two TNF homologues are primarily produced by monocytes, macrophages, and activated T cells. Their genes are located on human chromosome 6, approximately 1.1 kb apart in the major histocompatibility complex (MHC) II locus. Both ligands interact with either form of TNF receptors (p55 TNFR1 and p75 TNFR2), and both possess cytotoxic and proliferative activities, depending on their concentration and the target cell. These lymphokines exist as cell surface-bound or secreted molecules. The soluble forms of TNF and LT-α are both active as homotrimers. The cell surface form of TNF is a 26-kDa membrane-anchored precursor which after proteolytic cleavage yields the 17-kDa soluble form. LT-α was long considered to be only a secreted protein, but recent work has demonstrated more complexity (194,195). It is anchored to the cell surface by association with LT-β, a type II transmembrane member of the TNF ligand family (196). This work has developed the concept that LT-α–LT-β may represent interacting ligands that diversify receptor specificity and presumably signal transduction by altering subunit composition within the heteromeric complexes (189).

As mentioned earlier, there are two related TNF receptors, p55 TNFR1 (CD120a) and p75 TNFR2 (CD120b). Both p55 TNFR1 and p75 TNFR2 independently bind TNF-α and LT-α and are active in signal transduction. The p55 TNFR1 mediates signals for cytotoxicity and several other TNF activities in a variety of cell types (197). Signaling by p75 TNFR2 has thus far been confined to a small portion of TNF effects in certain lymphoid cells, including thymocyte proliferation and proliferation of the murine cytotoxic T-cell line CT6 (198). However, a role for p75 TNFR2 as a facilitator of p55 TNFR1 receptor signaling by increasing the local concentration of TNF at the cellular surface, has also been proposed. According to this "ligand-passing" model, p75 TNFR2 hands TNF over to active p55 TNFR1, thereby acting as an intermediary TNF-transfer protein (199).

The intracellular domains of p55 TNFR1 and p75 TNFR2 are structurally dissimilar, suggesting that the two receptors have distinct signaling mechanisms. Neither form contains intrinsic kinase activity. Mutagenesis studies demonstrated the presence of distinct functional domains in the cytoplasmic region of p55 TNFR1 (200,201). Deletion of amino acids 310–426 of p55 TNFR1 did not influence TNF binding, internalization, or degradation, but eliminated TNF-induced cytotoxicity. In addition, inducible receptor shedding was retained in receptors lacking most of the cytoplasmic domains. Similarly, inducible shedding was retained by truncated p75 TNFR2, although the intact form released its extracellular domain most efficiently (202). Alanine-scanning mutagenesis of the COOH-terminal region of the cytotoxic p55 TNFR1, indicated that several of the amino acids conserved between FAS, another receptor member with cytotoxic potential, and p55 TNFR1 are critical for a cytotoxic signal. This apoptosis domain is required for induction of antiviral activity and nitric oxide synthase by macrophages (186). Specific deletions of membrane-proximal segments of p55 TNFR1 blocked induction of nitric oxide synthase, but not the cytotoxic effect, indicating that another domain is required for full function of the cytoplasmic domain of p55 TNFR1.

The understanding of TNF receptor signal transduction is less clear than signaling by hematopoietin and interferon receptors. No general receptor-proximal effector mechanism has been identified. In principle, coupling to G-proteins, protein tyrosine kinases, or serine–threonine kinases with associated lipid hydrolysis constitute candidate initial signal generators, although novel paradigms are certainly possible. Figure 4 summarizes and speculates on the mechanisms involved. Receptor clustering or oligomerization induced by the multivalent oligomeric ligands appears to be the initial molecular event causing receptor activation. Of the two TNF receptors, the least is known about signaling by p75 TNFR2, although an involvement of phospholipases and protein kinase C (PKC) has been proposed

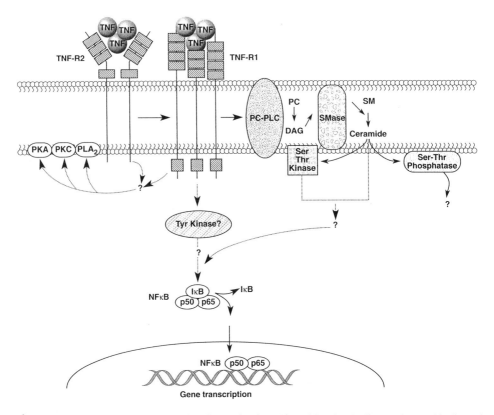

Figure 4   Model of TNF receptor signal transduction. The p55 TNFR1 oligomerize on binding of homotrimeric TNF (TNFα or LTα), causing phospholipid hydrolysis through an unknown coupling mechanism. Involvement of G-proteins or tyrosine kinases has been suggested. A serine–threonine protein kinase is rapidly activated by ceramide, one of the initial products of TNF-induced phospholipid hydrolysis. An involvement of the transcription factor NFκB has also been suggested. The p75 TNFR2 dimerize after binding of TNF, and limited evidence for activation of protein kinases and phospholipases has been presented. This receptor may also serve as an accessory protein to the p55 TNFR1 by effectively increasing the local concentration of TNF on the cell surface, and thereby making it more accessible for the p55 TNFR1. See text for discussion. PC, phosphatidylcholine; PC-PLC, phosphatidylcholine-specific phospholipase C; SMase, sphingomyelinase; DAG, diacylglycerol.

(203). On the other hand, a novel signal transduction pathway has been proposed for p55 TNFR1, involving sphingomyelinase-mediated phosphatidylcholine breakdown, producing ceramide, which is postulated to activate a ceramide-sensitive serine–threonine kinase (204–208). A possible involvement of protein tyrosine phosphorylation has also been suggested (209,210), which is associated with the potential for extensive recruitment of SH2 domain effector proteins. Furthermore, evidence for an involvement of G-proteins as key primary effectors has also been put forth (211–214). In HL-60 cells and a murine osteoblast cell line (MC3T3-E1) there is an increase in prostaglandin E_2 production when the cells are treated with TNF, thus indicating an activation of phospholipase A_2 (211,212). This activation was pertussis toxin-sensitive, suggesting G-protein involvement. The temporal order of these somewhat scattered biochemical events has not yet been established, and further work is needed to discern between principal signaling pathways and cross talk with parallel messenger systems.

Regardless of the nature of the initial key mechanism, regulatory protein phosphorylation occurs rapidly in response to TNF receptor activation. This includes both protein tyrosine and serine–threonine phosphorylation (207,209,210,215–217). Specifically, tyrosine phosphorylation of p42 and p44 MAP serine–threonine kinases, at least in fibroblasts and HL-60 cells, has been demonstrated (210). Moreover, an involvement of both protein kinases and protein phosphatases appears plausible (217).

A number of studies have been published on TNF-induced gene expression and the transcriptional factors involved. In short, TNF appears to activate NF-κB and induce synthesis of transcription factors AP-1, IRF-1, and IRF-2. These regulatory proteins, in turn, induce cell-specific sets of effector genes (for review, see Refs. 167,212).

CD40 and the CD40 Ligand

The CD40 ligand, CD40L, is a 30- to 39-kDa transmembrane protein expressed on activated T lymphocytes (172,218). The gene for CD40L is located on human chromosome X (219). A chimeric soluble form of CD40L has recently been produced to assist in the characterization of CD40L signal transduction (220).

CD40 is a 45-kDa glycoprotein expressed by B lymphocytes (185). Cross-linking of CD40 or activation by CD40L induces B-cell proliferation. On the other hand, if CD40 is not expressed, B cells undergo apoptosis (221). The presence or absence of CD40L on T cells may determine whether antigen-stimulated B cells are activated or killed, thereby illustrating the control of B-cell destiny by T cells. The signaling pathway mediating this activity is unknown, although it appears that CD40L signals independently of IL-6 and IL-4 (222,223) two separate lymphocyte growth factors that interact with receptors of the hematopoietin family. Stimulation of CD40 induces tyrosine phosphorylation of several cytoplasmic proteins, including a potential p46 MAP kinase. Serine–threonine protein phosphorylation is also stimulated and phospholipase (PLC) has been implicated in CD40 signaling (224). An initial mutagenesis study determined that a COOH-terminal deletion mutant, beginning at amino acid 232, could not transduce a signal, and that a point mutation of alanine-234 also abrogated signaling (225). This cytoplasmic region of CD40 is related to the apoptosis domain of p55 TNFR1 and Fas (186).

Fas and Fas Ligand

Fas is a 36-kDa receptor protein that transduces a cytotoxic signal to cells, and is expressed by myeloid cells, T cells, and fibroblasts (186). On the basis of sequence alignment with CD40 and TNFRp55, this activity is most likely associated with a 45-amino acid COOH-terminal region. The FAS ligand was recently cloned and is a type II transmembrane protein related to TNF (226). It is expressed in activated splenocytes and thymocytes, but also in nonlymphoid tissues, such as testis. The components of this signaling pathway have not yet been established, but one may speculate that the signal transduction is related to that used by p55 TNFR1.

CD30 and CD30 Ligand

The human and murine CD30 ligands (CD30L) have recently been cloned (171). The mRNA for CD30L is expressed by tonsillar T cells, LPS-activated monocytes, and can be induced in peripheral T cells by exposure to ionomycin and phorbol myristate acetate (PMA) (171). The CD30L is related to CD40L, TNF-α, and LT-α, and is a 40-kDa transmembrane glycoprotein. Similar to other members of this ligand family, the end effect of CD30L varies among target cells. It is a growth factor for purified peripheral T cells and CD30-positive lymphoma lines, but induces apoptosis in a CD30-positive non-Hodgkin's lymphoma cell line. This is particularly intriguing because CD30 does not contain the common domain involved in apoptosis that has been identified in CD40, Fas, and TNFRp55. The human gene encoding CD30L is located on chromosome 9q33.

The receptor for CD30L, CD30, is expressed on the cell surface of normal, activated T and B cells, but is also a cellular marker for Hodgkin's disease (184). Northern analysis of cells expressing CD30 demonstrated that there are two mRNA species, 3.8 and 2.6 kb. This cell marker is known to be inducibly phosphorylated on serine residues, but the mechanism is unknown. From limited cytoplasmic sequence homologies, it is speculated that CD30 signal mechanisms are similar to those of TNFRp55.

CD27 and CD27 Ligand

The CD27 ligand (CD27L) is a 50-kDa, membrane-anchored glycoprotein, expressed by monocytes, B cells, and T cells (170). Genetic analysis located CD27L on human chromosome 19p13. Similar to other members of this ligand family, CD27L has several functions. Activation of CD27 by antibody cross-linkage has been shown to enhance or inhibit T-cell proliferation, depending on the stage of T-cell maturity. Moreover, recombinant CD27L induced T-cell proliferation and cytotoxicity (170), suggesting that CD27L is both a growth factor and a differentiation agent for T cells.

CD27 is a 55-kDa transmembrane protein, usually expressed as a homodimer on resting T cells (183). A soluble form of the protein is expressed by activated T cells (227). Human CD27 is located on chromosome 12p13 (228). Little is known about the mechanism of CD27 signal transduction.

NGF and NGF Receptors

Nerve growth factor (NGF) plays an essential role in the development and survival of neurons. It is a functional homodimer composed of two 13-kDa subunits (229). Nerve growth factor and several related cytokines, including brain-derived neurotrophic factor (BDNF) and neurotrophin-3 (NT-3), interact with the low-affinity NGF receptor (171,230).

The 75-kDa, low-affinity receptor, p75 NGFR, binds NGF with an affinity characterized by a K_d of approximately 10^{-9} M (182). The high-affinity NGF receptor (K_d 10^{-11} M) is a heteromeric complex of the 140-kDa TRK and p75 NGFR. TRK belongs to the receptor tyrosine kinase family and has an intrinsic tyrosine kinase activity analogous to receptors for EGF and PDGF. Because of this apparently unique combination of two distinct receptor family members, it is difficult to distinguish which elements of NGF-signaling cascades are specifically mediated by p75 NGFR or TRK (for reviews, see Refs. 171,230). A recent deletional analysis of cytoplasmic regions indicated that the two receptor subunits may form a functional unit, which causes tyrosine phosphorylation of several cytoplasmic proteins (231). However, other studies indicate that p75 NGFR is not essential for TRK-mediated signal transduction (232). An NGF mutant that lost affinity for p75 NGFR, but retained ability to bind TRK, still induced TRK-mediated protein phosphorylation. The speculation has been put forth that p75 NGFR serves as an accessory protein that increases the local NGF concentration and provides TRK with NGF, analogous to the role of p75 TNFR2 for p55 TNFR1 activation (199). However, recent studies propose a more multifaceted involvement of p75 NGFR, indicating that this receptor is required for the survival of neural cells (233). There is an enhancement of cell death in serum-free medium by cells that solely express p75 NGFR. However, exposure to NGF reverses the effect, which may account for the dependence of certain neuronal cells on NGF for survival after differentiation. Similar observations have been made with the CD40 and CD40 ligand system.

OX-40, 4-1BB, VACC, and SFV-T2

Additional cloned members of the TNF receptor family include OX-40, 4-1BB, VACC, and SFV-T2. OX-40, which has been characterized in the rat, is a surface marker of activated T cells (187). 4-1BB is also a marker for T-cell activation. The predicted protein sequence would indicate a glycosylated 25-kDa protein expressed by human T cells (188). VACC is a vaccinia virus transcript that encodes a soluble TNF-receptor (191), and SFV-T2 is a Shope fibroma virus-encoded homologue (190,234).

The rate of cloning and identification of novel TNF-related receptors and their ligands seems to be leveling off, indicating that a completion of their membership records may be at hand. This will probably focus more attention and efforts toward the elucidation of the receptor-mediated signaling events over the next few years.

THE IMMUNOGLOBULIN RECEPTOR SUPERFAMILY

The immunoglobulin gene superfamily is composed of various cell surface molecules that have diverse roles in cell adhesion, neuronal function, and signal transduction. These proteins are characterized by the presence of a repeated series of motifs in their extracellular domains that are homologous to motifs found in classic immunoglobulins. Immunoglobulin superfamily members that function as signal transducers for growth factors and lymphokines are the receptors for platelet-derived growth factor (PDGF), fibroblast growth factor (FGF), interleukin-1 (IL-1), macrophage colony-stimulating factor (M-CSF or CSF-1), and stem cell factor (SCF). Within the context of lymphokines and the immune system, the receptors for IL-1, CSF-1, and SCF are of considerable importance.

Interleukin-1

The interleukin-1 family of ligands includes two agonistic lymphokines, designated IL-1α and IL-1β, as well as the IL-1 receptor antagonist, IL-1Ra. Interleukin-1α and IL-1β are encoded by different genes, and despite sharing only 25% homology at the amino acid level (235), they both bind with similar affinity to IL-1 receptors (236) and exert the same biological effects (237). Similarly, IL-1Ra competes with both IL-1α and IL-1β for binding to IL-1 receptors, but cannot elicit a biological response alone (reviewed in Ref. 238). Interleukin-1 is a pleiotrophic lymphokine, with effects on many cell types. With the exception of keratinocytes, epithelial cells, and some cells of the central nervous system, IL-1 is produced only in response to immune system challenge (reviewed in Ref. 239).

The biological effects of IL-1 are initiated by interaction of IL-1 with cell surface IL-1 receptors. Two distinct IL-1 receptors have been identified. T cells and fibroblasts express an 80-kDa receptor (type I), whereas B cells, monocytes, neutrophils, and bone marrow cells predominantly express a 60-kDa receptor (type II) (240). The difference between type I and type II receptors lies within their cytoplasmic domains, with type I receptors having a cytoplasmic domain of 215 amino acids, whereas type II receptors have only 29 (240). Both contain similar extracellular domains with characteristics of the immunoglobulin receptor superfamily (240).

Recent observations suggest that the biological effects of IL-1 are mediated exclusively through the 80-kDa type I receptor (241,242). Analysis of amino acid sequence of the type I receptor revealed that it does not possess catalytic activity. However, IL-1 rapidly induced the activity of protein kinase C (PKC) in T cells (243), fibroblasts (244), and mesangial cells (245); cAMP-dependent protein kinase (PKA) in the pre–B-cell line 70Z/3 (246) and human foreskin fibroblasts (247); both PKC and PKA in $T_H 2$ cells (248); and tyrosine kinase activity in mouse T cells (249), human fibroblasts (213), and other human and mouse cell lines (250). Furthermore, others have reported that IL-1 acts by G-protein recruitment, phospholipase activation, and ensuing phospholipid hydrolysis (reviewed in Ref. 239).

The mechanism by which the IL-1 receptor transduces signal to activate these and other second-messenger systems is unclear. However, much emphasis has been placed on the involvement of the large cytoplasmic portion of the type I receptor. A chimeric receptor consisting of the extracellular, IL-1-binding domain of the type II receptor, which does not transmit IL-1 signal, and the cytoplasmic domain of the type I receptor, produced a functional IL-1 receptor capable of inducing IL-8 gene expression in the human T-cell line, Jurkat (251). Mutations of the mouse type I receptor and analysis of signal transduction in a human cell line also revealed several regions of critical importance. Systematic COOH-terminal deletion mutations revealed that all except the COOH-terminal 28–42 amino acids are required for receptor function (252). Additionally, regions with some similarity to the homology box 1 and 2 of hematopoietin receptors are critical, since mutations in this region abolished IL-1 signaling (252).

Collectively, these experiments imply that the cytoplasmic portion of the type I receptor is essential for IL-1 signal transduction, probably by mediating an association with one or more signal-transducing molecules. Some evidence suggests that the sphingomyelin-signaling pathway is coupled to IL-1 receptor signal transduction. In EL4 cells, IL-1 rapidly stimulated sphingomyelin hydrolysis to ceramide, with an associated increase in ceramide-activated protein kinase activity (253). More importantly, coupling to the sphingomyelin-signaling pathway was attained by IL-1 in a cell-free system, indicating a tight association of this activity with IL-1–IL-1R complex formation. Although this suggests that the sphingomyelin pathway is activated very early in IL-1 signaling, it is not clear whether this is the most proximal receptor-associated event.

Interleukin-1 induces expression of many lymphokines, growth factors, and cellular proteins, such as IL-1 through IL-8, TNF-α and -β, G-CSF, GM-CSF, CSF-1, PDGF, (reviewed in 239); proto-oncogenes, such as c-*abl*, c-*fos* (248), c-*jun* (254), and c-*myc* (255); and transcription factors, such as *Egr*-1, NAK-1, and IRG-9 (256). A common mechanism by which cytokines control gene expression is by modulating the activity of specific DNA-binding proteins. Studies with IL-1 have shown that it is capable of inducing the DNA-binding activity of AP-1 (254), c/EBP, and NF-κB (257). The mechanism of activation of these factors remains obscure, although studies of NF-κB activation imply that protein kinases distinct from PKC are required, and that tyrosine kinase activation is essential (250). The activation of AP-1 appears to involve increasing the expression of the AP-1 constituents c-*fos*, and c-*jun*, and increasing the stability of c-*jun* mRNA (258).

Colony-Stimulating Factor-1

Colony-stimulating factor-1 (CSF-1) or macrophage colony-stimulating factor (M-CSF) controls the growth and survival of monocytes, macrophages, and their committed bone marrow precursors. These functions are initiated by the binding of CSF-1 to a single class of high-affinity receptors that are encoded by the c-*fms* proto-oncogene (259). Like other members of the immunoglobulin superfamily, Fms contains a series of immunoglobulin-like repeats in the extracellular domain. The cytoplasmic domain contains a tyrosine kinase motif interrupted by a short insertion sequence, characteristic of type III receptor tyrosine kinases (260).

Analogous to the action of PDGF and FGF, binding of CSF-1 to Fms results in receptor oligomerization, autophosphorylation, and receptor tyrosine kinase activation (260–262). Signal is then propagated by the tyrosine phosphorylation of numerous proteins (261,262), with a central involvement of SH2 domain proteins. A well-described target for Fms tyrosine kinase activity is phosphatidylinositol-3 (PI-3) kinase (263). Autophosphorylation of Fms facilitates association with PI-3 kinase, followed by tyrosine phosphorylation and PI-3 kinase activation. This results in increased levels of inositol-3 phosphate. The function of this molecule in signal transduction is not well understood, but it may be involved in receptor trafficking (264). A point mutation at tyrosine Y809 in Fms, which does not eliminate PI-3 kinase association, or the induction of c-*fos* or *junB*, does impair the ability of CSF-1 to elicit a proliferative response (265). This suggests that in addition to PI-3 kinase association and activation, the association of other, uncharacterized, effector molecules is essential for CSF-1-induced mitogenesis.

Similar to other lymphokines, CSF-1 signal transduction affects a variety of downstream pathways. CSF-1 increases GTP-binding and GTPase activity in human monocyte membranes (266), and modulates the function of Ras-signaling pathway (263). The CSF-1-dependent increases in diacylglycerol (DAG) turnover have been shown in human monocytes (267) and bone marrow-derived macrophages, but not in peritoneal macrophages, which show a poor proliferative response (268). This may suggest a role for CSF-1-induced DAG turnover in CSF-1-regulated mitogenesis. The mechanism by which CSF-1 increases DAG appears to be by activation of a phosphatidylcholine-specific phospholipase C (PC-PLC) and not by activation of phospholipase Cγ (268,269). Protein kinase C, which is activated by DAG, is activated by CSF-1 (267). However, there is also evidence for the activation of PKC-independent pathways. CSF-1 appears to decrease the intracellular levels of cAMP and thus antagonize cAMP-dependent protein kinase activity (270). The activity of the serine–threonine kinase Raf-1 is also stimulated by CSF-1 (271). Protein tyrosine phosphatase 1C (PTP1C or HCP) undergoes rapid tyrosine phosphorylation by CSF-1, indicating a possible role for phosphatase activity in CSF-1 signal transduction (272).

The CSF-1-dependent modulation of these signal transduction pathways results in the induced expression of several immediate early genes, including c-*fos*, *junB*, and c-*myc* (273,274). The direct mechanisms by which CSF-1 accomplishes this is not well understood. Recent results suggest that the induction of c-*fos* and *junB* transcripts is dependent on the activation of PC-PLC and is independent of PKC and Ras activation (275). Induction of c-*myc* appears to require a different signal transduction pathway.

Stem Cell Factor

Stem cell factor (SCF), also variably referred to as mast cell growth factor (MGF), Steel factor (SF or SLF), or kit ligand (KL), plays a critical role in the survival and proliferation of early hematopoietic stem cell progenitors by cooperating or synergizing with other hematopoietic cytokines (reviewed in Ref. 276).

The receptor for SCF has been identified as the proto-oncogene c-*kit* (277). This receptor shares a strong homology to the proto-oncogene c-*fms* (the receptor for CSF-1), as well as the PDGF receptor (278). All of these proteins belong to the immunoglobulin gene superfamily and contain a cytoplasmic tyrosine kinase domain with an internal insertion sequence typical of class III receptor tyrosine kinases (278). As with all members of this group, ligand binding to the receptor triggers receptor aggregation, autophosphorylation on tyrosine residues, and tyrosine kinase activation (279).

As discussed previously, receptor tyrosine phosphorylation induces the association of the receptor with proteins containing SH2 domains in many signal transduction systems. This is true for c-*kit*, and it appears that tyrosine phosphorylation within the kinase domain insert of c-*kit* is required for the association with, and subsequent activation of phosphatidylinositol-3 kinase (PI-3K) (280). Some evidence suggests that phospholipase Cγ also associates with c-*kit* (281,282). On the other hand, SCF does not induce an increase in inositol 1,4,5-triphosphate, indicating a lack of involvement of phosphatidylinositol-specific phospholipase C in SCF signal transduction (281,283). However, SCF has been shown to induce an increase in 1,2-diacylglycerol with an associated increase in choline release, suggesting that SCF acts by the activation of a phosphatidylcholine-specific phospholipase, perhaps phospholipase D (283). Association of an SH2 domain protein tyrosine phosphatase, hematopoietic cell phosphatase (HCP or PTP1C), has been shown with tyrosine phosphorylated c-*kit* (284). HCP can effectively dephosphorylate c-*kit* and may function by down-regulating SCF stimulation.

Stimulation of responding cells with SCF results in the rapid activation of additional signal transduction pathways. SCF induces the tyrosine phosphorylation of mitogen-activated protein (MAP) kinase (282,285,286), and serine phosphorylation and activation of the serine–threonine kinase Raf-1 (282,285,286). Stem cell factor also activates Ras without tyrosine phosphorylation of GAP (287). However, Ras activation requires tyrosine kinase activation and is not dependent on the activation of PKC (287).

Signal transduction events induced by SCF show considerable overlap with those stimulated by IL-3, GM-CSF, CSF-1, and other growth factors. Stem cell factor and the other factors induce tyrosine phosphorylation of many similar proteins identified by antiphosphotyrosine immunoblotting (282,285,286). Parallel overlap was seen with phosphorylation and activation of MAP kinase and Raf-1 (282,285,286). Furthermore, several experiments suggest that signal transduction by EGF receptors mimic certain aspects of SCF signaling. Expression of normal and mutant EGF receptors in the bone marrow of c-*kit* mutant heterozygous mice, restored normal mast cell development (288), and mice reconstituted with bone marrow containing the v-*erbB* oncogene developed lethal mast cell disease (289). These results indicate that SCF functions by stimulating signal transduction pathways shared by a growing number of cytokines.

As expected, SCF also induces the expression of several early response genes. In mouse bone marrow-derived mast cells, SCF induced expression of c-*fos*, c-*jun*, and *junB*, but had little effect on induction of *junD* (290). Interleukin-3 had similar, but not identical effects, in that it induced expression of c-*fos* and *junB* in mast cells (290). The mechanism by which SCF elicits this response is not well understood. However, owing to the similarity in signal transduction between SCF, IL-3, GM-CSF, and CSF-1, it is plausible that answers may be found by studying these signal transduction systems as well. Involvement of STAT proteins and other SH2 domain proteins probably accounts for considerable overlap (see foregoing).

THE CHEMOKINE RECEPTOR FAMILY

Extensive reviews have been written on the general topic of chemokines, also referred to as intercrines (291,292). Detailed reviews have also recently been published on individual chemokines, such as monocyte chemoattractant protein (MCP)-1 (293) and macrophage inflammatory protein (MIP) (294,295). This section of the review will focus on the structure of chemokines and their receptors, structural determinants of interaction specificity, and the proposed biochemical mechanisms of signal transduction.

Chemokines are traditionally defined as a subgroup of lymphokines that share a common role in the inflammatory response, the chemoattraction of specific leukocytes to the site of inflammation. In some cases, chemokines are also involved in subsequent activation of the recruited cells. Chemokines are produced in response to inflammatory stimuli, which usually are mediated by the proinflammatory cytokines IL-1 and IFN-γ, as described later. The assays for chemoattraction (296) and the ability to induce secretion of the chemokines were exploited in the isolation and discovery of the chemokine family members. Many chemokines were thus cloned from cDNA libraries generated by subtractive hybridization, or purified from media supernatants of lipopolysaccharide (LPS)-stimulated monocytes.

Chemokines can be grouped into two structural categories, based on the first pair of conserved cysteines in the mature protein, which are either adjacent in C–C chemokines, or separated by one amino acid in C–X–C chemokines. The C–C chemokines and the C–X–C chemokines appear to be not only structurally distinct, but differ also functionally in receptor interaction and the cells that they attract.

C–X–C Chemokines

The C–X–C chemokines include platelet factor 4, β-thromboglobulin, interleukin-8, GRO/MGSA, IP-10, mig, and ENA-78. Interleukin-8 was purified from human peripheral blood mononuclear cells, then cloned from these cells using degenerate oligonucleotide probes (297). β-Thromboglobulin is produced as part of a proteolytic-processing pathway that begins with the biologically inactive platelet basic protein (PBP) (298). The first nine residues are removed to yield connective tissue-activating protein (CTAP-3), which has another four residues removed to yield β-thromboglobulin. Proteolytic removal of an additional 11 amino acids produces the neutrophil attractant peptide (NAP-2). The *mig* (*m*onokine *i*nduced by *g*amma interferon) clone was obtained by differential hybridization of cDNA prepared from activated mouse macrophage cell line RAW 264.7 (299). Its gene product is predicted to have a translated size of 14.4 kDa, making *mig* one of the larger siblings in the chemokine family. ENA-78 was purified from IL-1β- or TNF-α-conditioned medium of the human epithelial A549 cell line (300). IP-10 was cloned from a cDNA library prepared from U937 cells stimulated by IFN-γ (301). GRO/MGSA was cloned from a human placental cDNA library (302), using oligonucleotide probes, based on the NH_2-terminal amino acid sequence of GRO/MGSA isolated from the human melanoma cell line Hs294T. All C–X–C chemokines that have been chromosomally mapped are located on human chromosome 4. These include platelet factor 4, mapped to 4q12-q21 (303); GRO/MGSA, mapped to 4q13-q21 (302); and GIP-10, mapped to 4q21 (304).

The tertiary structure of PF4 and of IL-8 have been determined by both nuclear magnetic resonance (NMR) spectroscopy and x-ray diffraction techniques. The solution of the structure of IL-8 revealed a dimer composed of monomers of three antiparallel β-sheets, with a long α-helical COOH-terminus superimposed at a 60° angle (305,306). Each monomer contains a pair of disulfide bonds (Cys7-Cys34 and Cys9-Cys50). The dimer is stabilized by intersubunit hydrogen bonding of the first β-sheet of each monomer.

Bovine platelet factor 4 (PF4) was crystallized after proteolytic removal of the first 13-amino acid residues, which contain a glycosylation site (307). The PF4 crystals formed a tetramer in which each subunit comprised an extended NH_2-terminal loop, a "Greek key" arrangement of three antiparallel β-sheets, and a COOH-terminal α-helix. Each monomer contains a pair of disulfide bonds (Cys25-Cys51 and Cys27-Cys67). Parameters that influence the monomer–dimer–tetramer equilibria include pH, ionic strength, and protein concentration, as determined by NMR spectroscopy (308).

C–C Chemokines

The C–C chemokines include macrophage inflammatory protein-1α, macrophage inflammatory protein-1β, I-309, RANTES, monocyte chemoattractant protein-1, monocyte chemoattractant protein-3 (MCP-3), HC-14, and C-10. RANTES (regulated on activation, normal T expresses, and presumably secreted) was cloned from a T- minus B-lymphocyte cDNA library (309). MCP-3 was purified from human osteosarcoma cell line MG-63 stimulated with IL-1β, then an MG-63 cDNA library was screened with degenerate oligonucleotide primers derived from MCP-3 peptide sequence data to yield a cDNA clone for MCP-3 (310). MCP-1 was cloned from the human glioma cell line U-105MG (311) and appears to be the human homologue of murine JE. I-309 was cloned from the Il-2-dependent T-cell line IDP2 (312). Macrophage inflammatory protein (MIP) was originally purified from media supernatants of LPS-stimulated murine macrophage RAW 264.7 cells (313), and distinct clones of MIP-1α (314) and MIP-1β (315) were subsequently isolated and characterized.

Human C–C chemokines have been chromosomally mapped to chromosome 17, including I-309 (316) and RANTES, which are located on 17q11.2-q12 (317). The murine chemokines MIP-1α and MIP-1β have been mapped to a cluster of cytokine genes on a region of mouse chromosome 11 (318).

High-resolution solution structure of the C–C chemokine MIP-1β revealed a homodimeric structure (319). However, the quaternary structure of MIP-1β differed markedly from that of the C–X–C chemokine IL-8. Whereas the IL-8 dimer was globular, the MIP-1β dimer was cylindrical, and entirely different residues were involved in the dimer interfaces of the respective chemokines. This may provide a structural basis for the absence of cross-binding and reactivity between members of the two chemokine families (319).

An interesting phenomenon common to several chemokines, especially members of the C–C class with acidic COOH-terminal tails, is the apparent aggregation of the elementary dimeric units into multimers with molecular mass in excess of 100 kDa (320). This tendency of self-association implies that these peptides may interact with their receptors as multimers. However, nonaggregating forms of MIP-1α, which had been created by deletion of acidic COOH-terminal amino acids and presumably exist in their native dimeric form, retained full activity (320).

Target Cells and Effects of Chemokines

The chemokines appear to recruit only a specific cell populations to areas of inflammation. For example, IL-8 attracts neutrophils, but does not attract monocytes. Conversely, MCP-1 attracts monocytes, but not neutrophils. In general, the C–X–C chemokines tend to attract neutrophils, and C–C chemokines preferentially attract monocytes. This is not a firm rule, however, since IP-10, a C–X–C chemokine, attracts stimulated T cells and human peripheral blood monocytes, but not neutrophils (321). Fibroblasts are most effectively attracted by PF4 and by β-thromboglobulin (322). I-309 attracts monocytes, but not neutrophils (323). RANTES, which attracts monocytes, but not neutrophils, also selectively attracts CD4+/UCHL1+ T lymphocytes, which are phenotypic memory T cells (309). Neither

MIP-1α nor MIP-β attract T lymphocytes before CD3 activation, but MIP-1α selectively attracts activated CD8$^+$ T cells, and MIP-β selectively attracts activated CD4$^+$ T cells (324).

Recent site-directed mutagenesis studies have helped define regions of the chemokines that may be important in determining target cell specificity. For instance, introduction of a double (Tyr28Leu, Arg30Val) mutation into MCP-1 decreases its monocyte chemotactic activity and introduces a neutrophil chemotactic activity (325). The Glu-Leu-Arg sequence preceding the C–X–C motif of IL-8 is required for binding of IL-8 to its receptor. Truncated forms of IL-8 containing mutations in this region can act as IL-8 antagonists (326). Moreover, introduction of this region into PF4 results in a modified protein with the capacity to chemoattract and activate neutrophils (327).

The common effect of chemokines is the induction of specific cells to migrate toward the ligand in a chemotactic fashion. In some of these recruited cells, other specific responses may be induced that include respiratory bursts, adhesive modulation (which relates to chemotaxis), expression of cell surface proteins, and proliferation. Some of these activation events will be discussed later under "Secondary Biochemical Events."

One of the chemokines, MIP-1, is noteworthy in that it is a pyrogen that is insensitive to monooxygenase inhibitors and is independent of prostaglandin E$_2$ (PGE$_2$) synthesis, thereby demonstrating the existence of a novel mechanism for febrile responses (328). Microinjection studies have implicated the anterior hypothalamic, preoptic region of the rat brain as the most sensitive region for inducing such a fever (329). Now that a cloned receptor for MIP-1α and MIP-1β has been discovered, determining the molecular mechanism of MIP-1 febrile response may be facilitated by the study of C–C chemokine receptor gene expression in this region of the brain.

Chemokine Receptor Structure

Tremendous progress has recently been made in the cloning and molecular characterization of chemokine receptors. Two distinct cDNA clones for human IL-8 receptors have been isolated, designated IL-8R1 (330) and IL-8R2 (331). Both receptors bind IL-8 and related C–X–C chemokines and independently mediated chemotaxis (332). The two genes have been mapped to band 2q35 of human chromosome 2 (333,334). A closely related receptor for IL-8 has also been cloned from rabbit (335). This receptor displays the essential chemokine-binding characteristics of the human type 1 receptor. Chimeric IL-8 receptors, built from human types 1 and 2 receptors, provide data to suggest that the NH$_2$-terminal region of IL-8R2 contains structural determinants that will allow binding of the GRO/MGSA ligand (336). This observation has been corroborated by studies of chimeric IL-8 receptors containing domains from rabbit type 1 and human type 2 (337); this study also indicates that the NH$_2$-terminal region of type 2 receptor confers promiscuous binding ability. Scanning-alanine mutagenesis has further defined regions of the receptor that are critical for ligand binding (338). In addition to confirming the importance of the NH$_2$-terminus, this study provides evidence that residues of the putative third extracellular loop, Glu-275 and Arg-280 of human IL-8R1, appear to reside in the IL-8-binding domain.

A receptor for the C–C chemokine subgroup, designated C–C CKR-1, has been cloned by two laboratories (339,340). This cDNA clone contains an open-reading frame of 1065 bases, encoding a protein of 355-amino acid residues with a predicted mass of 41 kDa. Neote and co-workers described the behavior of the expressed protein. Human kidney 293 cells transfected with C–C CKR-1 will bind RANTES, both human and murine MIP-1α,

MIP-β, and MCP-1, with apparent dissociation constants of 468, 6.5, 4.2, 232, and 122 nM, respectively. However, the binding affinities of these chemokines do not directly relate to their efficacy for receptor-mediated calcium mobilization, since 100 nM of RANTES will support calcium mobilization in C–C CKR-1-transfected cells, whereas 100 nM of human MIP-β or MCP-1 will not. Indeed, C–C CKR-1-mediated calcium mobilization is induced by as low as 1 nM of RANTES, despite the observation that the apparent K_d of the RANTES–C–C CKR-1 complex is 468 nM. Furthermore, receptor desensitization responds anomalously in that human MIP-1α will completely desensitize the receptor to RANTES, but RANTES will only partially desensitize the receptor to MIP-1α. Gao and colleagues obtained a clone containing additional noncoding regions and mapped the gene to band 3p21 of chromosome 3. Both groups propose that C–C CKR-1 may be the physiologically relevant receptor for MIP-1α.

Cloned receptors for the chemokines are unique among lymphokine receptors in that they are predicted to contain seven transmembrane helices, a motif common to ligand receptors that couple to G-proteins. However, the predicted structures of chemokine receptors differ from the predicted structures of traditional seven transmembrane-spanning helical receptors in that the extramembrane segments connecting the membrane-spanning domains are smaller in chemokine receptors, and the COOH-terminal domains of chemokine receptors are very short and lack potential palmitoylation sites.

It is of interest to note the apparent conservation of structure among chemokine receptors and receptors for chemotactic substances that are not traditionally classified as chemokines (Fig. 5). The complement anaphylatoxin C5a receptor was cloned from human HL-60 and cAMP-induced U937 libraries (341). A receptor for the chemotactic formylated bacterial tripeptide fMLP has been cloned from human HL-60 cells (342). These receptors are predicted to contain seven transmembrane helices and also apparently couple to G-proteins. Overall amino acid identity among the C–C CKR-1, C5a, and fMLP receptors is less than 24%, whereas IL-8R1, C5a, and fMLP receptors possess 29–34% amino acid identity. Interleukin-8R2 is more closely related to the rabbit receptor for fMLP (343), but has less than 30% amino acid identity with the human fMLP receptor.

"Orphan receptors" (i.e., receptors with as yet unidentified physiological ligands), possessing a high degree of similarity to chemokine receptors, have also been cloned. Such a putative seven-transmembrane segment receptor has been cloned from human spleen and mapped to chromosome 2q21 (344). Also, the open-reading frame US28 of cytomegalovirus encodes a C–C CKR-1 homologue that binds C–C, but not C–X–C chemokines (339), suggesting a mechanism whereby CMV-infected cells may evade immune defenses.

A novel, but as yet uncloned, chemokine receptor on erythrocytes has been biochemically characterized to bind both to C–C and to C–X–C chemokines (345). Interleukin-8 can be competitively displaced from erythrocyte ghosts by GRO/MGSA, MCP-1, or RANTES, but not by MIP-1α (346). The apparent molecular mass of this receptor is estimated to be 39 kDa, of which 5 kDa is contributed by glycosylation. Preincubation with GTP or [γS]GTP did not affect the affinity of this receptor for its ligands.

Parasitic invasion of host cells is sometimes mediated by binding of the parasite to surface receptors of the host cell. Such appears to be true for the malarial parasite *Plasmodium vivax*, which binds to the Duffy blood group antigen. The Duffy blood group antigen has recently been identified as the erythrocyte receptor for IL-8 and GRO/MGSA (347).

```
Humstsr    - - - - - - - M E G I S I Y T S D - - - N Y T E E M G S G D Y D S M K E P C F R E E N A N F N K I F    40
Humcccckr1 - - - - - - - M E G I S I Y T S D - - - N Y T E E M G S G D Y D S M K E P C F R E E N A N F N K I F    40
Rabil8r    M E V N V W N M T D L W T W F E D-E F A N A T - - - G M P P V E K D Y S P C L V V T Q T - L N K Y V    46
Humil8ra   - - - - M S N I T D P Q M W D F D D L - N F T - - - G M P P A D E D Y S P C M L E T E T - L N K Y V    41
Humil8rb   - - - - M E S D S F E D F W K G E D L S N Y S Y S S T L P P F L L D A A P C E P E S L E - I N K Y F    45
Humfmlr    - - - - - - - - - - - - - - - - - - - - M E T N S S L P T N I S G G T P A V S A G Y - L F L D I I    28
Humc5ar    - - - - - - - - M N S F N Y T T P D Y G H Y D D K D T L D L N T P V D K T - - S N T L - R V P D I L    39

Humstsr    L P T I Y S I I F L T G I V G N G L V I L V M G Y Q K K L R S M T D K Y R L H L S V A D L L F V I T    90
Humcccckr1 L P T I Y S I I F L T G I V G N G L V I L V M G Y Q K K L R S M T D K Y R L H L S V A D L L F V I T    90
Rabil8r    V V V I Y A L V F L L S L L G N S L V M L V I L Y S R S N R S V T D V Y L L N L A M A D L L F A L T    96
Humil8ra   V I I A Y A L V F L L S L L G N S L V M L V I L Y S R V G R S V T D V Y L L N L A L A D L L F A L T    91
Humil8rb   V V I I Y A L V F L L S L L G N S L V M L V I L Y S R V G R S V T D V Y L L N L A L A D L L F A L T    95
Humfmlr    T Y L V F A V T F V L G V L G N G L V I W V A G F - R M T H T V T T I S Y L N L A V A D F C F T S T    77
Humc5ar    A L V I F A V V F L V G V L G N A L V V W V T A F - E A K R T I N A I W F L N L A V A D F L S C L A    88

Humstsr    L P F W A V D A V A N - - W Y F G N F L C K A V H V I Y T V N L Y S S V L I L A F I S L D R Y L A I    138
Humcccckr1 L P F W A V D A V A N - - W Y F G N F L C K A V H V I Y T V N L Y S S V L I L A F I S L D R Y L A I    138
Rabil8r    M P I W A V S K E K G - - W I F G T P L C K V V S L V K E V N F Y S G I L L L A C I S V D R Y L A I    144
Humil8ra   L P I W A A S K V N G - - W I F G T F L C K V V S L L K E V N F Y S G I L L L A C I S V D R Y L A I    139
Humil8rb   L P I W A A S K V N G - - W I F G T F L C K V V S L L K E V N F Y S G I L L L A C I S V D R Y L A I    143
Humfmlr    L P F F M V R K A M G G H W P F G W F L C K F L F T I V D I N L F G S V F L I A L I A L D R C V C V    127
Humc5ar    L P I L F T S I V Q H H H W P F G G A A C S I L P S L I L L N M Y A S I L L L A T I S A D R F L L V    138

Humstsr    V H A T N S Q R P R K L L A E K V V Y V G V W I P A L L L T I P D F I F A N V - - S E A D D R Y I C    186
Humcccckr1 V H A T N S Q R P R K L L A E K V V Y V G V W I P A L L L T I P D F I F A N V - - S E A D D R Y I C    186
Rabil8r    V H A T R T L T Q K R H L V - K F I C L G I W A L S L I L S L P F F L F R Q V F S P N N S S P V C Y    193
Humil8ra   V H A T R T L T Q K R H L V - K F V C L G C W G L S M N L S L P F F L F R Q A Y H P N N S S P V C Y    188
Humil8rb   V H A T R T L T Q K R Y L V - K F I C L S I W G L S L L L A L P V L L F R R T V Y S S N V S P A C Y    192
Humfmlr    L H P V W T Q N H R T V S L A K K V I I G P W V M A L L L T L P V I I - R V T T V P G K T G T V A C    176
Humc5ar    F K P I W C Q N F R G A G L A W I A C A V A W G L A L L L T I P S F L Y R V V R E E Y F P P K V L C    188

Humstsr    D - - - - - - - - - - - R F Y P N D L - W V V V F Q F Q H I M V G L I L P G I V I L S C Y C I I I S    224
Humcccckr1 D - - - - - - - - - - - R F Y P N D L - W V V V F Q F Q H I M V G L I L P G I V I L S C Y C I I I S    224
Rabil8r    E - - - - - - - - - - - D L G H N T A K W R M V L R I L P H T F G F I L P L L V M L F C Y G F T L R    232
Humil8ra   E - - - - - - - - - - - V L G N D T A K W R M V L R I L P H T F G F I V P L F V M L F C Y G F T L R    227
Humil8rb   E - - - - - - - - - - - D M G N N T A N W R M L L R I L P Q S F G F I V P L L I M L F C Y G F T L R    231
Humfmlr    T F N F S P W T N D P K E R I N V A V A M L T V R G I I R F I I G F S A P M S I V A V S Y G L I A T    226
Humc5ar    G V D Y S H - - D K R R E R - - - A V A - - - - - - I V R L V L G F L W P L L T L T I C Y T F I L L    227

Humstsr    K L S H S K G H Q K R K A L K T T V I L I L A F F A C W L P Y Y I G I S I D S F I L L E I I K Q G C    274
Humcccckr1 K L S H S K G H Q K R K A L K T T V I L I L A F F A C W L P Y Y I G I S I D S F I L L E I I K Q G C    274
Rabil8r    T L F Q A H M G Q K H R A M R V I F A V V L I F L L C W L P Y N L V L L A D T L M R T H V I Q E T C    282
Humil8ra   T L F K A H M G Q K H R A M R V I F A V V L I F L L C W L P Y N L V L L A D T L M R T Q V I Q E T C    277
Humil8rb   T L F K A H M G Q K H R A M R V I F A V V L I F L L C W L P Y N L V L L A D T L M R T Q V I Q E T C    281
Humfmlr    K I H K Q G L I K S S P P L R V L S F V A A A F F L C W S P Y Q V V A L I A T V R I R E L L Q G M Y    276
Humc5ar    R T W S R R A T R S T K T L K V V V A V V A S F F I F W L P Y Q V T G I M - - M S F L E P S S P T F    275

Humstsr    E F E N T V H K W I S I T E A L A F F H C C L N P I L Y A F L G A K F K T S A Q H A L T S V S R G S    324
Humcccckr1 E F E N T V H K W I S I T E A L A F F H C C L N P I L Y A F L G A K F K T S A Q H A L T S V S R G S    324
Rabil8r    Q R R N D I D R A L D A T E I L G F L H S C L N P I I Y A F I G Q N F R N G F L K M L A A R G L I S    332
Humil8ra   E R R N N I G R A L D A T E I L G I L H S C L N P I I Y A F I G Q N F R H G F L K I L A M H G L V S    327
Humil8rb   E R R N H I D R A L D A T E I L G I L H S C L N P L I Y A F I G Q K F R H G L L K I L A I H G L I S    331
Humfmlr    K - - - E I G I A V D V T S A L A F F N S C L N P M L Y V F M G Q D F R E R L I H A L P A - - - - S    319
Humc5ar    L - - - L L N K L D S L C V S F A Y I N C C I N P I I Y V V A G Q G F Q G R L R K S L P S - - - - L    318

Humstsr    S L K I L S K G K R G G H S S V S T E S E S S S F H S S - - - - -    352
Humcccckr1 S L K I L S K G K R G G H S S V S T E S E S S S F H S S - - - - -    352
Rabil8r    K - E F L T R H R V T S Y T S S S T N V P S N L - - - - - - - - -    355
Humil8ra   K - E F L A R H R V T S Y T S S S V N V S S N L - - - - - - - - -    350
Humil8rb   K - D S L P K D S R P S F V G S S S G H T S T T L - - - - - - - -    355
Humfmlr    L E R A L T E D S - T Q T S D T A T N S T L P S A E V A L Q A K -    350
Humc5ar    L R N V L T E E S V V R E S K S F T R S T V D T M A Q K T Q A V -    350
```

Figure 5 Structural comparison of cloned chemokine receptors. Humstsr (340) and Humcccckr1 (339) are identical sequences encoding human C–C chemokine receptor CCKR-1; Rabil8r (335) encodes the rabbit IL-8 receptor; Humil8ra (330) encodes the type 1 human IL-8 receptor; Humil8rb (331) encodes the type 2 human IL-8 receptor; Humfmlr (342) encodes the human receptor for the bacterial formylated tripeptide, fMPL; Humc5ar (341) encodes the human anaphylatoxin C5a receptor. The analysis was performed using the PILEUP algorithm of the Sequence Analysis Software Package, ver. 7.0, by Genetics Computer, Inc., Madison, Wisconsin.

Receptor Activation and G-Protein-Coupled Signal Transduction

The understanding of the biochemical processes involved in chemokine receptor activation is limited. The apparent homodimeric structure of several chemokines examined so far implies an ability of these ligands to induce dimerization of their receptors, although oligomerization of chemokine receptors has not yet been demonstrated. However, evidence is accumulating for an involvement of G-proteins as a primary signaling event, with subsequent activation of phospholipases, particularly PLCγ, and possibly other G-protein-coupled enzyme reactions (Fig. 6). Activation of phospholipase C causes hydrolysis of phosphatidylinositol 4,5-diphosphate to inositol-triphosphate (IP_3) and diacylglycerol (DAG). The IP_3 production transiently increases intracellular calcium ion concentrations by the release of calcium from internal storage vesicles, and DAG activates protein kinase C (PKC), a serine–threonine kinase (348). It is widely observed that stimulation of a chemokine-sensitive cell with a cognate chemokine induces a rapid and transient elevation of intracellular free calcium levels. Since receptors for chemokines have only recently been characterized, a definitive universal-signaling pathway has not yet been established, as discussed in the following paragraph.

Transient increases in intracellular free calcium concentrations have been observed in human monocytic leukemia cell line THP-1 in response to stimulation by RANTES, MCP-1, and MIP-1α (349). Interleukin-8, RANTES, MCP-1, and MIP-1α also induce a transient rise in intracellular free calcium concentrations in basophils; pertussis toxin pretreatment prevents IL-8 from coupling to calcium mobilization and greatly inhibits MCP-1 from mobilizing calcium (350). Pertussis toxin can also block the chemokine-induced release of histamine, as discussed later. Cytoplasmic free calcium levels transiently rise in monocytes in response to I-309 stimulation (323). Some investigators have shown that the transient calcium increase in human monocytes responding to MCP-1 is coupled to extracellular, not intracellular, calcium sources (351). These investigators also showed that blocking of calcium influx also inhibited chemotaxis and, furthermore, that MCP-1 did not stimulate IP_3 production in human monocytes.

Interleukin-8 activates GTPase activity of human neutrophil plasma membranes and also stimulates high-affinity binding of [γS]GTP by such membranes (352). It induces a concentration- and time-dependent formation of IP_3 in human neutrophils (353) and enhances the activity of PKC in membranes from such cells. The IL-8Rα and IL-8Rβ can couple to PLC-β2 through $G_{\alpha16}$, $G_{\alpha14}$, and $G_{\alpha15}$, but not through $G_{\alpha11}$ or $G_{\alpha q}$ (354). $G_{\alpha16}$, which was cloned from human promyelocytic HL-60 cells, is expressed only in specific hematopoietic cells (355). $T_{\alpha16}$ is not expressed in the B-cell lines Raji (lymphoblast phenotype) and IM9 (plasmacytoma phenotype). $G_{\alpha16}$ lacks a potential site for ADP ribosylation by pertussis toxin and is a member of the G_q class of G-proteins, which activate phospholipase Cβ isozymes (356,357).

Given the diversity of signal transduction effectors, such as ion channels, phospholipase C, phospholipase A_2, adenylate cyclases, and phosphodiesterases, which may be modulated by specific G-protein family members (358), it is very likely that chemokine-signaling pathways will be significantly clarified by an improved definition of the cell-specific distributions of not only chemokine receptors, but also of the resident G-protein isoforms and effector isozymes. Indeed, several reports already point toward phospholipase A_2 activation as a parallel pathway, resulting in rapid release of arachidonic acid (358–361).

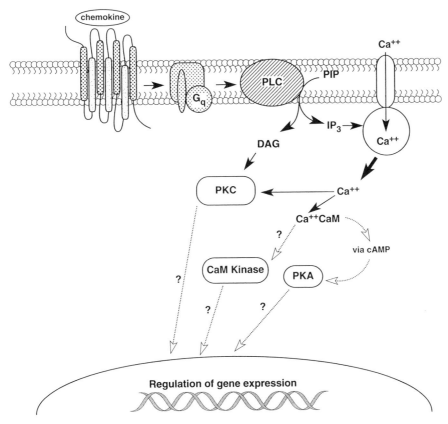

Figure 6 Model of chemokine receptor signal transduction. The chemokine receptor is displayed as a seven-transmembrane-spanning protein, which after ligand binding triggers G-protein-coupled signaling events. A proposed activation of phospholipase C (PLC), with ensuing diacylglycerol and phosphatidylinositol generation, is depicted. Subsequent activation of serine–threonine protein kinases, notably PKC, by DAG and the accompanying increase in intracellular Ca^{2+}, represent the next level of relayed signal. See text for discussion.

Secondary Biochemical Events

The process of cell recruitment involves not only the chemotactic response, per se, but includes adhesion events. Selectins and integrins (362) are cell surface macromolecules that play crucial roles in intercellular adhesion. CD11 and CD18 are subunits of leukocyte integrins (363), and LAM-1 is a selectin implicated in leukoycte "rolling" before endo-thelial attachment (364). MCP-1 induced expression of p150,95 (CD11c/CD18) and of Mac-1 (CD11b/CD18) in human monocytes, but no significant effect on LFA-1 (CD11a/CD18), nor on LAM-1 (365). There is evidence that RANTES up-regulates the expression of CD11b/CD18 on the surface of human eosinophils (366). It is unclear whether the regulation of integrin expression should truly be considered a response that is downstream from the G-protein–calcium mobilization cascade, or if it occurs through an independent mechanism. On the other hand, histamine release appears to be an immediate consequence of G-protein activation. Both MCP-1 and RANTES induce peak histamine release from human leukocytes within the first minute of stimulation, and the ability of these chemokines to trigger histamine release from human basophils is effectively blocked by pertussis toxin pretreatment (367).

There are also negative regulatory events mediated by chemokines. Interleukin-8 down-regulates the surface availability of its own receptor by receptor internalization (368), and cellular desensitization is broadly reported in the chemokine literature. GRO/MGSA and IL-8, but not RANTES, MIP-1α, nor MIP-1β, lead to a decreased collagen mRNA level in human fibroblasts (369).

Cloning of additional chemokine receptors and identification of their affiliated G-proteins and effector molecules will help clarify the signaling circuits used by different chemokines.

CONCLUDING REMARKS

In this chapter we have reviewed some of the exciting progress that has recently been made in the field of transmembrane signal transduction, with particular reference to lymphokine receptors. Although a variety of second messengers and effector molecules have been identified, the basic principles of transmembrane communication by extracellular factors appears to be few. Ligand-induced oligomerization of single-spanning transmembrane receptor components constitutes one standard concept. In fact, there is as yet no solid evidence for signal transmission across the cell membrane along a solitary protein chain (61). Moreover, a prerequisite for receptor oligomerization is polyvalency of the ligand. This is intuitively a feature of homodimeric and homotrimeric ligands, such as NGF and TNF. Studies of other factors, such as the monomeric growth hormone, unexpectedly revealed an inherent asymmetric bivalency toward its receptor, illustrating an innovative evolutionary twist on this theme.

One of the many questions that remains unanswered is how receptor oligomerization allows the cytoplasmic tails to cause activation of intracellular enzymes. In cases where the receptor itself possesses catalytic activity, such as receptors for EGF, PDGF, or SCF, with intrinsic tyrosine kinases, ligand-induced dimerization is believed to pairwise adjoin the catalytic sites, and activation takes place as a result of intermolecular, autoactivating tyrosine phosphorylation (60). A similar triggering mechanism is postulated for the JAK tyrosine kinases associated with hematopoietin and interferon receptors. Moreover, this general activation paradigm may be used by any autoactivating enzyme when its molecules are brought together by the aggregation of receptor domains, and not restricted to tyrosine kinases. However, because of the multiplicity of SH2 domain effector proteins, tyrosine kinases have proved especially versatile and powerful in initial signal transduction schemes. Tyrosine kinase activation and phosphorylation of ligand-specific receptor α-subunits, the cytoplasmic domains of which encode the recruitment of designated SH2 domain effectors, translate into ligand-characteristic messages inside the cell. As exemplified by several hematopoietin receptors, ligand-specific signals can be achieved despite an economical sharing of a limited number of receptor β-subunits and JAK kinases. This partial sharing of signaling components also explains overlapping effects of many lymphokines.

Although much has been learned about lymphokine-induced signal transduction over the past few years with landmark discoveries, especially within the field of hematopoietin and interferon receptor function, certain systems have remained elusive. Studies of the fascinating family of TNF receptors may reveal the next set of remarkable mechanisms of intercellular communication. We hope that the insight will bring along clinically useful strategies to correct disturbances of these delicate programs.

ACKNOWLEDGMENTS

We thank Drs. Paul D. Crowe, Todd L. VanArsdale, and Carl F. Ware at the University of California, Riverside, for their criticism and helpful suggestions on the review of TNF-receptor signal transduction. We also acknowledge the support and critical comments by Drs. Joost Oppenheim and Dan Longo. We thank the National Cancer Institute for allocation of computing time and staff support at the Frederick Biomedical Supercomputer Center of the Frederick Cancer Research and Development Center.

REFERENCES

1. Miyajima A, Kitamura T, Harada N, Yokata T, Arai K. Cytokine receptors and signal transduction. Annu Rev Immunol 1992; 10:295–331.
2. Bazan JF. A novel family of growth factor receptors: a common binding domain in the growth hormone, prolactin, erythropoietin and IL-6 receptors and the p75 IL-2 receptor β-chain. Biochem Biophys Res Commun 1989; 164:788–795.
3. Bazan JF. Structural design and molecular evolution of a cytokine receptor superfamily. Proc Natl Acad Sci USA 1990; 87:6934–6938.
4. Cosman D. The hematopoietin receptor superfamily. Cytokine 1993; 5:95–106.
5. Foxwell BM, Barrett K, Feldmann M. Cytokine receptors: structure and signal transduction. Clin Exp Immunol 1992; 90:161–169.
6. Miyajima A, Hara T, Kitamura T. Common subunits of cytokine receptors and the functional redundancy of cytokines. Trends Biochem Sci 1992; 17:378–382.
7. Patthy L. Homology of a domain of the growth hormone/prolactin receptor family with type III modules of fibronectin [letter]. Cell 1990; 61:13–14.
8. Kelly PA, Ali S, Rozakis M, et al. The growth hormone/prolactin receptor family. Recent Prog Horm Res 1993; 48:123–164.
9. Vigon I, Mornon JP, Cocault L, et al. Molecular cloning and characterization of MPL, the human homolog of the v-*mpl* oncogene: identification of a member of the hematopoietic growth factor receptor superfamily. Proc Natl Acad Sci USA 1992; 89:5640–5644.
10. Yoshimura A, Longmore G, Lodish HF. Point mutations in the exoplasmic domain of the erythropoietin receptor resulting in hormone-independent activation and tumorigenicity. Nature 1990; 348:647–649.
11. Chiba T, Amanuma H, Todokoro K. Tryptophan residue of Trp-Ser-X-Trp-Ser motif in extracellular domains of erythropoietin receptor is essential for signal transduction. Biochem Biophys Res Commun 1992; 184:485–490.
12. Yoshimura A, Zimmers T, Neumann D, Longmore G, Yoshimura Y, Lodish HF. Mutations in the Trp-Ser-X-Trp-Ser motif of the erythropoietin receptor abolish processing, ligand binding, and activation of the receptor. J Biol Chem 1992; 267:11619–11625.
13. Quelle DE, Quelle FW, Wojchowski DM. Mutations in the WSAWSE and cytosolic domains of the erythropoietin receptor affect signal transduction and ligand binding and internalization. Mol Cell Biol 1992; 12:4553–4561.
14. Tanaka M, Maeda K, Okubo T, Nakashima K. Double antenna structure of chicken prolactin receptor deduced from the cDNA sequence. Biochem Biophys Res Commun 1992; 188:490–496.
15. Itoh N, Yonehara S, Schreurs J, et al. Cloning of an interleukin-3 receptor gene: a member of a distinct receptor gene family. Science 1990; 247:324–327.

16. Colosi P, Wong K, Leong SR, Wood WI. Mutational analysis of the intracellular domain of the human growth hormone receptor. J Biol Chem 1993; 268:12617–12623.
17. Murakami M, Narazaki M, Hibi M, et al. Critical cytoplasmic region of the interleukin 6 signal transducer gp130 is conserved in the cytokine receptor family. Proc Natl Acad Sci USA 1991; 88:11349–11353.
18. O'Neal KD, Montgomery DW, Truong TM, Yu-Lee LY. Prolactin gene expression in human thymocytes. Mol Cell Endocrinol 1992; 87:R19–23.
19. Fukunaga R, Ishizaka-Ikeda E, Pan CX, Seto Y, Nagata S. Functional domains of the granulocyte colony-stimulating factor receptor. EMBO J 1991; 10:2855–2865.
20. Fukunaga R, Ishizaka E, Nagata S. Growth and differentiation signals mediated by different regions in the cytoplasmic domain of granulocyte colony stimulating factor receptor. Cell 1993; 74:1079–1087.
21. Miura O, Cleveland JL, Ihle JN. Inactivation of erythropoietin receptor function by point mutations in a region having homology with other cytokine receptors. Mol Cell Biol 1993; 13:1788–1795.
22. Hatakeyama M, Mori H, Doi T, Taniguchi T. A restricted cytoplasmic region of IL-2 receptor β chain is essential for growth signal transduction but not for ligand binding and internalization. Cell 1989; 59:837–845.
23. Hatakeyama M, Kono T, Kobayashi N, Kawahara A, Levin SD, Perlmutter RM, Taniguchi T. Interaction of the IL-2 receptor with the src-family kinase p56lck: identification of novel intermolecular association. Science 1993; 252:1523–1528.
24. Hatakeyama M, Kawahara A, Mori H, Shibuya H, Taniguchi T. c-fos gene induction by interleukin 2: identification of the critical cytoplasmic regions within the interleukin 2 receptor beta chain. Proc Natl Acad Sci USA 1992; 89:2022–2026.
25. Harada N, Yang G, Miyajima A, Howard M. Identification of an essential region for growth signal transduction in the cytoplasmic domain of the human interleukin-4 receptor. J Biol Chem 1992; 267:22752–22758.
26. D'Andrea AD, Yoshimura A, Youssoufian H, Zon LI, Koo JW, Lodish HF. The cytoplasmic region of the erythropoietin receptor contains nonoverlapping positive and negative growth-regulatory domains. Mol Cell Biol 1991; 11:1980–1987.
27. Koettnitz K, Kalthoff FS. Human interleukin-4 receptor signaling requires sequences contained within two cytoplasmic regions. Eur J Immunol 1993; 23:988–991.
28. Satoh T, Minami Y, Kono T, et al. Interleukin 2-induced activation of Ras requires two domains of interleukin 2 receptor beta subunit, the essential region for growth stimulation and Lck-binding domain. J Biol Chem 1992; 267:25423–25427.
29. Ziegler SF, Bird TA, Morella KK, Mosley B, Gearing DP, Baumann H. Distinct regions of the human granulocyte-colony-stimulating factor receptor cytoplasmic domain are required for proliferation and gene induction. Mol Cell Biol 1993; 13:2384–2390.
30. Asao H, Takeshita T, Ishii N, Kumaki S, Nakamura M, Sugamura K. Reconstitution of functional interleukin 2 receptor complexes on fibroblastoid cells: involvement of the cytoplasmic domain of the gamma chain in two distinct signaling pathways. Proc Natl Acad Sci USA 1993; 90:4127–4131.
31. Merida M, Williamson P, Kuziel WA, Greene WC, Gaulton GN. The serine-rich cytoplasmic domain of the interleukin-2 receptor β chain is essential for interleukin-2 dependent tyrosine protein kinase and phosphatidylinositol-3-kinase activation. J Biol Chem 1993; 1993:6765–6770.
32. Quelle DE, Wojchowski DM. Localized cytosolic domains of the erythropoietin receptor regulate growth signaling and down-modulate responsiveness to granulocyte–macrophage colony-stimulating factor. Proc Natl Acad Sci USA 1991; 88:4801–4805.
33. Sakamaki K, Miyajima I, Kitamura T, Miyajima A. Critical cytoplasmic domains of the common beta subunit of the human GM-CSF, IL-3 and IL-5 receptors for growth signal transduction and tyrosine phosphorylation. EMBO J 1992; 11:3541–3549.

34. DaSilva L, Rui H, Kirken RA, Farrar WL, Howard OMZ. Growth signal and JAK2 activation mediated by membrane-proximal regions of the cytoplasmic domain of prolactin receptors. J Biol Chem 1994; 269:18267–18270.

35. Taniguchi T, Minami Y. The IL-2/IL-2 receptor system: a current overview. Cell 1993; 73:5–8.

36. Stahl N, Yancopoulos GD. The alphas, betas, and kinases of cytokine receptor complexes. Cell 1993; 74:587–590.

37. Kishimoto T, Taga T, Akira S. Cytokine signal transduction. Cell 1994; 76:253–262.

38. Sato N, Miyajima A. Multimeric cytokine receptors: common versus specific functions. Curr Opin Gen Dev 1994; 4:174–179.

39. Leonard WJ, Depper JM, Crabtree GR, Rudikoff S, Pumphery J, Robb RJ, Kronke M, Svetlik PB, Peffer NJ, Waldmann TA, Greene WC. Molecular cloning and expression of cDNAs for the human interleukin-2 receptor. Nature 1984; 311:628–631.

40. Waldmann TA. The interleukin-2 receptor. J Biol Chem 1991; 266:2681–2684.

41. Grant AJ, Roessler E, Ju G, Tsudo M, Sugamura K, Waldmann TA. The interleukin 2 receptor (IL-2R): the IL-2R alpha subunit alters the function of the IL-2R beta subunit to enhance IL-2 binding and signaling by mechanisms that do not require binding of IL-2 to IL-2R alpha subunit. Proc Natl Acad Sci USA 1992; 89:2165–2169.

42. Russell SM, Keegan AD, Harada N, Nakamura Y, Noguchi M, Leland P, Friedmann MC, Miyajima A, Puri RK, Paul WE, Leonard WJ. Interleukin-2 receptor gamma chain: a functional component of the interleukin-4 receptor. Science 1993; 262:1880–1883.

43. Noguchi M, Nakamura Y, Russell SM, Ziegler SF, Tsang M, Cao X, Leonard WJ. Interleukin-2 receptor γ chain: a functional component of the interleukin-7 receptor. Science 1993; 262:1877–1880.

44. Kondo M, Takeshita T, Ishii N, Nakamura M, Watanabe S, Arai K-i, Sugamura K. Sharing of the interleukin-2 (IL-2) receptor γ chain between receptors for IL-2 and IL-4. Science 1993; 262:1874–1877.

45. Aversa G, Punnonen J, Cocks BG, et al. An interleukin 4 (IL-4) mutant protein inhibits both IL-4 or IL-13-induced human immunoglobulin G4 (IgG4) and IgE synthesis and B cell proliferation: support for a common component shared by IL-4 and IL-13 receptors. J Exp Med 1993; 178:2213–2218.

46. Zurawski SM, Vega F Jr, Huyghe B, Zurawski G. Receptors for interleukin-13 and interleukin-4 are complex and share a novel component that functions in signal transduction. EMBO J 1993; 12:2663–2670.

47. Skoda RC, Seldin DC, Chiang MK, Peichel CL, Vogt TF, Leder P. Murine c-*mpl*: a member of the hematopoietic growth factor receptor superfamily that transduces a proliferative signal. EMBO J 1993; 12:2645–2653.

48. Noguchi M, Yi H, Rosenblatt HM, Filipovich AH, Adelstein S, Modi WS, McBride OW, Leonard WJ. Interleukin-2 receptor γ chain mutation results in X-linked severe combined immunodeficiency in humans. Cell 1993; 73:147–157.

49. Voss SD, Hong R, Sondel PM. Severe combined immunodeficiency, interleukin-2 (IL-2), and the IL-2 receptor: experiments of nature continue to point the way. Blood 1994; 83:626–635.

50. Davis S, Aldrich TH, Valenzuela DM, et al. The receptor for ciliary neurotrophic factor. Science 1991; 253:59–63.

51. Hibi M, Murakami M, Saito M, Hirano T, Taga T, Kishimoto T. Molecular cloning and expression of an IL-6 signal transducer, gp130. Cell 1990; 63:1149–1157.

52. Yasukawa K, Futatsugi K, Saito T, et al. Association of recombinant soluble IL-6-signal transducer, gp130, with a complex of IL-6 and soluble IL-6 receptor, and establishment of an ELISA for soluble gp130. Immunol Lett 1992; 31:123–130.

53. Barnard R, Rowlinson SW, Waters MJ. Soluble forms of the rabbit adipose tissue and liver growth hormone receptors are antigenically identical, but the integral membrane forms differ. Biochem J 1990; 267:471–477.

54. Raines MA, Liu L, Quan SG, Joe V, DiPersio JF, Golde DW. Identification and molecular cloning of a soluble human granulocyte–macrophage colony-stimulating factor receptor. Proc Natl Acad Sci USA 1991; 88:8203–8207.

55. Narazaki M, Yasukawa K, Saito T, et al. Soluble forms of the interleukin-6 signal-transducing receptor component gp130 in human serum possessing a potential to inhibit signals through membrane-anchored gp130. Blood 1993; 82:1120–1126.

56. Fukunaga R, Seto Y, Mizushima S, Nagata S. Three different mRNAs encoding human granulocyte colony-stimulating factor receptor. Proc Natl Acad Sci USA 1990; 87:8702–8706.

57. Suzuki H, Yasukawa K, Saito T, et al. Serum soluble interleukin-6 receptor in MRL/lpr mice is elevated with age and mediates the interleukin-6 signal. Eur J Immunol 1993; 23:1078–1082.

58. Schoenhaut DS, Chua AO, Wolitzky AG, et al. Cloning and expression of murine IL-12. J Immunol 1992; 148:3433–3440.

59. Wolf SF, Temple PA, Kobayashi M, et al. Cloning of cDNA for natural killer cell stimulatory factor, a heterodimeric cytokine with multiple biologic effects on T and natural killer cells. J Immunol 1991; 146:3074–3081.

60. Schlessinger J, Ulrich A. Growth factor signalling by receptor tyrosine kinases. Neuron 1992; 9:383–391.

61. Wells JA. Structural and functional basis for hormone binding and receptor oligomerization. Curr Opin Gen Dev 1994; 4:163–173.

62. de Vos AM, Ultsch M, Kossiakoff AA. Human growth hormone and extracellular domain of its receptor: crystal structure of the complex. Science 1992; 255:306–312.

63. Ultsch M, de Vos AM, Kossiakoff AA. Crystals of the complex between human growth hormone and the extracellular domain of its receptor. J Mol Biol 1991; 222:865–868.

64. Fuh G, Cunningham BC, Fukunaga R, Nagata S, Goeddel DV, Wells JA. Rational design of potent antagonists to the human growth hormone receptor. Science 1992; 256:1677–1680.

65. Fuh G, Colosi P, Wood WI, Wells JA. Mechanism-based design of prolactin receptor antagonists. J Biol Chem 1993; 268:5376–5381.

66. Murakami M, Hibi M, Nakagawa N, Nakagawa T, Yasukawa K, Yamanishi K, Taga T, Kishimoto T. IL-6-induced homodimerization of gp130 and associated activation of a tyrosine kinase. Science 1993; 260:1808–1810.

67. Ip NY, Nye SH, Boulton TG, Davis S, Taga T, Li Y, Birren SJ, Yasukawa K, Kishimoto T, Anderson DJ, Stahl N, Yancopoulos GD. CNTF and LIF act on neuronal cells via shared signaling pathways that involve the IL-6 signal transducing receptor component gp130. Cell 1992; 69:1121–1132.

68. Davis S, Aldrich TH, Stahl N, et al. LIFR beta and gp130 as heterodimerizing signal transducers of the tripartite CNTF receptor. Science 1993; 260:1805–1808.

69. Elberg G, Kelly PA, Djiane J, Binder L, Gertler A. Mitogenic and binding properties of monoclonal antibodies to the prolactin receptor in Nb2 rat lymphoma cells. Selective enhancement by anti-mouse IgG. J Biol Chem 1990; 265:14770–14776.

70. Cunningham BC, Ultsch M, de Vos AM, Mulkerrin MG, Clauser KR, Wells JA. Dimerization of the extracellular domain of the human growth hormone receptor by a single hormone molecule. Science 1991; 254:821–825.

71. Cunningham BC, Wells JA. Rational design of receptor-specific variants of human growth hormone. Proc Natl Acad Sci USA 1991; 88:3407–3411.

72. Witthuhn BA, Quelle FW, Silvennoinen O, Yi T, Tang B, Miura O, Ihle JN. JAK2 associates with the erythropoietin receptor and is tyrosine phosphorylated and activated following stimulation with erythropoietin. Cell 1993; 74:227–236.

73. Argetsinger LS, Campbell GS, Yang X, et al. Identification of JAK2 as a growth hormone receptor-associated tyrosine kinase. Cell 1993; 74:237–244.

74. Wilks AF, Harpur AG, Kurban RR, Ralph SJ, Zurcher G, Ziemiecki A. Two novel protein-tyrosine kinases, each with a second phosphotransferase-related catalytic domain, define a new class of protein kinase. Mol Cell Biol 1991; 11:2057–2065.

75. Harpur AG, Andres AC, Ziemiecki A, Aston RR, Wilks AF. JAK2, a third member of the JAK family of protein tyrosine kinases. Oncogene 1992; 7:1347–1353.

76. Pritchard MA, Baker E, Callen DF, Sutherland GR, Wilks AF. Two members of the JAK family of protein tyrosine kinases map to chromosomes 1p31.3 and 9p24. Mamm Genome 1992; 3: 36–38.

77. Howard OM, Dean M, Young H, Ramsburg M, Turpin JA, Michiel DF, Kelvin DJ, Lee L, Farrar WL. Characterization of a class 3 tyrosine kinase. Oncogene 1992; 7:895–900.

78. Bernards A. Predicted *tyk2* protein contains two tandem protein kinase domains. Oncogene 1991; 6:1185–1187.

79. Firmbach-Kraft I, Byers M, Shows T, Dalla-Favera R, Krolewski JJ. *Tyk2*, prototype of a novel class of non-receptor tyrosine kinase genes. Oncogene 1990; 5:1329–1336.

80. Velazquez L, Fellous M, Stark GR, Pellegrini S. A protein tyrosine kinase in the interferon alpha/beta signaling pathway. Cell 1992; 70:313–322.

81. Yang X, Chung D, Cepko CL. Molecular cloning of the murine JAK1 protein tyrosine kinase and its expression in the mouse central nervous system. J Neurosci 1993; 13:3006–3017.

82. Silvennoinen O, Witthuhn BA, Quelle FW, Cleveland JL, Taolin Y, Ihle JN. Structure of the murine Jak2 protein-tyrosine kinase and its role in interleukin 3 signal transduction. Proc Natl Acad Sci USA 1993; 90:8429–8433.

83. Rui H, Kirken RA, Farrar WL. Activation of receptor-associated tyrosine kinase JAK2 by prolactin. J Biol Chem 1994; 269:5364–5368.

84. Stahl N, Boulton TG, Farruggella T, et al. Association and activation of Jak-Tyk kinases by CNTF-LIF-OSM-IL-6 beta receptor components. Science 1994; 263:92–95.

85. Kirken RA, Rui H, Evans GA, Farrar WL. Characterization of an interleukin-2 (IL-2)-induced tyrosine phosphorylated 116-kDa protein associated with the IL-2 receptor β-subunit. J Biol Chem 1993; 268:22765–22770.

86. Kirken RA, Rui H, Howard OMZ, Farrar WL. Involvement of JAK-family tyrosine kinases in hematopoietin receptor signal transduction. Prog Growth Factor Res 1994; 5:195–211.

87. Kawamura M, McVicar DW, Johnston JA, Blake TB, Chen YC, Lal BK, Lloyd AR, Kelvin DJ, Staples JE, Ortaldo JR, O'Shea JJ. Molecular cloning of ljk, a novel Janus family protein tyrosine kinases expressed in natural killer cells and activated leukocytes. Proc Natl Acad Sci USA 1994; 91:6374–6378.

88. Kirken RA, Rui H, Malabarba MG, Farrar WL. Identification of the IL-2 receptor-associated tyrosine kinase p116 as novel leukocyte specific Janus kinase. J Biol Chem 1994; 269:19136–19141.

89. Johnston JA, Kawamura M, Kirken RA, Chen Y-i, Blake TB, Ortaldo JR, McVicar DW, O'Shea JJ. Phosphorylation and activation of kinase in response to interleukin-2. Nature 1994; 370: 351–353.

90. Takahashi T, Shirasawa T. Molecular cloning of rat JAK3, a novel member of the JAK family of protein tyrosine kinases. FEBS Lett 1994; 342:124–128.

91. Cance WG, Craven RJ, Weiner TM, Liu ET. Novel protein kinases expressed in human breast cancer. Int J Cancer 1993; 54:571–577.

92. Sanchez MP, Tapley P, Saini SS, He B, Pulido D, Barbacid M. Multiple tyrosine protein kinases in rat hippocampal neurons: isolation of Ptk-3, a receptor expressed in proliferative zones of the developing brain. Proc Natl Acad Sci USA 1994; 91:1819–1823.

93. Kirken RA, Rui H, Malabarba MG, Howard OMZ, Kawamura M, O'Shea JJ, Farrar WL. Activation of JAK3, but not JAK1 is critical for IL2-induced proliferation and STAT5 recruitment by a COOH-terminal region of the IL2-receptor β-chain. Cytokine 1995; 7:689–700.

94. Campbell GS, Christian LJ, Carter-Su C. Evidence for involvement of the growth hormone receptor-associated tyrosine kinase in actions of growth hormone. J Biol Chem 1993; 268: 7427–7434.

95. Rui H, Djeu JY, Evans GA, Kelly PA, Farrar WL. Prolactin receptor triggering. Evidence for rapid tyrosine kinase activation. J Biol Chem 1992; 267:24076–24081.

96. Wang X, Moller C, Norstedt G, Carter-Su C. Growth hormone-promoted tyrosyl phosphorylation of a 121 kDa growth hormone receptor associated protein. J Biol Chem 1993; 268:3573–3579.

97. Da Silva L, Rui H, Erwin RA, Howard OMZ, Kirken RA, Malabarba MG, Hackett RH, Larner AC, Farrar WL. Prolactin recruits STAT1, STAT3, and STAT5 independent of conserved receptor tyrosines Tyr402, Tyr479, Tyr515, and Tyr580. Mol Cell Endocrinol 1996; in press.

98. Rui H, Lebrun J-J, Kirken RA, Kelly PA, Farrar WL. JAK2 activation and cell proliferation induced by antibody-mediated prolactin receptor dimerization. Endocrinology 1994; 135:1299–1306.

99. Rui H, Farrar WL. In preparation.

100. Schlessinger J. SH2/SH3 signalling proteins. Curr Opin Gen Dev 1994; 4:25–30.

101. Montminy M. Trying on a new pair of SH2s. Science 1993; 261:1694–1695.

102. Burns LA, Karnitz LM, Sutor SL, Abraham RT. Interleukin-2-induced tyrosine phosphorylation of p52shc in T lymphocytes. J Biol Chem 1993; 268:17659–17661.

103. Li W, Hu P, Skolnik EY, Ullrich A, Schlessinger J. The SH2 and SH3 domain-containing Nck protein is oncogenic and a common target for phosphorylation by different surface receptors. Mol Cell Biol 1992; 12:5824–5833.

104. Merida I, Diez E, Gaulton GN. IL-2 binding activates a tyrosine-phosphorylated phosphatidyl-inositol-3-kinase. J Immunol 1991; 147:2202–2207.

105. Damen J, Mui AL, Hughes P, Humphries K, Krystal G. Erythropoietin-induced tyrosine phosphorylations in a high erythropoietin receptor-expressing lymphoid cell line. Blood 1992; 80:1923–1932.

106. Remillard B, Petrillo R, Maslinski W, et al. Interleukin-2 receptor regulates activation of phosphatidylinositol 3-kinase. J Biol Chem 1991; 266:14167–14170.

107. Larner AC, David M, Feldman GM, et al. Tyrosine phosphorylation of DNA binding proteins by multiple cytokines. Science 1993; 261:1730–1733.

108. Silvennoinen O, Schindler C, Schlessinger J, Levy DE. Ras-independent growth factor signaling by transcription factor tyrosine phosphorylation. Science 1993; 261:1736–1739.

109. Sadowski HB, Shuai K, Darnell JE Jr, Gilman MZ. A common nuclear signal transduction pathway activated by growth factor and cytokine receptors. Science 1993; 261:1739–1744.

110. McCormick F. Activators and effectors of ras p21 proteins. Curr Opin Gen Dev 1994; 4:71–76.

111. Marshall MS. The effector interactions of p21^{ras}. Trends Biochem Sci 1993; 18:250–259.

112. Ravichandran KS, Burakoff SJ. The adapter protein Shc interacts with the interleukin-2 (IL-2) receptor upon IL-2 stimulation. J Biol Chem 1994; 269:1599–1602.

113. Cutler RL, Liu L, Damen JE, Krystal G. Multiple cytokines induce the tyrosine phosphorylation of Shc and its association with Grb2 in hemopoietic cells. J Biol Chem 1993; 268:21463–21465.

114. Marshall CJ. Map kinase kinase kinase, MAP kinase kinase and MAP kinase. Curr Opin Gen Dev 1994; 4:82–89.

115. Schindler C, Fu X-Y, Improta T, Aebersold R, Darnell JE Jr. Proteins of transcription factor ISGF-3: one gene encodes the 91- and 84-kDa ISGF-3 proteins that are activated by interferon α. Proc Natl Acad Sci USA 1992; 89:7836–7839.

116. Fu XY, Kessler DS, Veals SA, Levy DE, Darnell JE Jr. ISGF3, the transcriptional activator induced by interferon alpha, consists of multiple interacting polypeptide chains. Proc Natl Acad Sci USA 1990;87:8555–8559.

117. Brady-Kalnay SM, Tonks NK. Protein tyrosine phosphatases: from structure to function. Trends Biochem Sci 1994; 19:73–76.

118. Neel BG. Structure and function of SH2-domain containing tyrosine phosphatases. Semin Cell Biol 1993; 4:419–432.

119. Townley R, Shen SH, Banville D, Ramachandran C. Inhibition of the activity of protein tyrosine phosphate 1C by its SH2 domains. Biochemistry 1993; 32:13414–13418.

120. Lechleider RJ, Sugimoto S, Bennett AM, et al. Activation of the SH2-containing phospho-

tyrosine phosphatase SH-PTP2 by its binding site, phosphotyrosine 1009, on the human platelet-derived growth factor receptor. J Biol Chem 1993; 268:21478–21481.

121. Vogel W, Lammers R, Huang J, Ullrich A. Activation of a phosphotyrosine phosphatase by tyrosine phosphorylation. Science 1993; 259:1611–1614.

122. Feng GS, Hui CC, Pawson T. SH2-containing phosphotyrosine phosphatase as a target of protein-tyrosine kinases. Science 1993; 259:1607–1611.

123. Yi T, Mui AL, Krystal G, Ihle JN. Hematopoietic cell phosphatase associates with the inter-leukin-3 (IL-3) receptor beta chain and down-regulates IL-3-induced tyrosine phosphorylation and mitogenesis. Mol Cell Biol 1993; 13:7577–7586.

124. Boulton TG, Stahl NG, Yancopoulos GD. The CNTF/LIF/IL6/OSM family of cytokines induce tyrosine phosphorylation of a common set of proteins overlapping those induced by other cytokines and growth factors. J Biol Chem 1994; 269:11648–11655.

125. Kolb JP, Abadie A, Paul-Eugene N, Dugas B. Intracellular signaling events associated with the induction of DNA synthesis in human B lymphocytes. II. Different pathways triggered by IL-2 and IL-4. Cell Immunol 1993; 146:131–146.

126. Welham MJ, Duronio V, Schrader JW. Interleukin-4-dependent proliferation dissociates p44erk-1, p42 erk-2 and p21ras activation from cell growth. J Biol Chem 1994; 269:5865–5873.

127. Wang LM, Keegan AD, Li W, et al. Common elements in interleukin 4 and insulin signaling pathways in factor-dependent hematopoietic cells. Proc Natl Acad Sci USA 1993; 90:4032–4036.

128. Bazan F. Shared architecture of hormone binding domains in type I and type II interferon receptors. Cell 1990; 61:753–754.

129. Thoreau E, Petridou B, Kelly PA, Djiane J, Mornon JP. Structural symmetry of the extracellular domain of the cytokine/growth hormone/prolactin receptor family and interferon receptors revealed by hydrophobic cluster analysis. FEBS Lett 1991; 282:26–31.

130. Ho ASY, Liu Y, Khan TA, Hsu Dh, Bazan JF. A receptor for interleukin 10 is related to interferon receptors. Proc Natl Acad Sci USA 1993; 90:11267–11271.

131. Pestka S, Langer JA, Zoon KC, Samuel CE. Interferons and their actions. Annu Rev Biochem 1987; 56:727–777.

132. Moore KW, O'Garra A, de Waal Malefyt R, Vieira P, Mosmann TR. Annu Rev Immunol 1993; 11:165–190.

133. Pellegrini S, Schindler C. Early events in signalling by interferons. Trends Biochem Sci 1993; 18:338–342.

134. Hamblin AS. In: Male D, ed. Lymphokines. Oxford: IRL Press, 1988.

135. Auget M, Dembic A, Merlin G. Molecular cloning and expression of the human interferon-γ receptor. Cell 1988; 55:273–280.

136. Gray PW, Leong S, Fennie EH, Farrar MA, Pingel JT, Fernandez LJ, Schreiber RD. Cloning and expression of the cDNA for the murine interferon gamma receptor. Proc Natl Acad Sci USA 1989; 86:8497–8501.

137. Hemmi S, Peghini P, Metzler M, Merlin G, Dembic Z, Aguet M. Cloning of murine interferon gamma receptor cDNA: expression in human cells mediates high-affinity binding but is not sufficient to confer sensitivity to murine interferon gamma. Proc Natl Acad Sci USA 1989; 86:9901–9905.

138. Aguet M. Molecular cloning of interferon receptors: a short review. Br J Haematol 1991; 79 (suppl 1):6–8.

139. Uzé G, Lutfalla G, Gresser I. Genetic transfer of a functional interferon α receptor into mouse cells: cloning and expression of its cDNA. Cell 1990; 60:225–234.

140. Soh J, Donnelly RJ, Mariano TM, Cook JR, Schwartz B, Pestka S. Identification of a yeast artificial chromosome clone encoding an accessory factor for the human interferon gamma receptor: evidence for multiple accessory factors. Proc Natl Acad Sci USA 1993; 90:8737–8741.

141. Hibino Y, Kumar CS, Mariano TM, Lai DH, Pestka S. Chimeric interferon-gamma receptors

demonstrate that an accessory factor required for activity interacts with the extracellular domain. J Biol Chem 1992; 267:3741–3749.

142. Hemmi S, Bohni R, Stark G, Di Marco F, Auget M. A novel member of the interferon receptor family complements functionality of the murine interferon γ receptor in human cells. Cell 1994; 76:803–810.

143. Soh J, Donnelly RJ, Kotenko S, et al. Identification and sequence of an accessory factor required for activation of the human interferon gamma receptor. Cell 1994; 76:793–802.

144. Aguet M, Merlin G. Purification of human gamma interferon receptors by sequential affinity chromatography on immobilized monoclonal antireceptor antibodies and human gamma interferon. J Exp Med 1987; 165:988–999.

145. Arakawa T, Hsu Y-R. Acid unfolding and self-association of recombinant *Escherichia coli* derived human interferon-γ. Biochemistry 1987; 26:5428–5432.

146. Ealick SE, Cook WJ, Vijay-Kumar S, et al. Three-dimensional structure of recombinant human interferon-γ. Science 1991; 252:698–702.

147. Griggs ND, Jarpe MA, Pace JL, Russell SW, Johnson HM. The N-terminus and C-terminus of IFN-γ are binding domains for cloned soluble IFN-γ receptor. J Immunol 1992; 149:517–520.

148. Greenlund AC, Schreiber RD, Goeddel DV, Pennica D. Interferon-gamma induces receptor dimerization in solution and on cells. J Biol Chem 1993; 268:18103–18110.

149. Silvennoinen O, Ihle JN, Schlessinger J, Levy DE. Interferon-induced nuclear signalling by Jak protein tyrosine kinases. Nature 1993; 366:583–585.

150. Shuai K. Interferon-activated signal transduction to the nucleus. Curr Opin Cell Biol 1994; 6:253–259.

151. Colamonici OR, Uyttendaele H, Domanski P, Yan H, Krolewski JJ. p135tyk2, an interferon-alpha-activated tyrosine kinase, is physically associated with an interferon-alpha receptor. J Biol Chem 1994; 269:3518–3522.

152. Müller M, Briscoe J, Laxton C, et al. The protein tyrosine kinase JAK1 complements defects in interferon-α/β and -γ signal transduction. Nature 1993; 366:29–35.

153. Watling D, Guschin D, Müller M, et al. Complementation by the protein tyrosine kinase JAK2 of a mutant cell line defective in the interferon-γ signal transduction pathway. Nature 1993;366:166–70.

154. Cook JR, Jung V, Schwartz B, Wang P, Pestka S. Structural analysis of the human interferon gamma receptor: a small segment of the intracellular domain is specifically required for class I major histocompatibility complex antigen induction and antiviral activity. Proc Natl Acad Sci USA 1992; 89:11317–11321.

155. Farrar MA, Schreiber RD. The molecular cell biology of interferon-gamma and its receptor. Annu Rev Immunol 1993; 11:571–611.

156. Fu X-Y, Schindler C, Improta T, Aebersold R, Darnell JE. The proteins of ISGF-3, the interferon α-induced transcriptional activator, define a gene family involved in signal transduction. Proc Natl Acad Sci USA 1992; 89:7840–7843.

157. Zhong Z, Wen Z, Darnell JE. Stat3: A STAT family member activated by tyrosine phosphorylation in response to epidermal growth factor and Interleukin-6. Science 1994; 264:95–98.

158. Fu XY. A transcription factor with SH2 and SH3 domains is directly activated by an interferon alpha-induced cytoplasmic protein tyrosine kinase(s). Cell 1992; 70:323–335.

159. David M, Larner AC. Activation of transcription factors by interferon-alpha in a cell-free system. Science 1992; 257:813–815.

160. David M, Romero G, Zhang ZY, Dixon JE, Larner AC. In vitro activation of the transcription factor ISGF3 by interferon alpha involves a membrane-associated tyrosine phosphatase and tyrosine kinase. J Biol Chem 1993; 268:6593–6599.

161. Schindler C, Shuai K, Prezioso VR, Darnell JE Jr. Interferon-dependent tyrosine phosphorylation of a latent cytoplasmic transcription factor. Science 1992; 257:809–813.

162. Shuai K, Stark GR, Kerr IM, Darnell JE Jr. A single phosphotyrosine residue of Stat91 required for gene activation by interferon-gamma. Science 1993; 261:1744–1746.

163. Kanno Y, Kozak CA, Schindler C, et al. The genomic structure of the murine ICSBP gene reveals the presence of the gamma interferon-responsive element, to which an ISGF3 alpha subunit (or similar) molecule binds. Mol Cell Biol 1993; 13:3951–3963.

164. Shuai K, Horvath CM, Huang LHT, Qureshi SA, Cowburn D, Darnell JE. Interferon activation of the transcription factor Stat91 involves dimerization through SH2-phosphotyrosyl peptide interactions. Cell 1994; 76:821–828.

165. Smith CA, Farrah T, Goodwin RG. The TNF receptor superfamily of cellular and viral proteins: activation, costimulation, and death. Cell 1994; 76:959–962.

166. Ruddle NH. Tumor necrosis factor (TNFα) and lymphoid (TNFβ). Curr Opin Immunol 1992; 4:327–332.

167. Vilcek J, Lee TH. Tumor necrosis factor. J Biol Chem 1991; 266:7313–7316.

168. Rothe J, Gehr G, Loetscher H, Lesslauer W. Tumor necrosis factor receptors: structure and function. Immunol Res 1992; 11:81–90.

169. Goodwin RG, Anderson D, Jerzy R, et al. Molecular cloning and expression of the type 1 and type 2 murine receptors for tumor necrosis factor. Mol Cell Biol 1991; 11:3020–3026.

170. Goodwin RG, Alderson MR, Smith CA, et al. Molecular and biological characterization of a ligand for CD27 defines a new family of cytokines with homology to tumor necrosis factor. Cell 1993; 73:447–456.

171. Smith CA, Gruss HJ, Davis T, et al. CD30 antigen, a marker for Hodgkin's lymphoma, is a receptor whose ligand defines an emerging family of cytokines with homology to TNF. Cell 1993; 73:1349–1360.

172. Armitage RJ, Fanslow WC, Strockbine L, Sato TA, Clifford KN, Macduff BM, Anderson DM, Gimpel SD, Davis-Smith T, Maliszewski CR, Grabstein KH, Cosman D, Spriggs MK. Molecular and biological characterization of a murine ligand for CD40. Nature 1992; 357:80–82.

173. Gravestein LA, Blom B, Nolten LA, et al. Cloning and expression of murine CD27: comparison with 4-1BB, another lymphocyte-specific member of the nerve growth factor receptor family. Eur J Immunol 1993; 23:943–950.

174. Bradshaw RA, Blundell TL, Lapatto R, McDonald NQ, Murray-Rust J. Nerve growth factor revisited. Trends Biochem Sci 1993; 18:48–52.

175. Eck MJ, Ultsch M, Rinderknecht E, de Vos AM, Sprang SR. The structure of human lymphotoxin (tumor necrosis factor-β) at 1.9 A resolution. J Biol Chem 1992; 267:2119–2122.

176. Jones EY, Stuart DI, Walker NPC. Structure of tumour necrosis factor. Nature 1989; 338:225–228.

177. Jones EY, Stuart DI, Walker NPC. Crystal structure of TNF. In: Aggarwal BB, Vilcek J, eds. Tumor Necrosis Factors: Structure, Function, and Mechanism of Action. New York: Marcel Dekker, 1992; 93–127.

178. Banner DW, D'Arcy A, Janes W, Gentz R, van den Berghe H, Maryen P. Crystal structure of the soluble human 55 kd TNF receptor-human TNF beta complex: implications for TNF receptor activation. Cell 1993; 73:431–445.

179. Loetscher H, Pan Y-CE, Lahm HW, Gentz R, Brockhaus M, Tabuchi H, Lesslauer W. Cell 1990; 61:351–359.

180. Schall TJ, Lewis M, Koller KJ, Lee A, Rice GC, Wong GHW, Gatanaga T, Lentz R, Raab H, Kohr WJ, Goeddel DV. Molecular cloning and expression of a receptor for human tumor necrosis factor. Cell 1990; 61:361–370.

181. Smith CA, Davis T, Anderson D, et al. A receptor for tumor necrosis factor defines an unusual family of cellular and viral proteins. Science 1990; 248:1019–1023.

182. Johnson D, Lanahan A, Buck CR, Sehgal A, Morgan C, Mercer E, Bothwell M, Chao M. Expression and structure of the human NGF receptor. Cell 1986; 47:545–554.

183. Camerini D, Waltz G, Loenen WAM, Borst J, Seed B. The T cell activation antigen CD27 is a member of the nerve growth factor/tumor necrosis factor receptor gene family. J Immunol 1991; 147:3165–3169.

184. Durkop H, Latza U, Hummel M, Eitelbach F, Seed B, Stein H. Molecular cloning and expression of a new member of the nerve growth factor receptor family that is characteristic for Hodgkin's disease. Cell 1992; 68:421–427.

185. Stamenkovic I, Clark EA, Seed B. A B-lymphocyte activation molecule related to the nerve growth factor receptor and induced by cytokines in carcinomas. EMBO J 1989; 8:1403–1410.

186. Itoh N, Yonehara S, Ishii A, Yonehara M, Mizushima S-I, Sameshima M, Hase A, Seto Y, Nagata S. The polypeptide encoded by the cDNA for human cell surface antigen Fas can mediate apoptosis. Cell 1991; 66:233–243.

187. Mallet S, Fossum S, Barclay AN. Characterization of the MRC OX40 antigen of activated CD4 positive T lymphocytes—a molecule related to nerve growth factor receptor. EMBO J 1990; 9:1063–1068.

188. Kwon BS, Weissman SM. cDNA sequences of two inducible T-cell genes. Proc Natl Acad Sci USA 1989; 86:1963–1967.

189. Crowe PD, VanArsdale TL, Walter BN, Ware CF, Hession C, Ehrenfels B, Browning JL, Din W, Goodwin RG, Smith CA. A lymphotoxin-β-specific receptor. Science 1994; 264:707–710.

190. Upton C, DeLange AM, McFadden, G. Tumorigenic poxviruses: genomic organization and DNA sequence of the telomeric region of the Shope fibromavirus genome. Virology 1987; 160:20–30.

191. Howard ST, Chan YS, Smith GL. Vaccinia virus homologues of the Shope fibroma virus inverted terminal repeat proteins and a discontinuous ORF related to the tumor necrosis factor receptor family. Virology 1991; 180:633–647.

192. Marsters SA, Frutkin AD, Simpson NJ, Fendy BM, Ashkenazi A. Identification of cysteine-rich domains of the type 1 receptor involved in ligand binding. J Biol Chem 1992; 267:5747–5750.

193. Hsu KC, Chao MV. Differential expression and ligand binding properties of tumor necrosis factor receptor chimeric mutants. J Biol Chem 1993; 268:16430–16436.

194. Browning JL, Androlewicz MJ, Ware CF. Lymphotoxin and an associated 33-kDa glycoprotein are expressed on the surface of an activated human T cell hybridoma. J Immunol 1991; 147: 1230–1237.

195. Ware CF, Crowe PD, Grayson MH, Androlewicz MJ, Browning JL. Expression of surface lymphotoxin and tumor necrosis factor on activated T, B, and natural killer cells. J Immunol 1992; 149:3881–3888.

196. Browning JL, Ngam-ek A, Lawton P, et al. Lymphotoxin beta, a novel member of the TNF family that forms a heteromeric complex with lymphotoxin on the cell surface. Cell 1993; 72:847–856.

197. Tartaglia LA, Rothe M, Hu YF, Goeddel DV. Tumor necrosis factor's cytotoxic activity is signaled by the p55 TNF receptor. Cell 1993; 73:213–216.

198. Tartaglia LA, Goeddel DV. Two TNF receptors. Immunol Today 1992; 13:151–153.

199. Tartaglia LA, Pennica D, Goeddel DV. Ligand passing: the 75-kDa tumor necrosis factor (TNF) receptor recruits TNF for signaling by the 55-kDa TNF receptor. J Biol Chem 1993; 268:18542–18548.

200. Tartaglia LA, Ayres TM, Wong GH, Goeddel DV. A novel domain within the 55 kd TNF receptor signals cell death. Cell 1993; 74:845–853.

201. Brakebusch C, Nophar Y, Kemper O, Engelmann H, Wallach D. Cytoplasmic truncation of the p55 tumour necrosis factor (TNF) receptor abolishes signalling, but not induced shedding of the receptor. EMBO J 1992; 11:943–950.

202. Crowe PD, VanArsdale TL, Goodwin RG, Ware CF. Specific induction of 80-kDa tumor necrosis factor receptor shedding in T lymphocytes involves the cytoplasmic domain and phosphorylation. J Immunol 1993; 151:6882–6890.

203. Kalthoff H, Roeder C, Brockhaus M, Thiele HG, Schmiegel W. Tumor necrosis factor (TNF) up-regulates the expression of p75 but not p55 TNF receptors, and both receptors mediate, independently of each other, up-regulation of transforming growth factor alpha and epidermal growth factor receptor mRNA. J Biol Chem 1993; 268:2762–2766.

204. Wiegmann K, Schutze S, Kampen E, Himmler A, Machleidt T, Kronke M. Human 55-kDa receptor for tumor necrosis factor coupled to signal transduction cascades. J Biol Chem 1992; 267:17997–18001.

205. Schutze S, Potthoff K, Machleidt T, Berkovic D, Wiegmann K, Kronke M. TNF activates NF-kappa B by phosphatidylcholine-specific phospholipase C-induced acidic sphingomyelin breakdown. Cell 1992; 71:765–776.

206. Dressler KA, Mathias S, Kolesnick RN. Tumor necrosis factor-alpha activates the sphingomyelin signal transduction pathway in a cell-free system. Science 1992; 255:1715–1718.

207. Raines MA, Kolesnick RN, Golde DW. Sphingomyelinase and ceramide activate mitogen-activated protein kinase in myeloid HL-60 cells. J Biol Chem 1993; 268:14572–14575.

208. Yang Z, Costanzo M, Golde DW, Kolesnick RN. Tumor necrosis factor activation of the sphingomyelin pathway signals nuclear factor kappa B translocation in intact HL-60 cells. J Biol Chem 1993; 268:20520–20523.

209. Akimaru K, Utsumi T, Sato EF, Klostergaard J, Inoue M, Utsumi K. Role of tyrosyl phosphorylation in neutrophil priming by tumor necrosis factor-alpha and granulocyte colony stimulating factor. Arch Biochem Biophys 1992; 298:703–709.

210. Vietor I, Schwenger P, Li W, Schlessinger J, Vilcek J. Tumor necrosis factor-induced activation and increased tyrosine phosphorylation of mitogen-activated protein (MAP) kinase in human fibroblasts. J Biol Chem 1993; 268:18994–18999.

211. Yanaga F, Abe M, Koga T, Hirata M. Signal transduction by tumor necrosis factor alpha is mediated through a guanine nucleotide-binding protein in osteoblast-like cell line, MC3T3-E1. J Biol Chem 1992; 267:5114–5121.

212. Kronke M, Schutze S, Scheurich P, Pfizenmaier K. TNF signal transduction and TNF-responsive genes. Immunol Ser 1992; 56:189–216.

213. Branellec D, De CP, Barreau P, Calvo F, Chouaib S. Tumor necrosis factor-mediated cell lysis in vitro: relationship to cAMP accumulation and guanine nucleotide-binding proteins. Eur J Immunol 1992; 22:963–967.

214. Hayakawa M, Hori T, Shibamoto S, Tsujimoto M, Oku N, Ito F. Solubilization of human placental tumor necrosis factor receptors as a complex with a guanine nucleotide-binding protein. Arch Biochem Biophys 1991; 286:323–329.

215. Van Lint J, Agostinis P, Vandevoorde V, et al. Tumor necrosis factor stimulates multiple serine/threonine protein kinases in Swiss 3T3 and L929 cells. Implication of casein kinase-2 and extracellular signal-regulated kinases in the tumor necrosis factor signal transduction pathway. J Biol Chem 1992; 267:25916–25921.

216. Guy GR, Chua SP, Wong NS, Ng SB, Tan YH. Interleukin 1 and tumor necrosis factor activate common multiple protein kinases in human fibroblasts. J Biol Chem 1991; 266:14343–14352.

217. Guy GR, Cairns J, Ng SB, Tan YH. Inactivation of a redox-sensitive protein phosphatase during the early events of tumor necrosis factor/interleukin-1 signal transduction. J Biol Chem 1993; 268:2141–2148.

218. Noelle RJ, Roy M, Shepherd DM, Stamenkovic I, Ledbetter JA, Aruffo A. A 39-kDa protein on activated helper T cells binds CD40 and transduces the signal for cognate activation of B cells. Proc Natl Acad Sci USA 1992; 89:6550–6554.

219. Graf D, Korthauer U, Mages HW, Senger G, Kroczek RA. Cloning of TRAP, a ligand for CD40 on human T cells. Eur J Immunol 1992; 22:3190–3194.

220. Lane P, Brocker T, Hubele S, Padovan E, Lanzavecchia A, McConnell F. Soluble CD40 ligand can replace the normal T cell-derived CD40 ligand signal to B cells in T cell-dependent activation. J Exp Med 1993; 177:1209–1213.

221. Tsubata T, Wu J, Nojo T. B-cell apoptosis induced by antigen receptor crosslinking is blocked by a T-cell signalling through CD40. Nature 1993; 364:645–648.

222. Gascan H, Gauchat J-F, Aversa G, Vlasselaer PV, De Vries JE. Anti-CD40 monoclonal antibodies or CD4+ T cell clones and IL-4 induce IgG4 and IgE switching in purified human B cells via different signalling pathways. J Immunol 1991; 147:8–13.

223. Clark EA, Shu G. Association between IL-6 and CD-40 signalling: IL-6 induces phosphorylation of CD40 receptors. J Immunol 1990; 145:1400–1406.

224. Uckun FM, Schieven GL, Dibirdik I, Chandan-Langlie M, Tuel-Ahlgren L, Ledbetter JA. Stimulation of protein tyrosine phosphorylation, phosphoinositide turnover, and multiple previously unidentified serine/threonine-specific protein kinases by the Pan-B-cell receptor CD40/Bp50 at discrete developmental stages of human B-cell ontogeny. J Biol Chem 1991; 266:17478–17485.

225. Inui S, Kaisho I, Kikutani H, Stamenkovic I, Seed B, Clark EA, Kishimoto T. Identification of the intracytoplasmic region essential for signal transduction through a B cell activation molecule, CD40. Eur J Immunol 1990; 20:1747–1753.

226. Suda T, Takahashi T, Golstein P, Nagata S. Molecular cloning and expression of the Fas ligand, a novel member of the tumor necrosis factor family. Cell 1993; 75:1169–1178.

227. Hintzen RQ, de Jong R, Hack CE, Chamuleau M, de Vries EFR, ten Berge IJM, Borst J, van Lier RAW. A soluble form of the human T cell differentiation antigen CD27 is released after triggering of the TCR/CD3 complex. J Immunol 1991; 147:29–35.

228. Loenen WAM, Gravestein LA, Beumer S, Melief CJM, Hagemeijer A, Borst J. Genomic organization and chromosomal localization of the human CD27 gene. J Immunol 1992; 149:3937–3943.

229. McDonald NQ, Lapatto R, Murray-Rust J, Gunning J, Wlodawer A, Blundell TL. New protein fold revealed by a 2.3-A resolution crystal structure of nerve growth factor. Nature 1991; 354:411–414.

230. Yancopoulos GD, Maisonpierre PC, Ip NY, Belluscio L, Boulton TG, Cobb MH, Squinto SP, Furth. Neurotrophic factors, their receptors, and the signal transduction pathways they activate. Cold Spring Harbor Symp Quant Biol 1990; 55:371–379.

231. Berg MM, Sternberg DW, Hempstead BL, Chao MV. The low-affinity p75 nerve growth factor (NGF) receptor mediates NGF-induced tyrosine phosphorylation. Proc Natl Acad Sci USA 1991; 88:7106–7110.

232. Ibanez CF, Ebendal T, Barbany G, Murray-Rust J, Blundell TL, Persson H. Disruption of the low affinity receptor-binding site in NGF allows neuronal survival and differentiation by binding to the *trk* gene product. Cell 1992; 69:329–341.

233. Rabizadeh S, Oh J, Zhong LT, Yang J, Bitler CM, Butcher LL, Bredesen DE. Induction of apoptosis by the low-affinity NGF receptor. Science 1993; 261:345–348.

234. Smith CA, Davis T, Wignall JM, et al. T2 open reading frame from the Shope fibroma virus encodes a soluble form of the TNF receptor. Biochem Biophys Res Commun 1991; 176:335–342.

235. March CJ, Mosley B, Larsen A, Cerretti DP, Braedt G, Price V, Gillis S, Henney CS, Kronheim SR, Grabstein K, Conlon PJ, Hopp TP, Cosman D. Cloning, sequence and expression of two distinct human interleukin-1 complementary DNAs. Nature 1985; 315:641–647.

236. Dower SK, Kronheim SR, Hopp TP, Cantrell M, Deeley M, Gillis S, Henney CS, Urdal DL. The cell surface receptors for interleukin-1α and interleukin-1β are identical. Nature 1986; 324:266–268.

237. Dinarello CA. Interleukin-1 and its biologically related cytokines. Adv Immunol 1989; 44:153–205.

238. Dinarello CA, Thompson RC. Blocking IL-1: Interleukin 1 receptor antagonist in vivo and in vitro. Immunol Today 1991; 12:404–410.

239. Dinarello CA. Interleukin 1 and interleukin 1 antagonism. Blood 1991; 77:1627–1652.

240. McMahan CJ, Slack JL, Mosley B, Cosman D, Lupton SD, Brunton LL, Grubin CE, Wignall JM, Jenkins NA, Brannan CI, et al. A novel IL-1 receptor, cloned from B cells by mammalian expression, is expressed in many cell types. EMBO J 1991; 10:2821–2832.

241. Sims JE, Gayle MA, Slack JL, Alderson MR, Bird TA, Giri JG, Colotta F, Re F, Mantovani A, Shanebeck K, Grabstein KH, Dower SK. Interleukin 1 signaling occurs exclusively via the type I receptor. Proc Natl Acad Sci USA 1993; 90:6115–6159.

242. Stylianou E, O'Neill LA, Rawlinson L, Edbrooke MR, Woo P, Saklatvala J. Interleukin 1

induces NF-κB through its type I but not its type II receptor in lymphocytes. J Biol Chem 1992; 267:15836–15841.

243. McConkey DJ, Hartzell P, Chow SC, Orrenius S, Jondal M. Interleukin 1 inhibits T cell receptor-mediated apoptosis in mature thymocytes. J Biol Chem 1990; 265:3009–3011.

244. Donati D, Baldari CT, Macchia G, Massone A, Telford JL, Parente L. Induction of gene expression by IL-1 in NIH 3T3 cells. Possible requirement of protein kinase C activity and independence from arachidonic acid metabolism. J Immunol 1990; 145:4115–4120.

245. Kester M, Simonson MS, Mene P, Sedor JR. Interleukin-1 generates transmembrane signals from phospholipids through novel pathways in cultured rat mesangial cells. J Clin Invest 1989; 83:718–723.

246. Shirakawa F, Yamashita U, Chedid M, Mizel SB. Cyclic AMP—an intracellular second messenger for interleukin 1. Proc Natl Acad Sci USA 1988; 85:8201–8205.

247. Zhang YH, Lin JX, Yip YK, Vilcek J. Enhancement of cAMP levels and of protein kinase activity by tumor necrosis factor and interleukin 1 in human fibroblasts: role in the induction of interleukin 6. Proc Natl Acad Sci USA 1988; 85:6802–6805.

248. Munoz E, Zubiaga AM, Sims JE, Huber BT. IL-1 signal transduction pathways. I. Two functional IL-1 receptors are expressed in T cells. J Immunol 1991; 146:136–143.

249. Munoz E, Zubiaga A, Huang C, Huber BT. Interleukin-1 induces protein tyrosine phosphorylation in T cells. Eur J Immunol 1992; 22:1391–1396.

250. Joshi-Barve SS, Rangnekar VV, Sells SF, Rangnekar VM. Interleukin-1-inducible expression of gro-beta via NF-kappa B activation is dependent upon tyrosine kinase signaling. J Biol Chem 1993; 268:18018–18029.

251. Heguy A, Baldari CT, Censini S, Ghiara P, Telford JL. A chimeric type II/ type I interleukin-1 receptor can mediate interleukin 1 induction of gene expression in T cells. J Biol Chem 1993; 268:10490–10494.

252. Kuno K, Okamoto S, Hirose K, Murakami S, Matsushima K. Structure and function of the intracellular portion of the mouse interleukin 1 receptor (type I). Determining the essential region for transducing signals to activate the interleukin 8 gene. J Biol Chem 1993; 268:13510–13518.

253. Mathias S, Younes A, Kan CC, Orlow I, Joseph C, Kolesnick RN. Activation of the sphingomyelin signaling pathway in intact EL4 cells and in a cell-free system by IL-1β. Science 1993; 259:519–522.

254. Muegge K, Williams TM, Kant J, Karin M, Chiu R, Schmidt A, Siebenlist U, Young HA, Durum SK. Interleukin-1 costimulatory activity on the interleukin-2 promoter via AP-1. Science 1989; 246:249–251.

255. Lin JX, Vilcek J. Tumor necrosis factor and interleukin-1 cause a rapid and transient stimulation of c-*fos* and c-*myc* mRNA levels in human fibroblasts. J Biol Chem 1987; 262:11908–11911.

256. Rangneker VV, Waheed S, Rangnekar VM. Interleukin-1-inducible tumor growth arrest is characterized by activation of cell type-specific "early" gene expression programs. J Biol Chem 1992; 267:6240–6248.

257. Mukaida N, Mahe Y, Matsushima K. Cooperative interaction of nuclear factor-kappa B- and cis-regulatory enhancer binding protein-like factor binding elements in activating the interleukin-8 gene by pro-inflammatory cytokines. J Biol Chem 1990; 265:21128–21133.

258. Muegge K, Vila M, Gusella GL, Musso T, Herrlich P, Stein B, Durum SK. Interleukin 1 induction of the c-*jun* promoter. Proc Natl Acad Sci USA 1993; 90:7054–7058.

259. Sherr CJ, Rettenmier CW, Sacca R, Roussel MF, Look AT, Stanley ER. The c-*fms* proto-oncogene product is related to the receptor for the mononuclear phagocyte growth factor, CSF-1. Cell 1985; 41:665–676.

260. Ullrich A, Schlessinger J. Signal transduction by receptors with tyrosine kinase activity. Cell 1990; 61:203–212.

261. Downing JR, Rettenmier CW, Sherr CJ. Ligand-induced tyrosine kinase activity of the colony-stimulating factor 1 receptor in a murine macrophage cell line. Mol Cell Biol 1988; 8:1795–1799.

262. Sengupta A, Liu WK, Yeung YG, Yeung DC, Frackelton AR Jr, Stanley ER. Identification and subcellular localization of proteins that are rapidly phosphorylated in tyrosine in response to colony-stimulating factor 1. Proc Natl Acad Sci USA 1988; 85:8062–8066.

263. Reedijk M, Liu XQ, Pawson T. Interactions of phosphatidylinositol kinase, GTPase-activating protein (GAP), and GAP-associated proteins with the colony-stimulating factor 1 receptor. Mol Cell Biol 1990; 10:5601–5608.

264. Joly M, Kazlauskas A, Fay FS, Corvera S. Disruption of PDGF receptor trafficking of its PI-3 kinase binding sites. Science 1994; 263:684–687.

265. Roussel MF, Shurtleff SA, Downing JR, Sherr CJ. A point mutation at tyrosine-809 in the human colony-stimulating factor 1 receptor impairs mitogenesis without abrogating tyrosine kinase activity, association with phosphatidylinositol 3-kinase, or induction of c-*fos* and *junB* genes. Proc Natl Acad Sci USA 1990; 87:6738–6742.

266. Imamura K, Kufe D. Colony-stimulating factor 1-induced Na$^+$ influx into human monocytes involves activation of a pertussis toxin-sensitive GTP-binding protein. J Biol Chem 1988; 263:14093–14098.

267. Imamura K, Dianoux A, Nakamura T, Kufe D. Colony-stimulating factor 1 activates protein kinase C in human monocytes [published erratum appears in EMBO J 1990; 9:3413]. EMBO J 1990; 9:2423–2428, 2389.

268. Veis N, Hamilton JA. Colony stimulating factor-1 stimulates diacylglycerol generation in murine bone marrow-derived macrophages, but not in resident peritoneal macrophages. J Cell Physiol 1991; 147:298–305.

269. Bishop WR, Bell RM. Functions of diacylglycerol in glycerolipid metabolism, signal transduction and cellular transformation. Oncogene Res 1988; 2:205–218.

270. Vairo G, Argyriou S, Bordun AM, Whitty G, Hamilton JA. Inhibition of the signaling pathways for macrophage proliferation by cyclic AMP. Lack of effect on early responses to colony stimulating factor-1. J Biol Chem 1990; 265:2692–2701.

271. Baccarini M, Sabatini DM, App H, Rapp UR, Stanley ER. Colony stimulating factor-1 (CSF-1) stimulates temperature dependent phosphorylation and activation of the RAF-1 proto-oncogene product. EMBO J 1990; 9:3649–3657.

272. Yeung YG, Berg KL, Pixley FJ, Angeletti RH, Stanley ER. Protein tyrosine phosphatase-1C is rapidly phosphorylated in tyrosine in macrophages in response to colony stimulating factor-1. J Biol Chem 1992; 267:23447–23450.

273. Hamilton JA, Veis N, Bordun AM, Vairo G, Gonda TJ, Phillips WA. Activation and proliferation signals in murine macrophages: relationships among c-*fos* and c-*myc* expression, phosphoinositide hydrolysis, superoxide formation, and DNA synthesis. J Cell Physiol 1989; 141: 618–626.

274. Adachi K, Saito H. Induction of *junB* expression, but not c-*jun*, by granulocyte colony-stimulating factor or macrophage colony-stimulating factor in the proliferative response of human myeloid leukemia cells. J Clin Invest 1992; 89:1657–1661.

275. Xu XX, Tessner TG, Rock CO, Jackowski S. Phosphatidylcholine hydrolysis and c-*myc* expression are in collaborating mitogenic pathways activated by colony-stimulating factor 1. Mol Cell Biol 1993; 13:1522–1533.

276. Broxmeyer HE, Maze R, Miyazawa K, Carow C, Hendrie PC, Cooper S, Hangoc G, Vadhan-Raj S, Lu L. The kit receptor and its ligand, steel factor, as regulators of hemopoiesis. Cancer Cells 1991; 3:480–487.

277. Zsebo KM, Williams DA, Geissler EN, Broudy VC, Martin FH, Atkins HL, Hsu R, Birkett NC, Okino KH, Murdoch DC, Jacobsen FW, Langley KE, Smith KA, Takeishi T, Cattanach BM, Galli SJ, Suggs SV. Stem cell factor is encoded at the *Sl* locus of the mouse and is the ligand for the c-*kit* tyrosine kinase receptor. Cell 1990; 63:213–224.

278. Qiu F, Prabir R, Brown K, Barker PE, Jhanwar S, Ruddle FH, Besmer P. Primary structure of c-*kit*: relationship with the CSF-1/PDGF receptor kinase family—oncogenic activation of v-*kit* involves deletion of extracellular domain and C terminus. EMBO J 1988; 7:1003–1011.

279. Rottapel R, Reedijk M, Williams DE, Lyman SD, Anderson DM, Pawson T, Bernstein A. The *Steel/W* transduction pathway: kit autophosphorylation and its association with a unique subset of cytoplasmic signaling proteins is induced by steel factor. Mol Cell Biol 1991; 11:3043–3051.

280. Lev S, Givol D, Yarden Y. Interkinase domain of *kit* contains the binding site for phosphatidylinositol 3' kinase. Proc Natl Acad Sci USA 1992; 89:678–682.

281. Lev S, Givol D, Yarden Y. A specific combination of substrates is involved in signal transduction by the *kit*-encoded receptor. EMBO J 1991; 10:647–654.

282. Hallek M, Druker B, Lepisto EM, Wood KW, Ernst TJ, Griffin JD. Granulocyte–macrophage colony-stimulating factor and steel factor induce phosphorylation of both unique and overlapping signal transduction intermediates in a human factor-dependent hematopoietic cell line. J Cell Physiol 1992; 153:176–186.

283. Koike T, Hirai K, Morita Y, Nozawa Y. Stem cell factor-induced signal transduction in rat mast cells. Activation of phospholipase D but not phosphoinositide-specific phospholipase C in c-*kit* receptor stimulation. J Immunol 1993; 151:359–366.

284. Yi T, Ihle JN. Association of hematopoietic cell phosphatase with c-*kit* after stimulation with c-*kit* ligand. Mol Cell Biol 1993; 13:3350–3358.

285. Welham MJ, Schrader JW. Steel factor-induced tyrosine phosphorylation in murine mast cells. Common elements with IL-3-induced signal transduction pathways. J Immunol 1992; 149:2772–2783.

286. Miyazawa K, Hendrie PC, Kim YJ, Mantel C, Yang YC, Kwon BS, Broxmeyer HE. Recombinant human interleukin-9 induces protein tyrosine phosphorylation and synergizes with steel factor to stimulate proliferation of the human factor-dependent cell line, M07e. Blood 1992; 80:1685–1692.

287. Duronio V, Welham MJ, Abraham S, Dryden P, Schrader JW. p21ras activation via hemopoietin receptors and c-*kit* requires tyrosine kinase activity but not tyrosine phosphorylation of p21ras GTPase-activating protein. Proc Natl Acad Sci USA 1992; 89:1587–1591.

288. von Ruden T, Stingl L, Ullrich A, Wagner EF. Rescue of W-associated mast cell defects in W/Wv bone marrow cells by ectopic expression of normal and mutant epidermal growth factor receptors. Blood 1993; 82:1463–1470.

289. von Ruden T, Kandels S, Radaszkiewicz T, Ullrich A, Wagner EF. Development of a lethal mast cell disease in mice reconstituted with bone marrow cells expressing the v-*erbB* oncogene. Blood 1992; 79:3145–3158.

290. Tsai M, Tam SY, Galli SJ. Distinct patterns of early response gene expression and proliferation in mouse mast cells stimulated by stem cell factor, interleukin-3, or IgE and antigen. Eur J Immunol 1993; 23:867–872.

291. Oppenheim JJ, Zachariae COC, Mukaida N, Matsushima K. Properties of the novel proinflammatory supergene "intercrine" cytokine superfamily. Annu Rev Immunol 1991; 9:617–648.

292. Miller MD, Krangel MS. Biology and biochemistry of the chemokines: a family of chemotactic and inflammatory cytokines. Crit Rev Immunol 1992; 12:17–46.

293. Yoshimura T, Leonard EJ. Human monocyte chemoattractant protein-1: structure and function. Cytokines 1992; 4:131–152.

294. Lord BI, Heyworth CM, Woolford LB. Macrophage inflammatory protein: its characteristics, biological properties and role in the regulation of haemopoiesis. Int J Hematol 1993; 57:197–206.

295. Sherry B, Horii Y, Manogue KR, Widmer U, Cerami A. Macrophage inflammatory proteins 1 and 2: an overview. Cytokines 1992; 4:117–130.

296. Falk W, Goodwin RH, Leonard EJ. A 48-well micro chemotaxis assembly for rapid and accurate measurement of leukocyte migration. J Immunol Methods 1980; 33:239–247.

297. Matsushima K, Morishita K, Yoshimura T, Lavu S, Kobayashi Y, Lew W, Appella E, Kung HF, Leonard EJ, Oppenheim JJ. Molecular cloning of a human monocyte-derived neutrophil chemotactic factor (MDNCF) and the induction of MDNCF mRNA by interleukin 1 and tumor necrosis factor. J Exp Med 1988; 167:1883–1893.

298. Holt JC, Harris ME, Holt AM, Lange E, Henschen A, Niewiarowski S. Characterization of human platelet basic protein, a precursor form of low-affinity platelet factor 4 and β-thromboglobulin. Biochemistry 1986; 25:1988–1996.

299. Farber JM. A macrophage mRNA selectively induced by γ-interferon encodes a member of the platelet factor 4 family of cytokines. Proc Natl Acad Sci USA 1990; 87:5238–5242.

300. Walz A, Burgener R, Car B, Baggiolini M, Kunkel SL, Strieter RM. Structure and neutrophil-activating properties of a novel inflammatory peptide (ENA-78) with homology to interleukin 8. J Exp Med 1991; 174:1355–1362.

301. Luster AD, Unkelss JC, Ravetch JV. γ-Interferon transcriptionally regulates an early-response gene containing homology to platelet proteins. Nature 1985; 315:672–676.

302. Richmond A, Balentien E, Thomas HG, Flaggs G, Barton DE, Spiess J, Bordoni R, Francke U, Derynck R. Molecular characterization and chromosomal mapping of melanoma growth stimulatory activity, a growth factor structurally related to β-thromboglobulin. EMBO J 1988; 7: 2025–2033.

303. Griffin CA, Emanuel BS, LaRocco P, Schwartz E, Poncz M. Human platelet factor 4 is mapped to 4q12-q21. Cytogenet Cell Genet 1987; 45:67–69.

304. Luster AD, Jhanwar SC, Chaganti RSK, Kersey JH, Ravetch JV. Interferon-inducible gene maps to a chromosomal band associated with a (4;11) translocation in acute leukemia cells. Proc Natl Acad Sci USA 1987; 84:2868–2871.

305. Baldwin ET, Weber IT, St Charles R, Xuan J-C, Apella E, Yamada M, Matsushima K, Edwards BFP, Clore GM, Gronenborn AM, Wlodawer A. Crystal structure of interleukin-8: symbiosis of NMR and crystallography. Proc Natl Acad Sci USA 1991; 88:502–506.

306. Clore GM, Gronenborn AM. Comparison of the solution nuclear magnetic resonance and crystal structures of interleukin-8. J Mol Biol 1991; 217:611–620.

307. St Charles R, Walz DA, Edwards BFP. The three-dimensional structure of bovine platelet factor 4 at 3.0 Å resolution. J Biol Chem 1989; 264:2092–2099.

308. Mayo KH, Chen M-J. Human platelet factor 4 monomer–dimer–tetramer equilibria investigated by ^{1}H NMR spectroscopy. Biochemistry 1989; 28:9469–9478.

309. Schall TJ, Bacon K, Toy KJ, Goeddel DV. Selective attraction of monocytes and T lymphocytes of the memory phenotype by cytokine RANTES. Nature 1990; 347:669–671.

310. Opdenakker G, Froyen G, Fiten P, Proost P, Van Damme J. Human monocyte chemotactic protein-3: molecular cloning of the cDNA and comparison with other chemokines. Biochem Biophys Res Commun 1993; 191:535–542.

311. Yoshimura T, Yuhki N, Moore SK, Appella E, Lerman MI, Leonard EJ. Human monocyte chemoattractant protein-1 (MCP-1). FEBS Lett 1989; 244:487–493.

312. Miller MD, Hata S, Malefyt RDW, Krangel MS. A novel polypeptide secreted by activated human T lymphocytes. J Immunol 1989; 143:2907–2916.

313. Wolpe SD, Davatelis G, Sherry B, Beutler B, Hesse DG, Nguyen HT, Moldawer LL, Nathan CF, Lowry SF, Cerami A. Macrophages secrete a novel heparin-binding protein with inflammatory and neutrophil chemokinetic properties. J Exp Med 1988; 167:570–581.

314. Davatelis G, Tekamp-Olsen P, Wolpe SD, Hermsen K, Luedke C, Gallegos C, Coit D, Merryweather J, Cerami A. Cloning and characterization of a cDNA for murine macrophage inflammatory protein (MIP) a novel monokine with inflammatory and chemokinetic properties. J Exp Med 1988; 167:1939–1944.

315. Sherry B, Tekamp-Olsen P, Wolpe SD, Hermsen K, Luedke C, Gallegos C, Coit D, Merryweather J, Cerami A. Resolution of the two components of macrophage inflammatory protein 1 and cloning and characterization of one of those components macrophage inflammatory protein 1β. J Exp Med 1988; 168:2251–2259.

316. Miller MD, Wilson SD, Dorf ME, Seuanez HN, O'Brien SJ, Krangel MS. Sequence and chromosomal location of the I-309 gene. J Immunol 1990; 145:2737–2744.

317. Donlon TA, Krensky AM, Wallace MR, Collins FS, Lovett M, Clayberger C. Localization of a

human T-cell-specific gene RANTES (D17S136E), to chromosome 17q11.2-q12. Genomics 1990; 6:548–553.

318. Wilson SD, Billings PR, D'Eustachio P, Fournier REK, Geissler E, Lalley PA, Burd PR, Housman DE, Taylor BA, Dorf ME. Clustering of cytokine genes on mouse chromosome 11. J Exp Med 1990; 171:1301–1314.

319. Lodi PJ, Garrett DS, Kuszewski J, et al. High-resolution solution structure of the beta chemokine hMIP-1 beta by multidimensional NMR. Science 1994; 263:1762–1767.

320. Graham GJ, MacKenzie J, Lowe S, et al. Aggregation of the chemokine MIP-1 alpha is a dynamic and reversible phenomenon. Biochemical and biological analyses. J Biol Chem 1994; 269:4974–4978.

321. Taub DD, Lloyd AR, Conlon K, Wang JM, Ortaldo JR, Harada A, Matsushima K, Kelvin DJ, Oppenheim JJ. Recombinant human interferon-inducible protein 10 is a chemoattractant for human monocytes and T lymphocytes and promotes T cell adhesion to endothelial cells. J Exp Med 1993; 177:1809–1814.

322. Senior RM, Griffin GL, Huang JS, Walz DA, Deuel TF. Chemotactic activity of platelet alpha granule proteins for fibroblasts. J Cell Biol 1983; 96:382–385.

323. Miller MD, Krangel MS. The human cytokine I-309 is a monocyte chemoattractant. Proc Natl Acad Sci USA 1992; 89:2950–2954.

324. Taub DD, Conlon K, Lloyd AR, Oppenheim JJ, Kelvin DJ. Preferential migration of activated CD4$^+$ and CD8$^+$ T cells in response to MIP-1α and MIP-1β. Science 1993; 260:355–358.

325. Beall CJ, Mahajan S, Kolattukudy PE. Conversion of monocyte chemoattractant protein-1 into a neutrophil attractant by substitution of two amino acids. J Biol Chem 1992; 267:3455–3459.

326. Moser B, Dewald B, Barella L, Schumacher C, Baggiolini M, Clark-Lewis I. Interleukin-8 antagonists generated by N-terminal modification. J Biol Chem 1993; 268:7125–7128.

327. Clark-Lewis I, Dewald B, Geiser T, Moser B, Baggiolini M. Platelet factor 4 binds to interleukin 8 receptors and activates neutrophils when its N terminus is modified with Glu-Leu-Arg. Proc Natl Acad Sci USA 1993; 90:3574–3577.

328. Davatelis G, Wolpe SD, Sherry B, Dayer J-M, Chicheportiche R, Cerami A. Macrophage inflammatory protein-1: a prostaglandin-independent endogenous pyrogen. Science 1989; 243:1066–1068.

329. Minano FJ, Sancibrian M, Myers RD. Fever induced by macrophage inflammatory protein-1 (MIP-1) in rats: hypothalamic sites of action. Brain Res Bull 1991; 27:701–706.

330. Holmes WE, Lee J, Kuang W-J, Rice GC, Wood WI. Structure and functional expression of a human interleukin-8 receptor. Science 1991; 253:1278–1280.

331. Murphy PM, Tiffany HL. Cloning of complementary DNA encoding a functional human interleukin-8 receptor. Science 1991; 253:1280–1283.

332. Loetscher P, Seitz M, Clark-Lewis I, Baggiolini M, Moser B. Both interleukin-8 receptors independently mediate chemotaxis. Jurkat cells transfected with IL-8R1 or IL-8R2 migrate in response to IL-8, GROα and NAP-2. FEBS Lett 1994; 341:187–192.

333. Lloyd A, Modi W, Cevario S, Oppenheim J, Kelvin D. Assignment of genes for interleukin-8 receptors (IL8R) A and B to human chromosome band 2q35. Cytogenet Cell Genet 1993; 63:238–240.

334. Ahuja SK, Ozcelik T, Milatovitc A, Francke U, Murphy PM. Molecular evolution of the human interleukin-8 receptor gene cluster. Nature Genet 1992; 2:31–36.

335. Beckmann MP, Munger WE, Kozlosky C, VandenBos T, Price V, Lyman S, Gerard N, Gerard C, Cerretti DP. Molecular characterization of the interleukin-8 receptor. Biochem Biophys Res Commun 1991; 179:784–789.

336. LaRosa GJ, Thomas KM, Kaufmann ME, Mark R, White M, Taylor L, Gray G, Witt D, Navarro J. Amino terminus of the interleukin-8 receptor is a major determinant of receptor subtype specificity. J Biol Chem 1992; 267:25402–25406.

337. Gayle RB, Sleath PR, Srinivason S, Birks CW, Weerawarna KS, Cerretti DP, Kozlosky CJ,

Nelson N, Bos TV, Beckman MP. Importance of the amino terminus of the interleukin-8 receptor in ligand interactions. J Biol Chem 1993; 268:7283–7289.

338. Hebert CA, Chuntharapai A, Smith M, Colby T, Kim J, Horuk R. Partial functional mapping of the human interleukin-8 type A receptor. J Biol Chem 1993; 268:18549–18553.

339. Neote K, DiGregorio D, Mak JY, Horuk R, Schall TJ. Molecular cloning, functional expression, and signaling characteristics of a C–C chemokine receptor. Cell 1993; 72:415–425.

340. Gao J-L, Kuhns DB, Tiffany HL, McDermott D, Li X, Francke U, Murphy PM. Structure and functional expression of the human macrophage inflammatory protein 1α/RANTES receptor. J Exp Med 1993; 177:1421–1427.

341. Gerard NP, Gerard C. The chemotactic receptor for human C5a anaphylatoxin. Nature 1991; 349:614–617.

342. Boulay F, Tardif M, Brouchon L, Vignais P. Synthesis and use of a novel N-formyl peptide derivative to isolate a human N-formyl peptide receptor cDNA. Biochem Biophys Res Commun 1990; 168:1103–1109.

343. Thomas KM, Pyun HY, Navarro J. Molecular cloning of the fMet-Leu-Phe receptor from neutrophils. J Biol Chem 1990; 265:20061–20064.

344. Federspiel B, Melhado IG, Duncan AMV, Delaney A, Schappert K, Clark-Lewis I, Jirik FR. Molecular cloning of the cDNA and chromosomal localization of the gene for a putative seven-transmembrane segment (7-TMS) receptor isolated form human spleen. Genomics 1993; 16:707–712.

345. Neote K, Darbonne W, Ogez J, Horuk R, Schall TJ. Identification of a promiscuous inflammatory peptide receptor on the surface of red blood cells. J Biol Chem 1993; 268:12247–12249.

346. Horuk R, Colby TJ, Darbonne WC, Schall TJ, Neote K. The human erythrocyte peptide (chemokine) receptor. Biochemical characterization, solubilization, and development of a binding assay for the soluble receptor. Biochemistry 1993; 32:5733–5738.

347. Horuk R, Chitnis CE, Darbonne WC, Colby TJ, Rybicki A, Hadley TJ, Miller LH. A receptor for the malarial parasite *Plasmodium vivax*: the erythrocyte chemokine receptor. Science 1993; 261:1182–1184.

348. Berridge MJ, Irvine RF. Inositol phosphates and cell signalling. Nature 1989; 341:197–204.

349. Wang JM, McVicar DW, Oppenheim JJ, Kelvin DJ. Identification of RANTES receptors on human monocytic cells: competition for binding and desensitization by homologous chemotactic cytokines. J Exp Med 1993; 177:699–705.

350. Bischoff SC, Krieger M, Brunner T, Rot A, Tcharner VV, Baggiolini M, Dahinden CA. RANTES and related chemokines activate human basophil granulocytes through different G protein-coupled receptors. Eur J Immunol 1993; 23:761–767.

351. Sozzani S, Molino M, Locati M, Luini W, Cerletti C, Vecchi A, Mantovani A. Receptor-activated calcium influx in human monocytes exposed to monocyte chemotactic protein-1 and related cytokines. J Immunol 1993; 150:1544–1553.

352. Kupper RW, Dewald B, Jakobs KH, Baggiolini M, Gierschik P. G-protein activation by interleukin 8 and related cytokines in human neutrophil plasma membranes. Biochem J 1992; 282:429–434.

353. Smith RJ, Sam LM, Leach KL, Justen JM. Postreceptor events associated with human neutrophil activation by interleukin-8. J Leukocyte Biol 1992; 52:17–26.

354. Wu D, LaRosa GJ, Simon MI. G protein-coupled signal transduction pathways for interleukin-8. Science 1993; 261:101–103.

355. Amatruda TT, Steele DA, Slepak VZ, Simon MI. Ga16 a G protein a subunit specifically expressed in hematopoietic cells. Proc Natl Acad Sci USA 1991; 88:5587–5591.

356. Lee CH, Park D, Wu D, Rhee SG, Simon MI. Members of the G_q a subunit gene family activate phospholipase C b isozymes. J Biol Chem 1992; 267:16044–16047.

357. Taylor SJ, Chae HZ, Rhee SG, Exton JH. Activation of the b1 isozyme of phospholipase C by a subunits of the G_q class of G proteins. Nature 1991; 350;516–518.

358. Simon MI, Strathmann MP, Gautam N. Diversity of G proteins in signal transduction. Science 1991; 252:802–808.

359. Sozzani S, Rieppi M, Locati M, et al. Synergism between platelet activating factor and C–C chemokines for arachidonate release in human monocytes. Biochem Biophys Res Commun 1994; 199:761–766.

360. Sozzani S, Zhou D, Locati M, Rieppi M, Proost P, Magazin M, Vita N, van Damme J, Mantovani A. Receptors and transduction pathways for monocyte chemotactic protein-2 and monocyte chemotactic protein-3: similarities and differences with MCP-1. J Immunol 1994; 152:3615–3622.

361. Locati M, Zhou D, Luini W, Evangelista V, Mantovani A, Sozzani S. Rapid induction of arachidonic acid release by monocyte chemotactic protein-1 and related chemokines. Role of Ca^{2+} influx, synergism with platelet-activating factor and significance for chemotaxis. J Biol Chem 1994; 269:4746–4753.

362. Springer TA. Adhesion receptors of the immune system. Nature 1990; 346:425–434.

363. Arnaout MA. Structure and function of the adhesion molecules CD11/CD18. Blood 1990; 75:1037–1050.

364. Lawrence MB, Springer TA. Leukocytes roll on a selectin at physiologic flow rates: distinction from and prerequisite for adhesion through integrins. Cell 1991; 65:859–873.

365. Jiang Y, Beller DI, Frendl G, Graves DT. Monocyte chemoattractant protein-1 regulates adhesion molecule expression and cytokine production in human monocytes. J Immunol 1992; 148:2423–2428.

366. Alam R, Strafford S, Forsythe P, Harrison R, Faubion D, Lett-Brown MA, Grant JA. RANTES is a chemotactic and activating factor for human eosinophils. J Immunol 1993; 150:3442–3447.

367. Kuna P, Reddigari SR, Schall TJ, Rucinski D, Viksman MY, Kaplan AP. RANTES, a monocyte and T lymphocyte chemotactic cytokine releases histamine from human basophils. J Immunol 1992; 149:636–642.

368. Samanta AK, Oppenheim JJ, Matsushima K. Interleukin 8 (monocyte-derived neutrophil chemotactic factor) dynamically regulates its own receptor expression on human neutrophils. J Biol Chem 1990; 265:183–189.

369. Unemori EN, Amento EP, Bauer EA, Horuk R. Melanoma growth-stimulatory activity/GRO decreases collegen expression by human fibroblasts. J Biol Chem 1993; 268:1338–1342.

3

FcεRI, ε-BP, and FcεRII: Structure and Involvement in Allergic Disease

Daniel H. Conrad
Virginia Commonwealth University, Richmond, Virginia

INTRODUCTION

For many facets of cell growth and differentiation, signal transduction through cell surface receptors such as those specific for antigen, lymphokines, or immunoglobulins (Ig) continues to be subject to intense investigation. The group of receptors for immunoglobulins are called Fc receptors by virtue of their capacity to interact with the Fc region of Ig. The current nomenclature is exemplified by FcεRI, where the Ig class is indicated by the greek letter and a roman numeral is used when more than one receptor for that Ig class has been identified. The Fc receptors have been implicated in a variety of immune functions, including phagocytosis, antibody-dependent cell-mediated cytotoxicity, and release of inflammatory mediators. This review will deal primarily with Fc receptors for IgE (FcεRI and FcεRII), and some attention will be given to $Fc_\gamma R$ as they relate to the function of the FcεRI. The reader is also referred to other recent reviews for more detailed information on IgE and IgG Fc receptors (1–4).

HISTORICAL PERSPECTIVE

The now classic experiments of Prausnitz and Kustner, in 1921, demonstrated that the serum of allergic individuals contained a humoral factor that transferred specific allergen sensitiveness to a nonallergic individual (5). This serum factor, termed reagin, was subsequently shown to be IgE, and the demonstration of highly specific binding to mast cells and basophils soon followed (6). This selective binding provided a powerful early insight into the mechanism of allergic disease (i.e., that these receptors were likely to be responsible for degranulation and release of mediators associated with the effector phase of allergy). Although recent, as yet unexplained, observations have demonstrated FcεRI expression on other cell types, it is still thought that the primary function of this receptor deals with mediator release from mast cells and basophils.

Subsequent to the discovery of this high-affinity receptor, another IgE receptor was identified on lymphocytes (7), primarily B cells, and is termed FcεRII. Its binding affinity was much lower, similar to other Fc receptors. The high-affinity receptor was called FcεRI, and the low-affinity receptor was called FcεRII (see Ref. 1 for discussion of nomenclature). The low-affinity receptor is unlikely to be involved in mast cell and basophil degranulation, but may be an important element in isotype-specific regulation of IgE. Therefore, both the high- and low-affinity receptors for IgE play important, although very different, roles in the development of allergic disease; and in this chapter they are reviewed separately to cover not only their pathological significance, but also their more recently characterized potential roles in normal physiology.

IMMUNOGLOBULIN E: PRIMARY HOMOCYTOTROPIC ANTIBODY IN HUMANS

Biological Functions

Immunoglobulin E is exquisitely T-cell-regulated both before and after class switch; the cytokines implicated for induction of class switch to IgE are IL-4 and the closely related IL-13 (8). Immunoglobulin E does not remain long in serum or other free fluid because of its high catabolic rate (2.5-day half-life for IgE vs. 21 days for IgG). When bound to cell surface receptors it protects them from the rapid degradation seen with serum IgE, as seen in the long retention of IgE when bound to the FcεRI (9). These distinctions may indicate a more local, rather than a systemic, natural role for IgE.

Immunoglobulin E appears very late in evolution and is presumed to be teleologically justified for its role in immunity to chronic infection with parasites such as gut helminths; this concept is primarily a result of the strongly elevated IgE levels seen after such parasitic infections, both in humans and in animal models. In addition, the finding that mast cells respond to IgE immune complexes by making and releasing many cytokines (discussed later) is supportive for a positive role for IgE in immunity. In spite of this, although there is certainly some evidence to support a role for IgE in parasite immunity (see Refs. 10 and 11 for review and commentary), especially in developed countries where human parasitic diseases are infrequent, IgE is associated with immunological problems rather that protective immunity. Indeed, although there is still some controversy concerning IgG_4, in humans, IgE is clearly the primary antibody responsible for type I allergic disease. Thus, because of this centrality of IgE in the development of immediate hypersensitivity, there has been a concerted effort by research investigators to inhibit IgE responses, without affecting other isotypes.

Structure Considerations

Immunoglobulin E (MW = 188,000) is slightly larger than IgG (MW = 155,000) because it has a fifth domain on the COOH-terminus, and it is more heavily glycosylated (12% for IgE vs. 3% for IgG). From this aspect it is most similar to IgM. Both of these isotypes have this additional constant region heavy chain domain and lack a classic hinge region; the Cε2 (and corresponding $C_\mu 2$) domain acts as a primitive "hinge." Proteolytic digestion of human IgE with pepsin and papain revealed $F(ab')_2$ and Fab'/Fc fragments, respectively (12), in which Cε2 domain is found in both the $F(ab')_2$ and Fc fragments. Whereas $F(ab')_2$-like fragments can be produced from rodent IgE with a variety of proteases, production of Fcε has not been reproducible. Although two of the three IgE-binding molecules reviewed in the following have lectin domains theoretically capable of binding oligosaccharide side chains, the significance of IgE's increased glycosylation is unknown, since deglycosylated IgE binds to both FcεR.

Obviously, the site on IgE that interacts with FcεR is of some interest in view of the possible development of inhibitors of the IgE–FcεR interaction. Several approaches have been taken to map the FcεRI site, including limited proteolysis (13), energy transfer (14), and inhibition of IgE binding with a monoclonal antibody (MAb) anti-IgE (15). The studies indicate that the most likely site of interaction is in the Cε2–Cε3 domains and, indeed, the energy-transfer studies indicate that IgE adopts a "bent" configuration when bound to the FcεRI (13). There is some controversy over the smallest IgE fragment that has FcεRI-binding activity. One group found that a 76-amino acid recombinant peptide bridging the Cε2–Cε3 domains was capable of binding to the FcεRI (16), whereas other results were unable to reproduce this finding and found binding only with recombinant peptides comprising both the Cε3–Cε4 domains, and the active product was always dimeric (17). The site of interaction of FcεRII has been mapped by similar techniques (15,18,19), and the results indicate that the interaction site is in the Cε3 domain and is close to, but not identical with, the FcεRI interaction site. Significantly, only dimeric recombinant IgE peptides bound to the FcεRII (15,19), in line with the expected dual-point interaction for the FcεRII (see later discussion). Recently, an alternative approach to treating allergy has been suggested, based on the site of IgE–FcεR interaction. Namely, anti-IgE MAbs that are directed to this area (as mentioned previously, the two sites appear to be quite close) are effective blocking agents for IgE binding to either FcεR. Interestingly, such antibodies not only appear to block this interaction, but also have some inhibitory properties for IgE synthesis (20). Although the use of xenogeneic MAbs for such a purpose is certainly not practical, owing to the problems from the immune response to the MAbs themselves, the concept of humanizing the MAbs, such that only the CDR is still of mouse origin, is certainly an attractive idea.

FcεRI: HIGH-AFFINITY Fc RECEPTOR FOR IgE

Discovery

The two major categories of Fc receptors for IgE are based on their relative affinities for it. Although initially thought to be related, molecular cloning has demonstrated that the only similarity between the FcεRI and FcεRII is the sharing of a common ligand. The FcεRI was discovered by Ishizaka et al. (6), who demonstrated that radiolabeled human IgE preferentially bound to human basophils and, subsequently, to monkey mast cells. Much of the research has been in the rodent system, especially because of the availability of the rat basophilic cell line as well as cultured mouse mast cells. In addition, rodent IgE is also readily available, and several hybridoma lines producing IgE with a defined antigen specificity can easily be obtained.

Affinity

The FcεRI has the highest affinity for Ig of the known Fc receptors. Affinity measurements have been performed in both the human and rodent system and the affinity is in the range of 10^{10}–10^{12} M^{-1} (21,22). Reflected in this high affinity is an extremely low dissociation rate

$(k_{-1} < 10^{-5}\ s^{-1})$, resulting in retention of monomeric IgE on the mast cell or basophil surface for long periods. Early studies on the fate of IgE bound to FcεRI indicated that, although there is turnover and endocytosis of IgE dimers, trimers, and larger oligomers, significant residual IgE could be detected 3 days after loading, particularly if the IgE was not cross-linked (23,24).

Structure

The FcεRI is composed of three different protein subunits and is schematically illustrated in Figure 1. The three peptides making up the FcεRI are designated α, β, and γ, respectively; the stoichiometry is known to be $\alpha\beta\gamma_2$. The α-chain was the first discovered (25); it is a 55- to 60-kDa glycoprotein that can be easily radiolabeled by surface iodination procedures. The associated β- and γ-chains were first discovered using chemical cross-linking procedures (26) and, subsequently, it was shown that phospholipids were important to maintain the intact FcεRI structure (27). Cloning of the individual components has led to a better understanding of the individual structures and resulted in the concept of Fc receptor families.

FcεRIα Chain

The cDNA for the rat α-chain was the first to be isolated (28), and the subsequent analysis of the human α-chain indicated a quite homologous molecule (29). Early biochemical studies suggested that the α-chain was highly surface-exposed, and no evidence for a cytoplasmic tail was seen. However, the predicted amino acid sequence clearly indicated a single transmembrane sequence, followed by a short cytoplasmic tail containing charged amino acids. The region lacked tyrosine residues, explaining why it had not been found in the earlier biochemical studies, which depended on iodination of inside-out vesicles. The extracellular region contains two domains, with interchain disulfide bonds and amino acid homology, such that the α-chain is placed in the Ig gene superfamily. The extracellular portion of the α-chain is both necessary and sufficient for IgE binding (30). Indeed,

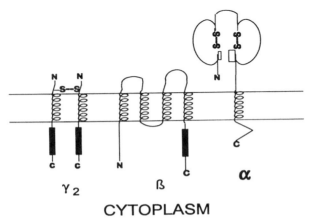

Figure 1 Schematic of the FcεRI and Fc$_\gamma$RIII as found on mast cells and basophils. The three different polypeptide components of these two receptors are illustrated; note that only the α-chain is unique between the FcεRI and Fc$_\gamma$RIII. The TAM motifs (see text) are shown as black boxes. The site of interaction of the FcεRI with IgE is discussed in the text. (Modified from Refs. 1,50.)

molecularly engineered soluble α-chain, in which the transmembrane and cytoplasmic regions have been deleted, will bind IgE with high affinity and, thus, block IgE binding to the mast cell or basophil (30). With use of chimeric recombinant proteins between the Fc$_\gamma$RII and the FcεRI, Hulett et al. (31) identified at least three different areas on the FcεRI that are important for the FcεRI–IgE interaction. Eventually, it may be possible to produce soluble α-chain constructs to provide an additional avenue for blocking allergic reactions.

FcεRIβ- and γ-Chains

The other two components of the FcεRI, termed the β- and γ-chains, are hydrophobic membrane proteins. The β-chain is predicted to traverse the membrane four times, meaning that both the NH_2- and COOH-termini are cytoplasmic (32). The β-chain was initially identified as part of the FcεRI on rat basophilic leukemia cells, and a highly homologous β-chain was seen in mouse mast cells (33). Identification in humans has only more recently been accomplished (34); the sequence divergence was sufficient to make cloning substantially more difficult. However, the predicted overall structure of the human β-chain is quite similar to the rodent counterpart.

The γ-chain is a 9-kDa disulfide-linked dimer, and its cloning allowed expression of the complete FcεRI (35). The predicted sequence is highly homologous with the ζ-chain of the T-cell receptor (TCR), which is a similar disulfide-linked dimer (36). Intriguingly, the γ-chain and ζ-chain are interchangeable in the human system, in that the γ-chain can be used in place of the ζ-chain in the TCR, and the ζ in place of the γ-chain in the FcεRI (reviewed in Ref. 37). This interchange is not as effective in the mouse, owing to changes in the transmembrane region (38). The γ-chain is also a component of some Fc receptors for IgG (Fc$_\gamma$R). Thus, the Fc$_\gamma$RIII, when expressed in the transmembrane form (see Ref. 1 for discussion of nomenclature) in humans, is associated with either γ-chain or ζ-chain (37). The Fc$_\gamma$RIII and FcεRI α-chains are highly homologous; especially in the transmembrane region, in which a sequence of eight amino acids is completely identical. Interestingly, one charged amino acid (aspartic acid) is found in this conserved sequence. Mutagenesis studies have confirmed the importance of the transmembrane regions of both the γ-chain, ζ-chain, and α-chain for their respective effective interaction (37).

Expression of the FcεRI and Fc$_\gamma$RIII

Efficient expression of the FcεRI and Fc$_\gamma$RIII is seen only if the appropriate associated chains are present. For the rodent FcεRI, transfection studies have demonstrated a requirement for both the γ- and β-chains (35). In cells transfected with α-chain alone, the newly synthesized protein is rapidly degraded and very little reaches the cell surface. Thus, one function of the associated chains is protection from intracellular degradation. In contrast, human FcεRI is expressed efficiently with only the γ-chain, as is both human and mouse Fc$_\gamma$RIII (37,39). The ζ-chain is completely interchangeable in humans with the γ-chain in all aspects, and thus, the ζ-chain will result in the same protection from degradation as the γ-chain. The cloning of the human β-chain has allowed expression studies to be performed in the human system using an entirely homologous system. These studies demonstrated that the human β-chain was indeed associated with the human FcεRI; however, expression was equally efficient in its absence (34). Since the β-chain can also be found in association with the Fc$_\gamma$RIII (40), present data are consistent with both the mast cell–basophil FcεRI and the Fc$_\gamma$RIII having the structure that is schematically illustrated in Figure 1, when the respective Fc receptor is on a mast cell or basophil. Some cell types that express the Fc$_\gamma$RIII (i.e., natural killer [NK] cells) do not show expression of the β-chain; thus, the expressed (and functional) Fc$_\gamma$RIII receptor consists of only the α- and γ- (or ζ)-chain proteins (37).

FcεRI and Fc$_\gamma$RIII Function

Early studies demonstrated that the FcεRI was intimately involved in the allergic mediator release process and that cross-linking of the FcεRI, in the absence of IgE, resulted in mast cell triggering (41). With the FcεRI, evidence for the importance of all three proteins (α, β, γ) is seen in mutagenesis studies. The mast cell-derived line P815 does not express FcεRI. Transfection of α-, β-, and γ-chains into these cells results in expression of a functional FcεRI, as measured by calcium translocation studies (42). Although the primary function of the α-chain appears to be IgE binding, specific mutations in either the β- or γ-chains resulted in defective signaling, suggesting that all three proteins play a role in the signaling process (42,43). Interestingly, transfection of COS cells (monkey kidney origin) with the three chains results in the expression of FcεRI, as evidenced by ligand binding; however, the COS-expressed receptor does not cause calcium translocation subsequent to aggregation (42), indicating that signaling is defective. Thus, these studies both emphasize the importance of all three proteins of the FcεRI for both expression and function and indicate that other, as yet unknown, mast cell-specific proteins are required for the signaling process.

The observation that both FcεRI and Fc$_\gamma$RIII utilize common proteins leads to the hypothesis that Fc$_\gamma$RIII is a triggering receptor for allergic reactions. At least in the rodent system, this has proved to be true. By using an MAb specific for the mouse Fc$_\gamma$RII and III, rat basophilic leukemia (RBL) cells transfected with the Fc$_\gamma$RIII α-chain, but not the Fc$_\gamma$RII, could be induced both to degranulate (44,45) and to produce tumor necrosis factor-alpha (TNF-α), after receiving the MAb-specific aggregation signal. Thus, at least in the rodent system, IgG antigen complexes are capable of inducing allergic mediator release. These studies demonstrate that it is Fc$_\gamma$RIII that is performing this function. The lack of expression of Fc$_\gamma$RIII on human mast cells or basophils presumably explains why IgG is less effective for this in humans. Given the observed capacity for the transfected Fc$_\gamma$RIII to trigger RBL cells, the recent observation that mice lacking the FcεRI expression were not susceptible to anaphylactic shock was somewhat surprising. By homologous recombination technology (i.e., *gene knockout*), either the FcεRIα (46) or FcεRI$_\gamma$ (47) chains were deleted, with this same result. This terminology refers to situations in which the gene for a respective component is interrupted by a stop codon by placing a DNA insert (usually a separate gene for antibiotic resistance is used for selection purposes) in the gene. The additional observations that the FcεRI$_\gamma$-deficient mice were generally abnormal in other Fc$_\gamma$R functions, such as phagocytosis (47), and that the FcεRI$_\gamma$ chain is coprecipitated with all three classes of transmembrane Fc$_\gamma$R (48) seems also somewhat incompatible with the Fc$_\gamma$RIII-transfected RBL studies (44,45). Potential explanations are limiting amounts of FcεRI$_\gamma$ chain, which may preferentially associate within the FcεRI complex, or lack of significant Fc$_\gamma$R expression on the mast cell and basophil populations responsible for the anaphylactic shock.

The mutagenesis studies just described indicated that the cytoplasmic portion of the γ-chain were important for FcεRI-induced signaling. The importance of the γ-chain in triggering was further emphasized by showing that the cytoplasmic domain of the γ-chain (or ζ-chain) could be linked to a separate molecule (the extracellular plus transmembrane domains of the p55 α-chain of the IL-2 receptor was used) and could cause signaling;

aggregation of this chimeric molecule with appropriate MAbs resulted in either T-cell activation or mast cell (RBL) mediator release. Latour et al. (49) made a chimeric molecule consisting of the Fc$_\gamma$RII extracellular plus transmembrane domains linked to the γ-chain cytoplasmic region. Expression of this chimeric molecule was achieved by appropriate transfection. Aggregation with anti-Fc$_\gamma$R MAb resulted in both serotonin and TNF-α release. Importantly, with these chimeric or mutant preparations, aggregation was a necessary step for signaling, consistent with the hypothesis that the cytoplasmic region of the γ- (or ζ-) chain is a crucial link in the allergic mediator release cascade, since aggregation is always required for the respective signaling of all the multichain immune recognition receptors (50).

New Pathways Involved in the FcεRI Triggering Mechanism

Characterization of events between FcεRI aggregation and mediator (or cytokine—see later) release continues to be an area of active investigation. As discussed earlier, the observation that signaling is seen only when the FcεRI is transfected into a mast cell line indicates the importance of other mast cell–basophil-specific components. Several pathways have been implicated in the FcεRI-signaling system; in general, these are also important in other receptor–ligand-signaling systems. The increase in cytoplasmic calcium and inositol phosphate metabolites has been known for some time (see Ref. 4 for review), although the exact role that these agents play in the mediator-release cascade remains unknown. A role for GTP-binding proteins has been suggested; however, the lack of effect of pertussis toxin on FcεRI signaling (51) indicated that a relatively novel G-protein would be required. The observation that the isoprenoid inhibitor lovastatin would block FcεRI signaling, but not GTP$_\gamma$S- (an irreversible activator of the GTP-binding protein system) mediated activation (52) is also suggestive that GTP-binding proteins do not play a major role in FcεRI-induced cell signaling. Interest has recently focused on the increased tyrosine kinase phosphorylation that is seen after FcεRI aggregation. The γ- and β-chains are specifically phosphorylated as a result of FcεRI aggregation (53). In addition, various other proteins are also phosphorylated by a tyrosine-specific kinase. Another component frequently implicated in cell-triggering phenomena (see Ref. 54 for review) is phospholipase C (PLC) which has several isoforms; PLC-$_{\gamma 1}$ is also phosphorylated after FcεRI aggregation (55), and phosphorylation is known to be important in the function of this enzyme (54). A difficulty in dissecting the events occurring subsequent to FcεRI cross-linking has always been the necessity of using intact cells to see any biological activity. The observation that protein-tyrosine kinase (PTK) activity could still be observed with isolated membrane preparations is promising for future analyses (56).

In a number of receptor–ligand systems, the tyrosine kinase involved is a member of the *src* family of nonreceptor associated kinases (see Refs. 57 and 58 for review). The association is weak and requires gentle detergent disruption conditions to be demonstrated. The NH$_2$-terminal attachment of myristic acid allows membrane association, whereas the SH2 domain usually interacts with the respective receptor cytoplasmic domain. The most well-characterized association of such a kinase with triggering is the p56*lck* (*lck*) kinase that is associated with the cytoplasmic domain of CD4 or CD8 on T cells (59). The importance of this association has been demonstrated in that when the *lck* gene was "knocked out," the resulting mice were severely T-cell–deficient (60). With FcεRI, the *src*-related kinases *lyn* or *yes* were associated with the FcεRI on RBL cells or on the mouse mast cell line PT-18, respectively (61). In addition, the mast cell has at least two unique (non–*src*-related family members) tyrosine kinases (62,63). Until the appropriate knockout animals

```
CONSENSUS                      D XXXXXXX D XX Y XX L XXXXXXX Y XX L
                               E         E                        I

FcεRIγ         RLKIQVRKA A IASREKA D AV Y TG L NTRSQET Y ET L KHEKPPQ
FcεRIß         YRIGQEL E -SKKVPD D RL Y EE L -NVYSPI Y SE L EDKGETSSPVDS
Ig-ß               DKD D GKAGMEE D HT Y EG L NIDQTAT Y ED I VTLRTGEVKWSVGEHPGQE
Ig-α       RKRWQNEKFGV D MPDDYED E NL Y EG L NLDDCSM Y ED I SRGLQGTYQDVGNLGIGDAQLEK
CD3γ        GQDGVRQSRAS D KQTLLQN E QL Y QP L KDREDDQ Y SH L QGNQLRRN
CD3δ        GHETGRPSGAA E VQALLKN E QL Y QP L RKREDTQ Y SS L GGNWPRNNKS
CD3ζ        ADAYSDIGTKG E RRRGKGH D GL Y QG L STATKDT Y DA L HMQTLAPR
```

Figure 2 Consensus structure of the TAM motif. As first noted by Reth (64), the cytoplasmic tails of a number of polypeptide components of "multichain immune recognition receptors" (50) share a consensus motif that has been variably termed "antigen receptor-associated motif (ARAM)" or "tyrosine-associated motif (TAM)" (65). The TAM motif is tyrosine phosphorylated on receptor aggregation in each situation. Identity of the molecules: Ig-β and Ig-α, associated with surface IgM and IgD on B cells; CD3γ, CD3δ, and CD3ζ, part of the CD3–T-cell receptor complex; FcεRIB/$_γ$ are discussed in the text.

are available, it is difficult to know which (if any) of the above-mentioned kinases are important for FcεRI- (or Fc$_γ$RIII)-induced cell activation.

Reth et al. (64) was the first to note that the cytoplasmic regions of the γ-chain and ζ-chain were similar in structure to a number of other "receptor-associated" proteins; in common with γ- and ζ-chains, these other proteins are also required for efficient expression of the "ligand-binding" subunit. These receptors, which have been termed *multichain immune recognition receptors* (MIRR; 50) include the FcεRI, Fc$_γ$RIII, the T-cell antigen receptor, and the B-cell antigen receptor; a listing of some of these proteins is shown in Figure 3, along with the alignment of the sequences to illustrate the consensus sequence shown at the top of the figure. This consensus motif is variably called a tyrosine-associated motif (TAM), or antigen receptor-associated motif (ARAM) (65). Current evidence indicates that the tyrosines in this motif become phosphorylated by an *src*-related kinase (53) when the corresponding receptor is activated by cross-linking (65). Various other proteins are also phosphorylated with kinetics similar to the FcεRI$_γ$- and β-chains. One of the most prominent phosphorylated bands is a 72-kDa protein, which has recently been identified as a PTK-related to the new *syk* kinase family (63). Subsequently, by the SH2 domains on this kinase, it becomes associated with the phosphorylated TAM (65,66). A schematic of the steps involved in activation of the *syk* kinase is shown in Figure 3. The importance of this *syk* PTK is seen in that a cross-linking of a chimeric protein, consisting of a CD16 extracellular and transmembrane domain linked to the *syk* kinase sequence, was capable of inducing a calcium and tyrosine phosphorylation response, similar to that seen with T-cell receptor cross-linking (67); note that the TCR and FcεRI both utilize the TAM motif pathway in cell activation (50). Thus, these studies indicate a commonality among MIRR receptors relative to the mechanism of signaling. Current work is aimed at elucidation of the events downstream of the *syk*-kinase; the aforementioned PLC-$_{γ1}$, and phosphatidyl-inositol-3-kinase (68) are two candidates for this.

Mast Cell Cytokine Production

The classic effect of FcεRI aggregation and mast cell activation is an allergic mediator release. In 1987, Brown et al. (69) noted that activated mast cells had high levels of mRNA for the cytokine interleukin-4 (IL-4). Subsequently, several groups have demonstrated that

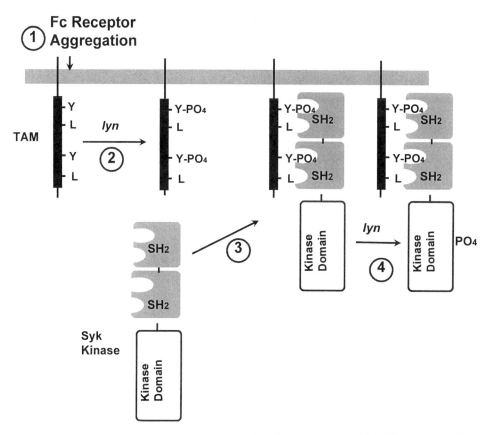

Figure 3 Model for kinase involvement in FcεRI triggering mechanism: (1) MIRR receptors such as the FcεRI are aggregated, for example, by antigen bound to IgE. (2) The TAM motifs (only a single motif is shown for simplicity) are tyrosine phosphorylated by an *src*-family kinase (lyn is shown in the figure); (3) the *syk* kinase binds to the phosphotyrosine by its SH2 domains; (4) the *src*-family kinase phosphorylates the *syk* kinase in the kinase domain, activating this kinase; (5) the activated *syk* kinase then functions in the additional triggering events (not shown). (Adapted from Ref. 65.)

a variety of cytokines are actually produced by these cells as a consequence of cell activation (reviewed in 70). The list includes IL-4, IL-5, IL-6, IL-3, interferon (IFN)-γ and TNF-α. The cytokine profile produced is quite similar to that produced by the T-helper phenotype, known as T_H2. This phenomenology has been used for the division of helper T cells (T_H) into two primary categories, T_H1 and T_H2, based on the cytokines that are produced after cell activation (71). The T_H2 cytokines are primarily involved in B-cell activation, whereas the T_H1 cytokines are especially important for cell-mediated immunity. Furthermore, the known requirement of IL-4 for IgE synthesis, given that IL-4 is made both by T_H2 cells and mast cells, indicates that mast cells can potentially be involved both at the effector phase (mediator release) and also the initiation phase (IgE synthesis) of allergic disease. Some evidence for the latter has been reported (72) in which non-B, non-T cells (these are presumably either mast cell precursors or basophils; 73) induced IgE synthesis after stimulation with IL-3.

Studies in mice have indicated that cytokine production may be seen at an early stage of mast cell development. Thus, spleen cell populations that were depleted of mature T and B cells (termed non-B, non-T cells) were enriched in cells capable of producing T_H2 profile cytokines on FcεRI or Fc$_\gamma$RIII aggregation (74). The number and activity of these cytokine-producing cells increases in murine animal models, associated with high IgE levels (75), an observation further suggesting their involvement in IgE production. Subsequently, the cytokine production was shown to be essentially confined to those cells capable of high-affinity binding of IgE and, therefore (presumably) expressing the FcεRI (76). The FcεRI-enriched population is enriched in mast cell precursors and in cells with basophilic morphology, indicating that both mast cell precursors and (mature?) basophils are present (76). It is not yet known which of the FcεRI$^+$ cells in the population are capable of producing cytokines. Huff and associates have suggested that this Fc receptor-induced cytokine production is associated not only with IgE synthesis, but also with mast cell development (77). This hypothesis is based on data indicating that the cell termed the "mast cell-committed progenitor" can be produced from appropriate bone marrow cells only if both Fc receptor aggregation and cytokine (IL-3) signals are present (77). Cytokines that are now recognized as important in mast cell development are IL-3, the recently identified stem cell factor (SCF; 78), and (to a lesser extent) IL-4. The SCF is primarily a product of fibroblasts or stromal cells. Important, and as yet unknown, for this hypothesis is whether the respective Fc receptor-induced (FcεRI or Fc$_\gamma$RIII) effect occurs *before* the necessity of cytokine involvement (and, thereby, causes cytokine production and autocrine mast cell development) or *because* of cytokine production by other cell types. Finally, all of the mast cell cytokine studies described in the foregoing have been in the mouse system, although the earlier discussed TNF-α production in RBL cells indicates a similar story for rats. An obvious important question is cytokine production by human mast cells or basophils and, although difficulties were initially encountered, data are emerging that show a similar situation in humans. One study found IL-4 mRNA after Fc receptor (presumably FcεRI) aggregation on human non-B, non-T cells (79), and this was recently confirmed in that IL-4 (protein) production by human basophils (80) and mast cells (81) was demonstrated. Overall, mast cell–basophil cytokine production has proved to be an intriguing story, and its potential importance in both IgE synthesis and mast cell development (see following) will make this a continued active area of investigation in both the human and murine systems.

ε-BINDING PROTEIN

A second IgE-binding protein, isolated and cloned from RBL cells during studies aimed at cloning of the FcεRI, has been identified and shown to bind rodent IgE (82). This protein, termed ε-binding protein (ε-BP), is now known to be a thiol-dependent (S-type) lectin with β-galactoside specificity. The ε-BP is highly homologous with a cytosolic protein known as carbohydrate-binding protein-35 and the macrophage surface protein Mac-2 (83). The human equivalent has also been cloned and shown to bind certain glycoforms (dependent on IgE carbohydrate) of human IgE (84). Expression at the surface of RBL cells suggested a possible involvement in allergic mediator release (85), and a direct activity of ε-BP in binding IgE and inducing mast cell activation has been reported (86). These results suggest a role for S-type animal lectins in allergic inflammation (reviewed in Ref. 87).

LOW-AFFINITY IgE RECEPTOR (FcεRII/CD23)

FcεRII Structure

The FcεRII was first described in 1976 on human lymphoblastoid cells by Lawrence et al. (7). The FcεRII is a member of the calcium-dependent animal lectin family; other members of this family include the asialoglycoprotein receptor, a protein known to bind carbohydrate, as well as adhesion molecules, such as endothelial leukocyte adhesion molecule-1 (ELAM-1); adhesion proteins that are members of this family have been termed *selectins* (88). Note that these proteins are not related to the S-type lectin family of which ε-BP is a member (see foregoing). A common property of this family is a shared lectin cassette. Calcium is required for the function of members of this family. Although calcium is required for IgE binding by the FcεRII (89), since deglycosylated IgE binds to the FcεRII, the role of carbohydrate on IgE binding remains equivocal (19). Another interesting possibility relates to FcεRII acting as an adhesion molecule, in common with other "selectins." The recent finding of an interaction between the FcεRII and CD21 is quite intriguing (see later discussion).

Between the transmembrane portion and COOH-terminal lectin homology region of FcεRII is a series (three in humans, four in mouse) of 20-amino acid regions that have homology with each other and presumably result from gene duplication. Indeed each of these regions is coded by a separate exon (90,91). Gould's laboratory (92) has noted that this region of the FcεRII, as well related regions of other members of the C-type animal lectin family, share a common structural motif with tropomyosin and has proposed a model in which these repetitive regions of the FcεRII interact in an α-helical coiled-coil complex involving two or three FcεRII molecules (93). The capacity of FcεRII to exhibit receptor–receptor association has been known for some time (94). Recent results have demonstrated that this association is crucial for normal IgE binding. A series of deletion mutants, in which different repetitive regions of the stalk were removed, were prepared. Whereas native FcεRII exhibits both a high- ($10^8\ M^{-1}$) and low- ($10^7\ M^{-1}$) affinity binding by Scatchard analysis, the mutant FcεRII exhibited only the low-affinity interaction. Furthermore, the mutant FcεRII did not exhibit the aforediscussed receptor–receptor association. These data provide additional support for the coiled-coil model, discussed earlier, and indicate that the FcεRII is an oligomeric protein that interacts in a multimeric manner with IgE, and (presumably) alternative FcεRII ligands, such as CD21. A current model for the FcεRII, based on this coiled-coil prediction and the demonstrated receptor–receptor association is shown in Figure 4.

FcεRII Expression and Isoforms

The FcεRII is cleaved at the cell surface in a potentially autoproteolytic manner, and the initial cleavage site is in this repetitive region (95). Binding of IgE by FcεRII inhibits this degradation, resulting in a ligand-specific up-regulation of the cell surface level of FcεRII (96). Below the repetitive region is a short stretch of amino acids, followed by the transmembrane and intracytoplasmic regions; since the FcεRII is a type II membrane protein, the NH_2-terminus is cytoplasmic. Kikutani et al. (97) demonstrated that in humans two forms of the FcεRII exist, termed FcεRIIa and FcεRIIb. The two forms utilize alternative transcription initiation sites, resulting in a different 5′ untranslated region and the first six amino acids. The two forms are both expressed on B cells; however, other

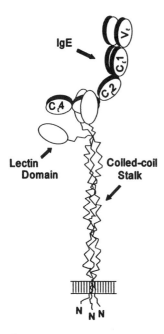

Figure 4   Current model for the FcεRII trimeric molecule would be expected to interact with two symmetric sites on the IgE molecule—the site of interaction is discussed in the text. (Based on Refs. 100,127.)

FcεRI$^+$ cell types, such as monocytes, T cells, and CD5$^+$ B cells, when examined in detail, express only the FcεRIIb. In mouse our studies failed to find evidence for alternative FcεRII forms (98), and this may explain the more restricted expression of FcεRII in the mouse, in which expression is limited to B cells and follicular dendritic cells (99).

The FcεRII is one of a number of proteins that have their expression levels elevated by the presence of IL-4 (reviewed in Ref. 100) and the related cytokine IL-13 (101,102). This increase is due to an increase in mRNA and protein levels; IL-4 has no effect on the stability of the FcεRII protein. The two FcεRII forms are regulated somewhat differently. Present evidence indicates that the FcεRIIa is specific for B cells, constitutively expressed, and up-regulated by IL-4; the expression of FcεRIIb requires IL-4 and, as indicated earlier, this form is not specific for B cells (97).

FcεRII Function

Since its discovery, FcεRII has been proposed to have a role in IgE regulation, either as the intact molecule or as the released, soluble FcεRII (termed sFcεRII). Early model systems for studying IgE regulation demonstrated a correlation between FcεRII levels and IgE synthesis; however, it is now realized that this correlation may be due to IL-4 production. Nelms et al. (103) have described an intriguing model in which IgE receptor$^+$ T cells are involved in suppression of ε-heavy chain production in certain IgE plasmacytomas. It is not yet clear whether this IgE receptor is the FcεRII, although studies with FcεRII-specific antibodies suggest a related molecule (104). Is the FcεRII directly involved in IgE regulation? The answer now depends on whether the mouse or human system is analyzed. The

IgE-binding factors involved in IgE regulation that were described by the Ishizaka laboratory (reviewed in Ref. 105) are not structurally related to the FcεRII. The substantially reduced affinity of sFcεRII for IgE makes targeting to an IgE-bearing B cell an unlikely model for function. Also, in the mouse, sFcεRII did not influence IgE synthesis in the LPS–IL-4 in vitro model (106). Finally, the recent analysis of FcεRII knockout mice have demonstrated that IgE production is not greatly altered in these animals (107,108), demonstrating that, at least in mice, FcεRII plays a limited role in IgE production.

Interestingly, in humans, evidence has accumulated in favor of a role for the FcεRII in IgE synthesis. Anti-FcεRII inhibits IgE synthesis, using IL-4-stimulated peripheral blood lymphocytes (PBL) (109), PBL from allergic patients, or the U266 IgE-producing cell line (110). This inhibition requires FcεRII cross-linking. The sFcεRII can potentiate IL-4-stimulated human IgE synthesis (reviewed in 3); since this activity can be seen with IgE[+] B cells that are FcεRII[−], Delespesse et al. (3) has suggested that the sFcεRII may work by interacting with an as yet unknown B-cell surface component; however, the low affinity of the sFcεRII for IgE makes B-cell surface IgE an unlikely target. The differences between these results in mouse and humans are not yet understood; one suggested possibility (3), that the absence of effect is due to the excess of sFcεRII that is already present in the in vitro murine models, seems unlikely in view of the results with FcεRII knockout animals.

FcεRII Role in Antigen Processing and Presentation

Kehry et al. (111) in mice and subsequently Pirron et al. (112) in humans, demonstrated a new function for the FcεRII: namely, to endocytose IgE complexes; this results in highly efficient antigen presentation by the respective FcεRII[+] B cells. Indeed, the efficiency of presentation is similar to that seen when the antigen is taken up by B-cell surface immunoglobulin. This suggests a new immunopotentiating role for IgE through FcεRII. This hypothesis is also supported by the observation that antigen–IgE–FcεRII complexes are found associated with germinal center follicular dendritic cells shortly after immunization of mice with antigen in complete Freund's adjuvant (99). We have taken advantage of this immunopotentiation by coupling antigen to anti-FcεRII and using this in immunization regimens. The anti-FcεRII–antigen conjugates greatly potentiate in vitro T- and B-cell proliferative response to antigen and, when tested in vivo, result in quite significant levels of antibody production (113). In addition, Heyman et al. (114) found that IgE complexes would potentiate the IgE response by this same enhancement of antigen processing mediated by the FcεRII. In FcεRII knockout mice, this IgE-mediated enhancement is completely abrogated (107), the only clear phenotype presently observed for these animals. Interestingly, Kikutani et al. (115) recently reported that there were differences in the function of the FcεRIIa and FcεRIIb. Thus, FcεRIIa exhibited increased endocytosis capacity, whereas FcεRIIb was capable of more efficient phagocytosis. Mutation analysis established which amino acids were important for the respective function.

FcεRII–CD21 Interaction

The sFcεRII has been reported to have several additional roles (reviewed in Refs. 3,100). When used in conjunction with IL-1, human sFcεRII promotes growth of myeloid and T-cell precursors (116) and inhibits apoptosis of germinal center B cells (117). Similar activities have not yet been found in the mouse system (118). Nonetheless, these provocative observations again point to specific interactions of sFcεRII with a cell receptor and, indeed, in support of this alternative ligand, the site on the FcεRII necessary for these activities is different from that of the IgE interaction site (119). By using intact FcεRII that was first incorporated into liposomes, Aubrey et al. (120) found that the FcεRII and CD21 are receptor ligand pair, and other studies have implicated this adhesion pair as being important, at least in the homotypic adhesion of human B cells (121). Also known as complement receptor type 2 (CR2) and the Epstein-Barr virus (EBV) receptor (reviewed in Ref. 122), this important finding may be involved in the various cytokine-like activities of the sFcεRII discussed earlier. The observation that some anti-CD21 MAbs would perform this same function in the rescue of germinal center B cells (123) is suggestive here. In addition, this group reported that sFcεRII will induce histamine release from human basophils and that this effect was mediated by CD21 on the basophils (124). Bonnefoy and co-workers have also found that a subset of anti-CD21 MAbs will stimulate human IgE production (125,126), thus providing a potential mechanism for how sFcεRII modulates human IgE production.

CONCLUSIONS AND FUTURE PERSPECTIVES

Progress in this area has continued to be rapid. With FcεRI, the recent exciting developments on the PTK activity associated with this receptor are being pursued extensively. At present, PTK activity is the only activity that has yet been seen (besides IgE binding) in membrane preparations from mast cells or basophils (127) and, perhaps, will provide a tool to begin in vitro "assembly" of the mediator–cytokine release pathway. Characterization and isolation of FcεRI and FcεRII in large amounts will potentially allow crystallization of the receptors or receptor–IgE complexes, which will ultimately allow sophisticated inhibitor design; the latter has the potential to specifically block either IgE synthesis (FcεRII) or IgE binding to mast cells and basophils (FcεRI). Clearly there is much work to be done, but as we look forward to the rapidly approaching 21st century, the goal of a general control of allergic disease appears ever more attainable.

REFERENCES

1. Ravetch JV, Kinet J-P. Fc receptors. Annu Rev Immunol 1991; 9:457–492.
2. Conrad DH. Murine CD23/FcεRII. Structure and function and comparison with the human counterpart. Monogr Allergy 1991; 29:9–27.
3. Delespesse G, Suter U, Mossalayi D, et al. Expression, structure, and function of the CD23 antigen. Adv Immunol 1991; 49:149–191.
4. Metzger H. The high affinity receptor for IgE on mast cells. Clin Exp Allergy 1991; 21:269–279.
5. Prausnitz D, Kustner H. Studien über die Ueberempfindlichkeit. Zentrabl Bakteriol [A] 1921; 86:160–175.
6. Ishizaka K, Tomioka H. Mechanisms of passive sensitization. I. Presence of IgE and IgG molecules on human leukocytes. J Immunol 1970; 105:1459–1467.
7. Lawrence DA, Weigle WO, Spiegelberg HL. Immunoglobulins cytophilic for human lymphocytes, monocytes, and neutrophils. J Clin Invest 1975; 55:268–275.
8. De Vries JE, Punnonen J, Cocks BG, De Waal Malefyt R, Aversa G. Regulation of the human IgE response by IL4 and IL13. Res Immunol 1993; 144:597–601.
9. Kulczycki A Jr, Metzger H. The interaction of IgE with rat basophilic leukemia cells. II. Quantitative aspects of the binding reaction. J Exp Med 1974; 140:1676–1695.
10. Capron M, Joseph M. The low affinity receptor for IgE on eosinophils and platelets. Monogr Allergy 1991; 29:63–75.
11. Thompson C. IgE declares war on parasites. Lancet 1994; 343:309–310.
12. Ishizaka K, Ishizaka T, Lee EH. Biologic function of the Fc fragments of E myeloma protein. Immunochemistry 1970; 7:687–702.

13. Perez-Montfort R, Metzger H. Proteolysis of soluble IgE–receptor complexes: localisation of sites on IgE which interact with the Fc receptor. Mol Immunol 1982; 19:1113–1125.
14. Holowka D, Conrad DH, Baird B. Structural mapping of membrane-bound immunoglobulin E–receptor complexes: use of monoclonal anti-IgE antibodies to probe the conformation of receptor-bound IgE. Biochemistry 1985; 25:6260–6267.
15. Keegan AD, Fratazzi C, Shopes B, Baird B, Conrad DH. Characterization of new rat anti-mouse IgE monoclonals and their use along with chimeric IgE to further define the site that interacts with FcεRII and FcεRI. Mol Immunol 1991; 28:1149–1154.
16. Helm B, Marsh P, Vercelli D, Padlan E, Gould H, Geha RS. The mast cell binding site on human immunoglobulin E. Nature 1988; 331:180–183.
17. Basu M, Hakimi J, Dharm E, et al. Purification and characterization of human recombinant IgE-Fc fragments that bind to the human high affinity IgE receptor. J Biol Chem 1993; 268:13118–13127.
18. Chretein I, Helm B, Marsh P, Padlan E, Wijdenes J, Banchereau J. A monoclonal anti-IgE antibody against an epitope (amino acids 367–376) in the CH3 domain inhibits IgE binding to the low affinity IgE receptor (CD23). J Immunol 1988; 141:3128–3134.
19. Vercelli D, Helm B, Marsh P, Padlan E, Geha RS, Gould H. The B-cell binding site on human immunoglobulin E. Nature 1989; 338:649–651.
20. Davis FM, Gossett LA, Pinkston KL, et al. Can anti-IgE be used to treat allergy. Springer Semin Immunopathol 1993; 15:51–73.
21. Ishizaka T, Dvorak AM, Conrad DH, Niebyl JR, Marquette JP, Ishizaka K. Morphologic and immunologic characterization of human basophils developed in cultures of cord blood mononuclear cells. J Immunol 1985; 134:532–540.
22. Rossi G, Newman SA, Metzger H. Assay and partial characterization of the solubilized cell surface receptor for immunoglobulin. J Biol Chem 1977; 252:704–711.
23. Isersky C, Rivera J, Mims S, Triche T. The fate of IgE bound to rat basophilic leukemia cells. J Immunol 1979; 122:1926–1936.
24. Isersky C, Rivera J, Segal DM, Triche T. The fate of IgE bound to rat basophilic leukemia cells. II. Endocytosis of IgE oligomers and effect on receptor turnover. J Immunol 1983; 131:388–396.
25. Conrad DH, Froese A. Characterization of the target cell receptor for IgE. II. Polyacrylamide gel analysis of the surface IgE receptor from normal rat mast cells and rat basophilic leukemia cells. J Immunol 1976; 116:319–326.
26. Holowka D, Hartmann H, Kanellopoulos JM, Metzger H. Association of the receptor for IgE with an endogenous polypeptide on rat basophilic leukemia cells. J Recept Res 1980; 1:41–68.
27. Rivnay B, Wang S, Poy G, Metzger H. Phospholipids stabilize the interaction between the alpha and beta subunits of the solubilized receptor for immunoglobulin E. Biochemistry 1982; 21:6922–6927.
28. Kinet J, Metzger H, Hakimi J, Kochan J. A cDNA presumptively coding for the α-subunit of the receptor with high affinity for immunoglobulin E. Biochemistry 1987; 26:4605–4610.
29. Shimizu A, Tepler I, Benfey PN, Berenstein EH, Siraganian RP, Leder P. Human and rat mast cell high-affinity immunoglobulin E receptors: characterization of putative α-chain products. Proc Natl Acad Sci USA 1988; 85:1907–1911.
30. Blank U, Ra C, Kinet J-P. Characterization of truncated α chain products from human, rat, and mouse high affinity receptor for immunoglobulin E. J Biol Chem 1991; 266:2639–2646.
31. Hulett MD, McKenzie IF, Hogarth PM. Chimeric Fc receptors identify immunoglobulin-binding regions in human Fc gamma RII and Fc epsilon RI. Eur J Immunol 1993; 23:640–645.
32. Kinet J, Blank U, Ra C, White K, Metzger H, Kochan J. Isolation and characterization of cDNAs coding for the B subunit of the high-affinity receptor for immunoglobulin E. Proc Natl Acad Sci USA 1988; 85:6483–6487.
33. Ra C, Jouvin M-HE, Kinet J. Complete structure of the mouse mast cell receptor for IgE (FcεRI) and surface expression of chimeric receptors (rat–mouse–human) on transfected cells. J Biol Chem 1989; 264:15323–15327.

34. Küster H, Zhang L, Brini AT, MacGlashan DWJ, Kinet J-P. The gene and cDNA for the human high affinity immunoglobulin E receptor β chain and expression of the complete human receptor. J Biol Chem 1992; 267:12782–12787.

35. Blank U, Ra C, Miller L, White K, Metzger H, Kinet J. Complete structure and expression in transfected cells of high affinity IgE receptor. Nature 1989; 337:187–189.

36. Orloff DG, Ra C, Frank SJ, Klausner RD, Kinet J. Family of disulphide-linked dimers containing the zeta and eta chains of the T cell receptor and the γ chain of Fc receptors. Nature 1990; 347:189–191.

37. Kinet J-P. The gamma–zeta dimers of Fc receptors as connectors to signal transduction. Curr Opin Immunol 1992; 4:43–48.

38. Kurosaki T, Gander I, Ravetch JV. A subunit common to an IgG Fc receptor and the T-cell receptor mediates assembly through different interactions. Proc Natl Acad Sci USA 1991; 88:3837–3841.

39. Miller L, Blank U, Metzger H, Kinet J. Expression of high-affinity binding of human immunoglobulin E by transfected cells. Science 1989; 244:334–337.

40. Kurosaki T, Gander I, Wirthmueller U, Ravetch JV. The β subunit of the FcεRI is associated with $Fc_\gamma RIII$ on mast cells. J Exp Med 1992; 175:447–451.

41. Ishizaka T, Ishizaka K. Triggering of histamine release from rat mast cells by divalent antibodies against IgE receptors. J Immunol 1978; 120:800–805.

42. Miller L, Alber G, Varin-Blank N, Ludowyke R, Metzger H. Transmembrane signaling in P815 mastocytoma cells by transfected IgE receptors. J Biol Chem 1990; 265:12444–12453.

43. Alber G, Miller L, Jelsema CL, Varin-Blank N, Metzger H. Structure–function relationships in the mast cell high affinity receptor for IgE. Role of the cytoplasmic domains and of the β subunit. J Biol Chem 1991; 266:22613–22620.

44. Alber G, Kent UM, Metzger H. Functional comparison of FcεRI, $Fc_\gamma RII$, and $Fc_\gamma RIII$ in mast cells. J Immunol 1992; 149:2428–2436.

45. Daeron M, Bonnerot C, Latour S, Fridman WH. Murine recombinant $Fc_\gamma RIII$, but not $Fc_\gamma RII$, trigger serotonin release in rat basophilic leukemia cells. J Immunol 1992; 149:1365–1373.

46. Dombrowicz D, Flamand V, Brigman KK, Koller BH, Kinet J-P. Abolition of anaphylaxis by targeted disruption of the high affinity immunoglobulin E receptor α chain gene. Cell 1993; 75:969–976.

47. Takai T, Li M, Sylvestre D, Clynes R, Ravetch JV. FcR gamma chain deletion results in pleiotrophic effector cell defects. Cell 1994; 76:519–529.

48. Masuda M, Roos D. Association of all three types of $Fc_\gamma R$ (CD64, CD32, and CD16) with a gamma-chain homodimer in cultured human monocytes. J Immunol 1993; 151:7188–7195.

49. Latour S, Bonnerot C, Fridman WH, Daëron M. Induction of tumor necrosis factor-α production by mast cells via $Fc_\gamma R$: role of the $Fc_\gamma RIII$ gamma subunit. J Immunol 1992; 149:2155–2162.

50. Keegan AD, Paul WE. Multichain immune recognition receptors: similarities in structure and signaling pathways. Immunol Today 1992; 13:63–68.

51. Saito H, Okajima F, Molski TFP, Sha'afi RI, Ui M, Ishizaka T. Effects of ADP-ribosylation of GTP-binding protein by pertussis toxin on immunoglobulin E-dependent and -independent histamine release from mast cells and basophils. J Immunol 1987; 138:3927–3934.

52. Deanin GG, Pfeiffer JR, Cutts JL, Fore ML, Oliver JM. Isoprenoid pathway activity is required for IgE receptor-mediated, tyrosine kinase-coupled transmembrane signaling in permeabilized RBL-2H3 rat basophilic leukemia cells. Cell Regul 1991; 2:627–640.

53. Paolini R, Jouvin M-H, Kinet J-P. Phosphorylation and dephosphorylation of the high-affinity receptor for immunoglobulin E immediately after receptor engagement and disengagement. Nature 1991; 353:855–858.

54. Rhee SG. Inositol phospholipid-specific phospholipase C: interaction of the gamma-1 isoform with tyrosine kinase. Trends Biochem Sci 1991; 16:297–301.

55. Fukamachi H, Kawakami Y, Takei M, Ishizaka T, Ishizaka K, Kawakami T. Association of protein–tyrosine kinase with phospholipase C-gamma1 in bone marrow-derived mouse mast cells. Proc Natl Acad Sci USA 1992; 89:9524–9528.

56. Pribluda VS, Metzger H. Transmembrane signaling by the high-affinity IgE receptor on membrane preparations. Proc Natl Acad Sci USA 1992; 89:11446–11450.

57. Brickell PM. Current status review: the c-*src* family of protein–tyrosine kinases. Int J Exp Pathol 1991; 72:97–108.

58. Pawson T, Gish GD. SH2 and SH3 domains: from structure to function. Cell 1992; 71:359–362.

59. Rudd CE. CD4, CD8 and the TCR-CD3 complex: a novel class of protein tyrosine kinase receptor. Immunol Today 1990; 11:400–405.

60. Molina TJ, Kishihara K, Siderovski DP, et al. Profound block in thymocyte development in mice lacking p56 (*lck*). Nature 1992; 357:161–164.

61. Eiseman E, Bolen JB. Engagement of the high-affinity IgE receptor activates *src* protein-related tyrosine kinases. Nature 1992; 355:78–80.

62. Kawakami T, Inagaki N, Takei M, et al. Tyrosine phosphorylation is required for mast cell activation by FcεRI cross-linking. J Immunol 1992; 148:3513–3519.

63. Hutchcroft JE, Geahlen RL, Deanin GG, Oliver JM. FcεRI-mediated tyrosine phosphorylation and activation of the 72-kDa protein–tyrosine kinase, PTK72, in RBL-2H3 rat tumor mast cells. Proc Natl Acad Sci USA 1992; 89:9107–9111.

64. Reth M. Antigen receptor tail clue. Nature 1989; 338:383–384.

65. Weiss A, Littman DR. Signal transduction by lymphocyte antigen receptors. Cell 1994; 76: 263–274.

66. Benhamou M, Ryba NJP, Kihara H, Nishikata H, Siraganian RP. Protein–tyrosine kinase p72^{syk} in high affinity IgE receptor signaling. Identification as a component of pp72 and association with the receptor gamma chain after receptor aggregation. J Biol Chem 1993; 268:23318–23324.

67. Kolanus W, Romeo C, Seed B. T cell activation by clustered tyrosine kinases. Cell 1993; 74:171–183.

68. Kanakaraj P, Duckworth B, Azzoni L, Kamoun M, Cantley LC, Perussia B. Phosphatidylinositol-3 kinase activation induced upon Fc$_\gamma$RIII–ligand interaction. J Exp Med 1994; 179:551–558.

69. Brown MA, Pierce JH, Watson CJ, Falco J, Ihle JN, Paul WE. B cell stimulatory factor-1 (interleukin-4) mRNA is expressed by normal and transformed mast cells. Cell 1987; 50: 809–819.

70. Gordon JR, Burd PR, Galli SJ. Mast cells as a source of multifunctional cytokines. Immunol Today 1990; 11:458–464.

71. Cherwinski HM, Schumacher JH, Brown KD, Mosmann TR. Two types of mouse helper T cell clone. III. Further differences in lymphokine synthesis between Th1 and Th2 clones revealed by RNA hybridization, functionally monospecific bioassays, and monoclonal antibodies. J Exp Med 1987; 166:1229–1244.

72. Ledermann F, Heusser C, Schlienger C, Le Gros G. Interleukin-3-treated non-B, non-T cells switch activated B cells to IgG$_1$/IgE synthesis. Eur J Immunol 1992; 22:2783–2787.

73. Seder RA, Paul WE, Dvorak AM, et al. Mouse splenic and bone marrow cell populations that express high-affinity Fcε receptors and produce interleukin 4 are highly enriched in basophils. Proc Natl Acad Sci USA 1991; 88:2835–2839.

74. Ben-Sasson SZ, LeGros G, Conrad DH, Finkelman FD, Paul WE. Cross-linking Fc receptors stimulate splenic non-B, non-T cells to secrete IL-4 and other lymphokines. Proc Natl Acad Sci USA 1990; 87:1421–1425.

75. Conrad DH, Ben-Sasson SZ, LeGros G, Finkelman FD, Paul WE. Infection with *Nippostrongylus brasiliensis* or injection of anti IgD antibodies markedly enhances Fc-receptor-mediated IL-4 production by non-B, non-T cells. J Exp Med 1990; 171:1497–1508.

76. Seder RA, Plaut M, Barbieri S, Urban J Jr, Finkelman FD, Paul WE. Purified FcεR$^+$ bone marrow and splenic non-B, non-T cells are highly enriched in the capacity to produce IL-4 in response to immobilized IgE, IgG2a, or ionomycin. J Immunol 1991; 147:903–909.

77. Ashman RI, Jarboe DL, Conrad DH, Huff TF. The mast cell-committed progenitor: in vitro generation of committed progenitors from bone marrow. J Immunol 1991; 146:211–216.

78. Zsebo KM, Williams DA, Geissler EM, et al. Stem cell factor is encoded at the SI locus of the mouse and is the ligand for the c-*kit* tyrosine kinase receptor. Cell 1990; 63:213–224.

79. Piccinni M-P, Macchia D, Parronchi P, et al. Human bone marrow non-B, non-T cells produce interleukin 4 in response to cross-linkage of Fcε and Fc$_\gamma$ receptors. Proc Natl Acad Sci USA 1991; 88:8656–8660.

80. Arock M, Merle-Béral H, Dugas B, et al. IL-4 release by human leukemic and activated normal basophils. J Immunol 1993; 151:1441–1447.

81. Bradding P, Feather IH, Howarth PH, et al. Interleukin 4 is localized to and released by human mast cells. J Exp Med 1992; 176:1381–1386.

82. Liu F, Albrandt K, Mendel E, Kulczycki A Jr, Orida NK. Identification of an IgE-binding protein by molecular cloning. Proc Natl Acad Sci USA 1985; 82:4100–4104.

83. Liu F. Molecular biology of IgE-binding protein, IgE-binding factors, and IgE receptors. CRC Crit Rev Immunol 1990; 10:289–306.

84. Robertson MW, Albrandt K, Keller D, Liu F. Human IgE-binding protein: a soluble lectin exhibiting a highly conserved interspecies sequence and differential recognition of IgE glyco-forms. Biochemistry 1990; 29:8093–8100.

85. Frigeri LG, Liu F-T. Surface expression of functional IgE binding protein, an endogenous lectin, on mast cells and macrophages. J Immunol 1991; 148:861–867.

86. Frigeri LG, Zuberi RI, Liu F-T. εBP, a β-galactoside-binding animal lectin, recognizes IgE receptor (FcεRI) and activates most cells. Biochemistry 1993; 32:7644–7649.

87. Liu FT. S-type mammalian lectins in allergic inflammation. Immunol Today 1993; 14:486–490.

88. Bevilacqua M, Butcher E, Furie B, et al. Selectins: a family of adhesion receptors. Cell 1991; 67:233.

89. Richards ML, Katz DH. The binding of IgE to murine FcεRII is calcium-dependent but not inhibited by carbohydrate. J Immunol 1990; 144:2638–2646.

90. Suter U, Bastos R, Hofstetter H. Molecular structure of the gene and the 5′-flanking region of the human lymphocyte immunoglobulin E receptor. Nucleic Acids Res 1987; 15:7295–7308.

91. Richards ML, Katz DH, Liu F-T. Complete genomic sequence of the murine low affinity Fc receptor for IgE: demonstration of alternative transcripts and conserved sequence elements. J Immunol 1991; 147:1067–1074.

92. Beavil AJ, Edmeades RL, Gould HJ, Sutton BJ. α-Helical coiled-coil stalks in the low-affinity receptor for IgE (FcεRII/CD23) and related C-type lectins. Proc Natl Acad Sci USA 1992; 89:753–757.

93. Gould H, Sutton B, Edmeades R, Beavil A. CD23/FcεRII: C-type lectin membrane protein with a split personality. Monogr Allergy 1991; 29:28–49.

94. Lee WT, Conrad DH. The murine lymphocyte receptor for IgE. III. Use of chemical cross-linking reagents to further characterize the B lymphocyte Fcε receptor. J Immunol 1985; 134:518–525.

95. Letellier M, Nakajima T, Pulido-Cejudo G, Hofstetter H, Delespesse G. Mechanism of formation of human IgE-binding factors (soluble CD23): III. Evidence for a receptor (FcεRII)-associated proteolytic activity. J Exp Med 1990; 172:693–700.

96. Lee WT, Rao M, Conrad DH. The murine lymphocyte receptor for IgE IV. The mechanism of ligand-specific receptor upregulation on B cells. J Immunol 1987; 139:1191–1198.

97. Yokota A, Kikutani H, Tanaka T, et al. Two species of human Fcε receptor II (FcεRII/CD23): tissue-specific and IL-4-specific regulation of gene expression. Cell 1988; 55:611–618.

98. Conrad DH, Kozak CA, Vernachio J, Squire CM, Rao M, Eicher EM. Chromosomal location and isoform analysis of mouse FcεRII/CD23. Mol Immunol 1993; 30:27–33.

99. Maeda K, Burton GF, Padgett DA, et al. Murine follicular dendritic cells (FDC) and low affinity Fc-receptors for IgE (FcεRII). J Immunol 1992; 148:2340–2347.

100. Conrad DH. FcεRII/CD23: the low affinity receptor for IgE. Annu Rev Immunol 1990; 8:623–645.

101. Zurawski G, De Vries JE. Interleukin 13, an interleukin 4-like cytokine that acts on monocytes and B cells, but not on T cells. Immunol Today 1994; 15:19–26.

102. Punnonen J, Aversa G, Cocks BG, et al. Interleukin 13 induces interleukin 4-independent IgG4 and IgE synthesis and CD23 expression by human B cells. Proc Natl Acad Sci USA 1993; 90:3730–3734.

103. Nelms K, Van Ness BG, Lynch RG, Mathur A. Enhancer mediated suppression of epsilon heavy-chain gene expression in a murine IgE-producing hybridoma. Mol Immunol 1991; 28:599–606.

104. Mathur A, Conrad DH, Lynch RG. Characterization of the murine T cell receptor for IgE (FcεRII). Demonstration of shared and unshared epitopes with the B cell FcεRII. J Immunol 1988; 141:2661–2667.

105. Ishizaka K. IgE-binding factors and regulations of the IgE antibody response. Annu Rev Immunol 1988; 6:513–534.

106. Keegan AD, Snapper CM, VanDusen R, Paul WE, Conrad DH. Superinduction of the murine B cell FcεRII by T helper cell clones. Role of interleukin-4. J Immunol 1989; 142:3868–3874.

107. Fujiwara H, Kikutani H, Suematsu S, et al. The absence of IgE antibody-mediated augmentation of immune responses in CD23-deficient mice. Proc Natl Acad Sci USA. In press.

108. Stief A, Texido G, Sansig G, Eibel H, Le Gros G, Van der Putten H. Mice deficient in CD23 reveal its modulatory role in IgE production but no role in T and B cell development. J Immunol 1994; 152:3378–3390.

109. Sarfati M, Delespesse G. Possible role of human lymphocyte receptor for IgE (CD23) or its soluble fragments in the in vitro synthesis of human IgE. J Immunol 1988; 141:2195–2199.

110. Sherr E, Macy E, Kimata H, Gilly M, Saxon A. Binding the low affinity FcεR on B cells suppresses ongoing human IgE synthesis. J Immunol 1989; 142:481–489.

111. Kehry MR, Yamashita LC. Fcε receptor II (CD23) function on mouse B cells: role in IgE dependent antigen focusing. Proc Natl Acad Sci USA 1989; 86:7556–7560.

112. Pirron U, Schlunck T, Prinz JC, Rieber EP. IgE-dependent antigen focusing by human B lymphocytes is mediated by the low-affinity receptor for IgE. Eur J Immunol 1990; 20:1547–1551.

113. Squire CM, Studer E, Lees A, Finkelman FD, Conrad DH. Antigen presentation is enhanced by targeting antigen to the FcεRII by antigen–anti-FcεRII conjugates. J Immunol 1994; 152:4388–4396.

114. Heyman B, Tianmin L, Gustavsson S. In vivo enhancement of the specific antibody response via the low-affinity receptor for IgE. Eur J Immunol 1993; 23:1739–1742.

115. Yokota A, Yukawa K, Yamamoto A, et al. Two forms of the low-affinity Fc receptor for IgE differentially mediate endocytosis and phagocytosis: identification of the critical cytoplasmic domains. Proc Natl Acad Sci USA 1992; 89:5030–5034.

116. Mossalayi MD, Dalloul AH, Fourcade C, Arock M, Debré P. Soluble CD23 is a potent cytokine for early human haematopoietic precursors. Bull Inst Pasteur 1991; 89:139–146.

117. Liu Y-J, Cairns JA, Holder MJ, et al. Recombinant 25-kDa CD23 and interleukin 1α promote the survival of germinal center B cells: evidence for bifurcation in the development of centrocytes rescued from apoptosis. Eur J Immunol 1991; 21:1107–1114.

118. Bartlett WC, Conrad DH. Murine soluble FcεRII: a molecule in search of a function. Res Immunol 1992; 143:431–436.

119. Mossalayi MD, Arock M, Delespesse G, et al. Cytokine effects of CD23 are mediated by an epitope distinct from the IgE binding site. EMBO J 1992; 11:4323–4328.

120. Aubry J-P, Pochon S, Graber P, Jansen KU, Bonnefoy J-Y. CD21 is a ligand for CD23 and regulates IgE production. Nature 1992; 358:505–507.

121. Björck P, Elenström-Magnusson C, Rosén A, Severinson E, Paulie S. CD23 and CD21 function as adhesion molecules in homotypic aggregation of human B lymphocytes. Eur J Immunol 1993; 23:1771–1775.

122. Fearon DT, Ahearn JM. Complement receptor type 1 (C3b/C4b receptor; CD35) and complement receptor type 2 (C3d/Epstein-Barr virus receptor; CD21). Curr Top Microbiol Immunol 1990; 153:83–98.

123. Bonnefoy JY, Henchoz S, Hardie D, Holder MJ, Gordon J. A subset of anti-CD21 antibodies promote the rescue of germinal center B cells from apoptosis. Eur J Immunol 1993; 23: 969–972.

124. Bacon K, Gauchat J-F, Aubry J-P, et al. CD21 expressed on basophilic cells is involved in histamine release triggered by CD23 and anti-CD21 antibodies. Eur J Immunol 1993; 23:2721–2724.

125. Henchoz S, Gauchat J-F, Aubry J-P, Graber P, Pochon S, Bonnefoy J-Y. Stimulation of human IgE production by a subset of anti-CD21 monoclonal antibodies: requirement of a co-signal to modulate ε transcripts. Immunology 1994; 81:285–290.

126. Bonnefoy J-Y, Pochon S, Aubry J-P, et al. A new pair of surface molecules involved in human IgE regulation. Immunol Today 1993; 14:1–2.

127. Metzger H. Transmembrane signaling: the joy of aggregation. J Immunol 1992; 149:1477–1487.

128. Sutton BJ, Gould HJ. The human IgE network. Nature 1993; 366:421–428.

4

Cell Adhesion Molecules in Allergic Diseases

Devendra K. Agrawal
Creighton University School of Medicine, Omaha, Nebraska

Arthur F. Kavanaugh
The University of Texas Southwestern Medical Center, Dallas, Texas

INTRODUCTION

Cell adhesion molecules (CAMs) are involved in cell–cell communication and cell–extracellular matrix adhesion interactions in various cells. Although many adhesion molecules were discovered in the early 1980s, recent studies from several groups have further delineated important aspects of the structure and function of these immune markers (1,2). Cell adhesion molecules allow cells to interact with their environment for such diverse purposes as intercellular communication, cell trafficking and immune surveillance, reactions to infectious organisms and other inflammatory responses, hemostasis and wound healing, and malignant transformation and metastasis. Cell adhesion molecules play a role in the tethering, triggering, adhesion, and migration of inflammatory cells into the sites of allergic reactions (3–5). To accomplish this, cell adhesion molecules bind to specific ligands expressed on the surface of other cells and on extracellular matrix constituents. By understanding how cells move throughout the body through the detection or measurement of cell adhesion molecules, researchers can begin to develop new diagnostic and therapeutic paradigms for allergic as well as other immunological and inflammatory diseases.

The field of cell adhesion molecules has made rapid strides in recent years. Because of intense investigations, there has been an exponential growth in our understanding of various cell adhesion molecules. Therefore, it is very difficult to present a comprehensive review of the entire field. However, in this chapter an attempt has been made to provide a brief overview of many cell adhesion molecules, their modulation and regulation by various soluble endogenous factors, and their role in allergic diseases, in particular, extrinsic allergic bronchial asthma.

CLASSIFICATION OF CELL ADHESION MOLECULES

Many adhesion receptors have currently been classified into four families on the basis of their structural similarities. These molecules include the *integrins*, *selectins*, *cadherins*, and the *immunoglobulin superfamily*. These groups are determined by structural similarities between the cell surface adhesion molecules. Several cell adhesion molecules that do not fit into the four families have been classified into other categories, such as vascular addressins and carbohydrate ligands (5). The best-known examples of the carbohydrate ligands include Lewis x (CD15) antigen and sialyl Lewis x (CD15s) that serve as counterreceptors for E-selectin (CD62E) and P-selectin (CD62P) (see following for further discussion).

Integrins

The integrins are a family of glycoproteins that are heterodimeric receptors consisting of two noncovalently associated polypeptide chains; the α- and β-subunits, which are products of separate genes. The integrin family now comprises 15α-subunits and 8 β-subunits (6–8). Each subunit contains a transmembrane domain and a short cytoplasmic segment, with the exception of the β_4-subunit of which the cytoplasmic domain is more than 1000 residues. However, α- and β-subunits are mutually interdependent for correct processing and surface expression. Integrins function in both cell–cell and cell–substratum adhesion.

Integrins belong to a major family of cell surface receptors that mediate attachment to the extracellular matrix components, such as fibronectin, laminin, collagens, tenascin, vitronectin, and fibrinogen, and to other cells, such as endothelial cells. Specific integrins are involved in cell–cell adhesive interactions, and transduce information from the outside to the inside of the cell by an increase in cytosolic free Ca^{2+} (9), partly by interaction with the cytoskeleton. In addition, integrins are capable of bidirectional signaling, as activation stimuli frequently alter the affinity of the integrins for their ligand. Indeed, although most integrins may be expressed on the surface of a resting cell, they demonstrate little constitutive avidity for their specific ligands. However, activation of the cell results in conformational changes of the integrins so that they are capable of binding their counterreceptors, thereby mediating adhesive interactions. The binding of ligands to integrins is mediated by RGD (Arg-Gly-Asp) sequences for several adhesive proteins (10). Integrins perform their functions by interacting with components of the insoluble extracellular matrix or surface proteins on other cells to form links with intracellular elements involved in bidirectional-signaling events. A list of various members of the integrin superfamily involved in leukocyte–endothelium interaction is given in Table 1.

Cadherins

The cadherin molecules are calcium-dependent, and their cytoplasmic domains interact directly or indirectly with cytoskeletal proteins through catenins. Cadherins bind to another molecule of the same cadherin on a neighboring cell, and this interaction is mediated by an "HAV (His-Ala-Val) motif" in the extracellular region of the cadherin. The main function of cadherins is to maintain tissue structural integrity. There are five different cadherins: N(neural)-cadherin, P(placental)-cadherin, T-cadherin, V-cadherin, and E(epithelial)-cadherin (11). Catenins are essential for the proper functioning of the adhesion protein E-cadherin. Nearly all epithelial tissues express E- and P-cadherins, although their cellular distributions are not identical. During development, transient expression of N-cadherins is

Table 1 Members of the Integrin Superfamily Involved in Leukocyte–Endothelium Interactions: Their Expression and Function

Receptor	Ligand(s)	Distribution	Regulation
β_1 (CD29) Very late activation (VLA) antigens			
$\alpha_1\beta_1$/VLA-1 (CD49a/CD29)	Laminin (Lm), collagen (Co)	Activated T cells, fibroblasts, mesangial cells, hepatic sinusoids	Expression increased by antigen or mitogen
$\alpha_2\beta_1$/VLA-2 (CD49b/CD29)	Co, Lm[a]	Activated T cells, EC platelets, basophils	Expression increased by antigen or mitogen
$\alpha_3\beta_1$/VLA-3 (CD49c/CD29)	Lm, Co fibronectin (Fn)[a]	Glomerular, thyroid, basement membrane, many cell lines	
$\alpha_4\beta_1$/VLA-4 (CD49d/CD29)	VCAM-1, Fn (CS-1 domain)	Lymphocytes, monocytes, eosinophils, basophils, mast cells, NK cells (not PMN)	Expression and activity increased by antigen or mitogen
α_5/β_1/VLA-5 (CD49e/CD29)	Fn[a]	Lymphocytes, monocytes, EC, basophils, mast cells, fibroblasts	Activity increased by antigen
α_6/β1/VLA-6	Lm	Platelets, T cells, eosinophils, monocytes	Activity increased by antigen
$\alpha_v\beta_1$ (CD 51)	Fn, vitronectin (Vn)[a]		
β_2 (CD18) Leukocyte integrins			
LFA-1 (CD11a/ CD18)	ICAM-1, 2, 3 E-selectin	All leukocytes	Activity increased by many stimuli (antigen, mitogen, and such)
CR3 (CD11b/ CD18)	ICAM-1, Fb, LPS iC3b, factor X	Monocytes, granulocytes, LGL	Expression and activity increased by cytokines, other stimuli
p150/95, CR4 (CD11c/CD18)	Fibrinogen (Fb), iC3b	Monocytes, granulocytes, LGL, B cell subset, platelets	Expression increased by TNF-α
α_D/CD18	ICAM-3	Tissue macrophages	Constitutive
β3 (CD61) Cytoadhesins			
gp IIb/IIIa CD41/ CD61	Fb, Vn, Fn, vWF,[a]	Platelets, EC	Expression increased by many stimuli
α_v/IIIa CD51/ CD61	Vn, Fb, vWF, Lm, Fn, thrombo-spondin,[a]	Platelets, many nonhematopoietic cells	Expression increased by various stimuli
β_7			
$\alpha_4\beta_7$, LPAM-1 CD49d/β7	MAdCAM-1, VCAM-1, Fn (CS-1 domain)	Subset of memory T cells, eosinophils, basophils, EC	
$\alpha_E\beta_7$ CD 103	E-cadherin	Intestinal intraepithelial lymphs (>95%)	Expression increased by TGF-β

[a]Binds the amino acid sequence RGD (Arg-Gly-Asp). The RGD motif is part of the recognition site for several extracellular matrix (ECM) molecules, including: Fn, Fb, vWF, Vn, and collagen.

observed in many tissues. However, adult neural and muscle cells distinctly express N-cadherin. Cadherins play an important role in such cellular processes as intercellular communication and morphogenesis, and alterations in adenomatous polyposis coli gene may lead to problems in adhesion that are associated with cancer.

Selectins

The selectin family of adhesion molecules share a common structure, consisting of a domain of short consensus repeats, with homology to complement-binding proteins, an epithelial growth factor (EGF)-like domain, and a terminal lectin domain that confers binding specificity for sialylated oligosaccharide structures on opposing cells. In addition to selectin structure, binding specificity is defined by the ligand carbohydrate moiety. Selectin have been classified into L(leukocyte)-selectin (CD62L), E(endothelial)-selectin (CD62E), and P(platelet)-selectin (CD62P) (12,13). The L-selectin is constitutively expressed on most leukocytes, whereas the expression of E-selectin and P-selectin typically requires activation by cytokines or other stimuli (Table 2). Recently, an interaction between P-selectin and monocytes has been reported wherein P-selectin-mediated adhesion regulates monocyte chemokine and cytokine secretion (14,15). In addition, a truncated version of L-selectin that lacks its cytoplasmic domain is still capable of binding its ligand, but is not capable of mediating rolling (16). These observations suggest selectins may be capable of transducing signals. Cytokines, including interleukin-1 (IL-1) and tumor necrosis factor-α (TNF-α) induce endothelial and platelet selectins. All three selectins have been implicated in recruitment of neutrophils, monocytes, and lymphocytes into inflammatory tissue sites. In fact, the role of selectins is crucial in the very initial step of rolling and tethering (Fig. 1), and under the influence of fluid shear forces, leukocytes contact and roll

Table 2 The Selectin Family of Cell Adhesion Molecules: Their Counterreceptors and Function

Receptor	Counterreceptor	Distribution	M_r (kDa)	Regulation
E-selectin CD62-E (ELAM-1)	Sialyl Lewis x (CD15s), L-selectin, CLA, LFA-1, Sialyl Lewis A, CD66, ESL-1, PSGL-1	Activated EC	115	Synthesized and expressed (h) by IL-1, TNF-α, LPS, IFN-γ
L-selectin CD62-L (LECAM-1, Leu-8, Mel-14 Ag)	GlyCAM-1 (sgp50;PNAd), CD34 (sgp90), MAdCAM-1, E-selectin, P-selectin, other ligands at inflammatory sites	Resting leukocytes (L-selectin expressed on the tips of microvilli may be most important)	74 (lymph) 90–100 (PMN)	Rapidly cleaved on activation
P-selectin CD62-P (GMP-140, PADGEM)	Sialyl Lewis x, L-selectin, Lewis x (CD15), PSGL-1	Activated EC Activated platelets	140	Rapidly redistributed to cell surface (mins) by PAF, thrombin, histamine, LTC$_4$, LTB$_4$

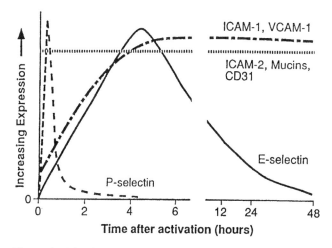

Figure 1   Kinetics of endothelial cell adhesion molecule expression after exposure to IL-1, TNF-α, or endotoxin (E-selectin, VCAM-1, ICAM-1), or to thrombin, histamine, terminal complement components, or hydrogen peroxide (P-selectin). ICAM-1 is also inducible by IFN-γ. In addition to the rapid redistribution of P-selectin from intracellular stores shown here, a slower, TNF-α-induced synthesis and expression similar to that of E-selectin has been observed. (From Ref. 17; reproduced, with permission, from the *Annual Review of Medicine*, vol. 45, © 1994; by Annual Reviews Inc.).

over the endothelial cells, followed by the arrest of rolling owing to firm adhesion. This will be discussed in detail in the subsequent section.

Immunoglobulin Superfamily

Molecules in the immunoglobulin superfamily have a characteristic extracellular immunoglobulin-like domain. In addition to immunoglobulins, other molecules included in this superfamily are T-cell receptors, major histocompatibility complex (MHC) class I and II molecules, and various adhesion molecules (Table 3). These cell adhesion molecules mediate cell–cell adhesion by homotypic (NCAM, NgCAM) and heterotypic (e.g., VCAM and ICAM) interactions (17). Other cell adhesion molecules in this group such as platelet–endothelial (PE)CAM (PECAM-1/CD31) may mediate both homotypic and heterotypic interactions (18). These cell adhesion molecules are found on various cells, including mononuclear cells, granulocytes, natural killer (NK) cells, fibroblasts, platelets, and endothelial cells. Circulating leukocytes that have slowed down sufficiently to be seen as rolling, on intravital microscopy, by interactions of the selectins may undergo firm adhesion to the endothelium followed by transendothelial migration. Firm adhesion and migration are typically mediated by interactions between members of the integrin family on the circulating leukocytes and immunoglobulin superfamily adhesion molecules on the endothelial cells. Among the various cell adhesion molecules in this superfamily, intracellular (I)CAM-1 (CD54), ICAM-2 (CD102), vascular (V)CAM-1 (CD106), and PECAM-1 (CD31) have been clearly associated with the firm adhesion and transmigration of leukocytes (Table 3). ICAM, VCAM, and PECAM are mainly involved in leukocyte trafficking, whereas the prominent function of neural (N)CAM is in neural development. PECAM-1 is constitutively expressed and concentrated on in the lateral borders between endothelial cells and is expressed on the surfaces of neutrophils, monocytes, platelets, and some T-cell

Table 3 The Immunoglobulin (Ig) Superfamily Adhesion Molecules: Their Counterreceptors and Function

Receptor	Counterreceptor	Distribution	Regulation
ICAM-1 (CD54) [5 Ig domains]	LFA-1 (CD11a/CD18), Mac-1 (CD11b/ CD18), CD43 (leukosialin)	Widespread: EC, fibroblasts, epithelial, monocytes, lymphocytes, dendritic cells, chondrocytes	Constitutive; expression increased by IL-1, TNF-α, IFN-γ, LPS, substance P
ICAM-2 (CD102) [2 Ig domains]	LFA-1	EC, lymphocytes, monocytes	Constitutive
ICAM-3 (CD50) [5 Ig domains]	LFA-1, α_D/CD18	Lymphocytes, monocytes, PMN, eosinophils, basophils	Expression increased by activation
VCAM-1 CD106 [6 or 7 Ig domains]	α_4/β_1 (VLA-4 CD49d/ CD29) α_4/β_7	EC, monocytes, fibroblasts, dendritic cells, bone marrow stromal cells, myoblasts	Expression increased by IL-1, TNF-α, IL-4, IL-13, LPS, oxidative stress
LFA-3, (CD58)	CD2	EC, leukocytes, epithelial cells	
PECAM-1 (CD31)	CD31, other	EC (at EC–EC junctions), T-cell subsets, platelets, PMN, monocytes, smooth-muscle cells	
NCAM	NCAM, heparan-SO$_4$	Neural cells [CD56 homologue]	
MAdCAM-1	$\alpha_4\beta_7$, L-selectin	Mucosal EC; HEV of Peyer patch and mesenteric lymph nodes	Expression increased by TNF-α, IL-1, IFN-γ
CD2	CD58, CD59, CD48	T lymphocytes	

subsets (18). The basal level of ICAM-1 on vascular endothelium is very low. However, under the influence of endotoxins, IL-1, and TNF-α, the expression of ICAM-1 on cultured endothelial cells dramatically rises and the upregulation of ICAM-1 persists for several days (see Fig. 1). VCAM-1 can also be up-regulated by endotoxins and cytokines, with a time course similar to that of ICAM-1 induction. In contrast with ICAM-1, ICAM-2 is constitutively expressed on endothelial cells, and its expression is not affected by inflammatory cytokines.

REGULATION AND MODULATION OF CELL ADHESION MOLECULES

In general, leukocyte–endothelial cell interactions that result in the extravasation of leukocytes might best be considered as a cascade that involves several integrated steps. During these steps, circulating leukocytes roll along the endothelium, adhere tightly, migrate between adjacent endothelial cells, and finally move through the extracellular matrix to perform effector functions in a given tissue. It appears that the soluble mediators, including cytokines and regulatory peptides, chemotactic factors, proinflammatory lipids, and cell adhesion molecules, are expressed in a programmed and interactive manner to create a specific inflammatory response.

The recruitment of leukocytes from the circulating blood to the tissue takes place in three sequential adhesion molecule events (19). In the initial step, constitutively expressed leukocyte adhesion molecules bind transiently and reversibly to specific ligands on endothelial cells, resulting in the adherence and rolling over of the leukocytes on the surface of endothelial cells in postcapillary venules (Fig. 2). This event, which is mediated mainly by selectins, activates the leukocyte and endothelial cells, that then release many soluble mediators. These soluble mediators, which include cytokines such as IL-1 and TNF-α, not only increase the expression of constitutive adhesion molecules, but they also express new so-called inducible adhesion molecules. Additionally, the mediators increase the avidity of leukocyte adhesion molecules, such as the β_2-integrins through soluble factors such as integrin-modulating factor. Finally, the activated leukocytes are able to adhere tightly to the activated endothelial cells, diapedese through the endothelium, and migrate into the extracellular matrix along a chemoattractant gradient (see Fig. 2).

In leukocyte–endothelial cell interaction, leukocyte components, such as L-selectin and sialyl Lewis x (sLe^x), are involved in the rolling phenomenon and the initial binding of leukocytes to activated endothelium. In fact, tetrasaccharide sLe^x and related terminal sugars, which are expressed on many leukocytes, can act as ligands for E-selectin (1,5,17).

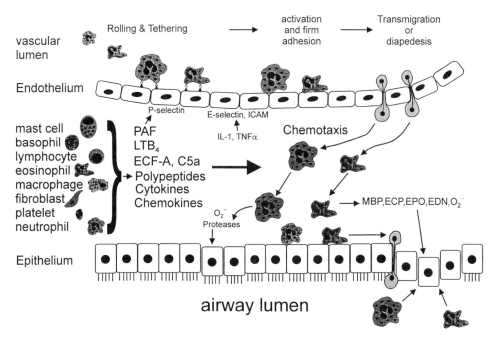

Figure 2 Molecular interactions involved in leukocyte adhesion to endothelial cells and the transmigration into the tissues. In the airway tissues, inflammatory cells might migrate through the extracellular matrix and traverse the basement membrane, leading to the desquamation of airway epithelium. The migration and activation of the cells are regulated under the influence of many chemoattractants and cytokines that are generated and released from various inflammatory cells. Many of these mediators may also induce the expression of cell adhesion molecules on endothelial and epithelial cells, as well as on leukocytes.

Sialyl Le^x has a low affinity for P-selectin and E-selectin, for which mucin-type molecules that contain multiple O-linked carbohydrates extending from a protein backbone, have been described as high-affinity ligands. Interestingly, a recent study demonstrated that nonsteroidal anti-inflammatory drugs, such as indomethacin and diclofenac, attenuated the neutrophil attachment to endothelial cells in vitro by decreasing the expression of L-selectin. The down-regulation of L-selectin was due to the rapid cleavage and shedding of the membrane L-selectin (20). This study further supports the crucial role of L-selectin in the very initial step involved in neutrophil adhesion to endothelial cells.

An endothelial glycoprotein, E-selectin, is also involved in the adhesion of neutrophils, eosinophils, monocytes, and lymphocytes. E-selectin is synthesized and expressed maximally within 4–6 h in response to IL-1, TNF-α, and bacterial endotoxins. However, within 2 days, the expression of E-selectin returns back to the basal level (see Fig. 1). P-selectin, an adhesion molecule transiently expressed on the surface of endothelial cells and platelets, increases the adhesion of neutrophils (PMN) under both static and flow conditions. P-selectin is constitutively synthesized and found in Weibel–Palade bodies of endothelial cells and in storage granules of platelets. Under the influence of various stimuli, including histamine, thrombin, complement factors, and cytokines, such as IL-1 and TNF-α, P-selectin is redistributed within minutes to the cell surface. Very recently, Lorant and colleagues (21) demonstrated that the distribution of ligands for P-selectin is influenced by cytoskeletal interactions, and that redistribution of these ligands may influence adhesive interactions. Furthermore, activation of polymorphonuclear leukocytes may cause loosening or disengagement of bonds between P-selectin and its ligands, facilitating transendothelial migration. Recently, Weyrich and colleagues (15) demonstrated the regulation of nuclear factor-κB (NF-κB) translocation to the monocyte nucleus by the tethering of monocytes to P-selectin. Additionally, these investigators observed an increase in secretion of TNF-α and monocyte chemotactic protein-1 (MCP-1). These data clearly suggest an important role of P-selectin in the infiltration of inflammatory cells to areas of acute and chronic inflammation. This could also be supported by the observations of Mayadas and colleagues (22) during which leukocyte rolling and extravasation were severely compromised in P-selectin-deficient mice.

Wein and colleagues (23) recently reported that the counterligand for P-selectin on human eosinophils is a sialylated glycoprotein just as it is for PMN, and despite the relatively low levels of sLe^x on eosinophils, they bind as well as PMN. Furthermore, activation of eosinophils and PMN with platelet-activating factor (PAF), but not with other stimuli, partially reduced P-selectin binding, suggesting that the function or expression of counterligands for P-selectin of human eosinophils can be altered after activation. Smith and colleagues (24) demonstrated the expression of L-selectin on unstimulated normodense eosinophils, and the expression of this cell adhesion molecule was rapidly lost from the cell surface, with a concomitant increase in CD11b/CD18 (Mac-1) expression after stimulation with PAF or calcium ionophore A23187. Anwer et al. (25) demonstrated that the survival of eosinophils was significantly enhanced after their adhesion to fibronectin. This may further support the possibility that the eosinophils might be activated during the journey from bloodstream to inflammatory tissues by adhesion to endothelial cells and fibronectin.

Expression of ICAM-1 is constitutive and also inducible by TNF-α, IL-1, and interferon (IFN)-γ. Unstimulated cells do not express either VCAM-1 or ELAM-1. One of the molecular mechanisms responsible for the adherence of leukocytes to human airway epithelial cells appears to be the binding of leukocyte integrins to ICAM-1 on the epithelium. ICAM-1 expression and PMNs adherence are increased after epithelial infection with

Table 4 Leukocyte and Endothelial Cell Components Involved in the Molecular Interactions During Leukocyte Adhesion to Endothelium

Component	Inflammatory stimulus	Rolling	Activation	Firm adhesion and transmigration	Chemotaxis; tissue retention
Leukocyte component		sLe^x, L-selectin, PSGL-1	Cytokine and chemokine receptors; CD31	β_2 integrins (also β_1 and β_7 integrins, CD31)	Chemokine receptors; β_1 integrins
Endothelial and tissue component	Histamine, thrombin, bradykinin, LPS, IL-1, TNF-α, various lipid and peptide mediators	P-selectin, E-selectin, GlyCAM-1, MAdCAM-1, PAF, VCAM-1	Chemokines, cytokines, CD31, PAF, C5a, FMLP	ICAM-1, 2 (also VCAM-1, CD31)	Chemokines, lipid mediators, ECM molecules

parainfluenza virus type-2 (26). Recently, two sulfated glycoprotein ligands, 50 and 90 kDa, have been identified with an L-selectin–IgG chimera, as ligands for L-selectin. The cDNA cloning of the 50-kDa sulfated glycoprotein (glycosylation-dependent cell adhesion molecule 1; glyCAM-1) has shown it to be a mucin-like scaffold that presents a carbohydrate ligand to the lectin domain of L-selectin (27). Mebius and colleagues (28) recently reported that a soluble or cellular component of afferent lymph regulates the expression of glyCAM-1 mRNA; which results in an increased adherence of lymphocytes to high endothelial venules.

Cytokines other than IL-1 and TNF-α also induce the expression of cell adhesion molecules. Interleukin-4 (IL-4) is derived primarily from T_H2 cells and stimulates IgE production by B lymphocytes. By itself IL-4 is a weak stimulus for VCAM-1 expression on endothelial cells in vitro. However, IL-4 synergistically up-regulates TNF-α-mediated induction of VCAM-1 (29). These data have been supported by the in vivo studies in baboon skin, when IL-4 injected concomitantly with TNF-α significantly increased VCAM-1 expression together with the infiltration of dermal T cells (30).

A serum adhesion factor, with molecular weight of more than 12,000, enhanced neutrophil adherence to airway epithelial cells in culture (31). The monoclonal antibodies, anti-CD18 and anti-CD11b attenuated the serum-induced neutrophil adherence. This factor is most likely serum complement fragment iC3b. These data, therefore, suggest a possible regulatory role of complement factors on cell adhesion molecules.

Increased expression of cell adhesion molecules has also been demonstrated in several viral infections. An up-regulation of ICAM-1 expression, together with increased neutrophil adhesion, were observed in epithelial cells following parainfluenza virus type-2 infection (26). Interestingly, it was recently reported (32) that recombinant adenovirus infection blunted IFN-induced up-regulation of ICAM-1 expression. This could be due to the effect of adenovirus on a postreceptor site involved in cytokine-induced signal transduction pathways. Thus, it appears that there could be a differential effect of viruses on the expression of cell adhesion molecules.

Subsets of T cells, as defined by distinct patterns of β_1 and β_7 integrins, have been observed in human bronchoalveolar lavage (BAL) fluid (33). It is speculated by the investigators that these T cells, which express different adhesion molecule repertoires, interact differently with other cells and with the extracellular matrix, and they may have distinct roles in the pulmonary immune response. Cells belonging to the $\alpha E \beta 7^+$ subset might, for example, adhere more tightly to epithelial cells, to collagen, and to epiligrin (an epithelial basement membrane-specific matrix protein). Indeed Lazaar and colleagues (34) recently reported that T lymphocytes initially adhere to airway smooth-muscle cells by integrins and CD44 and induce smooth-muscle DNA synthesis.

Mast cells and basophils play an important role in immediate allergic reactions and in the inflammatory aspect of the late-phase reaction of bronchial asthma (35). These cells contain high-affinity IgE receptors (Fc$_\epsilon$RI). In response to an allergic reaction, the aggregation of IgE bound to Fc$_\epsilon$RI on the surface of mast cells and basophils results in degranulation and the release of many preformed mediators, such as histamine and proteases, and newly synthesized mediators, such as leukotrienes, prostaglandins, and platelet-activating factor. In addition, cytokines such as TNF-α and IL-4 are also released. These cytokines modulate the expression of adhesion molecules on endothelial cells. Indeed, the release of TNF-α in response to mast cell degranulation induced E-selectin expression 4–6 h later, which correlated well with the timing of leukocyte infiltration that characterizes the cutaneous late-phase response after allergen-induced mast cell degranulation (36). In addition IL-4 and IL-5, cytokines preferentially released from the T_H2 subset of T-helper cells, have been demonstrated to increase the adherence of human eosinophils to endothelial cells (37,38).

Mast cells express fibronectin–receptor integrins on their cell surface, and these integrins are involved in cellular activation (35). Ra and colleagues (39) reported that rat and mouse mast cells adhered to fibronectin through VLA4 and VLA5 (β_1-integrin) and vitronectin receptor (β_3-integrin), and engagement of these receptors promoted cellular degranulation induced by cross-linking of high-affinity IgE receptors. This results in the hypersensitivity and increased activation of cells, leading to the prolonged survival of mast cells on fibronectin. The latter phenomenon is probably due to an autocrine or paracrine effect of IL-3. Thus, released cytokines at the site of injury may increase inflammatory cells, including mast cells and basophils, and the activated cells may lead to a chronic inflammatory response. For a further discussion on mast cells and basophils, see Chapter 8.

REGULATORY POLYPEPTIDES AND CELL ADHESION MOLECULES

Regulatory polypeptides play a significant role in various inflammatory conditions. We have recently reported that the polypeptides, endothelin-1, neurokinin-A, and substance P promoted the adherence of leukocytes to vascular endothelial cells (40). The effect of these peptides was more pronounced on the adherence of neutrophils and lymphocytes. These data suggest that neuropeptides are capable of modulating the expression of cell adhesion molecules on endothelial cells or on leukocytes. Zimmerman and colleagues (41) reported that the neuropeptide substance P (SP) and calcitonin gene-related peptide (CGRP) promote neutrophil adherence to venular endothelium, and that this neuropeptide-induced adhesion is not mediated by the adhesion molecules CD11/CD18, L-selectin, E-selectin, or ICAM-1. Sung and colleagues have also reported an increased adherence of U937 cells and neutrophils to HUVECs in response to calcitonin gene-related peptide (42) and neuropeptide Y (43). Neuropeptide Y, a 36-amino acid neuropeptide, which is colocalized and released with norepinephrine from sympathetic nerves, modulates the degranulation of mast cells and thus the release of histamine.

Smith and colleagues (44) also demonstrated the proinflammatory effects and the induction of cell adhesion molecules by sensory neuropeptides in normal human skin. In these studies, intradermal injections of substance P, vasoactive intestinal polypeptide (VIP), and calcitonin gene-related peptide up-regulated the expression of P-selectin and E-selectin in the skin, and the increased expression of the cell adhesion molecules paralleled the neutrophilic infiltration. There was no endothelial expression of VCAM-1. Because substance P induced a marked eosinophilic as well as neutrophilic infiltration without VCAM-1 expression, these data suggest that eosinophil recruitment does not require VCAM-1 expression.

Thus, various regulatory polypeptides might regulate the expression of cell adhesion molecules. Because most of the polypeptide hormones are released in conjunction with various cytokines, it is possible that there is a synergistic interaction in their effect on the induction and regulation of the cell adhesion molecules' expression. The complexity of these interactions between polypeptides, cytokines, and adhesion receptors highlights the integrated and cascade-like nature of immunological and inflammatory reactions. These issues need to be further explored.

CELL ADHESION MOLECULES IN
BRONCHIAL ASTHMA

Nonspecific airway hyperresponsiveness, which is a hallmark of asthma, is characterized by an exaggerated bronchoconstriction to a variety of endogenously released mediators such as histamine, acetylcholine, leukotrienes, platelet-activating factor, regulatory peptides, and soluble cytokines (45,46). The mechanisms underlying airway hyperresponsiveness are not yet fully known. However, airway inflammation is now considered to be closely associated with airway hyperresponsiveness. In an inflammatory response, the circulating effector cells communicate with the resident cells by the release of various soluble chemotactic factors and cytokines which, in turn, alter the expression of cell adhesion molecules. Thus, specific adhesion molecules play an important role in the recruitment of various inflammatory cells including eosinophils, in bronchial asthma.

Adhesion molecules play a significant role in the movement of inflammatory cells in the allergic inflammatory reactions (47–50). Cellular infiltrate and mediator release contribute to the clinical symptoms of late-phase reaction following allergen challenge. Cytokines and mediators attract various inflammatory cells. LFA-1, or CD11a/CD18, is a receptor that binds to ICAM-1, or CD54, a member of the immunoglobulin supergene family, widely expressed on activated mononuclear cells and granulocytes. An increased expression of E-selectin, ICAM-1, and VCAM-1 in allergic diseases, including bronchial asthma and atopic dermatitis, has been demonstrated by immunohistochemical studies. Indeed the role of various leukocyte adhesion molecules, including VLA-4, LFA-1, and Mac-1, has been demonstrated in allergic airway responses in the rat (51). Brown et al. (52) examined the role of cell adhesion molecules in the homotypic aggregation of rat alveolar macrophages after exposure to wool and grain dusts. Wool dusts collected from the air of British wool textile mills, and sieved grain dust formed aggregation of macrophages, and this process involved up-regulation of LFA-1α and LFA-1β and its key counterreceptor ICAM-1 (CD54). Protein kinase C inhibitors had no effect on this phenomenon. In another study, Ciprandi and colleagues (53) reported that CD54 expression on epithelial cells in allergic subjects may be considered a hallmark of the inflammation following allergic reaction, even in the absence of signs and symptoms, and is related to inflammatory cell infiltration during both early and late phases.

Several studies demonstrated the important role of ICAM-1 in leukocyte infiltration. ICAM-1 expression has been detected on inflamed endothelium and epithelium; in allergic inflammation the increased expression of CD54 was first demonstrated on epithelial cells and eosinophils of bronchial mucosa after allergen challenge in a monkey model of asthma. Increased expression of ICAM-1 was also reported in experimental rats (54).

Montefort and colleagues (55) examined the expression of ICAM-1 and ELAM-1 in normal subjects and symptomatic asthmatics. Expression of ICAM-1 was demonstrated in both the epithelium and the vasculature in normal subjects, asthmatics, and asthmatics who had received sufficient inhaled steroid to ameliorate the bronchial inflammation. Similar to ICAM-1, ELAM-1 expression was also found in the vasculature of both normal and asthmatic subjects. These investigators suggested that the recruitment of cells into the mucosa is a complex process, and one must investigate other critical steps that can be modulated by therapy other than those involving cell adhesion (56,57). However, in their follow-up study, Montefort and colleagues (58,59) examined the endobronchial subcarinal mucosal biopsy of asthmatic airways 5–6 h after local subsegmental challenge with allergen and saline. These investigators observed a marked increase in the expression of

E-selectin and ICAM-1, but not VCAM-1, following allergen challenge. Up-regulation of endothelial cell adhesion molecules was associated with a marked increase in the number of leukocytes expressing the β_2 integrin LFA-1 that correlated with ICAM-1 expression. The latter data support the thesis that allergen challenge produces up-regulation of E-selectin and ICAM-1, compared with the saline-challenge, in asthmatic subjects. These results were also supported by other investigators (60). Bochner et al. (61) reported that the variations in the E-selectin-mediated cell recruitment of neutrophils and eosinophils during inflammatory responses in vivo could be due to the differential expression of sLe^x-containing surface molecules on these cells; sialyl-dimeric Le^x being the most prominent E-selectin ligand on eosinophils, whereas neutrophils expressed significant levels of sLe^x and a sialylated dimeric form of the Le^x antigen.

Roche et al. (56) examined the expression of ICAM-1 and ELAM-1 in normal subjects and symptomatic asthmatics. These investigators detected ICAM-1 in both the epithelium and the vasculature in normal subjects, asthmatics, and asthmatics who had received sufficient inhaled steroid to reduce the inflammatory cell infiltrate in their bronchi. Similarly, there was ELAM-1 expression in the vasculature of normal and asthmatic subjects; however, corticosteroid treatment did not affect the ELAM-1 expression.

Increased expression of VCAM-1 and ICAM-1 was also observed on endothelial cells of nasal biopsies obtained from perennial allergic rhinitis subjects (62). However, the expression of the cell adhesion molecules did not correlate with the severity of the disease or the number of eosinophils in biopsy specimens.

Up-regulation of ICAM-1 has also been reported on peripheral blood T lymphocytes. De Rose and colleagues (63) recently demonstrated that, in dual asthmatic responders, ICAM-1 is up-regulated on peripheral blood immunoregulatory T lymphocytes and, particularly, on CD4$^+$ T lymphocytes. The up-regulation of ICAM-1 expression was related to the change in the 7-s forced expiratory volume (FEV$_1$) at the time of the late-phase reaction. These data suggest that T lymphocytes are in a higher state of activation in those asthmatics who show both early- and late-phase response, as compared with those who show only early response after allergen challenge.

Sedgwick and colleagues (64) have previously reported the presence of soluble ICAM-1 (sICAM-1) in bronchoalveolar lavage fluid only during the late-phase response in atopic patients who underwent segmental antigen challenge. An increased level of circulating sICAM-1 has also been observed in patients with acute asthma when compared with stable asthmatics and control subjects (65,66). Such an increase in sICAM-1 could be due to a shedding of ICAM-1 from activated cells. If it is true, the activated cells in asthmatics should show a decreased expression of cell adhesion molecules on their surface. Indeed, De Rose and colleagues (63) in their study observed a significant decrease in ICAM-1 expression in both CD4$^+$ and CD8$^+$ T-lymphocyte subsets in dual asthmatics responders. However, the possibility of the migration of activated T lymphocytes from the vascular compartment into the airways cannot be ruled out.

Muller (67) recently reported that PECAM-1 is important for mediating a final common event during transmigration that is shared by polymorphonuclear leukocytes and monocytes on the activated or unactivated human umbilical vein endothelial cells, as well as at sites of acute inflammation, irrespective of any adhesion molecule involved in rolling and tight adhesion to the apical surface. Thus, the unique position of PECAM-1 helps in fulfilling its role in transendothelial migration and in mediating multiple important cell–cell interactions.

Eosinophils play a key role in the pathogenesis of bronchial asthma. Infiltration of eosinophils is facilitated by the presence of several types of cell adhesion molecules that are expressed on the surface of eosinophils. These cell adhesion molecules interact with the counterreceptors on endothelial cells, thereby facilitating the diapedesis of eosinophils through the endothelial cells. Very late antigen (VLA-4), which is a ligand for VCAM-1, is highly expressed in eosinophils, but not in neutrophils (37,68,69). Therefore, VCAM-1 is considered an important molecule for selective eosinophil infiltration in asthmatic airways. However, VCAM-1 may not be the sole determinant for eosinophil recruitment. This could be supported by a study in allergic cutaneous inflammation in vivo, in which skin biopsies, taken 6 h after intradermal antigen in previously documented late-phase responders, showed marked eosinophil infiltration in the absence of significant VCAM-1 up-regulation (70). Indeed, E-selectin and P-selectin are also involved in the recruitment of eosinophils into the airway (71,72). Ohkawara and colleagues (73) recently examined the in situ expression of adhesion molecules in the bronchial mucosa and submucosa and correlated it with the airway narrowing in the patients with bronchial asthma. The immunohistochemical studies revealed a marked up-regulation of ICAM-1, VCAM-1, and E-selectin in vascular endothelial cells, and there was a good correlation between the increased expression of cell adhesion molecules and increased infiltration of eosinophils and mononuclear cells in epithelial lining and bronchial submucosa in asthmatic subjects. Immunoreactivity for Mac-1, LFA-1, and VLA-4 was strongly positive in eosinophils and mononuclear cells that had infiltrated in the bronchial tissues from asthmatic subjects with airflow limitation. Increased expression of ICAM-1, VCAM-1, and E-selectin is due to new synthesis of these molecules before spontaneous asthma attack, as demonstrated by increased mRNA expression by in situ hybridization.

Thus, it appears that the increased expression of various cell adhesion molecules on endothelial cells in conjunction with the integrins present on leukocytes facilitate the recruitment and adherence of eosinophils in the airways. Release of several soluble mediators and cytokines from mast cells, basophils, monocytes–macrophages, lymphocytes, especially T_H2-type, and endothelial cells may control the expression of cell adhesion molecules in allergic diseases such as bronchial asthma.

ADHESION RECEPTORS AS THERAPEUTIC TARGETS IN ALLERGIC DISEASE

In addition to the studies alluded to in the foregoing, a variety of studies targeting adhesion receptors as a means to modify various animal models of allergic disease have helped confirm the important role played by these molecules. In addition, successful modification of allergic inflammation in animal models raises the expectation that adhesion molecules might someday be important therapeutic targets for the treatment of human allergic diseases. There are several potential mechanisms by which adhesion receptor-directed therapies might exert beneficial therapeutic effects in allergic diseases. In the simplest paradigm, blocking a cell's adhesion receptors may prevent it from gaining access to a tissue site of allergic inflammation. For example, eosinophils may be prevented from accruing in the bronchial submucosa. Another means by which anti-adhesion therapy might interfere with the propagation of allergic inflammation is by inhibiting the activation of cells. Several adhesion receptors are capable of transducing signals. Therefore, inhibition of adhesion receptors might prevent a cell already present at the site of inflammation from becoming activated and contributing to the inflammatory response and tissue injury. Lastly, because the nature of the adhesion cascade requires the orchestrated involvement of diverse cell types, inhibition of the adhesion receptor on a given cell may inhibit other components

of the inflammatory response downstream. For example, adhesion receptor-directed therapies primarily targeting CD4$^+$ T-helper cells may preclude these cells from recruiting
eosinophils into an allergic inflammatory site. Individual adhesion receptor-directed therapies may involve one or several of these mechanisms.

In a monkey model of airway responsiveness related to repeated allergen inhalation, a
monoclonal antibody (MAb) against ICAM-1 was effective at decreasing both eosinophil
accrual into the airway as well as airway hyperresponsiveness (74). In a similar, but slightly
differently designed study, these same investigator showed that MAb to either ICAM-1 or
E-selectin were capable of inhibiting the allergic late-phase response (75). Of note when
considering the potential relevance of these studies to the treatment of human disease,
treatment with these agents was substantially less effective when given after allergen
exposure.

Because it is expressed on eosinophils and lymphocytes, but not on neutrophils, VLA-4
may be an attractive target for allergic disease. Theoretically, by sparing any inhibition of
neutrophils, VLA-4-directed therapies could exert substantial effects on allergic inflammation, while not causing a profound nonspecific immunosuppression. In a guinea pig model
of allergic asthma, MAb to VLA-4 inhibited the accrual of eosinophils as well as CD4$^+$ T
cells into the bronchial submucosa (76). Importantly, this inhibition of extravascular
cellular accumulation was accompanied by decreased airway hyperreactivity. With the
same MAb, other investigators assessed the effect of VLA-4 inhibition in a sheep model of
allergic airway disease (77). In this study, treatment was effective even when administered
by aerosol and after allergen challenge. Interestingly, although airway hyperreactivity was
diminished, treatment with the anti-VLA-4 MAb did not appear to inhibit the accrual of
eosinophils into the lung. This suggests that the effect of the antibody may have been more
at the level of preventing cellular activation, rather than preventing cellular accrual. Terada
and colleagues also demonstrated that an anti-VLA-4 MAb was able to prevent eosinophil
accumulation and activation in the guinea pig nasal mucosa (78).

The applicability of adhesion receptor-directed therapies to human disease has been
demonstrated in patients with rheumatoid arthritis (79). In that study, an anti-ICAM-1 MAb
effectively inhibited synovitis in a group of patients with long-standing refractory disease.
Of note, the efficacy of the anti-ICAM-1 MAb correlated with the induction of hyporesponsiveness among circulating T cells (80).

Finally, therapies directed at other components of the immune response may exert part
of their therapeutic benefit by altering adhesion molecule utilization. For example, therapies directed at the cytokine IL-4 inhibit the adherence of eosinophils to endothelium, an
effect mediated somewhat by interfering with the capacity of IL-4 to induce VCAM-1
expression by the endothelium (37). Van Oosterhout and colleagues (81) have also shown
that an anti-IL-5 MAb inhibited eosinophilia in bronchoalveolar lavage fluid as well as
airway hyperreactivity following antigen challenge in guinea pigs. In addition, corticosteroids, which presumably exert diverse immunomodulatory effects, primarily by
inhibition of cytokine production, inhibit ICAM-1 (CD54) expression by epithelial
cells (82).

CONCLUSIONS AND FUTURE DIRECTIONS

In the last decade there has been a tremendous growth in our understanding of the nature of
cell adhesion molecules, their role in various pathophysiological conditions, and the
regulatory and modulatory role of several soluble factors, especially cytokines. However,
many questions remain to be answered. In allergic diseases, such as bronchial asthma,

increased expression of cell adhesion molecules appears to correlate with the infiltration of various inflammatory cells, such as eosinophils, suggesting the possible therapeutic role of the inhibitors or antibodies to the cell adhesion molecules. However, airway inflammation involves a very complex regulatory interplay between cytokines, chemotactic factors, inflammatory cells, and the molecules required in leukocyte–epithelial and leukocyte–endothelial cell adhesion. Therefore, a detailed understanding of the underlying mechanisms in the regulation of cell adhesion molecules is required for the development of new therapeutic modalities for a better prognosis of allergic diseases. One area for future work is the role of phosphorylation and dephosphorylation of various intracellular molecules by tyrosine kinases and the regulatory effect of nuclear transcription factors on the gene transcription of cell adhesion molecules. Additionally, is there a differential expression and regulation of cell adhesion molecules on airway epithelium of allergic subjects in and out of the season? Finally, there appears to be a controversy on the effect of corticosteroids on the expression of cell adhesion molecules. Obviously, further studies are warranted on the effect of various bronchodilators and corticosteroids on cell adhesion molecules at the transcriptional, translational, and posttranslational levels.

REFERENCES

1. Bevilacqua MP. Endothelial–leukocyte adhesion molecules. Annu Rev Immunol 1993; 11: 767–804.
2. Springer TA. Adhesion receptors of the immune system. Nature 1990; 346:425–434.
3. Pober JS, Cotran RS. The role of endothelial cells in inflammation. Transplantation 1990; 50:537–544.
4. Abelda SM, Smith CW, Ward PA. Adhesion molecules and inflammatory injury. FASEB J 1994; 8:504–512.
5. Pilewski JM, Albelda SM. Adhesion molecules in the lung: an overview. Am Rev Respir Dis 1993; 148:S31–S37.
6. Albelda SM, Buck CA. Integrins and other cell adhesion molecules. FASEB J 1990; 4:2868–2880.
7. Hemler ME. VLA proteins in the integrin family: structures, functions and their role on leukocytes. Annu Rev Immunol 1990; 8:365–400.
8. Hynes RO. Integrins: versatility, modulation, and signaling in cell adhesion. Cell 1992; 69:11–25.
9. Jaconi MEE, Theler JM, Schlegel W, Appel RD, Wright SD, Lew PD. Multiple elevations of cytosolic-free Ca^{2+} in human neutrophils: initiation by adherence receptors of the integrin family. J Cell Biol 1991; 112:1249–1257.
10. Ruoslahti E, Pierschbacher MD. New perspectives in cell adhesion: RGD and integrins. Science 1987; 238:491–497.
11. Takeichi M. Cadherin cell adhesion receptors as a morphogenetic regulator. Science 1991; 251:1451–1455.
12. Lasky LA. Selectins: interpreters of cell-specific carbohydrate information during inflammation. Science 1992; 258:964–969.
13. Bevilacqua M, Butcher E, Furie B, Gallatin M, Gimbrone M, Harlan J, Kishimoto K, Lasky L, McEver R, Paulson J, Rosen S, Seed B, Springer T, Stoolman L, Tedder T, Varki A, Wagner D, Weissman I, Zimmerman G. Selectins: a family of adhesion receptors. Cell 1991; 67:233–244.
14. Wagner DD. P-selectin chases a butterfly [Editorial]. J Clin Invest 1995; 95:1955–1956.
15. Weyrich AS, McIntyre TM, McEver RP, Prescott SM, Zimmerman GA. Monocyte tethering by P-selectin regulates monocyte chemotactic protein-1 and tumor necrosis factor-α secretion. Signal integration and NF-κB translocation. J Clin Invest 1995; 95:2297–2303.

16. Hogg N, Berlin C. Structure and function of adhesion receptors in leukocyte trafficking. Immunol Today 1995; 16:327–330.

17. Bevilacqua MP, Nelson RM, Mannori G, Cecconi O. Endothelial–leukocyte adhesion molecules in human disease. Annu Rev Med 1994; 45:361–378.

18. DeLisser HM, Newman PJ, Albelda SM. Molecular and functional aspects of PECAM-1/CD31. Immunol Today 1994; 15:490–495.

19. Butcher EC. Leukocyte–endothelial cell recognition: three (or more) steps to specificity and diversity. Cell 1991; 67:1033–1937.

20. Diaz-Gonzalez F, Gonzalez-Alvaro I, Campanero MR, Mollinedo F, del Pozo MA, Munoz C, Pivel JP, Sanchez-Madrid F. Prevention of in vitro neutrophil–endothelial attachment through shedding of L-selectin by nonsteroidal antiinflammatory drugs. J Clin Invest 1995; 95:1756–1765.

21. Lorant DE, McEver RP, McIntyre TM, Moore KL, Prescott SM, Zimmerman GA. Activation of polymorphonuclear leukocytes reduces their adhesion to P-selectin and causes redistribution of ligands for P-selectin on their surfaces. J Clin Invest 1995; 96:171–182.

22. Mayadas TN, Johnson RC, Rayburn H, Hynes RO, Wagner DD. Leukocyte rolling and extravasation are severely compromised in P-selectin deficient mice. Cell 1993; 74:541–554.

23. Wein M, Sterbinsky SA, Bickel CA, Schleimer RP, Bochner BS. Comparison of human eosinophil and neutrophil ligands for P-selectin: ligands for P-selectin differ from those for E-selectin. Am J Respir Cell Mol Biol 1995; 12:315–319.

24. Smith CH, Barker JNWN, Lee TH. Adhesion molecules in allergic inflammation. Am Rev Respir Dis 1993; 148:S75–S78.

25. Anwer ARF, Moqbel R, Walsh A, Kay AB, Wardlaw AJ. Adhesion to fibronectin prolongs eosinophil survival. J Exp Med 1993; 177:839–843.

26. Tosi MF, Stark JM, Hamedani A, Smith CW, Gruenert DC, Infeld MD. ICAM-1-dependent and ICAM-1-independent adhesive interactions between PMN and human airway epithelial cells infected with parainfluenza virus type 2. J Immunol 1992; 149:3345–3349.

27. Imai Y, Singer MS, Fennie C, Lasky LA, Rosen SD. Identification of a carbohydrate-based endothelial ligand for a lymphocyte homing receptor. J Cell Biol 1991; 113:1213–1218.

28. Mebius RE, Dowbenko D, Williams A, Fennie C, Lasky LA, Watson SR. Expression of glyCAM-1, an endothelial ligand for L-selectin, is affected by afferent lymphatic flow. J Immunol 1993; 151:6769–6776.

29. Thornhill MH, Wellicome SM, Mahiouz DL, Lanchbury JS, Kyan-Aung U, Haskard DO. Tumor necrosis factor combines with IL-4 or IFN-gamma to selectively enhance endothelial cell adhesiveness for T cells. The contribution of vascular cell adhesion molecule-1 dependent and independent binding mechanisms. J Immunol 1991; 146:592–598.

30. Briscoe DM, Cotran RS, Pober JS. Effects of tumor necrosis factor, lipopolysaccharide, and IL-4 on the expression of vascular cell adhesion molecule-1 in vivo. Correlation with $CD3^+$ T cell infiltration. J Immunol 1992; 149:2954–2960.

31. Varsano S, Joseph-Lerner N, Reshef T, Frolkis I. Normal serum increases adhesion of neutrophils to tracheal epithelial cells by a CD11b/CD18-dependent mechanism. Am J Respir Cell Mol Biol 1994; 10:298–305.

32. Pilewski JM, Sott DJ, Wilson JM, Albelda SM. ICAM-1 expression on bronchial epithelium after recombinant adenovirus infection. Am J Respir Cell Mol Biol 1995; 12:142–148.

33. Erle DJ, Brown T, Christian D, Aris R. Lung epithelial lining fluid T cell subsets by distinct patterns of β_7 and β_1 integrin expression. Am J Respir Cell Mol Biol 1994; 10:237–244.

34. Lazaar AL, Albelda SM, Pilewski JM, Brennan B, Pure E, Panettieri RA. T lymphocytes adhere to airway smooth muscle cells via integrins and CD44 and induce smooth muscle cell DNA synthesis. J Exp Med 1994; 180:807–816.

35. Hamawy MM, Mergenhagen SE, Siraganian RP. Adhesion molecules as regulators of mast-cell and basophil function. Immunol Today 1994; 15:62–66.

36. Klein LM, Lavker RM, Matis WL, Murphy GF. Degranulation of human mast cells induces an endothelial antigen central to leukocyte adhesion. Proc Natl Acad Sci USA 1989; 86:8972–8976.
37. Schleimer RP, Sterbinsky SA, Kaiser J, Bickel CA, Klunk DA, Tomioka K, Newman W, Luscinskas FW, Gimbrone MA Jr, McIntyre BW. IL-4 induces adherence of human eosinophils and basophils but not neutrophils to endothelium. Association with expression of VCAM-1. J Immunol 1992; 148:1086–1092.
38. Weller PF. Role of eosinophils in allergy. Curr Opin Immunol 1992; 4:782–787.
39. Ra C, Yasuda M, Yagita H, Okumura K. Fibronectin receptor integrins are involved in mast cell activation. J Allergy Clin Immunol 1994; 94:625–628.
40. McGregor PE, Agrawal DK, Edwards JD. Differential effects of peptides on the adherence of white blood cells to endothelial cell monolayers. FASEB J 1994; 8:A323.
41. Zimmerman BJ, Anderson DC, Granger DN. Neuropeptides promote neutrophil adherence to endothelial cell monolayers. Am J Physiol 1992; 263:G678–G682.
42. Sung CP, Arleth AJ, Aiyar N, Bhatnagar PK, Lysko PG, Feuerstein G. CGRP stimulates the adhesion of leukocytes to vascular endothelial cells. Peptides 1992; 13:429–434.
43. Sung CP, Arleth AJ, Feuerstein GZ. Neuropeptide Y upregulates the adhesiveness of human endothelial cells for leukocytes. Circ Res 1991; 68:314–318.
44. Smith CH, Barker JNWN, Morris RW, MacDonald DM, Lee TH. Neuropeptides induce rapid expression of endothelial cell adhesion molecules and elicit granulocytic infiltration in human skin. J Immunol 1993; 151:1–6.
45. Agrawal DK. Platelet-activating factor receptors in the airways. In: Agrawal DK, Townley RG, eds. Inflammatory Cells and Mediators in Bronchial Asthma. Boca Raton, FL: CRC Press, 1991:171–206.
46. Agrawal DK, Numao T. Transmembrane signaling in eosinophils. In: Makino S, Fukuda T, eds. Eosinophils: Biological and Clinical Aspects. Boca Raton, FL: CRC Press, 1993:171–192.
47. Holtzman MJ, Look DC. Cell adhesion molecules as targets for unraveling the genetic regulation of airway inflammation. Am J Respir Cell Mol Biol 1992; 7:246–247.
48. Pilewski JM, Albelda SM. Cell adhesion molecules in asthma: homing, activation and airway remodeling. Am J Respir Cell Mol Biol 1995; 12:1–3.
49. Leung DYM, Pober JS, Cotran RS. Expression of endothelial–leukocyte adhesion molecule-1 in elicited late phase allergic reactions. J Clin Invest 1991; 87:1805–1809.
50. Hansel TT, Walker C. The migration of eosinophils into the sputum of asthmatics: the role of adhesion molecules. Clin Exp Allergy 1992; 22:345–356.
51. Rabb HA, Olivenstein R, Issekutz TB, Renzi PM, Martin JG, Pantano R, Seguin S. The role of the leukocyte adhesion molecules VLA-4, LFA-1, and Mac-1 in allergic airway responses in the rat. Am J Respir Crit Care Med 1994; 149:1186–1191.
52. Brown DM, Dransfield I, Wetherill GZ, Donaldson K. LFA-1 and ICAM-1 in homotypic aggregation of rat alveolar macrophages: organic dust-mediated aggregation by a non-protein kinase C-dependent pathway. Am J Respir Cell Mol Biol 1993; 9:205–212.
53. Ciprandi G, Pronzato C, Ricca V, Passalacqua G, Bagnasco M, Canonica GW. Allergen-specific challenge induces intercellular adhesion molecule 1 (ICAM-1 or CD54) on nasal epithelial cells in allergic subjects: relationships with early and late inflammatory phenomena. Am J Respir Crit Care Med 1994; 150:1653–1659.
54. Sun J, Elwood W, Haczku A, Barnes PJ, Hellewell PG, Chung KF. Contribution of intercellular adhesion molecule-1 in allergen-induced airway hyperresponsiveness and inflammation in sensitized brown-Norway rats. Int Arch Allergy Immunol 1994; 104:291–295.
55. Montefort S, Roche WR, Howarth PH, Djukanivic R, Gratziou C, Carroll M, Smith L, Britten KM, Haskard D, Lee TH, Holgate ST. Intercellular adhesion molecule-1 (ICAM-1) and endothelial leukocyte adhesion molecule-1 (ELAM-1) expression in the bronchial mucosa of normal and asthmatic subjects. Eur Respir J 1992; 5:815–823.
56. Roche WR, Montefort S, Baker J, Holgate ST. Cell adhesion molecules and the bronchial epithelium. Am Rev Respir Dis 1993; 148:S79–S82.

57. Morland CM, Wilson SJ, Holgate ST, Roche WR. Selective eosinophil recruitment by transendothelial migration and not by leukocyte–endothelial cell adhesion. Am J Respir Cell Mol Biol 1992; 6:557–566.
58. Montefort S, Gratziou C, Goulding D, Polosa R, Haskard DO, Howarth PH, Holgate ST, Carroll MP. Bronchial biopsy evidence for leukocyte infiltration and upregulation of leukocyte–endothelial cell adhesion molecules 6 hours after local antigen challenge of sensitized asthmatic airways. J Clin Invest 1994; 93:1411–1421.
59. Montefort S, Lai CKW, Kapahi P, Leung J, Lai KN, Chan HS, Haskard DO, Howarth PH, Holgate ST. Circulating adhesion molecules in asthma. Am J Respir Crit Care Med 1994; 149:1149–1152.
60. Bentley AM, Durham SR, Robinson DS, Menz G, Storz C, Cromwell O, Kay AB, Wardlaw AJ. Expression of endothelial and leukocyte adhesion molecules intercellular adhesion molecule-1, E-selectin, and vascular cell adhesion molecule-1 in the bronchial mucosa in steady-state and allergen-induced asthma. J Allergy Clin Immunol 1993; 92:857–868.
61. Bochner BS, Sterbinsky SA, Bickel CA, Werfel S, Wein M, Newman W. Differences between human eosinophils and neutrophils in the function and expression of sialic acid-containing counterligands for E-selectin. J Immunol 1994; 152:774–782.
62. Montefort S, Feather IH, Wilson SJ, Haskard DO, Lee TH, Holgate ST, Howarth PH. The expression of leukocyte–endothelial adhesion molecules is increased in perennial allergic rhinitis. Am J Respir Cell Mol Biol 1992; 7:393–398.
63. De Rose V, Rolla G, Bucca C, Ghio P, Bertoletti M, Baderna P, Pozzi E. Intercellular adhesion molecule-1 is upregulated on peripheral blood T lymphocyte subsets in dual asthmatic responders. J Clin Invest 1994; 94:1840–1845.
64. Sedgwick JB, Quan SF, Calhoun WJ, Jarjour N, Rothlein R, Wegner CD, Busse WW. Expression of ICAM-1 on human peripheral blood and airway eosinophils (EOS) and soluble ICAM-1 (sICAM1) in bronchoalveolar lavage fluid (BALF). Am Rev Respir Dis 1992; 145:A188.
65. Lai CK, Kapahi P, Haskard DO, Howarth PH, Holgate ST, Montefort S. Circulating ICAM-1, but not VCAM-1 is increased in the peripheral blood during acute asthma. Eur Respir J 1992; 5:399s.
66. Takahashi N, Liu MC, Proud D, Yu X-Y, Hasegawa S, Spannhake EW. Soluble intercellular adhesion molecule-1 in bronchoalveolar lavage fluid of allergic subjects following segmental antigen challenge. Am J Respir Crit Care Med 1994; 150:704–709.
67. Muller WA. The role of PECAM-1 (CD31) in leukocyte emigration: studies in vitro and in vivo. J Leukoc Biol 1995; 57:523–528.
68. Weller PF, Rand TH, Goelz SE, Chi-Rosso G, Lobb RR. Human eosinophil adherence to vascular endothelium mediated by binding to vascular cell adhesion molecule 1 and endothelial leukocyte adhesion molecule 1. Proc Natl Acad Sci USA 1991; 88:7430–7433.
69. Dobrina A, Menegazzi R, Carlos TM, Nardon W, Vramer R, Zucchi T, Harlan JM. Mechanisms of eosinophil adherence to cultured vascular endothelial cells: eosinophils bind to cytokine-induced endothelial ligand vascular cell adhesion molecule-1 via the very late activation antigen-4 integrin receptor. J Clin Invest 1991; 88:20–26.
70. Kyan-Aung U, Haskard DO, Poston RN, Thornhill MH, Lee TH. Endothelial leukocyte adhesion molecule-1 and intercellular adhesion molecule-1 mediate the adhesion of eosinophils to endothelial cells in vitro and are expressed by endothelium in allergic cutaneous inflammation in vivo. J Immunol 1991; 146:521–528.
71. Georas SN, Liu MC, Newman W, Beall LD, Stealey BA, Bochner BS. Altered adhesion molecule expression and endothelial cell activation accompany the recruitment of human granulocytes to the lung after segmental antigen challenge. Am J Respir Cell Mol Biol 1992; 7:261–269.
72. Vadas MA, Lucas CM, Gamble JR, Lopez AF, Skinner MP, Berndt MC. Regulation of eosinophil function by P selectin. In: Gleich GJ, Kay AB, eds. Eosinophils in Allergy and Inflammation. New York: Marcel Dekker, 1993; 69–84.
73. Ohkawara Y, Yamauchi K, Maruyama N, Hoshi H, Ohno I, Honma M, Tanno Y, Tamura G, Shirato K, Ohtani H. In situ expression of the cell adhesion molecules in bronchial tissues from

asthmatics with air flow limitation: in vivo evidence of VCAM-1/VLA-4 interaction in selective eosinophil infiltration. Am J Respir Cell Mol Biol 1995; 12:4–12.

74. Wegner CD, Gundel RH, Reilly P, Haynes N, Letts LG, Rothlein R. Intercellular adhesion molecules-1 (ICAM-1) in the pathogenesis of asthma. Science 1990; 247:456–459.

75. Gundel RH, Wegner CD, Torcellini CA, Clarke CC, Haynes N, Rothlein R, Smith CW, Letts LG. Endothelial leukocyte adhesion molecule-1 mediates antigen-induced acute airway inflammation and late-phase airway obstruction in monkeys. J Clin Invest 1991; 88:1407–1411.

76. Pretolani M, Ruffie C, Lapa e Silva JR, Joseph D, Lobb R, Vargaftig BB. Antibody to very late activation antigen-4 prevents antigen-induced bronchial hyperreactivity and cellular infiltration in guinea pig airways. J Exp Med 1994; 180:795–805.

77. Abraham WM, Sielczak MW, Ahmed A, Cortes A, Lauredo IT, Kim J, Pepinsky B, Benjamin CD, Leone DR, Lobb RR, Weller PF. α-4-Integrins mediate antigen-induced late bronchial responses and prolonged airway hyperresponsiveness in sheep. J Clin Invest 1994; 93:776–787.

78. Terada N, Konno A, Togawa K. Biochemical properties of eosinophils and their preferential accumulation mechanism in nasal allergy. J Allergy Clin Immunol 1994; 94:629–642.

79. Kavanaugh AF, Davis LS, Nichols LA, Norris SH, Rothlein R, Scharschmidt LA, Lipsky PE. Treatment of refractory rheumatoid arthritis with a monoclonal antibody to intercellular adhesion molecule-1 (ICAM-1). Arthritis Rheum 1994; 37:992–999.

80. Davis LS, Kavanaugh AF, Nichols LA, Lipsky PE. Induction of persistent T cell hyporesponsiveness in vivo by monoclonal antibody to ICAM-1 in patients with rheumatoid arthritis. J Immunol 1995; 154:3525–3537.

81. Van Oosterhout AJM, Ladenius ARC, Savelkoul HFJ, Van Ark I, Delsman KC, Nijkamp FP. Effect of anti-IL-5 and IL-5 on airway hyperreactivity and eosinophilia in guinea pigs. Am Rev Respir Dis 1993; 147:548–552.

82. Ciprandi G, Buscaglia S, Pesce GP, Ludice A, Bagnasco M, Canonica GW. Deflazacort protects late phase but not early phase events induced by allergen specific conjunctival provocation test. Allergy 1993; 48:421–430.

5

Immunological Basis for the Action of Immune-Reacting Substances

Mary E. Paul and Eric T. Sandberg
Baylor College of Medicine, Houston, Texas

William T. Shearer
Baylor College of Medicine and Texas Children's Hospital, Houston, Texas

INTRODUCTION

The immune system involves a complex network of cells and products of cells that afford protection against invaders. However, the immune response can also result in disease. A thorough understanding of the immune system is essential for an appreciation of both established and emerging therapies of allergic disease. The goal of this chapter is to provide an overview of the immune system to serve as a basis for the detailed discussions in subsequent chapters on different aspects of the immune response.

An important aspect of protective immunity is the capacity of the immune system to remember previous encounters with antigen. In the simplest scenario, reinfection with an organism elicits an immune response that prevents repetition of a symptomatic infection. T cells and B cells, as well as their interactions, contribute to immune memory. During maturation, T and B lymphocytes form unique receptors capable of antigen binding. Every receptor of a single B cell or T cell, and of the progeny of that cell, will have a particular antigen specificity. When exposed to appropriate antigen, the lymphocyte proliferates, forming clones with identical receptors. Some of these lymphocytes may persist as long-lived memory cells, with the capacity for more rapid and robust response when subsequently exposed to antigen.

In addition to memory, protective immunity depends on the ability to distinguish self from nonself. The complex mechanisms that allow generation of a tremendous diversity of antigen receptors must include a process that eliminates those receptors with the potential to recognize host antigens and mediate self-destruction. The capability to distinguish self from nonself is mediated predominantly through T lymphocytes and is obtained principally during T-lymphocyte development in the thymus gland. Other factors also contribute to the discrimination of self from nonself, and the term *immunological tolerance* refers to the multiple regulatory influences that prevent autoimmunity.

LYMPHOCYTES

Lymphocytes are small, round cells that have a large nucleus and densely packed chromatin; they constitute 25–45% of circulating leukocytes in normal adults. Lymphocytes originate in the bone marrow. A pluripotent stem cell in the bone marrow gives rise to both lymphoid and myeloid cell lines. It is believed that a lymphoid stem cell exists from which T cells, B cells, and possibly large granular lymphocytes, or natural killer (NK) cells, arise under the influence of the bone marrow microenvironment. B cells become mature, resting B cells in the bone marrow. T cells develop primarily in the thymus. Both B and T cells then migrate through the bloodstream to peripheral lymphoid organs, such as the spleen, lymph nodes, and tonsils, where final differentiation occurs. After final differentiation, lymphocytes are fully capable of responding to immunological challenge.

T Cells

T-Cell Development

Lymphoid stem cells that become T cells migrate from the bone marrow to the thymus, where maturation occurs by a process that is not completely defined. Within the thymus, these cells obtain surface antigens. Some of these surface markers are associated with specific effector functions. The cluster of differentiation (CD)3 antigen is found on all mature T cells. The CD3 molecule is an association of membrane proteins. The proteins forming CD3 are called γ, δ, ϵ, ζ (ζ sometimes exists as a heterodimer with a fifth polypeptide, η). Some mature T cells have CD4 surface glycoprotein markers. These T cells, sometimes called T helper (T_H) cells, recognize antigen when presented in association with the class II major histocompatibility complex (MHC) molecules. Other mature T cells have CD8 surface glycoprotein markers. These T cells, sometimes called cytotoxic or suppressor T (Tc) cells, recognize antigen when presented in association with the class I MHC molecules.

Another important T cell surface marker, the T-cell receptor (TCR), is a member of the immunoglobulin supergene family. The TCR recognizes processed antigen presented, in association with an MHC molecule, by an antigen-presenting cell (APC), such as a dendritic cell, a monocyte, or a macrophage. The TCR is a heterodimer formed of α- and β-glycoprotein chains (Fig. 1). An alternative form of TCR, comprising γ and δ polypeptide chains, exists on fewer than 10% of T cells. The TCR is expressed with CD3 on the surface of the T cell, and the resulting association is termed the TCR complex. [The γ and δ polypeptides forming the minority population of TCRs are not to be confused with the γ and δ peptides that contribute to CD3 formation.]

Early in the developmental process when the stem cell enters the thymic cortex, the cell expresses neither the TCR nor the effector function markers, CD4 or CD8 (Fig. 2). As the thymocyte matures, the cell has low expression of $\alpha\beta$-TCR and has both CD4 and CD8 on the surface. Through a process of positive and negative selection, TCRs are formed that recognize antigen in association with self-MHC molecules. Thymic APCs present peptides to a developing thymocyte. Failure of thymocytes to bind with low-level affinity to the self-MHC molecule expressed by the APC leads to programmed cell death (*apoptosis*). *Positive selection* refers to the survival of thymocytes with TCRs that bind MHC molecules with low affinity (1). The antigenic peptides expressed by the thymic APC are mostly self-proteins. Therefore, thymocytes that bind with very high affinity to the thymic APCs are potentially autoimmune. Thymocytes with receptors with high affinity for self-antigen

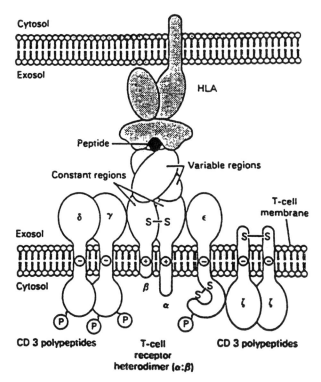

Figure 1 The TCR complex (lower half of the drawing) contains the association of the TCR heterodimer with the CD3 polypeptides. The TCR is activated by antigen when antigen is presented in association with the appropriate HLA molecule (HLA class I pictured) by the antigen-presenting cell (upper half of the drawing). (Modified from Ref. 36.)

presented with self-MHC molecules do not survive (*negative selection*) (2). Mature T cells emerging from the thymus express either CD4 or CD8, along with an αβ-TCR complex. T cells with γδ-TCR may or may not express either CD4 or CD8 and have an unknown function.

Mature T cells, as well as mature B cells, circulate to the secondary lymphoid organs and to sites of inflammation. The lymphocytes home to these sites by utilizing interactions between lymphocyte cell surface adhesion molecules and their corresponding ligands, or *addressins*, on vascular endothelial cells. The adhesion molecules, L-selectin and α4β7, an integrin, together mediate most of the circulation and recirculation of the lymphocytes into lymphoid organs independently of antigenic stimulation (3). For further discussion, see Chapter 9.

T-Cell Receptor Gene Rearrangement Diversity of the TCR is increased by pairing two polypeptide chains that are each the product of genes that have undergone rearrangement in the thymus. Both the α- and β-glycoprotein chains (as well as γ and δ) have an amino(NH_2)-terminal domain, with a variable amino acid sequence, termed the V region, and a carboxy(COOH)-terminal region of constant amino acid sequence, termed the C region. The C region domains secure the receptor to the T-cell membrane, and the V region domains are involved in antigen recognition. The gene that encodes the V region of the α-

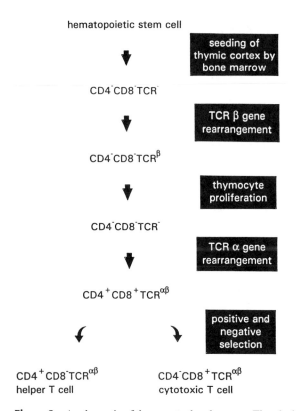

Figure 2   A schematic of thymocyte development. The pluripotent hematopoietic stem cell is seeded from the bone marrow to the thymic cortex. Proliferation of the maturing thymocyte occurs following gene rearrangement and surface expression of the β-chain of the TCR. Subsequent α-chain gene rearrangement allows expression of a functional TCR. Positive and negative selection of the T lymphocyte, based on interactions of the TCR with MHC molecules, results in further thymocyte maturation. Development of helper T cells generally requires MHC class II interactions and, likewise, cytotoxic T cells require MHC class I interactions.

and γ-chains is formed by rearrangement between a V and a J (joining) segment of the gene. Multiple V and J segments are available for recombination. The gene that encodes the V region of the β- and δ-chains is formed by joining a V, a D (diversity), and a J gene segment. After transcription, the message that encodes the VDJ region is brought together, by mRNA splicing, with a message encoding a C region. Studies have shown that β-chain rearrangement precedes α-chain rearrangement. The repertoire of TCRs formed from the gene rearrangements is diverse, permitting recognition of a vast number of antigens.

T-Cell Activation

Antigens processed and presented on the surface of APC in the context of the MHC molecule will be recognized by the appropriate TCR complex. This recognition requires direct cell–cell contact and is strengthened by accessory molecules, such as the adhesion molecule's lymphocyte function-associated antigen (LFA-1 and LFA-2). The ligands for these molecules are, respectively, intracellular adhesion molecules (ICAM-1, ICAM-2, and ICAM-3) for LFA-1, and LFA-3 (CD58) for LFA-2 (CD2). The binding of the processed antigen and MHC molecule to the TCR complex provides a stimulus for T-cell activation. An accessory molecule on the surface of the APC, B7 (CD80) provides a costimulus for T-cell activation. The B7 receptor on the T cell, CD28, generates a second signal within the T-cell for activation when bound by B7 (4). Other ligand–receptor pairs may also participate in T-cell activation.

Appropriate interaction between the T cell and the antigen-bearing APC leads to gene activation that results in cytokine production and T-cell proliferation. The T-cell activation signal is transduced by CD3 and either CD4 or CD8 (5). The biochemical interactions resulting in T-cell activation begin with hydrolysis of phosphatidylinositol biphosphate, a phospholipid in the lipid bilayer, into inositol triphosphate (IP_3) and diacylglycerol (DAG). Calcium moves into the cell partly through the action of IP_3. Calcium and DAG, in turn, activate protein kinase C. Tyrosine kinase is then phosphorylated and activated. Other protein kinases are also activated. Protein kinase activation results in phosphorylation of specific proteins that activate cytoplasmic transcription factors, such as nuclear factors of activated T and pre-B lymphocytes (NF-AT and NF-κB). The cytoplasmic transcription factors are then translocated to the nucleus, where they bind genes important to T-lymphocyte activation (6).

The Major Histocompatibility Complex

The T lymphocytes recognize antigens only when the antigens are presented in noncovalent association with MHC molecules. Cytokines can up-regulate the cell surface expression of MHC molecules; this serves as an important amplification step in the T-cell response. T cells do not interact with soluble, free antigen. Class I and class II MHC molecules are polymorphic membrane-bound proteins that are involved in T-cell recognition of antigen. The class I and class II MHC molecules are part of the HLA system. The designation HLA, which stands for human leukocyte antigen, was derived from studies of the leukocyte antibodies in transfused patients, from which the existence of the system was discovered.

The MHC refers to a region of highly polymorphic genes located on the short arm of chromosome 6: the MHC molecules are—with the exception of B_2-microglobulin, which makes up part of class I molecules—products of these MHC gene loci (Fig. 3) (7). The MHC encodes a variety of proteins in addition to the proteins in the HLA system. The MHC contains regions that encode particular proteins. The class I and class II regions encode the proteins in the HLA system. The class III region encodes C2, C4, and factor B of the complement system as well as heat-shock proteins, and the cytokines tumor necrosis factor (TNF), lymphotoxin B, and lymphotoxin.

The three class I MHC molecules and the three class II MHC molecules that are currently known to be involved in T-cell receptor recognition are HLA-A, HLA-B, and HLA-C; and HLA-DR, HLA-DQ, and HLA-DP, respectively. The genes encoding each of these HLA molecules exist in many different allelic forms in the human population. The *HLA* genes are inherited as a block (a person has one haplotype from each parent) and exhibit codominant expression. Therefore, every person has two different alleles at each locus and may, at a minimum, express six different class I and six different class II proteins.

Class I proteins, expressed on nearly all nucleated cells, are composed of a polymorphic, 44-kDa α-chain from *HLA-A*, *-B*, or *-C* loci and of a nonpolymorphic, 12-kDa polypeptide, $β_2$-microglobulin, encoded on chromosome 15 (Fig. 4). These polypeptide chains are noncovalently associated on the cell surface. The α-chain NH_2-terminal end has two polymorphic domains (α1 and α2) that form a cleft that serves as the antigen-binding site (8). The CD8$^+$ T lymphocyte recognizes antigen presented in association with class I HLA

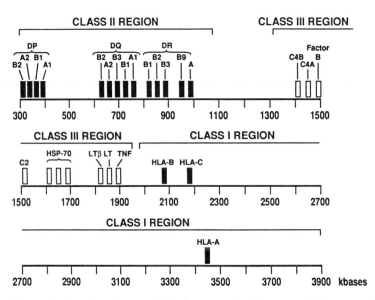

Figure 3 A molecular map of the human major histocompatibility complex. A large number of mostly uncharacterized genes are not depicted. The MHC regions encoding the three classes of proteins are indicated by the brackets. Class III proteins are not involved in antigen presentation. (Modified from Ref. 18, p. 108.)

molecules. Generally, antigen presented in association with class I HLA is endogenously derived, such as that from a viral infection. A third external domain in the α-chain of the class I molecule, α3, contains a nonpolymorphic region that serves as the binding site for CD8 (8).

Class II proteins, normally expressed on B lymphocytes, macrophages, dendritic cells, and endothelial cells, are composed of two noncovalently associated polypeptide chains, an α-chain and a β-chain. Each chain has two external domains, α1 and α2 for the α-chain and β1 and β2 for the β-chain. The NH$_2$-terminal domains, α1 and β1, are polymorphic and combine to form the antigen-binding cleft (9). The CD4$^+$ T lymphocyte recognizes antigen presented in association with class II MHC molecules. In general, antigen presented in association with class II HLA is exogenously derived, such as soluble bacterial antigen. The β2 domain may provide the binding site for CD4 (9).

B Cells

B-Lymphocyte Development

The B lymphocytes were so named because of their maturation in the bursa of Fabricius in birds. In humans, the B cell matures to the resting, inactive B-cell stage in the bone marrow or in the fetal liver. B cells are the only cell type to produce immunoglobulin. Resting B cells leave the bone marrow to further differentiate in specialized regions of peripheral lymphoid organs, such as the periarteriolar lymphoid sheath of the spleen and the germinal centers in lymph nodes. Antigen circulating through the peripheral lymphoid organs can bind specific surface immunoglobulin on the B cell, resulting in activation of the B cell and antibody production. Activated B cells can further differentiate into either plasma cells,

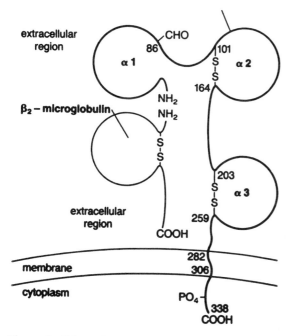

extracellular
region

β₂ – microglobulin

extracellular
region

membrane

cytoplasm

Figure 4   Schematic of the HLA class 1 molecule. The polymorphic α-chain has a transmembrane tail that anchors the molecule to the cell membrane and has three extracellular domains, α1, α2, and α3. α3 associates with β_2-microglobulin and α1 and α2 form a cleft for binding of processed foreign peptides for presentation to T cells. (From Ref. 20, p. 59.)

capable of antibody secretion, or into memory B cells. Memory B cells are cells that, on reexposure to antigen, are responsible for the secondary immune response.

B-cell maturation involves a series of DNA rearrangements, with the formation of cell surface immunoglobulin and other cell surface receptors (Fig. 5). Production of both heavy and light immunoglobulin chains are necessary for cell surface expression of immunoglobulin. The pre-B lymphocyte is the first cell type in B-cell maturation to synthesize an immunoglobulin gene product, the cytoplasmic μ heavy chain. Therefore, the μ heavy chain gene rearrangement and expression precedes light chain expression. The early expression of the μ heavy chain allows positive selection of pre-B lymphocytes (1). As the B cell matures, an immunoglobulin light chain type, κ or λ, is produced and IgM molecules are expressed on the cell surface. The first cells expressing cell surface IgM are called the immature B lymphocytes. These cells are unresponsive to antigen. The first antigen responsive B cell is the mature B cell, which expresses both membrane IgM and IgD. Mature B cells are activated to proliferate and further differentiate in the periphery on exposure to antigen. This further maturation can involve switching to the other heavy chain classes (isotype switching) such as γ, α, and ε. Isotype switching requires the influence of T lymphocytes. Activated B lymphocytes may secrete immunoglobulin, or may persist as immunoglobulin-expressing memory cells. Plasma cells are antibody-secreting cells formed from final differentiation of mature B cells or of memory B cells.

Cell surface markers other than immunoglobulin are present on the B cell at different stages of maturation. CD10, the common acute lymphoblastic leukemia antigen (CALLA),

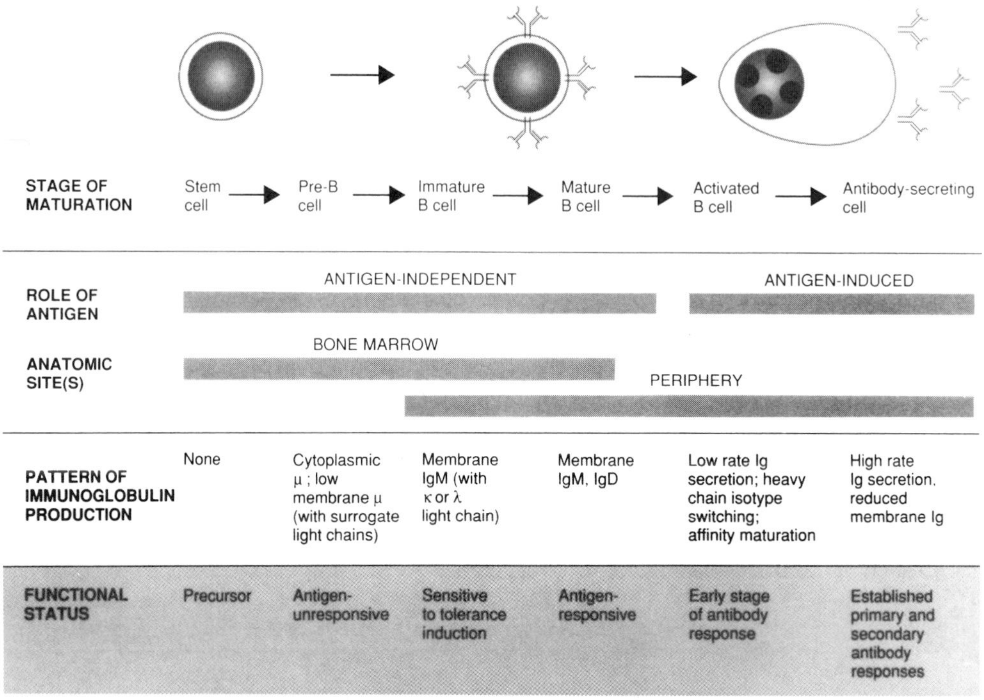
STAGE OF MATURATION
Stem cell
Pre-B cell
Immature B cell
Mature B cell
Activated B cell
Antibody-secreting cell
ROLE OF ANTIGEN
ANTIGEN-INDEPENDENT
ANTIGEN-INDUCED
ANATOMIC SITE(S)
BONE MARROW
PERIPHERY
PATTERN OF IMMUNOGLOBULIN PRODUCTION
None
Cytoplasmic μ ; low membrane μ (with surrogate light chains)
Membrane IgM (with κ or λ light chain)
Membrane IgM, IgD
Low rate Ig secretion; heavy chain isotype switching; affinity maturation
High rate Ig secretion, reduced membrane Ig
FUNCTIONAL STATUS
Precursor
Antigen-unresponsive
Sensitive to tolerance induction
Antigen-responsive
Early stage of antibody response
Established primary and secondary antibody responses

Figure 5 Schematic of B lymphocyte maturation. (From Ref. 18, p. 67.)

is present on the pre-B cell and is subsequently lost (10). First CD19 then CD20 are also found on the pre-B cell, but persist and are found on mature and activated B cells. Immature and mature (although not activated) B cells also express CD21, which is a receptor for a fragment of the complement component, C3 (11,12). CD23, the low-affinity Fc receptor for IgE, and CD25, the IL-2 receptor, are expressed on activated B cells (13). All B cells, except plasma cells, express MHC class II molecules.

Immunoglobulin Gene Rearrangement Immunoglobulins are composed of a heavy polypeptide chain, encoded on chromosome 14, and a light polypeptide chain (λ or κ, encoded on chromosomes 22 and 2, respectively). Each type of polypeptide chain has a variable region, which participates in antigen binding, and a constant region, which participates in other functions of the antibody. The formation of the variable region of the heavy chain requires two gene rearrangements (14) (Fig. 6). With the first, a D (diversity) segment of DNA is joined to a J (joining) segment. Next, one of many possible V (variable) genomic segments is joined to the rearranged DJ segment, and the resulting *VDJ* gene encodes the variable region of the heavy chain for that B cell. The genomic segments encoding each possible constant region follow the rearranged *VDJ* gene on the chromosome. The initial transcription produces a primary transcript that can be spliced to form RNA encoding either the δ or the μ heavy chain. Therefore, each heavy chain from a particular B cell has the same variable domain.

A change from the μ or δ heavy chain to another heavy chain class requires B-cell activation. This process, called *class switching*, involves either another DNA rearrangement to move a different heavy chain constant gene into the position adjacent to the *VDJ*

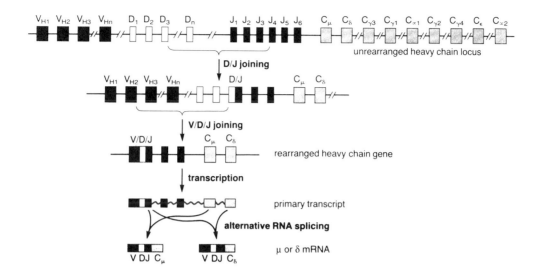

Figure 6 Schematic of the initial heavy chain immunoglobulin gene rearrangements. The DJ joining is followed by rearrangement of a variable (V) DNA sequence. Only C_μ and C_δ are initially transcribed. Class switching, or change from the μ or δ heavy chain to another heavy chain type, requires a third gene rearrangement. (From Ref. 37.)

gene, or alternative mRNA splicing (15). The VDJ region remains unchanged so that the antigen specificity of the immunoglobulin remains unchanged. The CD40 ligand on the B cell interacts with the CD40 ligand receptor on the T cell to enable this switch (16). The B-cell microenvironment can influence class switching. The environment in the Peyer's patches favors the switch to the heavy chain constant region of IgA, and IL-4 promotes the switch to IgE production (17).

Immunoglobulin light chain rearrangement follows the initial heavy chain rearrangement during B-cell maturation. The process is the same for the κ and λ light chains. Before rearrangement, the κ-chain locus contains a single constant segment (C_κ) with multiple V and J genomic segments. As with heavy chain rearrangement, a single V segment is juxtaposed with a single J segment to form the *VJ* gene encoding the variable region of the light chain. Splicing of mRNA results in the joining of the light chain constant region transcript to the variable region transcript. Whereas the κ light chain has only one genomic segment encoding the constant region of the polypeptide, the λ light chain has up to six constant genomic segments (producing various subtypes of λ polypeptide), each with nearby J regions.

The light chain genes are located on different chromosomes. V/J joining is attempted at each chromosome 2 or 22 in succession until a functional κ or λ gene is produced. Once a functional light chain gene is produced, V/J joining ceases so that a single B cell produces only one light chain type, a phenomenon called *allelic exclusion* (18). Although in a given individual, two chromosomes exist with loci for the heavy chain and two chromosomes exist with loci for each (κ or λ) light chain, the successful rearrangement of a single light chain or heavy chain gene prevents other genes of the same type from undergoing rearrangement in the same cell. Therefore, only one heavy chain gene and one light chain gene can give rise to expressed immunoglobulin in any given B cell. This phenomenon is termed *isotype exclusion*. As a given B lymphocyte divides, all progeny retain the original antigen specificity and light chain type. Diversity of antibody results, in part, from the large number of B-cell precursors undergoing independent gene rearrangement.

Core Immunoglobulin Structure   Immunoglobulin core design pairs two heavy chain polypeptides with two light chain polypeptides to form the four-chain basic immunoglobulin unit (Fig. 7). The heavy chain is linked to the light chain by noncovalent forces and by a single covalent disulfide bond. The NH$_2$-terminal end of the heavy and light chain pair—termed antigen-binding fragment (Fab)—contains the variable domains that associate to form the antigen-binding site. The four-chain complex contains two antigen-binding sites and is said to be divalent. Antigen binding occurs when antigen is paired with immunoglobulin that has a binding surface complementary to the antigen configuration. The COOH-terminal end of the basic unit, which contains only heavy chain constant regions, is termed the crystalline fragment (Fc) portion of the molecule. The Fc portion can function to bind cell surface receptors and, in certain immunoglobulin classes, to bind complement.

Immunoglobulin heavy chain type and light chain type are defined by the constant region of the polypeptide. Immunoglobulins with the same constant regions are called *isotypes*. Again, two light chain isotypes exist, κ and λ. Five heavy chain isotypes exist: α, γ, μ, ε, and δ. The specific heavy chain isotype confers conformation and function for the class of immunoglobulin: IgA, IgG, IgM, IgE, and IgD, respectively.

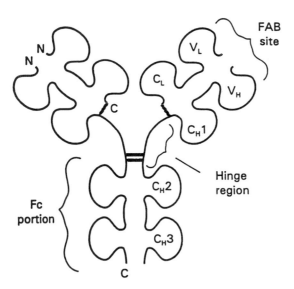

Figure 7   Schematic of the structure of the basic immunoglobulin unit. Immunoglobulin glycoproteins consist of two identical heavy chains and two identical light chains. The NH$_2$-terminal ends (N) are characterized by significant sequence variability in the heavy and light chain variable domains, referred to as V$_H$ and V$_L$, respectively. The association of the V$_H$ and V$_L$ forms the Fab site capable of antigen binding. The remaining portion of the molecule, including the COOH-terminus (C), has a relatively constant structure. The constant portion of the light chain is designated C$_L$ and the constant regions of the heavy chain are termed C$_H$1, C$_H$2, and C$_H$3. The hinge region is a site of protein flexibility, located between the C$_H$1 and C$_H$2 domains. The Fc portion is formed by the regions of the heavy chain that are below the hinge region. Interchain disulfide bonds (depicted by hatched lines) may vary between different immunoglobulin classes and subclasses. (From Ref. 38.)

Immunoglobulin Classes Immunoglobulin of all classes can exist in the membrane-bound or in the secreted form. The membrane-bound form is similar to the four-chain basic unit, with an additional transmembrane tail that anchors the immunoglobulin: IgG, IgA, IgE, and IgD can also be secreted in this basic form (i.e., can be secreted as a monomer). Immunoglobulin-A also exists as a dimer and, as a dimer with an additional secretory component, can be secreted onto mucosal surfaces. Secreted IgM exists as a pentamer. The J (joining) chain, which is a low molecular weight glycoprotein, facilitates polymerization of IgA and IgM.

Immunoglobulin-G is the predominant class of immunoglobulin in the serum. The average half-life of IgG is approximately 3 weeks. IgG exhibits multiple functions. During the secondary humoral immune response to invaders, such as microbes or toxins, IgG is the predominant class of immunoglobulin produced to bind antigen. It can also bind to cells with Fc receptors to function in antigen binding. Binding of secreted IgG onto Fc receptors on macrophages or natural killer cells allows these cells to bind antigen and carry out antibody-dependent cell-mediated cytotoxicity. Antibody-coated antigens are said to be *opsonized*. Opsonization enhances phagocytosis by the binding of opsonized particles through Fc receptors on phagocytes. IgG also activates complement through binding of the complement component, C1q. It is the only immunoglobulin to cross the placenta to provide antibody protection to newborn infants.

Within the IgG class, four different subclasses exist, IgG1, IgG2, IgG3, and IgG4, defined by small variations in the Fc portion of the heavy chain. The differences in the Fc portion of the heavy chain affect function (19). Immunoglobulin-G2 is transferred across the placenta less efficiently than the other IgG subclasses; IgG3 fixes complement most effectively (IgG3 > IgG1 > IgG2 > IgG4).

Immunoglobulin-A is a major component of immunity at mucosal surfaces, including those in the gastrointestinal, genitourinary, and respiratory tracts. Two subclasses, IgA1 and IgA2, are present in a 5:1 ratio in blood (20).

Immunoglobulin-M is the first antibody formed as a result of primary infection. It can activate complement by activation of the classic complement pathway. Isohemagglutinins, cold agglutinins, and heterophil antibodies all are IgM antibodies.

Immunoglobulin-E is the class of antibody that participates in immediate hypersensitivity reactions. It functions in atopy by attaching to mast cells, basophils, and eosinophils through binding of the Fc receptors and, then, by binding antigen. Mediators released from these cells when antigen is bound to attached IgE produce the symptoms of immediate hypersensitivity. IgE is normally present in small amounts in the serum; however, the amount of IgE in the serum may be increased in persons with atopy. With allergy to certain antigens, amounts of antigen-specific IgE may be increased in the peripheral blood.

The B-cell production of IgE is influenced by particular cytokines. Recent evidence supports the existence of a subset of $CD4^+$ T lymphocytes, T_H2 lymphocytes, that promotes B-cell formation of IgE through selective cytokine production (21,22). Interleukin-5 (IL-5) is known to stimulate B-lymphocyte heavy chain class switch to ϵ. T-lymphocyte regulation of IgE production will be discussed in detail in Chapter 9.

Immunoglobulin-D is present in very low concentration in the blood. The function of IgD is unclear.

B-Cell Activation

B-cell activation is initiated by the binding of antigen by immunoglobulin present on the B-cell surface. Antigen alone can activate B cells independent of T-cell help if the antigen is able to interact with multiple immunoglobulin proteins on the surface of the B cell, resulting in the cross-linking of surface immunoglobulin (i.e., with antigens, such as polymeric proteins or polysaccharides). Most antigens in nature do not cross-link surface immunoglobulin and activate B lymphocytes by binding surface immunoglobulin, with simultaneous stimulation of B cells by lymphokines secreted by nearby, activated T lymphocytes. Following the binding of antigen to the B-cell receptor, a series of G-proteins are activated that, in turn, activate phospholipase C. The resulting cascade of events results in increased intracellular calcium concentration, the phosphorylation and activation of protein kinase C, and the liberation of arachidonic acid from membrane phospholipids. Activation of B cells results in gene activation, in production of proteins, and in proliferation (23–25). An activated, proliferating B cell can differentiate into a plasma cell or can become a memory B cell.

Large Granular Lymphocytes

Large granular lymphocytes (LGLs) make up 2–5% of the lymphocytes in the peripheral blood. These lymphocytes lack most of the cell surface markers found on B or T lymphocytes, and they lack T-cell receptors. Markers found on LGLs include CD2, CD16, and CD56 (26). The LGLs have several functions. They are also called natural killer (NK) cells secondary to their ability to lyse a variety of tumor cells and virus-infected cells, without specific antigen stimulation. CD16 acts as an Fc receptor for IgG allowing LGLs to function in antibody-dependent cell-mediated cytotoxicity. The LGLs can be stimulated by IL-2 to become lymphokine-activated killer (LAK) cells, which have enhanced cytolytic function and are active in tumor surveillance.

MYELOID DERIVED CELLS

In contrast with lymphocytes, which provide specific, genetically determined immune response to antigen, immune cells derived from the myeloid progenitor cell provide nonspecific, controlled inflammatory response to antigen. Basophils, mast cells, and eosinophils are derived from the myeloid progenitor. The myeloid progenitor can also differentiate into the granulocyte–monocyte progenitor from which monocytes and neutrophils are derived.

All hemotopoiesis occurs under the influence of the surrounding microenvironment. Two families of polypeptide hormones, the interleukins (ILs) and the colony-stimulating factors (CSFs), serve a major role in control of hematopoiesis. Interleukin-3 and granulocyte–monocyte colony-stimulating factor (GM-CSF) enhance the production and maturation of all myeloid cell types. Specific maturation of granulocytes is enhanced by granulocyte colony-stimulating factor (G-CSF) and of monocytes by monocyte colony-stimulating factor (M-CSF). Interleukin-5 amplifies eosinophil maturation.

Neutrophils

Neutrophils function as the primary cell in the acute inflammatory response. Mature cells, also called polymorphonuclear leukocytes (PNLs), contain a multilobed nucleus and storage granules in the cytoplasm. The storage granules confer the ability to digest engulfed particles by means of intracellular degranulation. Neutrophils can also degranulate into the extracellular space. Extracellular degranulation allows targeting of particles that are too large to engulf. Storage granules include the characteristic azurophilic granules that contain acid hydrolases, myeloperoxidase, and lysozyme, and secondary granules that contain lactoferrin and lysozyme. Complement and IgG interact with the neutrophil through their ability to opsonize invading particles, particularly encapsulated bacteria. Neutrophils contain Fc receptors and complement receptors for binding and engulfment of opsonized particles.

Neutrophils have many surface receptors that permit their rapid recruitment to sites of tissue invasion or injury. Chemotactic factors are detected by neutrophils in the peripheral blood and by vessel endothelial cells, resulting in changes in cell membrane molecules that allow *margination*, or attachment of the neutrophil to the vessel wall, and *emigration*, or movement of the neutrophil through the vessel and into tissue. The selectin family of adhesion molecules participates in the initial tethering of the neutrophil to the vessel wall (27). Through a series of selectin–ligand attachments, the neutrophil is able to roll along the vessel wall in the direction of the blood flow. L-selectin is expressed on neutrophils; P-selectin and E-selectin are expressed on endothelial cell surfaces during inflammation. Firm adhesion of the neutrophil to the vessel wall is possible with expression and activation of the β_2-integrin family of adhesion molecules on the neutrophil surface. LFA-1 and Mac-1 are β_2-integrins on neutrophils that interact with appropriate ligands on endothelial cells. ICAM-1, which interacts with both LFA-1 and Mac-1, is one of a number of integrin ligands. Following firm adhesion, neutrophils migrate between endothelial cells and move up chemotactic factor gradients to sites of tissue injury or infection.

Monocytes and Macrophages

Mononuclear phagocytes reside in most tissues in the body. These residential phagocytes begin as circulating monocytes. Monocytes constitute 0–4% of circulating leukocytes in normal adults. Once out of the bloodstream and settled into tissue, monocytes are referred to as macrophages or histiocytes. Macrophages have specific names when residing in certain tissue: Langerhans cells in skin; Kupffer cells in liver; osteoclasts in bone; and microglia in the central nervous system. The mononuclear phagocytes function to promote inflammation through cytokine production, and they serve as antigen-presenting cells in addition to their role as phagocytes. The mononuclear phagocytes are activated for phagocytosis in multiple ways, including direct contact with certain antigens. These cells also have receptors for opsonins, such as complement and immunoglobulin. When serving as an antigen-presenting cell, the monocyte–macrophage processes the internalized antigen and presents a fragment of the antigen on its cell surface in association with the appropriate class MHC molecule. Mononuclear phagocytes express both MHC class I and II antigens and can present to either CD4+ or CD8+ lymphocytes.

Basophils and Mast Cells

Basophils and mast cells, which normally constitute 0–1% of the leukocytes in the peripheral blood, are characterized by the presence of high-affinity cell surface receptors for the Fc portion of IgE and play important roles in allergy. Basophils are circulating cells that stain blue with Wright stain; mast cells are found only in tissue. Both contain granules with histamine. Degranulation occurs, resulting in allergic symptoms when IgE is cross-linked on the cell surface by allergen.

Eosinophils

Eosinophils, which normally constitute 0–3% of the circulating leukocytes, are granulocytes with a bilobed nucleus and characteristic eosinophilic granules in the cytoplasm. Eosinophils participate in allergic disease and in the immune response to parasitic infection. Eosinophils express low affinity Fc receptors for IgE and are the principal effector cell of antibody-dependent cell-mediated cytotoxicity against helminthic infections. Eosinophils are also found in large numbers during the late phase of allergic reactions. Regulation of proliferation may be under the control of the $T_H 2$ subset of T cells that is thought to regulate IgE synthesis through selective cytokine production. The activated eosinophil appears larger and "hypodense" by microscopy. The major proteins in the eosinophilic granule are major basic protein and eosinophil cationic protein. The cytokine IL-5 activates the eosinophil and augments eosinophil production (for further discussion of eosinophils, see Chap. 10).

OTHER COMPONENTS OF THE IMMUNE RESPONSE

Complement

Complement is a term used to designate a group of proteins, derived from a cascade of cleavage events, that plays a vital role in the immune response. The early components in the cascade, which exist in the serum in an inactive form, are produced in the liver and, to a lesser extent, by fibroblasts and monocytes. The two major pathways of activation and cleavage—the classic pathway and the alternative pathway—result in proteins that are active in opsonization, as chemoattractants, in cell lysis, and as anaphylatoxins. Anaphylatoxins promote degranulation of mast cells and basophils with release of histamine and other vasoactive substances, causing capillary leakage, thereby promoting entry of inflammatory cells into the tissue compartment. Complement activation plays important roles in inflammation and clearance of foreign substances.

The Classic Pathway

The classic and alternative cascades differ in their initial phases, but share common components in the later part of the cascade (Fig. 8). The classic pathway is typically initiated by antigen–antibody complexes, whereas the alternative pathway is typically activated by bacteria, without antibody.

The classic cascade begins with the activation of C1, the first component of the pathway (28). Either a single molecule of IgM, or two molecules of IgG (of the subclass type that can activate complement), in a side-by-side association bound to antigen, can activate C1. C1 is composed of three different proteins, C1q and two chains each of C1r and C1s. C1q binds to the Fc portion of IgM or to the IgG Fc side-by-side arrangement (subclasses 1, 2, and 3 only). Certain bacteria and viruses can also bind C1q directly to result in initiation of this cascade. C1r and C1s are proteolytic enzymes: C1r activates C1s which, in turn, activates the next complement component, C4. C4 is cleaved by C1, and the smaller product, C4a is released; C4b is bound. C2 can bind C4b and is cleaved by C1 with the release of C2b. The C14b2a complex, called C3 convertase, can now bind and activate C3. C3a and C3b are formed by this activation, and C3a is released. C3b can bind to C4b2a and the cascade can continue, or the bound C3b can act as an opsonin. Instead of binding C4b, C3b can interact with other IgG molecules to provide opsonization. Particles opsonized with C3b can be cleared by cells carrying C3b receptors (called CR1). Unbound C3b is quickly inactivated by water in the tissue. The complexed C4b2a3b serves to cleave C5 and is called the classic pathway C5 convertase. C5a is released and C5b remains associated with the convertase.

The activity of C5b is the same in both pathways. As C5b has no covalent attachment to the antigen or to the complex, it is rapidly inactivated, unless bound by the next component, C6. Components C7, C8, and C9 are then bound in succession to form the membrane-attack

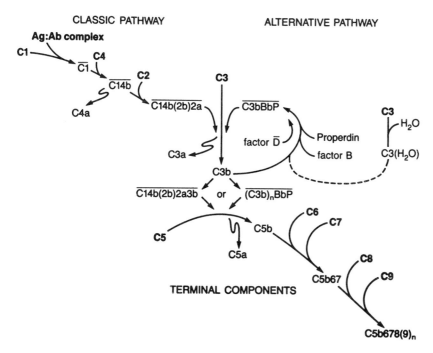

Figure 8   The complement cascade. See text for description. (From Ref. 28.)

complex (MAC) that causes cell lysis by creating a pore in the cell membrane. Multiple molecules of C9 may participate in the formation of the MAC [C5b678(9)$_n$].

The fragments released during cleavage include C3a, C4a, and C5a. These fragments act as anaphylatoxins. C5a can also act as a chemotactic factor.

The Alternative Pathway

The alternative pathway provides an important mechanism for complement activation independent of antibody. C3 can undergo hydrolysis and can bind water to form C3(H$_2$O). This hydrolysis may occur spontaneously at a low level. The C3(H$_2$O) then binds factor B. This complex is acted on by factor D, and factor B is cleaved. The remaining complex has C3 convertase activity and cleaves C3 to form highly active C3b. If foreign particles are present, the C3b formed can bind the particle and factor B can be bound and activated (by factor D activity). Then C3bBb is stabilized by binding another protein, properdin, forming the C3 convertase of the alternative pathway, C3bBbP. Attachment of additional C3b molecules forms the C5 convertase of the alternate pathway (C3b)$_n$BbP. C5 convertase cleaves C5 to initiate formation of the MAC.

Complement Control Mechanisms

Multiple factors in the complement system serve to regulate complement activity and control inflammation in attempt to prevent damage of self. C1 inhibitor (C1INH), also active in regulation in the kinin-generating system, inactivates C1r and C1s. C4b is inactivated by factor I. C4-binding protein enhances the C4b inactivation by factor I. Factor I, with a cofactor, factor H, also inactivates C3b and C3(H$_2$O). Degradation by factors H and I results in the formation of inactive C3b (iC3b), which can act as an opsonin. Further

Table 1 Cytokines: Their Sources and Effects

Cytokine	Principal cell source	Principal effects[a]
IL-1α and β	Macrophages, other APCs, other somatic cells	Costimulation of APCs and T cells; B-cell proliferation and IgG production; acute-phase response of the liver; phagocyte activation; inflammation and fever; hematopoiesis
IL-2	Activated T_H1 cells, cytotoxic T cells (Tc), NK cells	Proliferation of activated T cells; NK and Tc cell functions; B-cell proliferation and IgG2 expression
IL-3	T lymphocytes	Growth of early hematopoietic progenitors
IL-4	T_H2 cells, mast cells	B-cell proliferation, IgE expression, and class II MHC expression; T_H2 and Tc cell proliferation and functions; eosinophil and mast cell growth and function; inhibits macrophage activation and cytokine production
IL-5	T_H2 cells, mast cells	Eosinophil growth and production
IL-6	Activated T_H2 cells, APCs, other somatic cells	Synergistic effects with IL-1 or TNF to costimulate T cells; acute-phase response of the liver; B-cell proliferation and Ig production; thrombopoiesis
IL-7	Thymic and marrow stromal cells	B and T lymphopoiesis; Tc cell functions
IL-8	Macrophages, other somatic cells	Chemoattractant for neutrophils and T cells
IL-9	Cultured T cells	Some hematopoietic and thymopoietic effects
IL-10	Activated T_H2 cells, CD8 T cells, and B lymphocytes, macrophages	Inhibition of cytokine production by T_H1 cells, NK cells, and APCs; promotion of B-cell proliferation and antibody responses; suppression of cellular immunity; mast cell growth
IL-11	Stromal cells	Synergistic effects on hematopoiesis and thrombopoiesis
IL-12	B cells, macrophages	Proliferation and function of activated Tc cells and NK cells; IFN-γ production; T_H1 cell induction; suppression of T_H2 cell functions; promotion of cell-mediated immune responses
IL-13	T_H2 cells	IL-4-like effects
IL-14 (39)	T cells	B-cell proliferation; inhibits immunoglobulin secretion
IL-15 (40)	Monocytes, other somatic cells (41)	Proliferation of T lymphocytes
TNF-α	Activated macrophages, other somatic cells	IL-1-like effects; vascular thrombosis and tumor necrosis
TNF-β or lymphotoxin	Activated T_H1 cells	IL-1-like effects; vascular thrombosis and tumor necrosis
IFN-α and -β	Macrophages, neutrophils, other somatic cells	Antiviral effects; induction of class I MHC on all somatic cells; activation of macrophages and NK cells

Table 1 Continued

Cytokine	Principal cell source	Principal effects[a]
IFN-γ	Activated T_H1 cells and NK cells	Induction of class I MHC on all somatic cells; induction of class II MHC on APCs and somatic cells; activation of macrophages, neutrophils, and NK cells; promotion of cell-mediated immunity; promotion of changes in vascular endothelial cells favoring T-cell adhesion and extravasation; antiviral effects
TGF-β	Activated T lymphocytes, platelets, macrophages, other somatic cells	Anti-inflammatory; antiproliferative for macrophages and lymphocytes; promotion of B-cell expression of IgA; promotion of fibroblast proliferation and wound healing

[a]All of the listed processes are enhanced unless otherwise indicated.
Source: Modified from Ref. 42.

degradation forms C3dg which has immune regulatory properties. Another control protein, S protein (or vitronectin), inhibits the lysis of cells by the MAC (28). Cell lysis by complement is also inhibited by C8-binding protein and CD59.

Cytokines

The complex network of cells involved in immunity communicate through the activity of cytokines. Cytokines are, for the most part, soluble proteins that mediate specific immune and nonspecific inflammatory responses by acting as regulators and as stimulators of growth. General properties shared by cytokines include the following: a single cytokine can mediate multiple effector functions; a single cytokine can act on multiple cell types; multiple different cytokines can produce the same function; multiple sources can produce the same cytokine; and cytokines can influence the production and action of other cytokines. Several chapters in this book will detail the activity of specific cytokines and their relation to allergic diseases. The following discussion provides an overview of cytokines as mediators of nonspecific inflammation and as mediators of lymphocytes and specific immunity (Table 1).

Cytokines in Nonspecific Inflammation

Tumor necrosis factor (TNF) is the principal cytokine released in response to lipopolysaccharide (LPS), which is released during gram-negative bacterial infection (29). Two forms of TNF exist, TNF-α and TNF-β. The major source of TNF-α is the mononuclear phagocyte that has been activated by LPS, although T cells, NK cells, and mast cells can release TNF-α when activated. The exclusive source of TNF-β is the T cell. Both TNF-α and TNF-β promote inflammation by up-regulating adhesion molecules on vascular endothelial cells and by activating neutrophils. Also, TNF-α promotes inflammation by activating macrophages and eosinophils and by increasing the release of IL-1 and IL-6. Both TNF-α and TNF-β are important in the immune response to viruses and up-regulate MHC class I molecules on virally infected cells to promote lysis of these cells. TNF-α is an endogenous pyrogen and produces cachexia. It promotes shock by reducing cardiac contractility, decreasing vascular tone, and by promoting vascular thrombosis.

Interleukin-1 is similar in activity to TNF-α (30). It is primarily produced by activated mononuclear phagocytes, although IL-1 is also produced by endothelial and epithelial cells. It acts as an endogenous pyrogen and mediates septic shock.

Interferon (IFN)-α and IFN-β are cytokines important in immunity against viruses. Both inhibit viral replication and inhibit cell proliferation. Also, both increase the expression of class I MHC molecules, enhancing cytolytic T-cell activity, and inhibit class II MHC molecule expression. Interferon-α is principally produced by mononuclear phagocytes, and IFN-β is principally produced by fibroblasts.

Cytokines as Mediators of Lymphocytes and Specific Immunity

Interferon-γ also induces an antiviral state and increases class I MHC expression. However, IFN-γ differs from IFN-α and IFN-β in that IFN-γ increases the expression of class II MHC molecules promoting T-helper cell activation. It activates macrophages and also promotes the differentiation of T and B lymphocytes: IFN-γ promotes the activity of TNF.

The major cytokine stimulating T-cell growth is IL-2. This cytokine is released by T cells to stimulate proliferation of the producing as well as surrounding T cells. The activity of IL-2 is markedly enhanced following T-cell activation. This effect is partly mediated by the up-regulation of a protein that serves as a portion of the IL-2 receptor, namely, IL-2Rα, during T-cell activation (31). It also stimulates the growth and activity of B cells and NK cells.

Interleukin-4 is a major cytokine, promoting the allergic response. It promotes the proliferation of T cells, especially T_H2 cells, promotes class switch of B cells to production of IgE, and promotes mast cell growth (30). Interleukin-4 (as well as IL-10) inhibits macrophage activation and inhibits the effects of INF-γ on macrophages.

Transforming growth factor-β (TGF-β) acts as a negative regulator of immunity (32). It is produced by macrophages and T lymphocytes and has antiproliferative effects on T cells, B cells, macrophages, and endothelial cells.

Other cytokines important in inflammation include IL-5 and IL-12. Interleukin-5 is produced by T cells and functions mainly in stimulation of proliferation and activation of eosinophils. Interleukin-12 activates NK cells and promotes the proliferation of activated T cells.

T_H-Cell Subsets

Subsets of T_H cells exist that differ both in their pattern of cytokine production and in their response to certain cytokines (21,33). Two T_H subsets have now been delineated in humans. The pattern of cytokine production and the T_H subset response to specific cytokines orchestrates the immune response following presentation of the antigen to the T_H cell. T_H1 cells secrete IL-2 and IFN-γ and are associated with cell-mediated immune responses (21,33). T_H2 cells secrete IL-4 and IL-5 and are associated with allergy and antibody production (22,34). T_H0 cells, described in the murine model, can secrete all of the cytokines produced by T_H1 and T_H2 cells (35).

SUMMARY

Over 2 centuries ago, Edward Jenner discovered that a protective response against disease could be induced in a person through vaccination. Since that time, the study of the immune system has evolved. Current knowledge of the immune system is rapidly expanding in this era of high technology and deadly immunodeficiency. Relatively recent discoveries that have furthered our understanding of the immune mechanism have included the molecular mechanisms for diversity, cell markers enabling cell-to-cell communication, mechanisms for intracellular signal transduction, and the actions of certain cytokines. As basic knowledge of the immune system increases, so increases our ability to comprehend and treat dysfunction of the immune system, such as allergic disease.

REFERENCES

1. von Boehmer H. Positive selection of lymphocytes. Cell 1994; 76:219–228.
2. Nossal GJ. Negative selection of lymphocytes. Cell 1994; 76:229–239.
3. Weissman IL. Developmental switches in the immune system. Cell 1994; 76:207–218.
4. Jenkins MK, Taylor PS, Norton SD, Urdahl KB. CD28 delivers a costimulatory signal involved in antigen-specific IL-2 production by human T cells. J Immunol 1991; 147:2461–2466.
5. Beyers AD, Spruyt LL, Williams AF. Molecular associations between the T-lymphocyte antigen receptor complex and the surface antigens CD2, CD4, or CD8 and CD5. Proc Natl Acad Sci USA 1992; 89:2945–2949.
6. Weiss A, Littman DR. Signal transduction by lymphocyte antigen receptors. Cell 1994; 76: 263–274.
7. Campbell RD, Trowsdale J. Map of the human MHC. Immunol Today 1993; 14:349–352.
8. Matsumura M, Fremont DH, Peterson PA, Wilson IA. Emerging principles for the recognition of peptide antigens by MHC class I molecules. Science 1992; 257:927–934.
9. Brown JH, Jardetzky TS, Gorga JC, et al. Three-dimensional structure of the human class II histocompatibility antigen HLA-DR1. Nature 1993; 364:33–39.
10. Huston DP, Kavanaugh AF, Rohane PW, Huston MM. Immunoglobulin deficiency syndromes and therapy. J Allergy Clin Immunol 1991; 87:1–17.
11. Thornton BP, Vetvicka V, Ross GD. Natural antibody and complement-mediated antigen processing and presentation by B lymphocytes. J Immunol 1994; 152:1727–1737.
12. Ross GD, Winchester RJ, Rabellino EM, Hoffman T. Surface markers of complement receptor lymphocytes. J Clin Invest 1978; 62:1086–1092.
13. Banchereau J, Rousset F. Human B lymphocytes: phenotype, proliferation, and differentiation. Adv Immunol 1992; 62:125–262.
14. Schatz DG, Oettinger MA, Schlissel MS. V(D)J recombination: molecular biology and regulation. Annu Rev Immunol 1992; 10:359–383.
15. Esser C, Radbruch A. Immunoglobulin class switching: molecular and cellular analysis. Annu Rev Immunol 1990; 8:717–735.
16. Allen RC, Armitage RJ, Conley ME, et al. CD40 ligand gene defects responsible for X-linked hyper-IgM syndrome. Science 1993; 259:990–993.
17. Romagnani S. Regulation and deregulation of human IgE synthesis. Immunol Today 1990; 11:316–321.
18. Abbas AK, Lichtman AH, Pober JS. Cellular and Molecular Immunology. 2nd ed. Philadelphia: WB Saunders, 1994.
19. Spiegelberg HL. Biological activities of immunoglobulins of different classes and subclasses. Adv Immunol 1974; 19:259–294.
20. Goodman JW, Parslow TG. Immunoglobulin proteins. In: Stites DP, Terr AI, Parslow TG, eds. Basic and Clinical Immunology. 8th ed. Norwalk: Appleton & Lange, 1994:66–79.
21. Mosmann TR, Coffman RL. Heterogeneity of cytokine secretion patterns and functions of helper T cells. Adv Immunol 1989; 46:111–147.
22. Wierenga EA, Snoek M, deGroot C, et al. Evidence for compartmentalization of functional subsets of CD2+ lymphocytes in atopic patients. J Immunol 1990; 144(12):4651–4656.

23. Schulam PG, Shearer WT. Evidence for 5-lipoxygenase activity in human B cell lines. A possible role for arachidonic acid metabolites during B cell signal transduction. J Immunol 1990; 144:2696–2701.

24. Schulam PG, Kuruvilla A, Putcha G, Mangus L, Franklin-Johnson J, Shearer WT. Platelet-activating factor induces phospholipid turnover, calcium flux, arachidonic acid liberation, eicosanoid generation, and oncogene expression in a human B cell line. J Immunol 1991; 146:1642–1648.

25. Mazer B, Domenico J, Sawami H, Gelfand EW. Platelet-activating factor induces an increase in intracellular calcium and expression of regulatory genes in human B lymphoblastoid cells. J Immunol 1991; 146:1914–1920.

26. Trinchieri G. Biology of natural killer cells. Adv Immunol 1989; 47:187–376.

27. Springer TA. Traffic signals for lymphocyte recirculation and leukocyte emigration: the multistep paradigm. Cell 1994; 76:301–314.

28. Frank MM. Complement and kinin. In: Stites DP, Terr AI, Parslow TG, eds. Basic and Clinical Immunology. 8th ed. Norwalk: Appleton & Lange, 1994:124–136.

29. Vassalli P. The pathophysiology of tumor necrosis factors. Annu Rev Immunol 1992; 10: 411–452.

30. Arai KI, Lee F, Miyajima A, Miyatake S, Arai N, Yokota T. Cytokines: coordinators of immune and inflammatory responses. Annu Rev Biochem 1990; 59:783–836.

31. Minami Y, Kono T, Miyazaki T, Taniguchi T. The IL-2 receptor complex: its structure, function, and target genes. Annu Rev Immunol 1993; 11:245–268.

32. Palladino MA, Morris RE, Starnes HF, Levinson AD. The transforming growth factor-betas. A new family of immunoregulatory molecules. Ann NY Acad Sci 1990; 593:181–1887.

33. Mosmann TR. Cytokine patterns during the progression to AIDS. Science 1994; 265:193–194.

34. Robinson D, Hamid Q, Bentley A, Ying S, Kay AB, Durham SR. Activation of CD4+ T cells, increased T_H2-type cytokine mRNA expression, and eosinophil recruitment in bronchoalveolar lavage after allergen inhalation challenge in patients with atopic asthma. J Allergy Clin Immunol 1993; 92:313–324.

35. Firestein GS, Roeder WD, Laxer JA, et al. A new murine CD4+ T cell subset with an unrestricted cytokine profile. J Immunol 1989; 143:518–525.

36. Krensky AM, Weiss A, et al. T-lymphocyte–antigen interactions in transplant rejection. N Engl J Med 1990; 322:510–517.

37. Parslow TG. Immunoglobulin genes, B cells and the humoral immune response. In: Stites DP, Terr AI, Parslow TG, eds. Basic and Clinical Immunology, 8th ed. Norwalk: Appleton & Lange, 1994:83.

38. Sandberg E, Shearer WT. Normal immune responses. In: Bierman CW, Pearlman DS, Shapiro GE, Busse WW, eds. Allergy, Clinical Immunology, and Asthma Management in Infants, Children, and Adults, 3rd ed. Philadelphia: WB Saunders, 1996: 1–19.

39. Ambrus JL Jr, Pippin J, et al. Identification of a cDNA for a human-high-molecular-weight B-cell growth factor. Proc Natl Acad Sci USA 1993; 90:6330–6334.

40. Grabstein KH, Eisenman J, et al. Cloning of a T cell growth factor that interacts with the β-chain of the interleukin-2 receptor. Science 1994; 264:965–968.

41. Armitage RJ, Macduff BM, Eisenman J, Paxton R, Grabstein KH. IL-15 has stimulatory activity for the induction of B cell proliferation and differentiation. J Immunol 1995; 154:483–490.

42. Oppenheim JJ, et al. Cytokines. In: Stites DP, Terr AI, Parslow TG, eds. Basic and Clinical Immunology. 8th ed. Norwalk: Appleton & Lange, 1994:105–123.

6

Inflammatory Cell Differentiation and Maturation in Allergic Reactions

Judah A. Denburg and Brian F. Leber
McMaster University, Hamilton, Ontario, Canada

INTRODUCTION

The presence of specific types of granulocytes in inflammatory allergic type reactions is well known. Specifically, eosinophilic infiltration into tissues, such as the airways, in patients with allergic rhinitis and asthma constitutes a constant and almost pathognomonic feature. Likewise, the presence of mast cells in various types of allergic reactions in the skin and mucous membranes places this cell, as well as its related blood-borne counterpart, the basophil, in a unique position to carry out specific roles in allergic inflammation. How eosinophils, basophils, and mast cells get to tissue sites continues to be an area of fruitful exploration in the investigation of allergy's pathogenesis. Recent evidence that all three of these mature inflammatory cells are the targets not only of specific hematopoietic cytokines, but also produce an array of cytokines themselves after activation, has led to an awareness of the increasing complexity of the cytokine–inflammatory cell circuitry in allergic inflammation. A particular focus of the research done in our laboratory has been the differentiation and maturation of these effector cells and the contribution of these hematopoietic processes to the final inflammatory reaction in the tissues. In this chapter, general issues related to hematopoiesis and progenitor–progeny relationships will be raised, and then specifically applied to inflammatory cell (eosinophil, basophil, and mast cell) progenitors, and their differentiation and maturation into cells present during allergic reactions. A fundamental hypothesis is that the bone marrow produces an increased supply of progenitors of these inflammatory cells during allergic processes as a consequence of feedback mechanisms from local tissue sites.

GENERAL ISSUES IN HEMATOPOIESIS

Progenitors and Models of Differentiation

Early, Intermediate, and Late Progenitors

A large body of literature exists concerning the hierarchy of differentiation of granulocytes and other formed elements of the blood. In essence, in both animal and human systems, pluripotent progenitors that can give rise to myeloid, lymphoid, erythroid, or megakaryocytic lineages are present in the bone marrow (reviewed in 1,2). These develop in a series of steps during the differentiation process, which are marked by more restricted commitment, presumably as a result of deletion of specific programs for lineage commitment and persistence of others, or the specific activation of lineage-specific genes. Late progenitors, termed oligo- or unipotent, finally give rise to specific cells that themselves may exhibit considerable heterogeneity within each general lineage compartment, as shown in Figure 1.

What is not clear is the process whereby specific lineage commitment comes about: is it a result of random activation, or of events that are selected by the presence of specific growth factor(s)? Evidence from studies of single cells in tissue culture has been interpreted as supporting stochastic or random development of lineage programs (1). The strong interpretation of this model, however, is at variance with a large body of literature demonstrating that a variety of cytokines are able to support the growth and differentiation of pluripotent progenitor cells. What is unclear from these studies is whether lineage-specific growth factors are "forcing" stem cells to choose one pathway, or are simply selecting those cells that have already been randomly committed to the pathway. Recent work (3) with nonleukemic pluripotent cell lines that have been genetically engineered to survive without growth factors is most compatible with a hybrid model (4), with both stochastic and selective features. In this system, the immortalized cell line is capable of differentiation into all myeloid lineages in the absence of growth factors, but different

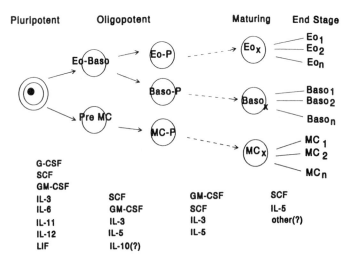

Figure 1 Progenitor hierarchies in allergic inflammatory cell differentiation: The notion depicted here is that at various stages of progenitor commitment, combinations of cytokines are preferentially active in determining subsequent maturational events.

subclones show distinct preferences (e.g., for erythroid, rather than neutrophilic, differentiation). However, an exposure to the appropriate combination of growth factors is capable of overriding the bias of individual subclones and of "forcing" them to differentiate into either red cells or neutrophils. Thus, the complicated processes of stem cell maintenance, proliferation, and differentiation are likely due to a complex mechanism whereby the interaction of cytokines with their receptors will depend on the preset genetic tendency of the target cell. This complexity is further emphasized by the multiple dissociable effects that individual cytokines have on progenitor cells (survival vs. proliferation vs. differentiation (5). Recent evidence indicates that these different effects may be mediated by distinct subdomains within a given cytokine receptor molecule (6). Despite the elegant results obtained with these experimental systems, it is still unclear whether or not pluripotent stem cells in their natural physiological environment are ever allowed to develop stochastically (i.e., without growth factor influence). For example, recent studies (7,8) of embryonic stem cells revealed that mRNAs for many cytokine receptor genes undergo a consistent, orderly pattern of induction and expression during differentiation; some mRNAs for the receptors are constitutively expressed, whereas others appear early or late in the process (7).

It is likely that early progenitors proceed through several intermediate stages and then to late stages of differentiation, and that this process is complemented by the capacity of specific groups of cytokines to act at different stages of differentiation: that is, cytokines, such as stem cell factor (SCF, also known as c-*kit* ligand or mast cell growth factor), act to initiate differentiation of early progenitors, whereas granulocyte–macrophage colony-stimulating factor (GM-CSF) or interleukin (IL)-3 act on intermediate progenitors, and IL-5 on late progenitors (stimulating eosinophil differentiation). This is clearly an oversimplification; the degree of redundancy in cytokines and their receptors on various stages of progenitors is complex, and may reveal specific biological functions that help determine the final outcome of a given response in a given context (2).

One can also attempt to group cytokines with hematopoietic activity in the same way as one can group progenitors, establish progenitor–cytokine complementarities (Fig. 2). This may be essentially subserved by expression of groups of cytokine receptors at different stages of differentiation (7) and linked to the biological redundancy of growth factor receptors themselves (2), or to the common downstream pathways that they activate (5). For example, the common beta (β)-subunit for the receptor for IL-3, IL-5, and GM-CSF is encoded on chromosome 5 (9; reviewed in 10), whereas IL-6, tumor necrosis factor (TNF), and leukemia inhibitory factor (LIF)—and, remotely, G-CSF—also share a common subunit, gp-130.

Place of Myeloid and Lymphoid Lineages at Hematopoiesis

Although the early steps in specific commitment to myeloid lineages are not fully understood, both early data and more recent observations (11,12) indicate that a common, multipotent lymphoid–myeloid progenitor can give rise to a more restricted myeloid progenitor cell during early stages of differentiation. Several of the cytokines with some "specific" hematopoietic progenitor activity (e.g., IL-4 for mast cells; IL-5 for eosinophils; and IL-6 for megakaryocytes) play additional roles in supporting the growth, differentiation, and maturation of lymphoid cells, including immunoglobulin isotype switching and plasma cell differentiation (13–16). Whether this is a fundamental biological process involving common signal transduction mechanisms within variously committed cell lineages in different body tissues, or is restricted to hematopoiesis is not fully clarified. Once

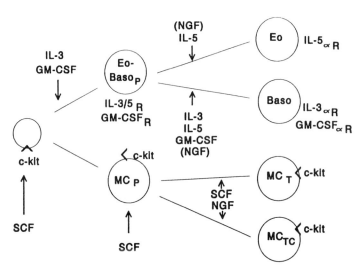

Figure 2 Progenitor–cytokine complementarities in allergic inflammatory cell differentiation: Committed progenitors are hypothesized to display different densities of cytokine receptors on their surfaces at several stages of maturation. The relevant cytokines for specific lineage commitment are depicted.

the commitment to myeloid or lymphoid lineages has been made, there are still several interactions that persist between these two systems of cellular differentiation: for example, T-cell-derived cytokines, derived from either T-helper type I (T_H1) as opposed to T_H2 cells (17), are important in various stages of myeloid cell differentiation. The involvement of a specific T-helper type may be critical in regulating the number and type of inflammatory cells—for example, IL-5 derived from T_H2 cell will specifically stimulate eosinophil differentiation, both in vitro (15) and in vivo (18). The implications of this will be discussed in the following.

Identification of Progenitors

Marker Studies of Progenitors

Within the last decade with the use of hybridoma technology, surface markers of hemato-poietic progenitors in both rodent and human systems have been identified. Hematopoietic progenitor cell antigens include CD34 (19–22), c-*kit* [the proto-oncogene cell product that binds SCF; (23–25)], CD33, CD38, and the common leukocyte antigen CD45 and its variants (21). The earliest progenitors appear to bear CD34 and the flt3/flk-2 tyrosine kinase receptor on their surface (26) and later acquire CD33, c-*kit*, CD38, CD45, or some combination thereof (21). Recent studies have pointed out the complexity of this system; depending on conditions for flow cytometry and cell sorting, various combinations of progenitors, with characteristics of early, intermediate, or late stages of commitment may be obtained (21). Although still controversial, a self-renewing pluripotent hematopoietic progenitor appears to be negative for most markers except CD34 (27,28), a now sequenced and cloned 120-kDa *O*-sialated glycoprotein (29) expressed on the surface of these cells as well as on vascular endothelium (29,30) and possibly other tissue structural cells (31).

Relationships of Markers to Differentiation

The relationships between hematopoietic progenitor cell antigens and cytokine receptors, their coexpression and signaling mechanisms (7), and their relation to lineage commitment are not yet clearly understood. A recent paper examined CD34 expression in the context of cytokine receptor gene expression (7) and concluded that the CD34 gene is induced at an intermediate stage of embryonic stem cell development, after induction of the common β-subunit of IL-3, IL-5, and GM-CSF receptor. CD34 may play an important role in progenitor cell adhesion and activation within the bone marrow stromal compartment, in a process involving carbohydrate interactions (32). How this then influences differentiation processes is totally unclear. From the practical point of view, marker studies combined with cell sorting have provided large quantities of purified progenitor populations accessible for study in vitro and for replenishment of bone marrow in vivo. A scheme for lineage commitment based on cell surface markers of progenitors is shown in Figure 3.

Progenitor Responses

Hematopoietic Cytokines and Differentiation

Depending on their cell target and the degree of differentiation of the latter, cytokines with hematopoietic activity can either be lineage-nonspecific or lineage-specific. This will be determined by the cytokine receptor array on the progenitor and the state of the progenitor at the time of introduction to the cytokine stimulant. In addition, cytokines acting on the cell may be either stimulatory or inhibitory; in fact, certain cytokines possess both of these properties, depending on the stage of commitment of the progenitor and receptors displayed on it.

Cytokine Receptors on Progenitors

Several groups of receptors may afford a degree of "redundancy" or allow for "subtlety" in the system (2), but may also direct specificity through mechanisms such as synergy, transactivation (33), or costimulation (2). For example gp-130, a common receptor for IL-6, LIF, TNF-α, and IL-11 (and partially, for IL-12 or G-CSF), may, at an early stage of differentiation, allow a given progenitor to receive a variety of different inputs, depending on the kind of cytokines available in the local microenvironment (marrow or other tissue). The end result may be stimulation or inhibition of further differentiation. The same can be said for the triad of IL-3, IL-5, and GM-CSF, which share a β-subunit with binding specificity related to an α-subunit, which, when bound to the β-subunit confers a high-affinity interaction with the specific cytokine–receptor (reviewed in Ref. 10). This is a key concept, because it implies that the availability of a given combination of cytokines at a given tissue site is what might ultimately determine intermediate, and then final, stages of differentiation. In the model of allergic inflammation to be proposed herein, the progenitor–cytokine profile of a given tissue is a key element in determining the final pattern of differentiation, which will determine the pattern of accumulation of inflammatory effector cells. Moreover, the systemic release of these cytokines may well underlie the feedback between tissues involved in allergic reactions and the bone marrow–peripheral blood axis for progenitors (Fig. 4).

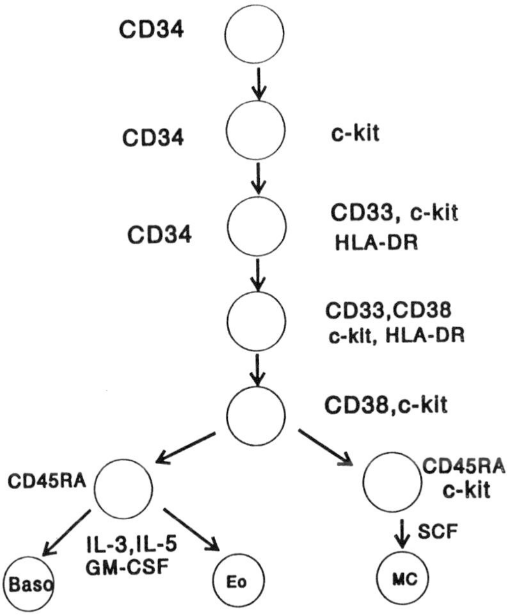

Figure 3 Cell surface immunophenotypes during hemopoietic differentiation: From in vitro studies of various sorted progenitor-enriched cell populations (see text), a scheme of immunophenotypic changes during and through final lineage commitment to eosinophil, basophil, and mast cell is shown.

SPECIFIC LINEAGE COMMITMENT AND EXPRESSION

Myeloid Lineages

Granulocyte Lineage Commitment

We will now focus on specific commitment in the myeloid lineage, based mostly on in vitro evidence using hematopoietic cell assay systems. Most authors would agree that neutrophil and monocyte–macrophage differentiation occur in tandem, whereas eosinophil and basophil differentiation form another pair, based on colony growth from single, committed progenitor cells in semisolid culture systems (1,2,34–38). Thus, specific types of leukocyte colonies grown in methylcellulose or agar, containing intermediate to late hematopoietic progeny from peripheral blood, cord blood, or bone marrow progenitor populations in the myeloid lineage, consist of mixtures of either neutrophils and monocytes, or of eosinophils and basophils. The colonies are recognizable by their appearance on inverted microscopy as well as by staining, and each can be formally shown to be derived of a single cell, thus proving at least an intermediate or late-stage common progenitor for each of these two pairs (1,35,36,39).

Mastopoiesis

The origin of mast cells has been controversial for quite some time. Although it can be formally demonstrated, both in vitro and in vivo in rodent systems, that mast cells are derived from the same pluripotent hematopoietic stem cell as the other granulocytes and formed elements of the blood (13,14), it is not yet fully clear at which stage of commitment of hematopoietic progenitors the mast cell lineage pathway splits off. Early reports, based

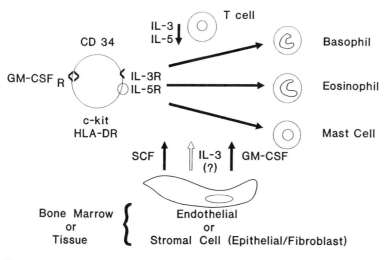

Figure 4 Microenvironmental determinants of inflammatory cell progenitor differentiation: The author and his co-workers have provided evidence for the production of an array of hematopoietic cytokines in allergic, inflamed tissues. These cytokines can be derived from T cells, or from the structural cells (endothelium, epithelium, fibroblasts) in the airways.

on mast cell growth from lymphoid tissues, such as lymph nodes, thymus, or spleen, in rodent systems favored a "lymphoid" cell origin (40), whereas more recent evidence would place the mast cell lineage as distinct (41) or as more closely related to that of monocytes—macrophages and, therefore, of "myeloid" derivation (42). However, precise experiments using purified hematopoietic progenitors and identifying these by stage of commitment as expressed through cytokine receptors or cell surface markers, have only recently been applied to the mast cell and other granulocyte lineages. A CD34(+)/CD14(−)/c-*kit*(+) cell gives rise to mast cells (33), whereas a CD34(−)CD11b/18(+)/CD33(+)/CD25(+) cell (in leukemic cell line HL-60 cultures) gives rise to basophils and eosinophils (43). Despite the preponderance of evidence that c-*kit* does not mediate basophil, but only mast cell, differentiation from human progenitors (41,42), there are some observations on leukemic cells suggesting the presence of c-*kit* on a common basophil–mast cell progenitor (37,43,44).

Basophil and Eosinophil Differentiation

Shared Progenitor–Cytokine Combinations   It is likely that all granulocytes, including monocytes–macrophages, are derived from an intermediate-stage progenitor under the influence of factors such as G-CSF, GM-CSF, and IL-3, in particular. Commitment to eosinophil and basophil lineages appears to be the result of more specific actions of cytokines at later stages of myeloid progenitor differentiation. Thus, eosinophil differentiation can be directed solely by IL-5 acting on a late-stage progenitor (15,45); nonetheless, IL-3 and GM-CSF also can be shown to play a role in the differentiation of eosinophil and basophil colonies in vitro (36,37). There is some evidence that IL-3 alone may support hematopoietic differentiation along the basophil lineage (42), although this cytokine clearly has more widespread hematopoietic activity (hence, the alternate name multi-CSF) and has not been shown to be as specific as IL-5. Binding studies reveal varying IL-3, IL-5,

GM-CSF, and SCF receptor expression on mature basophils and mast cells (37,42), but do not address the critical question of receptor expression on their respective progenitors. Furthermore, IL-5 has also been shown to have basophil differentiation-inducing activities in vitro (46), so that its supposedly unique specificity for eosinophils can be called into question here. These results are not surprising, given that eosinophils and basophils share a common, late ("committed") progenitor (38).

Lineage Interrelationships

Basophils, Eosinophils, and Mast Cells

Human mast cell growth can be stimulated almost exclusively by SCF both in vitro and in vivo (42,47,48); large numbers of differentiating mast cells in tissues can be elicited in several species using exogenous SCF (48–50). CD34-positive progenitors can give rise to mast cells under stimulation with SCF (40) and to mast cells and basophils using combinations of SCF and IL-3 (42,51,52). Stem cell factor, injected into primates or rodents, elicits a massive mastocytosis in vivo; SCF provided in cultures of human fetal liver cells, cord blood, or bone marrow can support the differentiation of mast cells (47,48,53,54).

The uniqueness and complexity of the mast cell lineage and its separability from the other granulocytic lineages is underscored by recent experiments done in a mast cell-deficient rat—a homologue of the mast cell-deficient W/W^V mouse—termed the W^S/W^S (or "white-spotting") rat. After nematode infestation, which induces mucosal mastocytosis in the normal rat, both basophils and mast cells are elicited in vivo (55,56), whereas in the W^S/W^S rat, only basophils are elicited, but not connective tissue-type mast cells, suggesting that there is a biological dissociation (and, therefore, different cytokines and cytokine receptors involved) between the two lineages (i.e., basophils and mast cells). Moreover, the number and function of mast cells in vivo can be related to the exact type of mutation in different c-*kit* receptor domains at the *W* locus in mice (57); likewise, the *W* locus in the rat is critical in determining the degree and type of mast cell differentiation into heterogeneous, mature phenotypes ("mucosal" and "connective tissue" mast cells; 58).

Nonetheless, there is still evidence in human systems of combinations of basophils and mast cells occurring in response to SCF, with or without IL-3 or GM-CSF, or even of hybrid basophil–mast cells in bone marrow disorders (59–62). Whether a specific progenitor for mast cells is clearly separable from the eosinophil–basophil progenitor still remains to be formally proved.

Lineage Restriction and Cytokine Effects on Mature Cell Phenotype

There are specific lineage factors and commitments for neutrophils (G-CSF) and macrophages (M-CSF), respectively. These probably act on late progenitors in each of these lineages, once they are "committed," just as IL-5 has apparent lineage restriction of eosinophil (late) progenitors. For each of these progenitor–cytokine combinations, effects carry over to the mature cell and are biologically read out as "activation" or "phenotype switching." Thus, IL-3, IL-5, and GM-CSF can activate and prolong the survival by preventing physiological apoptosis of basophils and eosinophils (54,63); G-CSF as well as GM-CSF can activate and prolong the survival of neutrophils (64). These effects on mature cells imply that these cells retain hematopoietic cytokine receptors on their surface (see Fig. 2). Given that these mature cells, when activated, can produce the very cytokines that target their progenitors, the complexity of possible interactions increases. Autocrine stimulation by each of these cells of their own differentiation or activation is thus likely; there is now direct evidence for the production of hematopoietic cytokines by both eosinophils and mast cells (48,65–71). The role of mature inflammatory effector cells in directing their own differentiation needs to be further explored (Fig. 5).

Evidence from Transgenic or Mutant Rodents

Interleukin-5   The analysis of the lineage specificity of cytokines involved in eosinophil, basophil, and mast cell differentiation, using transgenic mice or specific genetic mutations, has just begun. Sanderson et al. have described IL-5 transgenic mice, in which a massive eosinophilia in the peripheral blood and tissues was generated (15). Curiously, however, these mice do not have any major form of eosinophil-associated inflammatory disease. When challenged with cestoides nematodes, there is a paradoxical decrease in serum in IL-5 levels over time (15). This is accompanied by an inflammatory gastrointestinal response in the IL-5 transgenic animal.

W Locus Mutations   W/W^V and related mutant mice have been studied extensively because of their mast cell deficiency. The *W/W^V* and other *W* locus mutants have defects in c-*kit*, the receptor for SCF (23,48–50,58); various *W* locus mutations have been studied with relation to the functional derangements in mastopoiesis that are caused by different single-point mutations in the c-*kit* gene (57). Sl/Sl^d mice are also mast cell-deficient and have the same phenotype as the W/W^V; however, the Sl/Sl^d do not produce SCF (c-*kit* ligand); their fibroblasts and related cells are defective in this (49,50). Thus, mast cell deficiency can be observed whether c-*kit* is abnormal, or its ligand is missing, and each of these is sufficient to produce mast cell deficiency. A similar defect is seen in the W^S/W^S rat discussed earlier: various problems in pigmentation, other genetic abnormalities related to c-*kit* mutations, and mast cell deficiency are observed in these animals (55).

Stem Cell Factor In Vivo   Stem cell factor, when administered exogenously to normal primates or rodents, causes a massive mastocytosis, but also (as in IL-5 transgenics) does not necessarily engender a mast cell disease (48), as seen in the human (spontaneously occurring) counterpart. Antigenic challenge of sensitized SCF-treated animals causes abnormalities in various tissues related to mast cell degranulation, but these are not

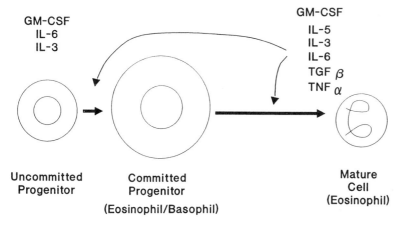

Figure 5   Proposed autocrine regulation of eosinophil differentiation: The eosinophil can produce a variety of cytokines with potential feedback hematopoietic activity on the committed eosinophil progenitor.

necessarily over and above those seen with SCF-treated mast cell-deficient animals (48,72). Recently, in vivo administration of SCF to humans subcutaneously has been reported (73): in these patients with cancer, SCF caused a wheal-and-flare reaction and pigmentation at the injection site, and increases in mast cells in the skin at distant sites.

Thus, in transgenic or mutant rodents, inflammatory cell progenitors or their cytokines express phenotypic abnormalities related to the cell lineage and cytokine in question, not necessarily accompanied by an inflammatory disease; in humans and primates, in vivo cytokine administration does not necessarily cause systemic allergic conditions. This raises the question of the "pathogenicity" or even therapeutic potential of any single cytokine: in the absence of an appropriate microenvironment (e.g., chronic inflammation); tissue susceptibility (e.g., airways smooth muscle); host factors (e.g., high specific IgE producer); and provocative stimulus (e.g., specific allergen), specific disease (e.g., asthma) may never eventuate, even with massive doses of IL-5 or SCF.

IN VIVO RELEVANCE AND CORRELATES OF INFLAMMATORY CELL PROGENITORS

Allergic Inflammation

In Vivo Models

Allergic Rhinitis and Asthma   A large body of evidence we have accumulated shows significant and relevant fluctuations in peripheral blood eosinophil–basophil progenitors in relation to allergic inflammation (34–39,74–78), Atopic patients in general have sponta-neously occurring increases in progenitors that are observed mainly out-of-season (76,77), but also early during natural allergen exposure (79), during exacerbations of asthma after corticosteroid withdrawal (74,75), or immediately after allergen provocation in a controlled setting (74,75). Topical therapy with corticosteroids to the airway, in very low to negligible doses systemically, causes reductions in peripheral blood progenitors (74,75). These studies highlight the dynamic relations that exist among allergen provocation (upper and lower), airway inflammation, corticosteroid therapy, and inflammatory cell progenitors.

Canine Allergen-Induced Airway Hyperresponsiveness   Recent experiments we have performed show that allergen provocation to the airway in a dog model of bronchial hyperreactivity and eosinophilic infiltration after parasite sensitization causes increases in bone marrow progenitors; treatment topically with budesonide, a potent corticosteroid that acts mainly, but not exclusively, on the airway, decreases bone marrow progenitor re-sponses (M. Woolley et al., submitted). Moreover, treatment of an asthma exacerbation in humans by reintroduction of corticosteroids causes a reversal in the increase of peripheral blood progenitors (74,75). These observations, taken together, indicate that the peripheral blood and bone marrow progenitor compartments, specifically colony-forming cells for eosinophils and basophils, respond to changes at local tissue inflammatory sites during allergen provocation or in natural allergen exposure. This suggests that the airway mucosa and related structural cells produce relevant lineage-specific cytokines for basophil, eosino-phil, and mast cell differentiation, and that these have "endocrine" effects distant from the tissue, acting on blood and bone marrow (Fig. 6).

In Vitro Models

Production of Hematopoietic Cytokines by Allergic Tissue Structural Cells   We have accumulated evidence that IL-3, IL-6, IL-8, G-CSF, M-CSF, GM-CSF, TNF-α, and SCF all

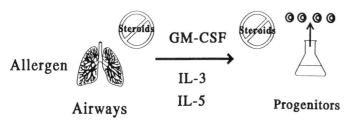

Figure 6 Endocrine effects of tissue cytokines in inflammatory cell differentiation: Topical cortico-steroids can suppress peripheral blood or bone marrow inflammatory cell progenitor responses to allergen. This is hypothesized to occur by blockade of tissue production of hematopoietic cytokines, with consequent systemic, endocrine-like effects.

are produced in increased amounts by the epithelial cells and fibroblasts of the airway during inflammatory processes (80–83). In particular, tissue structural cells taken from patients with nasal polyposis, allergic rhinitis, asthma, and pulmonary fibrosis, all have up-regulated gene expression and production of several of these cytokines (80–83; reviewed in 84). The concept that has emerged from these studies is that the tissue microenvironment creates a milieu that is conducive to lineage-specific, terminal differentiation of inflamma-tory cell progenitors participating in allergic inflammatory reactions. Whether provocation with allergen is necessary or sufficient for the increased production of these cytokines, and what regulatory influences are crucial in determining acute versus chronic inflammatory responses, are issues that should now be investigated. A current list of cytokines produced at allergic tissue sites, by all cells involved (including inflammatory cells), is given in Table 1. This list is continually expanding.

Inflammatory Cell Cytokines One possible modulatory (inhibitory?) cytokine for these hematopoietic responses is transforming growth factor-beta (TGF-β), which is produced in abundance by mature eosinophils in nasal polyp tissues (65) and by many other cell types. TGF-β is a hematopoietic inhibitor (85), and may specifically down-regulate eosinophilic differentiation as opposed to basophilic (86). Under different conditions, TNF-α, found in polyp eosinophils and mast cells (87,88), can play an inhibitory role (89). Again, the specific context of the cytokine in the tissues must be understood before one can reliably predict the direction and extent of the inflammatory response to allergen. Moreover, the contribution of cytokines derived from the inflammatory effector cells themselves (espe-cially eosinophils and mast cells) might be crucial in determining whether or not progeni-tors are recruited from the blood, what signals from the tissues go to the marrow to elicit a

Table 1 Cytokines
Produced by Inflamed
Allergic Tissues

GM-CSF	IL-3	TNF-α
G-CSF	IL-4	TGF-β
M-CSF	IL-5	SCF
IL-1	IL-6	IFN-γ
IL-2	IL-8	RANTES

progenitor response, and the intensity and duration of the final inflammatory reaction (see Fig. 5 and Table 1).

Evidence from Bone Marrow Transplantation

The contribution of the bone marrow to the allergic diathesis and response in tissues has been studied serendipitously through an analysis of transfer of allergic responses in bone marrow transplant situations (90). Nine of 12 nonatopic patients who received bone marrow from atopic donors converted to atopy, as measured by skin test responses to standard allergens; in a few patients asthmatic responses have also been transferred, together with IgE and skin test responsiveness (90). The hypothesis derived from these observations is that hematopoietic stem cells, both myeloid and lymphoid, may be involved in the transfer of IgE (owing to IL-4), basophilia (possibly owing to IL-3), mastocytosis (SCF), eosino-philia (IL-5), and related characteristic responses in an allergic reaction. Whether all this is due to the transfer of a T_H2 cell (91), sets of progenitors for specific lineages, or other factors that confer increased capacity to produce the inflammatory effector cells of allergy needs to be determined. Recent experiments we have performed strongly suggest that progenitors derived from the peripheral blood of atopics are not only increased in quantity, but also express programs for cytokines differently from progenitors from nonatopics. Specifically, the progeny in colonies of basophil–eosinophil progenitors in atopics produce far more GM-CSF than do nonatopic progeny (92). These observations are consistent with an "activated" state of the intermediate- to late-stage, committed progenitor in the atopic situation; they suggest that putatively stochastic processes in differentiation might be skewed in the atopic individual, perhaps even at the bone marrow stem cell level, or at intermediate stages of progenitor differentiation. Indeed, studies on cord blood for pre-dictors of allergic diathesis suggest that, in addition to IgE levels, the capacity for differen-tiation by progenitors to basophils and eosinophils may already be increased in those destined to become atopic (93).

Studies of Myeloproliferative Diseases

There are several experiments in nature affecting the bone marrow and recognized as syndromes or diseases in which specific lineage differentiation of the inflammatory effector cells of allergy occurs. Hypereosinophilic syndrome (HES) is one condition in which high levels of eosinophils and, in some cases, of eosinophil progenitors, exist. Although there is probable heterogeneity in HES, with some cases related to increased expression of IL-5 and consequent induction of eosinophilia and of activated eosinophils, others may simply reflect an increased demargination of eosinophils, rather than a bone marrow problem per se (94,95). Nonetheless, in a large proportion of HES patients, cytotoxic therapy directed at bone marrow progenitors can abrogate eosinophil responses and the consequent tissue damage by eosinophils, which appear to be activated and resistant to apoptosis. Part of this may be due to the autocrine stimulation by HES eosinophils, consequent on production of relevant cytokines such as IL-3, IL-5, and GM-CSF (66,96). A surprising parallel has been noted in eosinophils isolated from nasal polyps, which appear to be activated by autocrine stimulation: abrogation of spontaneous increased survival can be achieved by antibody to GM-CSF or GM-CSF receptors (84).

Mast cell diseases, including systemic mastocytosis and mast cell leukemia, appear to be related to the increased turnover and presence of mast cells in various organs. Whether or not systemic mastocytosis and related mast cell disease in humans is due to aberrant production or expression of SCF in tissues needs to be fully explored. Circumstantial evidence indicates that different tissues in patients with mast cell disease produce favorable environments for mast cell differentiation and phenotypic expression, especially of the serosal type mast cell that contains both chymase and tryptase (MC_{TC}). It would be of great interest to know the relation between cytokine (specifically SCF) expression and disease activity or severity in these patients.

Chronic myeloid leukemia and related myeloproliferative conditions often occur in relation to basophil proliferation and differentiation. This is especially seen closer to transformation to an acute form of leukemia, called "blast crisis." In these conditions, the specific cytokines involved in expression of the basophil lineage have not yet been delineated. However, large numbers of basophils, sometimes eosinophils, and sometimes mast cell-like cells (which appear morphologically to be hybrids between basophils and mast cells) can be seen in tissues and in blood (35,97). Blast cells can be observed to differentiate spontaneously to basophils and, sometimes, mast cells in vitro (59–61; reviewed in 36,37). Less frequently, acute myeloid leukemia, especially in those patients carrying the t(15;17) or t(6;9) translocations, has been associated with partial commitment to basophil differentiation (98,99), but the precise relation between the cytogenetic abnormality and the expression of this basophil lineage commitment has not yet been determined (99,100). The subject of myeloproliferative and bone marrow diseases in relation to lineage commitment and particularly in relation to basophil and mast cell lineages has been reviewed in detail elsewhere (37).

PREDICTIONS AND CONCLUSIONS

It is clear that inflammatory cell progenitors are present and fluctuate in clinically relevant ways during allergic inflammatory responses. The bulk of evidence from experimental and clinical data suggests that the progenitor contribution from local and bone marrow sources may be very important in determining the final outcome of an allergic response and, in fact, in determining whether or not allergy will occur. Dissection of cytokine–progenitor profiles in relation to the allergic diathesis and with specific interest in lineage commitment and terminal differentiation of eosinophils, basophils, and mast cells needs to be further examined. Certain predictions can be made on the basis of this; these are highlighted in Table 2.

Autocrine feedback through cytokines produced by mature inflammatory effector cells on their own progenitors also needs to be studied further. Of the array of cytokines that the mast cell, eosinophil, and basophil are known to produce, there appear to be sufficient and

Table 2 Predictions Derived from the Bone Marrow Hypothesis of Allergic Inflammation

Provocation by allergen elicits specific increases in bone marrow basophil and eosinophil progenitors.
Bone marrow and blood basophil and eosinophil progenitors traffic to sites of allergic inflammation.
Agents or factors (e.g., cytokines) that skew granulocyte lineage commitment away from basophil–eosinophil will have a beneficial (inhibitory) effect on allergic inflammation.
The inhibitory effects of corticosteroids on allergic inflammation involve direct and indirect modulation of hematopoietic cytokines involved in bone marrow basophil and eosinophil progenitor differentiation.
Allergic inflammation is primarily of bone marrow origin; abrogation of bone marrow basophil and eosinophil responses will greatly reduce allergic-type responses.

appropriate amounts for a hematopoietic microenvironment to exist in tissues at sites of inflammation, independent of bone marrow supply. Seen in this context, the bone marrow would provide the initial source for stem cells, which may already be activated or skewed toward differentiation in an allergic individual along specific lineages. However, the process may become autonomous within tissues once the progenitor supply is provided and ongoing signaling to the marrow, through the peripheral blood, occurs. The cytokines engendered during allergic reactions and by the tissues themselves may be sufficient to create a chronic allergic inflammatory condition, such as seen in asthma and nasal polyposis. Whether or not the bone marrow is necessary for this chronic inflammatory process to persist needs to be further substantiated. Moreover, the precise kinetics of progenitor traffic and differentiation, especially for eosinophil, basophil, and mast cell accumulation in tissues, can now be studied in several animal models. In any case, *the involvement of hematopoietic progenitors for inflammatory effector cells begins in the bone marrow and the allergic diathesis may well have its origin at that site.* Further studies in this field may shed new understandings of the allergic diathesis, possibly leading to more long-term solutions to its management.

REFERENCES

1. Ogawa M. Differentiation and proliferation of hematopoietic stem cells. Blood 1993; 81:2844–2853.
2. Metcalfe D. Hematopoietic regulators: redundancy or subtlety? Blood 1993; 82:3515–3523.
3. Fairbairn LJ, Cowling GJ, Reipert BM, Dexter TM. Suppression of apoptosis allows differentiation and development of a multipotent hemopoietic cell line in the absence of added growth factors. Cell 1993; 74:823–832.
4. Just U, Stocking C, Spooncer E, Dexter TM, Ostertag W. Expression of the GM-CSF gene after retroviral transfer in hematopoietic stem cell lines induces synchronous granulocyte–macrophage differentiation. Cell 1991; 64:1163–1173.
5. Bourette RP, Mouchiroud G, Ouazana R, Morle F, Godet J, Blanchet JP. Expression of human colony-stimulating factor-1 (CSF-1) receptor in murine pluripotent hematopoietic NFS-60 cells induces long-term proliferation in response to CSF-1 without loss of erythroid differentiation potential. Blood 1993; 81:2511–2520.
6. Fukunaga R, Ishizaka-Ikeda E, Nagata S. Growth and differentiation signals mediated by different regions in the cytoplasmic domain of granulocyte colony-stimulating factor receptor. Cell 1993; 74:1079–1087.
7. McClanahan T, Dalrymple S, Barkett M, Lee F. Hematopoietic growth factor receptor genes as markers of lineage commitment during in vitro development of hematopoietic cells. Blood 1993; 81:2903–2915.
8. Schmitt RM, Bruyns E, Snodgrass HR. Hematopoietic development of embryonic stem cells in vitro: cytokine and receptor gene expression. Genes Dev 1991; 5:728–740.
9. van Leeuwen BH, Martinson ME, Webb GC, Young IG. Molecular organization of the cytokine gene cluster, involving the human IL-3, IL-4, IL-5, and GM-CSF genes, on human chromosome 5. Blood 1989; 73:1142–1148.
10. Miyajima A, Mui AL-F, Ogorochi T, Sakamaki K. Receptors for granulocyte–macrophage colony-stimulating factor, interleukin-3, and interleukin-5. Blood 1993; 82:1960–1974.
11. Chen U, Kosco M, Staerz U. Establishment and characterization of lymphoid and myeloid mixed-cell populations from mouse late embryoid bodies, "embryonic-stem-cell fetuses." Proc Natl Acad Sci USA 1992; 89:2541–2545.
12. Hirayama F, Shih J-P, Awgulewitsch A, Warr GW, Clark SC, Ogawa M. Clonal proliferation of murine lymphohemopoietic progenitors in culture. Proc Natl Acad Sci USA 1992; 89:5907–5911.

13. Kitamura Y, Yokoyama M, Matsuda H, Ohno T, Mori KJ. Spleen colony-forming cell as common precursor for tissue mast cells and granulocytes. Nature 1981; 291:159–160.

14. Kitamura Y, Go S, Hatanaka K. Decrease of mast cells in W/W^V mice and their increase by bone marrow transplantation. Blood 1978; 52:447–452.

15. Sanderson CJ, Warren DJ, Strath M. Identification of a lymphokine that stimulates eosinophil differentiation in vitro. Its relationship to interleukin 3, and functional properties of eosinophils produced in culture. J Exp Med 1985; 162:60–74.

16. Paul WE. Interleukin-4: a prototypic immunoregulatory lymphokine. Blood 1991; 77:1859–1870.

17. Mosmann TR, Moore KW. The role of IL-10 in crossregulation of T_H1 and T_H2 responses. Immunol Today 1991; 12:A49–A53.

18. Cogan E, Schandene L, Crusiaux A, Cochaux P, Velu T, Goldman M. Clonal proliferation of type 2 helper T cell in a man with hypereosinophilic syndrome. N Engl J Med 1994; 330:535–538.

19. Civin CI, Strauss LC, Brovall C, Fackler MJ, Schwartz JF, Shaper JH. Antigenic analysis of hematopoiesis. III. A hematopoietic progenitor cell surface antigen defined by a monoclonal antibody raised against KG-1a cells. J Immunol 1984; 133:157–165.

20. Kato K, Radbruch A. Isolation and characterization of CD34$^+$ hematopoietic stem cells from human peripheral blood by high-gradient magnetic cell sorting. Cytometry 1993; 14:384–392.

21. Lansdorp PM, Sutherland JH, Eaves CJ. Selective expression of CD45 isoforms on functional subpopulations of CD34$^+$ hemopoietic cells from human bone marrow. J Exp Med 1990; 172:363–366.

22. Fritsch G, Buchinger P, Printz D, et al. Rapid discrimination of early CD34$^+$ myeloid progenitors using CD45-RA analysis. Blood 1993; 81:2301–2309.

23. Zsebo KM, Williams DA, Geissler EN, et al. Stem cell factor is encoded at the *Sl* locus of the mouse and is the ligand for the c-*kit* tyrosine kinase receptor. Cell 1990; 63:213–224.

24. Huang E, Nocka K, Beier DR, et al. The hematopoietic growth factor KL is encoded by the *Sl* locus and is the ligand of the c-*kit* receptor, the gene product of the *W* locus. Cell 1990; 63: 225–233.

25. Williams DE, Eisenman J, Baird A, et al. Identification of a ligand for the c-*kit* proto-oncogene. Cell 1990; 63:167–174.

26. Rosnet O, Schiff C, Pebusque M, Marchetto S, Tonnelle C, Toiron C, Birg F, Birnbaum D. Human *FLT3/FLK2* gene: cDNA cloning and expression in hematopoietic cells. Blood 1993; 82: 1110–1119.

27. Eaves CJ. Peripheral blood stem cells reach new heights. Blood 1993; 82:1957–1959.

28. Lapidot T, Sirard C, Vormoor J, Murdoch B, Hoang T, Cacaers-Cortes J, Minden M, Paterson B, Caligiuri M, Dick J. A cell initiating human acute myeloid leukemia after transplantation into SCID mice. Nature 1994; 367:645–648.

29. Fink L, Molgaard HV, Robertson D, et al. Expression of the CD34 gene in vascular endothelial cells. Blood 1990; 75:2417–2426.

30. Nickoloff BJ. The human progenitor cell antigen (CD34) is localized on endothelial cells, dermal dendritic cells, and perifollicular cells in formalin-fixed normal skin, and on proliferating endothelial cells and stromal spindle-shaped cells in Kaposi's sarcoma. Arch Dermatol 1991; 127:523–529.

31. Schligemann RD, Rietreld FJR, Waal RMW, et al. Leukocyte antigen CD34 is expressed by a subset of cultured endothelial cells and endothelial abluminal microprocesses in the tumor stroma. Lab Invest 1990; 62:690–696.

32. Majdic O, Stockl J, Pickl WF, et al. Signaling and induction of enhanced cytoadhesiveness via the hematopoietic progenitor cell surface molecule CD34. Blood 1994; 83:1226–1234.

33. Vadas MA, Lopez AF, Gamble JR, Elliot MJ. Role of colony-stimulating factors in leucocyte responses to inflammation and infection. Curr Opin Immunol 1991; 3:97–104.

34. Denburg JA, Dolovich J, Harnish D. Basophil mast cell and eosinophil growth and differentiation factors in human allergic disease. Clin Exp Allergy 1989; 19:249–254.

35. Denburg JA, Richardson M, Telizyn S, Bienenstock J. Basophil/mast cell precursors in human peripheral blood. Blood 1983; 61:775–780.

36. Denburg JA. Cytokine-induced human basophil/mast cell growth and differentiation in vitro. Springer Semin Immunopathol 1990; 12:401–414.

37. Denburg JA. Basophil and mast cell lineages in vitro and in vivo. Blood 1992; 79:846–860.

38. Denburg JA, Telizyn S, Messner H, et al. Heterogeneity of human peripheral blood eosinophil-type colonies: evidence for a common basophil–eosinophil progenitor. Blood 1985; 66: 312–318.

39. Denburg JA, Telizyn S, Belda A, Dolovich J, Bienenstock J. Increased numbers of circulating basophil progenitors in atopic patients. J Allergy Clin Immunol 1985; 76:466–472.

40. Ginsburg H, Lagunoff D. The in vitro differentiation of mast cells. Cultures of cells from immunized mouse lymph nodes and thoracic duct lymph on fibroblast monolayers. J Cell Biol 1967; 35:685–697.

41. Agis H, Willheim M, Sperr WR, et al. Identification of the circulating mast cell progenitor as a c-*kit*+, CD34+, CD14−, CD17−, LY−, colony forming cell [abstr]. Blood 1993; 82(suppl):102a.

42. Valent P, Ashman LK, Hinterberger W, et al. Mast cell typing: demonstration of a distinct hematopoietic cell type and evidence for immunophenotypic relationship to mononuclear phagocytes. Blood 1989; 73:1778–1785.

43. Wang C, DeCoteau J, Pinkerton PH, Reis MD. c-*kit* expression and response to kit–ligand by leukemic basophils from chronic myelogenous leukemia in basophilic transformation [abstr]. Blood 1993; 82(suppl):230a.

44. Wong DA, Switzer J, Ohtoshi T, Delespesse G, Dolovich J, Denburg J. CD23 expression on HL-60 cells: evidence for both basophilic and monocytic differentiation [abstr]. J Allergy Clin Immunol 1991; 87:305.

45. Clutterbuck EJ, Sanderson CJ. Human eosinophil hematopoiesis studied in vitro by means of murine eosinophil differentiation factor (IL-5): production of functionally active eosinophils from normal human bone marrow. Blood 1988; 71:646–651.

46. Denburg JA, Silver JE, Abrams JS. Interleukin-5 is a human basophilopoietin: induction of histamine content and basophilic differentiation of HL-60 cells and of peripheral blood basophil–eosinophil progenitors. Blood 1991; 77:1462–1468.

47. Irani A-M, Schwartz LB. In vitro development of MCT cells from human fetal liver [abstr]. J Allergy Clin Immunol 1990; 85:172.

48. Galli SJ. Biology of disease. New insights into "the riddle of the mast cells": microenvironmental regulation of mast cell development and phenotypic heterogeneity. Lab Invest 1990; 62: 5–33.

49. Jarboe DL, Huff TF. The mast cell-committed progenitor. II. W/W^V mice do not make mast cell-committed progenitors and Sl/Sl^d fibroblasts do not support development of normal mast cell-committed progenitors. J Immunol 1989; 142:2418–2423.

50. Jarboe DL, Marshall JS, Randolph TR, Kukolja A, Huff TF. The mast cell-committed progenitor. I. Description of a cell capable of IL-3-independent proliferation and differentiation without contact with fibroblasts. J Immunol 1989; 142:2405–2417.

51. Kirshenbaum AS, Kessler SW, Goff JP, Metcalfe DD. Demonstration of the origin of human mast cells from CD34+ bone marrow progenitor cells. J Immunol 1991; 146:1410–1415.

52. Kirshenbaum AS, Goff JP, Dreskin SC, Irani A-M, Schwartz LB, Metcalfe DD. IL-3-dependent growth of basophil-like and mast-like cells from human bone marrow. J Immunol 1989; 142:2424–2429.

53. Furitsu T, Saito H, Dvorak AM, et al. Development of human mast cells in vitro. Proc Natl Acad Sci USA 1989; 86:10039–10043.

54. Saito H, Hatake K, Dvorak AM, et al. Selective differentiation and proliferation of hematopoietic cells induced by recombinant human interleukins. Proc Natl Acad Sci USA 1988; 85:2288–2292.

55. Kasugai T, Okada M, Morimoto M, et al. Infection of *Nippostrongylus brasiliensis* induces normal increase of basophils in mast cell-deficient W^s/W^s rats with a small deletion at the kinase domain of c-*kit*. Blood 1993; 81:2521–2529.

56. Ebi Y, Kasugaí T, Seino Y, Onoue H, Kanemoto T, Kitamura Y. Mechanism of mast cell deficiency in mutant mice of *mi/mi* genotype: an analysis by co-culture of mast cells and fibroblasts. Blood 1990; 75:1247–1251.

57. Tsujimura T, Koshimizu U, Katoh H, et al. Mast cell number in the skin of heterozygotes reflects the molecular nature of c-*kit* mutation. Blood 1993; 81:2530–2538.

58. Tei H, Kasugai T, Tsujimura T, et al. Characterization of cultured mast cells derived from W^S/W^S mast cell-deficient rats with a small deletion at tyrosine kinase domain of c-*kit*. Blood 1994; 83:916–925.

59. Parkin JL, McKenna RW, Brunning RD. Philadelphia chromosome-positive blastic leukemia: ultrastructural and ultracytochemical evidence of basophil and mast cell differentiation. Br J Haematol 1982; 52:663–677.

60. Soler J, O'Brien M, deCastro JT, et al. Blast crisis of chronic granulocytic leukemia with mast cell and basophil precursors. Am J Clin Pathol 1985; 83:254–259.

61. Zucker-Franklin D. Ultrastructural evidence for the common origin of human mast cells and basophils. Blood 1980; 56:534–540.

62. Juhlin L, Michaelsson G. A new syndrome characterized by absence of eosinophils and basophils. Lancet 1977; 1:1233–1235.

63. Owen WF Jr, Rothenberg ME, Silberstein DS, et al. Regulation of human eosinophil viability, density and function by granulocyte/macrophage colony-stimulating factor in the presence of 3T3 fibroblasts. J Exp Med 1987; 166:129–141.

64. Gasson JC. Molecular physiology of granulocyte–macrophage colony-stimulating factor. Blood 1991; 77:1131–1145.

65. Ohno I, Lea RG, Flanders KC, et al. Eosinophils in chronically inflamed human upper airway tissues express transforming growth factor β1 gene (TGFβ1). J Clin Invest 1992; 89:1662–1668.

66. Ohno I, Lea R, Finotto S, et al. Granulocyte/macrophage colony-stimulating factor (GM-CSF) gene expression by eosinophils in nasal polyposis. Am J Respir Cell Mol Biol 1991; 5:505–510.

67. Wong DTW, Weller PF, Galli SJ, et al. Human eosinophils express transforming growth factor α. J Exp Med 1990; 172:673–681.

68. Desreumaux P, Janin A, Colombel JF, et al. Interleukin 5 messenger RNA expression by eosinophils in the intestinal mucosa of patients with coeliac disease. J Exp Med 1992; 175:293–296.

69. Moqbel R, Hamid Q, Ying S, et al. Expression of mRNA and immunoreactivity for the granulocyte/macrophage colony-stimulating factor in activated human eosinophils. J Exp Med 1991; 174:749–752.

70. Finotto S, Marshall JS, Irani A, et al. The effect of nasal polyp structural cell conditioned media on mast cell mediator expression [abstr]. FASEB J 1992; 6:A1723.

71. Bradding P, Feather IH, Howarth PH, et al. Interleukin 4 is localized to and released by human mast cells. J Exp Med 1992; 176:1381–1386.

72. Wershil BK, Wang Z-S, Gordon JR, Galli SJ. Recruitment of neutrophils during IgE-dependent cutaneous late phase reactions in the mouse is mast cell-dependent. J Clin Invest 1991; 87:446–453.

73. Costa JJ, Demetri GD, Harrist TJ, et al. Recombinant human stem cell factor (rhSCF) induces cutaneous mast cell activation and hyperplasia, and hyperpigmentation in humans in vivo [abstr]. J Allergy Clin Immunol 1994; 93:225.

74. Gibson PG, Manning PJ, O'Byrne PM, et al. Allergen-induced asthmatic responses: relationship between increases in airway responsiveness and increases in circulating eosinophils, basophils, and their progenitors. Am Rev Respir Dis 1991; 143:331–335.

75. Gibson PG, Dolovich J, Girgis-Gabardo A, et al. The inflammatory response in asthma exacerbation: changes in circulating eosinophils, basophils and their progenitors. Clin Exp Allergy 1990; 20:661–668.

76. Otsuka H, Dolovich J, Befus AD, Telizyn S, Bienenstock J, Denburg JA. Basophilic cell

progenitors, nasal metachromatic cells, and peripheral blood basophils in ragweed-allergic patients. J Allergy Clin Immunol 1986; 78:365–371.

77. Otsuka H, Dolovich J, Befus AD, Bienenstock J, Denburg JA. Peripheral blood basophils, basophil progenitors, and nasal metachromatic cells in allergic rhinitis. Am Rev Respir Dis 1986; 133:757–762.

78. Choudry NB, Watson R, Denburg J, O'Byrne PM. Time course of circulating inflammatory cells and their progenitors after allergen inhalation in asthmatic subjects [abstr]. Am Rev Respir Dis 1992; 145:A35.

79. Linden M, Svensson C, Andersson M, et al. Increased numbers of circulating leucocyte progenitors in patients with allergic rhinitis during natural allergen exposure [abstr]. Am J Respir Crit Care Med 1994; 149:A602.

80. Ohnishi M, Ruhno J, Bienenstock J, Dolovich J, Denburg JA. Hematopoietic growth factor production by cultured cells of human nasal polyp epithelial scrapings: kinetics, cell source, and relationship to clinical status. J Allergy Clin Immunol 1989; 83:1091–1100.

81. Ohtoshi T, Tsuda T, Vancheri C, et al. Human upper airway epithelial cell-derived granulocyte–macrophage colony-stimulating factor (GM-CSF) induces histamine-containing cell differentiation of human progenitor cells. Int Arch Allergy Appl Immunol 1991; 95:376–384.

82. Jordana M, Vancheri C, Ohtoshi T, et al. Hemopoietic function of the microenvironment in chronic airway inflammation. Agents Actions Suppl 1989; 28:85–95.

83. Denburg JA, Dolovich J, Ohtoshi T, Cox G, Gauldie J, Jordana M. The microenvironmental differentiation hypothesis of airway inflammation. Am J Rhinol 1990; 4:29–32.

84. Denburg JA, Dolovich J, Marshall J, et al. Eosinophil differentiation and cytokine networks in allergic inflammation. In: Gleich GJ, Kay AB, eds. Eosinophils in Allergy and Inflammation. New York: Marcel Dekker, 1993; 211–223.

85. Wahl SM. Transforming growth factor beta (TGF-beta) in inflammation: a cause and a cure. J Clin Immunol 1992; 12:61–74.

86. Sillaber C, Geissler K, Scherrer R, et al. Type beta transforming growth factors promote interleukin-3 (IL-3)-dependent differentiation of human basophils but inhibits IL-3 dependent differentiation of human eosinophils. Blood 1992; 80:634–641.

87. Finotto S, Ohno I, Lea R, et al. Tumor necrosis factorα [TNFα] gene expression by eosinophils in nasal polyp [NP] tissues [abstr]. Am Rev Respir Dis 1992; 145:A440.

88. Costa JJ, Matossian K, Resnick NB, et al. Human eosinophils can express the cytokines tumor necrosis factor-alpha and macrophage inflammatory protein-1 alpha. J Clin Invest 1993; 91:2673–2684.

89. Roodman, GD. TNF and hematopoiesis. In: Beutler B, ed. Tumor Necrosis Factor: The Molecules and Their Emerging Role in Medicine. New York: Raven Press, 1992:117–129.

90. Agosti JM, Sprenger JD, Lum LG, et al. Transfer of allergen-specific IgE-mediated hypersensitivity with allogeneic bone marrow transplantation. N Engl J Med 1988; 319:1623–1628.

91. Corrigan CJ, Kay AB. T cells and eosinophils in the pathogenesis of asthma. Immunol Today 1992; 13:501–507.

92. Denburg JA, Howie K, Girgis-Gabardo A. Expression of granulocyte macrophage-colony stimulating factor (GM-CSF) during maturation of eosinophils and basophils [abstr]. J Allergy Clin Immunol 1994; 93:194.

93. Bjorksten B, Gamrelidze A, Vanto T, Kjellman M. Seasonal variation of IgE synthesis in vitro by human peripheral blood mononuclear cells. Allergy 1990; 45:572–576.

94. Bjornson BH, Harvey JM, Rose L. Differential effect of hydrocortisone on eosinophil and neutrophil proliferation. J Clin Invest 1985; 76:924–929.

95. Spry CJ, Kay AB, Gleich GJ. Eosinophils 1992. Immunol Today 1992; 13:384–387.

96. Denburg J, Howie K, Dolovich J, Jordana M. Profile of eosinophil cytokine responses in hypereosinophilic syndrome (HES): lack of effect of granulocyte–macrophage colony-stimulating factor [abstr]. J Allergy Clin Immunol 1992; 89:160.

97. Denegri JF, Naiman SC, Gillen J, Thomas JW. In vitro growth of basophils containing the

Philadelphia chromosome in the acute phase of chronic myelogenous leukemia. Br J Haematol 1978; 40:351–352.

98. Le Beau MM, Lemons RS, Espinosa R III, Larson RA, Arai N, Rowley JD. Interleukin-4 and interleukin-5 map to human chromosome 5 in a region encoding growth factors and receptors and are deleted in myeloid leukemias with a del(5q). Blood 1989; 73:647–650.

99. Tallman MS, Hakimian D, Snower D, Rubin CM, Reisel H, Variakojis D. Basophilic differentiation in acute promyelocytic leukemia. Leukemia 1993; 7:521–526.

100. Lillington DM, MacCallum PK, Lister TA, Gibbons B. Translocation t(6;9) in acute myeloid leukemia without myelodysplasia or basophilia. Leukemia 1993; 7:527–531.

7

Innervation of Inflammatory Cells

Andrzej M. Stanisz and Ron H. Stead
McMaster University, Hamilton, Ontario, Canada

Ruth M. Williams
Eberhard-Karls-Universitat, Tubingen, Germany

INTRODUCTION

Until recently, the immune system was viewed as a discrete, compartmentalized, self-sufficient network of cells mediating humoral and cellular immunity. Traditionally, immune functions have been studied at the levels of T and B lymphocytes, macrophages, and granulocytic cells, focusing exclusively on the immune system per se. However, within the past few years, the interactions between the brain, endocrine, and immune systems have been shown to play important roles in health (and disease) of the organism. It is now generally accepted that the functions of lymphoid cells can be modulated by cells of nonlymphoid lineages and that the local microenvironment plays a crucial role in the initiation and maintenance of the immune response. The current view is not of a compartmentalized, functionally independent immune system, but one of integrated multiple cell functions that serve a common goal (i.e., response to a pathogen).

In contrast to the immune system, the inflammatory response in its classic form of dolor (pain), calor (heat), rubor (redness), and tumor (swelling) has been known for quite some time to be under neuroendocrine influence. Fundamental observations have now shown that adaptive immune responses can also be regulated by the nervous system. Thus, not only the immediate connective tissue responses to injurious stimuli, but also the capacity to mount antigen-mediated primary and secondary events, can be modulated by peripheral nerves.

In this chapter we would like to present some anatomical and functional data supporting neural regulation of the spectrum of inflammatory and immune reactions. In particular, we will review the evidence suggesting that mast cells, lymphocytes, macrophages, and eosinophils are found in close proximity to nerves in peripheral tissues, and the data that inflammatory cells can respond to nerve products both in vivo and in vitro (Table 1). We will also review changes in the proposed neuroimmune axes during inflammatory conditions and discuss the evidence for neuronal plasticity in such situations.

Table 1 The Known Effects of Neurotransmitter–Neuropeptides on Inflammatory Cells

Cell	Functional changes[a]
Mast cell	Degranulation
	Histamine release
	Serotonin release
	TNF-α release
B lymphocyte/plasma cells	Proliferation
	Immunoglobulin synthesis
T lymphocyte	Proliferation
	Cytokine production
	Lymphocyte migration
	Cytotoxic activity
Macrophages	Phagocytic activity
	Release of proinflammatory mediators
	Chemotaxis
Neutrophils	Phagocytic activity
	Release of proinflammatory mediators
	Chemotaxis

[a]Increased or decreased changes have been reported, depending on the specific neuropeptide or transmitter, dose, and tissue source of cells. For further details and references see text.

Over the past decade the number of publications on neuroimmune interactions has been growing exponentially. Accordingly, the literature in this field is now extensive. Space limitations do not permit an exhaustive and comprehensive review on all aspects of the innervation of inflammatory cells, which would warrant an entire volume. Therefore, we provide limited information in some sections, and refer the reader to relevant reviews for more details and additional references.

WHAT IS INNERVATION?

For there to be a direct interaction between the cells of the immune or inflammatory system and nerves or their products in vivo, various criteria must be met (Table 2). Nerve terminals should be found in the vicinity of the target cell(s); and following nerve stimulation, transmitter(s) should be released. For the transmitter to be active, specific receptors must be present on target cells. Occupancy of these receptors will activate second-messenger systems, resulting in a functional response. In this context, it is necessary to remember that indirect effects mediated by a chain reaction of neighboring cells could have profound consequences on inflammatory cell function, even though direct innervation of all inflammatory cells might not preexist.

It should be recognized that peripheral nerves do not necessarily form classic neuromuscular-type synapses or specialized membrane structures at their sites of communication with other cells. Rather, the neurotransmitters are stored in secretory vesicles that aggregate in swellings (varicosities) in preterminal axons of both sensory and autonomic nerves. It is now presumed that on stimulation these nerves exert their influence on various cell types by "en passant" release of neurotransmitters from varicosities (1). These are

Table 2   Criteria for Neuroeffector Function

1. Nerve fibers ending in close proximity to the target cell(s)
2. Release and availability of the neurotransmitter(s)
3. Presence of receptors on target cell(s)
4. Second messenger(s) linked to the target cell receptors
5. Functional response(s) by target cells

often separated from their targets by a distance of 200–300 nm (or up to 2 μm in some instances); therefore, membrane–membrane contact between the nerve and its target is not a prerequisite for communication. Nevertheless, the closer a target cell is to a nerve, the higher is the "dose" of the relevant transmitter to which it will be exposed. To our knowledge it is not known what local concentrations of neurotransmitters are released from varicosities, but, intuitively, these must be high enough to effect neurotransmission to any potential target expressing the appropriate response machinery (see Table 2). Dilution of the transmitters as they diffuse away from the varicosities (as well as degradation by specific enzymes) makes it unlikely that nerves mediate paracrine or endocrine effects. Thus, peripheral nerves may be considered as a system for targeted delivery of regulatory molecules. Viewed in reverse, regulatory cytokines released by cells of the immune system may impinge on the peripheral nervous system, providing such nerves have the appropriate receptors. Moreover, communication in either direction does not require stasis; transient cells may also activate nerves or be activated by local nerves.

WHAT IS NEUROGENIC INFLAMMATION?

Inflammation as an immediate defensive response to tissue injury, and invasion of the host by microorganisms is characterized by an accumulation and subsequent activation of leukocytes at the site of injury. This reaction also involves dilation of arterioles, capillaries, and venules; increased permeability and blood flow; and exudation of fluid and plasma proteins. Neurogenic inflammation was first described in the skin (2), where an inflammatory response to the application of mustard oil was prevented by nerve section distal, but not proximal, to the dorsal root ganglion (DRG). Many authors have confirmed that activation of selected nerves can induce vasodilation, vascular permeability, and other inflammatory changes. A significant part of nerve-induced inflammation is mediated by capsaicin-sensitive primary sensory neurons; that is, neurons containing substance P (SP) and other neuropeptides.

Neurogenic inflammation has been described in many organs and tissues (3–5), and the contribution of the nervous system to the pathophysiology of local inflammation is now a generally accepted concept. Studies on the mechanisms of neurogenic inflammation have shown a role for neuropeptides in the initiation, modulation, and perpetuation of immune and inflammatory events (6–10). Included in the array of peptides are SP, vasoactive intestinal peptide (VIP), somatostatin (SOM), and calcitonin gene-related peptide (CGRP). A variety of inflammatory cell populations express specific receptors for these neuropeptides, and there is considerable evidence for microanatomical associations of immune cells with autonomical and peptidergic nerve fibers (see later and 11–15). Furthermore, a number of neuropeptides are reported to be capable of causing significant metabolic changes in inflammatory cells (see later) and SP is established as a classic neurogenic inflammatory mediator (16).

Substantial evidence implicates mast cells in neurally mediated events; and this cell type might very well act as a relay between peripheral nerves and connective tissues in the "neurogenic" component of inflammatory responses. However, other immune cell types may also be innervated. Accumulating evidence has shown that neuropeptides influence the activity of granulocytes, monocytes–macrophages, and lymphocytes. Thus, leukocyte chemotaxis, leukocyte adhesion to the vessel wall, leukocyte migration into tissue, antibody production by lymphocytes, and the release of mediators from leukocytes may be under the control of neuropeptides released from nerve endings. In the following section we will review the evidence from microanatomical associations between nerves and immune cells; and the data suggesting inflammatory cells respond to neurotransmitters and peptides both in vivo and in vitro.

THE INNERVATION OF INFLAMMATORY CELLS

Mast Cells

Neurogenic inflammation expresses itself in diverse ways, many of which are mast cell-dependent. Traditionally, mast cells fulfill an important role in immediate hypersensitivity reactions by releasing numerous mediators, such as histamine, in response to immunoglobulin E (IgE) and specific antigen. The released mediators have pronounced biological effects, causing tissue edema and increased vascular permeability. Allergen binding is not the only stimulus capable of inducing mast cell degranulation (17), and research in recent years has suggested that neural mechanisms are involved in mast cell stimulation (12,15,18,19).

Morphological evidence, in many regions of the body, demonstrates that mast cells are in close apposition to autonomic, sensory, and neuropeptide-containing nerve terminals (Table 3; for a more complete review, see Ref. 20). For example, in the intestinal lamina propria, intestinal mucosal mast cells (IMMC) were found in close apposition to SP- and CGRP-containing nerves (Fig. 1; 13) and, similarly, in the respiratory tract (35). Studies in the rat lacrimal gland suggest close structural associations between mast cells and peptidergic nerves, in particular SP- and CGRP-immunoreactive (IR) fibers, which, although sparsely distributed in the gland, were invariably found close to mast cells (15). Mast cells have also been described in association with nerves in lymphoid tissues. For example, neuropeptide-containing nerve fibers have been demonstrated in the thymus, some of which were found in close apposition to mast cells. This association was particularly characteristic for tachykinin (TK)- and CGRP-IR nerves; however, VIP- and neuropeptide Y (NPY)-positive fibers have also been demonstrated in the thymus, localized to the vasculature, and near mast cells, occasionally making contact with the latter (36,37). This association with mast cells is similar to that described in the rat gut mucosa (13). Neuropeptides are also reported to interact with mast cells in lymph nodes (38). This association is regularly encountered, particularly with SP-, CGRP-, VIP-, and NPY-containing nerve fibers. The mast cells thus appear as a potential integrator of neural signals in lymphoid organs, as described in other tissues (13, 15).

Compelling functional evidence indicates that SP acts as a potent secretagogue for some mast cell mediators which, in turn, induce vasodilation and permeability. SP is known to induce histamine release from peritoneal mast cells (29,40) and skin mast cells (41–43). Other pharmacological studies (unpublished) have indicated SP as a potent serotonin (5-

Table 3   Morphological Evidence of Mast Cell–Nerve Associations

Species	Site	Nerve type	Data[a]	Ref.
Human	Colon	ACh ?	EM	21
Human	Small and large intestine	—	LM, EM	22
Human	Skin	NF (Ag)[b]	LM	23
Human	Glomus tumors	[c]	LM, EM	24, 25
Human	Arm	—	LM	26
Rat	Jejunum	SP, CGRP	LM, EM	13
Rat	Lacrimal gland	SP, CGRP	LM	15
Rat	Trachea	SP, CGRP	LM, EM	27
Rat	Lung	—	LM, EM	27
Rat	Ileum	—	EM	28
Rat	Colon	ACh	EM	29
Rat	Jejunum	—	EM	30
Rat	Duodenum	—	EM	32
Rat	Thymus	TK, CGRP, VIP, NPY	LM	36, 37
Rat	Lymph node	SP, CGRP, VIP, NPY	LM	38
Mouse	Ileum	—	LM	23
Dog	Colon	—	LM	34
Pig	Skin	SP, CGRP	IF	31
Cat	Duodenum	—	EM	32
Opossum	Stomach	—	EM	33

[a]LM, light microscopy; EM, electron microscopy; IF, immunofluorescence.
[b]Demonstrated using silver stains which localize neurofilaments.
[c]Abundant SP-containing nerves in glomus tumors.

hydroxytryptamine; 5-HT) liberator (for review, see Ref. 44). Interestingly, data from Levi-Schaffer and Shalit (45), using rat peritoneal mast cells, have shown that different mast cell secretagogues (antigen and neuropeptides) can cause differential release of histamine and prostaglandin D_2. Church et al. (43) have also commented on a similar differential activation of mast cells. Recently, Ansel et al. (46) have shown that low doses of SP cause selective release of tumor necrosis factor-α (TNF-α) from mast cells.

In addition to the neuropeptide secretagogue effects on mast cells, there is evidence that some neurotransmitters can modify mediator secretion induced by other stimuli. White et al. (47) showed that sympathetic stimulation through β-adrenoceptors inhibited antigen-induced mast cell degranulation. Acetylcholine (ACh) also appears to induce mast cell secretion, but there is heterogeneity in the reported mast cell responses (10).

The relationship of mast cells to the nervous system has led to the suggestion that mast cells might be considered as migrating unicellular glands, having diverse functions according to environmental conditions (20,48). Another important function proposed for mast cells in the neuroimmune connection is one of a "sensory transducer," receiving and transmitting information by primary sensory neurons and neuropeptides, to and from the brain. This bidirectional flux of information has been depicted in lymphoid tissue (37). It is suggested that mast cells release their mediators in response to sensory and autonomic neuropeptides which, in turn, transmit information to primary sensory neurons. By a cascade of sensory pathways, this information passes to the brain (37). Psychological conditioning experiments have suggested that mast cells may be modulated by the central nervous system (49), and psychological factors such as stress, hypnosis, and mental

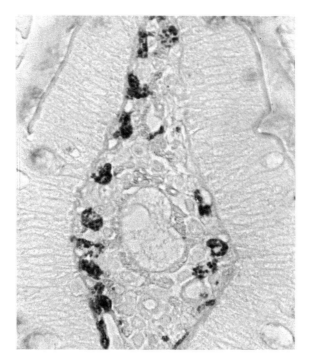

Figure 1   The close apposition of IMMCs and enteric nerves can be seen in this cross section of a rat jejunal villus. Note that some mast cells appear to enclose nerves (AB 0.5/NSE staining; ×425).

illnesses are thought to activate the sensory nervous system, resulting in an increased release of peptides in the periphery. Since neuropeptides activate mast cells, it is believed that such a sequence of events could initiate or block inflammatory systems, augmenting or perpetuating disease processes. Mast cells and nerves thus appear to function as an integrative network in the inflammatory processes.

Basophils

Basophils are physiologically very similar to mast cells. They bear receptors that bind IgE and participate in immunological reactions through the release of mediators that exert a variety of biological effects, including increased vascular permeability, smooth-muscle contraction, and enhancement of the inflammatory response. There are no reports describing the innervation of basophils. However, in light of existing knowledge supporting mast cell innervation and knowing, for example, that inflamed connective tissue can contain significant numbers of basophils and be richly innervated with sensory nerves housing a large array of neuropeptides, a close association of axons and recruited basophils might be predicted.

Macrophages

Macrophages are key players in the immune response, involved in antigen presentation and phagocytosis. The presence of nerve fibers in close proximity to macrophages appears to be a general neuroanatomical arrangement, particularly for sensory nerves. In the thymus gland, Muller and Weihe (50) described a spatial relation between peptidergic nerve fibers and macrophages. The majority of nerve–macrophage associations in the thymus involve the TK–CGRP fiber population. Associations with VIP- and vascular NPY-IR fibers were also observed, but less frequently. Similar relations were observed in tonsils (51), and nerve–macrophage contracts involving SP and CGRP were regularly encountered in the bronchus-associated lymphoid tissue (BALT) of the lung (52). In the chicken bursa of Fabricius, a close association between VIP-IR fibers and macrophages was observed (53). This was not observed for CGRP- and TK-IR fibers. In Peyer's patches, some evidence suggests that SP-containing nerve fibers infiltrate T-cell zones and associate with macrophages. Associations between CGRP and Langerhans cells, in esophageal mucosa, has been reported during inflammation (54). Using confocal laser microscopy CGRP-containing nerve fibers were observed in intimate association with Langerhans cells in human epidermis (55), and in functional assays, CGRP inhibited antigen presentation by Langerhans cells (55). Nerve–macrophage connections have also been encountered in other somatic and visceral tissues (for review, see Ref. 37). This microanatomical relation suggests the participation of macrophages in neurogenic inflammation.

Additional evidence supporting this proposition demonstrates neuropeptide receptors on macrophages and neuropeptide modulation of macrophage function. Jeurissem et al. (56) first demonstrated a non-NK receptor-binding site for SP on human monocytes, concluding that these are functionally linked to the reported effects of SP on cytokine production. Specific SP-binding sites on macrophages were isolated (57), occupation of which mediated macrophage activation. The VIP receptors have also been characterized on rat peritoneal macrophages (58), the physiological significance of which is unclear. However, the inhibition of monocyte function by VIP has been reported (59,60). Furthermore, a high proportion of CGRP receptors have been found on a macrophage-like cell line (61).

Neuropeptides, primarily SP, have been reported to modulate certain macrophage functions. Substance P, even at low concentrations, enhances the release of interleukin (IL)-1, IL-6, and TNF-α by blood monocytes (62–64) and induces the release of IL-1-like activity from a mouse macrophage cell line (65). Recently, endogenous norepinephrine was reported to regulate TNF-α production by macrophages in vitro (66). The generation of thromboxane A$_2$, oxygen free radicals, and hydrogen peroxide (H$_2$O$_2$), the down-regulation of membrane-associated 5′-nucleotidase and the stimulation of synthesis and release of arachidonic acid metabolites are also reported. Furthermore, there is evidence that SP enhances macrophage phagocytic activity (57,67). Generally, function of macrophages appears to be inhibited by CGRP, as evidenced by a reduction in their ability to produce the reactive oxygen metabolite, H$_2$O$_2$ and to present antigen (68). Collectively this evidence suggests macrophage function to be under modulatory influence of the nervous system.

Eosinophils

Eosinophils function as phagocytic cells in the inflammatory process. Furthermore, the eosinophil has been implicated as a putative cell of tissue injury, possibly through the release of its toxic compounds. In the gastrointestinal tract eosinophils are positioned for interaction with nerves. The lamina propria contains the greatest densities of nerves and immune effector cells in the intestinal mucosa. Arizono (1990) reported eosinophils in close proximity to non-myelinated nerve terminals or axons in the jejunal mucosa of rats. In studies conducted with Drs. Quinonez and Bramwell we also found extensive associations of eosinophils with nerves (69). Other studies have commented on the association of eosinophils with nerves in the intestinal mucosa. Felten and colleagues (70) observed noradrenergic terminals in the thymus, in close proximity to a variety of cell types including eosinophils, suggesting noradrenergic innervation to have influence over this cell type. To date, there is very little known regarding neuropeptide actions on eosinophil functions. The only report published to date is by Numao and Agrawal (164), where neuropeptides, including SP, NK-A, CGRP, and CCK had no effect by themselves, but potentiated the platelet-activating factor-induced eosinophil chemotaxis in allergic subjects. This suggests that neuropeptides can modulate eosinophil function in allergic inflammation.

Neutrophils

Increasing evidence suggests that SP and other tachykinins (TKs) are capable of regulating neutrophil function (70–73). Both SP and other TKs have been reported to function as neutrophil activators, causing the release of proinflammatory mediators (73), and SP has been reported to potentiate inflammation by priming neutrophils for an enhanced response to a second stimulus. However, the mechanisms of priming are unknown (70). There is no direct neurological evidence to support the existence of functional interactions between neutrophils and peptidergic nerves; however, we do not find this surprising. During an inflammatory response, circulating neutrophils migrate into tissue sites, a response that may be at least partially subject to nervous control. For example, it is known that SP can induce neutrophil migration (74), and the induction (by mast cells) or endothelial adhesion molecules may further promote neutrophil extravasation. We speculate that at sites of tissue repair neutrophils might form temporary interactions with neuropeptide-containing nerves.

T and B Lymphocytes or Plasma Cells

Lymphocytes are central cells in immunity, regulating a complex series of events that result in antibody and cell-mediated defenses. The cytokines produced by lymphocytes are capable of a wide range of biological activities, affecting many stages of inflammatory responses. Current evidence indicates that several of the cellular steps in the lymphocyte response can be regulated by neuropeptides, and that disturbances in neuropeptide signaling is an integral feature of inflammatory processes.

Primary and secondary lymphoid organs receive noradrenergic (NA), cholinergic, and peptidergic innervation (13,37,75–77). Cholinergic and sympathetic noradrenergic innervation has been investigated extensively; however, the importance of peptidergic innervation in nerve–lymphocyte dialogue is not fully understood. Yet, accumulating evidence indicates that both catecholamines and neuropeptides influence the functional capabilities of several lymphoid organs, including thymus, spleen, lymph nodes, and Peyer's patches in the intestine. Furthermore, specific neurotransmitter–peptide receptors have been identified on immune effector cells (78,79). In this section we describe the distribution of nerves in lymphoid tissues, and the effects of neurotransmitters and neuropeptides on lymphocytes.

Distribution of Nerves in Lymphoid Tissues

Both primary and secondary lymphoid tissues are extensively innervated by fibers of the sympathetic nervous system. In general, NA innervation is derived from postganglionic sympathetic neurons that synapse with preganglionic fibers originating in the thoracic and upper lumbar spinal cord (80). Sympathetic NA nerve fibers innervate lymphoid tissues in a distinct pattern: dense plexi surround blood vessels and extend into the parenchyma of T-cell and macrophage zones, terminating in close proximity to several cell types (81).

There is much controversy over cholinergic innervation of lymphoid tissue (82–85), and there is no definite evidence for parasympathetic innervation. Staining for acetylcholinesterase (AChE) has been predominantly non-neural, and neural AChE staining was observed in association with sympathetic non-noradrenergic nerves and nonadrenergic, nonvagal nerves (86).

A variety of neuropeptides are now known to innervate all lymphoid organs (36,52,53, 70,76,81,87,88). This peptidergic innervation is provided by NPY, SP, CGRP, VIP, and SOM (37,47); however, the exact origins, distribution patterns, and target relations of peptidergic nerves in various lymphoid tissues is still unclear. The likely origins of lymphoid peptidergic innervations, which appears to partly depend on their regional distribution, has been summarized (37), and, similar to noradrenergic fibers, neuropeptides are found adjacent to immune cells in some lymphoid tissues.

Innervation patterns of the spleen are the best characterized of all lymphoid organs. Noradrenergic innervation is highly compartmentalized (80,81,87,88). The NA fibers are distributed mainly in the white pulp along the central arteries and in the periarteriolar lymphatic sheaths (PALS), where they are found adjacent to and in contact with T lymphocytes. These nerve fibers are also localized in the marginal zones of the spleen, where they are found adjacent to macrophages and plasma cells. Close appositions between lymphocytes and tyrosine hydroxylase-positive nerve terminals have been demonstrated at the ultrastructural level (87). The spleens of rats, beluga whales, pigs, and cats are innervated with NPY-, SP-, SOM-, and VIP-containing nerve fibers (87,89–91). In the rat, NPY and NA are colocalized in the postganglionic sympathetic fibers, associated with lymphocytes and macrophages. In contrast, evidence suggests that SP, SOM, and VIP are not colocalized in NA nerves (87), but are generally associated with the vasculature (92).

The thymus is richly innervated by the sympathetic and parasympathetic nervous systems (75,93). The NA nerve fibers form networks around blood vessels and interlobular septae (76,86). From these regions fibers branch into the cortical region, where they are reported to associate with thymocytes.

The NA sympathetic nerve fibers enter lymph nodes at the hilar region and travel along the vasculature and in the subcapsular plexus. Individual fibers branch into the cortical and paracortical parenchyma surrounding the follicles. In these regions, NA varicosities and T lymphocytes are closely associated (86). Similar to the spleen, multiple neuropeptides are present in the lymph nodes of several species (38).

It is now recognized that an extensive nerve plexus innervates the intestinal lamina propria (1,94). Various neurotransmitters, including NA and ACh, and several neuropeptides (94) have been localized in these nerves. The intestinal lamina propria also houses numerous immune effector cells. However, Peyer's patches are relatively sparsely innervated, especially in the B-cell follicles. The NA and peptidergic nerves are present in the T-cell zones of Peyer's patches and are frequently seen in association with high endothelial venules (81).

Modulatory Effects of Neurotransmitters and Neuropeptides on Lymphocyte Function

The anatomical evidence for NA and peptidergic innervation of lymphoid organs suggests potential modulator roles for these neurotransmitters in immune function. Indeed, both catecholamines and neuropeptides influence several parameters of immune function.

Numerous functional studies have shown that catecholamines modulate immune functions, to a considerable degree, by inhibiting and enhancing lymphocyte responsiveness (for review, see Ref. 86). Several studies suggest that catecholamines, through the regulation of intracellular cAMP, alter lymphocyte activity by inducing changes in lymphocyte traffic, proliferation, and antibody secretion (86).

Substance P influences a large number of T- and B-lymphocyte functions through specific SP receptors. Payan and colleagues previously demonstrated specific surface membrane receptors for SP present on human lymphocytes (95). We have significantly extended this work to the murine system, for which we described SP receptors on both T and B cells (96). We also characterized the kinetics of SP-binding sites on these cells (96). Not only B- and T-lymphocyte proliferation, but also immunoglobulin synthesis, is significantly altered by SP. These effects are isotype- and organ-specific; that is, IgA synthesis is affected most, and lymphocytes from mucosal sites respond to a greater extent than those isolated from peripheral lymphoid organs (97). We were able to fully confirm these in vitro observations in vivo, using a constant delivery system of SP (by miniosmotic pumps; 98). In addition, both in vitro and in vivo, SP enhanced an antigen-specific (anti-SRBC) immunoglobulin response (99). Natural killer cell activity of lymphocytes from the compartmentalized population of intestinal epithelial lymphocytes (IEL), but not those isolated from spleens, was significantly enhanced by SP both in vivo and in vitro (100).

Recent investigations in murine infections with *Schistosoma mansoni* have shown that granulomas isolated from the liver express an authentic SP (NK-1) receptor. Interaction of granuloma SP with this receptor was observed to modulate IFN-γ and antibody production (101). Also, in this animal model, SP and SOM modulated antigen-induced IgG2a secretion (102). Again an NK-1 receptor was shown to mediate the SP effect, but not the SOM effect. Lymphoid cell migration is also affected by SP, and Moore et al. have shown SP to alter the flow of various populations of lymphocytes through sheep popliteal nodes (103). These results have important implications in disease processes, since the manipulation of the recruitment of various subsets of lymphocytes by neuropeptides could quantitatively and qualitatively modulate the inflammatory process and regulate humoral and cell-mediated immunity.

Plasma cells have been reported in association with nerves in intestinal, respiratory, and secretory gland mucosae (13,104). Also, lymphoid tissue plasma cells have been reported in close proximity to noradrenergic terminals (70). A direct activity for SP on plasma cells has been postulated by Helme and colleagues, who have shown that the plaque-forming response to sheep red blood cell antigen in draining lymph nodes is virtually abolished in neonatally capsaicin-treated animals (105). In these experiments, the ability to form antigen-specific plaques was restored following the local simultaneous injection of SP and antigen.

Vasoactive intestinal polypeptide (VIP), a potent vasodilator, is widely distributed in central and peripheral nerves, particularly those around blood vessels and in the gut (93,106–110). The presence of VIP receptors on lymphocytes or lymphocyte cell lines has been reported by a number of investigators (79,111–115). Initially, it was thought that only T cells could bind VIP, but in subsequent experiments, it was shown that B cells also bind and can be activated by VIP (116). O'Dorisio and her colleagues demonstrated a potent VIP effect on adenylate cyclase activity in lymphocytes (116), and this observation has now been confirmed by other investigators (117). Subsequently, it was shown that VIP stimulates activation of cAMP-dependent protein kinase A and increases protein phosphorylation (118). Mitogen-induced lymphocyte proliferation is inhibited by VIP (111,119), probably as a consequence of decreased IL-2 production (120,121). It is probable that VIP affects CD4$^+$ T cells, as these cells bear high numbers of VIP receptors. In contrast, CD8$^+$

suppressor T cells, which are relatively resistant to VIP, have correspondingly fewer VIP receptors (120). This maximum inhibition of mitogen-induced cellular proliferation was not cAMP-dependent and occurred within the first 24 h of incubation with VIP (121). Other research groups have found that the proliferation of lymphocytes isolated from the human colon is significantly inhibited by VIP (107), but that peripheral blood lymphocytes, or those isolated from the jejunum, are not affected by VIP (122). Interestingly, VIP modulates mouse mucosal and splenic lymphocyte immunoglobulin production, having both stimulatory and inhibitory effects (97). For example, IgA synthesis by murine Peyer's patch lymphocytes was inhibited by VIP, whereas IgM syntheses was enhanced. It is difficult to ascertain from these studies if VIP was acting directly on B cells, or whether its effects were mediated by macrophages or T cells (113,123). The increase in output of an IgA secretory component by rat lacrimal gland acinar cells was affected by VIP in a time- and dose-dependent manner (124). Natural killer activity of human lymphocytes generally was inhibited by VIP; however, under certain experimental conditions, an increase in NK activity was witnessed (125).

Elegant studies by Ottaway have suggested that VIP is involved in the control of lymphocyte trafficking (123). The expression of VIP receptors on mesenteric lymph node lymphocytes can be down-regulated in the presence of VIP. The subsequent adoptive transfer to those VIP-treated cells resulted in the decrease of their ability to localize in the gut. Also, preincubation of lymphocytes with VIP alters their capacity to bind to high endothelial venules in lymphoid tissues. Inhibition of lymphocyte migration out of popliteal lymph nodes in sheep was also observed in the presence of VIP (104,126). Collectively, these observations suggest that VIP may play an important role in immunity by affecting cell movement and localization.

Somatostatin is one of the most common neuropeptides. It is also known as growth hormone release-inhibiting hormone, and may function as a central and peripheral nervous system neurotransmitter (127,128). Somatostatin receptors have been described on various lymphocytes and lymphoid cell lines (129–132). Proliferation of mitogen-stimulated T lymphocytes and MOLT-4 T lymphoblasts, as well as human colonic lymphocytes and splenic and mucosal murine lymphocytes, is reduced in the presence of SOM (97,133,134). However, under certain conditions, particularly at high concentrations of SOM, an enhancing effect on cell proliferation has been reported (135,136). Similarly, SOM can both inhibit and enhance murine plasmacytoma MOPC 315 cell proliferation (131). In both in vitro and in vivo experiments, SOM has had an inhibitory effect on cell proliferation, immunoglobulin synthesis, and NK activity (97,134). On the other hand, rat T-cell cytotoxic activity was enhanced by SOM (137). Spontaneous IgA synthesis by the murine MOPC 315 plasmacytoma cell line can be either increased or decreased in the presence of SOM, depending on the experimental conditions (131). Given its general enhancement of cAMP, it seems reasonable to assume that, under normal physiological conditions, SOM has an inhibitory effect on cell proliferation and immunoglobulin synthesis both in vitro and in vivo. As yet there are no data on the effects of SOM on antigen-specific responses, and the mechanisms by which SOM exerts its immunomodulatory properties remain to be determined.

Calcitonin gene-related peptide (CGRP) has vasodilatory properties (138) similar to SP, and dual-probe immunocytochemical investigations have consistently shown colocalization of these two neuropeptides (139,140). Receptors for CGRP have been demonstrated on mouse splenocytes, macrophages, T cells, and on rat lymphocytes (141–143). In contrast to the stimulatory effects of SP, CGRP exerts predominantly inhibitory effects on lymphocytes; for example, phytohemagglutinin (PHA)- and concanavalin A (ConA)-induced lymphocyte proliferation is inhibited by CGRP; however, lipopolysaccharide (LPS)-induced cell proliferation is unaffected by incubation with CGRP (121,144). The CGRP effects on lymphocytes are probably mediated by cAMP, which is increased in T cells on activation with this neuropeptide (121,141,144). In view of its common colocalization with the immunostimulatory SP, and CGRP's mainly inhibitory function, we speculate that CGRP is a natural endogenous antagonist of the proinflammatory action of SP. Clearly, further investigation of CGRP-related immune events are warranted to elucidate the role of this neuropeptide and to confirm or refute this tentative hypothesis.

CHANGES IN THE LOCAL INNERVATION DURING INFLAMMATION

Data suggesting perturbation of the neuroimmune axis have been derived largely from animal models of inflammation in the gastrointestinal tract. Alterations in neuropeptide levels are reported in rodent enteritis models, such as *Trichinella spiralis* (Ts). In the rat, increased levels of SP are detected in the myenteric plexus of Ts-infected gut (145), which appears to be regulated by IL-1 (146). Similarly, in Ts-infected mice, significantly increased levels of SP in the serum and small intestine are detected, correlating well with the progress of inflammation (147). More recent studies show that by inhibiting SP synthesis or release, or by antagonizing the SP receptor, a significant reduction of the intestinal inflammation can be achieved. Somatostatin has physiological effects opposite those of SP in this model, and thus SOM may inhibit SP-mediated inflammation in the murine intestinal mucosa (148).

It now appears that the nerve plexus of the intestinal mucosa becomes damaged during inflammation (149,150). Rat jejunal mucosal nerve fibres were found to degenerate during the acute inflammatory phase of infection with *Nippostrongylus brasiliensis* (Nb), with subsequent regeneration during the recovery phase. It is likely that these effects are mediated by the activation of specific cell types as part of the inflammatory response. Since changes in the levels of neurotransmitters during inflammatory episodes also occur, these data suggest structural and phenotypic plasticity of nerves during intestinal inflammation.

Several neuropeptides, particularly SP, have been implicated in the pathogenesis of various chronic inflammatory conditions; for example, the idiopathic inflammatory bowel diseases (IBD): Crohn's disease (CD) and ulcerative colitis (UC). Although there are contradictory data, it appears that in both forms of IBD, VIP- and SOM-containing nerve fibers are decreased, and extractable quantities of VIP and SOM are also decreased in the mucosa (151). In contrast, SP levels are significantly enhanced in UC mucosae, which is not observed in CD (152). Furthermore, in both forms of IBD, the number of SP receptor-binding sites are significantly increased (1000–2000 times normal) by cells involved in mediating inflammatory and immune responses (153).

Rheumatoid arthritis (RA) is a chronic inflammatory condition in which nerves or peptide transmitters are thought to contribute to the pathogenesis. Of those neuropeptides thought to be involved, much work has focused on SP and its ability to functionally alter immune status. In RA patients, levels of SP in the synovial fluid and serum are significantly higher than in controls (154). The presence of SP-immunoreactive nerves in the synovium has been confirmed (155) in various animal models of arthritis. In rats, once the nerves containing SP are abolished by capsaicin treatment, the arthritic limb is spared an inflammatory bout; denervation appears to relieve the joint swelling and pain as well. To the contrary, worsening signs of arthritis in rats are seen after intra-articular instillation of SP. This can be prevented by cotreatment with an anti-SP antibody (156).

CONCLUSIONS AND PERSPECTIVES

Results from in vivo work, and in vitro studies employing impure or mixed cell populations, represent the net effects of both direct and indirect responses of the putative target cell to the added neuropeptide–transmitter. Also relatively high doses of neuropeptides–transmitters are often necessary to evoke a functional effect on inflammatory cells. Some of the described actions of neurally derived mediators could, therefore, easily be overinterpreted. To illustrate this point, we discuss the effects of substance P on immunoglobulin production in the gut.

Since SP receptors are expressed on lymphocytes and both T and B cells proliferate in vitro in the presence of SP, it is easy to presume that corresponding responses from in vivo administration are directly mediated. However, the proliferative zones of B cells in the intestines are the germinal centers of Peyer's patches (and other lymphoid aggregates) which are very sparsely innervated (Fig. 2); but Peyer's patch B cells both proliferate and

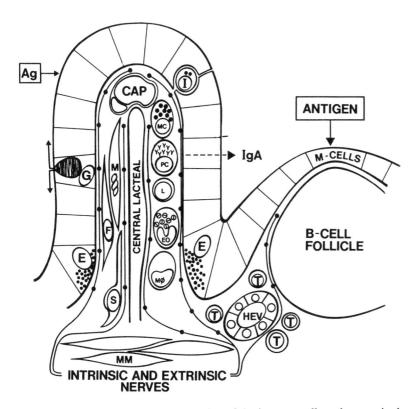

Figure 2 Highly schematic representation of the immune cells and nerves in the gastrointestinal mucosa. See text for discussion. Ag, antigen; cap, capillary; E, enteroendocrine cell; EO, eosinophil; F, fibroblast; G, goblet cell; HEV, high endothelial venule; I, intraepithelial leukocyte; L, lymphocyte; M, muscle cell; MC, mast cell; Mφ, monocyte; MM, muscularis mucosa; PC, plasma cell; S, Schwann cell; T, T lymphocyte.

produce increased amounts of IgA in response to SP. This suggests that little (if any) nerve-derived SP is available to act directly on the proliferating B-cell populations in germinal centers. Since SP is a late-acting cofactor, supporting IL-6-mediated IgA production (157), one might speculate that the effect of SP on B cells is postfollicular; that is, on B immunoblasts (plasmablasts). These plasma cell precursors leave Peyer's patches and migrate through the vasculature to the intestinal lamina propria. This part of the mucosa is densely innervated with SP-containing nerves, suggesting that true neurocrine actions are more likely to occur in the lamina propria per se than in lymphoid follicles. Interestingly, however, substance P receptor expression has been reported in lymphoid follicles in intestinal samples from IBD patients, but not in noninflamed bowel (153). Additionally, increased levels of tissue SP have been determined in inflamed intestines (145,147,152). These data suggest that SP receptors are possibly induced on follicular B cells in the presence of increased levels of SP. Clearly we need to gather more data in this area before we can begin to fully appreciate the role of nerves in regulating B-cell proliferation and differentiation. Moreover, such studies need expanding to encompass nerve-mediated commitment to IgE production, on which data are not available. Differential activation of T_H1 and T_H2 cells and stimulation of follicular dendritic cells must be studied in this context. This raises, once again, the issue of direct versus indirect effects.

The lamina propria of the small intestine is a good site to consider the multiple potential interactions between nerves and inflammatory or immune cells (see Fig. 2). This connective tissue element of the mucosa is packed with a mixture of inflammatory cells, and it is also densely innervated (one nerve fiber per 200 μm^2 of lamina propria in cross sections of rat jejunal villi; 150). Indeed, the mucosal nerve network secretes numerous peptides and classic neurotransmitters (128). This simple microanatomical evidence suggests that the lamina propria inflammatory cells might all be bathed in a mélange of nerve-derived molecules, including SP. Since most of the cell types present in the intestinal lamina propria (lymphocytes, plasma cells, macrophages, and mast cells) respond to SP, we must now ask which of the possible SP actions are more important; if some of the SP effects are inhibitory; or if SP primes an inflammatory cell to respond to a lower threshold of subsequent stimulation. We must also consider the "dose" of neurotransmitter, which might have a positive effect at low concentration and a negative effect at high concentration (or vice versa). Finally, we should also consider nonneural sources of neuropeptides, such as endocrine cells, as well as eosinophils and macrophages that are reported to synthesize SP (158), rat basophil leukemia cells that produce SOM (159) and truncated form of VIP (160), and neutrophils and eosinophils that also produce VIP (161).

In vivo, what are the main direct target cells for neuropeptides? Are they lymphocytes, macrophages, or connective tissue cells? All of these could be activated by neuropeptides. However, the mast cell seems to be a good candidate to play this role. It appears that mast cells in many tissues are in intimate association with nerves. These morphological data are supported by various functional studies that suggest bidirectional communication. The mast cell–nerve connection is worthy of additional study, since several perplexing questions remain unanswered concerning the complexity of mast cell–nerve associations. First, is this an obligatory functional unit, such that the release of neurotransmitters and peptides also results in mast cell activation? Do some nerve inputs inhibit mast cell secretion? Does mast cell activity influence neurotransmitter release? These questions are particularly important in the context of allergic reactions, during which mast cell degranulation occurs in response to antigen. Immunologically activated mast cells could potentially exert marked effects on nerve–immune cell interaction; or nerves could modulate the mast cell response to allergen. Second, how do mast cells recognize and respond to neuropeptide signals? The expression of cell surface receptors provides the means to receive such neuronal signals; however, the exact cellular mechanisms involved in mast cell activation are not fully understood. A receptor-independent pathway involving GTP-binding regulatory proteins (G-proteins) is one favored hypothesis for the mechanism of SP action on mast cells (56). However, Krumins and Broomfield (162) recently challenged this hypothesis, suggesting a receptor-mediated action for SP by apparent neurokinin (NK-1 and NK-2) receptors (162). Finally, are the relationships between mast cells and nerves altered during inflammation? We have commented on neural modeling in the gut mucosa during Nb infection. This appears to result in a 30% greater nerve density 7 weeks postinfection than in controls (150). At this time, both the mast cell density and degree of association with nerves are also increased (150,163). This implies a significantly greater connectivity between mucosal mast cells and nerves in the postinflammatory situation. In other words, the mast cell–nerve circuit is sensitized, which could result in a more rapid or augmented response from stimulation of either component. In contrast, during the acute inflammatory phase of Nb infection, mucosal mast cells are activated and mucosal nerves appear to degenerate (150). This suggests a period of disconnection, which would inhibit communication between these two cell types.

In this chapter we have provided substantial microanatomical and functional evidence for the innervation of inflammatory cells; yet, we are far from a complete understanding of the influence of neural signals on the initiation or perpetuation of the inflammatory–immune processes. Differences between normal and inflamed tissue must be detailed and the issues of augmentation, inhibition, priming, desensitization, and remodeling of both nerves and inflammatory cells carefully addressed. Over the next decade, we should be able to determine the importance of neuronal regulation of inflammatory processes.

ACKNOWLEDGMENTS

The authors' research is supported by the Medical Research Council (MRC) Canada, the Crohn's and Colitis Foundation of Canada (CCFC) and the Canadian Arthritis Society (CARS). We would like to thank Ms. Liz LaForme for her secretarial assistance.

REFERENCES

1. Cooke HJ. Neurobiology of the intestinal mucosa. Gastroenterology 1986; 90:1057–1081.
2. Bruce AN. Vasodilator axon reflexes. Q J Exp Physiol 1913; 6:339–354.
3. Kiernan JA. Pharmacological and histological investigation of the involvement of mast cells in cutaneous axon reflex vasodilation. Q J Exp Physiol 1975; 60:123–128.
4. Kowalski ML, Kaliner MA. Neurogenic inflammation, vascular permeability, and mast cells. J Immunol 1988; 140:3905–3911.
5. Levine JD, Dardick SJ, Basbaum AI, Scipio E. Reflex neurogenic inflammation: I. Contribution of the peripheral nervous system to spatially remote inflammatory responses that follow injury. Neuroscience 1985; 5:1380–1386.
6. Foreman JC, Jordan IC, Piotrowski W. Interaction of neurotensin with the substance P receptor mediating histamine release from rat mast cells and the flare in human skin. Br J Pharmacol 1982; 27:459–461.
7. Lembeck F, Holzer P. Substance P as a neurogenic mediator of antidromic vasodilatation and neurogenic plasma extravasation. Naunyn-Schmiedebergs Arch Pharmacol 1979; 310: 175–183.

8. Piotrowski W, Foreman JC. On the action of substance P, somatostatin and vasoactive intestinal polypeptide on rat peritoneal mast cells and human skin. Arch Pharmacol 1985; 331:364–368.

9. Foreman JC. Substance P and calcitonin gene-related peptide: effects on mast cells and in human skin. Int Arch Allergy Appl Immunol 1987; 82:366–371.

10. Befus AD. Reciprocity of mast cells–nervous system interactions. In: Tache BY, Wingate D, eds. Brain–Gut Interactions. Boca Raton, FL: CRC Press, 1994:315–329.

11. Shanahan F, Lee TD, Bienenstock J, Befus AD. The influence of endorphins on peritoneal and mucosal mast cell secretion. J Allergy Clin Immunol 1984; 74:449–504.

12. Shanahan F, Denburg JA, Fox J, Bienenstock J, Befus D. Mast cell heterogeneity: effects of neuroenteric peptides on histamine release. J Immunol 1985; 135:1331–1337.

13. Stead RH, Dixon MF, Bramwell NH, Riddell RH, Bienenstock J. Mast cells are closely apposed to nerves in the human gastrointestinal mucosa. Gastroenterology 1989; 97:575–585.

14. Stead RH, Tomioka M, Riddell RM, Bienenstock J. SP and/or CGRP are present in subepithelial enteric nerves apposed to intestinal mucosal mast cells. In: MacDermott RP, ed. Inflammatory Bowel Disease. New York: Excerpta Medica, 1988:43–48.

15. Williams RM, Singh J, Sharkey KA. Innervation and mast cells of the rat exorbital lacrimal gland: the effects of age. J Auton Nerv Syst 1994; 47:95–108.

16. Bienenstock JM, Blennerhassett M, Tomioka M, Marshall J, Perdue MH, Stead RH. Evidence for mast cell–nerve interactions. In: Goetzl EJ, Spector NH, eds. Neuroimmune Networks: Physiology and Diseases. New York: AR Liss, 1989:99–104.

17. Weshil BK, Galli SJ. Gastrointestinal mast cells. Gastroenterol Clin North Am 1991; 20: 613–627.

18. Foreman JC, Jordan CC, Oehme P, Remer H. Structure–activity relationships for some substance P-related peptides that cause wheal and flare reactions in human skin. J Physiol 1993; 335:449–465.

19. Barnes PJ. Regulatory peptides in the respiratory system. Experientia 1987; 43:832–839.

20. Stead RH, Perdue MH, Blennerhassett MG, Kakuta Y, Sestini P, Bienenstock J. The innervation of mast cells. In: Freier S, ed. The Innervation of Mast Cells: The Neuroendocrine–Immune Network. Boca Raton, FL: CRC Press, 1990:19–37.

21. Yonei Y. Autonomic nervous alterations and mast cell degranulation in the exacerbation of ulcerative colitis. Jpn J Gastroenterol 1987; 84:1045–1056.

22. Stead RH, Dixon MF, Bramwell NH, Riddell RH, Bienenstock J. Mast cells are closely apposed to nerves in the human gastrointestinal mucosa. Gastroenterology 1989; 97:575–585.

23. Heine H, Forster FJ. Histophysiology of mast cells in skin and other organs. Arch Dermatol Res 1975; 253:225–228.

24. Wiesner-Menzel L, Schulz B, Vakilzadeh F, Czarnetzki BM. Electron microscopical evidence for a direct contact between nerve fibres and mast cells. Acta Derm Venerol (Stockh) 1981; 61:465–469.

25. Kimura S. Mast cells in solitary glomus tumours: a possible allegenic role. Acta DermVenerol (Stockh) 1979; 59:415–419.

26. Eady RA, Cowen T, Marshall TF, Plummer V, Greaves MV. Mast cell population density, blood vessel density and histamine content in normal human skin. Br J Dermatol 1979; 100:623–633.

27. Kakuta Y, Stead RH, Perdue MH, Marshall JS, Bienenstock J. Microanatomical relationships of mast cells and nerves in rat lung and trachea. Am Rev Respir Dis 1989; 139:A118.

28. Newson B, Dahlstrom A, Enerback J, Ahlman H. Suggestive evidence for a direct innervation of mucosal mast cells. An electron microscopic study. Neuroscience 1983; 10:565–570.

29. Yonei Y, Oda M, Nakamura M, Watanabe HH, Tsuskada N, Komatsu HK, Akaiwa Y, Ichikawa E, Kanekook K, Asakura H, Fujiwara T, Tsuchiya M. Evidence for direct interaction between the cholinergic nerve and mast cells in the rat colonic mucosa. An electron microscope cytochemical and autoradiographic study. J Clin Electron Microsc 1985; 18:560–565.

30. Arizono W, Matsuda S, Hattori T, Kojima Y, Maeda T, Galli SJ. Anatomical variation in mast cell nerve associations in the rat small intestine, heart, lung and skin. Similarities of distances

between neural processes and mast cells, eosinophils or plasma cells in the jejunal lamina propria. Lab Invest 1990; 62:626–634.

31. Alving K, Sundstrom C, Matra R, Panula P, Hokfelt T, Lundberg JM. Association between histamine-containing mast cells and sensory nerves in the skin and airways of control and capsaicin-treated pigs. Cell Tiss Res 1991; 264:529–538.

32. Stack W. Uber die Nervengeflechte der Duodenalzotten: licht- und elektronen Mikroskopische-utersuchungen. Acta Anat 1973; 85:216.

33. Seelig LL, Schlusselberg DS, Smith WK, Woodward DJ. Mucosal nerves and smooth muscle relationships with gastric glands of the opossum: an ultrastructural and three-dimensional reconstruction study. Am J Anat 1985; 174:15–26.

34. Daley SJ, Rangachari PK, Stead RH. Mast cells are associated with PGP 9.5-immunoreactive nerves in the canine colonic mucosa: a compartmental analysis. In press.

35. Uddman R, Luts A, Sundler F. Occurrence and distribution of calcitonin gene-related peptide in the mammalian respiratory tract and middle ear. Cell Tissue Res 1985; 241:551–555.

36. Weihe E, Müller S, Fink T, Zentel MJ. Tachykinins, calcitonin gene-related peptide and neuropeptide Y in nerves of the mammalian thymus: interactions with mast cells in autonomic and sensory neuro-immunomodulation? Neuroscience 1989; 100:77–82.

37. Weihe E, Nohr D, Michel S, Müller S, Zentel MJ, Fink T, Krekel J. Molecular anatomy of the neuro-immune connection. Int J Neurosci 1991; 59:1–23.

38. Felten DL. Neurotransmitter signalling of cells of the immune system: important progress, major gaps. Brain Behav Immun 1991; 5:2–8.

39. Johnson AR, Erdös EG. Release of histamine from mast cells by vasoactive peptide. Proc Soc Exp Biol Med 1973; 142:1252–1256.

40. Pearce KL. Functional differences between mast cells from various locations. In: Befus AD, Bienenstock J, Denburg JA, eds. Mast Cell Differentiation and Heterogeneity. New York: Raven Press, 1986:215–222.

41. Hagermark O, Hokfelt T, Pernow B. Flare and itch induced by substance P in human skin. J Invest Dermatol 1978; 71:223–235.

42. Devillier P, Renoux M, Giroud JP, Regoli D. Peptides and histamine released from rat peritoneal mast cells. Eur J Pharmacol 1985; 117:89–96.

43. Church MK, Benyon RC, Rees RH. Functional heterogeneity of human mast cells. In: Galli SJ, Austen FK, eds. Mast Cell and Basophil Differentiation and Function in Health and Disease. New York: Raven Press, 1989:161.

44. Williams RM, Bienenstock J, Stead RH. The neuro-immune connection. In: Marone G, ed. Human Basophils and Mast Cells in Health and Disease. Basel: S Karger 1995: 208–235.

45. Levi-Schaffer F, Shalit M. Differential release of histamine and prostaglandin D_2 in rat peritoneal mast cells activated with peptides. Int Arch Allergy Appl Immunol 1989; 90:352–357.

46. Ansel JC, Braun JR, Payan DG, Brown MA. Substance P selectively activates TNF-α gene expression in murine mast cells. J Immunol 1993; 150:4478–4485.

47. White SR, Stimler-Gerard NP, Munoz WM, Popovion KJ, Murphy TM, Blake JS, Mack MM, Leff AR. Effect of beta-adrenergic blockade and sympathetic stimulation on canine bronchial mast cell response to immune degranulation in vivo. Am Rev Respir Dis 1989; 139:73–79.

48. Befus AD. Reciprocal interactions between mast cells and the endocrine system. In: Freier S, ed. The Neuroendocrine–Immune Network. Boca Raton, FL: CRC Press, 1990:39–52.

49. MacQueen G, Marshall JS, Siegal S, Perdue MH, Bienenstock J. Conditioned secretion of rat mast cell protease II release by mucosal mast cells. Science 1989; 243:83–85.

50. Müller S, Weihe E. Interaction of peptidergic innervation with mast cells and ED1-positive cells in rat thymus. Brain Behav Immun 1990; 5:55–72.

51. Weihe E, Krekel J. The neuroimmune connection in human tonsils. Brain Behav Immun 1991; 5:41–54.

52. Nohr D, Weihe E. The neuroimmune link in the bronchus-associated lymphoid tissue (BALT) of cat and rat: peptides and neural markers. Brain Behav Immun 1991; 5:84–101.

53. Zentel HJ, Weihe E. The neuro–B cell link of peptidergic innervation in the bursa Fabricii. Brain Behav Immun 1990; 5:132–147.
54. Singaram C, Segupta A, Stevens C, Spechler SJ, Goyal RK. Localisation of calcitonin gene-related peptide in human esophageal Langerhans cells. Gastroenterology 1991; 100:560–563.
55. Hosoi J, Murphy GF, Egan CL, Lerner EA, Grabbe S, Asahina A, Granstein RD. Regulation of Langerhans cell function by nerves containing calcitonin gene-related peptide. Nature 1993; 363:159–612.
56. Jeurissen F, Kavelaars A, Korstjens M, Brooke D, Franklin RA, Gelfand EW, Heijnen CJ. Monocytes express a non-neurokinin substance P receptor that is functionally coupled to MAP kinase. J Immunol 1994; 152:2987–2994.
57. Hartung HP, Wolters K, Toyka KV. Substance P binding properties and studies on cellular responses in guinea pig macrophages. J Immunol 1986; 136:3856–3863.
58. Segura JJ, Guerrero JM, Goberna R, Calvo JR. Characterization of functional receptors for vasoactive intestinal peptide (VIP) in rat peritoneal macrophages. Regul Peptides 1991; 33:133–143.
59. Wiik P. Vasoactive intestinal peptide inhibits the respiratory burst in human monocytes by a cyclic AMP mediated mechanism. Regul Peptides 1989; 25:187–197.
60. Wiik P, Haigen AH, Luhaug D, Byom A, Opstad PK. Effect of VIP on the respiratory burst in human monocytes ex vivo during prolonged strain and energy deficiency. Peptides 1989; 10:819–823.
61. Abello J, Kaiserlian P, Cuber JC, Revillard JP, Chayvialle JA. Characterisation of calcitonin gene-related peptide receptors and adenylate cyclase response in the murine macrophage cell line P388D1. Neuropeptides 1991; 19:43–49.
62. Lotz M, Vaughan JH, Carson DA. Effect of neuropeptides on production of inflammatory cytokines by human monocytes. Science 1988; 241:1218–1221.
63. Cowdery JS, Kemp JD, Ballas ZK, Weber SP. Interleukin-1 induces T cell mediated differentiation of murine Peyer's patch B cells to IgA secretion. Regul Immunol 1988; 1:9–14.
64. Beagley KW, Eldridge JH, Lee JH, Kiyono H, Everson MP, Koopman WJ, Hirano T, Kishimoto T, McGhee JR. Interleukins and IgA synthesis. Human and murine interleukin 6 induce high rate IgA secretion in IgA-committed B cells. J Exp Med 1989; 169:2133–2148.
65. Kimball ES, Persico FJ, Vaught JL. Substance P, neurokinin A, and neurokinin B induce generation of IL-1-like activity by P388D1 cells. J Immunol 1988; 141:3564–3569.
66. Spengler RN, Chensue SW, Giacherio DA, Blenk N, Kunkel SL. Endogenous norepinephrine regulates tumor necrosis factor-α production from macrophages in vitro. J Immunol 1994; 152:3024–3031.
67. Bar-Shavit Z, Goldman R, Stabinsky Y, Gottlieb P, Fridkin M, Teichborg VI, Blumberg S. Enhancement of phagocytosis—a newly found activity of substance P residing in its N-terminal tetrapeptide sequence. Biochem Biophys Res Commun 1980; 94:1445–1451.
68. Hanko J, Hardebo JE, Kahrstrom J, Owman C, Sundler F. Calcitonin gene-related peptide is present in mammalian cerebrovascular nerve fibers and dilates pial and peripheral arteries. Neurosci Lett 1985; 57:9195.
69. Quinonez G, Bramwell NH, Bienenstock J, Colley ECC, Riddell RH, Simon GT, Stead RH. Eosinophils are in intimate association with nerves in normal and nematode injected rat jejunal mucosae and in human small and large bowel mucosae. In preparation.
70. Felten DL, Felten SY, Carlson SL, Olschowka JA, Livnat S. Noradrenergic and peptidergic innervation of lymphoid tissue. J Immunol 1985; 135:755–765.
71. Wozniak A, McLennon G, Betts WH, Murphy GA, Scicchitano R. Activation of human neutrophils by substance P: effect on FMLP-stimulated oxidative and arachidonic acid metabolism on antibody-dependent cell-mediated cytotoxicity. Immunology 1989; 68:359–364.
72. Serra MC, Bazzoni F, Blanca VD, Greskowiak M, Rossi F. Activation of human neutrophils by substance P. J Immunol 1988; 141:2118–2124.
73. Wozniak A, Betts WH, McLennan G, Scicchitano R. Activation of human neutrophils by

tachykinins: effect on formyl-methionyl-leucyl-phenylalanine- and platelet-activating factor-stimulated superoxide anion production and antibody-dependent cell-mediated cytotoxicity. Immunology 1992; 78:629–634.

74. Matis WL, Lavker RM, Murphy GL. Substance P induces the expression of an endothelial-leukocyte adhesion molecule by microvascular endothelium. J Invest Dermatol 1990; 94: 492–495.

75. Felten SY, Felten DL, Belinger DL, Carlson SL, Ackerman KD, Madden KS, Olschowka JA, Livnat S. Noradrenergic sympathetic innervation of lymphoid organs. Prog Allergy 1988; 43:14–36.

76. Fink T, Weihe E. Multiple neuropeptides in nerves supplying mammalian lymph nodes: messenger candidates for sensory and autonomic neuroimmunomodulation? Neurosci Lett 1988; 90:39–44.

77. Weihe E. Neuropeptides in primary sensory neurons. In: Zenker W, Neuhuber W, eds. The Primary Afferent Neurone—A Survey of Recent Morpho-Functional Aspects. New York: Plenum Press, 1990:127–159.

78. O'Dorisio MS, Shannon BT, Fleshman DJ, Campolito LB. Identification of high affinity receptors for vasoactive intestinal peptide on human lymphocytes of B cell lineage. J Immunol 1989; 142:3533–3536.

79. Payan DG. Neuropeptides and inflammation: the role of substance P. Annu Rev Med 1989; 40:341–352.

80. Felten DL, Felten SY, Bellinger DL, Carlson SL, Ackerman KD, Madden KS, Olschowka JA, Livnat S. Noradrenergic sympathetic neural interactions with the immune system: structure and function. Immunol Rev 1987; 100:225–260.

81. Felten SY, Felten DL. Innervation of lymphoid tissue. In: Ader R, Felten DL, Cohen N, eds. Psychoneuroimmunology—II. San Diego: Academic Press, 1991:27–68.

82. Tollefson L, Bulloch K. Dual-label retrograde transport: CNS innervation of the mouse thymus distinct from other mediastinum viscera. J Neurosci Res 1990; 25:10–28.

83. Bullock K. A comparative study of the autonomic nervous system innervation of the thymus in the mouse and chicken. Int J Neurosci 1989; 40:129–140.

84. Nance DM, Hopkins DA, Bieger D. Re-investigation of the innervation of the thymus gland in mice and rats. Brain Behav Immun 1987; 1:134–147.

85. Bellinger DL, Felten SY, Felten DL. The origin of acetylcholinesterase-positive fibers or the spleen of young adult rats. Soc Neurosci 1988; 14:956–964.

86. Madden KS, Livnat S. Catecholamine action and immunologic reactivity. In: Ader R, Felten DL, Cohen N, eds. Psychoneuroimmunology. San Diego: Academic Press, 1991:283–310.

87. Felten SY, Olschowka JA. Noradrenergic sympathetic innervation of the spleen: II tyrosine-hydroxylase (TH)-positive nerve terminals form synaptic-like contacts on lymphocytes in the splenic white pulp. J Neurosci Res 1987; 18:37–48.

88. Fried G, Terenius L, Brodin E, Efendic S, Dockray G, Fahrenkrug J, Goldstein M, Hökfelt T. Neuropeptide Y, enkephalin and noradrenaline coexist in sympathetic neurons innervating the bovine spleen. Biochemical and histochemical evidence. Cell Tissue Res 1986; 243:495–508.

89. Olschowka JA, Felten SY, Bellinger DC, Lorton D, Felten DL. NPY-positive nerve terminals contact lymphocytes in the periarteriolar lymphatic sheath of the rat splenic white pulp (abstr). Soc Neurosci 1988; 14:1280.

90. Romano T, Olschowka JA, Felten SY, Felten DL. Tyrosine hydroxylase and neuropeptide Y positive nerve fibers in the spleen of the beluga whale. Proc Int Assoc Aquatic Anim Med 1989; 20:82.

91. Lundberg JM, Änggård A, Pernow J, Hökfelt T. Neuropeptide Y-, substance P-, and VIP-immunoreactive nerves in cat spleen in relation to autonomic vascular and volume control. Cell Tissue Res 1985; 239:9–18.

92. Lundberg JM, Felten SY, Carlson SL, Bellinger DL, Felten DL. Involvement of peripheral and central catecholamine systems in neural–immune interactions. J Neuroimmunol 1985; 10:5–30.

93. Williams JM, Peterson RG, Shea PA, Schmedtie JF, Bauer DC, Felten DL. Sympathetic innervation of murine thymus and spleen: evidence for a functional link between the nervous and immune systems. Brain Res Bull 1981; 6:83–94.

94. Davison JS. Innervation of the gastrointestinal tract. In: Christensen J, Wingate D, eds. A Guide to Gastrointestinal Motility. Bristol: Wright, 1983:1–47.

95. Payan DG, Brewster DR, Goetzl EJ. Stereo-specific receptors for substance P on cultured IM-9 lymphoblasts. J Immunol 1984; 133:3260–3265.

96. Stanisz AM, Scicchitano R, Dazin P, Bienenstock J, Payan DG. Distribution of substance P receptors on murine spleen and Peyer's patch T and cells. J Immunol 1987; 139:749–754.

97. Stanisz AM, Befus AD, Bienenstock J. Differential effect of vasoactive intestinal peptide, substance P and somatostatin on immunoglobulin synthesis and cell proliferation by lymphocytes from spleen, Peyer's patches and mesenteric lymph nodes. J Immunol 1986; 136:152–156.

98. Scicchitano R, Stanisz AM, Bienenstock J. In vivo immunomodulation by the neuropeptide substance P. Immunology 1988; 63:733–735.

99. Padol I, Agro A, Stanisz AM. Stimulatory effect of the neuropeptide substance P on antigen-specific immune response in mice. Prog Neuroendocrin-immunol 1990; 3:277–281.

100. Croitoru K, Ernst PB, Bienenstock J, Padol I, Stanisz AM. Selective modulation of the natural killer activity of murine intestinal intraepithelial leukocytes by the neuropeptide substance P. Immunology 1990; 71:196–201.

101. Cooke GA, Elliot D, Metwali A, Blum AM, Sandor M, Lynch R, Weinstock JV. Molecular evidence that granuloma T lymphocytes in murine schistosomiasis mansoni express an authentic substance P (NK-1) receptor. J Immunol 1994; 152:1830–1835.

102. Blum AM, Metwali AM, Mathew RC, Elliott D, Weinstock JV. Substance P and somatostatin can modulate the amount of IgG2a secreted in response to schistosome egg antigens in murine schistosomiasis mansoni. J Immunol 1993; 151:6994–7004.

103. Moore TC. Modification of lymphocyte traffic by vasoactive neurotransmitter substances. Immunology 1984; 52:511–518.

104. Walcott B, Keyser KT, Sibony PA. The association of nerves and plasma cells in a tear gland. Leukocytes Host Defense 1986; 2:227–232.

105. Helme RD, Eglezos A, Dandie GW, Andrews PV, Boyd RL. The effect of substance P on the regional lymph node antibody response to antigenic stimulation in capsaicin-pretreated rats. J Immunol 1987; 139:3470–3473.

106. Larsson LI, Fahrenkrug J, Schaffalitzky de Muckadell O, Sundler, F, Håkanson, Rehfeld J. Localization of vasoactive intestinal peptide (VIP) to central and peripheral neurons. Proc Natl Acad Sci USA 1976; 73:3197–3200.

107. Polak JM, Bloom SR. Distribution and tissue localization of VIP in the central nervous system and seven peripheral organs. In: Said SI, ed. Vasoactive Intestinal Peptide. New York: Raven Press, 1982:107–120.

108. McDonald TJ. Gastroenteropancreatic regulatory peptide structures: an overview. In: Daniel EE, ed. Neuropeptide Function in the Gastrointestinal Tract. Boca Raton, FL: CRC Press, 1991:19–86.

109. Ekblad E, Ekman R, Håkanson R, Sundler F. Projections of peptide-containing neurons in rat colon. Neuroscience 1988; 27:655–674.

110. Ottaway C, Lewis D, Asa S. Vasoactive intestinal peptide containing nerves in Peyer's patchers. Brain Behav Immun 1987; 1:148–158.

111. Wood CL, O'Dorisio MS. Covalent cross-linking of vasoactive intestinal polypeptide to its receptors on intact human lymphoblasts. J Biol Chem 1985; 260:1243–1247.

112. Finch RJ, Sreedharan SP, Goetzl EJ. High affinity receptor of vasoactive intestinal peptide on human myeloma cells. J Immunol 1989; 142:1977–1981.

113. Ottawa CA, Greenberg GR. Interaction of vasoactive intestinal peptide with mouse lymphocytes: specific binding and the modulation of mitogen responses. J Immunol 1984; 132:417–423.

114. Danek A, O'Dorisio MS, O'Dorisio TM, George JM. Specific binding sites for vasoactive intestinal polypeptide on nonadherent peripheral blood lymphocytes. J Immunol 1983; 131:1173–1177.

115. Beed EA, O'Dorisio MS, O'Dorisio TM, Gaginella TS. Demonstration of a functional receptor for vasoactive intestinal polypeptide on Molt 4b T lymphoblasts. Regul Peptides 1983; 6:1–12.

116. Ottaway CA, Jay T, Greenberg G. High affinity binding of vasoactive intestinal peptide to human circulating T cells, B cells and large granular lymphocytes. J Neuroimmunol 1990; 29:149–155.

117. Calvo JR, Guerrero JM, Molinero P, Blasco R, Goberna R. Interaction of vasoactive intestinal peptide (VIP) with human peripheral blood lymphocytes: specific binding and cyclic AMP production. Gen Pharmacol 1986; 17:185–189.

118. O'Dorisio MS, Wood CL, Wenger GD, Vassalo LM. Cyclic AMP-dependent protein kinase in Molt 4b lymphoblasts: identification by photo affinity labeling and activation in intact cells by vasoactive intestinal polypeptide (VIP) and peptidic histidine isoleuline (PHI). J Immunol 1985; 134:4078–4086.

119. O'Dorisio MS, Hermina NS, O'Dorisio TM, Balcerzak SP. Vasoactive intestinal polypeptide modulation of lymphocyte adenylate cyclase. J Immunol 1981; 127:2551–2554.

120. Ottaway CA. Selective effects of vasoactive intestinal peptide on the mitogenic response of murine T cells. Immunology 1987; 62:291–297.

121. Boudard F, Bastide M. Inhibition of mouse T-cell proliferation by CGRP and VIP: effects of these neuropeptides on IL-2 production and cAMP synthesis. J Neurosci Res 1991; 29:29–41.

122. Roberts AI, Panja A, Brolin RE, Ebert EC. Human intraepithelial lymphocytes: immunomodulation and receptor binding of vasoactive intestinal peptide. Dig Dis Sci 1991; 36: 341–396.

123. Ottaway CA. In vitro alteration of receptors for vasoactive intestinal peptide changes in the in vivo localization of mouse T cells. J Exp Med 1984:160:1054–1069.

124. Kelleher RS, Hann LE, Edwards JA, Sullivan DA. Endocrine, neural and immune control of secretory component output by lacrimal gland acinar cells. J Immunol 1991; 146:3405–3412.

125. Rola-Pleszczynski M, Bulduc D, St Pierre A. The effects of VIP on human NK cell function. J Immunol 1985; 135:2659–2673.

126. Moore TC, Spruck CH, Said SI. Depression of lymphocyte traffic in sheep by vasoactive intestinal peptide (VIP). Immunology 1988; 64:475–4781.

127. Wass JAH. Somatostatin. In: DeGroot JL, Besser GM, Cahill GF, eds. Endocrinology. Philadelphia: WB Saunders, 1990:152–153.

128. Ekblad E, Winther C, Ekman R, Håkanson R, Sundler F. Projections of peptide-containing neurons in rat small intestine. Neuroscience 1987; 20:169–188.

129. Bhathena SJ, Louie J, Schechter GP, Redman RS, Wahl L, Recant L. Identification of human mononuclear leukocytes bearing receptors for somatostatin and glucagon. Diabetes 1981; 30:127–131.

130. Nakamura H, Koike T, Hiruma T, Sato T, Tomioka H, Yoshida S. Identification of lymphoid cell lines bearing receptors for somatostatin. Immunology 1987; 62:655–658.

131. Scicchitano R, Dazin P, Bienenstock J, Payan DG, Stanisz AM. The murine IgA-secreting plasmacytoma MOPC-315 expresses somatostatin receptors. J Immunol 1988; 141:937–941.

132. Sreedharan SP, Kodama KT, Peterson KE, Goetzl EJ. Distinct subsets of somatostatin receptors on cultured human lymphocytes. J Biol Chem 1989; 264:949–952.

133. Agro A, Padol I, Stanisz AM. Immunomodulatory activities of the somatostatin analogue BIM 23014c: effects on murine lymphocyte proliferation and natural killer activity. Regul Peptides 1991; 32:129–135.

134. Payan DG, Hess CA, Goetzl EJ. Inhibition by somatostatin of the proliferation of T lymphocytes and Molt-4 lymphoblasts. Cell Immunol 1984; 84:433–438.

135. Pawlikowski M, Stepien H, Kunert Radek J, Zelazowski P, Schally AV. Immunomodulatory action of somatostatin. Ann NY Acad Sci 1987; 496:233–239.

136. Pawlikowski M, Stepien H, Kunert Radek J, Zelazowski P, Schally AV. Effect of somatostatin on the proliferation of mouse spleen lymphocytes in vitro. Biochem Biophys Res Commun 1985; 192:52–55.

137. Foris G, Gyimesi E, Komaromi I. The mechanism of antibody-dependent cellular cytotoxicity stimulation by somatostatin in rat peritoneal macrophages. Cell Immunol 1985; 90:217–225.

138. Brain SD, Williams TJ, Tippins JR, Morris HR, MacIntyre I. Calcitonin gene-related peptide is a potent vasodilator. Nature 1985; 313:54–56.

139. Clague JR, Sternini C, Brecha N. Localization of calcitonin gene-related peptide-like immuno-reactivity in neurons of the rat gastrointestinal tract. Neurosci Lett 1985; 56:63–68.

140. Hanko J, Hardebo JE, Kahrstrom J, Owman C, Sundler F. Calcitonin gene-related peptide is present in mammalian cerebrovascular nerve fibers and dilates pial and peripheral arteries. Neurosci Lett 1985; 57:91–95.

141. Abello J, Kaiserlain D, Cuber JC, Revillard JP, Chayvialle JA. Characterization of calcitonin gene-related peptide receptors and adenylate cyclase response in the murine macrophage cell line P388D1. Neuropeptides 1991; 19:43–49.

142. McGillis JP, Humphreys S, Reid S. Characterization of functional calcitonin gene-related peptide receptors on rat lymphocytes. J Immunol 1991; 147:3482–3485.

143. Umeda Y, Arisawa M. Characterization of the calcitonin gene-related peptide receptor in mouse T lymphocytes. Neuropeptides 1989; 14:237–242.

144. Umeda Y, Takamiya M, Yoshizaki H, Arisawa M. Inhibition of mitogen-stimulated T lympho-cyte proliferation by calcitonin gene-related peptide. Biochem Biophys Res Commun 1988; 154:227–235.

145. Swain MG, Agro A, Blennerhassett P, Stanisz A, Collins SM. Increased levels of substance P in the myenteric plexus of trichinella-infected rats. Gastroenterology 1992; 102:1913–1919.

146. Hurst S, Stanisz AM, Sharky K, Collins SM. Interleukin-1β induces increase in SP in rat myenteric plexus. Gastroenterology 1993; 105:1754–1760.

147. Agro A, Stanisz AM. Inhibition of murine intestinal inflammation by anti-substance P antibody. Regul Immunol 1993; 5:120–126.

148. Stanisz AM. Neuroimmunomodulation in the gastrointestinal tract. Ann NY Acad Sci 1994; 741:64–72.

149. Stead RH. Nerve remodelling during intestinal inflammation. Ann NY Acad Sci 1992; 664:443–455.

150. Stead RH, Kosecka-Janiszewska U, Oestreicher AB, Dixon MF, Bienenstock J. Remodelling of B-50 (GAP-43)- and NSE-immunoreactive mucosal nerves in the intestines of rats infected with *Nippostrongylus brasiliensis*. J Neurosci 1991; 11:3809–3821.

151. Koch T, Carney J, Govlin C. Distribution and quantitation of gut neuropeptides in normal and inflammatory bowel disease. Dig Dis Sci 1987; 32:369–376.

152. Goldin E, Karmeli F, Selinger Z, Rachmilewitz D. Colonic substance P levels are increased in ulcerative colitis and decreased in chronic severe constipation. Dig Dis Sci 1989; 34:754–757.

153. Mantyh CR, Gates TS, Zimmerman RP, Welton ML, Passaro EP, Vigna SR, Maggio JE, Kruger L, Mantyh PW. Receptor binding sites for substance P but not neuromedin K are expressed in high concentrations by arterioles, venules and lymph nodules in surgical specimens obtained from patients with ulcerative colitis and Crohn's disease. Proc Natl Acad Sci USA 1988; 85:3235–3239.

154. Marshall KW, Chiu B, Inman RD. Substance P and arthritis: analysis of plasma and synovial fluid levels. Arthritis Rheum 1990; 33:87–90.

155. Gronblad M, Konttinen YT, Korkala O, Liesi P, Hukkanen M, Polak JM. Neuropeptides in synovium of patients with rheumatoid arthritis and osteoarthritis. J Rheumatol 1988; 15:1807–1810.

156. Levine JD, Collier DH, Basbaum AI, Moskowitz MA, Helms CA. Hypothesis: the nervous system may contribute to the pathophysiology of rheumatoid arthritis. J Rheumatol 1985; 12:406–411.

157. Bost KL, Pascual DW. Substance P: a late-acting B lymphocyte differentiation cofactor. Am J Physiol 1992; 262:537–545.

158. Pascual DW, Bost KL. Substance P production by macrophage cell lines: a possible autocrine function for the peptide. J Immunol 1990; 71:52–56.

159. Goetzl EJ, Chernov-Rogan T, Cooke MP, Renold F, Payan DG. Endogenous somatostatin-like peptides of rat basophilic leukemia cells. J Immunol 1985; 135:207–2712.

160. Goetzl EJ, Sreedharan SP, Turck CW. Structurally distinctive VIP peptides from rat basophil leukemia cells. J Biol Chem 1988; 263:9083–9086.

161. Aliakbari J, Sreedharan SP, Turck CW, Goetzl EJ. Selective localisation of VIP and Substance P in human eosinophils. Biochem Biophys Res Commun 1987; 148:1440–1445.

162. Krumins SA, Broomfield CA. Evidence of NK1 and NK2 tackykinin receptors and their involvement in histamine release in a murine mat cell line. Neuropeptides 1992; 21:65–72.

163. Stead RH, Franks AJ, Goldsmith CH, Bienenstock J, Dixon MF. Mast cell, nerves and fibrosis in the appendix: a morphological study. J Path 1990: 161:209–219.

164. Numao T, Agrawal DK. Neuropeptides modulate human eosinophil chemotoxis. J Immunol 1992; 149:3309–3315.

8

Mast Cell and Basophil Development and Function

John J. Costa and Stephen J. Galli
Beth Israel Hospital and Harvard Medical School, Boston, Massachusetts

INTRODUCTION AND HISTORICAL PERSPECTIVE

Ehrlich (1) identified mast cells in human connective tissues on the basis of the metachromatic-staining properties of their prominent cytoplasmic granules. Ehrlich also described the basophil, a circulating leukocyte that contains cytoplasmic granules, with staining properties similar to those of the mast cell (2). Mast cells and basophils share several notable features besides staining properties (summarized in Table 1). Both cell types are derived from bone marrow progenitor cells, and both mast cells and basophils represent a major source of histamine and other potent chemical mediators that have been implicated in a wide variety of inflammatory and immunological processes, including allergic disorders with components of immediate hypersensitivity (reviewed in Refs. 3–8). In all mammalian species yet analyzed, both mast cells and basophils express plasma membrane receptors ($Fc_{\varepsilon}RI$) that specifically bind, with high affinity, the Fc portion of IgE antibody (9–12). Accordingly, mast cells and basophils are thought to represent critical effector cells in IgE-dependent host responses to parasites and allergic diseases (3–12). Several lines of evidence indicate that mast cells and basophils may also have important functions in a variety of other immunological, pathological, and perhaps physiological processes (3–8).

In light of their many similarities, it once was believed that basophils might represent the circulating precursor of mast cells, or that mast cells were "tissue basophils." However, current evidence greatly favors the view that mature basophils represent terminally differentiated granulocytes, and not circulating mast cell precursors (reviewed in Refs. 7,13). Thus, basophils are circulating granulocytes that can infiltrate tissues or appear in exudates during a variety of inflammatory or immunological processes. By contrast, morphologically identifiable mast cells do not normally circulate, but reside in virtually all normal vascularized tissues.

Furthermore, it is now appreciated that mature basophils and mast cells differ in many

Table 1 Natural History, Major Mediators, and Surface Membrane Structures of Human Mast Cells and Basophils

Characteristic	Basophils	Mast cells
Natural history		
Origin of precursor cells	Bone marrow	Bone marrow
Site of maturation	Bone marrow	Connective tissues; a few in the bone marrow
Mature cells in the circulation	Yes (usually $< 1\%$ of blood leukocytes)	No
Mature cells recruited into tissues from circulation	Yes (during immunological, inflammatory responses)	No
Mature cells normally residing in connective tissues	No (not detectable by microscopy)	Yes
Proliferative ability of morphologically mature cells	None reported	Yes (under certain circumstances)
Life span	Days (similar to other granulocytes)	Weeks to months (based on studies in rodents)
Mediators		
Major mediators stored preformed in cytoplasmic granules	Histamine, chondroitin sulfates, neutral protease with bradykinin-generating activity, β-glucuronidase, elastase, cathepsin G-like enzyme, major basic protein, Charcot–Leyden crystal protein	Histamine, heparin and/or chondroitin sulfates, neutral proteases (chymase and/or tryptase), many acid hydrolases, cathepsin G, carboxypeptidase
Major lipid mediators produced after appropriate activation	Leukotriene C_4 (LTC_4)	Prostaglandin D_2 (PGD_2), LTC_4, platelet-activating factor
Cytokines released after appropriate activation	IL-4	Tumor necrosis factor-α (mouse mast cells produce many more; see text)
Surface structures		
Ig receptors	$Fc_\varepsilon RI$, $Fc_\gamma RII$(CDw32)	$Fc_\varepsilon RI$
Cytokine/growth factor receptors for	IL-2(CD25), IL-3, IL-4, IL-5, IL-8, stem cell factor (SCF) [some basophils express low numbers of c-*kit* receptors (60)]	SCF (c-*kit* receptor)
Cell adhesion structures	LFA-1[a] α chain (CD11a), C43bi receptor (CD11b), gp150/95 (CD11c), LFA-1β chain (CD18), ICAM-1[b] (CD54), and CD44	

[a]LFA, lymphocyte function-associated antigen.
[b]ICAM, intercellular adhesion molecule.
Source: Ref. 8.

aspects of morphology, natural history, tissue distribution, mediator production, cell surface phenotype, growth factor requirements, and response to drugs (see Table 1). Nevertheless, mast cells and basophils share important functional characteristics. After sensitization with IgE, exposure to specific multivalent antigen triggers both cell types to undergo an integrated, noncytolytic series of biochemical (9–12) and ultrastructural (14–16) alterations, often referred to as anaphylactic degranulation or exocytosis, that results in the exposure of the matrices of the cytoplasmic granules to the external medium. These events are associated with the release of the preformed mediators, which are stored in the cytoplasmic granules (such as histamine, heparin, or other sulfated proteoglycans, and certain proteases), the de novo synthesis and release of such lipid mediators as prostaglandin D_2 or leukotriene C_4, and the release of multifunctional cytokines. A similar sequence of events may be initiated by antibodies to IgE or to the $Fc_\varepsilon RI$ itself. On the other hand, mast cells and basophils differ in their responsiveness to other potential activators of secretion, and also in the specific pattern of mediators that are released by the activated cells.

DEVELOPMENT AND DISTRIBUTION

Mast Cells

Distribution and Heterogeneity

Mast cells are ordinarily distributed throughout normal connective tissues, where they are often situated adjacent to blood and lymphatic vessels, near or within nerves, and beneath epithelial surfaces, such as those of the respiratory and gastrointestinal systems and the skin, that are exposed to the external environment (5–8,14–16). In some species, mast cells are also abundant in the fibrous capsules of internal organs and in physiological transudates, such as peritoneal fluid. Mast cells are also a normal, if numerically minor, component of the bone marrow and lymphoid tissues. However, unlike mature basophils, mature mast cells do not circulate in the blood.

In many mammalian species, including humans, mast cell numbers in normal tissues exhibit considerable variation according to anatomical sites (6,7). However, mast cell distribution can change during perturbations of homeostasis. For example, mast cells can appear within the respiratory or gastrointestinal epithelium and in secretions at these sites in association with certain inflammatory or immunological reactions (17). The numbers of mast cells at sites of chronic inflammation due to a variety of different causes can often be many times higher than in the corresponding normal tissues (5,15–18). In most cases, the extent to which such changes in mast cell number reflect proliferation of resident mast cell populations, as opposed to the recruitment and differentiation of mast cell precursors, remains to be determined.

Human basophils and mast cells exhibit several differences in morphology, particularly by transmission electron microscopy (TEN; Table 2). Figure 1 is an electron micrograph showing a human basophil adjacent to a human mast cell in the same tissue. The concept of mast cell heterogeneity is based on evidence derived from studies in humans and experimental animals, indicating that mast cells can vary in multiple aspects of phenotype, including morphology, histochemistry, mediator content, and response to drugs and stimuli of activation (6,7,19–22). These findings raise the possibility that mast cells of different phenotype might have different roles in health and disease and might respond differently to drugs used in clinical settings. Cells within a given population can be said to exhibit

Table 2 Morphological Features of Mature Basophils and Mast Cells in Humans

Characteristic	Basophils	Mast cells
Size	5–7 μm	6–12 μm
Surface	Irregular, short, thick processes	Numerous, rather uniformly distributed, elongated thin processes
Nucleus	Segmented	Nonsegmented (usually round to oval in electron micrographs)
Nuclear chromatin condensation	Marked	Moderate
Cytoplasmic granules	Fewer and larger than in mast cells; contain predominantly electron-dense particulate material with occasional membranous whorls	Smaller, more numerous, and generally more variable in appearance than in basophils; contain scroll-like structures, particles, or crystals, alone or in combination
Aggregates of cytoplasmic glycogen	Present	Absent
Cytoplasmic lipid bodies	Rare	Common (but not present in all cells)
Granule–granule fusion during "anaphylactic" degranulation	Rare (granule membranes usually fuse individually with plasma membrane)	Common

Source: Ref. 3.

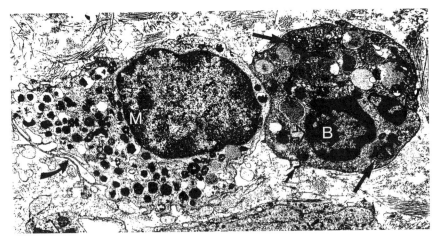

Figure 1   A basophil (B) adjacent to a mast cell (MC) in the ileal submucosa of patient with Crohn's disease. The basophil exhibits a bilobed nucleus (open arrows), whose chromatin is strikingly condensed beneath the nuclear membrane. The basophil surface is relatively smooth with a few blunt processes (small arrow). Some of the basophil's cytoplasmic granules contain membrane figures (solid arrows). The mast cell nucleus is larger and its chromatin less condensed than that of the basophil. The mast cell's granules are smaller, more numerous, and more variable in shape and content than those of the basophil. The mast cell surface has numerous elongated, thin folds (curved arrow). (Original magnification, × 9000). (From Ref. 180.)

heterogeneity once a certain minimal (but generally undefined) level of variation in one or more of their characteristics has been demonstrated. Thus, this is a purely descriptive term. For example, a particular cell type can be said to exhibit heterogeneity in ultrastructural appearance, mediator content, or other characteristics taken alone or in combination.

The distinction between rodent connective tissue-type mast cells (CTMC) and mucosal-type mast cells (MMC) subsets is the classic example of mast cell heterogeneity. Human mast cells also exhibit variation in phenotype. Human pulmonary mast cells vary in cytoplasmic granule ultrastructure, size, and response to stimuli of degranulation, and human intestinal mast cells exhibit variation in histochemistry (e.g., in the sensitivity of their staining to formalin fixation) (6,15,22). However, the separation of mast cell populations into distinct mucosal and connective tissue subclasses is not as clear in humans as it is in mice and rats. For example, most anatomical sites in humans contain some mast cells (MC_T) that express immunoreactivity for tryptase (localized to scroll-containing cytoplasmic granules), but no detectable chymase (< 0.04 pg/cell), and other mast cells (MC_{TC}) that contain immunoreactivity for both tryptase and chymase (localized to crystal-containing cytoplasmic granules) (6,23). It is not yet clear whether MC_T entirely lack chymase or have small amounts that are undetectable with current techniques. However, it is possible to classify human mast cells in multiple anatomical sites, on the basis of their predominant protease content, as MC_T or MC_{TC} (6,23). Thus, MC_T predominate in lung and small-intestinal mucosa and MC_{TC} predominate in skin and small-intestinal submucosa (6,23).

Tissue densities of intestinal mucosal and submucosal MC_T, but not MC_{TC}, are reduced in patients with either congenital combined immunodeficiency diseases or the acquired immunodeficiency syndrome (AIDS), consistent with a T-cell-dependent requirement for generation or maintenance of normal populations of MC_T (24). In this context, MC_T seem similar to rat or mouse MMC, and MC_{TC} resemble murine (CTMC). However, other properties of MC_T or MC_{TC} are not predictable based on the properties of rat MMC and CTMC. For example, in the rat, CTMC are much more sensitive than MMC to stimulation with basic compounds, such as substance P, as well as to inhibition of degranulation by disodium cromoglycate (DSCG; reviewed in 18,25). By contrast, Church et al. (26) reported that partially purified preparations of human skin mast cells (> 85% MC_{TC}) were very sensitive to stimulation by substance P and other basic secretagogues, but not to inhibition by DSCG, whereas mast cells isolated from lung (< 10% MC_{TC}) and from colon mucosa or muscle (60% MC_{TC}) were insensitive to substance P stimulation, but demonstrated inhibition of histamine release by DSCG.

As discussed in detail elsewhere (7), mast cell phenotypic variation theoretically might reflect the following mechanisms, acting alone or in combination: (1) the existence of distinct mast cell lineages, (2) the process of cellular maturation–differentiation, (3) the functional status of the cell, and (4) the influence of microenvironmental factors.

Mast Cell Development in Mice and Rats

Maintenance of normal mouse hematopoietic cells in vitro in media containing interleukin-3 (IL-3) yields an essentially homogeneous population of growth factor-dependent immature mast cells (7). When they have been derived from mouse bone marrow cells, such mast cells will be designated herein as IL-3-derived, bone marrow-derived cultured mast cells (IL-3-derived BMCMC). Table 3 compares some of the phenotypic characteristics of IL-3-derived BMCMC with those of mouse CTMC and MMC.

Although IL-3-derived BMCMC share some phenotypic characteristics with mouse

Table 3 Phenotypic Characteristics of Mast Cell Populations in the Mouse

Characteristic	Connective tissue or serosal (peritoneal) mast cells	Mucosal mast cells	Growth factor-dependent, bone marrow-derived cultured mast cells[a] (BMCMC)
Cytoplasmic granule ultrastructure	Uniformly electron-dense	Variably electron dense	Variably electron dense
T-cell dependence	No	Yes	Yes
Major granule-associated proteoglycan	Heparin	Chondroitin sulfates	Chondroitin sulfates
Staining with the heparin-binding dye, berberine sulfate	Yes	No	No
Staining with alcian blue	Yes	Yes	Yes
Staining with safranin	Yes	No	No
Histamine content	High	Low (by histochemistry)	Low
Serotonin content	Variable	Low (by histochemistry)	High
Surface expression of globopentaosylceramide	High	Not determined	Low
High-affinity surface receptors for IgE	Yes	Yes	Yes
Sensitivity to stimulation with compound 48/80	High	Low	Low

[a]The characteristics that are listed are those for BMCMC that have been generated in IL-3 containing medium. The phenotypic characteristics of these cells can become more like those of CTMC when they are maintained in the presence of mouse 3T3 fibroblasts or soluble rrSCF in vitro, or after they have been transferred to certain tissues of W/W^v mast cell-deficient mice in vivo (see text).

MMC, both in vivo and in vitro studies indicate that, in appropriate circumstances, these cells can acquire phenotypic features that are more similar to those of CTMC. The first demonstration of this point was achieved using genetically mast cell-deficient mice. Mutations at *W*, the dominant white-spotting locus on mouse chromosome 5, or *Sl*, the steel locus on mouse chromosome 10, affect several important developmental programs, including gametogenesis, pigmentation, hematopoiesis, and mast cell development. Thus, many *W* or *Sl* mutations render the homozygous mutant animals sterile, devoid of coat pigmentation, anemic, and profoundly mast cell-deficient (20,27–29).

The *W* or *Sl* mutant mice most commonly used in studies of mast cell development and function are WBB6F$_1$–*W/W^v*(*W/W^v*) or WCB6F$_1$–*Sl/Sl^d*(*Sl/Sl^d*) mice (reviewed in Refs. 7,20,27–29). The *W/W^v* and *Sl/Sl^d* mice are virtually devoid of mature, morphologically identifiable mast cells in all organs and anatomical sites examined. The mast cell deficiency of *W/W^v* mice reflects a defect intrinsic to cells in the mast cell lineage, whereas the mast cell deficiency of the *Sl/Sl^d* mouse reflects a problem in the microenvironments necessary for normal mast cell development. Combined in vitro and in vivo studies have shown that injection of either IL-3-derived BMCMCs expanded in vitro, or purified mouse peritoneal mast cells, into *W/W^v* recipients can give rise to progeny with biochemical, morphological, and histochemical characteristics similar to those of either CTMC or MMC (30,31). Furthermore, studies with single clonal populations derived from mouse peritoneal mast cells have demonstrated that these features exhibit bidirectional and reversible alteration, depending on the specific conditions that are experienced by the population in vitro or in vivo (32).

From the in vitro work, it is clear that fibroblasts represent one source of factors that can promote IL-3-derived BMCMC to develop features of CTMC (33). Subsequent work, discussed later, indicated that stem cell factor (SCF) represents a major fibroblast-derived factor that can induce BMCMC to acquire phenotypic characteristics of CTMC. However, several other cytokines can also influence mast cell development or proliferation in the mouse (reviewed in Ref. 34). For example, IL-4, IL-9, or IL-10, when combined with IL-3, can enhance the proliferation of IL-3-derived BMCMC (34). By contrast, when used as the only exogenous growth factor, these cytokines have little or no ability to induce BMCMC proliferation. The combination of IL-3 and IL-4 also triggers the proliferation of purified mouse peritoneal mast cells grown in methylcellulose. By contrast, it has been reported that either granulocyte–macrophage colony-stimulating factor (GM-CSF) or transforming growth factor-β1 (TGF-β1) can inhibit mouse BMCMC proliferation in response to IL-3 (34).

Stem Cell Factor and c-kit

Recent work demonstrated that the mast cell deficiency and other phenotypic abnormalities expressed by mice with *W* or *Sl* mutations reflect the consequences of these mutations on the production or function of the stem cell factor receptor (SCFR; CD117), which is encoded at the *W* locus in the mouse by the c-*kit* protooncogene, or the production or function of SCF, the ligand for this receptor, which is encoded at the *Sl* locus in the mouse (reviewed in Refs. 29,35,36). In general, SCFR expression diminishes with the progressive maturation of lymphohematopoietic lineages, although mature mast cells continue to express high levels of the SCFR (29,35,36). By contrast, studies of human basophils indicate that these cells express few or no SCFRs (37,38).

Although the tissues of W/W^v mice express normal levels of c-*kit* mRNA, which is normal in size, the SCFR that is expressed in W/W^v tissues retains little, if any, kinase activity owing to the structural alteration of the gene product (29,35,36). Specifically, the W^v mutation results in an amino acid substitution in the kinase domain, which dramatically reduces the kinase activity, whereas *W* comprises a deletion of the region of c-*kit* that encodes the transmembrane part of the SCFR, thereby preventing cell surface expression of the receptor (29,35,36).

Demonstration that the SCFR is the *W* gene product greatly assisted in the identification of the c-*kit* ligand, a novel growth factor that is the product of the *Sl* locus (reviewed in Refs. 29,35,36). Although several names have been proposed for this c-*kit* ligand, including stem cell factor (SCF), kit ligand (KL), mast cell growth factor (MGF), and steel factor, we will use the designation SCF. The *Sl* mutation represents a deletion of all SCF-coding sequences while the Sl^d allele encodes an abundant, smaller-than-normal SCF transcript (29,35,36). Two forms of the SCF protein have been identified: a transmembrane form, comprising the full-length translation product and a soluble factor, comprising the first 164 or 165 amino acids of the extracellular domain, which is derived from the larger cell-associated precursor by proteolysis (29,35,36).

The most dramatic effects of SCF in hematopoiesis generally reflect its actions as a survival factor for early hematopoietic progenitors and its ability to synergize with other growth factors to regulate the proliferation and differentiation of cells in multiple hemato-poietic lineages (29,35,36). However, the effects of SCF on mast cell development are notable both for their diversity and for their importance in the natural history of this particular hematopoietic lineage. Repeated injection of recombinant rat SCF into the skin of *Sl/Sl^d* mice resulted in the local development of a large number of mast cells with phenotypic characteristics of CTMC (39,40), and many of the mast cells in these sites were undergoing proliferation (40). As previously stated, *Sl/Sl^d* mouse skin ordinarily contains no detectable mast cell precursors (20,28). Thus, these experiments and others have shown that SCF influenced the recruitment, retention, and survival of mast cell precursors at the injection sites, as well as promoted the proliferation and maturation of these cells (39,40). The effects on recruitment of mast cell precursors probably reflected the ability of these cells to recognize the extracellular domain of SCF, which can be assessed as mast cell adherence or chemotaxis in vitro (29,35,36). The effect of SCF on mast cell survival is most likely mediated by suppression of mast cell apoptosis, which has been demonstrated both in vitro (41,42) and in vivo (42).

Stem cell factor represents the only cytokine that can promote significant proliferation of either immature mouse mast cells or mature mouse CTMC (39,40,43), as well as the only cytokine that can induce IL-3-derived BMCMC to acquire multiple phenotypic characteris-tics of CTMC, including a substantially higher histamine content (43), significant ability to synthesize and store heparin (43), and a CTMC-like protease phenotype (44). On the other hand, IL-3-derived BMCMC maintained in SCF do not acquire phenotypic characteristics identical with those of freshly isolated peritoneal mast cells (PMC), and PMC maintained in SCF have a substantially lower histamine content and, as a population, exhibit less mature histochemical characteristics than do freshly isolated PMC (43). These findings might reflect the lack of an additional factor(s) which, together with SCF, could induce or maintain full CTMC maturation in vitro. Both in vivo (40) and in vitro (45) studies in rats, and in vitro studies in mice (44), indicate that the phenotypic characteristics of the mast cells that develop in the presence of SCF can be significantly influenced by other factors in the cells' microenvironment, particularly IL-3 (44,45). Alternatively, the observation that BMCMC or PMC maintained in SCF differ in phenotype from freshly isolated PMC also may reflect, at least in part, consequence of the active proliferation of the mast cell populations that are maintained in SCF.

Beyond its effects on mast cell proliferation and maturation, under certain circumstances SCF can directly induce mouse mast cell degranulation and mediator release (46,47) and can enhance the mast cell mediator release that is observed with IgE-dependent activation of the cells (47). In contrast, the long-term administration of SCF to mice in vivo can *diminish* the mast cell's responsiveness to stimulation by IgE and antigen, and can also *decrease* the severity of IgE-dependent passive anaphylaxis (48). Although the explanation for these in vivo findings remains to be determined, the results certainly indicate that the effects of SCF on mast cell function may be quite complex.

Impressive SCF-induced mast cell hyperplasia can be observed not only in rodents, but it also occurs in nonhuman primates. In cynomolgus monkeys, treatment with rhSCF at 6.0 mg/kg per day for 21 days resulted in increased numbers of mast cells at all sites examined except the CNS, with increases ranging from 3-fold, in the heart, to 1500-fold, in the spleen (49). When rhSCF was given at 100 μg/kg per day, significant elevations of mast cell numbers occurred in the skin at the injection sites, bone marrow, mesenteric lymph nodes, liver, and spleen (49). Remarkably, in both groups of monkeys, mast cell numbers in most sites declined to the baseline numbers observed in vehicle-treated control monkeys by 15 days after cessation of rhSCF administration. Moreover, the rhSCF-treated monkeys appeared to be clinically well, not only throughout the course of treatment, but also during the period when mast cell populations were declining precipitously to normal levels (49).

Mast Cell Development in Humans

Unlike murine mast cells and human basophils, human mast cells have been difficult to culture from blood or bone marrow in sufficient numbers for studying their growth and differentiation. Human mononuclear cells separated by density sedimentation from adult peripheral blood, umbilical cord blood, or bone marrow, and then grown in short-term liquid suspension cultures with IL-3, give rise to cultures rich in basophils, rather than mast cells (reviewed in Refs. 3,6,7). Similarly, single-lineage and mixed colony-forming units (CFUs) containing basophils, but not mast cells, were observed when mononuclear cells were cultured in methylcellulose in the presence of IL-3. Small numbers of mast cells (1–3% of cultured cells) have been identified by histochemistry in cultures of human bone marrow-derived mononuclear cells suspended over agar or agarose in the presence of rhIL-3 (50). From experiments employing immunomagnetic selection approaches, the bone marrow progenitor for human mast cells resides in the CD34$^+$ population of hematopoietic progenitor cells (51).

Mast cells that express phenotypic characteristics of mature human mast cells can be derived by culturing appropriate progenitor cells together with mouse 3T3 fibroblasts (52). These mast cells coexpress cell surface IgE receptors and cytoplasmic granules that contain tryptase. In addition, they express a variety of cytoplasmic granule morphologies, including the scroll, mixed, reticular, dense core, or homogeneous patterns found in the mature human mast cells that occur within normal tissues (53).

The observations that mouse 3T3 fibroblasts can promote human mast cell development in vitro, and that the human SCFR can bind mouse SCF (39), suggested that SCF may promote mast cell development in humans, as it does in murine rodents and experimental primates. When CD34$^+$ human bone marrow cells were cultured in vitro in rhSCF plus IL-3, both mast cells and many other hematopoietic lineages developed (54). As a result, the cultures did not exhibit a net enrichment for mast cells. By contrast, rhSCF used as the only exogenous cytokine favored the development of mast cells from populations of human bone marrow or peripheral blood mononuclear cells (55), human umbilical cord blood mononuclear cells (56), or human fetal liver cells (57). However, the human mast cells that develop in cultures supplemented with soluble rhSCF appear to represent only a subset of the human mast cell phenotypes that are observed in vivo. For example, these rhSCF-derived human mast cells express little or no cytoplasmic granule-associated chymase (56,57). Whether membrane-associated forms of SCF might differ from soluble SCF in promoting human mast cell development remains to be determined.

Costa et al. (58) recently quantified mast cell numbers in skin biopsies obtained from patients enrolled in a phase I study of rhSCF. Treatment of these subjects with rhSCF at 5–50 µg/kg per day for 14 days resulted in an approximate 60% increase in the number of dermal mast cells in skin distant from the SCF injection sites. These represent the first data indicating that rhSCF can induce mast cell hyperplasia in vivo in humans.

The systemic expansion of mast cell numbers in mice, rats, monkeys, or humans receiving *exogenous* SCF suggests that changes in the level of expression of *endogenous* SCF may explain, at least in part, some of the striking alterations in mast cell numbers that have been noted in association with a variety of reparative responses, immunological reactions, and disease processes (29,49). Moreover, it is likely that the wide variation in the numbers of mast cells that ordinarily are present in different normal tissues may largely reflect differences in the levels of endogenous SCF bioactivity that are expressed at the various anatomical sites (29,49).

Basophils

Basophils, similar to other granulocytes, differentiate and mature in the bone marrow and then circulate in the blood. Basophils are not normally found in connective tissues. In humans, the basophil is the least common blood granulocyte, with a prevalence of approximately 0.5% of total leukocytes and approximately 0.3% of nucleated marrow cells (13). Because the normal frequency of blood and bone marrow basophils is so low, accurate basophil determinations ordinarily require absolute counting methods. The basophil's prominent, metachromatic cytoplasmic granules permit it to be identified easily in Wright–Giemsa-stained preparations of peripheral blood or bone marrow cells. Both cytogenetic evidence and in vitro studies (13,59) indicate that basophils share a common precursor with other granulocytes and monocytes. Specifically, in humans, basophils are derived from pluripotent $CD34^+$ hematopoietic progenitor cells (51). Human basophils appear to exhibit kinetics of production and peripheral circulation similar to that of eosinophils (13). However, unlike the eosinophil, the basophil ordinarily does not occur in peripheral tissues in significant numbers. Basophils can infiltrate sites of many immunological or inflammatory processes (often in association with eosinophils) and participate in the reactions to some tumors (14,60). In such cases, the basophils are readily distinguishable from mast cells residing in the same tissues (61). The ultrastructural features of human basophils are summarized in Table 2 and are illustrated in Figure 1.

Maintenance of human bone marrow cells or umbilical cord blood cells in suspension cultures in the presence of IL-3 generates populations that are highly enriched in basophils (25% or more), with the remaining cells consisting of neutrophils, eosinophils, monocytes, and rare mast cells (50,62,63). Moreover, high-affinity binding sites for IL-3 have been identified on the human basophil surface (64), and basophil numbers are slightly increased in the blood of patients who are treated with rhIL-3 (65). Although these findings indicate that IL-3 is an important growth factor for human basophils, other cytokines can also contribute to the development of this lineage (reviewed in 66,67). GM-CSF, but not G-CSF or M-CSF, can enhance the growth of basophils from peripheral blood. Interleukin-5 and nerve growth factor (NGF) may also synergize with other growth factors to enhance basophil development in vitro (68). Although basophils also express receptors for several other cytokines, including IL-2 (CD25), IL-4, and IL-8, neither these cytokines, IL-1, nor IL-6 appear to promote significant basophil differentiation (66,67).

MEDIATORS

Mast cells and basophils contain, or elaborate on appropriate stimulation, a diverse array of potent, biologically active mediators (3–6). Some of these products are stored preformed in the cells' cytoplasmic granules (e.g., proteoglycans, proteases, histamine); others are synthesized on activation of the cell by IgE and antigen or other stimuli (e.g., products of arachidonic acid oxidation through the cyclooxygenase or lipoxygenase pathways), and, in some cells, PAF. Cytokines represent the most recently identified group of mast cell and basophil mediators, at least one of which (TNF-α) can be both preformed and stored, as well as newly synthesized by activated cells (reviewed in Refs. 34,69). These agents can mediate a diverse array of effects in inflammation, immunity, and tissue remodeling, and can also influence the clotting, fibrinolytic, complement, and kinin systems.

Preformed Mediators

Those mediators that are stored preformed in the cytoplasmic granules include histamine, proteoglycans, serine proteases, carboxypeptidase A, and small amounts of sulfatases and exoglycosidases. Mast cells and basophils form histamine by the decarboxylation of histidine, and store histamine as an ionic complex, with the highly charged carboxyl or sulfate groups of the glycosaminoglycan side chains of the proteoglycans which constitute much of the matrix of the secretory granules. Mast cells isolated from human lung, skin, lymphoid tissue, or small intestine contain about 3–8 pg of histamine per cell, whereas human basophils contain about 1–2 pg/cell (3,6). Studies in genetically mast cell-deficient and congenic normal mice indicate that mast cells account for nearly all of the histamine stored in normal tissues, with the exception of the glandular stomach and the central nervous system (70). Basophils are the source of most of the histamine present in normal human blood (71). Mouse and rat mast cells contain significant quantities of serotonin, but this amine has not been detected in populations of human mast cells or basophils (4,5).

Human mast cell populations contain variable mixtures of heparin (~60 kDa) and chondroitin sulfate proteoglycans (72,73). Although the sulfated glycosaminoglycans of normal human blood basophils have not been characterized, chondroitin sulfates account for most of the proteoglycans in the basophils of patients with myelogenous leukemia (74). Proteoglycans are composed of a central protein core with extended unbranched carbohydrate side chains (glycosaminoglycans) of repeating disaccharide subunits (reviewed in Ref. 75). The central protein core of heparin has numerous serine–glycine repeating residues that, besides conferring protease resistance to the proteoglycan, form the attachment points for glycosaminoglycans. Each disaccharide of the glycosaminoglycans has between zero and, in heparin, three sulfate groups, the high charge of which contributes to many of the characteristic physicochemical properties of these molecules (6,75).

Basophil and mast cell proteoglycans probably express multiple biological functions, both within and outside of the cells. By ionic interactions, they bind histamine, neutral proteases and carboxypeptidases, and may contribute to the packaging and storage of these molecules within the secretory granules. When the granule matrices are exposed to physiological conditions of pH and ionic strength during the process of degranulation, the various mediators associated with the proteoglycans dissociate at different rates, histamine very rapidly, but tryptase and chymase much more slowly (6). In addition to regulating the kinetics of release of mediators from the granule matrices, proteoglycans can also regulate the activity of some of the associated mediators. For example, heparin stabilizes tryptase in a configuration that is required for its normal enzymatic activity (6,76).

Heparin and other mast cell- or basophil-derived proteoglycans may have a number of other functions as well. Heparin can bind and protect from degradation many growth factors, such as basic fibroblast growth factor (bFGF) and certain hematopoietic factors (77); can bind to (and alter the activity of) leukocyte products, such as eosinophil major basic protein (75); can influence the biological properties of extracellular matrix proteins, such as laminin, fibronectin, and vitronectin (75,77); and, through its ability to bind to antithrombin III, can function as an anticoagulant (5,75). However, the extent to which each of these functions is actually expressed at sites of mast cell activation in vivo is unknown.

Neutral proteases represent the major protein component of mast cell secretory granules.

Both basophils and mast cells contain enzymes with tosylargininemethylesterase (TAME) activity, which can be used as a marker of mast cell or basophil activation in vivo. By weight, tryptase is the major enzyme stored in the cytoplasmic granules of human mast cells, and this neutral protease has been detected in all human mast cell populations that have been examined (6). Human mast cell tryptase is a serine endopeptidase that exists in the granule in active form as a tetramer of 134 kDa, containing subunits of 31–35 kDa, each of which contains an active site (6). Negligible amounts of tryptase have been identified in normal human basophils by immunoassay (23). Because this enzyme appears to be unique to the human mast cell, measurements of mast cell tryptase in biological fluids, such as plasma, serum, or inflammatory exudates, have been used to assess mast cell activation in these settings (78). Tryptase is stored in the cytoplasmic granules in the active tetrameric form as a complex that is stabilized by its association with heparin and perhaps other proteoglycans within the mast cell granule (76). Although the function of mast cell tryptase in vivo is unknown, it can selectively cleave human C3 to its component peptides, C3b and C3a, and, while complexed with heparin, can degrade C3a to inactive peptides. Mast cell chymase is also a serine protease that is stored in active form in the mast cell granule, but as a monomer with a molecular mass of 30 kDa (79,80). Human mast cell chymase is present in 85% of the mast cells of the skin and intestinal submucosa, but some mast cells present within the intestinal mucosa and lung do not stain with monoclonal antibodies directed against the protease (23). Other components of the mast cell granule stored in complex with proteoglycans are the carboxypeptidases A and B, the former in rodent mast cells and the latter in human mast cells (3,6). Human basophils, like eosinophils, can form Charcot–Leyden crystals and contain Charcot–Leyden crystal protein (lysophospholipase) in quantities similar to that of eosinophils (81). This protein has been localized ultrastructurally to the major cytoplasmic granule population of basophils (82).

Newly Synthesized Lipid Mediators

Activation of mast cells with appropriate stimuli not only causes the secretion of preformed granule-associated mediators, but also can initiate the de novo synthesis of certain lipid-derived substances. Of particular importance are the cyclooxygenase and lipoxygenase metabolites of arachidonic acid, which possess potent inflammatory activities and may also play a role in modulating the release process itself (83). The major cyclooxygenase product of mast cells is prostaglandin D_2 (PGD_2), whereas the major lipoxygenase products derived from mast cells and basophils are the sulfidopeptide leukotrienes (LT): LTC_4, LTD_4, and LTE_4 (83). The substrate for the formation of both prostaglandins and leukotrienes, as well as for the third class of lipid mediator, platelet-activating factor (PAF), is arachidonic acid, which is released from the phospholipids constituting the membranes and, in some cells, lipid bodies, of mast cells and basophils by various phospholipase A_2 enzymes (15,83). However, the specific products of arachidonic acid metabolism that are produced by different populations of mast cells or by blood basophils vary considerably (3,4,83). For example, mast cells isolated from a variety of different human tissues release both LTC_4 and PGD_2, whereas peripheral blood basophils release LTC_4, but no detectable PGD_2.

The primary prostaglandin synthesized by murine or human mast cells PGD_2 is generated very rapidly after IgE-dependent mast cell activation (3,6,83). It enhances venular permeability, leukocyte adherence to vascular endothelial cells, and pulmonary vasoconstriction, and also acts as a peripheral vasodilator (3,6,83). Prostaglandin D_2 is also a potent inhibitor of platelet aggregation; it is chemokinetic for human neutrophils and, in conjunction with LTD_4, it can induce the accumulation of neutrophils in human skin (3,6,83). High levels of PGD_2 metabolites have been detected in the urine of patients with mastocytosis, and PGD_2 is believed to contribute to hypotension in such patients (84).

The primary products of the 5-lipoxygenase pathway of arachidonic acid metabolism that are generated by mast cells and basophils are the sulfidopeptide leukotrienes. Studies with purified cells show that basophils and mast cells produce only LTC_4; although in mixed cell preparations and certainly in vivo, LTC_4 is rapidly metabolized to LTD_4 and LTE_4 (3,83). Through interactions with their receptors on smooth-muscle cells, these products, formerly known as "slow-reacting substance of anaphylaxis (SRA-A)," induce a prolonged cutaneous wheal-and-flare reaction and, in the respiratory system, prolonged bronchoconstriction (3,83). These products also can enhance venular permeability, enhance bronchial mucous secretion, and induce constriction of arterial, arteriolar, and intestinal smooth muscle (3,83). Accordingly, the sulfidopeptide leukotrienes are considered important mediators of some of the pathophysiological hallmarks of late-phase reactions (see later), both in the airways in patients with asthma, as well as in other sites.

Human mast cells, but not human basophils, also can produce LTB_4, albeit in much smaller quantities than PGD_2 or the sulfidopeptide leukotrienes (3,5,83). There are three patterns of release of products of arachidonic acid metabolism by human mast cells and basophils: (1) gut or lung mast cells produce similar amounts of LTC_4 and PGD_2; (2) skin mast cells produce largely PGD_2; and (3) basophils generate only LTC_4.

Platelet-activating factor [PAF, more recently designated PAF-acether or alkylglyceryl-etherphosphorylcholine (AGEPC)] has been detected in mouse bone marrow-derived mast cells, rabbit basophils, and human mast cells, but not following activation of human basophils (3,83). It can aggregate and degranulate platelets, induce wheal-and-flare reactions on injection into human skin, increase lung resistance, and lead to systemic hypotension, suggesting a potential role for this mediator in systemic anaphylaxis (3,83). Platelet-activating factor is produced in large quantities by lung mast cells (as well as many other cells, including human neutrophils) but, with the mast cell, the mediator is not significantly released by these cells in vitro (3). However, PAF and its inactive derivative, lyso-PAF, appear in biological fluids after antigen challenge (85). Although the cellular source of the PAF that is detected in such settings has not yet been identified, this mediator may contribute to the prolonged increase in human bronchial reactivity that is observed with antigen challenge in asthmatic subjects (86).

Cytokines

The recent demonstration of cytokine production by mast cells and basophils has greatly expanded the possible mechanisms by which these cells might contribute to the pathophysiology of allergic and immunological diseases or host defense (reviewed in Refs. 34,69). Studies with virally transformed mouse mast cell lines revealed that these cells expressed mRNA or bioactivity for GM-CSF, IL-4, and IL-3 (34,69). Subsequent studies showed that IL-3-dependent in vitro-derived mouse mast cells, or mast cell lines that had been activated by the $Fc_\varepsilon RI$, contained increased levels of mRNA for many cytokines (IL-1α, IL-3, IL-4, IL-5, IL-6, and GM-CSF, as well as the chemokines MIP-1α and β, JE, and TCA3), and also secreted substances with the corresponding bioactivities (IL-1, IL-3, IL-4, IL-6, GM-CSF) (87–89).

The first cytokine bioactivity to be clearly associated with normal mast cells was tumor necrosis factor (TNF-α; cachectin) (90,91). Gordon and Galli demonstrated that unstimulated mouse peritoneal mast cells constitutively contain approximately twice as much TNF-α bioactivity as do LPS-stimulated mouse peritoneal macrophages (91), and that the TNF-α that is released from mouse mast cells with appropriate stimulation reflects cytokine that is rapidly released from these preformed stores, as well as even larger amounts of newly synthesized TNF-α, which is released over a period of hours after cell activation (91,92). Thus, the biological effects of mast cell-derived TNF-α can be expressed immediately after IgE-dependent activation of these cells and can be sustained for long intervals thereafter.

Table 4 summarizes the key concepts that have been derived from these and other studies of nonhuman mast cells. Currently, little information is available on the mechanism(s) of cytokine gene induction in mast cells. However, a requirement for prolonged receptor cross-linkage and extracellular calcium has been demonstrated (93), and a major component of the IL-3 and GM-CSF inductional response reflects posttranscriptional stabilization of mRNA (94).

Human mast cells and basophils also elaborate cytokines. Mast cells from a variety of anatomical sites, including the bone marrow (95), skin (96,97), and lung (98), all contain TNF-α mRNA and immunoreactive or bioactive protein product, and enhanced production of TNF-α has been demonstrated after Fc$_ε$RI cross-linking (99). Moreover, in skin organ culture systems, IgE-dependent activation of human skin mast cells results in the expression of the adherence molecule E-selectin (ELAM-1) on adjacent vascular endothelial cells, and this expression can be partially blocked by antibodies to TNF-α (96) or to TNF-α and IL-1 (100).

Interleukin-4 has been demonstrated in human skin and lung mast cells by immunohistochemistry, and these cells release both histamine and IL-4 bioactivity into culture

Table 4 Features of Mast Cell Cytokine Production[a]

1. Mast cells can transcribe and translate many different cytokines, including IL-1, -3, -4, -6, GM-CSF, TNF-α, IFN-γ, TGF-β, and the chemokines MIP-1α, MIP-1β, TCA3, and JE.
2. Mast cell cytokine genes can be differentially regulated, in that different signals can have distinct effects on the species, amounts, and kinetics of cytokine production.
3. In resposne to cellular activation (e.g., through the Fc$_ε$RI), mast cells can release at least one cytokine, TNF-α, from both preformed and stored as well as newly synthesized pools.
4. It is not yet clear whether all subpopulations of mast cells can produce the same spectrum of cytokines.
5. The pattern of mast cell cytokine production can vary depending on the stimulus used to activate the cells and can be regulated by cytokines and other microenvironmental factors that can influence mast cell phenotype.
6. Induction of cytokine mRNA in mast cells is not always accompanied by release of detectable cytokine bioactivity.
7. Under some circumstances, induction or release of mast cell cytokines can occur in response to stimuli that do not induce detectable release of histamine.
8. Release of some cytokines (e.g., TNF-α) can continue for hours after initial Fc$_ε$RI-dependent mast cell activation.
9. Mast cell cytokine mRNA expression or cytokine release can be inhibited by cyclosporine or dexamethasone.

[a]Most of these points so far have been established primarily by analyses of various mouse mast cell populations (see text).

supernatants after anti-IgE challenge (101). Immunohistochemical analysis has revealed that some mast cells in nasal turbinate specimens from patients with allergic rhinitis or from nonatopic volunteers display immunoreactivity for IL-4, IL-5, or IL-6, or a combination thereof (102).

Several lines of evidence indicate that mouse basophils can produce IL-4 on stimulation through the $Fc_\varepsilon RI$ (103,104). More recently, mature human basophils isolated from peripheral blood have been shown to release IL-4 in response to $Fc_\varepsilon RI$-dependent activation (105,106); and such release can be enhanced in basophils that have been exposed to IL-3, but not to IL-5, GM-CSF, or nerve growth factor (105,106). Interleukin-4 that is derived from mast cells or basophils at sites of allergic inflammation may play a role in T-cell differentiation toward a T_H2 phenotype. Recent findings indicate that human basophils and mast cells also express the CD40 ligand, and thus may be able to contribute to IgE production by promoting immunoglobulin class switching (107).

Mast Cell–Leukocyte Cytokine Cascades

We have proposed that the expression of many IgE-dependent reactions, as well as other responses in which mast cells play an important role, reflects the activities of a "mast cell–leukocyte cytokine cascade" (8,69,108). In this hypothesis, mast cell activation has an essential or important role in the initiation of the response, in part through the release of TNF-α and other cytokines that can directly or indirectly influence the recruitment or function of additional effector cells (neutrophils, eosinophils, basophils, lymphocytes, monocytes, and platelets). These recruited cells then importantly influence the progression of the response by providing additional sources of certain cytokines also produced by mast cells (e.g., TNF-α), and new sources of some cytokines (e.g., eosinophil-derived TGF-α; 109,110) that are not produced by the mast cell. As the reactions progress further, cytokines from mast cells and other resident cells, and from recruited (leukocyte) sources, exert complex effects on resident cells, such as vascular endothelial cells, fibroblasts, epithelial cells, nerves, and mast cells. These contribute to the vascular and epithelial changes, as well as to the tissue remodeling, angiogenesis, and fibrosis, that are so prominent in many disorders associated with mast cell activation and leukocyte infiltration. At certain points in the natural history of these processes, mast cell- or eosinophil-derived cytokines may also contribute to the down-regulation of the response.

MECHANISMS OF ACTIVATION

$Fc_\varepsilon RI$

The best understood cellular event that underlies expression of basophil or mast cell function is the process of degranulation, a stereotyped constellation of stimulus-activated biochemical and morphological events that result in the fusion of the cytoplasmic granule membranes with the plasma membrane (with external release of granule-associated mediators), associated with the generation and release of products of arachidonic acid oxidation and the release of stored or newly generated cytokines (4–12,14,15). Although a variety of agents can initiate basophil or mast cell degranulation, the best-studied pathway of stimulation is that transduced through $Fc_\varepsilon RI$ expressed on the basophil or mast cell surface (9–12). Human basophils generated in vitro express about 2.7×10^5 $Fc_\varepsilon RI$ per cell, which bind monovalent IgE immunoglobulin with a K_A of 2.8×10^9 mol/L (111). Similar values have been obtained for the $Fc_\varepsilon RI$ of rat and mouse mast cells (11). The $Fc_\varepsilon RI$ consists of one α, one β, and two identical disulfide-linked γ chains, all components of which have been cloned and sequenced (9,10). When adjacent Fc$_\varepsilon$RIs are bridged, either by bivalent or multivalent antigen interacting with receptor-bound IgE, or by antibodies directed against either receptor-bound IgE or the receptor itself, the cells are rapidly activated for the release of stored and newly generated mediators. This process is energy- and temperature-dependent; requires the mobilization of calcium, resulting in increased levels of free calcium in the cytosol; and occurs without evidence of toxicity to the responding cell. The bridging of only a few hundred pairs of IgE molecules are necessary to trigger human basophil histamine release (112). Moreover, the number of IgE–IgE bridges necessary to trigger release in the basophils of individual subjects apparently is not normally distributed; a subset of donors appears to be exceedingly sensitive to this stimulus (113). Because so few of a basophil's or mast cell's Fc$_\varepsilon$RI must be bridged to initiate the degranulation response, these cells may be sensitized simultaneously with IgE antibodies of many different specificities and, therefore, can react to stimulation by many different antigens. The IgE- and antigen-dependent activation represent the basis for the immunologically specific expression of mast and basophil function in IgE-dependent immune responses and allergic disorders.

Nonimmunological Direct Activation

In addition to IgE and specific antigen, a variety of biological substances (including products of complement activation and certain cytokines), chemical agents, and physical stimuli can elicit release of basophil or mast cell mediators (Table 5). However, the

Table 5 Stimuli of Human Basophil or Mast Cell Histamine Release

	Basophils		Mast cells	
Stimulus	Direct release	Enhance IgE-mediated release	Direct release	Enhance IgE-mediated release
C5a	+	ND	+[b]	ND
f-Met Leu Phe	+	ND	+[b]	ND
Mannitol (hyperosmolar)	+	ND	+	ND
Substance P	−	ND	+[b]	ND
Morphine	−	ND	+[b]	ND
IL-1	±[a]	+	±	+
IL-3	+	+	−	ND
IL-5	−	+	−	ND
GM-CSF	+	+	−	ND
Stem cell factor (SCF)	±	+	+	+
MCAF	+	+	ND	ND
MIP-1α	+	ND	+	ND
RANTES	+	ND	ND	ND
NAP-1	+	ND	ND	ND
CTAP-III	+	ND	ND	ND

ND, not determined.
[a]Some studies yes, some no.
[b]Cutaneous mast cells are much more sensitive to these stimuli than are mast cells derived from other sites.

responsiveness of human basophils and different populations of human mast cells to individual stimuli varies. For example, cutaneous mast cells appear to be much more sensitive to stimulation by neuropeptides than are pulmonary mast cells (3,26). Moreover, these stimuli can induce a pattern of mediator release that differs from that associated with IgE-dependent mast cell activation. For example, human cutaneous mast cells activated by substance P release about the same amounts of preformed mediators as do mast cell stimulated through the $Fc_{\varepsilon}RI$, but produce smaller amounts of lipid mediators (3,26).

In addition to neuropeptides, several other classes of small peptides of potential biological significance can induce basophil or mast cell mediator release. The best studied are the anaphylatoxins, products of complement activation, and the bacterial peptides, f-Met-Leu-Phe and its congeners (3,26). Both C5a and f-Met peptides release histamine from human basophils. However, f-Met-Leu-Phe is a more complete secretagogue, in that it induces release of both histamine and leukotrienes, whereas C5a produces a response that is largely limited to histamine release. Nevertheless, C5a-derived peptides provoke a sequence of ultrastructural changes in basophils that are similar to those induced by anti-IgE and specific antigen (3,26). Neither of these peptides is effective in causing mediator release from human lung or gut mast cells, but C5a and f-Met-Leu-Phe can induce histamine release from human skin mast cells (3,26).

Narcotics, such as morphine, represent examples of pharmacological agents that can induce mast cell mediator release, but predominantly from skin mast cells (3,26). In this respect, the agents are similar to neuropeptides, which can trigger mediator release from human skin mast cells, but not significantly from human basophils or gut or lung mast cells (see foregoing). Therefore, it is of some interest that the intravenous infusion of large doses of morphine regularly causes an increase in plasma histamine levels and often results in shock (3). Since the only mast cell in the body that seems to respond to morphine, including those from the heart, is the skin mast cell, these findings indicate that the rather selective activation of cutaneous mast cells may be sufficient to induce clinically significant systemic responses. The human skin mast cell also differs from other human mast cells or basophils in exhibiting responsiveness to the classic secretogogue of rat peritoneal mast cells; compound 48/80 (3,26).

Induction or Modulation of Basophil or Mast Cell Mediator Release by Cytokines

A considerable body of evidence now indicates that cytokines can directly release or augment IgE-stimulated mediator release in mast cells and basophils, but often with markedly different responses in each cell type. Among these agents, members of the chemokine cytokine superfamily and stem cell factor (SCF) appear to be particularly important. Chemokines, which can be produced by T cells, B cells, macrophages, mast cells, and eosinophils, as well as other cell types, are basic heparin-binding polypeptides that share significant structural similarities and have potent proinflammatory biological activities (114). Members of both the C–C branch of this family [including macrophage inflammatory protein (MIP-1α and β), monocyte chemotactic and activating factor (MCAF), RANTES, and I-309], as well as the C–X–C branch of this group (including connective tissue-activating peptide (CTAP)-III, and its derivative, neutrophil-activating peptide (NAP)-2)] are potent basophil secretagogues (115–120). MCAF, MIP-1α, CTAP-III, and NAP-2, all cause direct, dose-dependent histamine release from basophils (115–120), and some of them also enhance anti-IgE-induced basophil mediator release. MIP-1α also has been reported to induce histamine release from mouse mast cells, but only in certain mouse strains (120).

Recently, MCAF, RANTES, and IL-3 have been demonstrated to be the predominant constituents of mononuclear cell supernatants that exhibit histamine-releasing activity for basophils, suggesting that chemokines may account for a significant fraction of the bioactivities that have previously been attributed to uncharacterized "histamine-releasing factors" (121). Interestingly, another member of the C–X–C group, IL-8, can *inhibit* the release of histamine from basophils in response to certain stimuli (122).

Also, GM-CSF, IL-1, 3, or IL-5 can cause basophil histamine release directly, or enhance the basophil histamine release that is observed in response to other stimuli. Interleukin-3 or GM-CSF can directly induce the release of histamine and LTC_4 from basophils. Preincubation of purified human lung mast cells with IL-1α can prime these cells for enhanced IgE-dependent release of leukotriene C_4 and prostaglandin D_2 (34). The in vivo relevance of these observations is not yet clear.

Stem cell factor, perhaps the most important regulator of mast cell development in vivo, also can induce mediator release from some populations of mouse mast cells (47) or rat mast cells in vitro (123), can augment the magnitude of mouse peritoneal mast cell mediator release in response to IgE-dependent activation in vitro (47), and can trigger mast cell activation and a mast cell-dependent inflammatory response when injected intradermally in mice in vivo (46). Also, SCF can augment IgE-dependent mediator release from human mast cells (38,124) and, at concentrations higher than those from human basophils (38), can directly promote mediator release from human mast cells in vitro (38). It can also induce anaphylactic degranulation from human cutaneous mast cells in vivo (125).

In mice, activation of dermal mast cells by SCF in vivo is c-*kit*-dependent and occurs at doses of cytokine as low as 140 fmol/site (46). We recently reported preliminary data that suggest that administration of rhSCF in humans in vivo may produce similar effects. In phase I trials, daily subcutaneous administration of rhSCF (10–50 μg/kg per day) for 14 days resulted in an approximate 50% increase in urine methylhistamine concentrations, but little or no change in circulating levels of mast cell tryptase (58). However, wheal-and-flare reactions commonly occurred at rhSCF injection sites (125,126), and electron microscopic evaluation revealed extensive anaphylactic degranulation of cutaneous mast cells at these sites (125). Other adverse events suggestive of mast cell activation and mediator release included upper airway symptoms, such as cough, hoarseness, or laryngeal spasm and, in one patient, transient hypotension (126).

THE ROLES OF MAST CELLS AND BASOPHILS IN HEALTH AND DISEASE

In the absence of information derived from patients with isolated abnormalities of basophil or mast cell numbers or function, concepts of the roles of these cells in human health and disease have been developed based on more indirect lines of evidence, including animal experiments. This work indicates that the major roles of basophils and mast cells in host defense are in the orchestration of local immunological and inflammatory reactions, and that their major role in disease is to represent an important source of the mediators responsible for many reactions of immediate hypersensitivity and related disorders (3–8). The roles of basophils and mast cells are expressed primarily by the release to the exterior of preformed, cytoplasmic, granule-associated, cytokines or newly generated (lipid) mediators.

We have utilized mast cell-deficient mice that have been locally or systemically reconstituted by adoptive transfer of in vitro-derived cultured mast cells ("mast cell knock-in mice") as a model to search for differences in the expression of biological responses in anatomical sites or in whole animals that differ only in that one site or set of animals contains mast cells, whereas the control sites or animals remain profoundly mast cell-deficient (27,30; reviewed in Ref. 127). This general approach is summarized in Table 6.

Studies employing mast cell-reconstituted W/W^v mice have identified three patterns of mast cell involvement in biological responses (reviewed in Ref. 127). In some reactions, mast cells appear to have an essential role, in that the responses are not detectably expressed in the absence of the mast cell. In other responses, mast cells appear to regulate the intensity or kinetics of the response, but the reactions can be detectably expressed in the absence of mature mast cells. In yet other responses, no specific mast cell-dependent contribution has been identified. For example, this approach has established that virtually all of the inflammation associated with IgE-dependent reactions elicited in mouse skin (128,129) or stomach (130) is mast cell-dependent, that immune resistance to the cutaneous feeding of larval *Haemaphysalis longicornis* ticks in mice requires IgE and mast cells (131), and that mast cells are responsible for the bronchial hyperresponsiveness to methacholine observed after anti-IgE challenge in mice (132). Essentially all of the inflammation produced by intradermal injection of substance P is also mast cell-dependent (133,134), whereas mast cells can significantly augment, but are not essential for, the inflammation induced by PMA (135) or immune complexes (136). By contrast, most analyses have detected no impairment of the expression of T-cell-mediated contact hypersensitivity reactions in the skin of mast cell-deficient mice (137).

Immediate Hypersensitivity

The immediate hypersensitivity reaction is the pathophysiological hallmark of allergic rhinitis, allergic asthma, and anaphylaxis, and the central role of the mast cell in the pathogenesis of these disorders is widely accepted (3–12). The signs and symptoms that

---

Table 6   General Scheme for Investigating Mouse Mast Cell Function In Vivo

1. Search for quantitative differences in the expression of biological responses in genetically mast cell-deficient WBB6F$_1$-W/W^v and WCB6F$_1$-Sl/Sl^d mice and the congenic normal (+/+) mice.
   Note: Such studies should include appropriate histological analysis, since certain biological responses can result in the appearance of increased numbers of mast cells in the tissues of W/W^v (but not Sl/Sl^d) mice (see Refs. 8, 29, 127).
2. Compare the responses in W/W^v mice and in W/W^v mice that have received bone marrow transplantation from congenic +/+ mice.
   Note: This determines whether the response that is abnormally expressed in W/W^v mice is influenced by mast cells or other cells derived from hematopoietic precursors.
3. Analyze the response in W/W^v mice that have been *selectively* reconstituted with mast cells ("mast cell knock-in mice").
   Note: This determines whether the response which is abnormally expressed in W/W^v mice has a mast cell-dependent component.
4. Define the mechanism(s) by which mast cells contribute to the response.

Source: Modified from Ref. 7.

develop at the site of antigen exposure within the first few minutes of a (type I) immediate hypersensitivity reaction reflect the biological activities of the mast cell or basophil-derived mediators, which are released immediately after the activation of these cells. In sites that do not contain basophils, such as normal skin, these mediators are derived largely, perhaps exclusively, from mast cells. Thus, in most allergic patients, intradermal challenge with specific antigen or anti-IgE induces an immediate wheal-and-flare reaction, accompanied by intense pruritus, which reaches a maximum 15–30 min later (3,6). Such immediate allergic reactions are usually accompanied by an increase in local levels of LTC_4 and PGD_2, as well as the liberation of histamine and tryptase (3,6). Although there are several possible cellular sources for some of these mediators, tryptase is thought to be strictly mast cell-derived, providing the strongest biochemical evidence implicating mast cells in these responses in humans.

Studies in mast cell knockin mice showed that essentially all of the augmented vascular permeability, tissue swelling, and deposition of cross-linked ^{125}I-fibrin associated with IgE-dependent passive cutaneous anaphylaxis reactions (128), or IgE-dependent reactions in the stomach wall (138), were mast cell-dependent. In humans, mast cell participation in the immediate phase of type I reactions in multiple anatomical sites has been clearly established by several lines of evidence, including studies that have demonstrated release of both histamine and tryptase, with a strong correlation between levels of these two mediators in the nasal secretions or skin blister fluids that were induced by exposure to allergen (139). Such findings support the concept that mast cells may be essential for the expression of IgE-dependent immediate-phase responses in humans, as well as in mice.

Late-Phase Responses

In many allergic patients, the immediate reaction to cutaneous antigenic challenge is followed 4–8 h later by a period of persistent swelling and leukocyte infiltration, termed the late-phase reaction (LPR; 140). It is now clear that a LPR may develop following IgE-dependent reactions in the respiratory tract, nose, and other anatomical locations, as well as in the skin. Moreover, many of the clinically significant consequences of IgE-dependent reactions, both in the respiratory tract and in the skin, are now thought to reflect the actions of the leukocytes that are recruited to these sites during LPRs, rather than the direct effects of the mediators released by mast cells at early intervals after antigen challenge (3,8,140). Several lines of evidence, derived from both clinical and animal studies, suggest that the leukocyte infiltration associated with LPRs occurs as a result of mast cell degranulation. Thus, studies in mast cell knockin mice have demonstrated that both the early phase of tissue swelling associated with IgE-dependent cutaneous reactions, as well as the subsequent influx of leukocytes at these sites (which reached maximal levels 6–12 h after antigen challenge), are entirely mast cell-dependent (129). Furthermore, the injection of anti-TNF-α antisera at sites of IgE-dependent cutaneous mast cell activation diminished the leukocyte infiltration observed at the reactions by approximately 50% (129).

The leukocytes that are recruited to sites of late-phase responses in humans include basophils, eosinophils, neutrophils, and macrophages; all of these cells may influence the reactions by providing additional proinflammatory mediators and cytokines. The recruitment of basophils to late-phase reactions provides these responses with an $Fc_\varepsilon RI^+$ cell type, and analysis of nasal lavage or bronchoalveolar lavage (BAL) fluids obtained several hours after antigen challenge demonstrates elevations in histamine, TAME-esterase activity, and

LTC_4, but not PGD_2 or tryptase (141–143). Basophil recruitment into sites of tissue inflammation is thought to reflect the actions of chemotactic factors (such as C5a or cytokines of the chemokine group; see earlier discussion, and 144,145), as well as inter-actions between complementary adhesion molecules expressed on the surface of the basophil (e.g., VLA-4, CD 11/18, and glycoproteins that contain the sialyl-Lewis[x] moiety) and vascular endothelial cells [e.g., VCAM-1, ICAM-1, and E-selectin (ELAM-1)] (146). The expression of these molecules is subject to complex regulatory mechanisms in vivo, which probably include effects of cytokines (e.g., TNF-α, IL-1) and other products derived from activated mast cells.

Thus, the traditional concept of the "self-limited allergic reaction," which was thought to reflect the release of mast cell mediators, the biological half-lives of which were measured in minutes or hours, must now be recognized as incomplete. Indeed, the complex and temporally prolonged consequences of cytokine expression, when considered together with the potential long-term effects of some of the cells' other mediators, suggest that mast cell activation may contribute importantly to many of the chronic features of allergic diseases and other disorders that are associated with mast cell activation. For example, in patients with allergic asthma, evidence of mast cell degranulation is provided by elevated levels of histamine and tryptase in the BAL fluid of patients with moderately symptomatic asthma (147) and in BAL fluids after endobronchial allergen challenge (148). Moreover, a recent study of 17 children with mild to moderate chronic asthma showed a strong correlation between bronchial hyperresponsiveness to histamine and levels of mast cell tryptase in their BAL fluid (149). However, in contrast to earlier reports, recent studies with highly specific monoclonal antibodies have *not* demonstrated any significant differences in the numbers of MC_T or MC_{TC} mast cells in the airway mucosa of atopic asthmatics, atopic nonasthmatics, or healthy control subjects (150). This finding indicates that significant mast cell hyperplasia is unlikely to have an important role in the etiology of allergic asthma.

Many other factors probably also contribute to the chronicity of allergic inflammation, including prolonged or repeated exposure to relevant allergens and perhaps the diminished threshold for mast cell activation that can be observed in vivo after even a single antigenic challenge. In addition, in patients with chronic atopic diseases, including allergic rhinitis and atopic dermatitis, the sites of lesions contain complex inflammatory infiltrates that include T cells (particularly those that produce the T_H2-type pattern of cytokines that can promote allergic responses; 151,152), monocytes–macrophages, eosinophils, and neutro-phils, as well as mast cells and basophils. It is likely that all of these participants signifi-cantly influence the course of these disorders and, in aggregate, contribute to the local development of the pathological manifestations associated with these conditions.

Parasitic Diseases

Several lines of evidence support the concept that mast cells or basophils participate in adaptive immunological responses against parasites. Infection with helminthic parasites is associated with increased levels of parasite-specific IgE and nonspecific IgE, as well as mast cell hyperplasia (153,154). Moreover, the ability of worm antigens to cause de-granulation of mast cells obtained from parasite-infected animals, as well as the toxic properties of some mast cell mediators on these parasites, are well documented (153,154). Finally, some mast cell- or basophil-derived mediators, including histamine and serotonin, have physiological effects on vascular permeability, intestinal ion and mucous secretion, and gut motility, which might enhance local expressions of host defense against parasites (153,154). Accordingly, it has been hypothesized that mast cell and basophil sensitization by parasite-specific IgE, followed by mast cell and basophil degranulation in response to exposure to the parasite's antigens, promotes the expulsion of the parasites (153,154).

Consistent with this hypothesis, studies of *Trichinella spiralis* or *Strongyloides ratti* infections, as well as some experiments with the roundworm *Nippostrongylus brasiliensis*, showed that the duration of these experimental parasitic infections was prolonged in mast cell-deficient mice, when compared with the results in normal animals (reviewed in Ref. 155). However, the impairment of immunity in mast cell-deficient mice was never as severe as in athymic nude mice and, in each instance, the mast cell-deficient mice eventually were able to resolve the infection (155). Moreover, the successful elimination of parasites in the absence (or virtual absence) of a specific IgE response has also been reported (156,157). Thus, several lines of evidence indicate that mucosal mast cell hyperplasia and activation may contribute to host defense against certain helminthic infections, but, usually, mast cells may not represent an essential component of these immune responses.

The most compelling evidence for a role for mast cells or basophils in defense against parasites is in immune responses to ectoparasites, such as ticks. However, the relative importance of basophils or mast cells as effectors in these reactions to ticks may vary according to the species of host and the species of tick. Studies utilizing mast cell knockin mice have demonstrated that IgE and mast cells are essential for the expression of immune resistance to the cutaneous feeding of larval *Haemaphysalis longicornis* ticks (131). In contrast, basophils may be more important than mast cells in immune resistance to the feeding of a different tick species (*Dermacentor variabilis*) in mice (158), and both basophils and eosinophils appear to be required for immune resistance to the feeding of larval *Amblyomma americanum* ticks in guinea pigs (159). Finally, there has been a single report of a patient who lacked basophils and eosinophils (and expressed an IgA deficiency), who suffered from severe scabies (160). These and other findings support the concept that resident mast cells and recruited basophils may have similar, overlapping, or complementary functions in immune responses to ectoparasites, worms, and perhaps other parasites, with the relative contributions of each cell type varying according to the type of parasite, species of host animal, or other factors (60).

Arthritis

Mast cells are present in normal human synovium, but their numbers can be increased one- to tenfold in a variety of arthritides, including those associated with syphilis or tuberculosis, juvenile rheumatoid arthritis, adult rheumatoid arthritis, systemic lupus erythematosus, mixed connective tissue disease, osteoarthritis, psoriatic arthritis, postintestinal bypass arthropathy, and chronic villonodular synovitis (161–163). Mast cells are also present in the synovial fluid during some of these conditions (164,165). Given the biological effects of mast cell-derived mediators, it has been suggested that mast cells might contribute to the inflammation and tissue remodeling that is observed in these disorders (163). Indeed, Malone and Metcalfe have recently demonstrated that mast cells may participate in the development of experimental arthritis in rats by an IgE-dependent mechanism (166). On the other hand, the relative importance of mast cells, as opposed to other cell types, in the pathogenesis of rheumatoid arthritis or other naturally occurring arthritides remains to be determined.

Nerve–Mast Cell Interactions

The biological significance of potential interactions between nerves and mast cells has been the subject of considerable speculation (18,167,168). Morphological studies have documented a very close anatomical association between mast cells and nonmyelinated nerves, particularly in the gastrointestinal tract; in many instances, such nerves contain substance P, CGRP, or other neuropeptides (reviewed in 18,167–169). Several lines of evidence indicate that the close anatomical relation between mast cells and certain nerves may be functionally significant. Antidromic electrical stimulation (ES) of sensory nerves in the rat induces dilation and augmented permeability of cutaneous blood vessels, and also results in degranulation of cutaneous mast cells (170). Direct neural stimulation can result in degranulation of mucosal mast cells in rat glandular stomach or ileum (18,167), and systemic release of rat gastrointestinal mast cell proteases (172) can be elicited in appropriately sensitized animals after Pavlovian conditioning (172). Such findings have supported the concept that some of the psychological factors that can result in the exacerbation of allergic asthma and other atopic disorders may reflect, at least in part, the effects of neural activity on mast cell function (18,167,172).

Several different neuropeptides that can induce alterations in vascular tone or permeability when injected in vivo can also stimulate degranulation of a variety of human and rodent mast cell populations in vitro or in vivo (reviewed in Ref. 134). Cutaneous mast cells are particularly sensitive to stimulation by substance P, which can induce a wheal-and-flare response when injected into human skin in doses as low as 10 pmol. Pharmacological studies indicate that this flare response is largely mediated by histamine, suggesting that such effects may reflect neuropeptide-dependent mast cell degranulation. In accord with this hypothesis, studies in genetically mast cell-deficient and reconstituted mice indicate that all of the augmented vascular permeability, tissue swelling, fibrin deposition, and leukocyte infiltration associated with the intradermal injection of substance P is mast cell-dependent (133,134). However, the more prolonged wheal component of the reaction in humans occurs through a combination of histamine-dependent and histamine-independent mechanisms (reviewed in Refs. 173,174).

Several lines of evidence now indicate that mast cell products also might down-regulate certain vascular changes induced by release of neuropeptides. The rat CTMC protease RMCP I can effectively hydrolyze a variety of polypeptides in vitro, including neurotensin (175,176). In vivo studies indicate that degranulated rat cutaneous mast cells may be able to degrade the potent vasodilator calcitonin gene-related peptide (CGRP) (177), which can occur together with substance P in the same nerves. Moreover, the duration of vasodilation that follows injection of CGRP into rat or human skin is markedly diminished when substance P is injected at the same time, suggesting that substance P-induced mast cell degranulation can result in attenuation of CGRP-induced vasodilation (177).

These examples by no means exhaust the potentially important interactions between neuropeptides, mast cells, and the nervous system (18,167). Indeed, certain populations of mast cells may themselves be able to generate molecules similar to neuropeptides (178). Nor do we wish to imply that all aspects of "neurogenic inflammation" are mast cell-dependent, as this is very unlikely (179). However, the available evidence does illustrate how particular phenotypic characteristics of individual populations of mast cells may permit them to participate in both the augmentation and the subsequent down-regulation of certain manifestations of neuropeptide-induced inflammation.

ACKNOWLEDGMENTS

We thank Dr. Ann M. Dvorak for providing the electron micrographs. Some of the work reviewed in this chapter was supported by United States Public Health Service grants AI 22674, AI 23990, AI 31982, AI 33372, and HL 02240, by AMGEN, Inc., or by the Beth Israel Hospital Pathology Foundation.

REFERENCES

1. Ehrlich P. Beiträge zur Theorie und Praxis der histologischen Färbung. Thesis. Leipzig, 1878.
2. Ehrlich P. Über die spezifischen Granulationen des Blutes. Arch Anat Physiol Abt 1879; p. 571.
3. Galli SJ, Lichtenstein LM. Biology of mast cells and basophils. In: Middleton E Jr, Reed CE, Ellis EF, Adkinson NF Jr, Yunginger JW, eds. Allergy, Principles and Practice. 3rd ed. St. Louis: CV Mosby, 1988:106–134.
4. Holgate ST, Robinson C, Church MK. Mediators of immediate hypersensitivity. In: Middleton E Jr, Reed CE, Ellis EF, Adkinson NF Jr, Yunginger JW, Busse WW, eds. Allergy, Principles and Practice. 4th ed. St. Louis: CV Mosby, 1993:267–301.
5. Metcalfe DD, Kaliner M, Donlon MA. The mast cell. CRC Crit Rev Immunol 1981; 2:23–74.
6. Schwartz L, Huff T. Biology of mast cells and basophils. In: Middleton E Jr, Reed CE, Ellis EF, Adkinson NF Jr, Yunginger JW, Busse WW, eds. Allergy, Principles and Practice. 4th ed. St. Louis: CV Mosby, 1993:135–168.
7. Galli SJ. New insights into "the riddle of mast cells": microenvironmental regulation of mast cell development and phenotypic heterogeneity. Lab Invest 1990; 62:5–33.
8. Galli SJ. New concepts about the mast cell. N Engl J Med 1993; 328:257–265.
9. Beaven MA, Metzger H. Signal transduction by Fc receptors: the Fc epsilon RI case. Immunol Today 1993; 14:222–226.
10. Kinet JP. The high-affinity receptor for IgE. Curr Opin Immunol 1990; 2:499–505.
11. Ishizaka T. Mechanisms of IgE-mediated hypersensitivity. In: Middleton E Jr, Reed CE, Ellis EF, Adkinson NF Jr, Yunginger JW, eds. Allergy, Principles and Practice. 3rd ed. St. Louis: CV Mosby, 1988:71.
12. Benhamou M, Siraganian RP. Protein-tyrosine phosphorylation: an essential component of $Fc_\varepsilon RI$ signaling. Immunol Today 1992; 13:195–197.
13. Galli SJ, Dvorak AM. Production, biochemistry, and function of basophils and mast cells. In: Beutler E, Lichtman MA, Coller BS, Kipps TJ, eds. Williams Hematology. 5th ed. New York: McGraw-Hill. In press.
14. Galli SJ, Dvorak AM, Dvorak HF. Basophils and mast cells: morphologic insights into their biology, secretory patterns and function. Prog Allergy 1984; 34:1–141.
15. Dvorak AM. Blood cell biochemistry. In: Basophil and Mast Cell Degranulation and Recovery. Vol 4. New York: Plenum Press, 1991.
16. Selye H. The mast cells. Washington: Butterworth, 1965.
17. Enerbäck L, Pipkom U, Aldenborg F, Wingren U. Mast cell heterogeneity in man: properties and function of human mucosal mast cells. In: Galli SJ, Austen KF, eds. Mast Cell and Basophil Differentiation and Function in Health and Disease. New York: Raven Press, 1989:27–37.
18. Bienenstock J, Blennerhassett M, Kakuta Y, et al. Evidence for central and peripheral nervous system interaction with mast cells. In: Galli SJ, Austen KF, eds. Mast Cell and Basophil Differentiation and Function in Health and Disease. New York: Raven Press, 1989:275–284.
19. Enerbäck L. Mast cell heterogeneity: the evolution of the concept of a specific mucosal mast cell. In: Befus AD, Bienenstock J, Denburg JA, eds. Mast Cell Differentiation and Heterogeneity. New York: Raven Press, 1986:1–26.
20. Kitamura Y. Heterogeneity of mast cells and phenotypic changes between subpopulations. Annu Rev Immunol 1989; 7:59–76.

21. Miller HRP, Huntley JF, Newlands GFJ, et al. Mast cell granule proteases in mouse and rat: a guide to mast cell heterogeneity and activation in the gastrointestinal tract. In: Galli SJ, Austen KF, eds. Mast Cell and Basophil Differentiation and Function in Health and Disease. New York: Raven Press, 1989:81–91.

22. Bienenstock J, Befus AD, Denburg JA. Mast cell heterogeneity: basic questions and clinical implications. In: Befus AD, Bienenstock J, Denburg JA, eds. Mast Cell Differentiation and Heterogeneity. New York: Raven Press, 1986:391–402.

23. Irani AA, Schechter NM, Craig SS, et al. Two human mast cell subsets with distinct neutral protease compositions. Proc Natl Acad Sci USA 1986; 83:4464–4468.

24. Irani AA, Craig SS, DeBlois G, et al. Deficiency of the tryptase-positive, chymase-negative mast cell type in gastrointestinal mucosa of patients with defective T lymphocyte function. J Immunol 1987; 138:4381–4386.

25. Pearce FL. Functional differences between mast cells from various locations. In: Befus AD, Bienenstock J, Denburg JA, eds. Mast Cell Differentiation and Heterogeneity. New York: Raven Press, 1986:215–222.

26. Church MK, Benyon RC, Rees PH, et al. Functional heterogeneity of human mast cells. In: Galli SJ, Austen KF, eds. Mast Cell and Basophil Differentiation and Function in Health and Disease. New York: Raven Press, 1989:161–171.

27. Galli SJ, Kitamura Y. Animal model of human disease. Genetically mast cell-deficient W/W^v and Sl/Sl^d mice: their value for the analysis of the roles of mast cells in biological responses in vivo. Am J Pathol 1987; 127:191–198.

28. Kitamura Y, Nakayama H, Fujita J. Mechanism of mast cell deficiency in mutant mice of W/W^v and Sl/Sl^d genotype. In: Galli SJ, Austen KF, eds. Mast Cell and Basophil Differentiation and Function in Health and Disease. New York: Raven Press, 1989:15–25.

29. Galli SJ, Zsebo KM, Geissler EN. The kit ligand, stem cell factor. Adv Immunol 1994; 55:1–96.

30. Nakano T, Sonoda T, Hayashi C, et al. Fate of bone marrow-derived cultured mast cells after intracutaneous intraperitoneal and intravenous transfer into genetically mast cell-deficient W/W^v mice. Evidence that cultured mast cells can give rise to both connective tissue-type and mucosal mast cells. J Exp Med 1985; 162:1025–1043.

31. Sonoda S, Sonoda T, Nakano T, et al. Development of mucosal mast cells after injection of a single connective tissue-type mast cell in the stomach mucosa of genetically mast cell-deficient W/W^v mice. J Immunol 1986; 137:1319–1322.

32. Kanakura Y, Thompson H, Nakano T, et al. Multiple bidirectional alterations of phenotype and changes in proliferative potential during the in vitro and in vivo passage of clonal mast cell populations derived from mouse peritoneal mast cell. Blood 1988; 72:877–885.

33. Levi-Schaffer F, Austen KF, Gravallese PM, et al. Co-culture of interleukin 3-dependent mouse mast cells with fibroblasts results in a phenotypic change of the mast cells. Proc Natl Acad Sci USA 1986; 83:6485–6488.

34. Costa JJ, Burd PR, Metcalfe DD. Mast cell cytokines. In: Kaliner MA, Metcalfe DD, eds. The Role of the Mast Cell in Health and Disease. New York: Marcel Dekker, 1992:433–466.

35. Williams DE, de Vries P, Namen AE, et al. The steel factor. Dev Biol 1992; 151:368–376.

36. Besmer P. The kit ligand encoded at the murine steel locus: a pleiotropic growth and differentiation factor. Curr Opin Cell Biol 1991; 3:939–946.

37. Lerner NB, Nocka KH, Cole SR, et al. Monoclonal antibody YB5.B8 identifies the human c-kit protein product. Blood 1991; 78:876–1883.

38. Columbo M, Horowitz EM, Botana LM, et al. The recombinant human c-kit receptor ligand, rhSCF, induces mediator release from human cutaneous mast cells and enhances IgE-dependent mediator release from both skin mast cells and peripheral blood basophils. J Immunol 1992; 149:599–608.

39. Zsebo KM, Williams DA, Geissler EN, et al. Stem cell factor (SCF) is encoded at the Sl locus of the mouse and is the ligand for the c-kit tyrosine kinase receptor. Cell 1990; 63:213–224.

40. Tsai M, Shih L, Newlands GFJ, et al. The rat c-kit ligand, stem cell factor, induces the

development of connective tissue-type and mucosal mast cells in vivo. Analysis by anatomical distribution, histochemistry and protease phenotype. J Exp Med 1991; 174:125–131.

41. Mekori YA, Oh CK, Metcalfe DD. IL-3-dependent murine mast cells undergo apoptosis on removal of IL-3. J Immunol 1993; 151:3775–3784.

42. Iemura A, Tsai M, Ando A, et al. The c-*kit* ligand, stem cell factor, promotes mast cell survival by suppressing apoptosis. Am J Pathol 1994; 144:321–328.

43. Tsai M, Takeishi T, Thompson H, et al. Induction of mast cell proliferation, maturation and heparin synthesis by the rat c-*kit* ligand, stem cell factor. Proc Natl Acad Sci USA 1991; 88:6382–6386.

44. Gurish MF, Childyal N, Arm J, et al. Cytokine mRNA are preferentially increased relative to secretory granule protein mRNA in mouse bone marrow-derived mast cells that have undergone IgE-mediated activation and degranulation. J Immunol 1991; 146:1527–1533.

45. Haig DM, Huntley JF, MacKellar A, et al. Effects of stem cell factor (kit-ligand) and inter-leukin-3 on the growth and serine proteinase expression of rat bone marrow-derived or serosal mast cells. Blood. In press.

46. Wershil BK, Tsai M, Geissler EN, et al. The rat c-*kit* ligand, stem cell factor, induces c-*kit* receptor-dependent mouse mast cell activation in vivo. Evidence that signaling through the c-*kit* receptor can induce expression of cellular function. J Exp Med 1992; 175:245–255.

47. Coleman JW, Holliday MR, Kimber I, et al. Regulation of mouse peritoneal mast cell secretory function by stem cell factor, IL-3 or IL-4. J Immunol 1993; 150:556–562.

48. Ando A, Martin TR, Galli SJ. Effects of chronic treatment with the c-*kit* ligand, stem cell factor, on immunoglobulin E-dependent anaphylaxis in mice: genetically mast cell-deficient *Sl/Sl^d* mice acquire anaphylactic responsiveness, but the congenic normal mice do not exhibit aug-mented responses. J Clin Invest 1993; 92:1639–1649.

49. Galli SJ, Iemura A, Garlick DS, et al. Reversible expansion of primate mast cell populations in vivo by stem cell factor. J Clin Invest 1993; 91:148–152.

50. Kirshenbaum AS, Goff JP, Dreskin SA, et al. Interleukin 3-dependent growth of basophil-like and mast-like cells from human bone marrow. J Immunol 1989; 42:2424–2429.

51. Kirshenbaum AS, Kessler SW, Goff JP, Metcalfe DD. Demonstration of the origin of human mast cells from CD34$^+$ bone marrow progenitor cells. J Immunol 1991; 146:1410–1415.

52. Furitsu T, Saito H, Dvorak AM, et al. Development of human mast cells in vitro. Proc Natl Acad Sci USA 1989; 86:10039–10043.

53. Dvorak AM, Furitsu T, Ishizaka T. Ultrastructural morphology of human mast cell progenitors in sequential cocultures of cord blood cells and fibroblasts. Int Arch Allergy Immunol 1993; 100:219–229.

54. Kirshenbaum AS, Goff JP, Kessler SW, et al. Effect of IL-3 and stem cell factor on the appearance of human basophil and mast cells from CD34$^+$ pluripotent progenitor cells. J Immunol 1992; 148:772–777.

55. Valent P, Spanblöchl E, Sperr WR, et al. Induction of differentiation of human mast cells from bone marrow and peripheral blood mononuclear cells by recombinant human stem cell factor/*kit*-ligand in long-term culture. Blood 1992; 80:2237–2245.

56. Mitsui H, Furitsu T, Dvorak AM, et al. Development of human mast cells from umbilical cord blood cells by recombinant human and murine c-*kit* ligand. Proc Natl Acad Sci USA 1993; 90:735–739.

57. Irani A-MA, Nilsson G, Mettinen U, et al. Recombinant human stem cell factor stimulates differentiation of mast cells from dispersed fetal liver cells. Blood 1992; 80:3009–3021.

58. Costa JJ, Demetri GD, Hayes DF, et al. Increased skin mast cells and urine methyl histamine in patients receiving recombinant methionyl human stem cell factor (abstr). Proc Am Assoc Cancer Res 1993; 34:211.

59. Dvorak AM, Ishizaka T, Galli SJ. Ultrastructure of human basophils developing in vitro. Evidence for the acquisition of peroxidase by basophils, and for different effects of human and

murine growth factors on human basophil and eosinophil maturation. Lab Invest 1985; 53: 57–71.

60. Galli SJ, Askenase PW. Cutaneous basophil hypersensitivity. In: Abramoff P, Phillips SM, Escobar MR, eds. The Reticuloendothelial System: A Comprehensive Treatise. New York: Plenum Press, 1986:321–369.

61. Dvorak AM, Dvorak HF, Galli SJ. Ultrastructural criteria for identification of mast cells and basophils in humans, guinea pigs, and mice. Am Rev Respir Dis 1983; 128:S49–S52.

62. Aglietta M, Camussi G, Piacibello W. Detection of basophils growing in semisolid agar culture. Exp Hematol 1981; 9:95–100.

63. Valent P, Schmidt G, Besemer J, et al. Interleukin-3 is a differentiation factor for human basophils. Blood 1989; 73:1763–1769.

64. Valent P, Besemer J, Muhm M, et al. Interleukin-3 activates human blood basophils via high affinity binding sites. Proc Natl Acad Sci USA 1989; 86:5542–5546.

65. Ganser A, Lindemann A, Seipelt G, et al. Effects of recombinant human interleukin-3 patients with normal hematopoiesis and in patients with bone marrow failure. Blood 1990; 76:666–676.

66. Denburg JA. Cytokine-induced human basophil/mast cell growth and differentiation in vitro. Springer Semin Immunopathol 1990; 12:401–414.

67. Valent P, Bettelheim P. The human basophil. Crit Rev Oncol Hematol 1990; 10:327–352.

68. Tsuda T, Wong DA, Dolovich J, et al. Synergistic effects of nerve growth factor and granulocyte–macrophage colony-stimulating factor on human basophilic cell differentiation. Blood 1991; 77:971–979.

69. Gordon JR, Burd PR, Galli SJ. Mast cells as a source of multifunctional cytokines. Immunol Today 1990; 11:458–464.

70. Yamatodani A, Maeyama K, Watanabe T, et al. Tissue distribution of histamine in a mutant mouse deficient in mast cells: clear evidence for the presence of non–mast-cell histamine. Biochem Pharmacol 1982; 31:305–309.

71. Porter JF, Mitchell RGL. Distribution of histamine in human blood. Physiol Rev 1972; 52:361–381.

72. Stevens RL, Fox CC, Lichtenstein LM, Austen KF. Identification of chondroitin sulfate E proteoglycans and heparin proteoglycans in the secretory granules of human lung mast cells. Proc Natl Acad Sci USA 1988; 85:2284–2287.

73. Thompson HL, Schulman ES, Metcalfe DD. Identification of chondroitin sulfate E in human lung mast cells. J Immunol 1988; 140:2708–2713.

74. Metcalfe DD, Bland CE, Wasserman SI. Biochemical and functional characterization of proteoglycans isolated from basophils of patients with chronic myelogenous leukemia. J Immunol 1984; 132:1943–1950.

75. Kjellen L, Lindahl U. Proteoglycans: structures and interactions. Annu Rev Biochem 1991; 60:443–475.

76. Schwartz LB, Bradford TM. Regulation of tryptase from human lung mast cells by heparin stabilization of the active tetramer. J Biol Chem 1986; 261:7372–7379.

77. Ruoslahti E, Yamaguchi Y. Proteoglycans as modulators of growth factor activities. Cell 1991; 64:867–869.

78. Schwartz LB, Metcalfe DD, Miller JS, et al. Tryptase levels as an indicator of mast cell activation in systemic anaphylaxis and mastocytosis. N Engl J Med 1987; 316:1622–1626.

79. Schechter NM, Franki JE, Geesin JC, Lazarus GS. Human skin chymotryptic proteinase. Isolation and relation to cathepsin G and rat mast cell protease. J Biol Chem 1983; 258:2973–2978.

80. Johnson LA, Moon KE, Eisenberg M. Purification to homogeneity of the human skin chymotryptic proteinase "chymase." Anal Biochem 1986; 155:358–364.

81. Ackerman SJ, Corrette SE, Rosenberg HF, et al. Molecular cloning and characterization of human eosinophil Charcot–Leyden crystal protein (lysophospholipase). Similarities to IgE binding proteins and the S-type animal lectin superfamily. J Immunol 1993; 150:456–468.

82. Dvorak AM, Ackerman SJ. Ultrastructural localization of the Charcot–Leyden crystal protein (lysophospholipase) to granules and intragranular crystals in mature human basophils. Lab Invest 1989; 60:557–567.

83. Valone FH, Boggs JM, Goetzl EJ. Lipid mediators of hypersensitivity and inflammation. In: Middleton E Jr, Reed CE, Ellis EF, Adkinson NF Jr, Yuninger JW, Busse WW, eds. Allergy: Principles and Practice. 4th ed. St. Louis: CV Mosby, 1993:302–319.

84. Roberts LJ II, Sweetman BJ, Lewis RA, et al. Increased production of prostaglandin D_2 in patients with systemic mastocytosis. N Engl J Med 1980; 303:1400–1404.

85. Miadonna A, Tedeschi A, Arnoux B, et al. Evidence of PAF-acether metabolic pathway activation in antigen challenge of upper respiratory airways. Am Rev Respir Dis 1989; 140:142–147.

86. Cass FM, Dixon CM, Barnes PJ. Inhaled platelet-activating factor causes bronchoconstriction and increased bronchial reactivity in man. Am Rev Respir Dis 1986; 133:A212.

87. Plaut M, Pierce HJ, Watson CJ, et al. Mast cell lines produce lymphokines in response to cross-linkage of $Fc_\varepsilon RI$ or to calcium ionophores. Nature 1989; 339:64–67.

88. Wodnar-Filipowicz A, Heusser CH, Moroni C. Production of the haemopoietic growth factors GM-CSF and interleukin-3 by mast cells in response to IgE receptor-mediated activation. Nature 1989; 339:150–152.

89. Burd PR, Rogers HW, Gordon JR, et al. Interleukin 3-dependent and -independent mast cells stimulated with IgE and antigen express multiple cytokines. J Exp Med 1989; 170:245–257.

90. Young JD-E, Liu C-C, Butler G, et al. Identification, purification, and characterization of a mast cell-associated cytolytic factor related to tumor necrosis factor. Proc Natl Acad Sci USA 1987; 84:9175–9179.

91. Gordon JR, Galli SJ. Mast cells as a source of both preformed and immunologically inducible TNF-α/cachectin. Nature 1990; 346:274–276.

92. Gordon JR, Galli SJ. Release of both preformed and newly synthesized tumor necrosis factor α (TNF-α)/cachectin by mouse mast cells stimulated by the $Fc_\varepsilon RI$. A mechanism for the sustained action of mast cell-derived TNF-α during IgE-dependent biological responses. J Exp Med 1991; 174:103–107.

93. Plaut M, Kagey-Sobotka A, Niv Y, et al. Regulation of mast cell lymphokine production [abstr]. FASEB J 1990; 4:A1705.

94. Wodnar-Filipowicz A, Moroni C. Regulation of interleukin 3 mRNA expression in mast cells occurs at the posttranscriptional level and is mediated by calcium ions. Proc Natl Acad Sci USA 1990; 87:777–781.

95. Steffen M, Abboud M, Potter GK, et al. Presence of tumour necrosis factor or a related factor in human basophil/mast cells. Immunology 1989; 66:445–450.

96. Klein LM, Lavker RM, Matis, WL, et al. Degranulation of human mast cells induces an endothelial antigen central to leukocyte adhesion. Proc Natl Acad Sci USA 1989; 86:8972–8976.

97. Walsh LJ, Trinchieri G, Waldorf HA, et al. Human dermal mast cells contain and release tumor necrosis factor α which induces endothelial leukocyte adhesion molecule-1. Proc Natl Acad Sci USA 1991; 88:4220–4224.

98. Ohkawara Y, Yamauchi K, Tanno Y, et al. Human lung mast cells and pulmonary macrophages produce tumor necrosis factor-α in sensitized lung tissue after IgE receptor triggering. Am J Respir Cell Mol Biol 1992; 7:385–392.

99. Benyon RC, Bissonnette EY, Befus AD. Tumor necrosis factor-α dependent cytotoxicity of human skin mast cells is enhanced by anti-IgE antibodies. J Immunol 1991; 147:2253–2258.

100. Leung DYM, Pober JS, Cotran RS. Expression of endothelial–leukocyte adhesion molecule-1 in elicited late phase allergic reactions. J Clin Invest 1991; 87:1805–1809.

101. Bradding P, Feather IH, Howarth PH, et al. Interleukin 4 is localized to and released by human mast cells. J Exp Med 1992; 176:1381–1386.

102. Bradding P, Feather IH, Wilson S, et al. Immunolocalization of cytokines in the nasal mucosa of normal and perennial rhinitic subjects. J Immunol 1993; 151:3853–3865.

103. Seder RA, Paul WE, Dvorak AM, et al. Mouse splenic and bone marrow cell populations that express high-affinity Fc_ε receptors and produce interleukin 4 are highly enriched in basophils. Proc Natl Acad Sci USA 1991; 88:2835–2839.

104. Dvorak AM, Seder RA, Paul WE, et al. Ultrastructural characteristics of $Fc_\varepsilon R$-positive basophils in the spleen and bone marrow of mice immunized with goat anti-mouse IgD antibody. Lab Invest 1993; 68:708–715.

105. Brunner T, Heusser CH, Dahinden CA. Human peripheral blood basophils primed by interleukin 3 (IL-3) produce IL-4 in response to immunoglobulin E receptor stimulation. J Exp Med 1993; 177:605–611.

106. Arock M, Merle-Béral H, Dugas B, et al. IL-4 release by human leukemic and activated normal basophils. J Immunol 1993; 151:1441–1447.

107. Gauchat J-F, Henchoz S, Mazzel G, et al. Induction of human IgE synthesis in B cells by mast cells and basophils. Nature 1993; 365:340–343.

108. Galli SJ, Gordon JR, Wershil BK. Cytokine production by mast cells and basophils. Curr Opin Immunol 1991; 3:865–873.

109. Wong DTW, Weller PF, Galli SJ, et al. Human eosinophils express transforming growth factor-alpha. J Exp Med 1990; 172:673–681.

110. Liu M, Matossian K, Wong DTW, et al. Expression of mRNA for transforming growth factor-α (TGF-α) by eosinophils at sites of segmental airway challenge with antigen in allergic asthmatic subjects (abstr). Am Rev Respir Dis 1992; 145:A452.

111. Ogawa M, Nakahata T, Leary AG, et al. Suspension culture of human mast cells/basophils from umbilical cord blood mononuclear cells. Proc Natl Acad Sci USA 1983; 80:4494–4498.

112. Dembo M, Goldstein B, Sobotka AK, et al. Degranulation of human basophils: quantitative analysis of histamine release and desensitization, due to a bivalent penicilloyl hapten. J Immunol 1979; 123:1864–1872.

113. MacGlashan DW Jr, Lichtenstein LM. Characteristics of human basophil sulfidopeptide leukotriene release: releasability defined as the ability of the basophil to respond to dimeric crosslinks. J Immunol 1986; 136:2231–2239.

114. Oppenheim JJ, Zachariae COC, Mukaida N, Matsushima K. Properties of the novel proinflammatory supergene "intercrine" cytokine family. Annu Rev Immunol 1991; 9:617–648.

115. Dahinden C, Kurimoto Y, de Weck AL, et al. The neutrophil-activating peptide NAF/NAP-1 induces histamine and leukotriene release by interleukin 3-primed basophils. J Exp Med 1989; 170:1787–1792.

116. Reddigari SR, Kuna P, Miragliotta GF, et al. Connective tissue-activating peptide-III and its derivative, neutrophil-activating peptide-2, release histamine from human basophils. J Allergy Clin Immunol 1992; 89:666–672.

117. Kuna P, Reddigari SR, Rucinshi D, et al. Monocyte chemotactic and activating factor is a potent histamine-releasing factor for human basophils. J Exp Med 1992; 175:489–493.

118. Bischoff SC, Krieger M, Brunner T, Dahinden CA. Monocyte chemotactic protein 1 is a potent activator of human basophils. J Exp Med 1992; 175:1271–1275.

119. Alam R, Lett-Brown MA, Forsythe PA, et al. Monocyte chemotactic and activating factor is a potent histamine-releasing factor for basophils. J Clin Invest 1992; 89:723–728.

120. Alam R, Forsythe PA, Stafford S, et al. Macrophage inflammatory protein-1α activates basophils and mast cells. J Exp Med 1992; 176:781–786.

121. Kuna P, Reddigari SR, Schall TJ, et al. Characterization of the human basophil response to cytokines, growth factors, and histamine releasing factors of the intercrine/chemokine family. J Immunol 1993; 150:1932–1943.

122. Kuna P, Reddigari SR, Kornfeld D, Kaplan AP. IL-8 inhibits histamine release from human basophils induced by histamine releasing factors, connective tissue activating peptide III, and IL-3. J Immunol 1991; 147:1920–1924.

123. Nakajima K, Hirai K, Yamaguchi M, et al. Stem cell factor has histamine releasing activity in rat connective tissue-type mast cells. Biochem Biophys Res Commun 1992; 183:1076–1083.

124. Bischoff SC, Dahinden CA. c-*kit* ligand, a unique potentiator of mediator release by human lung mast cells. J Exp Med 1992; 175:237–244.

125. Costa JJ, Demetri GD, Harrist TJ, et al. Recombinant human stem cell factor (rhSCF) induces cutaneous mast cell activation and hyperplasia, and hyperpigmentation in humans in vivo. J Allergy Clin Immunol 1994. In press.

126. Demetri G, Costa J, Hayes D, et al. A phase I trial of recombinant methionyl human stem cell factor (SCF) in patients with advanced breast carcinoma pre- and post-chemotherapy (CHEMO) with cyclophosphamide (C) and doxorubicin (A) [abstr]. Proc Am Soc Clin Oncol 1993; 12:A367.

127. Galli SJ, Geissler EN, Wershil BK, et al. Insights into mast cell development and function derived from analyses of mice carrying mutations at beige, *W*/c-*kit* or *Sl*/SCF (c-*kit* ligand) loci. In: Kaliner MA, Metcalfe DD, eds. The Role of the Mast Cell in Health and Disease. New York: Marcel Dekker, 1992:129–202.

128. Wershil BK, Mekori YA, Murakami T, Galli SJ. ^{125}I-fibrin deposition in IgE-dependent immediate hypersensitivity reactions in mouse skin. Demonstration of the role of mast cells using genetically mast cell-deficient mice locally reconstituted with cultured mast cells. J Immunol 1987; 139:2605–2614.

129. Wershil BK, Wang Z-S, Gordon JR, Galli SJ. Recruitment of neutrophils during IgE-dependent cutaneous late phase responses in the mouse is mast cell dependent: partial inhibition of the reaction with antiserum against tumor necrosis factor-alpha. J Clin Invest 1991; 87:446–453.

130. Wershil BK, Wang Z-S, Galli SJ. Evidence of mast cell-dependent neutrophil infiltration during IgE-dependent gastric inflammation in the mouse: does this represent a gastric late phase reaction (LPR) [abstr]? Gastroenterology 1991; 100:A625.

131. Matsuda H, Watanabe N, Kiso Y, et al. Necessity of IgE antibodies and mast cells for manifestation of resistance against larval *Haemaphysalis longicornis* ticks in mice. J Immunol 1990; 144:259–262.

132. Martin TR, Takeishi T, Katz HR, et al. Mast cell activation enhances airway responsiveness to methacholine in the mouse. J Clin Invest 1993; 9:1176–1182.

133. Matsuda H, Kawakita K, Kiso Y, et al. Substance P induces granulocyte infiltration through degranulation of mast cells. J Immunol 1989; 142:927–931.

134. Yano H, Wershil BK, Arizono N, Galli SJ. Substance P-induced augmentation of cutaneous vascular permeability and granulocyte infiltration in mice is mast cell dependent. J Clin Invest 1989; 84:1276–1286.

135. Wershil BK, Murakami T, Galli SJ. Mast cell-dependent amplification of an immunologically nonspecific inflammatory response. Mast cells are required for the full expression of cutaneous acute inflammation induced by phorbol 12-myristate 13-acetate. J Immunol 1988; 140:2356–2360.

136. Ramos BF, Qureshi R, Olsen KM, Jakschik BA. The importance of mast cells for the neutrophil influx in immune complex-induced peritonitis in mice. J Immunol 1990; 145:1868–1873.

137. Galli SJ, Hammel I. Unequivocal delayed hypersensitivity in mast cell-deficient and beige mice. Science 1984; 226:710–713.

138. Wershil BK, Galli SJ. ^{125}I-fibrin deposition in IgE-dependent gastric reactions in the mouse: the role of mast cells (MCs) [abstr]. FASEB J 1989; 3:A789.

139. Alter SC, Schwartz LB. Tryptase: an indicator of mast cell-mediated allergic reactions. Prov Chall Proc 1989; pp. 167–183.

140. Lemanske RF Jr, Kaliner MA. Late phase allergic reactions. In: E Middleton Jr, Reed CE, Ellis EF, Adkinson NF Jr, Yunginger JW, Busse WW, eds. Allergy: Principles and Practice. 4th ed. St. Louis: CV Mosby, 1993:320–361.

141. Bascom R, Wachs M, Naclerio RM, et al. Basophil influx occurs after nasal antigen challenge: effects of topical corticosteroid pretreatment. J Allergy Clin Immunol 1988; 81:580–589.

142. Liu MC, Hubbard WC, Proud D, et al. Immediate and late inflammatory responses to ragweed antigen challenge of the peripheral airways in allergic asthmatics: cellular, mediator, and permeability changes. Am Rev Respir Dis 1991; 144:51–58.
143. Guo C-B, Liu MC, Galli SJ, et al. Identification of IgE bearing cells in the late phase response to antigen in the lung as basophils. Am J Respir Cell Mol Biol. In press.
144. Lett-Brown MA, Boetcher DA, Leonard EJ. Chemotactic responses of normal human basophil to C5a and to lymphocyte-derived chemotactic factor. J Immunol 1976; 117:246–252.
145. Ward PA, Dvorak HF, Cohen S, et al. Chemotaxis of basophils by lymphocyte-dependent and lymphocyte-independent mechanisms. J Immunol 1975; 4:1523–1531.
146. Bochner BS, Peachell PT, Brown KE, Schleimer RP. Adherence of human basophils to cultured umbilical vein vascular endothelial cells. J Clin Invest 1988; 81:1355–1363.
147. Broide DH, Gleich GJ, Cuomo AJ, et al. Evidence of ongoing mast cell and eosinophil degranulation in symptomatic asthma airway. J Allergy Clin Immunol 1991; 88:637–648.
148. Wenzel SE, Fowler AA III, Schwartz LB. Activation of pulmonary mast cells by bronchoalveolar allergen challenge. In vivo release of histamine and tryptase in atopic subjects with and without asthma. Am Rev Respir Dis 1988; 137:1002–1008.
149. Ferguson AC, Whitelaw M, Brown H. Correlation of bronchial eosinophil and mast cell activation with bronchial hyperresponsiveness in children with asthma. J Allergy Clin Immunol 1992; 90:609–613.
150. Bradley BL, Azzawi M, Jacobson M, et al. Eosinophils, T-lymphocytes, mast cells, neutrophils, and macrophages in bronchial biopsy specimens from atopic subjects with asthma: comparison with biopsy specimens from atopic subjects without asthma and normal control subjects and relationship to bronchial hyperresponsiveness. J Allergy Clin Immunol 1991; 88:661–674.
151. Kay AB. "Helper" (CD4+) T cells and eosinophils in allergy and asthma. Am Rev Respir Dis 1992; 145:S22–S26.
152. Romagnani S. Human TH$_1$ and TH$_2$ subsets: doubt no more. Immunol Today 1991; 12: 256–257.
153. Jarrett EEE, Miller HRP. Production and activities of IgE in helminth infections. Prog Allergy 1982; 31:178–233.
154. Askenase PW. Immunopathology of parasitic diseases: involvement of basophils and mast cells. Springer Semin Immunopathol 1980; 2:417–442.
155. Reed ND. In: Galli SJ, Austen KF, eds. Mast Cell and Basophil Differentiation and Function in Health and Disease. New York: Raven Press, 1989:205–215.
156. Jacobson RH, Reed ND, Manning DD. Expulsion of Nippostrongylus brasiliensis from mice lacking antibody production potential. Immunology 1977; 32:867–874.
157. Watanabe N, Katakura K, Kobayashi A, et al. Protective immunity and eosinophilia in IgE-deficient SJA/9 mice infected with Nippostrongylus brasiliensis and Trichinella spiralis. Proc Natl Acad Sci USA 1988; 85:4460–4462.
158. Steeves EB, Allen JR. Basophils in skin reactions of mast cell-deficient mice infested with Dermacentor variabilis. Int J Parasitol 1990; 20:655–667.
159. Brown SJ, Galli SJ, Gleich GJ, et al. Ablation of immunity to Amblyomma americanum by anti-basophil serum: cooperation between basophils and eosinophils in expression of immunity to ectoparasites (ticks) in guinea pigs. J Immunol 1982; 129:790–796.
160. Juhlin L, Michaelsson G. A new syndrome characterized by absence of eosinophils and basophils. Lancet 1977; 1:1233–1235.
161. Okada Y. The mast cell in synovial membrane of patients with joint disease. Jpn J Orthop Surg 1973; 47:657–662.
162. Godfrey HP, Ilardi C, Engber W, et al. Quantitation of human synovial mast cells in rheumatoid arthritis and other rheumatic diseases. Arthritis Rheum 1984; 27:852–856.
163. Woolley DE, Bartholomew JS, Taylor DJ, Evanson JM. Mast cells and rheumatoid arthritis. In: Galli SJ, Austen KF, eds. Mast Cell and Basophil Differentiation and Function in Health and Disease. New York: Raven Press, 1989:183–193.

164. Freemont AJ, Denton J. Disease distribution of synovial fluid mast cells and cytophagocytic mononuclear cells in inflammatory arthritis. Ann Rheum Dis 1985; 44:312–315.
165. Malone DG, Irani A-M, Schwartz LB, et al. Mast cell numbers and histamine levels in synovial fluids from patients with diverse arthritides. Arthritis Rheum 1986; 29:956–963.
166. Malone DG, Metcalfe DD. Demonstration and characterization of transient arthritis in rats following sensitization of synovial mast cells with antigen-specific IgE and parenteral challenge with specific antigen. Arthritis Rheum 1988; 31:1063–1067.
167. Stead RH, Perdue MH, Blennerhassett MG, et al. The innervation of mast cells. In: Freir S, ed. The Neuroendocrine–Immune Network. Boca Raton FL: CRC Press, 1990. In press.
168. Arizono N, Matsuda S, Hattori T, et al. Anatomical variation in mast cell nerve associations in the rat small intestine, heart, lung, and skin. Similarities of distances between neural processes and mast cells, eosinophils, or plasma cells in the jejunal lamina propria. Lab Invest 1990; 62:626–634.
169. Stead RH, Dixon MF, Bramwell NH, et al. Mast cells are closely opposed to nerves in the human gastrointestinal mucosa. Gastroenterology 1989; 97:575–585.
170. Kiernan JA. Study of chemically induced acute inflammation in the skin of the rat. Q J Exp Physiol 1977; 62:151–156.
171. Woodbury RG, Le Trong H, Cole K, et al. Rat mast cell proteases. In: Galli SJ, Austen KF, eds. Mast Cell and Basophil Differentiation and Function in Health and Disease. New York: Raven Press, 1989:71–79.
172. MacQueen G, Marshall J, Perdue M, et al. Pavlovian conditioning of rat mucosal mast cells to secrete rat mast cell protease II. Science 1989; 243:83–85.
173. Foreman JC, Jordan CC. Histamine release and vascular changes induced by neuropeptides. Agents Actions 1983; 13:105–116.
174. Foreman JC. Substance P and calcitonin gene-related peptide: effects on mast cells and in human skin. Int Arch Allergy Appl Immunol 1987; 82:366–371.
175. Le Trong H, Neurath H, Woodbury RG. Substrate specificity of the chymotrypsin-like protease in secretory granules isolated from rat mast cells. Proc Natl Acad Sci USA 1987; 84:364–367.
176. Caughey GH, Leidig F, Viro NF, Nadel JA. Substance P and vasoactive intestinal peptide degradation by mast cell tryptase and chymase. J Pharmacol Exp Ther 1988; 244:133–137.
177. Brain SD, Williams TJ. Substance P regulates the vasodilator activity of calcitonin gene-related peptide. Nature 1988; 335:73–75.
178. Wershil BK, Turck CW, Sreedharan SP, et al. Variants of vasoactive intestinal peptide in mouse mast cells and rat basophilic leukemia cells. Cell Immunol 1993; 151:369–378.
179. Kowalski ML, Kaliner MA. Neurogenic inflammation, vascular permeability, and mast cells. J Immunol 1988; 140:3905–3911.
180. Dvorak AM, Monahan RA, Osage JF, Dickersin GR. Hum Pathol 1980; 11:606.

9

Lymphocytes

E. Maggi and S. Romagnani
Institute of Clinica Medica III, University of Florence, Florence, Italy

INTRODUCTION

The immune system can evoke different mechanisms for attacking pathogens, but not all of these are activated after either infection or immunization. Most studies are devoted to investigating the mechanisms involved in the recognition of a given substance as "foreign," to the sequence of events that follows such recognition and leads to the stimulation of different immune competent cells, and to the different pathways through which the offending agent is eliminated by specific and nonspecific mechanisms. Studies with both animal and human models have shown that immune responses can be broadly subdivided into antibody-mediated (humoral) and cell-mediated (cellular) immunity. Antibodies are effective against soluble toxins and extracellular microorganisms, whereas cell-mediated immunity is more important for the elimination of intracellular agents. Furthermore, it has long been recognized that a reciprocal relationship exists between delayed-type hypersensitivity (DTH)—a typical feature of cell-mediated immunity—and humoral immunity. In spite of its broad practical usefulness, this compartmentalization of the immune response is an obvious oversimplification, and it is now clear that there is a tight interplay between the humoral and cellular arms of the immune system. Antibodies are effective against soluble toxins and extracellular microorganisms, whereas cell-mediated immunity is more important for the elimination of intracellular agents.

Atopy is a genetically determined disorder characterized by an increased ability of B lymphocytes to synthesize IgE antibodies specific for certain groups of ubiquitous antigens that can activate the immune system after inhalation or ingestion, and perhaps after penetration through the skin (allergens).

The increasing incidence and the clinical relevance of allergic diseases of the respiratory tract are well known; hence, the great research effort to solve problems related to the pathogenesis of these syndromes. The interaction between environmental allergens and the immune system is critical to the development of human allergy. This interaction is presumably initiated by uptake and presentation of allergens by MHC class II-positive accessory cells to helper T (T_H) lymphocytes. Activated T_H cells then induce B lymphocytes to produce allergen-specific antibodies, mainly belonging to the IgE class. However, the origin of the preferential IgE antibody production in individuals who are genetically determined to recognize allergen epitopes is still unclear. In the last few years great progress has been achieved toward the knowledge of the cellular and molecular signals responsible for IgE antibody synthesis and for the induction of allergic inflammation. There is a general consensus that T-cell-derived interleukin (IL)-4 and interferon (IFN)-γ are the main regulatory cytokines of IgE production, with opposite effects. Their pathophysiological role in atopy has been clearly established by both in vitro and in vivo studies. Convincing evidence is also accumulating to suggest that T_H lymphocyte subsets producing IL-4 and IL-5, but none or limited amounts of IFN-γ, accumulate in the blood or target organs of patients with helminth infections or atopic disorders. These cells can account for the IgE antibody formation and eosinophilia observed in these patients. The presence of T cells at sites of allergic inflammation and the recruitment of T cells in disease models both suggest that T cells as well as interactions among mediators, cytokines, neuropeptides, and neurotransmitters are involved in triggering the local expression of allergic inflammation (1–5). In this chapter we will first describe the mechanisms involved in allergen presentation to T helper cells, the regulation of human IgE synthesis, as well as the alterations responsible for their deregulation in allergic disorders. Then we will analyze the functional characteristics of T_H1 and T_H2 response and how allergens selectively expand T cells with a T_H2 profile. The cytokine profile of T cells infiltrating the target organs of allergic inflammation and the modulatory signals able to inhibit the T_H2 response in allergic patients will finally be examined.

ALLERGEN PRESENTATION TO T HELPER CELLS

Allergens, as are many other antigens, are processed by dendritic cells of the skin and of the respiratory and gastrointestinal mucosa. For simplicity we will analyze the events that probably occur in the respiratory tract. Once allergens are inhaled, the first step of their interaction with the immune system is the uptake of soluble allergen components by the major histocompatibility complex (MHC) class II-positive antigen-presenting cells (APC), followed by their presentation to allergen-specific T_H cells. Indeed, in contrast with the B-cell antigen receptor that directly recognizes unprocessed native antigens, the T-cell receptor (TCR) recognizes only small amino acids stretches (epitopes) on linear peptide fragments of protein antigens (6). Peptides have to be presented into a cleft formed by one of the various molecules encoded by the MHC. The TCR simultaneously recognizes the specific antigen epitope and a constant domain of a particular MHC molecule expressed on the surface of autologous APC (6). The molecular basis of allergen recognition has been extensively investigated in the last few years (7,8). The precise nature of APC involved in allergen recognition, processing, and presentation is still unknown. Several cell types have been positively identified as expressing MHC class II antigens in healthy or diseased lungs: B cells, activated T cells, fibroblasts, dendritic cells (DCs), and macrophages (9). Low molecular weight, soluble antigens, such as those derived from pollen degradation, may be expected to be readily translocated to intraepithelial or submucosal microenvironments by intracellular (pinocytic) or intercellular pathways and, thereby, gain access to all the potential APC populations listed in the foregoing. However, the relevant APC require at least two additional properties to act as efficient APC and to induce a primary immune response in a naive host. The first is the capacity to migrate selectively to T-cell areas in draining lymph nodes; the second is the ability to provide T_H cells with both the signal represented by the interaction between the peptide complexed with surface MHC class II and the TCR, and a simultaneous "costimulatory" signal. Recent data strongly suggest that cells possessing the B7/BB1 molecule, which interacts with the CD28 molecule, can efficiently costimulate T_H cells. From these statements, DCs appear to be more suitable for allergen presentation to T_H cells than other APC present in human parenchymal tissue. The DCs have indeed been estimated to constitute up to 25% of the overall MHC class II-positive cell population resident in the normal lung parenchyma, but they comprise the only MHC class II-positive resident cell population within the normal airway epithelium (9).

The DCs that are present in nonlymphoid tissue possess phagocytic activity and FcγRII, are capable of processing exogenous antigens, and are actively synthesize MHC class II molecules. However, similar to Langerhans cells present in the skin, they do not constitutively express the B7/BB1 costimulatory molecule. This type of DCs have been designed as *immature* DCs to discriminate them from DCs present in draining lymphoid tissues, designed as *mature* DCs. These latter also express surface MHC class II antigens, but lack phagocytic activity and FcγRII, as well as the ability to process antigens and to continuously synthesize MHC class II molecules. However, they exhibit the expression of the B7/BB1 costimulatory molecule on their surface. Thus, it is reasonable to speculate that, in the primary response to aeroallergens, the immature DCs present in normal airway epithelium are the professional APC that encounter and process grass pollen allergens. They then probably migrate through afferent lymphatic vessels to draining lymph nodes, where they acquire the mature phenotype. Mature DCs are able to present the processed peptide to the specific T_H cells and to provide the costimulatory signal by B7/BB1–CD28 interaction. This results in grass-specific T_H-cell activation and proliferation.

The result of antigen–MHC binding to T cells (plus the accessory molecule signals) elicits several intracellular events, including membrane phospholipid breakdown, elevated protein kinase C (PKC) activity, a rise in cytoplasmic calcium, and phosphorylation of several proteins. These messengers stimulate the activation of a second wave of nuclear factors acting on promoter elements for the transcription of those genes required for the proliferative and effector responses of T cells.

The ability of peripheral blood mononuclear cells (PBMC) to proliferate in response to aeroallergens or their extract components was first demonstrated 25 years ago by Girard et al. (10) and then confirmed in subsequent years by a number of investigators. In 1973, we examined the proliferative response of PBMC from three groups of subjects (untreated grass-sensitive; grass-sensitive treated with specific immunotherapy; and nonatopic) to an aqueous extract of *Holcus lanatus* (11). The PBMC from the great majority of atopic patients exhibited strong proliferative responses to an aqueous *H. lanatus* (HL) extract, and the response was significantly higher in the atopic than in the nonatopic group. Interestingly, the proliferative response to HL was also significantly higher in untreated grass-sensitive patients in comparison with those who had been treated with specific immunotherapy. On the basis of these data, we suggested that this proliferative response was mainly due to HL-specific circulating T lymphocytes present in higher concentrations in atopic than in nonatopic persons. Furthermore, a still unknown tolerogenic mechanism was suspected to be responsible for the reduced proliferative response of T cells from both nonatopic subjects and grass-sensitive patients treated with specific immunotherapy. Controversial results have been reported on this topic. Great progress in the knowledge of T-cell responses to allergens was made 10 years later, when in collaboration with Lanzavecchia, we established the first T-cell lines and T-cell clones specific for purified grass pollen allergen (*Lolium perenne* group I or Lol p I). These lines and clones were antigen-specific (i.e., responded to the allergen used to raise them and not to other antigens) and were MHC-restricted (12). Surface marker analysis revealed that Lol p I-specific lines comprised mainly cells with a CD4[+] phenotype, although a few CD8[+] cells could also be present. The introduction of T-cell cloning technology also proved to be crucial for the understanding of mechanisms that regulate the allergen-induced IgE antibody synthesis.

To better understand the molecular basis of T-cell responses to grass pollen allergens, the nature of epitopes recognized by different grass pollen-specific T-cell clones is now being analyzed. T-cell clones against purified Lol p I were generated from the PBMC of ryegrass-allergic individuals and, subsequently, screened for their reactivity against other ryegrass allergens, such as Lol p II and Lol p III, as well as a set of other grass species. Moreover, T-cell clones specific for Lol p I or Poa p IX were also screened for their reactivity against a set of overlapping peptides, the sequence of which was derived from the cDNA clones and covered the entire Lol p I or Poa p IX molecule.

Most of the 24 Lol p I-specific T-cell clones derived from four different donors responded to only Lol p I, but the others (37%) were stimulated, in addition, by either Lol p III, Lol p II, or both. In some of the later clones the response to Lol p III was relatively higher than that to Lol p II (13). Together, these results demonstrate the cross-reactivity among the Lol p proteins at the level of T-cell recognition, although, in general, the cross-reactivity to Lol p II was relatively less pronounced. Interestingly, seven of the nine Lol p I-specific clones reactive to Lol p II and Lol p III also exhibited cross-recognition of the recombinant Poa p IX allergen rKBG.2 (14). One of these cross-reactive clones was also examined for its proliferative response to eight different pollen extracts, and it was found to be reactive to Kentucky blue, Orchard, Redtop, and Smooth brome grasses (14). These results are taken to indicate that major allergens of different grass pollens share cross-reacting T-cell epitopes.

The observed cross-reactivity can be explained on the structural analysis of the three Lol p proteins that reveal several homologous segments among them. A recent report identifies one such segment in Lol p I (residues 191–210) as the immunodominant peptide for T-cell response (15). However, our data rather favor the view that different peptides, present all along the Lol p I molecule, are able to stimulate specific T cells. Therefore, it is possible that although some of these peptides will induce unique T-cell response, others will induce T cells that might cross-react with the other Lol p, as well as the other grass species, proteins.

In the mouse, inhalation of the allergen ovalbumin (OVA) has induced an IgE anti-OVA response associated with the selective expansion of Vβ8.1/8.2 T cells in local draining lymph nodes, leading to immediate cutaneous hypersensitivity and airways responsiveness. Since OVA-reactive Vβ2 T cells inhibited these effects, it has been suggested that T cells bearing different Vβ elements are differentially involved in the in vitro and in vivo regulation of IgE response.

Recently, it has been shown that those T-cell clones recognizing specific epitopes on Der p I molecule share any TCR Vα and Vβ gene products. However, in our laboratory, we found that the Vα genes of nine out of ten individual clones specific for cross-reactive T-cell epitopes of grass pollens (belonging to group I, II, III, and IX), utilize Vα 13, but different Jα genes. These studies indicate that the common Vα gene usage may explain the cross-reactive proliferation of T-cell clones.

CELLS AND FACTORS INVOLVED IN THE INDUCTION
AND REGULATION OF HUMAN IgE SYNTHESIS

In the last decade, a pathway of IgE regulation, essentially based on the reciprocal activity of interleukin-4 (IL-4) and interferon gamma (IFN-γ), has been discovered in mice (2). More recent studies, including those performed in our laboratory, have provided substantial information on the mechanisms that regulate IgE synthesis in humans.

At the beginning of 1980, several attempts to induce IgE production in vitro by stimulating PBMC with polyclonal activators, antigens, T-cell supernatants, or cytokines were performed, but all proved to be unsuccessful, because under these experimental conditions, only spontaneously synthesized IgE could be detected (16). The unambiguous demonstration that IgE production could be induced by signals delivered in vitro was provided by coculturing B cells with selected alloreactive, autoreactive, or phytohemagglutinin (PHA)-induced T-cell clones (16). By assaying the activity of large numbers of PHA-induced T-cell clones (TCCs) derived from different lymphoid organs, we then showed that human IgE synthesis was strictly regulated by the production of certain cytokines. The first demonstration that T_H-cell subsets, producing IL-4 or IFN-γ, play a reciprocal role in the regulation of human IgE synthesis was provided when a significant positive correlation was found between helper function for IgE and production of IL-4 by a wide series of mitogen-induced T-cell clones (16). In contrast, a significant inverse correlation was found between the IgE helper activity of TCCs (or their supernatants) and their ability to secrete IFN-γ (16). These findings were confirmed by the observations that human recombinant IL-4 can induce IgE synthesis in unfractionated mononuclear cells, and that this effect is inhibited by addition of human recombinant IFN-γ. The opposite regulatory role of IL-4 and IFN-γ in the synthesis of human IgE was confirmed by the observations that recombinant IL-4, as well as IL-13, can induce the synthesis of IgE in peripheral blood mononuclear cells, and this effect is inhibited by addition of recombinant IFN-γ, IFN-α, IL-12, or prostaglandin E_2 (PGE2) (17,18).

Even though necessary, IL-4 alone was not sufficient for the induction of human IgE synthesis, as shown by the use of highly purified B cells (16). In such experiments, however, IL-4-dependent IgE synthesis was restored by the readdition of appropriate concentrations of autologous or allogeneic T cells. Direct evidence that physical interaction between T and B cells is required for IL-4-dependent IgE synthesis was provided by assaying IgE production in a double-chamber system in which T and B cells were separated by a microporous membrane. In this system, IgE production occurred only when T and B cells were cultured in the same chamber (17). This and several other data confirmed our first observations that IgE synthesis is dependent on two main signals delivered by CD4$^+$ T cells to B cells: the first signal is due to soluble T-cell factors, such as IL-4 and IL-13, acting on the same receptor and inducing a sterile ε-germ line transcript on B cells. The second signal (leading to a productive ε-transcript) is mediated by T–B cell-to-cell, MHC class II-unrestricted, physical contact, mainly owing to the interaction of CD40L (on activated T cells) and CD40 molecules (on B cells) (18). Very recently, it has been described that mast cells or basophils, through CD40L molecule on their surface and IL-4 production, can also directly support the two signals for IgE synthesis by B cells (19). However, other molecule(s) are certainly involved in such noncognate activation signal; membrane tumor necrosis factor (TNF)-α (on T cells)–TNF-α receptor (on B cells) interaction, Epstein–Barr virus (EBV) infection of B cells, and corticosteroids can mimic the in vitro effect of CD40L–CD40 signal (20,21). All these findings strongly suggest that T_H cells, mainly those with a particular cytokine profile, play a role in mechanisms of induction and regulation of human IgE synthesis and, more importantly, also in the pathogenesis of allergic disorders.

FUNCTIONS OF HUMAN T_H1 AND T_H2 CELLS

Very recently, it has become clear that T-helper (T_H) lymphocytes, which are required for both cell-mediated and humoral immune responses, are composed of distinct subsets, distinguished by different patterns of cytokine production. In the mouse, CD4$^+$ T cells can be subdivided into at least two main groups, called T_H1 and T_H2, differing in their cytokine profile. The initial observation by Mossman et al. (22) that repeated stimulation of murine CD4$^+$ T_H lymphocytes in vitro with given antigens results in the development of a restricted and stereotyped pattern of cytokine production that frequently falls into T_H1 or T_H2 phenotype has been widely confirmed in both murine and human systems (23).

Because no highly specific surface marker is yet available to phenotypically identify the different CD4$^+$ T-cell subsets, both murine and human T_H1 and T_H2 cells are currently recognized on the basis of their cytokine secretion profile and effector functions. In murine systems T_H1 cells produce IL-2, IFN-γ, and lymphotoxin (TNF-β) and promote macrophage activation that results in delayed-type hypersensitivity (DTH), antibody-dependent cell cytotoxicity, and production of opsonizing antibodies, particularly of the IgG2a class, required for clearance of infection caused by intracellular organisms. The T_H2 cells secrete IL-4, IL-5, IL-6, IL-10, and IL-13, provide optimal help for production of antibodies, mainly of IgE and IgG1 isotypes, and mucosal immunity, through production of growth and differentiation factors for mast cells and eosinophils and for facilitation to IgA synthesis (22).

Human T_H1 and T_H2 cells were first evidenced by establishing CD4$^+$ T-cell clones specific for peculiar antigens. Most T cell clones, derived from normal donors and specific for purified protein derivative (PPD) of *Mycobacterium tuberculosis*, secreted IL-2 and IFN-γ, but not IL-4 and IL-5, following stimulation with either specific antigen or phorbol myristate acetate plus anti-CD3 monoclonal antibody, whereas under the same experimental conditions, most T-cell clones specific for the *Toxocara canis* excretory–secretory antigen (TES), derived from the same healthy donors, secreted IL-4 and IL-5, but not IL-2 or IFN-γ (24). The cytokines IL-6, IL-10, and IL-13 tend to segregate less clearly among human CD4$^+$ subsets than in the mouse (24). In the absence of clear polarizing conditions leading to stereotyped T_H1 or T_H2 patterns, human CD4$^+$ T-cell subsets, with a less differentiated lymphokine profile than those producing both T_H1- and T_H2-type cytokines, designed T_H0, usually arise, which are responsible for intermediate effects, depending on the ratio of cytokines produced and the nature of responding cells (25).

Human T_H1 and T_H2 clones differ not only in their profiles of cytokine secretion, but also in their responsiveness to cytokines. Interleukin-4 potentiated the antigen-induced proliferation and cytokine production of T_H2, but not that of T_H1, clones. In contrast, IFN-γ selectively inhibited the proliferative response and cytokine production by T_H2 clones. Unlike in the murine system, IL-10 significantly inhibited the proliferation and the cytokine production of both T_H1 and T_H2 human T-cell clones in response to either the specific antigen or PHA (26). Finally, human T_H1 and T_H2 clones also differ in their cytolytic potential and mode of providing help for B-cell antibody synthesis. T_H2 clones, which usually lack cytolytic potential, induce IgM, IgG, IgA, and IgE synthesis by autologous B cells in the presence of the specific antigen, with an immunoglobulin response that is proportional to the number of T_H2 cells added to B cells (27). In contrast, T_H1 clones (which are usually cytolytic) provide B-cell help for IgM, IgG, IgA (but not IgE) synthesis at low T-cell/B-cell ratios. At T-cell/B-cell ratios higher than 1:1, a decline in B-cell help could be observed, that was related to T_H1 lytic activity against autologous antigen-presenting B cells (27). This may represent a mechanism for the down-regulation of antibody responses in vivo as well. The failure of T_H2 cells to express antigen-dependent cytolytic activity against autologous APC may at least partly, account for the long-term ongoing IgE antibody responses seen in patients with atopy or helminthic infections.

HIGH INCIDENCE OF T_H2-LIKE CELL SUBSET IN PATIENTS WITH DEREGULATED IgE PRODUCTION

To evaluate the alterations of IgE-regulatory mechanisms that were involved in the genesis of human diseases characterized by hyperproduction of IgE, we first examined the ability to produce cytokines of mitogen-induced TCC from the PB of four patients with hyper-IgE (Buckley's) syndrome. Such patients had significantly lower proportions of circulating T_H1 cells, but not of T_H2 cells, than found in controls (28). The major immunological hallmarks of helminthic infections are eosinophilia, elevated serum IgE levels, and, occasionally, mastocytosis, which are stimulated by T_H2-derived cytokines. Earlier studies have implicated eosinophils and IgE as major effector elements in the protective immunity against several different helminths. A reevaluation of the question has recently led to a more complicated view on the role of these T_H2-dependent responses in helminthic immunity. Human T-cell clones, specific for excretory–secretory antigen of *Toxocara canis*, with a T_H2 profile were derived from the PB of healthy subjects (24). Likewise, patients affected by toxocariasis, filariasis, strongyloidiasis, or onchocerciasis showed in their PB an increased prevalence of IL-4- and IL-5-producing cells and increased production of IL-4 or IL-5 in response to mitogen stimulation (29). However, the increased proportion of T_H2 cells in the PB of patients with toxocariasis normalized after appropriate treatment (29). Interestingly, the ability of PB lymphocytes to produce IFN-γ was reduced in patients with toxocariasis or schistosomiasis, suggesting a worm-induced down-regulation of T_H1-type reactions (30).

Given the aforementioned findings, as well as the knowledge that IL-5 (another T-cell-derived cytokine) acts as a selective differentiation factor for eosinophils, it was reasonable to suggest that both atopic patients and patients with helminthisis may harbor T_H cells resembling the T_H2 murine subset in their ability to produce IL-4 and IL-5, but not IFN-γ. To test this possibility, we first investigated the profile of cytokine production of PHA-induced TCC established from the PB of patients with helminthiasis or severe atopic diseases. Significantly higher proportions of IL-4 producing and significantly lower proportions of IFN-γ-producing TCC were recovered from the PB of both groups of patients, in comparison with healthy controls (31). Furthermore, PHA-induced TCC derived from the conjunctival infiltrates of three patients with vernal conjunctivitis (VC) were examined. The great majority of TCC obtained from VC infiltrates were CD4 T cells that were inducible to the production of high concentrations of IL-4 and able to provide helper function for IgE synthesis by B cells. In contrast, even after maximal stimulation, such as that delivered by PMA plus anti-CD3 antibody, only a few TCC expressed IFN-γ mRNA could produce IFN-γ (32). By using a different experimental approach, strong IL-5, but poor IL-2 and no IFN-γ, message has recently been found in T cells present in bronchial biopsies of patients with allergic asthma (33).

Taken together, these data suggest that, in patients with helminth infections or atopy, both production of IgE and eosinophilia probably result from the expansion of T_H2-like cells that preferentially accumulate in target organs.

ALLERGENS SELECTIVELY EXPAND T CELLS SHOWING T_H2 CELLS

An attractive hypothesis to explain the increased production of allergen-specific IgE is that it may result from modified regulation of cytokines derived from T cells. This view is supported by the analysis of cytokine production by allergen-specific T cells. In contrast to T-cell clones specific for bacterial antigens derived from PB of atopic donors who showed a prevalent T_H0/T_H1 phenotype, the great majority of allergen-specific $CD4^+$ T-cell clones derived from the same donors expressed a T_H2/T_H0 phenotype, with high production of IL-4, and no (or low) production of IFN-γ (34). Why allergens preferentially expand T_H2-like $CD4^+$ T cells is still unclear; one possibility is their peculiar physicochemical structure. Some determinants are coexpressed by major allergens and parasitic antigens: helminths, that usually induce T_H2 responses, release proteolytic enzymes, and some allergens are also proteases. However, the allergen structure per se does not explain the induction of T_H2-like responses. Allergen-specific T-cell clones derived from nonatopic donors preferentially express a T_H1/T_H0 profile (34). On the other hand, $CD4^+$ T cells from atopic subjects are able to produce IL-4 and IL-5, even in response to bacterial antigens, such as PPD or streptokinase, that usually evoke responses with a restricted T_H1 profile in nonatopic individuals (35). Furthermore, allergen-specific T-cell clones, derived from polysensitized patients with severe atopy, produced very high amounts of IL-4 that were highly related to the amounts of IL-5, IL-3, and granulocyte–macrophage colony-stimulating factor (GM-CSF), suggesting that a deregulation of these cytokines' gene expression, clustered on chromosome 5, can be responsible for the atopic phenotype (36). Indeed, a sequence homology has been described between promoter elements of IL-4 and IL-5 genes. Finally, cord blood T lymphocytes consistently proliferate in response to Der p I, suggesting the possibility of an in utero sensitization to this allergen (37). Interestingly, $CD4^+$ T-cell clones derived from cord blood showed a different cytokine profile, depending of the atopic status of newborns' parents. The Der p I-specific T-cell clones derived from cord blood of newborns with nonatopic parents showed a prevalent T_H1 profile, whereas when both parents were atopic newborn $CD4^+$ T-cell clones exhibited a T_H0 or T_H2 profile (Piccinni MP, unpublished data).

Taken together, these data suggest that, in addition to the structure of allergens and the type of allergen-presenting cells, the genetic overexpression of some cytokine genes favor the preferential T_H2 response in atopic individuals. Further studies are required to clarify whether a deregulation leading to overexpression of the IL-4 (and other cytokine) gene is present at the level of intracellular signaling pathways, transcription factors, promoter elements, or some combination thereof.

T_H2-LIKE CELLS ACCUMULATE IN TARGET ORGANS OF ALLERGIC INFLAMMATION

Most T-cell clones derived from the conjunctival infiltrates of patients with vernal conjunctivitis express the T_H2 cytokine profile (32). With an in situ hybridization technique,

T cells showing mRNA for T_H2-type, but not the T_H1, cytokines were found at the site of late-phase reactions in skin biopsies from atopic patients (33), in mucosal bronchial biopsies or bronchoalveolar lavage from asthmatics (38,39) and, after local allergen challenge, in nasal mucosa of allergen-induced rhinitis. Likewise, increased levels of IL-4 and IL-5 were measured in the bronchoalveolar lavage fluid of allergic asthmatics, whereas in nonatopic asthmatics, IL-2 and IL-5 were predominant (39). More recently, to assess whether the T-cell response to inhaled allergens induced activation and recruitment of allergen-specific T_H2 cells in the airway mucosa of patients with respiratory allergy, biopsy specimens were obtained from the bronchial mucosa of patients with grass pollen-induced asthma 48 h after positive provocation test with the relevant allergen. About one-third of $CD4^+$ clones derived from stimulated mucosae of grass-allergic patients were specific for grass allergens, and most of them exhibited a definite T_H2 profile; furthermore, they induced IgE production by autologous B cells in the presence of the specific allergen (40). Taken together, these data suggest that allergen-specific T_H2 cells, through their ability to produce the IL-4 and IL-5 involved in IgE production and eosinophil response, respectively, may play an important role in the pathophysiology of allergic respiratory disorders. In contrast, the role of $CD4^+$ T cells and T-cell-derived cytokines in the pathogenesis of atopic dermatitis (AD) is still controversial. More than 80% of patients with AD have been described as exhibiting elevated levels of serum IgE, with specificity to several allergens. High proportions of T_H2-like $CD4^+$ T-cell clones specific for *Dermatophagoides pteronyssinus* (Dp) allergen(s) were obtained from the skin lesions of patients with AD, indicating accumulation or expansion of such T cells in the affected organ (41). Furthermore, Dp-specific T_H2-like clones were also derived from biopsy specimens of intact skin taken after contact challenge with Dp, suggesting that percutaneous sensitization to aeroallergens may play a role in the induction of skin lesions in patients with AD (42). However, most T-cell clones derived from the lesional skin of patients with active AD had a T_H0-like phenotype, and few of them were specific for Dp. Most TCC from lesional skin also exhibited IFN-γ production, and several of them appeared to be specific for bacterial antigens, suggesting that bacterial infections may complicate the pattern of T-cell responses in affected skin. Finally, the presence of both Dp-specific and T_H2-like cells in the skin of AD patients did not always correlate with the presence in the serum of Dp-specific IgE antibody or elevated serum IgE levels (Virtanen T, unpublished data). Thus, it is possible to speculate that T_H2-like responses against Dp at skin level may be involved in the initiation of skin lesions, but the relation between aeroallergen sensitization and the onset of full-blown lesions remains unclear.

MODULATORY SIGNALS ABLE TO INHIBIT THE T_H2 RESPONSE

Although in principle T_H1 and T_H2 cells might arise from distinct precursors, experiments with homogeneous populations of cells from T-cell receptor (TCR) transgenic mice, strongly suggest that a single precursor can differentiate into either a T_H1 or T_H2 phenotype (43,44). The recent paper of Reiner and colleagues (45), showing that T cells from mice infected with *Leishmania major* express a restricted TCR repertoire in both progressive infection and protective immunity, regardless of histocompatibility haplotypes, further supports this possibility. According to this model, naive T_H precursor (T_Hp) cells produce mainly IL-2, and progress into early-memory T_H0 effector cells following a first activation by the specific antigen. These cells would then terminally differentiate into T_H1 or T_H2 cells after repeated antigen stimulations (46). However, the mechanisms responsible for the differentiation of naive T_H cells into the T_H1 or T_H2 phenotype have not yet been completely clarified. Investigations have been focused first on the possibility that the type of TH response depends on the nature of the APC or their products. However, the type of APC per se does not critically influence the differentiation of T_H precursors into one or another phenotype. It more clearly appears that the role of cytokines—released by APC or other cell types during antigen exposure—is in determining the development of the specific T_H1 or T_H2 response. The use of naive, ovalbumin-specific TCR transgenic T cells, has shown that heat-killed *Listeria monocytogenes* induced T_H1 development in vitro through macrophage production of IL-12. The activity of IL-12 is probably related to its ability to promote IFN-γ production by natural killer (NK) cells in a T-cell–independent manner (47) and, in turn, IFN-γ favors the development of T_H1 cells. In contrast, early IL-4 production at the time of antigen presentation seems to be critical for the maturation of naive TH cells into T_H2 cells (47).

The signals that regulate the development of human T_H1 and T_H2 clones have been extensively investigated in our laboratory by using peripheral blood lymphocytes cultured with PPD, TES, or allergens, in the presence, or in the absence of exogenous cytokines or anticytokine antibody. The addition of IL-4 in bulk cultures of PB mononuclear cells stimulated with PPD shifted the differentiation of PPD-specific T cells from a T_H1 to a T_H0, or even T_H2, phenotype (48). Moreover, IL-4, added in bulk culture before cloning, inhibited not only the T_H1 differentiation of PPD-specific T cells, but also the development of their cytolytic potential (48). In contrast, early addition of both IFN-γ and anti-IL-4 antibody induced most of allergen- or TES-specific T cells to differentiate into cytolytic T_H0 and T_H1, instead of noncytolytic T_H2, clones (48), suggest that the presence of IL-4 or IFN-γ at the time of antigen stimulation of resting T cells has remarkable regulatory effects on their subsequent in vitro development into T_H1 or T_H2 clones. Even though IL-1 apparently does not play any role in the antigen-induced proliferative response of already established human CD4$^+$ T-cell clones, it is required for the in vitro development of T_H2 clones. Indeed, removal of IL-1 from bulk culture before cloning shifted the differentiation of allergen-specific T cells from the T_H2/T_H0 to the T_H0/T_H1 profile (49). It is not yet clear whether IL-1 exerts its effect by stimulating early IL-4 production which, in turn, induces the T_H2 development, or whether it synergizes the effects of IL-4 in regulating the T_H cell development.

More recently, we have looked at both the cytokine profile of CD8$^+$ human T-cell clones and the mechanisms involved in their development. Although most CD8$^+$ T-cell clones derived from the peripheral blood of normal individuals showed the same cytokine profile as T_H1-type CD4$^+$ T-cell clones, several CD8$^+$ T-cell clones exhibiting a T_H0-, or even a clear-cut T_H2-type, profile could be derived from Kaposi's sarcoma skin lesions and even from unharmed skin of human immunodeficiency virus (HIV)-infected patients (50). This finding may be consistent with recent observations suggesting association of HIV infection with a T_H1 to T_H2 switch (51). However, the most interesting observation was that IL-4 addition in bulk culture before cloning favored high proportions of CD8$^+$ T cells to shift (similar to the CD4$^+$ ones) from the T_H1- to the T_H0/T_H2-like phenotype. Interestingly, CD8$^+$ T_H2-like T cell clones also showed significantly lower cytolytic capacity than CD8$^+$ T_H1-like T-cell clones derived in the absence of IL-4 (Maggi E, unpublished data). Recently, IL-4-producing, noncytolytic, CD8$^+$ T-cell clones have also been derived from the skin lesions of patients with lepromatous leprosy (52) and from the peripheral blood of HIV-infected individuals showing a Job's-like syndrome (53). Thus, the presence of increased IL-4 concentrations at the time of antigen stimulation may be a critical factor in determining a bias of both CD4$^+$ and CD8$^+$ T cells toward the T_H2 pathway and might account for the reduced resistance to infections seen in patients with lepromatous leprosy or acquired immunodeficiency syndrome (AIDS).

On the other hand we have recently shown that IFN-α and IL-12 have regulatory activity opposite that of IL-4 on the in vitro differentiation of human CD4$^+$ T cells by favoring their development into T_H1 clones. The inhibitory activity of IL-12 on the development of allergen-specific CD4$^+$ T cells into T_H2 cells could be partially prevented by removal from bulk cultures before cloning of CD3–CD16$^+$ (NK) cells (54), whereas the inhibitory activity of IFN-α was not prevented by NK cell removal. Since IFN-α and IL-12 are produced primarily by macrophages—cells devoted in the processing and presentation of antigen to T_H cells—it is reasonable to suggest that, given the capacity of viruses and intracellular bacteria to stimulate macrophage production of IL-12 (which induces IFN-γ secretion by both T_H cells and NK cells), T_H cells may be simultaneously presented with processed antigen plus cytokines that induce them to differentiate toward a T_H1 phenotype (54). These findings suggest that endogeneous IL-12 and IFN-α favor the T_H1 development through at least partially different mechanisms.

In human models, only secondary responses to common environmental antigens can be explored. Thus, the question of whether changes induced in vitro by cytokines on the profile of antigen-specific human T-cell clones reflect shifting of a common precursor to one or another phenotype, or merely result from selective suppression of clones with an already established phenotype, remains open. However, even data obtained in the human models are in favor of a critical regulatory role of cytokines produced by cells of the natural immunity system in determining the nature of the subsequent specific immune response (55). Data obtained indicate that the availability of IL-4 and the absence (or low concentrations) of IFN-γ at the time of antigen stimulation are both essential for the development of T_H2 responses. How environmental allergens promote the differentiation of T_H precursors into T_H2 effector cells is less clear. A possible explanation would be that allergens and some parasite antigens fail to induce IFN-α and IL-12 production by macrophages and are poor stimulators of NK cells. Under these conditions, a T_H1-type response would be hampered, and the differentiation of specific T_H2 cells would be made possible, provided that some IL-4 is available. Because T cells seem to be unable to differentiate into IL-4-producing cells in the absence of IL-4 (55), IL-4 production by other cell types may be involved. Evidence has been obtained that a small subset of early thymic emigrants in mouse and non-T, non-B cells from both mouse spleen and human bone marrow—probably belonging to the mast cell–basophil lineage—can synthesize IL-4 (56). Indeed, IL-4 production by murine non-T, non-B cells is extraordinarily increased during *Nippostrongylus brasiliensis* infection or systemic treatment with anti-IgD antibody (57), suggesting that these cells may be involved in cytokine production during helminth infections or other situations associated with increased production of IgE antibodies. Although the role of naive T cells, FcϵRI$^+$ non-T cells (58), or mast cells has been suggested, the nature of the cell that provides the IL-4 that is critical at the time of antigen presentation and recognition in shifting the balance toward the development of T_H2 cells, still remains unclear.

The possibility to convert already established T-cell clones to another cytokine profile was also investigated. Whereas IL-4, IL-5, and IL-10 do not exert any effect, incubation with IL-12 induced mRNA expression for, and production of, detectable amounts of IFN-γ in established T_H2 clones stimulated with insolubilized anti-CD3 antibody. However, this change was transient, for IFN-γ production declined following removal of IL-12 (59). A stable change in the cytokine profile of already-established TCC can be also obtained after growth transformation by herpesvirus saimiri (HVS), an oncogenic virus of New World monkeys (60), able to transform human T cells and thymocytes to continuous growth. When established human T_H1 or T_H2 clones were immortalized with HSV, the cytokine activity of T_H1 clones was retained and enhanced, whereas T_H2 clones were switched to a T_H0 profile (60). These data suggest that a given T_H phenotype can be converted into another phenotype; the relevance of these findings in view of possible therapeutic manipulations of T_H1- or T_H2-mediated disorders is obvious.

CYTOKINE GENE EXPRESSION IN ATOPIC INDIVIDUALS

There is a general consensus that IL-4 has to be considered the only cytokine regulating the T_H2 development in humans. Even though microenvironmental cytokines and factors can influence such a process, no evidence has been reported for an impaired production of these molecules in atopic persons. On the contrary, there is a bulk of evidence from our and other laboratories that suggests that IL-4 synthesis is constitutively increased in these patients. In fact, in atopic individuals, there is an increased ability of T-cell clones to produce IL-4 and IL-5, even in response to antigens other than allergens (35). Moreover, T-cell clones derived from polysensitized patients with severe atopy produce high amounts of not only IL-4, but also of IL-5, IL-3, IL-13, and GM-CSF—proteins coded by genes located within the some cluster (36). In bronchial biopsies from atopic subjects with respiratory symptoms, IL-4 and IL-5 transcripts have been consistently found by in situ hybridization techniques (38). Finally, as discussed earlier, cord blood (CB) T lymphocytes consistently proliferate in response to Der p I, suggesting the possibility of an in utero sensitization to this allergen (37). Even though indirectly, all these data support the concept that in atopics the IL-4 gene and, possibly, clustered (IL-5, IL-13, IL-3, GM-CSF) genes on chromosome 5, are overexpressed. It is possible that the so-called IgE-regulating genes of some years ago, operating independently with HLA markers and determining the overall IgE responsiveness, really may be these clustered cytokine genes. Thus, in the next future the primary issue that remains to be solved is related to the mechanisms able to regulate the T-cell–specific and T_H2-restricted pattern of IL-4 gene expression. Promoter elements and transcriptional factors involved in IL-4 gene regulation have been extensively studied in the last few years. A homology has been found between IL-4 and IL-5 promoter genes. In addition, IL-4 and IL-2 genes are not regulated in a coordinate manner and several promoter elements seem to act together in regulating (positively or negatively) IL-4 gene transcription (61). Sib-pair analysis of several subjects from Amish families revealed a linkage between five markers (IL-4 and IL-13 included) in chromosome 5 and total IgE serum levels (62). Indeed, no current definitive explanations for T_H2-specific IL-4 regulation has been given, and no unambiguous evidence has yet been provided for the subset-specific nature of regulatory elements in human T cells. Also, it cannot be excluded that overexpression of IL-4 and of other cytokine gene transcription is due in some way to an impaired production of factors possessing down-regulatory activity on T_H2 development, such as IL-12, IFN-α, or TGF-β, or their soluble receptors.

CONCLUDING REMARKS

Cellular and molecular signals responsible for the regulation of human IgE synthesis have been achieved in the last few years. It is generally accepted that IL-4 and IFN-γ are the main regulatory cytokines of IgE production, with opposite effects; however, a contact signal, probably from CD40L–CD40 interaction, is needed to induce productive ε-transcripts, leading to IgE synthesis by purified B cells in the presence of IL-4 or IL-13. Convincing evidence is also accumulating to suggest that T_H cells producing IL-4 and IL-5, but not, or only limited amounts of, IFN-γ that resemble murine T_H2 cells accumulate in the blood or target organs of patients with helminthic infections or atopic disorders. In addition these cells are easily recruited and expanded by allergen in the airway mucosa and probably play a crucial role in the induction and maintenance of allergic inflammation. In fact, these cells can account for both IgE antibody formation and eosinophilia seen in these patients.

The mechanisms responsible for the preferential expansion of T_H2 cells in atopic patients and in patients with helminthic infections are currently under investigation. We have shown that virtually all TCC specific for TES and for purified allergens display the T_H2 phenotype of cytokine secretion, whereas the totality of PPD-specific TCC established from the same donors belong to the T_H1 cell subset. This finding suggests that different antigens may influence, in opposite ways, the profile of cytokine secretion of T_H cells. It remains to be established whether the preferential ability of helminth component(s) and allergens to expand T_H2 cells is related to their molecular structure, to the type of APC involved in their processing, to other microenvironmental influences at the site of immunization, or to a combination of these factors.

Why environmental allergens induce IgE antibody responses, but only in few individuals (so-called atopics), represents a still more complex question. At least two genetic traits seem to be implied in the control of IgE antibody responses in atopic subjects. First, the responsiveness to individual allergens is controlled by *Ir* genes linked to the MHC complex. This means that T_H cells able to recognize allergen epitopes can be activated only in persons who possess appropriate individual sequences in the MHC class II products of APC. This might explain why allergen-specific T-cell clones can be easily derived from allergen-sensitive patients, but not from randomly selected nonatopic people. Once recognized, allergens induce the preferential differentiation of T_H cells into the T_H2 phenotype of cytokine secretion, and this may be due to particular features of their structure, to the type of APC involved in their processing, or to other, still unknown, microenvironmental influences.

The role in the genesis of atopy of additional genes not linked to MHC that control the total serum IgE levels reflecting overall IgE responsiveness has also been suggested; the nature of these genes (probably those for cytokines are involved), as well as the mechanisms by which they exert their activity, are still unknown. Although indirectly, several findings on TCC, derived from atopic subjects and from newborns with atopic parents, suggest that a deregulation in the production of IL-4 may be responsible for the increase of overall IgE responses in atopic individuals.

Finally, clear-cut evidence from studies with both animal and human models suggest that IL-4 can strongly influence activated $CD4^+$ and $CD8^+$T cells to differentiate into cells that produce the T_H2 set of cytokines. In contrast, IFN-α and IL-12 (partly by induction of IFN-γ) appear to exert an opposite regulatory effect by favoring the development of T_H1-like cells. This suggests that a balance between IL-4 and IFN-α–IFN-γ–IL-12 at the triad (APC–Antigen–T_H cell) recognition level might play a critical role in determining the cytokine profile of the specific immune response. The better knowledge of factors modulating the T_H2 development provides a means for therapeutical interventions in IgE-mediated disorders through successful transformation of a T_H2-like into a T_H1-like response.

REFERENCES

1. Marsh DG, Freidhof LR, Meyers DA, Roebber M, Norman PS, Kautzky EE, Hsu SH, Bias WB. A genetic marker for human immune response to short ragweed pollen allergen Ra5. II. Response following ragweed immunotherapy. J Exp Med 1983; 155:1452.
2. Coffman RL, Carty JA. T cell activity that enhances polyclonal IgE production and its inhibition by interferon-γ. J Immunol 1986; 136:949.
3. Djukanovic R, Roche WR, Wilson JW, Beasley CRW, Twentyman OP, Howarth PH, Holgate ST. Mucosal inflammation in asthma. Am Rev Respir Dis 1990; 142:434.
4. Galli SJ, Lichtenstein LM. Biology of mast cells and basophils. In: Middleton E, Reed CE, Ellis EF, Adkinson NF, Yunginger JWS, eds. Allergy. Principles and Practice. St Louis: CV Mosby, 1988:106.
5. Romagnani S. Regulation and deregulation of human IgE synthesis. Immunol Today 1990; 1:316.
6. Pene J, Rousset F, Briere F, Chretien I, Bonnefoy J-Y, Spits H, Yokota T, Arai N, Arai K-I, Banchereau J, de Vries J. IgE production by normal human lymphocytes is induced by interleukin 4 and suppressed by interferons γ and α and prostaglandin E_2. Proc Natl Acad Sci USA 1988; 85:6880.
7. Abbas AK, Lichtman AH, Pober JS. Cellular and Molecular Immunology. Philadelphia: WB Saunders, 1991.
8. March DG, Lockart A, Holgate ST. The Genetics of Asthma. Oxford: Blackwell Scientific, 1993.
9. Schon-Hegrad MA, Oliver J, McMenamin PG, Holtr PG. Studies on the density, distribution and surface phenotype of intraepithelial class II MHC antigen (Ia)-bearing dendritic cells (DC) in the conducting airways. J Exp Med 1991; 173:1345.
10. Girard JP, Rose NR, Kunz ML, Kobayashi S, Arbesman C. In vitro lymphocyte transformation in atopic patients induced by antigens. J Allergy 1967; 39:65.
11. Romagnani S, Biliotti G, Passaleva A, Ricci M. In vitro lymphocyte response to pollen extract constituents in grass pollen-sensitive individuals. Int Arch Allergy Appl Immunol 1973; 44:40.
12. Lanzavecchia A, Santini P, Maggi E, Del Prete GF, Falagiani P, Romagnani S, Ferrarini M. In vitro selective expansion of allergen specific T cells from atopic patients. Clin Exp Immunol 1993; 52:21.
13. Baskar S, Parronchi P, Mohapatra S, Romagnani S, Ansari AA. Human T cell responses to purified pollen allergens of the grass, *Lolium perenne*. J Immunol 1992; 148:2378.
14. Mohapatra SS, Mohapatra S, Yang M, Sehon AH, Ansari AA, Parronchi P, Maggi E, Romagnani S. Molecular basis of cross-reactivity among allergen-specific human T cells: T cell receptor Vα gene usage and epitope structure. Immunology 1994; 81:15.
15. Perez M, Ishioka GY, Walker LE, Chestnut RW. cDNA cloning and immunological characterization of the rye grass allergen, Lol p I. J Biol Chem 1990; 264:16210.
16. Del Prete G-F, Maggi E, Parronchi P, Chretien I, Tiri A, Macchia D, Ricci M, Banchereau J, de Vries J, Romagnani S. IL-4 is an essential factor for the IgE synthesis induced in vitro by human T cell clones and their supernatants. J Immunol 1988; 140:4193.
17. Gauchat J-F, Lebman D, Coffman RL, Gascan H, de Vries JE. Structure and expression of germline E transcripts in human B cells induced by interleukin 4 to switch to IgE production. J Exp Med 1990; 172:463.
18. Jabara HH, Fu SM, Geha RS, Vercelli D. CD40 and IgE: synergism between anti-CD40 monoclonal antibody and interleukin 4 in the induction of IgE synthesis by highly purified B cells. J Exp Med 1990; 172:1861.
19. Gauchat J-F, Henchoz S, Mazzel G, Aubry J-P, Brunner T, Blasey H, Life P, Talabot D, Fores-

Romo L, Thompson J, Kishl K, Butterfield J, Dahinden C, Bonnefoy J-Y. Induction of human IgE synthesis in B cells by mast cells and basophils. Nature 1993; 365:340.

20. Macchia D, Almerigogna F, Parronchi P, Ravina A, Maggi E, Romagnani S. Membrane tumor necrosis factor α is involved in the polyclonal B-cell activation induced by HIV-infected human T cells. Nature 1993; 363:464.

21. Thyphronitis G, Tsokos GC, June CH, et al. IgE secretion by Epstein–Barr virus-infected purified B lymphocytes is stimulated by interleukin 4 and suppressed by interferon γ. Proc Natl Acad Sci USA 1989; 86:5580.

22. Mosmann TR, Coffman RL. Heterogeneity of cytokine secretion pattern and functions of helper T cells. Adv Immunol 1989; 46:11.

23. Romagnani S. Human T_H1 and T_H2: doubt no more. Immunol Today 1991; 12:256.

24. Del Prete GF, De Carli M, Mastomauro C, Macchia D, Biagiotti R, Ricci M, Romagnani S. Purified protein derivative of *Mycobacterium tuberculosis* and excretory–secretory antigen(s) of *Toxocara canis* expand in vitro human T cells with stable and opposite (type 1 T helper or type 2 T helper) profile of cytokine production. J Clin Invest 1991; 88:346.

25. Salgame P, Abrams JS, Clayberger C, Goldstein H, Convitt J, Modlin RL, Bloom BR. Differing lymphokine profiles and functional subsets of human CD4 and CD8 T cell clones. Science 1991; 254:279.

26. Del Prete GF, De Carli M, Almerigogna F, Giudizi M-G, Biagiotti R, Romagnani S. Human IL-10 is produced by both type 1 helper (Th1) and type 2 helper (Th2) T cell clones and inhibits their antigen-specific proliferation and cytokine production. J Immunol 1993; 150:1.

27. Del Prete G-F, De Carli M, Ricci M, Romagnani S. Helper activity for immunoglobulin synthesis of T_H1 and T_H2 human T cell clones: the help of T_H1 clones is limited by their cytolytic capacity. J Exp Med 1991; 174:809.

28. Del Prete GF, Tiri A, Maggi E, De Carli M, Macchia D, Parronchi P, Rossi ME, Pietrogrande MC, Ricci M, Romagnani S. Defective in vitro production of γ-interferon and tumor necrosis factor-α circulating T cells from patients with the hyperimmunoglobulin E syndrome. J Clin Invest 1989; 84:1830.

29. De Carli M, Romagnani S, Del Prete GF. Human T-cell response to excretory-secretory antigens of *Toxocara canis*. A model of preferential in vitro and in vivo activation of Th2 cells. In: *Toxocara* and Toxocariasis: Clinical Epidemiological and Molecular Perspectives. Lewis JW, Maizels RM, eds. Birmingham: Birbeck & Sons, 1993:141–148.

30. Ribeiro de Jesus AM, Almeida RP, Bacellar O, Araujo MI, Demeure C, Bina JC, Dessein AJ, Carvalho EM. Correlation between cell-mediated immunity and degree of infection in subjects living in an endemic area of schistosomiasis. Eur J Immunol 1993; 23:152.

31. Romagnani S, Del Prete GF, Maggi E, Parronchi P, Tiri A, Macchia D, Giudizi MG, Almerigogna F, Ricci M. Role of interleukins in induction and regulation of human IgE synthesis. Clin Immunol Immunopathol 1989; 50:S13.

32. Maggi E, Biswas P, Del Prete G-F, Parronchi P, Macchia D, Simonelli C, Emmi L, De Carli M, Tiri A, Ricci M, Romagnani, S. Accumulation of Th2-like helper T cells in the conjunctiva of patients with vernal conjunctivitis. J Immunol 1991; 146:1169.

33. Kay AB, Ying S, Varney V, Gaga M, Durham SR, Moqbel R, Wardlaw AJ, Hamid Q. Messenger RNA expression of the cytokine gene cluster, interleukin (IL)-3, IL-4, IL-5, and granulocyte/macrophage colony-stimulating factor, in allergen-induced late-phase cutaneous reactions in atopic subjects. J Exp Med 1991; 173:775.

34. Parronchi P, Macchia D, Piccinni M-P, Biswas P, Simonelli C, Maggi E, Ricci M, Ansari AA, Romagnani, S. Allergen- and bacterial antigen-specific T-cell clones established from atopic donors show a different profile of cytokine production. Proc Natl Acad Sci USA 1991; 88:4538.

35. Parronchi P, De Carli M, Manetti R, Simonelli C, Piccinni MP, Macchia D, Maggi E, Del Prete GF, Ricci M, Romagnani S. Aberrant interleukin (IL)-4 and IL-5 production in vitro by CD4 helper T cells from atopic subjects. Eur J Immunol 1992; 22:1615.

36. Parronchi P, Manetti R, Simonelli C, Santoni Rugiu F, Piccinni M-P, Maggi E, Romagnani S.

Cytokine production by allergen (Der pl)-specific CD4 T cell clones derived from a patient with severe atopic disease. Int J Clin Lab Res 1991; 21:186.

37. Piccinni M-P, Mecacci F, Sampognaro S, Manetti R, Parronchi P, Maggi E, Romagnani S. Aeroallergen sensitization can occur during fetal life. Int Arch Allergy Immunol 1993; 102:301.

38. Hamid Q, Azzawi M, Ying S, Moqbel R, Wardlaw AJ, Corrigan CJ, Bradley B, Durham SR, Collins JV, Jeffery PK, Quint DJ, Kay AB. Expression of mRNA for interleukin-5 in mucosal bronchial biopsies from asthma. J Clin Invest 1991; 87:1541.

39. Robinson DS, Hamid Q, Ying S, Tsicopoulos A, Barkans J, Bentley AM, Corrigan C, Durham SR, Kay AB. Predominant Th2-like bronchoalveolar T-lymphocyte population in atopic asthma. N Engl J Med 1992; 326:298.

40. Del Prete G-F, De Carli M, Maestrelli P, Ricci M, Fabbri L, Romagnani S. Allergen exposure induces the activation of allergen-specific Th2 cells in the airway mucosa of patients with allergic respiratory disorders. Eur J Immunol 1993; 23:1445.

41. van der Heijden FL, Wierenga EA, Bos JD, Kapsenberg ML. High frequency of IL-4-producing CD4$^+$ allergen-specific T lymphocytes in atopic dermatitis lesional skin. J Invest Dermatol 1991; 97:389.

42. van Reijsen FC, Bruijnzeel-Koomen CAFM, Kalthoff FS, Maggi E, Romagnani S, Westland JKT, Mudde GC. Skin-derived aero-allergen specific T cell clones of T_H2 phenotype in patients with atopic dermatitis. J Allergy Clin Immunol 1992; 2:184.

43. Swain SL. Regulation of the development of distinct subsets of CD4$^+$ T cells. Immunol Res 1991; 142:14.

44. Seder RA, Paul WE, Davis MM, Fazekas de St. Groth BF. The presence of interleukin 4 during in vitro priming determines the lymphokine producing potential of CD4$^+$ T cell from T cell receptor transgenic mice. J Exp Med 1992; 176:1091.

45. Reiner SL, Wang Z-E, Hatam F, Scott P, Locksley RM. Th1 and Th2 cell antigen receptors in experimental leishmaniasis. Science 1993; 259:1457.

46. Coffman RL, Chatelain R, Leal LMCC, Varkila K. *Leishmania major* infection in mice: a model system for the study of CD4$^+$ T-cell subset differentiation. Res Immunol 1991; 142:36.

47. Maggi E, Parronchi P, Manetti R, Simonelli C, Piccinni M-P, Santoni Rugiu F, De Carli M, Ricci M, Romagnani S. Reciprocal regulatory role of IFN-γ and IL-4 on the in vitro development of human T_H1 and T_H2 clones. J Immunol 1992; 148:2142.

48. Parronchi P, De Carli M, Piccinni MP, Macchia D, Maggi E, Del Prete G-F, Romagnani S. IL-4 and IFNs exert opposite regulatory effects on the development of cytolytic potential by T_H1 or T_H2 human T cell clones. J Immunol 1992; 149:2977.

49. Manetti R, Barak V, Piccinni M-P, Sampognaro S, Parronchi P, Maggi E, Dinarello CA, Romagnani S. Interleukin 1 favours the in vitro development of type 2 T helper (Th2) human T cell clones. Res Immunol 1994; 145:93.

50. Maggi E, Mazzetti M, Ravina A, Annunziato F, De Carli M, Piccinni M-P, Manetti R, Carbonari M, Pesce AM, Del Prete GF, Romagnani S. Ability of HIV to promote a Th1 to Th0 shift and to replicate preferentially in Th2 and Th0 cells. Science 1994; 265:244.

51. Clerici M, Hakim FT, Venzon DJ, Blatt S, Hendrix CW, Wynn TA, Shearer GM. Changes in interleukin-2 and interleukin-4 production in asymptomatic, human immunodeficiency virus-seropositive individuals. J Clin Invest 1993; 91:759.

52. Salgame P, Abrams JS, Clayberger C, Goldstein H, Convitt J, Modlin RL, Bloom BR. Differing lymphokine profiles and functional subsets of human CD4$^+$ and CD8$^+$ T cell clones. Science 1991; 254:279.

53. Maggi E, Giudizi MG, Biagiotti R, Annunziato F, Manetti R, Piccinni M-P, Parronchi P, Sampognaro S, Giannarini L, Zuccati G, Romagnani S. Th2-like CD8$^+$ T cells showing B cell helper function and reduced cytolytic activity in human immunodeficiency virus type 1 infection. J Exp Med 1994; 180:89.

54. Manetti R, Parronchi P, Giudizi MG, Piccinni M-P, Maggi E, Trinchieri G, Romagnani S. Natural killer cell stimulatory factor (NKSF/IL-12) induces Th1-type specific immune responses and inhibits the development of IL-4-producing cells. J Exp Med 1993; 177:1199.

55. Romagnani S. Induction of T_H1 and T_H2 response: a key role for the "natural" immune response? Immunol Today 1992; 13:379.

56. Zlotnik A, Godfrey DI, Fischer M, Suda T. Cytokine production by mature and immature CD4-CD8- T cells. αβ-T cell receptor+ CD4-CD8- T cells produce IL-4. J Immunol 1992; 149:1211.

57. Conrad DH, Ben Sasson SZ, LeGros G, Finkelman FD, Paul WE, Infection with *Nippostrongylus brasiliensis* or injection of anti-IgD antibodies markedly enhances Fc-ε receptor-mediated interleukin-4 production by non-B, non-T cells. J Exp Med 1990; 171:1497.

58. Piccinni M-P, Macchia D, Parronchi P, Giudizi M-G, Bani D, Alterini R, Grossi A, Ricci M, Maggi E, Romagnani S. Human bone marrow non-B, non-T cells produce interleukin 4 in response to cross-linkage of Fcε and Fcγ receptors. Proc Natl Acad Sci USA 1991; 88:8656.

59. Manetti R, Gerosa F, Giudizi MG, Biagiotti R, Parronchi P, Piccinni M-P, Sampognaro S, Maggi E, Romagnani S, Trinchieri G. Interleukin 12 induces stable priming for interferon γ (IFN-γ) production during differentiation of human T helper (Th) cells and transient IFN-γ production in established Th2 cell clones. J Exp Med 1994; 179:1273.

60. De Carli M, Berthold S, Fickenscher H, Fleckenstein IM, D'Elios M, Gao O, Biagiotti R, Giudizi MG, Kalden JR, Fleckenstein B, Romagnani S, Del Prete GF. Immortalization with herpesvirus saimiri modulates the cytokine secretion profile of established Th1 and Th2 human T cell clones. J Immunol 1993; 151:5022.

61. Todd MD, Grusby MJ, Lederer JA, Lacy E, Lichtman AH, Glimcher LH. Transcription of the interleukin 4 gene is regulated by multiple promoter elements. J Exp Med 1993; 177:1663.

62. March DG, Neely JD, Breazeale DR, Ghosh B, Friedhoff LR, Ehrlich-Kautzky E, Schou C, Krishnaswamy G, Beaty TH. Linkage analysis of IL-4 and other chromosome 5q31.1 markers and total serum immunoglobulin E concentrations. Science 1994; 264:1152.

10

Eosinophils

Julie B. Sedgwick and William W. Busse
University of Wisconsin, Madison, Wisconsin

INTRODUCTION

The complete role of eosinophils in asthma has not yet been defined, but the presence of an eosinophilic infiltration of the airways has led to the presumption that these cells are an essential and fundamental component of asthma (1). In allergic asthma, antigen provocation results in an immediate response of bronchoconstriction caused by release of mast cell-derived mediators. Several hours later this is followed by a late reaction that is characterized by renewed bronchial obstruction; enhanced airway hyperresponsiveness; and eosinophil influx, activation, and mediator release (2–4). Many researchers now believe that airway inflammation is required for the hyperresponsiveness observed in asthma, and that eosinophil infiltration of the airways is an important factor of the process (5). Since eosinophils appear to be crucial to the pathophysiology of asthma, a more complete understanding of the mechanisms of eosinophilic recruitment and function is important. The processes involved in the accumulation, priming, and activation of eosinophils in the airways are yet to be fully determined. However, it is the selectivity of eosinophilic recruitment to the airways that makes for both an intriguing area of research and, possibly, a unique insight into mechanisms by which the disease course can be altered.

Pharmacological manipulation of the eosinophils' participation in asthma development and progression not only provides a means for therapeutic modulation of the disease, but is also an important method to define mechanisms of eosinophilic participation in this process. By establishing the effects of specific drugs, with defined pathways of action, the processes in eosinophilic participation may be clarified. However, in vitro modulation of eosinophils' function with various drugs must be cautiously interpreted. In vivo treatment with the same drug may have profoundly different or additional effects on noneosinophil factors that directly affect the disease process (i.e., vascular permeability or smooth-muscle contraction), as well as indirect effects on subsequent eosinophilic function and recruitment (i.e., activation of T-lymphocyte cytokine production).

This chapter will review mechanisms by which eosinophils participate in allergic inflammation and the present knowledge of pharmacological manipulation to modify this participation.

EOSINOPHIL MEDIATORS

Although the eosinophil appears to be a quiescent cell when it is present in the circulation of healthy subjects, it can be stimulated in vitro and in vivo by a wide variety of agonists (see section on eosinophil agonists) to release a multitude of potent inflammatory mediators. These mediators provide eosinophils with potential mechanisms to injure many types of cells through degranulation, the respiratory burst, arachidonic acid metabolism, and cytokine generation (Table 1). All of these inflammatory mediators have been implicated in airway damage and may even contribute to airway hyperresponsiveness. The major mediators released by eosinophils following activation are briefly discussed in the following.

Granule Proteins

Eosinophils are characterized by a specific granule that comprises four highly basic proteins (3,6). The distinctive crystalline core is composed of major basic protein (MBP), whereas the noncore matrix includes eosinophil peroxidase (EPO), eosinophil cationic protein (ECP), and eosinophil-derived neurotoxin (EDN). For the most part, these basic proteins are confined to eosinophil granules and can be released immediately on cell stimulation by a variety of agonists (see following). Degranulation of eosinophil granule proteins at the sites of airway inflammation can result in tissue damage by various

Table 1 Eosinophil Mediators of Inflammation

Granule proteins	Major basic protein
	Eosinophil peroxidase
	Eosinophil cationic protein
	Eosinophil derived neurotoxin
Oxygen metabolites of the respiratory burst	O_2^-
	H_2O_2
	$^1O_2$
	$\cdot OH$
	BrO^-, ClO^-
Arachidonic acid metabolites	Platelet-activating factor
	Leukotriene C_4
Cytokines	Interleukins (see Table 2)
	GM-CSF
	TGF-α, TGF-β
Adhesion proteins	VLA-4, VLA-6
	CD11a/CD18, CD11b/CD18
	L-selectin, P-selectin
	CD4
Antigen-presenting molecules	HLA-DR
	ICAM-1

mechanisms. All of these basic proteins have both cytotoxic and noncytotoxic properties that could promote airway inflammation (7). When blood eosinophils from asthma patients were activated in vitro, the release of ECP and EDN was increased when compared with healthy control subjects (8). Moreover, increased peripheral eosinophil levels and serum concentration of eosinophil basic proteins were associated with allergen-induced late-phase asthmatic responses (9). Finally, we have demonstrated elevated MBP, EPO, EDN, and ECP levels in bronchoalveolar lavage (BAL) fluid collected 48 h after segmental broncho-provocation (SBP) with allergen (10). These observations suggest that the release of toxic eosinophil granule proteins is enhanced in asthma and that such a process is operative in allergen-induced models of asthma.

Major basic protein appears to be the primary bioactive bronchoconstricting protein released from eosinophils. It has been identified in the lung tissue of patients with bronchial asthma and is localized to the airway epithelium and mucosa (11). No MBP receptor has been reported; this suggests that MBP act on tissues by its high negative charge (1). Although its mechanism of action is unknown, MBP appears to have a potent twofold effect on airway epithelium: (1) in the *early phase* (minutes to hours); when the epithelium is intact, in vivo (12–14) and in vitro (15) exposure of the epithelium to MBP results in the release of unidentified factors that increase smooth-muscle contraction, thereby promoting airway obstruction. At this stage, MBP also increases epithelium production of prostaglandin (PG)E$_2$ (16) to affect airway tone and ion transport (17). (2) The *later phase* of MBP–epithelium interaction occurs after 12 h and results in epithelial cell death, decreased ciliary activity and, possibly, this is where changes in bronchial responsiveness begin (18,19).

Eosinophil peroxidase is distinct from neutrophil myeloperoxidase (MPO) (20). The combination of EPO, H$_2$O$_2$ from the eosinophil respiratory burst, and halide ion forms a very potent cytotoxic system (21–24). The EPO–H$_2$O$_2$–halide (preferably Br$^-$) system damages nasal sinus mucosa (25) and endothelial cells of the heart (26). This system is the first described physiological function of bromide anion and in vivo generation of singlet oxygen, not observed with the neutrophil MPO–H$_2$O$_2$–chloride system (27,28). Noncytotoxic effects of EPO include stimulation of mast cell degranulation (29), increase in neutrophil adhesion (through decreased receptor-mediated activation; 30,31), and inactivation of lipid mediators (32).

The last two major granule constituents, ECP and EDN, have RNase activity (33,34). Eosinophil cationic protein is detected by immunoblot techniques in bronchial tissues of asthma patients (35,36) and is cytotoxic to mammalian cells (37). The sputum of asthma patients has been reported to contain up to 10^{-5} M ECP (38). Effective in vitro cytotoxic concentrations of ECP are comparable with physiological levels of 10^{-6}–10^{-9} M (7). The noncytotoxic effects of ECP include stimulation of airway mucous secretion, as may occur in asthma (39), and alteration of T-lymphocyte function by inhibiting cell proliferation (40). Although the exact mechanism of ECP activity in allergic disease is unknown, Peterson and Venge (41) have proposed that ECP may bind to heparin or α_2-macroglobulin and, thus, initiate physiological effects.

Eosinophil-derived neurotoxin inhibits T-lymphocyte proliferation in a noncytotoxic manner, similar to ECP (40); however, this granule protein is a ribonuclease 100 times more potent than ECP (33).

Oxygen Metabolites

Similar to the neutrophil and monocyte–macrophage, the eosinophil is able to transform molecular oxygen into highly reactive and inflammatory metabolites, including superoxide anion (O_2^-), hydrogen peroxide (H_2O_2), singlet oxygen ($^1O_2$), hydroxyl radical (OH·), and hypohalous anion (XO^-, where $X = Br^-$ or Cl^-). All of these oxygen metabolites can promote tissue damage; the interaction of H_2O_2 with EPO and halide ion forms a very potent cytotoxic system.

Although some similarities exist, the eosinophil respiratory burst is distinct in its magnitude of response and activators from that observed in neutrophils. Normal peripheral eosinophils generate more O_2^- than corresponding neutrophils (42). Moreover, both normal and hypodense circulating eosinophils from patients with asthma generated higher levels of phorbol myristate acetate (PMA)-stimulated O_2^- than control eosinophils (43). Differences in the eosinophil respiratory burst were also observed when airway eosinophils, isolated from BAL fluid obtained 48 h after SBP with allergen, were found to have increased formyl f-Met-Leu-Phe (FMLP)-activated O_2^- production, compared with the corresponding blood cells (44). All of these changes in eosinophilic O_2^- were dependent on specific stimulus to the cell, not necessarily a generalized functional increase.

Arachidonic Acid Metabolites

Eosinophils are also capable of generating inflammatory lipid mediators. The two most prevalent of this class are platelet-activating factor (PAF) and the sulfidopeptide leukotriene C_4 (LTC_4). The PAF may play a role in the selective recruitment of eosinophils to sites of airway inflammation. Eosinophils are a rich source of PAF, production of which is further enhanced in hypodense eosinophils from asthma patients (45). PAF has a multitude of direct effects on eosinophils themselves as well as on other leukocytes and airway tissue. For example, it is selectively chemotactic for eosinophils in vitro (46–48) and in vivo (49–52), and can activate and prime eosinophil functions, such as degranulation (53,54), LTC_4 generation (55), and the respiratory burst (56,57). Finally, PAF is spasmogenic and can directly affect airway responsiveness (58–60).

Leukoteriene C_4 is a sulfidopeptide generated from arachidonic acid by a 5-lipoxygenase pathway. Activated peripheral eosinophils can release LTC_4, which causes smooth-muscle contraction and muscarinic hyperresponsiveness independently of granule proteins and the respiratory burst (61).

Cytokines

Cytokines that affect eosinophils' survival and function have been identified in bronchial biopsies and associated with bronchial disease (62–65). It is only recently that eosinophils themselves have been found to be a potential source of cytokines. Peripheral blood eosinophils express mRNA and protein for a variety of cytokines, which are detected either constitutively or after activation (Table 2). Airway eosinophils collected by BAL spontaneously express mRNA for interleukin (IL)-5 and granulocyte–macrophage colony-stimulating factor (GM-CSF) (66). Similarly, eosinophils have been demonstrated to have mRNA for GM-CSF (67) and transforming growth factor (TGF)-β (68) in nasal polyposis; IL-5, in biopsies of intestinal mucosa from celiac disease (69); and IL-3, IL-4, IL-5, and GM-CSF, in allergen-induced late-phase cutaneous reactions (70).

Wong and co-workers (72) demonstrated that human peripheral eosinophils from patients with hypereosinophilia express mRNA for TGF-α (71) and TGF-β. In addition, Walz et al. (73) reported that 100% of circulating eosinophils from healthy subjects express TGF-α mRNA and appear responsible for the production and release of mature, soluble TGF-α. No other white blood cells appear to have these properties. This suggests that

Table 2 Eosinophil Cytokine
Production: mRNA or Protein

Cytokine	Source[a]		
	Blood	BAL	Tissue
IL-3	233,234		70
IL-4			70
IL-5		66	69,70
IL-6	235		
IL-8	236		
GM-CSF	233,234	66	67,237
TGF-α	71,73		
TGF-β	72		68,238

[a]Reference number.

eosinophils specifically produce a product that can bind to endothelial cell TGF-α-receptors and, thereby, promote the eosinophil's adhesion and migration to the airways.

Unlike the production of hematopoietins, which appear to promote eosinophilic inflammatory function, eosinophils from patients with hypereosinophilia syndrome (72), or in chronically inflamed airway tissue (68), also express TGF-β mRNA. TGF-β has recently been found to inhibit eosinophil survival, generation of IL-5 and GM-CSF, and release of EPO (74). These findings suggest that TGF-β can inhibit the selective function and survival of mature eosinophils. Moreover, such observations are an example of how cytokines may down-regulate eosinophil activity in asthma and allergic disease. Therefore, by the production of cytokines, eosinophils are not only able to affect their own function (by positive- or negative-feedback loops), but are also likely to affect the function and participation of other airway cells (lymphocytes, macrophages, endothelial, and epithelial). Thus, eosinophils are capable of exerting both pro- and anti-inflammatory roles in airway disease.

Survival

Eosinophil participation in inflammatory reactions can be promoted by an inhibition of *apoptosis*, or programmed cell death. In vitro eosinophil survival is dramatically enhanced by the addition of IL-3, IL-5, and GM-CSF to the culture medium (75–79). In contrast, TGF-β inhibits the effects of these cytokines and actually promotes apoptosis (74). By extending the survival of eosinophils in tissues, these cells have a prolonged opportunity to respond to inflammatory mediators by activating the release of additional preformed and newly generated inflammatory mediators.

Adhesion Molecules

Eosinophils possess cell surface membrane adhesion molecules, such as CD11b/CD18 and L-selectin, similar to those of neutrophils (80). However, through the expression of the integrin adhesion molecule very late activation antigen (VLA)-4 (α4β1, CD49d/CD29), eosinophils have yet another means of selective infiltration into the airways. Although VLA-4 is present on eosinophil and mononuclear leukocyte surface membranes, it has not been detected on neutrophils (81,82). It is a homing molecule for lymphocytes and binds to the vascular cell adhesions molecule (VCAM) receptor on endothelial cells, such as those that may line the pulmonary vasculature (82–84). In vitro, the increased expression of VCAM-1 by endothelial cells treated with IL-4 or tissue-necrosis-factor (TNF)-α results in enhanced eosinophil adhesion; this effect is inhibited by either anti-VLA-4 (85) or anti-VCAM-1 antibodies (86). In an in vivo guinea pig model, cutaneous accumulation of eosinophils, following intradermal challenge with various inflammatory mediators, was inhibited when eosinophils were pretreated with anti-VLA-4 antibody (87). Moreover, in patients with either intrinsic or extrinsic asthma, the expression of intracellular adhesion molecule (ICAM)-1 and VCAM-1 significantly correlated with numbers of eosinophils in bronchial biopsies (88). These data suggest that VLA-4 is an important molecule in the selective recruitment of eosinophils during allergic inflammation.

Similar to T lymphocytes and monocytes, but not neutrophils, eosinophils also express the adhesion molecule, CD4 (89,90). Although the expression of CD4 is low, it appears that all eosinophils have this marker (90). In vitro, CD4 expression on peripheral blood eosinophils is enhanced during culture with IL-3, GM-CSF, and fibroblast monolayers (91). IL-16 (lymphocyte chemattractant factor) binds to CD4 (92,93) and is capable of promoting eosinophil migration at much lower concentrations than either C5a or PAF (90). This may be another mechanism for selective recruitment of eosinophils to the airways of asthma patients.

Antigen Presentation

Macrophages and monocytes are accepted as the predominant antigen-presenting cells to activate T lymphocytes. It has been reported that eosinophil infiltrates in inflamed airways also have this potential. Under certain in vivo and in vitro (cytokine-induced) conditions, eosinophils can be stimulated to express HLA-DR and ICAM-1, components of the T-cell receptor (94–98). Eosinophils from sputum (94), peritoneum (99), and bronchoalveolar lavage fluid (44) express detectable HLA-DR. Although normal peripheral eosinophils express little ICAM-1 or HLA-DR, several groups (95,100,101) report that culture of these cells with various cytokines or cytokine combinations results in the expression of these membrane markers. Hansel and co-workers (95) have reported that eosinophils expressing ICAM-1 have increased adhesion to autologous T lymphocytes. Moreover, eosinophil expression of both ICAM-1 and HLA-DR mediate antigen-specific proliferation of auto-logous, MHC-restricted T cells. This property suggests that eosinophils can participate in antigen uptake, processing, and presentation. Similar studies (100,101) conclude that eosinophils are capable of promoting T-lymphocyte activation by acting as antigen-presenting cells.

EOSINOPHIL ACTIVATORS

Eosinophil function can be modulated by a wide variety of agonists (Table 3). An agonist's effect can be threefold: (1) *activation*—cell functional activity can be initiated and sustained; (2) *priming*—the cell can be up-regulated so that subsequent exposure to a different agonist results in enhanced function compared with the effect of the final agonist alone; and (3) *desensitization*—activation and priming by an agonist that desensitizes the cell's ability to respond to a second exposure to the agonist. As assessed by in vitro testing, eosinophil agonists can be categorized as activators alone (calcium ionophore A23187), primers (certain cytokines), or combined activator–primer (PAF). The action of this last category is

Table 3 Eosinophil Agonists

Agonist	Function/activation
Physiological	
Histamine	Chemotaxis, O_2^-
PAF	Chemotaxis, O_2^-, adhesion, degranulation
LTB$_4$	Chemotaxis, O_2^-
PGD$_2$	Chemotaxis
IgA	Degranulation, O_2^-, cytokine production
IgG	Degranulation, cytokine production
C3b (STZ)	Degranulation, LTC$_4$, O_2^-, adhesion
C5a	Chemotaxis
IL-2	Chemotaxis
IL-3	Survival, cytokine production
IL-5	Chemotaxis, survival, degranulation, cytokine production
GM-CSF	Survival, cytokine production
RANTES	Chemotaxis
LCF	Chemotaxis
TGF-β	Apoptosis
IFN-γ	HLA-DR expression
Substance P	Degranulation, migration
TNF	ICAM-1 expression
Nonphysiological	
PMA	Adhesion, O_2^-
FMLP	Degranulation, O_2^-, chemotaxis, LTC$_4$
Ionomycin	Cytokine production
A23187	O_2^-, adhesion, LTC$_4$

dependent on the concentration of the agonist, the eosinophil function assessed, and possibly, the presence of other primers.

Functional Specificity

As advances in technology have promoted the study of peripheral and airway eosinophil function, it has become increasingly obvious that leukocyte functional activation (as well as functional priming) is highly specific in several ways (Table 4). Although eosinophils share many of the same functions with their fellow granulocyte, the neutrophil, it has been repeatedly demonstrated that the two cell types respond to different agonists and in different ways to the same agonist. For example, eosinophils generate significantly higher levels of O_2^- when activated with PMA or A23187 (42). Moreover, PAF can stimulate the eosinophil's, but not the neutrophil's, respiratory burst (56). Finally, the expression of the adhesion molecule CD11b/CD18 from intracellular pools is regulated differently in the two types of granulocytes (80,102). Although eosinophils have a greater total pool of CD11b/CD18, neutrophils are more responsive to bacteria-like agonists, such as FMLP, lipopolysaccharide (LPS), and C5a, whereas eosinophils are selectively stimulated by IL-5 (102). In contrast, L-selectin is decreased on both populations of granulocytes by PAF and FMLP (80).

A single agonist can stimulate multiple cell functions by different signal transduction pathways; LTB$_4$ initiates both eosinophil intracellular calcium ($[Ca^{2+}]_i$) mobilization and

Table 4 Determinants of Leukocyte Functional Specificity

Factor	Example
Agonist	Receptor-dependent vs. -independent (FMLP, PAF vs. PMA, calcium ionophore)
Function	Degranulation vs. chemotaxis vs. respiratory burst
Agonist concentration	1. PAF: Chemotaxis vs. respiratory burst
	2. PAF: Activation vs. priming
Cell type	Eosinophils vs. neutrophils
	Normal vs. hypodense eosinophils
Cell source	Healthy vs. asthma vs. HES
	Blood vs. airways vs. tissue
Species	Human vs. guinea pig vs. dog vs. rat
System	In vivo vs. in vitro

O_2^- as unrelated events (103). Another possibly important physiological stimulus that has multiple effects on eosinophils is PAF. This cytokine is produced by eosinophils and other cells that participate in the airway inflammation of asthma (e.g., endothelium; 60). Moreover, PAF is a poor activator of neutrophils, but can affect multiple eosinophilic functions independently and differentially, depending on its concentration in the system. At low doses (1 nM), PAF can activate eosinophil $[Ca^{2+}]_i$ mobilization (57), transmigration (104), and degranulation (53,54), as well as priming for subsequent activation of the cell's respiratory burst (57). However, at a higher dose (1 μM), PAF alone can activate the respiratory burst (56), chemotaxis (105), and LTC$_4$, but not neutrophil LTB$_4$ (55,106). Moreover, the eosinophil can express more than one receptor for an agonist; two distinct forms of PAF receptors, initiating different signal transduction pathways, appear to be expressed on eosinophils (107). This would account for the ability to selectively inhibit individual cell functions. Therefore, this single agonist provides eosinophils with both specificity and a wide range of functional activities, all of which could be important in asthma airway inflammation.

Finally, the source of eosinophils will determine the type of agonist that is an effective stimulator as well as the specific function activated. As stated above, peripheral eosinophils, from patients with asthma generate more O_2^- than cells from healthy controls (43), while eosinophils isolated by BAL 48 h after SBP of allergic subjects with allergin have an enhanced respiratory burst when compared to their corresponding peripheral cells (44).

Activators

Eosinophil agonists can be divided into two general categories: receptor-mediated or receptor-independent.

Receptor-Mediated

Agonists such as FMLP, PAF, IgG, IgA, C5a, and IL-5, all initiate eosinophil functions by a specific cell membrane receptor. Therefore, the efficacy of the stimulus can be affected by changes in receptor number and affinity. For example, IL-5 stimulation of eosinophils selectively augmented the appearance of new or stored adhesion molecules, such as Cd11b/CD18 (80,102,108). Agonist binding can also initiate different signal-transduction pathways, including the activation of G-proteins, phospholipases, protein kinases, and calcium channels (107,109–111). This versatility helps explain the diverse and numerous responses of eosinophils to activation and priming, and provides several possible approaches for pharmacological modulation.

One in vivo receptor-mediated agonist that may be particularly important in asthma is secretory IgA. Although neutrophils normally express more IgA receptors (FcαR) than eosinophils, these receptors are up-regulated on eosinophils from allergic subjects (112). Thus far, no difference between normal and allergic individuals has been reported in neutrophil expression of FcαR. In vitro, eosinophil expression of FcαR can be up-regulated in a time- and dose-dependent manner by calcium ionophore A23187 (112). Furthermore, IgA is an activator of eosinophil cytokine production (113), degranulation (114), and the respiratory burst (Sedgwick JB, personal observation).

Eosinophil function is also affected in a variety of ways by specific cytokines, of which IL-3, IL-5, and GM-CSF, have been extensively studied. The cell membrane receptors for these cytokines are heterodimers composed of a shared β-chain and a distinct α-chain (115,116). The binding of cytokine to its eosinophil receptor can activate or prime many cell functions (117), including the very important enhancement of cell survival (75,78,79,118). The effects of IL-5 on survival and function are specific to eosinophils; unlike GM-CSF, IL-5 does not appear to interact with neutrophils (119–121). Moreover, IL-5 is selectively chemotactic in vitro (119) and can recruit eosinophils to sites of inflammation in vivo (122–125). Therefore, this cytokine may be crucial for selective eosinophil recruitment to the airways or other organs. Elevated serum levels of IL-5 have been observed in patients with eosinophilia and either eosinophilic gastritis (126) or episodic angioedema (127). Finally, in vitro incubation of eosinophils with IL-5, at concentrations that enhance cell survival, has little effect on cell adherence or respiratory burst (128). These observations suggest that the process by which IL-5 promotes cell proliferation and survival is not only eosinophil-specific, but may be independent of other effects on cell function, such as activation or priming.

Finally, cross-linking of adhesion receptors may also stimulate eosinophil function. Laudanna and co-workers (129) have observed that cross-linking of β-1 or β-2 subfamilies of integrin adhesion molecules results in the stimulation of the eosinophil respiratory burst. From adhesion studies of eosinophils and fibronectin, these researchers used monoclonal antibodies to VLA-4 (CD49d/CD29), LFA-1 (CD11a/CD18), CR3 (CD11b/CD18), or the common β_2-subunit (CD18) to activate O_2^- generation in eosinophils. Neutrophils, in contrast, were stimulated only by anti-CD18 antibody. Although the levels of eosinophil activation in these conditions were low, such findings show that integrin-mediated adhesion of the β_1- and β_2-integrins is capable of initiating functional activity in a selective, cell-specific manner.

Receptor-Independent

In contrast, there is a group of agonists that stimulate eosinophils in the absence of a specific cell surface receptor. These include PMA, which becomes incorporated in the membrane and directly activates protein kinase C, and calcium ionophores, which create membrane channels for the entry of extracellular calcium. Such agonists utilize different mechanisms of signal transduction and, again, demonstrate the multiplicity of eosinophils' responses. Although not necessarily physiologically relevant, these agonists provide probes to study different mechanisms of eosinophil signal transduction and are very helpful in elucidating methods of modulating cell participation in asthma.

Care must be taken when projecting in vitro effects of a specific agonist on eosinophil function to an in vivo system. A single agonist may affect multiple cells in vivo or be ineffective because of the presence of an inhibitor or blocker. Moreover, agonists that are effective eosinophil activators in vitro may be irrelevant to a real-life situation, owing to their being nonphysiological (PMA, A23187) or requiring unrealistically high, nonphysiological concentrations. Similarly, it is by no means certain that all of the possibly relevant in vivo agonists have been identified.

IMMUNOPHARMACOLOGY OF EOSINOPHILS

From studies of granulocyte function, it is apparent that the specific cell response is influenced by multiple factors. Examples of these have already been presented and are listed in Table 4. Such factors must be taken into account when developing an effective therapy for modulation of eosinophil participation in asthma. Eosinophil participation may be altered or inhibited at several points, and by different mechanisms (Table 5). Finally, it is not necessary for the modulating agent to interact directly with eosinophils to affect subsequent function. By altering the function of other inflammatory cells, such as lymphocytes and endothelium, production of cytokines and other inflammatory mediators necessary for eosinophil participation can be regulated. The inhibition of a single cell function may have little effect on the eosinophil's overall ability to participate in airway inflammation and, therefore, would be insufficient to have a therapeutic effect. Conversely, a therapy that completely eliminates granulocyte function would be detrimental to the patient owing to loss of neutrophil bactericidal activity. Therefore, an optimal immunopharmacological therapy should be selective for eosinophils and should prevent cell recruitment to the inflammatory reaction in the airways, as opposed to altering their function once in the airways. Several types of pharmacological agents that have been applied to asthma therapy are listed in Table 6, and studies on their effects on eosinophil function are reviewed in the following.

Table 5 Mechanisms of Drug Interaction

Inhibit eosinophil
  Specificity
  Recruitment
  Priming
  Activation
Mechanism
  Agonist binding: receptor number, receptor affinity
  Stimulus–response coupling
  Cytokine production (+/−)
Cell affected
  Direct effect: eosinophil
  Indirect effect
    T-lymphocyte
    monocyte–macrophage
    endothelium
    epithelium

Table 6 Effect of Drugs on Eosinophil Function

Pharmacological agent	Effect
Glucocorticoids	Inhibit cell generation
	Inhibit survival
	Inhibit cytokine production
Nedocromil sodium	Inhibit cell recruitment
	Inhibit chemotaxis
	Inhibit cytotoxicty
	Inhibit LTC_4 production
Adrenergic agonists	Inhibit chemotaxis
	Inhibit degranulation
	Inhibit respiratory burst
Antihistamines	Inhibit adhesion
	Inhibit cell recruitment
	Inhibit chemotaxis
Adenosine	Inhibit adhesion?
	Inhibit respiratory burst?
	Inhibit degranulation?
	Enhance chemotaxis?
Phosphodiesterase inhibitors	Inhibit cell recruitment
	Inhibit respiratory burst
	Inhibit Ca^{2+} mobilization
	Activate cAMP protein kinase
Antiadhesion antibodies	Inhibit cell recruitment
	Inhibit adhesion
Anticytokine antibodies	Inhibit cell recruitment
	Inhibit survival

Glucocorticoids

Corticosteroids are frequently administered as a therapy for severe asthma and are potent inhibitors of the late asthma response. One of the major effects of glucocorticoids on asthma is the inhibition of cell infiltration into the airways. Charlesworth et al. (130) have observed that pretreatment of atopic subjects with prednisone decreased eosinophil and basophil, but not neutrophil, accumulation following allergen challenge of skin chambers. In the airways, large numbers of eosinophils are present in the bronchoalveolar lavage fluid following segmental or whole-lung allergen challenge (10,131,132), an event that is profoundly inhibited by glucocorticoid therapy (133). There are at least three major points at which steroids have an effect (134):

Inhibition of Eosinophil Generation

Two levels of action can contribute to these drugs' effect on eosinophils production. Short-term or even single-dose administration of corticosteroids decreases circulating eosinophils (135,136). This occurs without loss of resident eosinophils in the bone marrow and tissues (137,138). In contrast, prolonged corticosteroid therapy results in a progressive decrease of eosinophils in the bone marrow and tissues (137,138). Inhaled budesonide decreased not only the number of circulating eosinophils, but also hypodense eosinophils, which may be a subpopulation of cells more responsive to inflammatory stimuli (139). Furthermore, the decrease in circulating eosinophils correlated with decreased methacholine responsiveness of the airways. Interestingly, it appears that glucocorticoids are more effective in reducing eosinophils in patients with increased numbers of eosinophils than in healthy subjects (140). This effect is possibly due to the inhibition of generation of growth-promoting cytokines, such as IL-5, IL-3, and GM-CSF, rather than a direct effect on progenitor cells (141,142).

Inhibition of Eosinophil Priming and Recruitment by Eosinophil-Activating Cytokines (IL-3, IL-5, and GM-CSF)

Glucocorticoids are also capable of affecting mature eosinophil function. Several groups have reported that corticosteroids inhibit cytokine-enhanced in vitro eosinophil survival (143–146). This effect was dependent on both cytokine and corticosteroid derivative concentrations, suggesting that this is not a direct cytotoxic drug effect.

Although eosinophils express high -affinity receptors for corticosteroids (147), there is little in vitro evidence of a direct glucocorticoid effect on eosinophil functions other than survival (148). In vivo administration of glucocorticoids inhibited subsequent in vitro adhesion and chemotaxis of eosinophils (149,150). Moreover, inhaled budesonide completely inhibited the allergen-induced increase in nasal ECP and the late-occurring nasal symptoms, suggesting that this drug may exert its effect on eosinophil influx or degranulation (151,152). In contrast, in vitro incubation of eosinophil with glucocorticoids did not affect adhesion to endothelial cells which, in some experiments, were pretreated with cytokines to increase adhesion molecules (134,153). However, glucocorticoids may effectively inhibit the release of adhesion activators or alter postadhesion eosinophil function. Similarly, Kita and co-workers (154) report that in vitro incubation with glucocorticoids, except methylprednisolone, did not affect IgA-induced, IL-5-enhanced degranulation of EDN. Again, these data suggest that corticosteroid treatment had no direct effect on eosinophil function.

Cytokines, which are important promoters of eosinophil survival, are also factors that modulate cell function, particularly adhesion, migration, and chemotaxis (155). They may potentiate eosinophil degranulation, cytotoxicity, and mediator release (155). Although the mechanism of corticosteroid effects on airway inflammation is unclear, it may be partly due to the ability of such drugs to inhibit production and release of cytokines (156). A direct inhibition of IL-5 (157–159), IL-3 (160), and GM-CSF (160) gene expression or production by glucocorticoids has been reported. Therefore, inhibition of cytokine production could have an effect on eosinophil participation in inflammation. Eosinophils obtained from corticosteroid-treated subjects do not adhere to nylon fibers or migrate to a chemotactic stimulus (161). In parasite-infected mice, treatment with dexamethasone reduced both eosinophil numbers and serum IL-5 levels (52); eosinopenia in these animals was thought to be the result of diminished IL-5 production.

Inhibition of Eosinophil Recruitment by Endothelial-Activating Cytokines (IL-1β, IL-4, and TNFα)

Adhesion molecules are increased by exposure of endothelial cells to cytokines; IL-1β, IL-4, and TNF-α enhance endothelial expression of ICAM-1, E-selectin, and VCAM-1 (162–164). This process is insensitive to treatment with glucocorticoids. In an in vitro study, budesonide did not directly inhibit stimulus-driven adhesion of eosinophil to endothelial cells (153). These data suggest that corticosteroids do not act directly on endothelial cells, but rather, are inhibitors of the generation or release of endothelial-activating cytokines including IL-1β, IL-4, and TNF-α (134). It is at this site that corticosteroids may have a wide range of effects, including an indirect effect on eosinophil accumulation.

Nedocromil Sodium

Although corticosteroids may be the most potent antiasthma drugs (165), nedocromil sodium also reduces bronchial hyperresponsiveness and airway inflammation (see Ref. 166 for review). Nedocromil sodium is an anti-inflammatory, antiasthma prophylactic medication similar to, but more potent than cromolyn sodium (sodium cromoglycate) (167). Nedocromil sodium also has the preferential property of stabilizing mast cells located on mucosal surfaces (168). Pretreatment with nedocromil prevents the early and late reaction to antigen challenge in patients with asthma (169,170). Moreover, nedocromil sodium can inhibit a dual response when it occurs in exercised-induced asthma (171). Finally, it inhibits the in vivo accumulation of inflammatory cells (172–176) and in vitro mobilization of eosinophils (177).

Both in vivo and in vitro studies of nedocromil sodium on eosinophil function and recruitment have been reported. Perfused lungs isolated from ovalbumin-sensitized, nedocromil sodium-treated guinea pigs demonstrated less bronchoconstriction in response to PAF; similarly nedocromil sodium-treated animals had decreased numbers of BAL eosinophils compared with untreated animals (178). In vitro, nedocromil sodium has been reported to inhibit human eosinophil FMLP- and PAF-induced cytotoxicity (179,180), A23187- and IgG-induced LTC_4 generation (180,181), PMA-induced degranulation (182), and cytokine-primed and PAF-induced chemotaxis (177,183,184). However, the in vitro effects of nedocromil sodium treatment are not always consistent. Burke et al. (185) reported that pretreatment with nedocromil sodium had no significant effect on A23187-induced or on opsonized zymosan-induced generation of PAF or LTC_4 by human eosinophils.

Although nedocromil sodium also affects in vitro neutrophil function, it is not always similar to its effect on eosinophils, introducing specificity to the cell–drug interaction. Nedocromil sodium inhibited opsonized zymosan-induced chemotaxis of neutrophils, but not eosinophils (177). Conversely, it inhibited A23187 and opsonized zymosan activation of leukotriene generation by eosinophils, but not neutrophils (186). It also inhibited PAF-stimulated neutrophil O_2^- generation (187), but did not affect FMLP, PMA, and opsonized zymosan activation (187,188). In contrast, nedocromil sodium did not affect FMLP-, PMA-, or PAF-induced eosinophil O_2^- production (181). These data indicate agonist- and cell-specific effects of nedocromil sodium on granulocyte function.

Adrenergic Agonists

β-Adrenergic agonists are important drugs in the management of bronchial asthma by their ability to activate β_2-adrenoceptors on airway smooth muscle and cause bronchodilation. Whether these drugs also have an anti-inflammatory effect is uncertain. Guinea pig blood eosinophils have β-adrenoceptors on their surface (189). To assess the in vitro effect of adrenergic agents on guinea pig eosinophil function, Masuyama and Ishikawa (190) found that β-adrenergic agonists inhibited guinea pig eosinophil chemotaxis and degranulation. In contrast, α-adrenergic agonists stimulated eosinophil phagocytosis, the opposite of their effect on neutrophil and macrophage phagocytosis. Both α- and β-stimulants inhibited the eosinophil respiratory burst, as measured by nitroblue tetrazolium (NBT) reduction. More recently, Yukawa et al. (189) extended in vitro studies on guinea pig peritoneal eosinophils and observed that albuterol (salbutamol) had no effect on PMA- or opsonized zymozan-stimulated O_2^- generation. In contrast, Rabe and co-workers (191) found that the β_2-adreno-ceptor agonists albuterol and formoterol, but not salmeterol, inhibited LTB_4-induced H_2O_2 generation. Moreover, treatment of guinea pigs with formoterol before antigen challenge resulted in inhibited BAL eosinophil O_2^- generation (192). Interestingly, the mechanism of this effect did not appear to be through formoterol's interaction with the cell's β_2-adreno-ceptors because BAL macrophages were not similarly affected. Finally, formoterol is a more potent inhibitor than albuterol of PAF- and FMLP-induced eosinophil chemotaxis and degranulation of ECP (193). This process was enhanced by isobutyl methylxanthine (IBMX) and not abolished by propranolol, again suggesting that the effect is due to direct inhibition by a non–β-adrenoceptor-mediated process. These data suggest that formoterol can more effectively prevent eosinophil-mediated inflammation of the late asthma reaction, compared with more conventional β_2-adrenergic agonists. Differences between these studies may reflect different incubation times and, possibly most important, different functional stimuli: eosinophil responses are very dependent on the specific activator.

Finally, β-adrenergic agonists can modulate eosinophil accumulation. Inhaled β-adrenergic agonists markedly inhibited BAL eosinophil infiltration following aerosolized antigen (194,195). This effect may be more relevant than actions on individual cell functions and prevent the participation of eosinophils in the allergic reaction. One concern with β-agonist effects on eosinophil function is the development of tachyphylaxis. This property may explain why β-receptor agonist inhibition of the eosinophil respiratory burst occurs only with very short incubation (191). These observations suggest that β-adrenergic agonists may be of limited value to modulate chronic or extended airway inflammation.

Antihistamines

Some of the newer H_1-antihistamines not only act as inhibitors of histamine release, but also affect the recruitment and function of airway eosinophils (196,197). Cetirizine is a specific H_1-receptor antagonist that is used in the treatment of allergic disease and provides dose-dependent protection against histamine-induced bronchoconstriction (198). Studies have shown that cetirizine inhibits not only eosinophil accumulation in the skin after allergen challenge of atopic subjects (199–201), but also in vitro eosinophil chemotaxis (202). Rédier and associates (203) treated allergic asthma patients with cetirizine for 8 days. These patients were then challenged with allergen and underwent BAL 24 h later. Although cetirizine-treatment had no significant effect on the late asthma reaction (LAR) 7 h after challenge, it did markedly reduce the number of eosinophils in the BAL 24 h after challenge when compared with subjects treated with placebo. Although cetirizine did not appear to directly affect the development of the LAR, it may influence future responses to allergen by its effect on eosinophil accumulation in the airways. Cetirizine has also been reported to inhibit the late eosinophil influx into PAF- or compound 48/80-challenged rat pleural cavities (204) and into allergen-challenged skin windows (205). The initial step in the recruitment of eosinophils to the airways following an allergen challenge is cell adhesion to the vascular endothelium; it may be at this level that cetirizine affects eosinophil influx. High concentrations of cetirizine significantly inhibit eosinophil adhesion to endothelial cell monolayers when either cell type was stimulated (FMLP for eosinophils; IL-1 for endothelial cells; 206). In contrast, cetirizine had no effect on neutrophil adhesion in this system. These results suggest that cetirizine may have important and specific eosinophil activity, possibly by its ability to inhibit VLA-4/VCAM-1 interaction.

Adenosine and Phosphodiesterase Inhibitors

The observation of increased levels of adenosine in the BAL fluid following bronchial challenge with either inhaled allergen or methacholine suggests the release of this nucleoside during an asthmatic response (88). Although the cellular origin and role of adenosine in bronchoconstriction is unclear, adenosine inhibitors modulate neutrophil functions in vitro. Physiological concentrations of adenosine inhibit activation of the receptor-dependent neutrophil respiratory burst (207,208), adhesion (209), endothelial cell cytotoxicity (209), and degranulation (207,210). Interestingly, adenosine actually enhanced cell chemotaxis (211). Burkey and Webster (212) proposed a mechanism of adenosine action: this nucleoside inhibits the G-protein–dependent pathway of receptor stimulation by uncoupling G-proteins from cell surface receptor-mediated signals. Whether these same effects occur in eosinophils has not been reported.

Phosphodiesterase (PDE) inhibitors regulate cycle nucleotide activity and appear to have two important mechanisms in the treatment of asthma, both of which are mediated by potentiation of cAMP or cGMP levels. Although PDE inhibitors can relax smooth muscle under certain conditions and, hence, can inhibit bronchoconstriction, their most important role may be as anti-inflammatory agents. Both human and guinea pig eosinophils appear to have membrane-bound PDE IV, a regulator of cAMP (213,214). The cAMP acts as a second messenger in the signal transduction pathways of many leukocyte functions. In guinea pig peritoneal eosinophils, PDE inhibitors have been reported to inhibit agonist-specific activation of the respiratory burst, thromboxane synthesis, Ca^{2+} mobilization, and to activate cAMP-dependent protein kinase (213–215). Similarly, human eosinophils are sensitive to PDE inhibitors; rolipram and zardaverine inhibit opsonized zymosan-activated H_2O_2 generation (215).

The infiltration of proinflammatory cells into the airway lumen has been evaluated in a series of in vivo studies of sensitized guinea pigs challenged with PAF or allergen (216–218). Treatment with either the PDE inhibitor zardaverine or dexamethasone reduced allergen-induced recruitment of proinflammatory leukocytes into the airway lumen (216). The BAL fluids from these treated guinea pigs were significantly lower in eosinophils, neutrophils, and macrophages. Similar results were reported with PDE III/IV inhibition by benzafentrine of PAF-induced cellular infiltration (217,218). The inhibition of inflammatory cell infiltration, however, was not associated with a reduction in airway responsiveness. In contrast, when guinea pigs were pretreated with rolipram, this particular PDE IV inhibitor reduced both antigen-induced bronchoconstriction and recruitment of inflammatory cells to the airways and airway epithelium (219). Similarly, rolipram inhibited eosinophil infiltration in guinea pig conjunctiva following topical histamine or leukotriene challenge (220). Finally, in vitro increases in bovine pulmonary microvessel endothelial cell cAMP levels (as observed with PDE inhibitors) decrease human neutrophil permeability and are protective of granulocyte cytotoxicity, a process that may minimize endothelial injury after cell activation (221).

However, the effects of PDE inhibitors are not always straightforward. Methylxanthines, such as theophylline and aminophylline, are PDE inhibitors with a biphasic effect on neutrophil function. At low concentrations, these drugs potentiate FMLP-stimulated degranulation, O_2^- generation, and aggregation (222). At higher concentrations, which inhibit PDE activity, they also inhibit these granulocyte functions. Schmeichel and Thomas (222) concluded that this dichotomy is the result of competition between the methylxanthines and endogenously produced adenosine for the granulocyte adenosine receptors. These studies suggest that asthma therapy with the commonly prescribed methylxanthine theophylline may actually have proinflammatory actions at certain in vivo concentrations. Proof of this concept will require further study.

Immunotherapy

Although immunotherapy has long been a treatment for allergic disease, its exact mechanism of action is still unclear. Immunotherapy of a group of pollen-allergic patients resulted in a complete loss of heat-labile eosinophil and neutrophil chemotactic activity in the patients' sera (223). The reduction of these chemotactic factors may contribute to decreased granulocyte accumulation in the lungs and, thereby, a diminished inflammatory response. In a subsequent study, Rak and co-workers (224) found that immunotherapy inhibited eosinophil chemotactic activity as well as eosinophil number and ECP levels in both serum and BAL fluid during pollen season. Moreover, treated patients showed no increase in bronchial hyperresponsiveness during pollen season compared with untreated patients. Finally, Furin et al. (225) demonstrated a parallel between in vivo provocation and seasonal exposure to allergen for the effects of immunotherapy on influx of nasal eosinophils. Immunotherapy before ragweed antigen provocation decreased the number of infiltrating nasal eosinophils. Similarly, ragweed-allergic patients receiving long-term immunotherapy had fewer eosinophils in their nasal washes during pollen season; the levels of eosinophils correlated negatively with the duration of therapy. These data demonstrate that in vivo antigen provocation is a useful model of seasonal allergy, and that one mechanism to explain the efficacy of immunotherapy is its ability to prevent eosinophil accumulation and activation.

Antiadhesion and Anticytokine Antibodies

In an eloquent series of studies, Wegner and co-workers (see Ref. 226 for review) demonstrated, in both a primate and murine model of airway inflammation, that adhesion molecules play an important role in the recruitment, retention, and site-specific activation of inflammatory cells within the airways. In monkeys, infusion of a monoclonal antibody against ICAM-1 inhibited influx of eosinophils following repeated antigen challenge (227). Similarly, anti-α_4-integrin (VLA-4) antibodies inhibited the chemotactic factor-induced accumulation of eosinophils in guinea pig skin (87). Finally, in a sheep model of asthma, anti-α_4-integrin antibodies inhibited an antigen-induced late bronchial response and airway hyperresponsiveness. These antibodies were effective whether given intravenously or as an aerosol. Although anti-α_4 antibodies would be expected to inhibit VLA-4/VCAM adhesion and, hence, cell recruitment of eosinophils and lymphocytes, the exact mechanism of its effect is unclear and interaction with other integrins is possible.

The efficacy of these types of antiadhesion antibodies is currently limited (156). Production of these antibodies in a different species results in a short half-life and the possible production of host antibodies to the foreign protein. Alternatively, soluble forms of the adhesion molecules may modify and suppress airway inflammation (156). It would be expected that these mechanisms would modulate eosinophil participation in asthma.

Similar to antiadhesion molecule antibodies, anticytokine antibodies have been proposed as a method to modulate eosinophil participation in asthma. This path could be very useful, since IL-5 interacts so specifically with eosinophils. In a mouse model, administration of intraperitoneal anti-IL-5 antibody inhibited influx of eosinophils into the BAL fluid of parasite-infected mice (123). Similarly, anti-IL-5 treatment decreased BAL and tissue eosinophilia in a guinea pig model following substance P challenge (228). Interestingly, higher concentrations of anti-IL-5 were also able to inhibit airway hyperresponsiveness. Finally, anti-IL-5 antibodies inhibited eosinophilia and airway hyperresponsiveness in chronic ovalbumin-exposed guinea pigs (124).

Although anti-IL-5 antibodies may provide an eosinophil-specific modulation of asthma, they have the same limitations as antiadhesion antibodies. Because it appears that T lymphocytes are a major source of IL-5 (123), methods to regulate T-cell production of this cytokine may be preferable, if not as selective. Interestingly, certain cytokines may counteract the effects of eosinophil-promoting cytokines such as IL-5. TGF-β, which is produced by eosinophils, can promote natural cell apoptosis as well as inhibit cytokine-enhanced survival (229). It is also possible that stimulation of the T_H1 lymphocyte population and its subsequent cytokine production may modulate the T_H2-like production of cytokines normally observed in asthma airway inflammation (230,231). Interleukin-5 is produced by T_H2 lymphocytes. Nakajima and associates (232) used IFN-γ, a product of T_H1 lymphocytes, to prevent antigen-induced eosinophil recruitment in the mouse trachea.

SUMMARY

The eosinophil is a key cell in the development of active asthma symptoms; there are many ways and means by which eosinophils may be selectively elicited to participate in asthma. Therefore, the actions of the eosinophil and its many inflammatory mediators present a highly visible target in the asthma process. In designing therapeutics to modify eosinophil participation in airway inflammation, it will be helpful to keep the pharmacological regulation as eosinophil-specific as possible. Such an approach will allow the host to retain normal neutrophil function and prevent a modification of normal host defense mechanisms.

ACKNOWLEDGMENT

Supported in part by a grant from the NIH, AI23181.

REFERENCES

1. Leff AR. Immunopharmacology of the eosinophils in asthma. In: Jolles G, Karlsson J-A, Taylor J, eds. T-Lymphocytes and Inflammatory Cell Research in Asthma. New York: Academic Press, 1993:193–220.
2. Barnes PJ, Chung KF, Page CP. Inflammatory mediators and asthma. Pharmacol Rev 1988; 40:49–84.
3. Gleich GJ. The eosinophil and bronchial asthma: current understanding. J Allergy Clin Immunol 1990; 85:422–436.
4. Holgate ST, Roche WR, Church MK. The role of the eosinophil in asthma. Am Rev Respir Dis 1991; 143:S66–S70.
5. Leff AR, Hamann KJ, Wegner CD. Inflammation and cell–cell interactions in airway hyperresponsiveness. Lung Cell Mol Physiol 1991; 4:L189–L206.
6. Weller PF. The immunobiology of eosinophils. N Engl J Med 1991; 324:1110–1118.
7. Venge P. Eosinophil-derived inflammatory mediators. In: Jolles G, Karlsson J-A, Taylor J, eds. T-Lymphocyte and Inflammatory Cell Research in Asthma. New York: Academic Press, 1993:133–149.

8. Carlson M, Håkansson L, Peterson C, Stålenheim G, Venge P. Secretion of granule proteins from eosinophils and neutrophils is increased in asthma. J Allergy Clin Immunol 1991; 87: 27–33.

9. Durham SR, Loegering DA, Dunnette S, Gleich GJ, Kay AB. Blood eosinophils and eosinophil-derived proteins in allergic asthma. J Allergy Clin Immunol 1989; 84:931–936.

10. Sedgwick JB, Calhoun WJ, Gleich GJ, Kita H, Abrams JS, Schwartz LB, Volovitz B, Ben-Yaakov M, Busse WW. Immediate and late airway response of allergic rhinitis patients to segmental antigen challenge. Characterization of eosinophil and mast cell mediators. Am Rev Respir Dis 1991; 144:1274–1281.

11. Filley WV, Holley KE, Kephart GM, Gleich GJ. Identification by immunofluorescence of eosinophil granular major basic protein in lung tissues of patients with bronchial asthma. Lancet 1982; 2:11–16.

12. Brofman JD, White SR, Blake JS, Munoz NM, Gleich GJ, Leff AR. Epithelial augmentation of trachealis contraction caused by MBP of eosinophils. J Appl Pathol 1989; 66:1867–1873.

13. Gundel RH, Letts LG, Wegner CD. Human eosinophil major basic protein induces airway constriction and airway hyperresponsiveness in primates. J Clin Invest 1991; 87:1470–1473.

14. White SR, Ohno S, Munoz NM, Gleich GH, Abrahams C, Solway J, Leff AR. Epithelium-dependent contraction of airway smooth muscle caused by eosinophil MBP. Am J Physiol 1990; 259:L294–L303.

15. Flavahan NA, Slifman NA, Gleich GJ. Human major basic protein causes hyperreactivity of respiratory smooth muscle. Am Rev Respir Dis 1988; 138:685–688.

16. White SR, Sigrist KS, Spaethe SM. Prostaglandin secretion by guinea pig tracheal epithelial cells caused by eosinophil major basic protein. Am J Physiol 1993; 265:L234–L242.

17. Jacoby DB, Ueki IF, Widdicombe JH, Loegering DA, Gleich GJ, Nadel JA. Effect of human eosinophil major basic protein on ion transport in dog tracheal epithelium. Am Rev Respir Dis 1988; 137:13–16.

18. Frigas E, Loegering DA, Gleich GJ. Cytotoxic effects of guinea pig eosinophil major basic protein on tracheal epithelium. Lab Invest 1980; 42:35–43.

19. Ayars GH, Altman LC, Gleich GJ, Loegering DA, Baker CB. Eosinophil- and eosinophil granule-mediated pneumocyte injury. J Appl Pathol 1985; 76:595–604.

20. Mayeno AN, Currant AJ, Roberts RL, Foote CS. Eosinophils preferentially use bromide to generate halogenating agents. J Biol Chem 1989; 264:5660–5668.

21. Jong EC, Klebanoff SJ. Eosinophil-mediated mammalian tumor cell cytotoxicity: role of the peroxidase system. J Immunol 1980; 124:1949–1953.

22. Klebanoff SJ, Agosti JM, Jörg A, Waltersdorph AM. Comparative toxicity of the horse eosinophil peroxidase–H_2O_2 halide system and granule basic proteins. J Immunol 1989; 143:239–244.

23. Hamann KJ, Gleich GJ, Checkel JL, Loegering DA, McCall JW, Barker RL. In vitro killing of microfilaria of Brugia pahangi and Brugia malayi by eosinophil granule proteins. J Immunol 1990; 144:3166–3173.

24. Agosti JM, Altman LC, Ayars GH, Loegering DA, Gleich GJ, Klebanoff SJ. The injurious effect of eosinophil peroxidase, hydrogen peroxide, and halides on pneumocytes in vitro. J Allergy Clin Immunol 1987; 79:496–504.

25. Hisamatsu K, Ganbo T, Nakazawa T, Murakami Y, Gleich GJ, Makiyama K, Koyama H. Cytotoxicity of human eosinophil granule major basic protein to human nasal sinus mucosa in vitro. J Allergy Clin Immunol 1990; 86:52–63.

26. Slugaard A, Mahoney JR Jr. Bromide-dependent toxicity of eosinophil peroxidase for endo-thelium and isolated working rat hearts: a model for eosinophilic endocarditis. J Exp Med 1991; 173:117–126.

27. Weiss SJ, Test ST, Eckmann CM, Roos D, Regaini S. Brominating oxidants generated by human eosinophils. Science 1986; 234:200–203.

28. Kanofski JB, Hoogland H, Wever R, Weiss SJ. Singlet oxygen production by human eosinophils. J Biol Chem 1988; 263:9692–9696.

29. Chi EY, Henderson WR. Ultrastructure of mast cell degranulation induced by eosinophil peroxidase. J Histochem Cytochem 1993; 32:332–341.

30. Zabucchi G, Menegazzi R, Soranzo MR, Patriarca P. Uptake of human eosinophil peroxidase by human neutrophils. Am J Pathol 1986; 124:510–518.

31. Zabucchi G, Menegazzi R, Cramer R, Nardon E, Patriarca P. Mutual influence between eosinophil peroxidase (EPO) and neutrophils: neutrophils reversibly inhibit EPO enzymatic activity and EPO increases neutrophil adhesiveness. Immunology 1990; 69:580–587.

32. Henderson WR, Jorg A, Klebanoff SJ. Eosinophil peroxidase-mediated inactivation of leukotrienes B_4, C_4, and D_4. J Immunol 1982; 128:2609–2613.

33. Gullberg U, Widegren B, Arneson U, Egesten A, Olsson I. The cytotoxic eosinophil cationic protein (ECP) has ribonuclease activity. Biochem Biophys Res Commun 1986; 139:1239–1242.

34. Slifman NR, Loegering DA, McKean DJ, Gleich GJ. Ribonuclease activity associated with human eosinophil-derived neurotoxin and eosinophil cationic protein. J Immunol 1986; 137:2913–2917.

35. Dahl R, Venge P, Fredens K. The eosinophil. In: Barnes PJ, Rodger I, Thomson N, eds. Asthma: Basic Mechanisms and Clinical Management. New York: Academic Press, 1988:115–130.

36. Fredens K, Dybdahl H, Dahl R, Baandrup U. Extracellular deposit of the cationic proteins ECP and EPX in tissue infiltrations of eosinophils related to tissue damage. APMIS 1988; 96:711–719.

37. Young JO, Peterson CG, Venge P, Cohn ZA. Mechanism of membrane damage mediated by human eosinophil cationic protein. Nature 1986; 321:613–616.

38. Hällgren R, Bjelle A, Venge P. Eosinophil cationic protein in inflammatory synovial effusions as evidence of eosinophil involvement. Ann Rheum Dis 1984; 43:556–562.

39. Lundgren JD, Davey RT Jr, Lundgren B, Mullol J, Marom Z, Logun C, Baraniuk J, Kaliner MA, Shelhamer JH. Eosinophil cationic protein stimulates and major basic protein inhibits airway mucus secretion. J Allergy Clin Immunol 1991; 87:689–698.

40. Peterson CG, Skoog V, Venge P. Human eosinophil cationic proteins (ECP and EPX) and their supportive effects on lymphocyte proliferation. Immunobiology 1986; 171:1–13.

41. Peterson CG, Venge P. Interaction and complex formation between the eosinophil cationic protein (ECP) and α_2-macroglobulin. Biochem J 1987; 245:781–787.

42. Sedgwick JB, Vrtis RF, Gourley MF, Busse WW. Stimulus-dependent differences in superoxide anion generation by normal human eosinophils and neutrophils. J Allergy Clin Immunol 1988; 81:876–883.

43. Sedgwick JB, Geiger KM, Busse WW. Superoxide generation by hypodense eosinophils from patients with asthma. Am Rev Respir Dis 1990; 142:120–125.

44. Sedgwick JB, Calhoun WJ, Vrtis RF, Bates MB, McAllister PK, Busse WW. Comparison of airway and blood eosinophil function after in vivo antigen challenge. J Immunol 1992; 149:3710–3718.

45. Lee T, Lenihan DJ, Malone B, Roddy LL, Wasserman SI. Increased biosynthesis of platelet-activating factor in activated human eosinophils. J Biol Chem 1984; 259:5526–5530.

46. Morita DJ, Schröder J-M, Christophers E. Differential sensitivities of purified human eosinophils and neutrophils to defined chemotaxins. Scan J Immunol 1989; 29:709–716.

47. Sigal CE, Valone FH, Holtzman MJ, Goetzl EJ. Preferential human eosinophil chemotactic activity of the platelet-activating factor (PAF) 1-O-hexadecyl-2-acetyl-sn-glyceryl-3-phosphocholine (AGEPC). J Clin Immunol 1987; 7:179–184.

48. Håkansson L, Westerlund D, Venge P. New method for the measurement of eosinophil migration. J Leukoc Biol 1987; 42:689–696.

49. Henocq E, Vargaftig BB. Skin eosinophils in atopic patients. J Allergy Clin Immunol 1988; 81:691–695.

50. Arnoux B, Page CP, Denjean A, Nolibe D, Morley J, Benveniste J. Accumulation of platelets and eosinophils in baboon lung after PAF-acether challenge. Am Rev Respir Dis 1988; 137:855–860.

51. Denjean A, Arnoux B, Benveniste J. Effect of PAF-acether in non-primates. Prog Clin Biol Res 1988; 263:81–90.

52. Lellouch-Tubiana A, Lefort J, Simon M-T, Pfister A, Vargaftig BB. Eosinophil recruitment into guinea pig lungs after PAF-acether and allergen administration. Modulation by prostacyclin, platelet depletion and selective antagonists. Am Rev Respir Dis 1988; 137:948–954.

53. Kroegel C, Yukawa T, Dent G, Venge P, Fan Chung K, Barnes PJ. Platelet-activating factor induces eosinophil peroxidase release from purified human eosinophils. Immunology 1988; 64:559–562.

54. Kroegel C, Yukawa T, Dent G, Venge P, Chung KF, Barnes PJ. Stimulation of degranulation from human eosinophils by platelet-activating factor. J Immunol 1989; 142:3518–3526.

55. Bruijnzeel PLB, Kok PTM, Hamelink ML, Kijne AM, Verhagen J. Platelet-activating factor induces leukotriene C_4 synthesis by purified human eosinophils. Prostaglandins 1987; 34: 205–214.

56. Zoratti EM, Sedgwick JB, Vrtis RF, Busse WW. The effect of platelet-activating factor on the generation of superoxide anion in human eosinophils and neutrophils. J Allergy Clin Immunol 1991; 81:749–758.

57. Zoratti E, Sedgwick JB, Bates ME, Vrtis RF, Geiger K, Busse WW. Platelet-activating factor priming of human eosinophil generation of superoxide. Am J Respir Cell Mol Biol 1992; 6: 100–106.

58. Townley RG, Hopp RJ, Agrawal DK, Bewtra AK. Platelet-activating factor and airway reactivity. J Allergy Clin Immunol 1989; 83:997–1010.

59. Smith LJ, Rubin A-HE, Patterson R. Mechanism of platelet activating factor-induced bronchoconstriction in humans. Am Rev Respir Dis 1988; 137:1015–1019.

60. Barnes PJ, Chung KF, Page CB. Platelet activating factor as a mediator of allergic disease. J Allergy Clin Immunol 1988; 81:919–934.

61. Hamann KJ, Strek ME, Baranowski SL, Munoz NM, Williams FS, White SR, Vita A, Leff AR. Effects of activated eosinophils cultured from human umbilical cord blood on guinea pig trachealis. Am J Physiol 1993; 265:L301–L307.

62. Hamid Q, Azzawi M, Ying S, Moqbel R, Wardlaw AJ, Corrigan CJ, Bradley B, Durham SR, Collins JV, Jeffery PK, Quint DJ, Kay AB. Expression of mRNA for interleukin-5 in mucosal bronchial biopsies from asthma. J Clin Invest 1991; 87:1541–1546.

63. Bentley AM, Meng Q, Robinson DS, Hamid Q, Kay AB, Durham SR. Increases in activated T lymphocytes, eosinophils, and cytokine mRNA expression for interleukin-5 and granulocyte/macrophage colony-stimulating factor in bronchial biopsies after allergen inhalation challenge in atopic asthmatics. Am J Respir Cell Mol Biol 1993; 8:35–42.

64. Robinson DS, Ying S, Bentley AM, Meng Q, North J, Durham SR, Kay AB, Hamid Q. Relationships among numbers of bronchoalveolar lavage cells expressing messenger ribonucleic acid for cytokines, asthma symptoms, and airway methacholine responsiveness in atopic asthma. J Allergy Clin Immunol 1993; 92:397–403.

65. Robinson D, Hamid Q, Bentley A, Ying S, Kay AB, Durham SR. Activation of CD4 T cells, increased T_H2-type cytokine mRNA expression, and eosinophil recruitment in bronchoalveolar lavage after allergen challenge in patients with atopic asthma. J Allergy Clin Immunol 1993; 92:313–324.

66. Broide DH, Paine MM, Firestein GS. Eosinophils express interleukin 5 and granulocyte macrophage-colony stimulating factor mRNA at sites of allergic inflammation in asthmatics. J Clin Invest 1992; 90:1414–1424.

67. Ohno I, Lea R, Finotto S, Marshall J, Denburg J, Dolovich J, Gauldie J, Jordana M. Granulocyte/macrophage colony-stimulating factor (GM-CSF) gene expression by eosinophils in nasal polyposis. Am J Respir Cell Mol Biol 1991; 5:505–510.

68. Ohno I, Lea RG, Flanders KC, Clark DA, Banwatt D, Dolovich J, Denburg J, Harley CB, Gauldie J, Jordana M. Eosinophils in chronically inflamed human upper airway tissues express transforming growth factor β1 gene (TGF-β1). J Clin Invest 1992; 89:1662–1668.

69. Desreumaux P, Janin A, Colombel JF, Prin L, Plumas J, Emilie D, Torpier G, Capron A, Capron M. Interleukin 5 messenger RNA expression by eosinophils in the intestinal mucosa of patients with coeliac disease. J Exp Med 1992; 175:293–296.

70. Kay AB, Ying S, Varney V, Gaga M, Durham SR, Moqbel R, Wardlaw AJ, Hamid Q. Messenger RNA expression of the cytokine gene cluster, interleukin 3 (IL-3), IL-4, IL-5, and granulocyte/macrophage colony-stimulating factor, in allergen-induced late-phase cutaneous reactions in atopic subjects, J Exp Med 1991; 173:775–778.

71. Wong DT, Weller PF, Galli SJ, Elovic A, Rand TH, Gallagher GT, Chiang T, Chou MY, Matossian K, McBride J, Todd R. Human eosinophils express transforming growth factor α. J Exp Med 1990; 172:673–681.

72. Wong DT, Elovic A, Matossian K, Nagura N, McBride J, Chou MY, Gordon JR, Rand TH, Galli SJ, Weller PF. Eosinophils from patients with blood eosinophilia express transforming growth factor β1. Blood 1991; 78:2702–2707.

73. Walz TM, Nishikawa BK, Maim C, Wasteson A. Production of transforming growth factor α by normal blood eosinophils. Leukemia 1993; 7:1531–1537.

74. Alam R, Forsythe P, Stafford S, Fukuda Y. Transforming growth factor β abrogates the effects of hematopoietins on eosinophils and induces their apoptosis. J Exp Med 1994; 179:1041–1045.

75. Rothenberg ME, Owen WF Jr, Silberstein DS, Woods J, Soberman RJ, Austen KF, Stevens RL. Human eosinophils have prolonged survival, enhanced functional properties, and become hypodense when exposed to human interleukin 3. J Clin Invest 1988; 81:1986–1992.

76. Owen WF Jr, Petersen J, Austen KF. Eosinophils altered phenotypically and primed by culture with granulocyte/macrophage colony-stimulating factor and 3T3 fibroblasts generate leukotriene C_4 in response to FMLP. J Clin Invest 1991; 87:1958–1963.

77. Her E, Frazer J, Austen KF, Owen WF Jr. Eosinophil hematopoietins antagonize the programmed cell death of eosinophils. Cytokine and glucocorticoid effects on eosinophils maintained by endothelial cell-conditioned medium. J Clin Invest 1991; 88:1982–1987.

78. Rothenberg ME, Petersen J, Stevens RL, Silberstein DS, McKenzie DT, Austen KF, Owen WF Jr. IL-5 dependent conversion of normodense human eosinophils to the hypodense phenotype uses 3T3 fibroblasts for enhanced viability, accelerated hypodensity, and sustained antibody-dependent cytotoxicity. J Immunol 1989; 143:2311–2316.

79. Owen WF, Rothenberg ME, Silberstein DS, Gasson JC, Stevens RL, Austen KF, Soberman RJ. Regulation of human eosinophil viability, density, and function by granulocyte/macrophage colony-stimulating factor in the presence of 3T3 fibroblasts. J Exp Med 1987; 166:129–141.

80. Neeley SP, Hamann KJ, White SR, Baranowski SL, Burch RA, Leff AR. Selective regulation of expression of surface adhesion molecules Mac-1, L-selectin, and VLA-4 on human eosinophils and neutrophils. Am J Respir Cell Mol Bio 1993; 8:633–639.

81. Weller PF, Rand TH, Goelz SE, Chi-Rosso G, Lobb RR. Human eosinophil adherence to vascular endothelium mediated by binding to vascular cell adhesion molecule 1 and endothelial leukocyte adhesion molecule 1. Proc Natl Acad Sci USA 1991; 88:7430–7433.

82. Walsh GM, Mermod JJ, Hartnell A, Kay AB, Wardlaw AJ. Human eosinophil, but not neutrophil, adherence to IL-1-stimulated human umbilical vascular endothelial cells is α4β1 (very late antigen-4) dependent. J Immunol 1991; 146:3419–3423.

83. Schleimer RP, Sterbinsky SA, Kaiser J, Bickel CA, Klunk DA, Tomioka K, Newman W, Luscinskas FW, Gimbrone MA Jr, McIntyre BW, Bochner BS. IL-4 induces adherence of human eosinophils and basophils but not neutrophils to endothelium. Association with expression of VCAM-1. J Immunol 1992; 148:1086–1092.

84. Elices MJ, Osborn L, Takada Y, Crouse C, Luhowskyj S, Hemler ME, Lobb RR. VCAM-1 on activated endothelium interacts with the leukocyte integrin VLA-4 at a site distinct from the VLS-/fibronectin binding site. Cell 1990; 60:577–584.

85. Chanez P, Dent G, Yukawa T, Barnes PJ, Chung KF. Generation of oxygen free radicals from blood eosinophils from asthma patients after stimulation with PAF or phorbol ester. Eur Respir J 1990; 3:1002–1007.

86. Kyan-Aung U, Haskard DO, Lee TH. Vascular cell adhesion molecule-1 and eosinophil adhesion to cultured human umbilical vein endothelial cells in vitro. Am J Respir Cell Mol Biol 1991; 5:445–450.

87. Weg VB, Williams TJ, Lobb RR, Nourshargh S. A monoclonal antibody recognizing very late activation antigen-4 inhibits eosinophil accumulation in vivo. J Exp Med 1993; 177:561–566.

88. Mann JS, Holgate ST, Renwick AG, Cushley MJ. Airway effects of purine nucleosides and nucleotides and release with bronchial provocation in asthma. J Appl Pathol 1986; 61:1667–1676.

89. Lucey DR, Dorsky DI, Nicholson-Weller A, Weller PF. Human eosinophils express CD4 protein and bind HIV-1 GP120. J Exp Med 1989; 169:327–332.

90. Rand TH, Cruikshank WW, Center DM, Weller PF. CD4-mediated stimulation of human eosinophils: lymphocyte chemoattractant factor and other CD4-binding ligands elicit eosinophil migration. J Exp Med 1991; 173:1521–1528.

91. Riedel D, Lindemann A, Brach M, Mertelsmann R, Herrmann F. Granulocyte–macrophage colony-stimulating factor and interleukin-3 induce surface expression of interleukin-2 receptor p55-chain and CD4 by human eosinophils. Immunology 1990; 70:258–261.

92. Cruikshank WW, Berman JS, Theodore AC, Bernardo J, Center DM. Lymphokine activation of T4+ lymphocytes and monocytes. J Immunol 1987; 138:3817–3823.

93. Cruikshank WW, Greenstein JL, Theodore AC, Center DM. Lymphocyte chemotactant factor (LCF) induces CD4-dependent intracytoplasmic signaling in lymphocytes. J Immunol 1991; 146:2928–2934.

94. Hansel TT, Braunstein JB, Walker C, Blaser K, Bruijnzeel PL, Virchow JC Jr., Virchow C. Sputum eosinophils from asthmatics express ICAM-1 and HLA-DR. Clin Exp Immunol 1991; 86:271–277.

95. Hansel TT, DeVries JM, Carballido JM, Braun RK, Carballido-Perrig N, Rihs S, Blaser K, Walker C. Induction and function of eosinophil intercellular adhesion molecule-1 and HLA-DR. J Immunol 1992; 149:2130–2136.

96. Lucey DR, Nicholson-Weller A, Weller PF, Mature human eosinophils have the capacity to express HLA-DR. Proc Natl Acad Sci USA 1989; 86:1348–1351.

97. Czech W, Krutmann J, Budnik A, Schöpf E, Kapp A. Induction of intercellular adhesion molecule 1 (ICAM-1) expression in normal human eosinophils by inflammatory cytokines. J Invest Dermatol 1993; 100:417–423.

98. Beninati W, Derdak S, Dixon PF, Grider DJ, Strollo DC, Hensley RF, Lucey DR. Pulmonary eosinophils express HLA-DR in chronic eosinophilic pneumonia. J Allergy Clin Immunol 1993; 92:442–449.

99. Roberts RL, Ank BJ, Salusky IB, Stiehm ER. Purification and properties of peritoneal eosinophils from pediatric dialysis patients. J Immunol Methods 1990; 126:205–211.

100. Del Pozo V, De Andres B, Martin E, Cardaba B, Fernandez JC, Gallardo S, Tramon P, Leyva-Cobian F, Palomino P, Lahoz C. Eosinophil as antigen-presenting cell: activation of T cell clones and T cell hybridoma by eosinophils after antigen processing. Eur J Immunol 1992; 22:1919–1925.

101. Weller PF, Rand TH, Barrett T, Elovic A, Wong DTW, Finberg RW. Accessory cell function and human eosinophils. J Immunol 1993; 150:2554–2562.

102. Lundahl J, Haliden G, Hed J. Differences in intracellular pool and receptor-dependent mobilization of the adhesion-promoting glycoprotein Mac-1 between eosinophils and neutrophils. J Leukoc Biol 1993; 53:336–341.

103. Subramanian N. Leukotriene B_4 induced steady state calcium rise and superoxide anion generation in guinea pig eosinophils are not related events. Biochem Biophys Res Commun 1992; 187:670–676.

104. Morland CM, Wilson SJ, Holgate ST, Roche WR. Selective eosinophil leukocyte recruitment by transendothelial migration and not by leukocyte–endothelial cell adhesion. Am J Respir Cell Mol Biol 1992; 6:557–566.

105. Wardlaw AJ, Moqbel R, Cromwell O, Kay AB. Platelet-activating factor: a potent chemotactic and chemokinetic factor for human eosinophils. J Clin Invest 1986; 78:1701–1706.

106. Tamura N, Agrawal DK, Townley RG. Leukotriene C_4 production from human eosinophils in vitro: role of eosinophil chemotactic factors on eosinophil activation. J Immunol 1988; 141:4291–4297.

107. Kroegel C, Warner JA, Giembycz MA, Matthys H, Lichtenstein LM, Barnes PJ. Dual trans-membrane signalling mechanisms in eosinophils: evidence for two functionally distinct receptors for platelet activating factor. Int Arch Allergy Immunol 1992; 99:226–229.

108. Walsh GM, Wardlaw AJ, Hartnell A, Sanderson CJ, Kay AB. Interleukin-5 enhances the in vitro adhesion of human eosinophils, but not neutrophils, in a luecocyte integrin (CD11/18)-dependent manner. Int Arch Allergy Appl Immunol 1991; 94:174–178.

109. Koenderman L, Tool ATJ, Roos D, Verhoeven AJ. Priming of the respiratory burst in human eosinophils is accompanied by changes in signal transduction. J Immunol 1990; 145:3883–3888.

110. Cromwell O, Bennett JP, Hide I, Kay AB, Gomperts BD. Mechanisms of granule enzyme secretion from permeabilized guinea pig eosinophils. J Immunol 1991; 147:1905–1911.

111. Aizawa T, Kakuta Y, Yamauchi K, Ohkawara Y, Maruyama N, Nitta Y, Tamura G, Sasaki H, Takishima T. Induction of granule release by intracellular application of calcium and guanosine-5'-O-(3-thiotriphosphate) in human eosinophils. J Allergy Clin Immunol 1992; 90:789–795.

112. Monteiro RC, Hostoffer RW, Cooper MD, Bonner JR, Gartland GL, Kubagawa H. Definition of immunoglobulin A receptors on eosinophils and their enhanced expression in allergic individuals. J Clin Invest 1993; 92:1681–1685.

113. Dubucquoi S, Desreumaux P, Janin A, Klein O, Goldman M, Tavernier J, Capron A, Capron M. Interleukin 5 synthesis of eosinophils: association with granules and immunoglobulin-dependent secretion. J Exp Med 1994; 179:703–708.

114. Abu-Ghazaleh RE, Fujisawa T, Mestecky J, Kyle RA, Gleich GJ. IgA-induced degranulation. J Immunol 1989; 142:2393–2400.

115. Miyajima A, Kitamura T, Harada N, Yokota T, Arai K. Cytokine receptors and signal transduction. Annu Rev Immunol 1992; 10:295–331.

116. Migita M, Yamaguchi N, Mita S, Higuchi S, Hitoshi Y, Yoshida Y, Tomonaga M, Matsuda I, Tominaga A, Takatsu K. Characterization of the human IL-5 receptors on eosinophils. Cell Immunol 1991; 133:484–497.

117. Fabian I, Kletter Y, Mor S, Geller-Bernstein C, Ben-Yaakov M, Volovitz B, Golde DW. Activation of human eosinophil and neutrophil functions by haematopoietic growth factors: comparisons of IL-1, IL-3, IL-5 and GM-CSF. Br J Haematol 1992; 80:137–143.

118. Tai P-C, Sun L, Spry CJF. Effects of IL-5, granulocyte/macrophage colony-stimulating factor (GM-CSF) and IL-3 on the survival of human blood eosinophils in vitro. Clin Exp Immunol 1991; 85:312–316.

119. Wang JM, Rambaldi A, Biondi A, Chen ZG, Sanderson CJ, Mantovani A. Recombinant human interleukin 5 is a selective eosinophil chemoattractant. Eur J Immunol 1989; 19:701–705.

120. Sanderson CJ. The biological role of interleukin 5. Int J Cell Cloning 1990; 8(suppl 1):147–153.

121. Lopez AF, Sanderson CJ, Gamble JR, Campbell HD, Young IG, Vadas MA. Recombinant human interleukin 5 is a selective activator of human eosinophil function. J Exp Med 1988; 167:219–224.

122. Terada N, Konno A, Natori T, Tada H, Togawa K. Interleukin-5 preferentially recruits eosinophils from vessels in nasal mucosa. Acta Otolaryngol Suppl 1993; 506:57–60.

123. Okudaira H, Nogami M, Matsuzaki G, Dohi M, Suko M, Kasuya S, Takatsu K. T-cell-dependent accumulation of eosinophils in the lung and its inhibition by monoclonal anti-interleukin-5. Int Arch Allergy Appl Immunol 1991; 94:171–173.

124. Van Oosterhout AJM, Ladenius ARC, Savelkoul HFJ, Van Ark I, Delsman KC, Nijkamp FP. Effect on anti-IL-5 and IL-5 on airway hyperreactivity and eosinophils in guinea pigs. Am Rev Respir Dis 1993; 147:548–552.

125. Van Oosterhout AJM, Ladenius ARC, Savelkoul HFJ, Van Ark I, Nijkamp FP. Anti-IL-5 inhibits airway hyperresponsiveness and eosinophilia in chronic ovalbumin exposed guinea pigs. Am Rev Respir Dis 1993; 147:A1013.

126. Quan SF,Sedgwick JB, Nelson MV, Busse WW. Corticosteroid resistance in eosinophilic gastritis-relation to in vitro eosinophil survival and interleukin 5. Ann Allergy 1993; 70: 256–260.

127. Butterfield JH, Leiferman KM, Abrams J, Silver JE, Bower J, Gonchoroff N, Gleich GJ. Elevated serum levels of interleukin-5 in patients with the syndrome of episodic angioedema and eosinophilia. Blood 1992; 79:688–692.

128. Sedgwick JB, Quan SF, Calhoun WJ, Busse WW. Effect of interleukin-5 and granulocyte macrophage colony stimulating factor: comparison with airway eosinophils. J Allergy Clin Immunol 1995; 96:375–85.

129. Laudanna C, Melotti P, Bonizzato C, Piacenttini G, Boner A, Serra MC, Berton G. Ligation of members of the β1 or the β2 subfamilies of integrins by antibodies triggers eosinophil respiratory burst and spreading. Immunology 1993; 80:273–280.

130. Charlesworth EN, Kagey-Sobotka A, Schleimer RP, Norman PS, Lichtenstein LM. Prednisone inhibits the appearance of inflammatory mediators and the influx of eosinophils and basophils associated with the cutaneous late-phase response to allergen. J Immunol 1991; 146:671–676.

131. DeMonchy JGR, Kauffman HF, Venge P, Koeter GH, Jansen HK, Sluiter HJ, DeVries K. Bronchoalveolar eosinophilia during allergen-induced late asthmatic reactions. Am Rev Respir Dis 1985; 131:373–376.

132. Liu MC, Hubbard WC, Proud D, Stealey B, Galli S, Kagey-Sobotka A, Bleecker ER, Lichtenstein LM. Immediate and late inflammatory responses to ragweed antigen challenge of the peripheral airways in asthmatics: cellular, mediator, and permeability changes. Am Rev Respir Dis 1991; 144:51–58.

133. Schleimer RP. Glucocorticosteroids: their mechanisms of acton and use in allergic diseases. In: Middleton EJ, Reed CE, Ellis EF, Adkinson NFJ, Yunginger JW, eds. Allergy: Principles and Practice. St Louis: CV Mosby, 1988:739–765.

134. Schleimer RP, Kaiser J, Tomioka K, Ebisawa M, Bochner BS. Studies on the mechanisms by which glucocorticoids inhibit tissue eosinophilia in allergic reactions. Int Arch Allergy Immunol 1992; 99:289–294.

135. Kellgren JH, Janus O. The eosinopenic response to cortisone and ACTH in normal subjects. Br Med J 1951; 2:1183–1187.

136. Dunsky EH, Zweiman B, Fischler E, Levy DA. Early effects of corticosteroids on basophils, leukocyte histamine and tissue histamine. J Allergy Clin Immunol 1979; 64:426–432.

137. Beeson PB, Bass DA. Mechanisms of accelerated eosinophil production. In: Beeson PA, Bass DA, eds. The Eosinophil. (Major Problems in Internal Medicine Series (vol 14). Philadelphia: WB Saunders, 1977:79–89.

138. Butterfield JH, Gleich GJ. In: Schleimer RP, Claman HW, Oronsky A, eds. Anti-inflammatory Steroid Action: Basic and Clinical Aspects. London: Academic Press, 1989:151–197.

139. Evans PM, O'Conner BJ, Fuller RW, Barnes PJ, Chung KF. Effect of inhaled corticosteroids on peripheral blood eosinophil counts and density profiles in asthma. J Allergy Clin Immunol 1993; 91:643–650.

140. Butterfield MDJH, Ackerman SJ, Weiler MS, Eisenbrey AB, Gleich GJ. Effects of glucocorticoids on eosinophil colony growth. J Allergy Clin Immunol 1986; 78:450–457.

141. Gibson PG, Dolovich J, Girgis-Gabardo A, Morris MM, Anderson M, Hargreave FE, Denburg JA. The inflammatory response in asthma exacerbation: changes in circulating eosinophils, basophils, and their progenitors. Clin Exp Allergy 1990; 20:661–668.

142. Ebsworth KJ, Lawrence CE, DeBrito FB. Glucocorticoids inhibit interleukin-5 induced maturation of eosinophils. Clin Exp Allergy 1992; 22:125.

143. Lamas AM, Marcotte GV, Schleimer RP. Human endothelial cells prolong eosinophil survival. Regulation by cytokines and glucocorticoids. J Immunol 1989; 142:3978–3984.

144. Lamas AM, Leon OG, Schleimer RP. Glucocorticoids inhibit eosinophil responses to granulocyte-macrophage colony-stimulating factor. J Immunol 1991; 147:254–259.

145. Wallen N, Kita H, Weiler D, Gleich GJ. Glucocorticoids inhibit cytokine-mediated eosinophil survival. J Immunol 1991; 147:3490–3495.

146. Hallsworth MP, Litchfield TM, Lee TH. Glucocorticoids inhibit granulocyte–macrophage colony-stimulating factor-1 and interleukin-5 enhanced in vitro survival of human eosinophils. Immunology 1992; 75:382–385.

147. Peterson AP, Altman LC, Hill JS, Gosney K, Kadin ME. Glucocorticoid receptors in normal human eosinophils: comparison with neutrophils. J Allergy Clin Immunol 1981; 68:212–217.

148. Schleimer RP. Effects of glucocorticoids on inflammatory cells relevant to their therapeutic applications in asthma. Am Rev Respir Dis 1992; 141:S59–S69.

149. Altman LC, Hill JS, Hairfield WM, Mullarkey MF. Effects of corticosteroids on eosinophil chemotaxis and adherence. J Clin Invest 1981; 67:28–36.

150. Håkansson L, Carlson M, Stålenheim G, Venge P. Migratory responses of eosinophil and neutrophil granulocytes from patients with asthma. J Allergy Clin Immunol 1990; 85:743–750.

151. Bisgaard H, Gronborg H, Mygind N, Dahl R, Lindqvist N, Venge P. Allergen-induced increase of eosinophil cationic protein in nasal lavage fluid: effect of the glucocorticoid budesonide. J Allergy Clin Immunol 1990; 85:891–895.

152. Klementsson W, Svensson C, Andersson M, Venge P, Pipkorn U, Persson CG. Eosinophils, secretory responsiveness and glucocorticoid-induced effects on the nasal mucosa during a weak pollen season. Clin Exp Allergy 1991; 21:705–710.

153. Kaiser J, Bickel CA, Bochner BS, Schleimer RP. T he effects of the potent glucocorticoid budesonide on adhesion of eosinophils to human vascular endothelial cells and on endothelial expression of adhesion molecules. J Pharmacol Exp Ther 1993; 267:245–249.

154. Kita H, Abu-Ghazaleh R, Sanderson CJ, Gleich GJ. Effect of steroids on immunoglobulin-induced eosinophil degranulation. J Allergy Clin Immunol 1991; 87:70–77.

155. Silberstein DS, Austen KF, Owen WF. Hematopoietins for eosinophils. Glycoprotein hormones that regulate the development of inflammation in eosinophilia-associated disease. Hematol Oncol Clin North Am 1989; 3:511–533.

156. Wein M, Bochner BS. Adhesion molecule antagonists: future therapies for allergic disease? Eur Respir J 1994; 6:1239–1242.

157. Rolfe FG, Hughes JM, Armour CL, Sewell WA. Inhibition of interleukin-5 gene expression by dexamethasone. Immunology 1992; 77:494–499.

158. Hughes JM, Rolfe FG, Sewell WA, Black JL, Armour CL. Corticosteroid inhibition of interleukin-5 expression in peripheral blood mononuclear cells. Immunology 1992; 77:494–499.

159. Mirza S, DeBrito FB. Cyclosporin A and FK-506 inhibit cytokine secretion from T-helper-2 lymphocytes. Clin Exp Immunol 1992; 22:125.

160. Culpepper JA, Lee F. Regulation of IL-3 expression by glucocorticoids in cloned murine T lymphocytes. J Immunol 1985; 135:3191–3197.

161. DeBrito FB, Lawrence CE, Karlsson J-A. The role of cytokines in eosinophilia and modulatory effects of glucocorticoids. In: Jolles G, Karlsson J-A, Taylor J, eds. T-Lymphocytes and Inflammatory Cell Research in Asthma. New York: Academic Press, 1993:167–191.

162. Thornhill MH, Haskard DO. IL-4 regulates endothelial cell activation by IL-1, tumor necrosis factor, or IFN-γ. J Immunol 1990; 145:865–872.

163. Masinovsky B, Urdal D, Gallatin WM. IL-4 acts synergistically with IL-1β to promote lymphocyte adhesion to microvascular endothelium by induction of vascular cell adhesion molecule-1. J Immunol 1990; 145:2886–2895.

164. Kyan-Aung U, Haskard DO, Poston RN, Thornhill MH, Lee TH. Endothelial leukocyte adhesion molecule-1 and intercellular adhesion molecule-1 mediate the adhesion of eosinophils to endothelial cells in vitro and are expressed by endothelium in allergic cutaneous inflammation in vivo. J Immunol 1991; 146:521–528.

165. Woolcock AJ, Salome CM, Keena VA. Therapy for bronchial hyperreactivity. Reducing the severity of bronchial hyperresponsiveness. Am Rev Respir Dis 1991; 143:S75–S77.

166. Brogden RN, Sorkin EM. Nedocromil sodium: an updated review of its pharmacological properties and therapeutic efficacy in asthma. Drugs 1993; 45:693–715.

167. Richards R, Phillips GD, Holgate ST. Nedocromil sodium is more potent than sodium cromoglycate against AMP-induced bronchoconstriction in atopic asthmatic subjects. Clin Exp Immunol 1989; 19:285–291.

168. Wells E, Jackson GG, Harper ST, Mann J, Eady RP. Characterisation of primate bronchoalveolar mast cells. II. Inhibition of histamine, LTC_4 and PGD_2 release from primate bronchoalveolar mast cells and a comparison with rat peritoneal mast cells. J Immunol 1986; 127:3941–3945.

169. Crimi E, Brusasco V, Crimi P. Effect of nedocromil sodium on the late asthmatic reaction to bronchial antigen challenge. J Allergy Clin Immunol 1989; 83:985–990.

170. Twentyman OP, Sams VR, Holgate ST. Albuterol and nedocromil sodium affect airway and leukocyte responses to allergen. Am Rev Respir Dis 1993; 147:1425–1430.

171. Speelberg B, Verhoeff NPLG, van den Berg NJ, Oosthoek CHA, van Herwaarden CLA, Bruijnzeel PLB. Nedocromil sodium inhibits the early and late asthmatic response to exercise. Eur Respir J 1992; 5:430–437.

172. Pretolani M, Lefort J, Silva P, Malachere E, Dumarey C, Bachelet M, Vargaftig BB. Protection by nedocromil sodium of active immunization-induced bronchopulmonary alterations in the guinea pig. Am Rev Respir Dis 1990; 141:1259–1265.

173. Hutson PA, Holgate ST, Church MK. Effect of cromolyn sodium and albuterol on early and late phase bronchoconstriction and airway leukocyte infiltration after allergen challenge of non-anesthetized guinea pigs. Am Rev Respir Dis 1988; 138:1157–1163.

174. Church MK, Hutson PA, Holgate ST. Effect of nedocromil sodium on early and late responses to allergen challenge on the guinea pigs. Drugs 1989; 37:101–108.

175. Abraham WM. Effect of nedocromil sodium on antigen-induced airway responses in allergic sheep. Drugs 1989; 37(suppl 1):78–86.

176. Schellenberg RR, Ishida K, Thomson RJ. Nedocromil sodium inhibits airway hyperresponsiveness an eosinophilic infiltration induced by repeated antigen challenge in guinea pigs. Br J Pharmacol 1991; 103:1842–1846.

177. Bruijnzeel PLB, Warringa RAJ, Kok PTM, Kreukniet J. Inhibition of neutrophil and eosinophil induced chemotaxis by nedocromil sodium and sodium cromoglycate. Br J Pharmacol 1990; 99:798–802.

178. Pretolani M, Lefort J, Vargaftig BB. Inhibition by nedocromil sodium of recombinant human interleukin-5 induced lung hyperresponsiveness to platelet activating factor in actively sensitized guinea pigs. J Allergy Clin Immunol 1993; 91:809–816.

179. Moqbel R, Cromwell O, Walsh GM, Wardlaw AJ, Kurlak L, Kay AB. Effects of nedocromil sodium (Tilade) on the activation of human eosinophils and neutrophils and the release of histamine from mast cells. Allergy 1988; 43:268–276.

180. Moqbel R, Cromwell O, Kay AB. The effect of nedocromil sodium on human eosinophil activation. Drugs 1989; 37(suppl 1):19–22.

181. Sedgwick JB, Bjornsdottir U, Geiger KM, Busse WW. Inhibition of eosinophil density change and leukotriene C_4 generation by nedocromil sodium. J Allergy Clin Immunol 1992; 90:202–209.

182. Davalia JL, Sapsford RJ, Rusznak C, Davies RJ. The effect of human eosinophils on cultured human nasal epithelial cell activity and the influence of nedocromil sodium in vitro. Am J Respir Cell Mol Biol 1992; 7:270–277.

183. Warringa RAJ, Mengelers HJJ, Koenderman L, Maikoe T, Bruijnzeel PLB. Inhibition of cytokine-primed eosinophil chemotaxis by nedocromil sodium. J Allergy Clin Immunol 1993; 91:802–809.

184. Bruijnzeel PL, Warringa RA, Kok PT, Hamelink ML, Kreukniet H, Koenderman L. Effects of nedocromil sodium on in vitro induced migration, activation, and mediator release from human granulocytes. J Allergy Clin Immunol 1993; 92:159–164.

185. Burke LA, Crea AEG, Wilkinson JRW, Arm JP, Spur BW, Lee TH. Comparison of the generation of platelet-activating factor and leukotriene C_4 in human eosinophils stimulated by unopsonized zymosan and by the calcium ionophore A23187: the effects of nedocromil sodium. J Allergy Clin Immunol 1990; 85:26–35.

186. Bruijnzeel PLB, Hamelink ML, Kok PTM, Kreukniet J. Nedocromil sodium inhibits the A23187- and opsonized zymosan-induced leukotriene formation by human eosinophils but not by human neutrophils. Br J Pharmacol 1989; 96:631–636.

187. Rubin RP, Thompson RH, Naps MS. Differential inhibition by nedocromil sodium of superoxide generation elicited by platelet activating factor in human neutrophils. Agents Actions 1990; 31:237–242.

188. Rand TH, Lopez AF, Gamble JR, Vadas MA. Nedocromil sodium and cromolyn (sodium cromoglycate) selectively inhibit antibody-dependent granulocyte-mediated cytoxicity. Int Arch Allergy Appl Immunol 1988; 87:151–158.

189. Yukawa T, Ukena D, Kroegel C, Chanez P, Dent G, Chung KF, Barnes PJ. β_2-adrenergic receptors on eosinophils. Binding and functional studies. Am Rev Respir Dis 1990; 141:1446–1452.

190. Masuyama K, Ishikawa T. Direct interaction of guinea pig eosinophils and adrenergic agents. Int Arch Allergy Appl Immunol 1985; 78:243–248.

191. Rabe KF, Giembycz MA, Dent G, Perkins RS, Evans P, Barnes PJ. Salmeterol is a competitive antagonist at β-adrenoceptors mediating inhibition of respiratory burst in guinea-pig eosinophils. Eur J Pharmacol 1993; 231:305–308.

192. Okada C, Sugiyama H, Eda R, Miyagawa H, Hopp RJ, Bewtra AK, Townley RG. Effect of formoterol on superoxide anion generation from bronchoalveolar lavage cells after antigen challenge in guinea pigs. Am J Respir Cell Mol Biol 1993; 8:509–517.

193. Eda R, Sugiyama H, Hopp RJ, Okada C, Bewtra AK, Townley RG. Inhibitory effects of formoterol on platelet-activating factor induced eosinophil chemotaxis and degranulation. Int Arch Allergy Immunol 1993; 102:391–398.

194. Fugner A. Formation of oedema and accumulation of eosinophils in the guinea pig lung. Int Arch Allergy Appl Immunol 1989; 88:225–227.

195. Sanjar S, McCabe PJ, Reynolds LH, Johnson M. Salmeterol inhibits antigen-induced eosinophil accumulation in the guinea pig lung. Fundam Clin Pharmacol 1991; 5:402.

196. Rafferty P. Antihistamines in the treatment of clinical asthma. J Allergy Clin Immunol 1990; 86:647–650.

197. Townley RG. Antiallergic properties of the second-generation H_1 antihistamines during the early and late reactions to antigen. J Allergy Clin Immunol 1992; 90:720–725.

198. Campoli-Richards DM, Buchley MM, Fitton A, Cetirizine. A review of its pharmacological properties and clinical potential in allergic rhinitis, pollen-induced asthma, and chronic urticaria. Drugs 1990; 40:762–781.

199. Fadel R, Herpin-Richard N, Henocq E. Inhibitory effect of cetirizine on eosinophil migration in vivo. Clin Allergy 1987; 17:373–379.

200. Fadel R, David B, Herpin-Richard N, Borgnon A, Rassemont R, Rihoux JP. In vivo effects of cetirizine on cutaneous reactivity and eosinophil migration induced by platelet-activating factor (PAF-acether) in man. J Allergy Clin Immunol 1990; 86:314–320.

201. Townley RG, Okada C. Use of cetirizine to investigate non-H_1 effects of second generation antihistamines. Ann Allergy 1992; 68:190–196.

202. De Vos C, Joseph M, Leprovost C, Vorng H, Tomassini M, Capron M. Inhibition of human eosinophil chemotaxis and of the IgE-dependent stimulation of human blood platelets by cetirizine. Int Arch Allergy Appl Immunol 1989; 88:212–215.

203. Rédier H, Chanez P, De Vos C, Rifai N, Clauzel A, Michel FB, Godard P. Inhibitory effect of cetirizine on the bronchial eosinophil recruitment induced by allergen inhalation challenge in allergic patients with asthma. J Allergy Clin Immunol 1992; 90:215–224.

204. Martins MA, Pasquale CP, Silva PM, Pires AL, Ruffie C, Rihoux JP, Cordeiro RS, Vargaftig BB. Interference of cetirizine with the late eosinophil accumulation induced by either PAF or compound 48/80. Br J Pharmacol 1992; 105:176–180.

205. Snyman JR, Sommers DK, Gregorowski MD, Boraine H. Effect of cetirizine, ketotifen and chloropheniramine on the dynamics of the cutaneous hypersensitivity reaction: a comparative study. Eur J Clin Pharmacol 1992; 42:359–362.

206. Kyan-Aung U, Hallsworth M, Haskard D, De Vos C, Lee TH. The effects of cetirizine on the adhesion of human eosinophils and neutrophils to cultured human umbilical vein endothelial cells. J Allergy Clin Immunol 1992; 90:270–272.

207. McGarrity ST, Stephenson AH, Webster RO. Regulation of human neutrophil functions by adenine nucleotides. J Immunol 1989; 142:1986–1994.

208. Meltzer S, Goldberg B, Lad P, Easton J. Superoxide generation and its modulation by adenosine in the neutrophils of subjects with asthma. J Allergy Clin Immunol 1989; 83:960–966.

209. Cronstein BN, Levin RI, Belanoff J, Weissmann G, Hirschhorn R. Adenosine: an endogenous inhibitor of neutrophil-mediated injury to endothelial cells. J Clin Invest 1985; 78:760–770.

210. Richter J. Effect of adenosine analogues and cAMP-raising agents on TNF-, GM-CSF-, and chemotactic peptide-induced degranulation in single adherent neutrophils. J Leukoc Biol 1992; 51:270–275.

211. Rose FR, Hirschhorn R, Weissmann G, Cronstein BN. Adenosine promotes neutrophil chemotaxis. J Exp Med 1988; 167:1186–1194.

212. Burkey TH, Webster RO. Adenosine inhibits fMLP-stimulated adherence and superoxide anion generation by human neutrophils at an early step in signal transduction. Biochim Biophys Act 1993; 1175:312–318.

213. Dent G, Giembycz MA, Rabe KF, Barnes PJ. Inhibition of guinea pig eosinophil cyclic nucleotide PDE activity and opsonized zymosan-stimulated respiratory burst by "type IV"-selective PDE inhibitors. Br J Pharmacol 1991; 103:1339–1346.

214. Souness JE, Carter CM, Diocee BK, Hassall GA, Wood LJ, Turner NC. Characterization of guinea pig eosinophil phosphodiesterase activity. Assessment of its involvement in regulating superoxide generation. Biochem Pharmacol 1991; 42:937–945.

215. Giembycz MA, Dent G. Prospects for selective cyclic nucleotide phosphodiesterase inhibitors in the treatment of bronchial asthma. Clin Exp Allergy 1992; 22:337–344.

216. Schudt C, Winder S, Eltze M, Kilian U, Beume R. Zardaverine: a cyclic AMP specific PDE III/IV inhibitor. Agents Actions Suppl 1991; 34:379–402.

217. Sanjar S, Aoki S, Boubeckeur K, Chapman ID, Smith D, Kings MA, Morley J. Eosinophil accumulation in pulmonary airways of guinea pigs induced by exposure to an aerosol of platelet activating factor: effect of anti-asthma drugs. Br J Pharmacol 1990; 99:267–272.

218. Sanjar S, Aoki S, Kristersson A, Smith D, Morley J. Antigen challenge induces pulmonary airway eosinophil accumulation and airway hyperreactivity in sensitized guinea pigs: the effect of anti-asthma drugs. Br J Pharmacol 1990; 99:679–686.

219. Underwood DC, Osborn RR, Novak LB, Matthews JK, Newsholme SJ, Undem BJ, Hand JM, Torphy TJ. Inhibition of antigen-induced bronchoconstriction and eosinophil infiltration in the guinea pig by the cyclic AMP-specific phosphodiesterase inhibitor, rolipram. J Pharmacol Exp Ther 1993; 266:306–313.

220. Newsholme SJ, Schwartz L. cAMP-specific phosphodiesterase inhibitor, rolipram, reduces eosinophil infiltration evoked by leukotrienes or by histamine in guinea pig conjunctiva. Inflammation 1993; 17:25–31.

221. Siflinger-Birnboim A, Bode DC, Malik AB. Adenosine 3′,5′-cyclic monophosphate attenuates neutrophi-mediated increase in endothelial permeability. Am J Physiol 1993; 264:370–375.
222. Schmeichel CJ. Methylxanthine bronchodilators potentiate multiple human neutrophil functions. J Immunol 1987; 138:1896–1903.
223. Rak S, Håkanson L, Venge P. Immunotherapy abrogates the generation of eosinophil and neutrophil chemotactic activity during pollen season. J Allergy Clin Immunol 1990; 86:706–713.
224. Rak S, Bjornson A, Håkanson L, Sorenson S, Venge P. The effect of immunotherapy on eosinophil accumulation and production of eosinophil chemotactic activity in the lung of subjects with asthma during natural pollen exposure. J Allergy Clin Immunol 1991; 88: 878–888.
225. Furin MJ, Norman PS, Creticos PS, Proud D, Kagey-Sobotka A, Lichtenstein LM, Naclerio RM. Immunotherapy decreased antigen-induced eosinophil cell migration into the nasal cavity. J Allergy Clin Immunol 1991; 88:27–32.
226. Churchill L, Gundel RH, Letts G, Wegner CD. Contribution of specific cell-adhesive glycoproteins to airway and alveolar inflammation and dysfunction. Am Rev Respir Dis 1993; 148: 583–587.
227. Wegner CD, Gundel RH, Reilly P, Haynes N, Letts LG, Rothlein R. Intercellular adhesion molecule-1 (ICAM-1) in the pathogenesis of asthma. Science 1990; 247:456–459.
228. Mauser PJ, Pitman A, Witt A, Fernandez X, Zurcher J, Kung T, Jones H, Watnick AS, Egan RW, Kreutner W, Adams GK III. Inhibitory effect of the TRFK-5 anti IL-5 antibody in a guinea pig model of asthma. Am Rev Respir Dis 1993; 148:1623–1627.
229. Roberts RL, Ank BJ, Stiehm ER. Human eosinophils are more toxic than neutrophils in antibody-independent killing. J Allergy Clin Immunol 1991; 87:1105–1115.
230. Walker C, Virchow JC, Bruijnzeel PLB, Blaser K. T cells and asthma. Int Arch Allergy Appl Immunol 1991; 94:248–250.
231. Kay AB. T lymphocytes and their products in atopic asthma. Int Arch Allergy Appl Immunol 1991; 94:189–193.
232. Nakajima H, Iwamoto I, Yoshida S. Aerolized recombinant interferon-γ prevents antigen-induced eosinophil recruitment on mouse trachea. Am Rev Respir Dis 1993; 148:1102–1104.
233. Kita H, Ohnishi T, Okubo Y, Weiler D, Abrams JS, Gleich GJ. Granulocyte/macrophage colony-stimulating factor and interleukin 3 release from human peripheral blood eosinophils and neutrophils. J Exp Med 1991; 174:745–748.
234. Moqbel R, Hamid Q, Ying S, Barkans J, Hartnell A, Tsicopoulos A, Wardlaw AJ, Kay AB. Expression of mRNA and immunoreactivity for the granulocyte/macrophage colony-stimulating factor in activated human eosinophils. J Exp Med 1991; 174:749–752.
235. Melani C, Mattia GF, Silvani A, Care A, Rivoltini L, Parmiani G, Colombo MP. Interleukin-6 expression in human neutrophil and eosinophil peripheral blood granulocytes. Blood 1993; 81:2744–2749.
236. Braun RK, Franchini M, Erard F, Ribs S, De Vries IJM, Blaser K, Hansel TT, Walker C. Human peripheral blood eosinophils produce and release interleukin-8 on stimulation with calcium ionophore. Eur J Immunol 1993; 23:956–960.
237. Thorne KJI, Richardson BA, Taverne J, Williamson DJ, Vadas MA, Butterworth AE. A comparison of eosinophil-activating factor (EAF) with other monokines and lymphokines. Eur J Immunol 1986; 16:1143–1149.
238. Redington AE, Djukanovic R, Howarth P, Holgate ST. Transforming growth factor β is localized to eosinophils in bronchial biopsies from asthmatics. Am Rev Respir Dis 1993; 147:A785.

11

Monocytes and Macrophages in Asthma

Jean Bousquet, Pascal Chanez, Bernard Arnoux, François-Bernard Michel, and Philippe Godard
INSERM, Hopital Arnaud de Villeneuve, Montpellier, France

A. Maurizio Vignola
Istituto di Fisiopatologia Respiratoria, Palermo, Italy

Marcelle Damon
INSERM, Montpellier, France

INTRODUCTION

The mononuclear phagocyte system consists of a migratory, specialized family of cells, derived from hematopoietic precursors, that circulate in blood as monocytes and are widely distributed as macrophages in tissues and body fluids. Mononuclear phagocytes have always been the scavenger cells of the body. Although this traditional role remains critical, it became evident after 1970 that these cells had a much wider function in biology and pathology. By virtue of their specialized plasma membrane receptors and versatile biosynthetic and secretory responses, macrophages play a major role in inflammation, in repair, and in specific immunity, by their accessory cell function.

Airway macrophages are among the cells involved in the chronic inflammatory processes underlying bronchial asthma. Alveolar macrophages obtained by bronchoalveolar lavage (BAL) from asthmatic patients differ functionally and metabolically from those obtained from healthy subjects and are in an activated stage or postactivated stage. In bronchial biopsies, the number of macrophages is significantly increased in asthmatic patients, and these cells are activated. However, the exact role of airway macrophages is still incompletely understood.

CELLS OF THE MONOCYTE–MACROPHAGE LINEAGE

Cell Lineage

In adult life, monocytes are formed only in the bone marrow. The most immature cell of the mononuclear cell line is the monoblast, derived from the granulocyte–monocyte progenitor cell (1). The production and maturation of monocytes in vivo is controlled by interleukin (IL)-3, granulocyte–macrophage colony-stimulating factor (GM-CSF), and M-CSF, which stimulate the production of monocytes, and by prostaglandin (PG)E$_2$ and interferon

(IFN)-α/β, which are inhibitory mediators. Monocytes enter the circulation within 24 h of their formation and are then distributed over a circulating pool and a marginating pool. The latter cells are localized close to the endothelium and are ready to migrate from the vessels to tissue to become macrophages (2). The movement of monocytes from the blood circulation into sites of inflammation requires cooperative interactions between signaling and adhesion molecules. Selectins mediate the initial rolling contacts of monocytes with the endothelium. Following monocyte activation, integrins (intracellular adhesion molecules; ICAMs) strengthen adhesion and then direct migration beneath the endothelium as well as their activation. Unique combinations of signaling and adhesion molecules regulate the subsets of monocytes that are recruited into specific tissues (3,4).

The origin of tissue macrophages, however, is more complex (5). Animal studies, using steady-state conditions, suggest that most macrophages derive from monocytes that have migrated to tissues and differentiated. However, a smaller population of macrophages apparently derive from locally dividing cells (6–8). During inflammation, the number of DNA-synthesizing macrophages undergoes a transient rise (9), indicating a temporary rise in the local production of macrophages, although the share taken by local production is relatively small (10).

Monocytes and macrophages show heterogeneity in morphology, cytochemistry, expression of surface markers, and metabolic activity (11,12). Different subsets of macrophages have been identified.

Pulmonary Macrophages

In the past, lung macrophages were usually equated with alveolar macrophages (AM). However, in the lung, macrophages are present in the bronchi (13), alveoli, connective tissue (14), and capillaries (15). Bronchial macrophages are found from the large to the small airways in the connective tissue of submucosa, between epithelial cells, and in the mucus. Cells recovered by BAL are called AM and originate from the alveoli and the surface of the bronchi. They should be distinguished from macrophages present in the pulmonary interstitium, which represent immediate precursors of AM (16). Connective tissue macrophages represent a large population of cells approximating, equaling, or exceeding, the number of AM. They increase in number during inflammation (17). It is interstitial macrophages—not AM—that are in direct contact with extracellular matrix (ECM), and the metabolic effects of these macrophages may have a greater effect than those released by their sisters in the airspaces. Pulmonary intravascular macrophages are not simply adherent monocytes (18). They are large and mature macrophages that reside in the pulmonary capillaries. Scavenging activity appears to be their main function (19).

The alveolar macrophages are of bone marrow origin (20,21). Moreover, a local replication of macrophages appears to exist in the human lung. In sarcoidosis, pulmonary fibrosis, and to a lesser extent, in smokers, AM display an enhanced mitotic activity, and an increased number of cells were found to be in the $G_2 + M$ phase of the cell cycle (22,23).

Little is known about the fate of macrophages. Lung macrophages leave the body through the airways or migrate to local lymph nodes where they are likely to die (1). The lifespan of AM appears to be about 150–180 days.

Function of Macrophages

Mononuclear phagocytes are ubiquitous cells involved in all phases of inflammation and the healing following the inflammatory response (24). They have always been known as the scavenger cells of the body since the time of Metchnikoff, in 1900 (25). In inflammation they are very abundant after the very early stage, when they phagocytose and digest foreign particles, debris from injured red cells, proteins that have leaked out, and even their predecessors, the neutrophils, after the latter have finished their own job of their ingestion. Macrophages, however, have much wider functions in biology and pathology (26). They have the fundamental role in specific immunity through a relationship within lymphocytes (27) and possess wide metabolic properties (28). Tissue macrophages present a very large number of functions, which are dependent on their microenvironment, state of activation, and differentiation, that make them very versatile (29).

Activated macrophages have the potential to secrete a wide variety of products, many of which are active in inflammation. The spectrum of biological activities induced is phenomenal for a single cell (26,30,31). Furthermore, the versatility of the macrophage is such that secretions of their products can be regulated (increased or decreased) by interactions between the cells and their environment; other cells; extracellular matrix (ECM) components, such as fibronectin and serum (complement); as well as exogenous agents. Thus, macrophages may become "deactivated" favoring the resolution of the inflammatory response. One of the known deactivators is transforming growth factor (TGF)-β.

Among the important classes of macrophage products are the following (26,30):

Proteases, such as collagenase and elastase, which degrade connective tissue components and plasminogen activator

Chemotactic factors for other lymphocytes

Both cyclooxygenase and lipoxygenase products of arachidonic acid

Reactive oxygen metabolites

Complement components of both pathways

Coagulation factors, such as factor V and thromboplastin

Growth-promoting factors for fibroblasts, blood vessels, and myeloid progenitor cells, including platelet-derived growth factor (PDGF) and TGFs

Cytokines, such as IL-1, tissue necrosis factor (TNF), IL-6, GM-CSF, IL-8, IL-10, macrophage inflammatory factor (MIP)-1, and others

Other biologically active agents that cause inflammation platelet-activating factor (PAF-acether) or have antiviral activity (interferons).

Although many of these factors and properties are beneficially responding to injurious agents, unregulating macrophage activation might have a deleterious effect and, indeed, macrophages may play a role in the pathogenesis of many chronic lung diseases, including asthma.

Role of Macrophages in Inflammation

Inflammation is divided into acute and chronic patterns (24). Acute inflammation is of relatively short duration, lasting for a few minutes to 1–2 days, and its main characteristics are exudation of fluid and plasma protein (edema) and the emigration of leukocytes, predominantly neutrophils. Regardless of the nature of the injurious agent, acute inflammation is more or less stereotypic. Chronic inflammation, on the other hand, is less uniform. Of longer duration, chronic inflammation is associated histologically with the presence of lymphocytes and macrophages and with the proliferation of blood vessels and connective tissue. Many of the vascular cellular responses of inflammation are mediated by chemical factors derived from the action of the inflammatory stimulus on plasma or cells and on the outcome of inflammation.

Chronic inflammation in various organs arise in one of three ways. (1) It may follow acute inflammation, either because of the persistence of the offending stimulus (e.g., organisms), or because of some interference in the normal process of healing. However, persistence of these organisms or their products lead to tissue destruction, the smoldering inflammation. (2) Repeated bouts of acute inflammation may also be responsible. In this type, histological examination will show evidence of acute inflammation, healing between attacks, and chronic inflammation. (3) More curiously, chronic inflammation may begin insidiously as a low-grade smoldering response that does not follow classic symptomatic acute inflammation. This last form includes some of the most common and disabling diseases of humans, such as chronic lung diseases.

The macrophage is the central figure in chronic inflammation because of the great number of biologically active products it can produce. Some of these products are toxic for tissues (enzymes, oxygen metabolites, or protease), others cause influx of other cell types (lymphocytes, metachromatic cells, or eosinophils), and still others cause fibroblast proliferation and collagen deposition. Therefore, macrophages are central cells in the repair of tissue injury. It is likely that macrophages participate in most processes of healing from acute and chronic inflammation through angiogenesis (32), proliferation of endothelial and mesenchymal cells, and the regulation of ECM synthesis and degradation, possibly leading to fibrosis (33).

METHODS FOR THE STUDY OF MACROPHAGES IN ASTHMA

Different methods can be used to investigate inflammation in asthma (34).

Bronchial Biopsies

The first pathological observations on patients who died of an asthma attack were made in the 19th century. However, until 1980 few pathological studies were done in living asthmatics, and it was uncertain about whether postmortem findings represented a common feature in all asthmatic patients because (1) in almost all cases they were done on the most severe asthmatic patients who died of an asthma attack; (2) there was no detailed clinical information for these patients; (3) it was not known if the asthma attack leading to death was precipitated by a viral infection able to alter the bronchial epithelium; (4) the smoking status was usually unknown, and some patients may have suffered from asthma and chronic bronchitis; (5) the classification of chronic obstructive pulmonary disease (COPD) has changed over the years; and (6) most studies were carried out using conventional histological methods.

In the 1980s, fiberoptic bronchoscopy made it possible to have an easier access to bronchi, and techniques such as electron microscopy, immunohistochemistry, or in situ hybridization, have significantly improved our knowledge. However, specimens from biopsies may not be completely adequate to quantitate the inflammation of asthma because (1) they examine only pathological abnormality of large airways; (2) their size is very small; (3) they do not recognize the possible heterogeneity of the lesions; (4) submucosal edema (caused by asthma or the biopsy procedure) is often present and makes quantitation impossible; and (5) the specimens may be altered by the biopsy procedure.

Bronchoalveolar Lavage

Bronchoalveolar lavage (BAL) was initiated in asthmatics in the early 1980s (35) and largely improved our understanding of asthma. It examines a segment of the lung, including small and large airways as well as alveoli, such that, although the heterogeneity of the lesions is taken into account, cells and mediators recovered originate from ill-defined sites of the lung (36,37). Since asthma is a bronchial disease, attempts have been made to obtain fluid derived from the bronchi, which is called a bronchial sample. The best technique is to perform a true bronchial lavage in an isolated airway segment, using a double-balloon bronchoscope or a double-balloon–tipped catheter inserted through a double-lumen bronchoscope (38–40). In the bronchial wash, there is a higher percentage of neutrophils and epithelial cells than in BAL. These techniques are of great interest because the fluid recovered comes from the airways and because they make it possible to recover cells and mediators before and after bronchoprovocation from the airways of asthmatics. However, these techniques are more difficult to carry out than classic BAL, their safety is not fully assessed, and they cannot be performed on a large scale. Thus, other investigators have proposed to fractionate the lavage, the first aliquot being more related to a bronchial sample and other aliquots coming from more distal parts, including small airways and alveoli (so-called alveolar sample) (41–44). Whatever technique is used, it is important to define it precisely, because the results obtained are not identical.

Quantitative measures are easy, but BAL fluid (BALF) analysis represents only an indirect measure of bronchial inflammation. (1) Mediators may be degraded or released only in situ; therefore, they may be undetectable in BALF (cytokines, except IL-1 and TNF, are usually undetectable in unconcentrated BALF, whereas they can be detected in biopsies). (2) The dilution of the fluid is poorly known and the use of markers, such as albumin or urea, is still under evaluation.

By combining results of BALF and biopsies for similar markers using immunohistochemistry, electron microscopy, and molecular biology-based techniques, a new area of clinically important informations has been opened. It has now become possible to directly examine the presence of bronchial inflammation and to study its cellular component in patients with varying severity of asthma.

Bronchial Brushing

The bronchial brushing technique allows the examination of mainly epithelial cells and is not appropriate to study macrophages.

Sputum

Sputum is easy to study but its examination requires a perfect specimen that is difficult to obtain except with highly precise techniques (45). Cells and mediators can be studied. The presence of macrophages is an indicator of cells recovered from the deep lung.

Peripheral Blood

Many studies have been performed in peripheral blood because of the lineage of monocytic cells. It may be of importance to determine precisely the phenotype of monocytes to better understand the traffic of these cells from the bone marrow to the tissues where they differentiate into macrophages.

MACROPHAGES IN ASTHMA

Demonstration of Macrophage Involvement in Asthma

Bronchoalveolar Lavage

Alveolar macrophages (AM) recovered by BAL have been extensively studied in asthma, and most studies revealed an increased AM activation (46–50). The activation of AM assessed by chemiluminescence induced by luminol (51) or lucigenin (52) is significantly correlated with the severity of asthma. By using Percoll density fractionation, it was shown that AM of asthmatics are hypodense by comparison with those of normal subjects (53). Electron microscopic studies showed that low-density AM of both asthmatic and normal subjects appear to have morphological characteristics of activated cells, by comparison with high-density AM that present characteristics of quiescent cells in both asthmatic and normal subjects. The density of AM was correlated with periods of recent instability of the asthma, but not with its severity. Hypodense AM did not appear to be hyperresponsive in vitro and may have been already committed into the airways.

Challenge Studies

Local challenge studies with allergen have revealed the activation of AM (54–57). In the first study, Tonnel et al. (54) showed that *Dermatophagoides pteronyssinus* challenge induced an immediate release of macrophage β-glucuronidase into the lavage fluid, demonstrating an activation of macrophages. Metzger et al. (58,59) studied the late-phase allergic reaction following local allergen challenge. Neutrophils and eosinophils increased significantly at 48 h after challenge, as did helper T lymphocytes. Characteristically, at 96 h, neutrophil counts returned to normal values, whereas eosinophil and helper T cell counts remained elevated. Peroxidase-staining cells (macrophages) were also elevated at 48 h after local allergen challenge. Electron microscopy revealed degranulation of mast cells and eosinophils, both immediately and later (48 and 96 h), after local allergen challenge. Macrophages were highly activated and had phagocytosed partially intact granules from both eosinophils and mast cells. The activation of AM during segmental allergen challenge has been further studied. The AM activation occurs immediately after antigen challenge, and the late airway response to antigen is characterized by the appearance of high-density AM, which have potentiated superoxide anion release (60). This study suggests the recruitment of monocytes that become rapidly activated in the airways.

In red cedar asthma, bronchial lavage was carried out in 44 patients at different time intervals after bronchial challenge with plicatic acid (61). The late-phase reaction was associated with an increase in eosinophils in the lavage fluid, an increase in sloughing of bronchial epithelial cells, and an increase in degenerate cells consisting mainly of degenerate epithelial cells and alveolar macrophages.

During allergen challenge (62,63) or challenge with toluene diisocyanate (64), peripheral blood monocytes of sensitized asthmatics are activated.

Acute Asthma

In asthmatics recovering from a recent exacerbation, AM are often necrotic whereas in stable asthmatics these patterns of cell death were not detected (Figs. 1–3). Necrosis was correlated with eosinophil numbers in BAL fluid (Vago P, Chanez P, and Bousquet P, unpublished data).

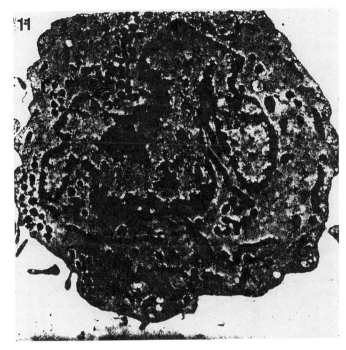

Figure 1 Monocytoid macrophage recovered by BAL from a stable asthmatic patient.

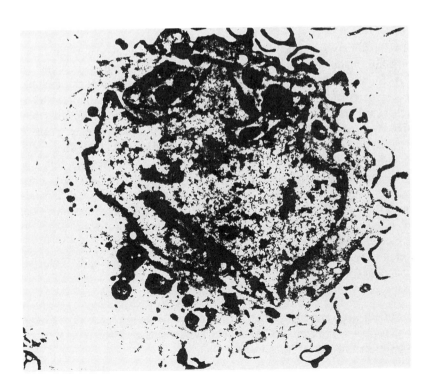

Figure 2 Activated macrophage recovered by BAL from an unstable asthmatic patient.

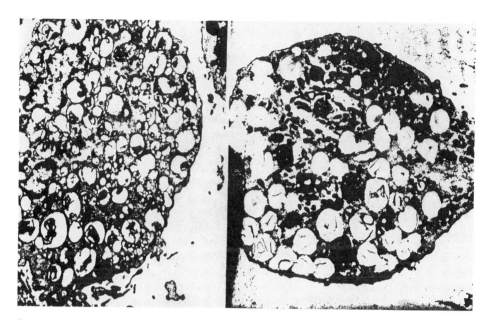

Figure 3 Macrophages undergoing necrosis recovered by BAL from an asthmatic patient 24 h after an exacerbation.

Bronchial Biopsies in Chronic Asthma

Studies using BAL indirectly suggested the involvement of macrophages in asthma, but until recently, little information was available on monocytes and macrophages in bronchial biopsies (65–70). By using immunohistochemical methods with different monoclonal antibodies, it was shown that in asthma (1) macrophages are increased in numbers (pan-macrophage marker), (2) many of these cells bear monocytic markers, suggesting that they are recently derived from blood monocytes, and (3) the number of class II antigen-positive macrophages is increased, suggesting that they are in an activated stage (Fig. 4). These cells were found mainly beneath the basement membrane and among epithelial cells. Some of them had a foamy appearance and resembled the "hypodense" cells that represent most BAL macrophages of asthmatics (53). Macrophages are present even in mild asthmatics (Bousquet J, unpublished observations) and in patients with newly diagnosed asthma (71). By electron microscopy, Beasley et al. (65) found eosinophils, monocytes, and platelets, in contact with the vascular endothelium, with emigration of eosinophils and monocytes in asthmatic subjects. These changes were found in stable asthmatics or after bronchial challenge with allergen.

Conclusions

Studies performed with BAL and biopsies clearly demonstrate the presence of activated macrophages in the airways of asthmatics. These cells often bear the phenotype of blood monocytes, suggesting an increased recruitment.

Fate and Kinetics of Cells of Monocyte–Macrophage Lineage in Asthma

The origin of macrophages in asthma is still under investigation. It appears that the replication of macrophages is no greater than that in normal subjects (72). In asthma, an increased expression of various adhesion molecules has been observed on endothelial cells (73–75); therefore, it is likely that there is an increased recruitment of monocytes into the bronchi (65). Monocytes are activated in asthma, as demonstrated by their release of increased amounts of oxygen free radicals (62,76). An active recruitment of activated monocytes has been observed after segmental allergen challenge (56,59), but analysis of the phenotype of monocytes in steady-state asthma does not show increased levels of adhesion molecules (Bousquet J, et al., unpublished data). However, it is possible that monocytes from asthmatics may present increases in the functional properties of integrins.

In the BAL fluid, the number of AM is not increased in asthma. These cells are less viable in stable asthmatics than in normal subjects (46) and, after an asthma exacerbation, AM are often necrotic (Vago P, Bousquet J, Godard P, unpublished data). These data combined with those of bronchial biopsies suggest that there may be an increased turnover of macrophages in asthma.

Activation and Role of Macrophages in Asthma

Phenotype of Macrophages

In asthmatics, the number of AM recovered in BALF expressed CD11 (LFA-1) CD33, HLA-DR, CD23 (Fc$_\epsilon$RII), CD44 (homing receptor), CD54 (ICAM-1) is greater than in control subjects (50,77,78).

Release of Eicosanoids

In asthma of various causes, it has been consistently shown that AM released, spontaneously or after activation, increased levels of PGE_2, $PGF_{2\alpha}$, TXB_2, or LTC_4/D_4, and 5-hydroxyeicosatetraeonic acid (5-HETE) (35,50,79–82).

The modulation of arachidonic acid activation in AM is complex. Alveolar macrophages from asthmatic patients and healthy volunteers were compared for their respective capacities to produce lipoxins and leukotrienes when stimulated by the calcium ionophore A23187, with or without 15 (S)-HETE. Without 15-HETE, AM from asthmatics produced

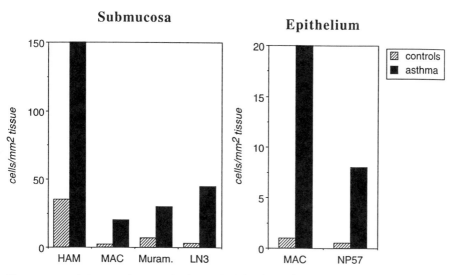

Figure 4 Individual cell counts in bronchial biopsies. Abbreviations: HAM: pan macrophage monoclonal antibody; MAC: MAC387: anti-monocyte monoclonal antibody; MURAM: polyclonal antibody against muramidase; NP57: anti-HLA-DR monoclonal antibody. From Ref. 68.

more LTB$_4$ and 5-HETE than those from controls. In the presence of 15-HETE, human AM were able to produce 5,15-diHETE and lipoxins. Moreover, the total amount of lipoxins synthesized by AM from asthmatics was twofold higher than that synthesized by AM from controls, thereby showing an enhanced cell activation by the 5-lipoxygenase (5-LO) pathway (83) and a possible interaction with epithelial cells, since 15-HETE is the major eicosanoid released both in normal subjects and asthmatics (84). Pretreatment with methyl-prednisolone inhibited A23187-induced synthesis of immunoreactive cyclooxygenase products to a greater extent than immunoreactive leukotrienes (79). However, dexa-methasone has a variable effect on arachidonic acid metabolites in AM from normal subjects or asthmatics (85).

The release of eicosanoids by macrophages may have some relevance in the patho-genesis of asthma (86). Sulfidopeptide leukotrienes increase microvascular flow and per-meability, leading to local accumulation of plasma-derived proteins and leukocytes, includ-ing eosinophils (71). These eicosanoids are also smooth-muscle constrictors, induce cough, and increase the secretion of mucus. Leukotriene B$_4$ is a potent chemoattractant for neutro-phils, but the exact role of these cells in asthma remains to be elucidated.

Release of Platelet-Activating Factor

Stimulation of human blood monocytes from asthmatics or healthy subjects with ionophore A23187 induced the release of platelet-activating factor (PAF-acether). This release was also observed after phagocytosis of zymosan and bacteria (*Bordetella pertussis*). The AM did not release PAF-acether after zymosan phagocytosis; AM, but not monocytes, were stimulated to release PAF-acether by a specific allergen challenge or IgE–anti-IgE (87,88). These studies indicate that the release of PAF-acether depends on the state of activation of cells of the monocytic lineage.

The significance of PAF-acether release by cells of the monocytic lineage needs further study, but animal studies (89) and a controversial human study (90) have shown that inhalation of this autacoid can increase nonspecific bronchial hyperreactivity. In animals, PAF-acether inhalation induces eosinophil infiltration in the airways.

Release of Oxygen Free Radicals

The lung is particularly exposed to oxidant stresses, such as those that can be brought about by oxygen-derived free radicals (91). They mainly result from the monovalent reduction of molecular oxygen. Free radicals are highly reactive species, normally produced by cellular metabolism. Their target molecules are proteins, DNA, and polyunsaturated fatty acids, the alterations of which can lead to cell death. Activated AM generate highly reactive toxic species of oxygen in many pulmonary disorders, including asthma. Chemiluminescence induced by luminol (51), lucigenin (52), and the production of superoxidate anion (60,92) was increased in AM from asthmatics. There was a significant correlation between the activation of AM and eosinophils (51); the greater the activation of AM, the more severe the asthma (51,52). Superoxide anion release was significantly enhanced during segmental allergen challenge (56,60).

Monocytes in peripheral blood can release superoxidate anion, and there is an increased release in cells from untreated asthmatics (76), whereas cells from asthmatics receiving inhaled corticosteroids had a decreased activity (Fig. 5).

Release of Cytokines

Unstimulated AM from asthmatics spontaneously release greater amounts of IL-1, TNF-α, IL-6, IL-8, or GM-CSF than those of normal subjects (50,93–98). Interleukin-1, TNF-α, and IL-6 can be released by AM from normal subjects after lipopolysaccharide (LPS)

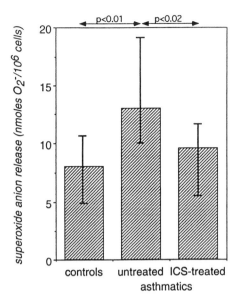

Figure 5 Levels of superoxide anion release by blood monocytes of control subjects and asthmatics. ICS: inhaled corticosteroids, results expressed in medians and 95% confidence intervals; statistical analysis: Wilcoxon W test and Bonferroni's correction. From Campbell et al., unpublished data.

stimulation (99). Moreover, TNF-α and IL-6 are released by AM stimulated by anti-IgE obtained from asthmatics. Patients who developed a late-phase reaction after allergen challenge had a greater cytokine release (94,95). In asthmatics, the release of IL-6 is significantly correlated with TNF-α in AM stimulated by anti-IgE (95) or LPS (Chanez P, Vignola M, Bousquet P, unpublished data), suggesting common regulatory pathways. Corticosteroids administered some hours before BAL reduce the release of IL-1β by AM (97).

Unstimulated monocytes from asthmatics and normal subjects usually do not spontaneously release cytokines (100). After in vitro allergen challenge monocytes from asthmatics released IL-1 (100). Lipopolysaccharide induces the release of cytokines from monocytes of normal subjects and asthmatics (101).

Proinflammatory cytokines such as IL-1, TNF-α, and IL-6 produce several effects in common. They are pyrogenic, can induce the synthesis of acute-phase proteins, and amplify the immune and inflammatory reactions by the activation of lymphocytes, granulocytes, and structural cells (102–104). Interleukin-1β, TNF, and IL-6 released by mononuclear phagocytes are involved in the modulation of cellular immunity, as well as in recruitment and activation of inflammatory or structural cells (103,104). These cytokines, therefore, may be involved in the asthmatic bronchial inflammation. Tissue necrosis factor-α is a potent in vivo and in vitro chemoattractant and cell activator, that is also able to activate AM in an autocrine pathway, leading to an increase in their phagocytic activities (105). It may be an important cytokine in asthma. In animals, inhalation of TNF-α causes bronchial hyperreactivity (106). This cytokine may cause a recruitment of inflammatory cells by at least two mechanisms. It is chemotactic for monocytes, and TNF-α released by AM recovered in BALF during the late-phase allergic reaction increased the expression of adhesion molecules on endothelial cells (107). Interleukin-6 is involved in the control of many cell functions, including IgE antibody synthesis, T-cell cytotoxicity, stem cell differentiation, and acute-phase protein synthesis (108). It can inhibit the proliferation of macrophages (109), and its spontaneous release by AM of asthmatics may explain the lack of proliferation of AM we have recently described (72). Granulocyte–macrophage colony-stimulating factor is a multipotent cytokine regulating the growth, maturation, and differentiation of several cell types, including the monocyte lineage. Moreover, GM-CSF can increase the metabolism of eosinophils (98) or monocytes and AM (110). Incubation of eosinophils with AM supernatants isolated from asthmatic subjects, followed by stimulation with the calcium ionophore A23187, resulted in enhancement of the capacity of eosinophils to elaborate LTC_4, whereas the supernatants of AM from controls failed to induce such an activation. GM-CSF is responsible for eosinophil priming (98).

Release of Products Regulating Extracellular Matrix

Alveolar macrophages can also synthesize and secrete a group of metalloproteases having the capacity to degrade various extracellular matrix macromolecules, including elastin (111). Macrophages may also be involved in the regulation of airway inflammation through the secretion of cytokines and growth factors, such as PDGF or TGF-β that are likely to be involved in fibrosis. However, such properties have yet to be characterized in cells from asthmatics.

Immunological Properties of Macrophages

The activation of T cells recognizing specific antigens is a crucial and early event in the development of an immune response, but T cells cannot respond to antigens without help of a second cell type, called accessory cells or antigen-presenting cells. The potential role of individual cell populations in regulation of local T-cell–dependent immune reactions in the lung and airways depends on a variety of additional factors, including their precise localization; migration characteristics; expression of T-cell "costimulatory" signals; responsiveness to inflammatory stimuli, in particular cytokines; host immune status; and the nature of the antigen challenge. Pulmonary dendritic cells and Langerhans cells, similar to their counterparts in other tissues, are potent accessory cells in the lung (112). Recent evidence suggests that the induction of primary immunity to inhaled antigens is normally controlled by specialized populations of dendritic cells, which perform a surveillance role within the epithelia of the upper and lower respiratory tract; in the presensitized host, a variety of other cell populations (both bone marrow-derived and mesenchymal) may participate in restimulation of "memory" T lymphocytes (113). In normal subjects and animals, macrophages recovered in the BAL fluid (AM) or by digestion of the lung parenchyma (airways macrophages) are suppressive of lymphocyte proliferation in response to mitogen, alloantigen, and antigen, when cultured with lymphocytes at ratios approaching the relationship between these cells in the airways (114). However, in the human lung, a large degree of heterogeneity exists within the macrophage population (115), and variable effects on T cells may be expected, depending on the balance between the monocyte versus the mature macrophage cell population, the latter one being suppressive (116,117). Inflammation induces changes in the lung antigen-presenting cell populations, and in sarcoidosis or idiopathic pulmonary fibrosis, there is an enhanced alveolar macrophage-mediated antigen-induced T-lymphocyte proliferation in sarcoidosis (118).

Alveolar macrophages from asthmatics present a decreased in vitro T-cell inhibitory activity when compared with cells recovered in normal subjects. These effects of AM were observed on lymphoproliferative responses to polyclonal T-cell mitogens (119) or after antigen-specific stimulation. The capacity of peripheral blood monocytes and alveolar macrophages (AM) obtained by bronchoalveolar lavage (BAL) to present recall antigens, namely, tuberculin purified protein derivative (PPD) or streptokinase–streptodornase (SKSD), to highly purified autologous T cells has been compared in asthmatic and normal subjects. In the asthmatic group, AM accessory cell function was variable, and most subjects were unable to present either recall antigen as effectively as blood monocytes, although one asthmatic subject demonstrated larger proliferative responses than blood monocytes for both antigens. The AM accessory cell activity was not antigen-specific. In the normal subjects; AM were also unable to act effectively as accessory cells for the presentation of PPD and SKSD in most subjects (120).

Regulation of Macrophages in Asthma

Airway macrophages of asthmatics appear to be in an activated state and spontaneously release greater amounts of vasoactive mediators and cytokines. The activation patterns of AM have been extensively studied, whereas the regulation of the activation of AM is still poorly understood.

Immunological Activation of Macrophages

Airway macrophages bear low-affinity IgE receptors ($Fc_\epsilon RII$ or CD23). An early study (47), showed that AM from nonatopic donors were passively sensitized with allergen-specific IgE antibody from the serum of asthmatic patients. A selective release of 4–8% of the lysosomal β-glucuronidase of these cells occurred within 30 min of contact with the related allergen or with antihuman IgE antibody in the absence of any mast cells or basophils. The cell reactivity was dependent on the interaction of macrophages with IgE, as shown by the disappearance of the allergen-induced enzyme release after either heating or IgE immune adsorption of the sensitizing serum, but not after IgG adsorption. Alveolar macrophages from asthmatic patients behaved similarly to passively sensitized normal macrophages. Contact with the related allergen or with anti-IgE antibody induced the same percentage of enzyme release, demonstrating that these cells possess allergen-specific IgE bound on their surface. The presence of IgE-specific receptors on the macrophage surface was demonstrated at the ultrastructural level by immunoperoxidase labeling. In other studies AM sensitized with human myeloma IgE and challenged with anti-IgE were able to release LTB_4, $PGF_{2\alpha}$, TB_2, and N-acetyl-β-glucosaminidase (121,122), IL-1β, TNF-α or IL-6 (77,94,95).

Monocytes and AM from asthmatics present an increased expression of CD23. Stimulation of CD23 expression on monocytes is an activity of IL-4, GM-CSF, IFN-α, IFN-γ, and M-CSF, but not of IL-2, IL-6, or TNF-α. Expression of CD23 by these cytokines was associated with the induction of specific mRNA transcripts. Instillation of allergen in the asthmatic's airway up-regulated CD23 on AM (123). Up-regulation of CD23 in atopic individuals, therefore, may reflect allergen-induced exposure of mononuclear phagocytes to one or more of these cytokines.

Activation of Macrophages by Cytokines

Mutual interactions between cytokines and cells of the monocytic lineage involve both the effects of cytokines on cell function and the production of cytokines by these cells. They play a significant role in inflammatory processes and immune reactions and are likely to be of importance in asthma. Among all cytokines that may be of importance in the regulation of macrophages in asthma, few have been studied.

In most instances, IL-4 down-regulates AM from normal subjects. It decreases the production of cytokines such as IL-1, TNF-α, IL-6 (124), oxygen free radicals (125), and metalloproteases (126). The AM appear to be differentially regulated in normal subjects and asthmatics, as IL-4 was far more effective in reducing the release of cytokines by AM from normal subjects than from asthmatics (101). The differences in the response of AM from asthmatics to IL-4 may be due to different possible mechanisms. The local inflammation surrounding AM might alter their potential response to the inhibitory effect of IL-4. These findings suggest a constant activation of AM in asthma and a lower sensitivity of these cells to physiological suppressive factors. Alternatively, this lack of response may be due to a decreased number or affinity of IL-4 receptors, or to the rapid degradation of IL-4 because of the high potential proteolytic activity of AM. In asthmatics, therefore, it appears that IL-4 cannot play its major role as a suppressor of immune and inflammatory responses of mononuclear phagocytes, leading to the amplification of the deleterious effects of AM to the airways.

Interferon-γ, IL-10 (127), IL-13 (128), and GM-CSF (129) regulate cells of the monocytic lineage, but there is no data on their regulatory effect on AM from asthmatics.

Activation of Macrophages by Proinflammatory Mediators

In asthma, the bronchial microenvironment may play a key role in the regulation and function of resident cells, including the cooperation between macrophages and other cells of the bronchi (130). Mast cells and macrophages are in close proximity in the airways, and cooperation between these two cell types may be important. Histamine modulates macrophage activation. The H_1-receptors have been found in AM (131). Moreover, histamine can increase the metabolism of AM and the expression of surface markers (LFA-1, ICAM-1, CD23b) (132).

Interactions between eosinophils and macrophages have been examined. Alveolar macrophages can engulf eosinophil granules that activate AM, or may even induce cytotoxicity. Moreover, an increased expression of heat-shock protein in AM from asthmatics has been associated with eosinophil numbers in the BAL fluid (Vignola M, Chanez P, Polla, Bousquet P, unpublished observation).

Activation of Macrophages by Neuropeptides

The role of substance P in the pathogenesis of asthma is unclear. Animal studies suggest that it may be important, whereas human studies do not confirm this. Alveolar macrophages stimulated by LPS were activated poorly, or not at all, by substance P (133).

Signal Transduction and Cyclic Nucleotides

Activation of AM is different at the transduction level in asthmatics and normal subjects. Activation of phosphatidylinositol (PI) phosphate (134) and the translocation of protein kinase C toward membranes (135) are increased in asthma. Phosphatidylethanolamine methylation was increased in AM membranes from asthmatics, when compared with control subjects (136).

Cyclic nucleotides appear to be abnormally regulated in AM from asthmatics. Alveolar macrophages from asthmatics accumulated less AMP and presented a lower adenylate cyclase activity when exposed to isobutyl methylxanthine, albuterol (salbutamol), or prostaglandin E_2, by comparison with cells from control subjects without asthma. The degree of the hyporesponsiveness was related to the severity of asthma. The refractoriness observed in patients with asthma was not accounted for by a specific β-adrenergic desensitization at the adenylate cyclase receptor level, but rather, should be explained by a AMP-dependent postreceptor mechanism (137). However, there may be an additive hyporesponsiveness of β-adrenoceptors linked to the exposure to cytokines, such as GM-CSF, that reduced the activity of the receptor (138). The adenylate cyclase stimulator forskolin was able to reduce the release of TXB_2, LTB_4, and superoxide from AM stimulated by opsonized zymosan. On the other hand, these inhibitory effects were not observed with isoprenaline or the phosphodiesterase inhibitor Ro-20 1724 (48). The adenylate cyclase responsiveness to PGE_2, histamine, and the β-adrenoceptor agonist albuterol (salbutamol) was significantly impaired in AM from asthmatics, and an intrinsic desensitization was suggested to occur in AM from these patients (139). The AMP, GMP phosphodiesterase, and phospholipid N-methyltransferase activities were significantly decreased in monocytes from asthmatic patients compared with the control group (140).

Pharmacological Regulation of Macrophages

In Vitro Studies

Several studies have examined the in vitro effects of antiasthma drugs on the activation of AM and monocytes.

Nedocromil inconsistently reduced monocyte or AM activation. In AM stimulated by IgE–anti-IgE complexes nedocromil sodium was unable to block the release of IL-1β or IL-6 (141). It produced an inhibition of IgE-mediated generation of cytotoxic molecules from monocytes, with a concomitant inhibition of their oxidative metabolism, measured by chemiluminescence. In addition, nedocromil sodium reduced the ability of AM to synthesize and release β-glucuronidase (142). The effects of nedocromil sodium were studied on the metabolism of arachidonic acid released from AM in healthy and asthmatic subjects. The only effect observed in this study was a slight decrease in LTD_4 synthesis by ATMs from asthmatic patients (80). The AM from asthmatics incubated in the presence of LTC_4 or LTE_4, generated LTB_4 and 5-HETE. Nedocromil sodium decreased LTB_4 releasability and intracellular 5-HETE concentrations in zymosan-stimulated AM from asthmatic patients, and decreased the LTC_4-4 or LTE_4-promoted formation of LTB_4 and 5-HETE (143).

Cromolyn sodium (disodium cromoglycate) decreased the IgE-dependent activation of AM, including the release of neutrophil chemotactic factor, chemiluminescence and β-glucuronidase release and synthesis (144). One site of action of cromolyn sodium may be at the GTP-binding protein of the PI pathway (145).

In Vivo Studies

Except in the study of corticosteroid-resistant asthma, very few in vivo studies have been carried out.

Macrophages in Corticosteroid-Dependent Asthma Glucocorticoids are used as antiinflammatory and immunosuppressive drugs (146). They act on the many functions of macrophages, mainly by modulating the production of inflammatory mediators, such as cytokines, phospholipid-derived mediators, proteases, and oxygen metabolites. For inducing these effects, glucocorticoids interact with their receptors–transcription factors that recognize specific genomic sequences, the glucocorticoid-responsive elements (GRE). Glucocorticoids modulate the transcription of genes in association with other transcription factors, such as Fos, Jun, or CREB. These combinatorial associations—differing according to the differentiation or activation state of the cell—may, therefore, produce a fine-tuning of the induction or repression of genes.

Although the definition of corticosteroid resistance is still vague (147), it is clear that some patients do not respond favorably to oral corticosteroids (148). Several studies have found that patients with corticosteroid resistance had impaired mononuclear phagocyte functions. In asthmatics who responded clinically to corticosteroids, monocyte–complement receptor expression reversed to normal levels following treatment with prednisolone, whereas, in those asthmatics who failed to improve clinically, the levels of complement receptor expression remained elevated (149). Cells from patients known to be clinically sensitive to glucocorticoid therapy did not differ significantly from those of clinically resistant patients in terms of their immunophenotype or the number of colonies generated by culture in the presence of phytohemagglutinin. Methylprednisolone, at low concentration (10 nmol/L), inhibited colony growth from cells of glucocorticoid-sensitive patients, whereas there was much less inhibition of colony growth from resistant patients' cells (150). The source of resistance to corticosteroids was more related to monocytes than to lymphocytes (151). The effects of monocytes from asthmatics on granulocytes differ according to the clinical effects of corticosteroids. A 3-kDa neutrophil-priming activity derived from peripheral blood monocytes is suppressed by glucocorticoid treatment of monocytes derived from individuals with corticosteroid-sensitive, but not from those with corticosteroid-resistant asthma (152). These results suggest that monocytes of corticosteroid-resistant asthmatics can increase the inflammatory potential of neutrophils and that they are hyperactive, as indicated by increased cytokine production and enhanced expression of activation markers, despite the presence of corticosteroids (153). The characteristics of corticosteroid receptors on monocytes is similar in patients sensitive or resistant to corticosteroids (152), and the release of cytokines by LPS-stimulated monocytes was inhibited in a similar fashion in corticosteroid-sensitive and corticosteroid-resistant asthmatics (154). Different results were observed by Vecchiarelli et al. (155), who found that LPS-induced TNF secretion was reduced in blood monocytes obtained from corticosteroid-sensitive asthmatics after a treatment course of prednisolone, whereas monocytes from corticosteroid-resistant asthmatics released the same amount of TNF before and during treatment.

Other In Vivo Effects of Drugs   The expression of IgG-Fc receptor and complement receptor is significantly reduced in asthmatics treated with oral corticosteroids by comparison with patients receiving inhaled corticosteroids (156). The numbers of AM with the phenotype of antigen-presenting cells and of cells expressing HLA-DR were reduced in six patients after a treatment with inhaled steroids (157)

CONCLUSIONS

Monocytes and macrophages are likely to be important cells in the generation and regulation of airways inflammation in asthma. In normal subjects, macrophages play a central role as a first-line immune defense. In asthma, macrophages are activated rapidly in the airways after allergen challenge and, in chronic asthma, their activation state is correlated with the severity of the disease. The regulation of macrophagic inflammation in the airways of asthmatics is still poorly known, but it appears that these cells are less sensitive to normal inhibitors than those of normal subjects. The role of macrophages appears to be deleterious by the release of lipid mediators, oxygen-reactive species, and toxic cytokines, such as TNF. Macrophages may also be potent regulators of airways' inflammation, but more data are needed to fully understand their role in remodeling. In immune defense, the normal suppressive effect of macrophages may be reduced, possibly explaining why immune mechanisms are persistent in the airways of asthmatics. Finally, the pharmacological modulation of macrophages may have some relevance for a better understanding of the treatment of asthma, because corticosteroid-resistance may be at least partly related to monocytic cells.

REFERENCES

1. van-Furth R. Production and migration of monocytes and kinetics of macrophages. In: van-Furth R, ed. Mononuclear Phagocytes. Dordrecht: Kluwer Academic Publishers, 1992:3–12.
2. Rabinovits S, Cybulsky M, Kume N, Gimbrone MJ. Endothelial-dependent mechanisms of monocyte adhesion. In: van-Furth R, ed. Mononuclear Phagocytes. Dordrecht: Kluwer Academic Publishers, 1992:89–91.
3. Hogg N, Landis RC. Adhesion molecules in cell interactions. Curr Opin Immunol 1993; 5: 383–390.
4. McEver RP. Leukocyte–endothelial cell interactions. Curr Opin Cell Biol 1992; 4:840–849.
5. van-Furth R. Phagocytic cells: development and distribution of mononuclear phagocytes in normal steady state and inflammation. In: Gallin J, Goldstein I, Snyderman R, ed. Inflammation, Basic Principles and Clinical Correlates. New York: Raven Press, 1988:281–295.
6. Volkman A. Disparity in the origin of mononuclear phagocyte populations. J Reticuloendothel Soc 1976; 19:249–268.
7. van-oud-Alblas AB, van-Furth R. Origin, kinetics, and characteristics of pulmonary macrophages in the normal steady state. J Exp Med 1979; 149:1504–1518.
8. Coggle JE, Tarling JD. The proliferation kinetics of pulmonary alveolar macrophages. J Leukoc Biol 1984; 35:317–327.
9. Blusse-van-Oud-Alblas A, van-der-Linden-Schrever B, van-Furth R. Origin and kinetics of pulmonary macrophages during an inflammatory reaction induced by intravenous administration of heat-killed bacillus Calmette-Guerin. J Exp Med 1981; 154:235–252.
10. Brandes ME, Finkelstein JN. The production of alveolar macrophage-derived growth-regulating proteins in response to lung injury. Toxicol Lett 1990; 54:3–22.
11. Zembala M, Asherson G. Human monocytes. London: Academic Press, 1989:553.
12. van-Furth R. Mononuclear phagocytes. In: Biology of Monocytes and Macrophages. Dordrecht, NL: Kluwer Academic Publishers, 1992:667.
13. Brain JD, Gehr P, Kavet RI. Airway macrophages. The importance of the fixation method. Am Rev Respir Dis 1984; 129:823–826.
14. Holt PG, Degebrodt A, Venaille T, et al. Preparation of interstitial lung cells by enzymatic digestion of tissue slices: preliminary characterization by morphology and performance in functional assays. Immunology 1985; 54:139–147.
15. Brain JD. Mechanisms, measurement, and significance of lung macrophage function. Environ Health Perspect 1992; 97:5–10.
16. Bowden D, Adamson I. The pulmonary interstitial cell as immediate precursor of the alveolar macrophage. Am J Pathol 1972; 78:521–536.
17. Barry BE, Miller FJ, Crapo JD. Effects of inhalation of 0.12 and 0.25 parts per million ozone on the proximal alveolar region of juvenile and adult rats. Lab Invest 1985; 53:692–704.
18. Warner AE, Brain JD. The cell biology and pathogenic role of pulmonary intravascular macrophages. Am J Physiol 1990; 258:L1–12.
19. Dehring DJ, Wismar BL. Intravascular macrophages in pulmonary capillaries of humans. Am Rev Respir Dis 1989; 139:1027–1029.
20. Thomas E, Ramberg R, Sale G, Sparkes R, Golde D. Direct evidence for a bone marrow origin of the alveolar macrophage in man. Science 1976; 192:1016–1018.
21. Hoffman RM, Dauber JH, Paradis IL, Griffith BP, Hardesty RL. Alveolar macrophage migration after lung transplantation. Am Rev Respir Dis 1991; 143:834–838.
22. Arnoux B, Masse R, Chrétien J. Evidence of an increased persistent mitotic activity in cells recovered by bronchoalveolar lavage in sarcoidosis. In: Chrétien J, Marsac J, Saltiel J, eds. Sarcoidosis and Other Granulomatous Disorders. New York: Pergamon Press, 1983.

23. Bitterman PB, Saltzman LE, Adelberg S, Ferrans VJ, Crystal RG. Alveolar macrophage replication. One mechanism for the expansion of the mononuclear phagocyte population in the chronically inflamed lung. J Clin Invest 1984; 74:460–469.
24. Cotran R, Kumar V, Robin S. Inflammation and repair. In: Cotran R, Kumar V, Robin S, eds. Robbins Pathologic Basis of Disease. Philadelphia: WB Saunders, 1989:39–87.
25. Celada A, Nathan C. Macrophage activation revisited. Immunol Today 1994; 15:100–102.
26. Johnston R Jr. Current concepts: immunology. Monocytes and macrophages. N Engl J Med 1988; 318:747–752.
27. Unanue ER, Cerottini JC. Antigen presentation. FASEB J 1989; 3:2496–2502.
28. Sibille Y, Reynolds HY. Macrophages and polymorphonuclear neutrophils in lung defense and injury. Am Rev Respir Dis 1990; 141:471–501.
29. Stein M, Keshav S. The versatility of macrophages. Clin Exp Allergy 1992; 22:19–27.
30. Nathan CF. Secretory products of macrophages. J Clin Invest 1987; 79:319–326.
31. Werb Z, Underwood J, Rappolee D. The role of macrophage-derived growth factors in tissue repair. In: van-Furth R, ed. Mononuclear Phagocytes. Dordrecht: Kluwer Academic Publishers, 1992:404–409.
32. Sunderkötter C, Steinbrink K, Goebeler M, Bhardawaj R, Sorg C. Macrophages and angiogenesis. J Leukoc Biol 1994; 55:410–422.
33. Shaw RJ. The role of lung macrophages at the interface between chronic inflammation and fibrosis. Respir Med 1991; 85:267–273.
34. Bousquet J, Chanez P, Campbell AM, et al. Inflammatory processes in asthma. Int Arch Allergy Appl Immunol 1991; 94:227–232.
35. Godard P, Chaintreuil J, Damon M, et al. Functional assessment of alveolar macrophages: comparison of cells from asthmatics and normal subjects. J Allergy Clin Immunol 1982; 70:88–93.
36. Reynolds H. Bronchoalveolar lavage. State of art. Am Rev Respir Dis 1987; 135:250–263.
37. Fabbri L, DeRose V, Godard P, Boschetto P, Rossi G. Guidelines and recommendations for the clinical use of bronchoalveolar lavage in asthma. Eur Respir Rev 1992; 2:114–120.
38. Eschenbacher WL, Gravelyn TR. A technique for isolated airway segment lavage. Chest 1987; 92:105–109.
39. Rankin JA, Marcy T, Rochester CL, et al. Human airway macrophages. A technique for their retrieval and a descriptive comparison with alveolar macrophages. Am Rev Respir Dis 1992; 145:928–933.
40. Zehr BB, Casale TB, Wood D, Floerchinger C, Richerson HB, Hunninghake GW. Use of segmental airway lavage to obtain relevant mediators from the lungs of asthmatic and control subjects. Chest 1989; 95:1059–1063.
41. Davis GS, Giancola MS, Costanza MC, Low RB. Analyses of sequential bronchoalveolar lavage samples from healthy human volunteers. Am Rev Respir Dis 1982; 126:611–616.
42. Lam S, Leriche JC, Kijek K, Phillips D. Effect of bronchial lavage volume on cellular and protein recovery. Chest 1985; 88:856–859.
43. Kirby JG, Hargreave FE, Gleich GJ, O'Byrne PM. Bronchoalveolar cell profiles of asthmatic and nonasthmatic subjects. Am Rev Respir Dis 1987; 136:379–383.
44. Van-Vyve T, Chanez P, Lacoste JY, Bousquet J, Michel FB, Godard P. Comparison between bronchial and alveolar samples of bronchoalveolar lavage fluid in asthma. Chest 1992; 102: 356–361.
45. Gibson PG, Girgis-Gabardo A, Morris MM, et al. Cellular characteristics of sputum from patients with asthma and chronic bronchitis. Thorax 1989; 44:693–699.
46. Godard P, Damon M, Chaintreuil J, Flandre O, Crastes-de-Paulet A, Michel FB. Functional assessment of alveolar macrophages in allergic asthmatic patients. Adv Exp Med Biol 1982; 155:667–671.
47. Joseph M, Tonnel AB, Torpier G, Capron A, Arnoux B, Benveniste J. Involvement of immunoglobulin E in the secretory processes of alveolar macrophages from asthmatic patients. J Clin Invest 1983; 71:221–230.

48. Fuller RW, O'Malley G, Baker AJ, MacDermot J. Human alveolar macrophage activation: inhibition by forskolin but not beta-adrenoceptor stimulation or phosphodiesterase inhibition. Pulmon Pharmacol 1988; 1:101–106.

49. Rankin JA. The contribution of alveolar macrophages to hyperreactive airway disease. J Allergy Clin Immunol 1989; 83:722–729.

50. Catena E, Mazzarella G, Peluso GF, Micheli P, Cammarata A, Marsico SA. Phenotypic features and secretory pattern of alveolar macrophages in atopic asthmatic patients. Monaldi Arch Chest Dis 1993; 48:6–15.

51. Cluzel M, Damon M, Chanez P, et al. Enhanced alveolar cell luminol-dependent chemiluminescence in asthma. J Allergy Clin Immunol 1987; 80:195–201.

52. Kelly C, Ward C, Stenton CS, Bird G, Hendrick DJ, Walters EH. Number and activity of inflammatory cells in bronchoalveolar lavage fluid in asthma and their relation to airway responsiveness. Thorax 1988; 43:684–692.

53. Chanez P, Bousquet J, Couret I, et al. Increased numbers of hypodense alveolar macrophages in patients with bronchial asthma. Am Rev Respir Dis 1991; 144:923–930.

54. Tonnel AB, Joseph M, Gosset P, Fournier E, Capron A. Stimulation of alveolar macrophages in asthmatic patients after local provocation test. Lancet 1983; 1:1406–1408.

55. Metzger WJ, Zavala D, Richerson HB, et al. Local allergen challenge and bronchoalveolar lavage of allergic asthmatic lungs. Description of the model and local airway inflammation. Am Rev Respir Dis 1987; 135:433–440.

56. Calhoun WJ, Reed HE, Moest DR, Stevens CA. Enhanced superoxide production by alveolar macrophages and air-space cells, airway inflammation, and alveolar macrophage density changes after segmental antigen bronchoprovocation in allergic subjects. Am Rev Respir Dis 1992; 145:317–325.

57. Calhoun WJ, Jarjour NN, Gleich GJ, Stevens CA, Busse WW. Increased airway inflammation with segmental versus aerosol antigen challenge. Am Rev Respir Dis 1993; 147:1465–1471.

58. Metzger WJ, Nugent K, Richerson HB, et al. Methods for bronchoalveolar lavage in asthmatic patients following bronchoprovocation and local antigen challenge. Chest 1985; 87:16S–19S.

59. Metzger WJ, Richerson HB, Worden K, Monick M, Hunninghake GW. Bronchoalveolar lavage of allergic asthmatic patients following allergen bronchoprovocation. Chest 1986; 89:477–483.

60. Calhoun WJ, Stevens CA, Lambert SB. Modulation of superoxide production of alveolar macrophages and peripheral blood mononuclear cells by beta-agonists and theophylline. J Lab Clin Med 1991; 117:514–522.

61. Lam S, LeRiche J, Phillips D, Chan-Yeung M. Cellular and protein changes in bronchial lavage fluid after late asthmatic reaction in patients with red cedar asthma. J Allergy Clin Immunol 1987; 80:44–50.

62. Durham SR, Carroll M, Walsh GM, Kay AB. Leukocyte activation in allergen-induced late-phase asthmatic reactions. N Engl J Med 1984; 311:1398–1402.

63. Carroll MP, Durham SR, Walsh G, Kay AB. Activation of neutrophils and monocytes after allergen- and histamine-induced bronchoconstriction. J Allergy Clin Immunol 1985; 75: 290–296.

64. Siracusa A, Vecchiarelli A, Brugnami G, Marabini A, Felicioni D, Severini C. Changes in interleukin-1 and tumor necrosis factor production by peripheral blood monocytes after specific bronchoprovocation test in occupational asthma. Am Rev Respir Dis 1992; 146:408–412.

65. Beasley R, Roche WR, Roberts JA, Holgate ST. Cellular events in the bronchi in mild asthma and after bronchial provocation. Am Rev Respir Dis 1989; 139:806–817.

66. Poulter LW, Power C, Burke C. The relationship between bronchial immunopathology and hyperresponsiveness in asthma. Eur Respir J 1990; 3:792–799.

67. Bradley BL, Azzawi M, Jacobson M, et al. Eosinophils, T-lymphocytes, mast cells, neutrophils, and macrophages in bronchial biopsy specimens from atopic subjects with asthma: comparison with biopsy specimens from atopic subjects without asthma and normal control subjects and relationship to bronchial hyperresponsiveness. J Allergy Clin Immunol 1991; 88:661–674.

68. Poston RN, Chanez P, Lacoste JY, Litchfield T, Lee TH, Bousquet J. Immunohistochemical characterization of the cellular infiltration in asthmatic bronchi. Am Rev Respir Dis 1992; 145: 918–921.

69. Bentley AM, Menz G, Storz C, et al. Identification of T lymphocytes, macrophages, and activated eosinophils in the bronchial mucosa in intrinsic asthma. Relationship to symptoms and bronchial responsiveness. Am Rev Respir Dis 1992; 146:500–506.

70. Laitinen LA, Laitinen A, Haahtela T. Airway mucosal inflammation even in patients with newly diagnosed asthma. Am Rev Respir Dis 1993; 147:697–704.

71. Laitenen LA, Laitinen A, Haahtela T, Vilkka V, Spur BW, Lee TH. Leukotriene E_4 and ganulocytic infiltration into asthmatic airways. Lancet 1993; 341:989–990.

72. Chanez P, Vago P, Demoly P, et al. Airway macrophages from patients with asthma do not proliferate. J Allergy Clin Immunol 1993; 92:869–877.

73. Montefort S, Roche WR, Howarth PH, et al. Intercellular adhesion molecule-1 (ICAM-1) and endothelial leucocyte adhesion molecule-1 (ELAM-1) expression in the bronchial mucosa of normal and asthmatic subjects. Eur Respir J 1992; 5:815–823.

74. Montefort S, Holgate ST, Howarth PH. Leucocyte–endothelial adhesion molecules and their role in bronchial asthma and allergic rhinitis. Eur Respir J 1993; 6:1044–1054.

75. Bentley AM, Durham SR, Robinson DS, et al. Expression of endothelial and leukocyte adhesion molecules, interacellular adhesion molecule-1, E-selectin, and vascular cell adhesion molecule-1 in the bronchial mucosa in steady-state and allergen-induced asthma. J Allergy Clin Immunol 1993; 92:857–868.

76. Vachier I, Damon M, Le-Doucen C, et al. Increased oxygen species generation in blood monocytes of asthmatic patients. Am Rev Respir Dis 1992; 146:1161–1166.

77. Borish L, Mascali JJ, Rosenwasser LJ. IgE-dependent cytokine production by human peripheral blood mononuclear phagocytes. J Immunol 1991; 146:63–67.

78. Chanez P, Vignola A, Lacoste P, Michel F, Godard P, Bousquet J. Increased expression of adhesion molecules (ICAM-1 and LFA-1) on alveolar macrophages from asthmatic patients. Allergy 1993; 48:576–580.

79. Balter MS, Eschenbacher WL, Peters-Golden M. Arachidonic acid metabolism in cultured alveolar macrophages from normal, atopic, and asthmatic subjects. Am Rev Respir Dis 1988; 138:1134–1142.

80. Damon M, Chavis C, Crastes-de-Paulet A, Michel FB, Godard P. Effect of nedocromil sodium on TXB_2, LTB_4 and LTD_4 synthesis by alveolar macrophages from asthmatic patients. Eur J Respir Dis Suppl 1986; 147:206–209.

81. Damon M, Chavis C, Crastes-de-Paulet A, Michel FB, Godard P. Arachidonic acid metabolism in alveolar macrophages. A comparison of cells from healthy subjects, allergic asthmatics, and chronic bronchitis patients. Prostaglandins 1987; 34:291–309.

82. Chavis C, Godard P, Michel FB, Crastes-de-Paulet A, Damon M. Sulfidopeptide leukotrienes contribute to human alveolar macrophage activation in asthma. Prostaglandins Leukot Essent Fatty Acids 1991; 42:95–100.

83. Chavis C, Godard P, Crastes-de-Paulet A, Damon M. Formation of lipoxins and leukotrienes by human alveolar macrophages incubated with 15(S)-HETE: a model for cellular cooperation between macrophages and airway epithelial cells. Eicosanoids 1993; 5:203–211.

84. Campbell AM, Chanez P, Vignola AM, et al. Functional characteristics of bronchial epithelium obtained by brushing from asthmatic and normal subjects. Am Rev Respir Dis 1993; 147: 529–534.

85. Lans DM, Rocklin RE. Dysregulation of arachidonic acid release and metabolism by atopic mononuclear cells. Clin Exp Allergy 1989; 19:37–44.

86. Valone F, Boggs J, Goetzl E. Lipid mediators of hypersensitivity and inflammation. In: Middleton EJ, Reed C, Ellis E, Adkinson NJ, Yunginger J, Busse W, eds. Allergy, Principles and Practice, 4th ed. St Louis: CV Mosby, 1993:302–319.

87. Arnoux B, Jouvin-Marche E, Arnoux A, Benveniste J. Release of PAF-acether from human blood monocytes. Agents Actions 1982; 12:713–716.
88. Arnoux B, Joseph M, Simoes MH, et al. Antigenic release of PAF-acether and beta-glucuronidase from alveolar macrophages of asthmatics. Bull Eur Physiopathol Respir 1987; 23: 119–124.
89. Arnoux B, Denjean A, Page CP, Nolibe D, Morley J, Benveniste J. Accumulation of platelets and eosinophils in baboon lung after PAF-acether challenge. Inhibition by ketotifen. Am Rev Respir Dis 1988; 137:855–860.
90. Cuss FM, Dixon CM, Barnes PJ. Effects of inhaled platelet activating factor on pulmonary function and bronchial responsiveness in man. Lance 1986; 2:189–192.
91. Housset B. Biochemical aspects of free radicals metabolism. Bull Eur Physiopathol Respir 1987; 23:287–290.
92. Damon M, Cluzel M, Chanez P, Godard P. Phagocytosis induction of chemiluminescence and chemoattractant increased superoxide anion release from activated human alveolar macrophages in asthma. J Biolumin Chemilumin 1989; 4:279–286.
93. Gosset P, Lassalle P, Tonnel AB, et al. Production of an interleukin-1 inhibitory factor by human alveolar macrophages from normals and allergic asthmatic patients. Am Rev Respir Dis 1988; 138:40–46.
94. Gosset P, Tsicopoulos A, Wallaert B, et al. Increased secretion of tumor necrosis factor alpha and interleukin-6 by alveolar macrophages consecutive to the development of the late asthmatic reaction. J Allergy Clin Immunol 1991; 88:561–571.
95. Gosset P, Tsicopoulos A, Wallaert B, Joseph M, Capron A, Tonnel AB. Tumor necrosis factor alpha and interleukin-6 production by human mononuclear phagocytes from allergic asthmatics after IgE-dependent stimulation. Am Rev Respir Dis 1992; 146:768–774.
96. Pujol JL, Cosso B, Daures JP, Clot J, Michel FB, Godard P. Interleukin-1 release by alveolar macrophages in asthmatic patients and healthy subjects. Int Arch Allergy Appl Immunol 1990; 91:207–210.
97. Borish L, Mascali JJ, Dishuck J, Beam WR, Martin RJ, Rosenwasser LJ. Detection of alveolar macrophage-derived IL-1 beta in asthma. Inhibition with corticosteroids. J Immunol 1992; 149: 3078–3082.
98. Howell CJ, Pujol JL, Crea AE, et al. Identification of an alveolar macrophage-derived activity in bronchial asthma that enhances leukotriene C_4 generation by human eosinophils stimulated by ionophore A23187 as a granulocyte–macrophage colony-stimulating factor. Am Rev Respir Dis 1989; 140:1340–1347.
99. Kotloff RM, Little J, Elias JA. Human alveolar macrophage and blood monocyte interleukin-6 production. Am J Respir Cell Mol Biol 1990; 3:497–505.
100. Enk C, Mosbech H. Interleukin-1 production by monocytes from patients with allergic asthma after stimulation in vitro with lipopolysaccharide and Dermatophagoides pteronyssinus mite allergen. Int Arch Allergy Appl Immunol 1988; 85:308–311.
101. Chanez P, Vignola A, Paul-Eugène N, et al. Modulation by IL-4 of cytokine release from mononuclear phagocytes in asthma. J Allergy Clin Immunol 1994; 94:997–1005.
102. Le J, Vilcek J. Tumor necrosis factor and interleukin 1: cytokines with multiple overlapping biological activities. Lab Invest 1987; 56:234–248.
103. Urban JL, Shepard HM, Rothstein JL, Sugarman BJ, Schreiber H. Tumor necrosis factor: a potent effector molecule for tumor cell killing by activated macrophages. Proc Natl Acad Sci USA 1986; 83:5233–5237.
104. Le JM, Vilcek J. Interleukin 6: a multifunctional cytokine regulating immune reactions and the acute phase protein response. Lab Invest 1989; 61:588–602.
105. Witsell AL, Schook LB. Tumor necrosis factor alpha is an autocrine growth regulator during macrophage differentiation [published erratum appears in Proc Natl Acad Sci USA 1993 May 15;90:4763]. Proc Natl Acad Sci USA 1992; 89:4754–4758.

106. Kips JC, Tavernier JH, Joos GF, Peleman RA, Pauwels RA. The potential role of tumour necrosis factor alpha in asthma. Clin Exp Allergy 1993; 23:247–250.

107. Lassalle P, Gosset P, Delneste Y, et al. Modulation of adhesion molecule expression on endothelial cells during the late asthmatic reaction: role of macrophage-derived tumor necrosis factor-alpha. Clin Exp Immunol 1993; 94:105–110.

108. Sanceau J, Wijdenes J, Revel M, Wietzerbin J. IL-6 and IL-6 receptor modulation by IFN-gamma and tumor necrosis factor-alpha in human monocytic cell line (THP-1). Priming effect of IFN-gamma. J Immunol 1991; 147:2630–2637.

109. Riedy MC, Stewart CC. Inhibitory role of interleukin-6 in macrophage proliferation. J Leukoc Biol 1992; 52:125–127.

110. Rivier A, Chanez P, Pène J, et al. Modulation of phenotypic and functional properties of normal human mononuclear phagocytes by GM-CSF. Int Arch Allergy Immunol 1994; 104:27–32.

111. Senior RM, Connolly NL, Cury JD, Welgus HG, Campbell EJ. Elastin degradation by human alveolar macrophages. A prominent role of metalloproteinase activity. Am Rev Respir Dis 1989; 139:1251–1256.

112. Hance AJ. Pulmonary immune cells in health and disease: dendritic cells and Langerhans' cells [see comments]. Eur Respir J 1993; 6:1213–1220.

113. Holt PG. Regulation of antigen-presenting cell function(s) in lung and airway tissues. Eur Respir J 1993; 6:120–129.

114. Holt PG. Down-regulation of immune responses in the lower respiratory tract: the role of alveolar macrophages. Clin Exp Immunol 1986; 63:261–270.

115. Elias JA, Schreiber AD, Gustilo K, et al. Differential interleukin 1 elaboration by unfractionated and density fractionated human alveolar macrophages and blood monocytes: relationship to cell maturity. J Immunol 1985; 135:3198–3204.

116. Mackanness G. The induction and expression of cell-mediated hypersensitivity in the lung. Am Rev Respir Dis 1971; 104:813–826.

117. Holt PG. Inhibitory activity of unstimulated alveolar macrophages on T-lymphocyte blastogenic response. Am Rev Respir Dis 1978; 118:791–793.

118. Venet A, Hance AJ, Saltini C, Robinson BW, Crystal RG. Enhanced alveolar macrophage-mediated antigen-induced T-lymphocyte proliferation in sarcoidosis. J Clin Invest 1985; 75: 293–301.

119. Aubas P, Cosso B, Godard P, Michel FB, Clot J. Decreased suppressor cell activity of alveolar macrophages in bronchial asthma. Am Rev Respir Dis 1984; 130:875–878.

120. Gant V, Cluzel M, Shakoor Z, Rees PJ, Lee TH, Hamblin AS. Alveolar macrophage accessory cell function in bronchial asthma. Am Rev Respir Dis 1992; 146:900–904.

121. Fuller RW, MacDermot J. Stimulation of IgE sensitized human alveolar macrophages by anti-IgE is unaffected by sodium cromoglycate. Clin Allergy 1986; 16:523–526.

122. Fuller RW, Morris PK, Richmond R, et al. Immunoglobulin E-dependent stimulation of human alveolar macrophages: significance in type 1 hypersensitivity. Clin Exp Immunol 1986; 65: 416–426.

123. Williams J, Johnson S, Mascali JJ, Smith H, Rosenwasser LJ, Borish L. Regulation of low affinity IgE receptor (CD23) expression on mononuclear phagocytes in normal and asthmatic subjects. J Immunol 1992; 149:2823–2829.

124. Yanagawa H, Sone S, Sugihara K, Tanaka K, Ogura T. Interleukin-4 downregulates interleukin-6 production by human alveolar macrophages at protein and mRNA levels. Microbiol Immunol 1991; 35:879–893.

125. Bhaskaran G, Nii A, Sone S, Ogura T. Differential effects of interleukin-4 on superoxide anion production by human alveolar macrophages stimulated with lipopolysaccharide and interferon-gamma. J Leukoc Biol 1992; 52:218–223.

126. Lacraz S, Nicod L, Galve-de-Rochemonteix B, Baumberger C, Dayer JM, Welgus HG. Suppression of metalloproteinase biosynthesis in human alveolar macrophages by interleukin-4. J Clin Invest 1992; 90:382–388.

127. Moore KW, O'Garra A, de-Waal-Malefyt R, Vieira P, Mosmann TR. Interleukin-10. Annu Rev Immunol 1993; 11:165–190.

128. de-Waal-Malefyt R, Figdor CG, Huijbens R, et al. Effects of IL-13 on phenotype, cytokine production, and cytotoxic function of human monocytes. Comparison with IL-4 and modulation by IFN-gamma or IL-10. J Immunol 1993; 151:6370–6381.

129. Hamilton JA. Colony stimulating factors, cytokines and monocyte-macrophages—some controversies. Immunol Today 1993; 14:18–24.

130. Rock MJ, Despot J, Lemanske R Jr. Mast cell granules modulate alveolar macrophage respiratory-burst activity and eicosanoid metabolism. J Allergy Clin Immunol 1990; 86: 452–461.

131. Cluzel M, Liu MC, Goldman DW, Undem BJ, Lichtenstein LM. Histamine acting on a histamine type 1 (H_1) receptor increases beta-glucuronidase release from human lung macrophages. Am J Respir Cell Mol Biol 1990; 3:603–609.

132. Vignola A, Chanez P, Paul-Lacoste P, Paul-Eugène N, Godard P, Bousquet J. Phenotypic and functional modulation of normal human alveolar macrophages by histamine. Am J Respir Cell Mol Biol 1994. In press.

133. Pujol JL, Bousquet J, Grenier J, et al. Substance P activation of bronchoalveolar macrophages from asthmatic patients and normal subjects. Clin Exp Allergy 1989; 19:625–628.

134. Damon M, Vial H, Crastes-de-Paulet A, Godard P. Phosphoinositide breakdown and superoxide anion release in formyl–peptide-stimulated human alveolar macrophages. Comparison between quiescent and activated cells. FEBS Lett 1988; 239:169–173.

135. Godard P, Radeau T, Parant M, Vial H, Damon M. Protein kinase C activation in human unstimulated alveolar macrophage. Am Rev Respir Dis 1991; 143:A12.

136. Pacheco Y, Fonlupt P, Macovschi O, et al. Phosphatidyl ethanolamine methylation in membrane from bronchoalveolar lavage mononuclear cells, in asthmatic patients: a new marker of macrophage activity. Biomed Pharmacother 1983; 37:398–401.

137. Bachelet M, Vincent D, Havet N, et al. Reduced responsiveness of adenylate cyclase in alveolar macrophages from patients with asthma. J Allergy Clin Immunol 1991; 88:322–328.

138. van-Oosterhout AJ, Nijkamp FP. Effect of lymphokines on beta-adrenoceptor function of human peripheral blood mononuclear cells. Br J Clin Pharmacol 1990; 30:150S–152S.

139. Beusenberg FD, Van-Amsterdam JG, Hoogsteden HC, et al. Stimulation of cyclic AMP production in human alveolar macrophages induced by inflammatory mediators and beta-sympathicomimetics. Eur J Pharmacol 1992; 228:57–62.

140. Prigent AF, Fonlupt P, Dubois M, et al. Cyclic nucleotide phosphodiesterases and methyltransferases in purified lymphocytes, monocytes, and polymorphonuclear leucocytes from healthy donors and asthmatic patients. Eur J Clin Invest 1990; 20:323–329.

141. Borish L, Williams J, Johnson S, Mascali JJ, Miller R, Rosenwasser LJ. Anti-inflammatory effects of nedocromil sodium: inhibition of alveolar macrophage function. Clin Exp Allergy 1992; 22:984–990.

142. Joseph M, Thorel T, Tsicopoulos A, Tonnel AB, Capron A. Nedocromil sodium inhibition of IgE-mediated activation of human mononuclear phagocytes and platelets from asthmatics. Drugs 1989; 1:32–36.

143. Radeau T, Godard P, Chavis C, Michel FB, Descomps B, Damon M. Effect of nedocromil sodium on sulfidopeptide leukotrienes-stimulated human alveolar macrophages in asthma. Pulmon Pharmacol 1993; 6:27–31.

144. Tsicopoulos A, Lassalle P, Joseph M, et al. Effect of disodium cromoglycate on inflammatory cells bearing the Fc epsilon receptor type II (Fc epsilon RII). Int J Immunopharmacol 1988; 10:227–236.

145. Holian A, Hamilton R, Scheule RK. Mechanistic aspects of cromolyn sodium action on the alveolar macrophage: inhibition of stimulation by soluble agonists. Agents Actions 1991; 33: 318–325.

146. Russo-Marie F. Macrophages and the glucocorticoids. J Neuroimmunol 1992; 40:281–286.

147. Woolcock AJ. Steroid resistant asthma: what is the clinical definition? Eur Respir J 1993; 6: 743–747.

148. Carmichael J, Paterson IC, Diaz P, Crompton GK, Kay AB, Grant IW. Corticosteroid resistance in chronic asthma. Br Med J Clin Res 1981; 282:1419–1422.

149. Kay AB, Diaz P, Carmicheal J, Grant IW. Corticosteroid-resistant chronic asthma and monocyte complement receptors. Clin Exp Immunol 1981; 44:576–580.

150. Poznansky MC, Gordon AC, Douglas JG, Krajewski AS, Wyllie AH, Grant IW. Resistance to methylprednisolone in cultures of blood mononuclear cells from glucocorticoid-resistant asthmatic patients. Clin Sci 1984; 67:639–645.

151. Poznansky MC, Gordon AC, Grant IW, Wyllie AH. A cellular abnormality in glucocorticoid resistant asthma. Clin Exp Immunol 1985; 61:135–142.

152. Lane SJ, Lee TH. Glucocorticoid receptor characteristics in monocytes of patients with corticosteroid-resistant bronchial asthma. Am Rev Respir Dis 1991; 143:1020–1024.

153. Wilkinson JR, Lane SJ, Lee TH. Effects of corticosteroids on cytokine generation and expression of activation antigens by monocytes in bronchial asthma. Int Arch Allergy Appl Immunol 1991; 94:220–221.

154. Lane SJ, Wilkinson JR, Cochrane GM, Lee TH, Arm JP. Differential in vitro regulation by glucocorticoids of monocyte-derived cytokine generation in glucocorticoid-resistant bronchial asthma. Am Rev Respir Dis 1993; 147:690–696.

155. Vecchiarelli A, Siracusa A, Cenci E, Puliti M, Abbritti G. Effect of corticosteroid treatment on interleukin-1 and tumour necrosis factor secretion by monocytes from subjects with asthma. Clin Exp Allergy 1992; 22:365–370.

156. Gin W, Kay AB. The effect of corticosteroids on monocyte and neutrophil activation in bronchial asthma. J Allergy Clin Immunol 1985; 76:675–682.

157. Burke C, Power CK, Norris A, Condez A, Schmekel B, Poulter LW. Lung function and immunopathological changes after inhaled corticosteroid therapy in asthma. Eur Respir J 1992; 5:73–79.

12

Roles of Epithelial Cells and Fibroblasts in Allergic Diseases

John R. Spurzem, Debra J. Romberger, and Stephen I. Rennard
University of Nebraska Medical Center, Omaha, Nebraska

INTRODUCTION

The idea that epithelial cells and mesenchymal cells play important roles in the immuno-pharmacology of allergic diseases might have seemed a bit far-fetched just a few years ago. Considering all the attention given to cells of the immune system and the newly discovered cytokines, students of immunology might have appropriately assumed that epithelial cells and mesenchymal cells were passive, uninteresting cells. However, there has been an explosion of information in recent years suggesting that epithelial cells and fibroblasts are not just passive bystanders during immunological processes. Epithelial dysfunction is now thought to be a very important contributor to disorders such as asthma. The burgeoning interest in the airway epithelium was highlighted by the recent publication in 1991 of a text in the Lung Biology in Health and Disease series, *The Airway Epithelium. Physiology, Pathophysiology, and Pharmacology* (1).

Conferences have been devoted to epithelial cell biology and airway disease (2). The amount of information generated in the past 2 years might warrant another text devoted to the airway epithelium. Similarly, a large amount of information is now available about keratinocytes and their involvement in inflammatory reactions of the epidermis (3,4) and also about gut mucosal immunity (5). Fibroblasts have not been ignored and are now thought to release relevant inflammatory cytokines and to participate in immunological processes. This review will be organized around four themes. First, epithelial and mesenchymal cells are important sources of proinflammatory and regulatory cytokines and participate in inflammatory reactions through direct interactions with inflammatory cells. Second, epithelial cells have important metabolic functions that are involved in the degradation of mediators such as neuropeptides. Third, epithelial cells participate in the control of airway tone. Fourth, repair and restitution of the normal epithelium is important for the resolution of airway disorders such as asthma.

287

EPITHELIAL AND MESENCHYMAL CELLS PARTICIPATE IN INFLAMMATORY REACTIONS

Release of Inflammatory Mediators

The idea that epithelial cells and mesenchymal cells participate in inflammatory processes by the release of mediators is now a well-developed concept. When agents are inhaled into the lung, the airway epithelial cells are likely the first cells to encounter toxins or pathogens, and the ability to initiate a response would seem to be an important defense mechanism (6). Similarly, it has been proposed that keratinocytes and enterocytes play a role as "sentinel cells" that are capable of transmitting signals (3,4). Epithelial cells also release mediators more associated with chronic inflammation. A survey of inflammatory mediators from several families of mediators is described in Table 1. Work from several animal species is represented. The absence of a reference for some mediators in a cell type may not necessarily indicate that the cell type is incapable of producing the mediator. Rather, it may be that it has not been examined. Eicosanoid metabolism in airway epithelial cells has been extensively studied and reviewed (19), but less has been published about eicosanoid metabolism in keratinocytes and enterocytes. Keratinocytes are capable of producing arachidonic acid and may participate in eicosanoid cascades in the skin, but specific leukotrienes have not been described as being produced form cultured keratinocytes (48). Intestinal mucosa and colon cancer tissues contain eicosanoids, such as prostaglandin $(PG)E_2$ and leukotriene $(LT)B_4$, but the cell sources are not clear (49,50). Of the newly described chemokine family of chemotactic cytokines only interleukin (IL)-8 is listed, as there is good evidence that epithelial cells are capable of producing IL-8. It may be possible that epithelial cells are also capable of producing other chemokines, such as RANTES. Murine renal tubular epithelium expresses an MuRANTES (51,52).

The idea that epithelial cells function as a first line of defense is supported by the observations that epithelial cells are capable of releasing mediators relatively quickly after

Table 1 Inflammatory Mediators Released by Epithelial Cells[a]

Mediators	Bronchial epithelial cells	Keratinocytes	Enterocytes
G-CSF	7, 41	24	
GM-CSF	7–9, 15	21–24	
Il-1	10	21, 22, 25–27	40
IL-3		28–30, 38	
IL-5		22	
IL-6	10, 15, 39, 41, 42	22, 31	43
IL-7		22, 32, 33	
IL-8	11, 15, 39, 41, 77	34, 35	44
TGF-β	12–14, 37	37	45, 46
TNF-α	20	21, 22, 36	47
Eicosanoids			
LTB_4	18–20		
Di-HETES	18–20		
PGE_2	16–19		

[a]The numbers refer to publications as referenced at the end of the chapter.

stimulation or damage. Koyama et al. (20) have shown that cultured bovine bronchial epithelial cells release arachidonate metabolites, including LTB_4, within 1 h of exposure to endotoxin. Other chemotactic activities for neutrophils and monocytes were released at later time points (20). The release of arachidonate metabolites may be a rather general, early response of airway epithelial cells to injury, as many stimuli will elicit LTB_4 release from bovine bronchial epithelial cells in primary culture. Viral infection and ozone are just two of the described stimuli (17,53). There may be significant species differences in the array of arachidonate metabolites produced by airway cells (19). Some of the reported differences may also relate to differences in cell preparation and culture methods. Keratinocytes also respond quickly to external stimuli. After acute perturbation of skin, the epidermis produces tissue necrosis factor (TNF)-α within several hours (21,36).

Epithelial cells also participate in more chronic inflammatory processes. Some hours after stimulation, airway epithelial cells release very potent chemotactic factors for neutrophils, which likely play roles in the chronic attraction of leukocytes. The cytokine with perhaps the most potent chemotactic activity for neutrophils is IL-8 (54). Interleukin-8 is thought to have a relatively long half-life (54). It is now considered to be one member of a family of similarly sized (8–10 kDa) chemokines. These peptides are important in the biology of the epidermis (34,35), gut mucosa (44,55), as well as the airway epithelium (11,15,39). Another family of closely related chemokines is the C-C family which includes RANTES and macrophage inflammatory protein (MIP)-1. These chemokines have more activity on macrophages (56). Epithelial cells may also release RANTES, as the gene is expressed in renal tubular epithelium (51). Epithelial cells also release mediators that are involved in the maturation and activation of leukocytes. Airway cells release granulocyte–macrophage colony-stimulating factor (GM-CSF) in vitro (7–9,15), which is capable of promoting survival and activation of eosinophils, stimulating neutrophils, and stimulating macrophage proliferation. Ohtoshi et al. (8) have demonstrated that GM-CSF released by human upper airway epithelial cells induces histamine-containing cell differentiation of progenitor cells. The same group has also shown that epithelial cells from inflamed tissues release more GM-CSF than the cells from normal tissues (8). Analogously, keratinocytes are reported to release colony-stimulating factors and IL-1, IL-6, and IL-8, and enterocytes are reported to release IL-1, IL-6, and IL-8. Thus, epithelial cells from inflamed tissues release factors that recruit, activate, and differentiate leukocytes (Fig. 1).

The foregoing emphasis on epithelial cells is not to ignore mesenchymal cells. Recent reviews have discussed the roles of fibroblasts in the interactions with inflammatory cells (57,58). Clearly, fibroblasts are capable of releasing relevant cytokines, such as GM-CSF (59,60) and IL-6 (61,62) and IL-8 (63). Fibroblasts also release monocyte chemoattractant protein-1 (MCP-1; 64,65) and are thought to express MIP-1α in interstitial lung disease (56). Both MCP-1 and MIP-1α are members of the C-C family of chemokines. The expression of cytokines by fibroblasts is modulated by other mediators including substance P, IL-1, TNF-α and transforming growth factor (TGF)-β (57–65). The capability of fibroblasts and epithelial cells to modulate inflammatory cell functions leads to the concepts that cells in the epidermis and mucosal surfaces are central players in controlling the inflammatory processes in localized areas and participate in cytokine cascades, discussed further later.

Epithelial cells and fibroblasts are also capable of producing mediators that down-regulate inflammatory processes. Many cells are potential producers of TGF-β, including macrophages (66), epithelial cells (12–14,37,45,46), and fibroblasts (37,67). TGF-β is present in the epithelial lining fluid of the lung (68) and also in the epithelium of damaged

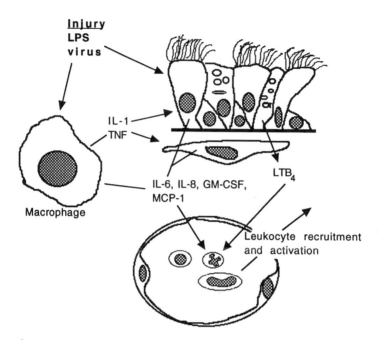

Figure 1 Cytokine cascades in the airway epithelium. Initial stimuli, such as endotoxin or viral infection, initiate alarm mediators such as LTB_4 from epithelial cells and IL-1 and TNF-α from macrophages. In response to mediators released by macrophages, epithelial and mesenchymal cells further augment the inflammatory response by releasing additional mediators that recruit and activate leukocytes.

lung (69). It plays important roles in tissue repair and can function as a chemoattractant for leukocytes (70,71). Interestingly, TGF-β also has anti-inflammatory properties, such as the ability to inhibit IL-2-dependent proliferation of T lymphocytes (72). It also inhibits cytokine production by mononuclear cells (73). Among the arachidonate metabolism products released by epithelial cells (20) and fibroblasts (74), PGE_2 has a number of anti-inflammatory effects. It reduces the production of neutrophil chemoattractants by macrophages, for example (75). Interleukin-6 is capable of reducing inflammation in several models of inflammation, including an in vivo model of pulmonary inflammation (76). In the context that IL-6 also has well-documented proinflammatory effects, such cytokines may be *bifunctional*, with differing activities dependent on the inflammatory setting.

An important aspect of inflammatory responses is thought to be the amplification of response through cytokine cascades. Epithelial cells and fibroblasts likely play an important role in the cascade effect, especially for IL-8 and MCP-1. Tumor necrosis factor-α (TNF-α) is a potent stimulator of IL-8 expression in airway epithelial cells (11,41) and MCP-1 in fibroblasts (64). It is thought that TNF-α released from macrophages, followed by IL-8 and MCP-1 release, constitutes an important cytokine network effect in the lung (11). It has also been reported that treatment of an airway epithelial cell line, derived from a cystic fibrosis patient, with IL-1β increases secretion of IL-6 and IL-8 (39). The expression of IL-6 and IL-8 is also regulated in intestinal epithelial cell lines by other cytokines (43,44). Thus, epithelial cells and fibroblasts participate in cycles of cytokine cascades that accelerate or perpetuate the inflammatory process. However, some of the released mediators have inhibitory effects on inflammation, as described earlier. Thus, epithelial cells and fibroblasts may produce the critical proinflammatory or anti-inflammatory cytokines that control the progress of inflammatory events. Denburg et al. (78) have proposed that these structural cells play the central role in creating a web of cytokines that control chronic inflammation in a tissue microenvironment, a compartment consisting of the epithelium.

Cell–Cell Adhesion Molecules

In addition to the ability to produce important inflammatory mediators, epithelial cells and fibroblasts express surface molecules that enhance interactions with leukocytes. The ability of epithelial and mesenchymal cells to directly interact with T cells, for example, may be another mechanism to amplify immune responses. Several investigations have emphasized the importance of the expression of intercellular adhesion molecule-1 (ICAM-1) by epithelial cells (79–81). ICAM-1 is the ligand for lymphocyte function-associated antigen (LFA)-1 on leukocytes (82). The interaction of ICAM-1 with LFA-1 is thought to strengthen the cell–cell adhesion mechanisms during activities such as antigen presentation and target recognition (83–85). The expression of ICAM-1 is enhanced on airway epithelial cells, keratinocytes, enterocytes, and fibroblasts by proinflammatory cytokines (79–81,86,87). Interleukin-1β, TNF-α, and interferon gamma (IFN-γ) are the cytokines that are implicated with the expression-enhancing activity. The expression and function of adhesion molecules, such as ICAM-1, are also modulated by inflammatory injury and viral infection (53,81). The ability of the cells to express ICAM-1 in the setting of a viral infection may be an important component of the defense mechanism to clear such infections. The regulation of ICAM-1 expression on epithelial cells is a potentially important target for pharmacological intervention in inflammatory processes.

The importance of ICAM-1 expression has been explored in a primate model of asthma (80). Eosinophils infiltrating into the epithelium were found in association with ICAM-1-expressing epithelial cells. Daily intravenous treatment of the animals with antibodies to ICAM-1 antagonized the induction of airway hyperresponsiveness and eosinophil infiltration. Certainly, the effect of the antibodies may have been to disrupt the interactions between leukocytes and epithelial cells, thereby disrupting eosinophil recruitment. Perhaps disruption of the interactions between eosinophils and other cells, including fibroblasts and epithelial cells, also plays a role. Certainly, ICAM-1 expression would be important for the cytotoxic injury of epithelial cells and fibroblasts.

Epithelial cells also express major histocompatibility complex (MHC) antigens (88–93). Expression of MHC antigens allows cells to directly interact with lymphocytes and raises the possibility that epithelial cells can present antigen to lymphocytes. Both MHC class I (HLA-A, B, C, in humans) and MHC class II (HLA-DR, DQ, DP, in humans) antigens' expression is regulated on a variety of epithelial cell types. The most potent stimulant for expression is likely IFN-γ (90–93), but TNF-α may potentiate the effect in some settings (93). Expression of MHC antigens can confer the ability to stimulate lymphoblasts in mixed lymphocyte reactions. This has been demonstrated for bronchial epithelial cells (92) and keratinocytes (89,90). Bronchial epithelial cells that had been stimulated with IFN-γ were more potent stimulators of such allogenic lymphocyte reactions (92). Keratinocytes, however, are not good stimulators of allogenic reactions, even after MHC class II antigens have been induced.

The presence of MHC antigens on epithelial cells is essential for them to be targets of immune reactions. The regulation of MHC expression on epithelial cells is considered to be an important aspect in pathogenesis of the graft-versus-host reactions that affect epithelial organs (87,90). Increased expression of MHC antigens on epithelial cells has been documented in graft-versus-host reactions (94). The MHC expression is also critical for organ rejection (97,98). The increase in expression of MHC antigens on bronchial epithelial cells can be reduced by corticosteroids in vitro, but not by cyclosporine (93). Thus, the difference in effects of corticosteroids and cyclosporine on epithelial cells may be a partial explanation for the more marked beneficial effects of corticosteroids in treating bronchiolitis obliterans, a manifestation of rejection, that occurs after lung transplantation (95).

The ability of epithelial cells to interact with T cells has implications for other disorders. Nickoloff and Turka (3) have presented the thesis that keratinocytes are targets of skin-specific T cells. Activation of keratinocytes with subsequent amplification of the recruitment of T cells may enlarge psoriasis lesions. As we mentioned earlier, activation of epithelial cells and expression of ICAM-1 may be critical to the successful immune response to viral infection (53,81). The issue has been examined by several investigators for papillomavirus infections. It has been observed that T cells become activated when they enter the epidermal compartment of papillomas (96).

Antigen Presentation by Epithelial Cells

The presence of cell surface molecules, such as MHC antigens, raises the question of whether epithelial cells are capable of presenting antigen to T cells. The MHC-expressing epithelial cells can act as alloantigens in mixed lymphocyte reactions, but there is some difference between cell types, as keratinocytes appear to be less stimulatory than airway epithelial cells. Keratinocytes, however, are capable of presenting superantigens and act as accessory cells in some situations (99,100). There also appear to be differences between the different types of epithelial cells in their ability to present soluble antigens. Enterocytes, from both rat and human preparations, have demonstrated antigen-presenting and accessory cell activities (101,102). Keratinocytes and airway epithelial cells appear to be inefficient processors and presenter of soluble antigen (91). The reasons for these cells' lack of ability to present soluble antigen are unclear. There is some evidence that bronchial epithelial cells and keratinocytes can produce IL-1β, but a lack of accessory signals may be a reason. The presence of dendritic–Langerhans cells in the epithelium may be necessary for sufficient production of IL-1β and accessory cell signals. The ability to process small peptides and associate them with the MHC cell surface complex of proteins may be lacking in keratinocytes and airway epithelial cells.

Dendritic–Langerhans Cells and Other Specialized Tissues

It is clear that the epithelia of various organs are not made up of uniform populations of cells. Langerhans cells and their precursors, dendritic cells, are found scattered in epithelia (103–107). Dendritic cells are thought to be derived from γδT cells (107). Under the influence of cytokines or other differentiating factors, dendritic cells mature into Langerhans cells and acquire a different phenotype of surface markers (108). Dendritic cells are $CD3^+$, $CD45^+$, $CD4^-$, $CD8^-$, and generally $CD1a^-/CD1c^+$. Langerhans cells in the skin are thought to acquire CD1a and lose CD1c positivity (104). These cells are considered to be resident antigen-presenting cells in epithelia. They are 10- to 100-fold more potent in stimulating lymphocyte proliferation than are monocyte lineage cells (102,107). Langerhans and dendritic cells, derived from both human and murine epidermis, are reported to produce a broad spectrum of cytokines, including GM-CSF, IL-1, IL-2, IL-3, IL-4, IL-6, IL-7, IFN-γ, TNF-α, TNF-β, and MIP-1α (105,106). Matsue et al. (108) propose that Langerhans cells are potential targets of the cytokines produced by dendritic cells, thus, there is an integrated immune surveillance system in the epidermis. The roles of these $\gamma\delta$T-cell–derived cells in disease states are being addressed by various investigators. The pulmonary disorder histiocytosis X may be an uncontrolled immune response initiated by Langerhans cells (104).

Other specialized cells in epithelia include M cells that overlie Peyer's patches in intestinal mucosa (5). These cells may function as portals for entry of certain antigens. The roles of Peyer's patches as specialized lymphoid organs will not be further discussed in this review. Other specialized lymphoid tissues found in epithelia include mucosa-associated lymphoid tissue (MALT), and bronchus-associated lymphoid tissue (BALT) (109). The presence of such tissue in the lungs of some species, such as rats and rabbits, is well documented, but the corresponding tissues in humans are not as well developed. BALT also has specialized overlying epithelium that contains lymphoid cells.

The rarest pulmonary epithelial cell has been considered to be the neuroendocrine cell. The neuroendocrine cell has been attracting attention recently, and the attention has generated a workshop conference (110). Pulmonary neuroendocrine cells are found near the basement membrane, either as sparse cells or in groups of cells. The clusters of cells are called neuroepithelial bodies. Neuroepithelial bodies have associations with nerve endings, and acetylcholine causes release of granules from these bodies. Neuroendocrine cells contain several hormonal peptides of interest, including gastrin-releasing peptide, calcitonin, calcitonin gene-related peptide, enkephalin, somatostatin, cholecystokinin, substance P, and endothelin (110). Obviously, a plethora of effects could be expected to result from the release of such mediators. The peptides are known to influence airway tone, vasoconstriction, and mucous secretion, stimulate J receptors, and act as growth factors for epithelial cells. The role of hormonal peptides in disease states is being investigated (110). Hyperplasia of neuroendocrine cells occurs with pulmonary inflammation in humans and can be induced in experimental animals.

Production of Nitric Oxide

One of the more exciting discoveries of the past few years has been the recognition of nitric oxide (NO) as an important mediator of cellular responses. Progress in the characterization of the factor released by endothelial cells that caused relaxation of vascular smooth muscle had been difficult until the identification of the gas NO as the likely mediator of the effect (111,112). There has been an explosion of interest in the implications for drug development.

Various cells are capable of producing NO, including macrophages (113,114); the epithelium likely produces NO. In vitro airway epithelial cells metabolize L-arginine to L-citrulline by nitric oxide synthase, a pathway for NO production (115). Two forms of nitric oxide synthase have been described, and bronchial epithelial cells are thought to contain, or can be induced to express, both types (116). The expression of inducible nitric oxide synthase is increased by inflammatory mediators (TNF, IL-1 and IFN-γ) (117), suggesting a mechanism whereby the epithelium responds to inflammation and contributes to cascades of mediators. Nitric oxide is detected in the exhaled air of normal human subjects and, interestingly, expired NO concentrations are higher during asthmatic exacerbations and decline with clinical improvement (117–119). The role of NO in the pathogenesis of asthma is unclear. There is some evidence that inhalation of NO at high concentrations (80 ppm vs. the 80 ppb found in exhale of normals) is a mild bronchodilator in asthma, but not in chronic obstructive pulmonary disease (COPD) or in normal persons (120). There is also some evidence that NO modulates leukocyte function (111,112). The precise role of NO in the inflammatory response and the relevant sources of NO during inflammation are unclear.

METABOLISM BY EPITHELIAL CELLS

Epithelial cells contain several enzymes that inactivate inflammatory mediators. Airway epithelial cells may be particularly important for the metabolism and inactivation of neuropeptides, such as bradykinin, substance P, and neurokinin A. Airway epithelia express several peptidases, including membrane-associated neutral endopeptidase, previously called enkephalinase, and angiotensin-converting enzyme (121). The use of neutral endo-peptidase inhibitors has shown augmentation of airway responsiveness in several animal models (122). The loss of neutral endopeptidase activity when epithelium is shed has been hypothesized as a major mechanism of airway hyperresponsiveness and neurogenic inflam-mation in asthma (122–124). Angiotensin-converting enzyme also inactivates bradykinin and substance P. Angiotensin-converting enzyme inhibitors have caused cough and airway hyperreactivity in some patients, and it has been suggested that the effect is mediated by a reduction in the metabolism of neuropeptides (125).

Histamine, released from mast cells and basophils, is an important mediator of broncho-constriction and epithelial permeability. Enzymes that degrade histamine have been de-scribed, including histamine N-methyltransferase (HMT) and histaminase (diamine oxidase; DAO). Several groups have characterized the activity of histamine-degrading enzymes in the lung (126–129). Epithelial cells are a rich source of HMT. The possibility that histamine-degrading activity modulates allergic responses appears worthy of further investigation.

Airway epithelial cells are thought to play important roles in the metabolism of xeno-biotics. These cells are capable of phase I metabolism by means of cytochromes P-450 (130,131) and phase II or conjugative enzymes such as glutathione transferases and sulfo-transferases (132,133). The role of these metabolic pathways in allergic diseases has not been defined, but there are several possibilities; for example, sulfation is a predominant mechanism for the inactivation of catecholamines (135). Airway epithelial cells may be partly responsible for the metabolism of inhaled catecholamines. Recent studies by Beck-mann et al. (133) demonstrated greatest expression of phenol sulfotransferases in the nonciliated secretory epithelial cells of the bronchioles, with lower levels of expression in the larger airways. It is not yet known whether phenol sulfotransferase expression is regulated in airway epithelial cells. If, however, sulfotransferase activity is modulated, this might have consequences for the fate of inhaled catecholamines.

AIRWAY TONE

Bronchial epithelial cells are capable of altering airway smooth muscle by several mecha-nisms. Airway epithelial cells inactivate several mediators that are thought to be involved in neurogenic inflammation and bronchoconstriction. Bronchial epithelial cells also release substances with bronchoconstricting and bronchodilating action. Bronchial epithelial cells release arachidonic acid-derived lipoxygenase products, including PGE_2, which has a bronchodilatory effect (135). Bronchial epithelial cells also release endothelin, which is a direct bronchoconstrictor (135).

The influence of intact epithelium on airway responsiveness has been studied in models of smooth-muscle contraction in multiple species. The subject has been extensively reviewed (135,136). The original observation was that removal of the airway epithelium caused a significant leftward shift of the concentration–effect curve for several bronchoconstrictors. It was hypothesized that the epithelium was capable of providing an "epithelium-derived inhibitory factor" that reduced responsiveness to various bronchoconstrictors. A clear-cut identification of the inhibitory factor has not been achieved, and several factors likely account for the inhibitory activity. Some of the activity is probably PGE_2 (135). It is tempting to hypothesize that NO is the inhibitory activity, as it has already been identified as the endothelium-derived relaxing factor, and NO has some relaxing activity on airway smooth muscle (136). Careful studies (137) have shown that endogenous NO is produced during acetylcholine-induced contractions. However, endogenous NO did not appear to be the major factor involved in epithelium-derived inhibition of contractions.

INJURY AND REPAIR OF THE EPITHELIUM

Injury of the epithelium is a major feature of allergic disorders such as asthma. Laitinen et al. (138) have clearly documented the desquamation of epithelial cells, leaving a bare basement membrane in some instances, in asthma. There are various mechanisms by which the epithelial cells are injured. Activated eosinophils and neutrophils release a considerable armamentarium of proteases, oxidants, and toxic molecules. The major constituent of eosinophil granules, major basic protein (MBP), is toxic to epithelial cells in culture (139,140). Neutrophil elastase is capable of causing epithelial cell detachment from the underlying matrix in in vitro assays (141). Acute inflammation is also associated with vasodilation, leakage of fluid, and possible increases in hydrostatic forces (142,143). Hydrostatic forces could also contribute to epithelial damage.

Damaged epithelium likely plays a role in the processes of inflammation and allergic diseases in multiple ways: The presence of intact epithelium provides an inhibitory factor that reduces the bronchoconstrictor response to many agents. The absence of intact epithelium and its neutral endopeptidase is thought to prolong neurogenic inflammation and to be a major mechanism of airway hyperresponsiveness. Thus, restoration of normal, intact epithelium may be seen as a major mechanism for the resolution of allergic, inflammatory responses.

Restoration of the epithelium has been extensively described at the electron microscopic level in both in vitro and in vivo models of repair. In models of intestinal, epidermal, or airway repair, cells at the edge of the wound migrate into the provisional matrix that forms in the wound (144–148). Once the epithelium is intact, the cells differentiate into the mature cell types. Interestingly, there are conflicting data on which of the cells of the normal bronchial airway are responsible for the migration into the wound. It appears that the basal cells are not necessarily the progenitors of all the other cell types. Secretory cells, or an intermediatory cell, may flatten out at the edge of a wound and start the migration process (149). The rest of the discussion will focus on several aspects of the reepithelialization process. First, the formation of the matrix in a wound site is likely influenced by epithelial cells and fibroblasts; second, the migrating cells respond to attractants in the wound with the matrix components functioning as attractants; and third, inflammatory mediators likely modify the processes.

The provisional matrix in wounds in various tissues includes fibrin, fibronectin, vitronectin, collagens, various proteoglycans, and likely, remnants of the basement membrane, such as type IV collagen and laminin (150–153). In animal epidermal-wounding models, the major components that underlie the migrating keratinocytes appear to be fibrin and fibronectin (150,151). The adjacent epithelial cells and underlying fibroblasts appear to be able to contribute matrix proteins and proteoglycans to the mix. Bronchial epithelial cells are capable of producing fibronectin (154,155). Epithelial-derived fibronectin may represent a form of the protein, produced by either differential splicing of the gene or by posttranslational modifications, that results in some biological differences compared with plasma-derived fibronectin (156). The structural organization of the fibronectin gene and protein has been reviewed (152,156). Alternative splicing of three different regions can occur. The first two regions are called extra domains (ED-A and ED-B; also known as EIII-A and EIII-B). Each of them can undergo cassette splicing of entire exons. The third region, CS-III, has several splice donor and acceptor sites within the exon. Tissue-specific splice variants have been described. Bronchial epithelial cells are also likely able to produce type IV collagen (155), but the extent of matrix proteins produced by normal bronchial epithelial cells has not been fully evaluated. Similarly, keratinocytes produce fibronectin and other matrix components (157). Fibroblasts underlying wounds are thought to be important sources of collagens, fibronectin, and proteoglycans after injury (158).

Production of matrix after injury is modulated by at least several mediators. Transforming growth factor-β is an important mediator of wound repair and has been the subject of a recent review (159). One of the major effects of TGF-β is the accumulation of collagen and increasing wound strength (160); it also modulates the alternative splicing of fibronectin in some cells (152). Production of fibronectin by bronchial epithelial cells is also increased by TGF-β (154). When bronchial epithelial cells were examined for their ability to produce factors that subsequently modulated matrix production by fibroblasts in vitro, both stimulatory and inhibitory factors were found (161). The stimulatory factor is composed in part of TGF-β. The inhibitory activity produced by bronchial epithelial cells appeared to be PGE_2, capable of inhibiting collagen production by fibroblasts. Thus, mediator "networking" is likely operating in the control of matrix production in epithelia. Other mediators of relevance to matrix production in the lung include PDGF, bFGF, IGF-1, TNF-α, IL-1, and IL-6 (152).

The migration of epithelial cells in wounds has been described in several animal models. Similar to that described for keratinocytes, bronchial epithelial cells and enterocytes flatten out and migrate as a sheet to rapidly cover small wounds (144–148). Various potential attractants are likely present in wounds (Fig. 2). The matrix components themselves are capable of stimulating epithelial cell migration in both chemotaxis and haptotaxis assays. Fibronectin and collagens are potent stimulators of bronchial epithelial cell migration in modified Boyden chamber assays (162); laminin is a less potent attractant. Keratinocytes will also migrate to gradients of fibronectin and collagen, but not as well to laminin (163–165).

For migrating cells to interact with and attach to the underlying matrix, specific receptors are used. Most of the cell surface receptors for matrix proteins that have been described are members of the integrin family of receptors. Integrins are heterodimers consisting of α- and β-chains (166–168). Some β-chains and some α-chains interact with multiple other chains so that families of integrins have been described (Table 2). Some integrins likely function solely as matrix receptors, whereas some are also involved in cell–cell adhesion. Some integrins interact primarily with matrix components of basement membrane (collagen and laminin), whereas others interact primarily with inflammatory matrix proteins

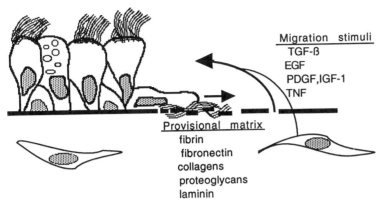

Figure 2 (Spurzem) injury. The matrix components themselves and cytokines are capable of stimulating migration.

(fibronectin, vitronectin, or fibrinogen) (168). Epithelial cells and fibroblasts may have characteristic patterns of integrin expression that are different from each other and from other cell types (166,167). The migrating cells use specific receptors to attach to matrix and can form focal contacts. Focal contacts are contact points at which integrins interact with several cytoplasmic proteins and the actin cytoskeleton (169). The formation of the focal contacts is essential for the anchoring of the matrix to the cytoskeleton (170). The aggregation of some integrins to focal contacts is influenced by the underlying matrix. Different

Table 2   Extracellular Matrix Receptors

Integrin receptor families	
$\alpha1/\beta1$	Laminin, collagen
$\alpha2/\beta1$	Collagen, laminin
$\alpha3/\beta1$	Laminin, collagen, fibronectin
$\alpha4/\beta1$	Fibronectin
$\alpha5/\beta1$	Fibronectin
$\alpha6/\beta1$	Laminin
$\alpha7/\beta1$	Laminin
$\alpha8/\beta1$	?
$\alpha6/\beta4$	Laminin
$\alpha4/\beta7$	Fibronectin
$\alpha v/\beta1$	Fibronectin
$\alpha v/\beta3$	Vitronectin, fibrinogen, VWF
$\alpha v/\beta5$	Vitronectin
$\alpha v/\beta6$	Fibronectin
$\alpha v/\beta8$	?
Nonintegrin matrix receptors	
69 kDa	Laminin
CD44	Hyaluronic acid
Syndecan	Collagen, fibronectin

Source: Adapted from Refs. 166–168.

integrins may subserve different functions during attachment and migration. Integrins containing either the α_2- or α_3 chains have affinity for collagen (168). However, antibodies to α_2 inhibit keratinocyte migration to collagen, and antibodies to α_3 may enhance migration (163,164). Control of the expression and function of integrins is an active area of research. Transforming growth factor-β can alter the spectrum of integrins expressed on many cell types (171,172). It increases the attachment of bronchial epithelial cells to matrix-coated dishes and is associated with increased expression of fibronectin receptors (173). Interestingly, the increase in adhesion was associated with decreased migration. The balance between adhesion and mobility may be delicate. It has recently been reported that smooth-muscle cell migration is maximal when attachment strength is more moderate (174).

In addition to matrix proteins themselves, other stimuli for epithelial and mesenchymal cell migration have been described. TGF-β has been described as a chemoattractant for fibroblasts and bronchial epithelial cells (173,175). This effect may be in contrast with the in vitro effects of TGF-β on epithelial cells, described earlier. The effect of TGF-β in in vivo models is thought to be one of cellular accumulation, particularly the accumulation of fibroblasts (159). Hence, its effects may then be multiphasic, with initial effects on increasing cell accumulation in wounds, followed by later effects that alter morphology of the cells (176) and increase cell attachment and wound strength. Bronchial epithelial cells also respond to insulin, IGF-1, and epidermal growth factor (EGF) (177,178), which has been described as increasing enterocyte migration (179,180). Epidermal growth factor might also affect sheet migration of epithelial cells through effects on cell proliferation.

Transforming growth factor-β has multiple important effects on epithelial and mesenchymal cells during epithelial healing. Possible sources of TGF-β in the tissues include macrophages, eosinophils, fibroblasts, and epithelial cells (12,13,66,181). Macrophages produce primarily the TGF-β_1 isoform, whereas, in some circumstances, bronchial epithelial cells produce TGF-β_2 (12). At least five isoforms of TGF-β have been described (159). TGF-β_1 and TGF-β_2 have similar activities on cells in vitro, thus, it is unclear what significance the isoforms have. There is extraordinary conservation of sequence of the different isoforms across species, underlining their importance, but the reasons for different forms remain puzzling. TGF-β is present in the epithelial lining fluid of normal lungs (68) and can be produced by multiple cell types. Immunohistochemistry studies have shown increased staining of TGF-β in the epithelium and matrix of the lung in several injury models (69). Disordered or excessive expression of TGF-β is now suspected to be a cause of fibrotic disorders (159). Understanding the control of TGF-β in epithelial repair may be important for the understanding of airway inflammatory diseases and in proposing possible therapeutic approaches. Anti-TGF-β therapy may be on the horizon. Decorin, a small proteoglycan, binds TGF-β and has reduced fibrosis in a model of glomerulosclerosis (159). It is not yet known whether neutralizing TGF-β and its effects will be beneficial or detrimental for airway healing, as the effects of TGF-β are so varied.

There are several lines of evidence to suggest that the process of epithelial and mesenchymal cell migration in wound healing can be modulated by inflammatory cytokines and mediators. Certainly, leukocyte migration is modulated by inflammatory mediators and pharmacological agents (182,183), and it appears that some of the same mechanisms of activation of migration may also act on epithelial cells and fibroblasts. Agents that modulate leukocyte migration, and that may also be active on epithelial cells, include TNF-α, IL-1β, IFN-γ, PGE$_2$, and phorbol esters (184). The subject of cell mobility and possible mechanisms of activation have been recently reviewed (182,185). Stimuli that interact with receptors that activate the inositol phospholipid pathway appear to switch on actin assembly. Various proteins are likely important, including the myristoylated alanine-rich C kinase substrate (MARCKS) (182). MARCKS is well described as a protein kinase C (PKC) substrate that is induced by TNF-α and LPS in macrophages and neutrophils. When MARCKS in phosphorylated by PKC it shuttles between the cell membrane and the cytosol and binds to actin, possibly facilitating motility. Although epithelial and mesenchymal cells are less well studied relative to activation of motility, it appears that TNF-α is also able to stimulate bronchial epithelial cell motility, and the effects are PKC mediated (184). Other stimuli for epithelial migration include insulin, insulin-like growth factor (IGF), platelet-derived growth factor (PDGF), and epidermal growth factor (EGF). The receptors for these mediators belong to a family of similar growth factor receptors that have tyrosine protein kinase activity.

One recent observation that could be relevant to airway repair and the current therapeutic agents we commonly use in asthma is the observation that theophylline inhibits the migration of neutrophils (186). The mechanism of the effects of theophylline are unknown, but perhaps the effects of theophylline on cyclic nucleotides and calcium flux are important, as cAMP and cGMP levels and calcium flux are involved in the polarization of chemotaxis, actin polymerization, and motility of neutrophils (183). Since many aspects of cellular migration are similar between multiple eukaryotic cells (185), it is entirely possible that some of the effects described in leukocytes will be similar to those in epithelial and mesenchymal cells. There is preliminary evidence that PGE_2, which increases fibroblast cAMP levels, inhibits fibroblast chemotaxis to fibronectin (187). Other agents that increase fibroblast cAMP levels—vasoactive intestinal polypeptide (VIP) and isoproterenol—had similar inhibiting effects (187). Bronchial epithelial cells have β-adrenergic agonist receptors (188), so it is not unreasonable to hypothesize that bronchial epithelial cells might be similarly affected by isoproterenol or the other agents.

SUMMARY

It is increasingly clear that epithelial cells and fibroblasts are not passive bystanders in allergic and inflammatory processes. These structural cells have a broad array of capabilities that allow them to communicate with more traditional immune cells. Epithelial cells and fibroblasts may help direct the inflammatory response and contribute to cytokine cascades in epithelia by producing chemotactic cytokines and cytokines with effects on granulocytic and monocytic cell differentiation and activation. Epithelial and mesenchymal cells may then be viewed as potential targets for pharmacological intervention. Epithelial cells are responsive to agents such as corticosteroids. Epithelial repair and fibrosis might also be viewed as processes that are amenable to pharmacological intervention. Factors that enhance epithelial repair and reduce fibrosis would seem important in the resolution of airway hyperresponsiveness and reduction of airway anatomical distortion. Knowledge of the mediators controlling cellular migration, proliferation, differentiation, and matrix production should lead to insights into repair and fibrosis. Agents to modify the actions of cytokines, such as TGF-β, should provide important new information and possibly lead to therapeutic intervention.

REFERENCES

1. Farmer SG, Hay D. The Airway Epithelium. New York: Marcel Dekker. 1991:1–582.
2. 34th Annual Thomas L. Petty Aspen Lung Conference. Chest 1992; 101:2S–85S.

3. Nickoloff BJ, Turka LA. Keratinocytes: key immunocytes of the integument. Am J Pathol 1993; 143:325–331.

4. Barker JNWN, Mitra RS, Griffiths CEM, Dixit VM, Nickoloff BJ. Keratinocytes as initiators of inflammation. Lancet 1991; 337:211–214.

5. Kagnoff MF. Immunology of the intestinal tract. Gastroenterology 1993; 105:1275–1280.

6. Jordana M, Clancy R, Dolovich J, Denburg J. Effector role of the epithelial compartment in inflammation. Ann NY Acad Sci 1992; 664:180–189.

7. Ohtoshi T, Vancheri C, Cox G, Gauldie J, Dolovich J, Denburg JA, Jordana M. Monocyte–macrophage differentiation induced by human upper airway epithelial cells. Am J Respir Cell Mol Biol 1991; 4:255–263.

8. Ohtoshi T, Tsuda T, Vancheri C, Abrams JS, Gauldie J, Dolovich J, Denburg JA, Jordana M. Human upper airway epithelial cell-derived granulocyte–macrophage colony-stimulating factor induces histamine-containing cell differentiation of human progenitor cells. Int Arch Allergy Appl Immunol 1991; 95:376–384.

9. Marini M, Soloperto M, Mezzetti M, Fasoli A, Mattoli S. Interleukin-1 binds to specific receptors on human bronchial epithelial cells and upregulates granulocyte/macrophage colony-stimulating factor synthesis and release. Am J Respir Cell Mol Biol 1991; 4:519–524.

10. Mattoli S, Miante S, Calabrò F, Mezzetti M, Fasoli A, Allegra L. Bronchial epithelial cells exposed to isocyanates potentiate activation and proliferation of T-cells. Am J Physiol 1990; 259:L320–L327.

11. Standiford TJ, Kunkel SL, Basha MA, Chensue SW, Lynch JP III, Toews GB, Westwick J, Strieter RM. Interleukin-8 gene expression by a pulmonary epithelial cell line: a model for cytokine networks in the lung. J Clin Invest 1990; 86:1945–1953.

12. Sacco O, Romberger D, Rizzino A, Beckmann JD, Rennard SI, Spurzem JR. Spontaneous production of transforming growth factor-$\beta2$ by primary cultures of bronchial epithelial cells: effects on cell behavior in vitro. J Clin Invest 1992; 90:1379–1385.

13. Steigerwalt RW, Rundhaug JE, Nettesheim P. Transformed rat tracheal epithelial cells exhibit alterations in transforming growth factor-β secretion and responsiveness. Mol Carcinog 1992; 5:32–40.

14. Pelton RW, Johnson MD, Perkett EA, Gold LI, Moses HL. Expression of transforming growth factor-β_1, -β_2, and -β_3 mRNA and protein in the murine lung. Am J Respir Cell Mol Biol 1991; 5:522–530.

15. Mattoli S, Marini M, Fasoli A. Expression of the potent inflammatory cytokines, GM-CSF, IL6, and IL8, in bronchial epithelial cells of asthmatic patients. Chest 1992; 101(suppl): 27S–29S.

16. Churchill L, Chilton FH, Resau JH, Bascom R, Hubbard WC, Proud D. Cyclooxygenase metabolism of endogenous arachidonic acid by cultured human tracheal epithelial cells. Am Rev Respir Dis 1989; 140:449–459.

17. Leikauf GD, Driscoll KE, Wey HE. Ozone-induced augmentation of eicosanoid metabolism in epithelial cells from bovine trachea. Am Rev Respir Dis 1988; 137:435–442.

18. Holtzman MJ, Hansbrough JR, Rosen GD, Turk J. Uptake release and novel species-dependent oxygenation of arachidonic acid in human and animal airway epithelial cells. Biochim Biophys Acta 1988; 963:401–413.

19. Holtzman MJ. Epithelial cell regulation of arachidonic acid oxygenation. New York: Marcel Dekker, 1991:65–115.

20. Koyama S, Rennard SI, Leikauf GD, Shoji S, VonEssen S, Claassen L, Robbins RA. Endotoxin stimulates bronchial epithelial cells to release chemotactic factors for neutrophils. J Immunol 1991; 147:4293–4301.

21. Wood LC, Jackson SM, Elias PM, Grunfeld C, Feingold KR. Cutaneous barrier perturbation stimulates cytokine production in the epidermis of mice. J Clin Invest 1992; 90:482–487.

22. Matsue H, Cruz PD Jr, Bergstresser PR, Takashima A. Cytokine expression by epithelial cell subpopulations. J Invest Dermatol 1992; 99:42S–45S.

23. Kapp A, Danner M, Luger TA, Hauser C, Schöpf E. Granulocyte-activating mediators (GRAM). II. Generation by human epidermal cells—relation to GM-CSF. Arch Dermatol Res 1987; 279:470–477.

24. Denburg JA, Sauder DN. Granulocyte colony stimulating activity derived from human keratinocytes. Lymphokine Res 1986; 5:261–274.

25. Lee SW, Morhenn VB, Ilnicka M, Eugui EM, Allison AC. Autocrine stimulation of interleukin-1α and transforming growth factor α production in human keratinocytes and its antagonism by glucocorticoids. J Invest Dermatol 1991; 97:106–110.

26. Hauser C, Saurat J-H, Schmitt A, Jaunin F, Dayer J-M. Interleukin 1 is present in normal human epidermis. J Immunol 1986; 136:3317–3323.

27. Kupper TS, Ballard DW, Chua AO, McGuire JS, Flood PM, Horowitz MC, Langdon R, Lightfoot L, Gubler U. Human keratinocytes contain mRNA indistinguishable from monocyte interleukin 1α and β mRNA. J Exp Med 1986; 164:2095–2100.

28. Danner M, Luger TA. Human keratinocytes and epidermoid carcinoma cell lines produce a cytokine with interleukin 3-like activity. Invest Dermatol 1987; 88:353–361.

29. Luger TA, Köck A, Kirnbauer R, Schwarz T, Ansel JC. Keratinocyte-derived interleukin 3. Ann NY Acad Sci 1988; 548:253–261.

30. Gallo RL, Staszewski R, Sauder DN, Knisely TL, Granstein RD. Regulation of GM-CSF and IL-3 production from the murine keratinocyte cell line PAM 212 following exposure to ultraviolet radiation. J Invest Dermatol 1991; 97:203–209.

31. Kupper TS, Min K, Sehgal P, Mizutani H, Birchall N, Ray A, May L. Production of IL-6 by keratinocytes. Implications for epidermal inflammation and immunity. Ann NY Acad Sci 1989; 557:454–464.

32. Matsue H, Bergstresser PR, Takashima A. Keratinocyte-derived IL-7 serves as a growth factor for dendritic epidermal T cells in mice. J Immunol 1993; 151:6012–6019.

33. Heufler C, Young D, Peschel C, Schuler G. Murine keratinocytes express interleukin-7 (abstr). J Invest Dermatol 1990; 94:534A.

34. Larsen CG, Anderson AO, Oppenheim JJ, Matsushima K. Production of interleukin-8 by human dermal fibroblasts and keratinocytes in response to interleukin-1 or tumour necrosis factor. Immunology 1989; 68:31–36.

35. Barker JNWN, Sarma V, Mitra RS, Dixit VM, Nickoloff BJ. Marked synergism between tumor necrosis factor-α and interferon-γ in regulation of keratinocyte-derived adhesion molecules and chemotactic factors. J Clin Invest 1990; 85:605–608.

36. Köck A, Schwarz T, Kirnbauer R, Urbanski A, Perry P, Ansel JC, Luger TA. Human keratinocytes are a source of tumor necrosis factor α: evidence for synthesis and release upon stimulation and endotoxin or ultraviolet light. J Exp Med 1990; 172:1609–1614.

37. Thompson NL, Flanders KC, Smith JM, Ellingsworth LR, Roberts AB, Sporn MB. Expression of transforming growth factor-β1 in specific cells and tissues of adult and neonatal mice. J Cell Biol 1989; 108:661–669.

38. Peterseim UM, Sarkar SN, Kupper TS. Production of IL-3 by non-transformed primary neonatal murine keratinocytes: evidence for constitutive IL-3 gene expression in neonatal epidermis. Cytokine 1993; 5:240–249.

39. Ruef C, Jefferson DM, Schlegel-Haueter SE, Suter S. Regulation of cytokine secretion by cystic fibrosis airway epithelial cells. Eur Respir J 1993; 6:1429–1436.

40. Radema SA, VanDeventer SJH, Cerami A. Interleukin 1β is expressed predominantly by enterocytes in experimental colitis. Gastroenterology 1991; 100:1180–1186.

41. Levine SJ, Larivèe P, Logun C, Angus CW, Shelhamer JH. Corticosteroids differentially regulate secretion of IL-6, IL-8, and G-CSF by a human bronchial epithelial cell line. Am J Physiol 1993; 265:L360–L368.

42. Noah TL, Paradiso AM, Madden MC, McKinnon KP, Devlin RB. The response of a human bronchial epithelial cell line to histamine: intracellular calcium changes and extracellular release of inflammatory mediators. Am J Respir Cell Mol Biol 1991; 5:484–492.

43. McGee DW, Beagley KW, Aicher WK, McGhee JR. Transforming growth factor-β and IL-1β act in synergy to enhance IL-6 secretion by the intestinal epithelial cell line, IEC-6. J Immunol 1993; 151:970–978.
44. Eckmann L, Jung HC, Schurer-Maly C, Panja A, Morzycka-Wroblewska E, Kagnoff MF. Differential cytokine expression by human intestinal epithelial cell lines: regulated expression of interleukin 8. Gastroenterology 1993; 105:1689–1697.
45. Koyama S, Podolsky DK. Differential expression of transforming growth factors α and β in rat intestinal epithelial cells. J Clin Invest 1989; 83:1768–1773.
46. Barnard JA, Beauchamp RD, Coffey JR, Moses HL. Regulation of intestinal epithelial cell growth by transforming growth factory type β. Proc Natl Acad Sci USA 1989; 86:1578–1582.
47. Keshav S, Lawson L, et al. Tumor necrosis factor mRNA localized to Paneth cells of normal murine intestinal epithelium by in situ hybridization. J Exp Med 1990; 171:327–332.
48. Kast R, Furstenberger G, Marck F. Phorbol ester TPA- and bradykinin-induced arachidonic acid release from keratinocytes is catalyzed by a cytosolic phospholipase A_2 ($cPLA_2$). J Invest Dermatol 1993; 101:567–572.
49. Pothoulakis C, Karmeli F, Kelly CP, Eliakim R, Joshi MA, O'Keane J, Castagliuolo I, LaMont JT, Rachmilewitz D. Ketotifen inhibits Clostridium difficile toxin A-induced enteritis in rat ileum. Gastroenterology 1993; 105:701–707.
50. Rigas B, Goldman IS, Levine L. Altered eicosanoid levels in human colon cancer. J Lab Clin Med 1993; 122:518–523.
51. Heeger P, Wolf G, Meyers C, Sun MJ, O'Farrell SC, Krensky AM, Neilson EG. Isolation and characterization of cDNA from renal tubular epithelium encoding murine RANTES. Kidney Int 1992; 41:220–225.
52. Nelson PJ, Kim HT, Manning WC, Goralski TJ, Krensky AM. Genomic organization and transcriptional regulation of the RANTES chemokine gene. J Immunol 1993; 151:2601–2612.
53. Raz M, Robbins RA, Kelling CL, Stine LC, Leikauf GD, Rennard SI, Spurzem JR. Viral infection of bovine bronchial epithelial cells induces increased neutrophil chemotactic activity and neutrophil adhesion. Clin Sci 1993; 85:753–760.
54. Baggiolini M, Walz A, Kunkel SL. Neutrophil-activating peptide-1/interleukin 8, a novel cytokine that activates neutrophils. 1989; 84:1045–1049.
55. Izzo RS, Witkon K, Chen AI, Hadjiyane C, Weinstein MI, Pellecchia C. Interleukin-8 and neutrophil markers in colonic mucosa from patients with ulcerative colitis. Am J Gastroenterol 1992; 87:1447–1452.
56. Standiford TJ, Rolfe MW, Kunkel SL, Lynch JJP III, Burdick MD, Gilbert AR, Orringer MB, Whyte RI, Strieter RM. Macrophage inflammatory protein-1 α expression in interstitial lung disease. J Immunol 1993; 151:2852.
57. Denburg JA, Gauldie J, Dolovich J, Ohtoshi T, Cox G, Jordana M. Structural cell-derived cytokines in allergic inflammation. Arch Allergy Appl Immunol 1991; 94:127–132.
58. Gauldie J, Jordana M, Cox G, Ohtoshi T, Dolovich J, Denburg J. Fibroblasts and other structural cells in airway inflammation. Am Rev Respir Dis 1992; 145:S14–S17.
59. Vancheri C, Gauldie J, Bienenstock J, Cox G, Scicchitano R, Stanisz A, Jordana M. Human lung fibroblast-derived granulocyte–macrophage colony stimulating factor (GM-CSF) mediates eosinophil survival in vitro. Am J Respir Cell Mol Biol 1989; 1:289–295.
60. Vancheri C, Ohtoshi T, Cox G, Xaubet A, Abrams JS, Gauldie J, Dolovich J, Denburg J, Jordana M. Neutrophilic differentiation induced by human upper airway fibroblast-derived granulocyte/macrophage colony-stimulating factor (GM-CSF). Am J Respir Cell Mol Biol 1991; 4:11–17.
61. Zitnik RJ, Zheng T, Elias JA. cAMP inhibition of interleukin-1-induced interleukin-6 production by human lung fibroblasts. Am J Physiol 1993; 264:L253–L260.
62. Elias JA, Lentz V, Cummings PJ. Transforming growth factor-beta regulation of IL-6 production by unstimulated and IL-1-stimulated human fibroblasts. J Immunol 1991; 146:3437–3443.
63. Rolfe MW, Kunkel SL, Standiford TJ, Chensue SW, Allen RM, Evanoff HL, Phan SH, Strieter

RM. Pulmonary fibroblast expression of interleukin-8: a model for alveolar macrophage-derived cytokine networking. Am J Respir Cell Mol Biol 1991; 5:493–501.

64. Standiford TJ, Kunkel SL, Phan SH, Rollins BJ, Strieter RM. Alveolar macrophage-derived cytokines induce monocyte chemoattractant protein-1 expression from human pulmonary type II-like epithelial cells. J Biol Chem 1991; 266:9912–9918.

65. Rolfe MW, Kunkel SL, Standiford TJ, Orringer MB, Phan SH, Evanoff HL, Burdick MD, Strieter RM. Expression and regulation of human pulmonary fibroblast-derived monocyte chemotactic peptide-1. Am J Physiol 1992; 263:L536–L545.

66. Assoian RK, Fleurdelys BE, Stevenson HC, Miller PJ, Madtes DK, Raines EW, Ross R, Sporn MB. Expression and secretion of type β transforming growth factor by activated human macrophages. Proc Natl Acad Sci USA 1987; 84:6020–6024.

67. Danielpour D, Dart LL, Flanders KC, Roberts AB, Sporn MB. Immunodetection and quantitation of the two forms of transforming growth factor-beta (TGF-β1 and TGF-β2) secreted by cells in culture. J Cell Physiol 1989; 138:79–86.

68. Yamauchi K, Martinet Y, Basset P, Fells GA, Crystal RG. High levels of transforming growth factor-β are present in the epithelial lining fluid of the normal human lower respiratory tract. Am Rev Respir Dis 1988; 137:1360–1363.

69. Khalil N, O'Connor RN, Unruh HW, Warren PW, Flanders KC, Kemp A, Bereznay OH, Greenberg AH. Increased production and immunohistochemical localization of transforming growth factor-β in idiopathic pulmonary fibrosis. Am J Respir Cell Mol Biol 1991; 5:155–162.

70. Adams DH, Hathaway M, Shaw J, Burnett D, Elias E, Strain AJ. Transforming growth factor-β induces human T lymphocyte migration in vitro. J Immunol 1991; 147:609–612.

71. Brandes ME, Uwe E, Mai H, Ohura K, Wahl SM. Type I transforming growth factor-β receptors on neutrophils mediate chemotaxis to transforming growth factor-β. J Immunol 1991; 147:1600–1606.

72. Kehrl JH, Wakefield LM, Roberts AB, Jakowlew S, Alvarez-Mon M, Derynck R, Sporn MB, Fauci A. Production of transforming growth factor β by human T lymphocytes and its potential role in the regulation of T cell growth. J Exp Med 1986; 163:1037–1050.

73. Espevik T, Figari IS, Shalaby MR, Lackides GA, Lewis GD, Shepard M, Paladino MA Jr. Inhibition of cytokine production by cyclosporin A and transforming growth factor β. J Exp Med 1987; 166:571–576.

74. Diaz A, Varga J, Jimenez SA. Transforming growth factor-β stimulation of lung fibroblast prostaglandin E$_2$ production. J Biol Chem 1989; 264:11554–11557.

75. Christman JW, Christman BW, Shepherd VL, Rinaldo JE. Regulation of alveolar macrophage production of chemoattractants by leukotrine B$_4$ and prostaglandin E$_2$. Am J Respir Cell Mol Biol 1991; 5:297–304.

76. Ulich TR, Yin S, Guo K, Yi ES, Remick D, delCastillo J. Intratracheal injection of endotoxin and cytokines. II. Interleukin-6 and transforming growth factor-β inhibit acute inflammation. Am J Pathol 1991; 138:1097–1101.

77. Nakamura H, Yoshimura K, McElvaney NG, Crystal RG. Neutrophil elastase in respiratory epithelial lining fluid of individuals with cystic fibrosis induces interleukin-8 gene expression in a human bronchial epithelial cell line. J Clin Invest 1992; 89:1478–1484.

78. Denburg JA, Dolovich J, Ohtoshi T, Cox G, Gauldie J, Jordana M. The microenvironmental differentiation hypothesis of airway inflammation. Am J Rhinol 1990; 4:29–34.

79. Rothlein R, Czajkowski M, O'Neill MM, Marlin SD, Mainolfi E, Merluzzi VJ. Induction of intercellular adhesion molecule 1 on primary and continuous cell lines by pro-inflammatory cytokines. J Immunol 1988; 141:1665–1669.

80. Wegner CD, Gundel RH, Reilly P, Haynes N, Letts LG, Rothlein R. Intercellular adhesion molecule-1 (ICAM-1) in the pathogenesis of asthma. Science 1990; 2:456–459.

81. Tosi MF, Stark JM, Hamedani A, Smith CW, Gruenerts DC, Huang YT. Intercellular adhesion molecule-1 (ICAM-1)-dependent and ICAM-1-independent adhesive interactions between

polymorphonuclear leukocytes and human airway epithelial cells infected with parainfluenza virus type 2. J Immunol 1992; 149:3345–3349.

82. Marlin SD, Springer TA. Purified intercellular adhesion molecule-1 (ICAM-1) is a ligand for lymphocyte function-associated antigen 1 (LFA-1). Cell 1987; 51:813–819.

83. Krensky AM, Sanchez-Madrid F, Robbins E, Nagy JA, Springer TA, Burakoff SJ. The functional significance, distribution, and structure of LFA-1, LFA-2, and LFA-3: cell surface antigens associated with CTL-target interactions. J Immunol 1983; 131:611–616.

84. Davignon D, Martz E, Reynolds T, Kürzinger K, Springer TA. Monoclonal antibody to a novel lymphocyte function-associated antigen (LFA-1): mechanism of blockade of T lymphocyte-mediated killing and effects on other T and B lymphocyte functions. J Immunol 1991; 127: 590–595.

85. Fischer A, Durandy A, Sterkers G, Griscelli C. Role of the LFA-1 molecule in cellular interactions required for antibody production in humans. J Immunol 1986; 136:3198–3203.

86. Dustin ML, Singer KH, Tuck DT, Springer TA. Adhesion of T lymphoblasts to epidermal keratinocytes is regulated by interferon γ and is mediated by intercellular adhesion molecule 1 (ICAM-1). J Exp Med 1988; 167:1323–1340.

87. Norris DA. Cytokine modulation of adhesion molecules in the regulation of immunologic cytotoxicity of epidermal targets. J Invest Dermatol 1990; 95:111S–120S.

88. Aubcock J, Niederwieser D, Romani N, Fritsch P, Huber C. Human interferon-gamma induces expression of HLA-DR on keratinocytes and melanocytes. Arch Dermatol Res 1985; 277: 270–275.

89. Niederwieser D, Aubcock J, Troppmair J, Herold M, Schuler G, Boeck G, Lotz J, Fritsch P, Huber C. IFN-mediated induction of MHC antigen expression on human keratinocytes and its influence on in vitro alloimmune responses. J Immunol 1988; 140:2556–2564.

90. Gaspari AA, Katz SI. Induction and functional characterization of class II MHC (Ia) antigens on murine keratinocytes. J Immunol 1988; 140:2956–2963.

91. Taylor PM, Rose ML, Yacoub MH. Expression of MHC antigens in normal human lungs and transplanted lungs with obliterative bronchiolitis. Transplantation 1989; 48:506–510.

92. Rossi GA, Sacco O, Balbi B, Oddera S, Mattioni T, Corte G, Ravazzoni C, Allegra L. Human ciliated bronchial epithelial cells: expression of the HLA-DR antigens and of the HLA-DR alpha gene, modulation of the HLA-DR antigens by gamma-interferon, and antigen-presenting function in the mixed leukocyte reaction. Am J Respir Cell Mol Biol 1990; 3:431–439.

93. Spurzem JR, Sacco O, Rossi GA, Beckmann JD, Rennard SI. Regulation of major histocompatibility complex class II gene expression on bovine bronchial epithelial cells. J Lab Clin Med 1992; 120:94–102.

94. Sviland L, Pearson ADJ, Green MA, Eastham EJ, Malcolm AJ, Proctor SJ, Hamilton PJ. Expression of MHC class I and II antigens by keratinocytes and enterocytes in acute graft-versus-host disease. Bone Marrow Transplant 1989; 4:233–238.

95. Glanville AR, Baldwin JC, Burke CM, Theodore J, Robin ED. Obliterative bronchiolitis after heart–lung transplantation: apparent arrest by augmented immunosuppression. Ann Intern Med 1987; 107:300–304.

96. Okabayashi M, Angell MG, Budgeon LR, Kreider JW. Shope papilloma cell and leukocyte proliferation in regressing and progressing lesions. Am J Pathol 1993; 142:489–496.

97. Yousem SA, Curley JM, Dauber J, Paradis I, Rabinowich H, Zeevi A, Duquesnoy R, Dowling R, Zenati M, Hadesty R, Griffith BP. HLA-class II antigen expression in human heart-lung allografts. Transplantation 1990; 49:991–995.

98. Burke CM, Glanville AR, Theodore J, Robin ED. Lung immunogenicity, rejection, and obliterative bronchiolitis. Chest 1987; 92:547–549.

99. Nickoloff BJ, Mitra RS, Green J, Shimizu Y, Thompson C, Turka LA. Accessory cell function of keratinocytes for superantigen: dependence on LFA-1/ICAM-1 interaction. J Immunol 1993; 150:2148–2159.

100. Udey MC, Peck RD, Pentland AP, Schreiner GF, Lefkowith JB. Antigen-presenting cells in

essential fatty acid-deficient murine epidermis: keratinocytes bearing class II (Ia) antigens may potentiate the accessory cell function of Langerhans cells. J Invest Dermatol 1991; 96: 950–958.

101. Bland PW, Warren LG. Antigen presentation by epithelial cells of the rat small intestine. I. Kinetics, antigen specificity and blocking by anti-Ia antisera. Immunology 1990; 171:327–332.

102. Mayer L, Shlien R. Evidence for function of Ia molecules on gut epithelial cells in man. J Exp Med 1987; 166:1471–1483.

103. Tazi A, Bouchonnet F, Grandsaigne M, Boumsell L, Hance AJ, Soler P. Evidence that granulocyte–macrophage colony-stimulating factor regulates the distribution and differentiated state of dendritic cells/Langerhans cells in human lung and lung cancers. J Clin Invest 1993; 91:566–576.

104. Tazi A, Bonay M, Grandsaigne M, Battesti J-P, Hance AJ, Solder P. Surface phenotype of Langerhans cells and lymphocytes in granulomatous lesions from patients with pulmonary histiocytosis X. Am Rev Respir Dis 1993; 147:1531–1536.

105. Schreiber S, Kilgus O, Payer E, Kutil R, Elbe A, Mueller C, Stingl G. Cytokine pattern of Langerhans cells isolated from murine epidermal cell cultures. J Immunol 1992; 149:3525–3534.

106. Matsue H, Cruz PD Jr, Bergstresser PR, Takasha A. Profiles of cytokine mRNA expressed by dendritic epidermal T cells in mice. J Invest Dermatol 1993; 101:537–542.

107. Steinman RM. The dendritic cell system and its role in immunogenicity. Annu Rev Immunol 1991; 9:271–296.

108. Matsue H, Bergstresser PR, Takashima A. Reciprocal cytokine-mediated cellular interactions in mouse epidermis: promotion of γδ T-cell growth by IL-7 and TNFα and inhibition of keratinocyte growth by γIFN. J Invest Dermatol 1993; 101:543–548.

109. Berman JS, Beer DJ, Theodore AC, Kornfeld H, Bernardo J, Center DM. Lymphocyte recruitment to the lung. Am Rev Respir Dis 1990; 142:238–257.

110. Becker KL. The coming of age of a bronchial epithelial cell. Am Rev Respir Dis 1993; 148:1166–1168.

111. Moncada S, Higgs EA. Endogenous nitric oxide: physiology, pathology and clinical relevance. Eur J Clin Invest 1991; 21:361–374.

112. Moncada S, Higgs A. The L-arginine–nitric oxide pathway. N Engl J Med 1993; 329:2002–2010.

113. Iyengar R, Stuehr DJ, Marletta MA. Macrophage synthesis of nitrite, nitrate, and N-nitrosamines: precursors and role of the respiratory burst. Proc Natl Acad Sci USA 1987; 84:669–673.

114. Lowenstein CJ, Alley EW, Raval P, Snowman AM, Snyder SH, Russell ST, Murphy WJ. Macrophage nitric oxide synthase gene: two upstream regions mediate induction by interferon γ and lipopolysaccharide. Proc Natl Acad Sci USA 1993; 90:9730–9734.

115. Robbins RA, Hamel FG, Floreani AA, Gossman GL, Nelson KJ, Belenky S, Rubinstein I. Bovine bronchial epithelial cells metabolize L-arginine to L-citrulline: possible role of nitric oxide synthase. Life Sci 1993; 52:709–716.

116. Robbins RA, Warren JW, Springall DR, Kwon OJ, Wilson A, Robichaud A, Buttery L, Adcock IM, Geller D, Polak J, Barnes PJ. Inducible nitric oxide synthase is increased in murine lung epithelial cells by cytokine stimulation. Submitted.

117. Borland C, Yolande C, Higenbottam T. Measurement of exhaled nitric oxide in man. Thorax 1993; 48:1160–1162.

118. Gustafsson LE, Leone AM, Persson MG, Wiklund NP, Moncada S. Endogenous nitric oxide is present in the exhaled air of rabbits, guinea pigs and humans. Biochem Biophys Res Commun 1991; 181:852–857.

119. Kharitonov SA, Yates D, Robbins RA, Logan-Sinclair, Shinebourne EA, Barnes PJ. Increased nitric oxide in exhaled air of asthmatic patients. Lancet 1994; 343:133–135.

120. Höhman M, Frostell CG, Hedenström G. Inhalation of nitric oxide modulates adult human bronchial tone. Am Rev Respir Dis 1993; 148:1474–1478.

121. Bunnett NW. Release and breakdown. Postsecretory metabolism of peptides. Am Rev Respir Dis 1987; 136:S27–S34.
122. Casale TB. Neuropeptides and the lung. J Allergy Clin Immunol 1991; 88:1–14.
123. Barnes PJ. Asthma as an axon reflex. Lancet 1986; 1:242–245.
124. Nadel JA. Regulation of neurogenic inflammation by neutral endopeptidase. Am Rev Respir Dis 1992; 145:S48–S52.
125. Ujiie Y, Sekizawa K, Aikawa T, Sasaki H. Evidence for substance P as an endogenous substance causing cough in guinea pigs. Am Rev Respir Dis 1993; 148:1628–1632.
126. Ohrui T, Yamauchi K, Sekizawa K, Ohkawara Y, Maeyama K, Sasaki M, Tekemura M, Wada H, Watanabe T, Sasaki H, Takishima T. Histamine N-methyltransferase controls the contractile response of guinea pig trachea to histamine. J Pharmacol Exp Ther 1992; 261:1268–1272.
127. Sekizawa K, Nakazawa T, Ohrui T, Yamauchi K, Ohkaware Y, Maeyama K, Watanabe T, Sasaki H, Takishima T. Histamine N-methyltransferase modulates histamine- and antigen-induced bronchoconstriction in guinea pigs in vivo. Am Rev Respir Dis 1993; 147:92–96.
128. Abe Y, Ogino S, Irifune M, Imamura I, Liu QY, Fukui H, Matsunaga T. Histamine content, synthesis and degradation in nasal mucosa and lung of guinea-pigs treated with toluene diisocyanate (TDI). Clin Exp Allergy 1993; 23:512–517.
129. Ignesti G, Banchelli G, Raimondi L, Pirisino R, Buffoni F. Histaminase activity in rat lung and its comparison with intestinal mucosal diamine oxidase. Agents Actions 1992; 35:192–199.
130. Nemoto N. Glutathione, glucuronide, and sulfate transferase in polycyclic aromatic hydrocarbon metabolism. Polycyclic Hydrocarbons Cancer 1981; 3:213–258.
131. Sims P, Grover PL. Epoxides in polycyclic aromatic hydrocarbon metabolism and carcinogenesis. Adv Cancer Res 1974; 20:165–274.
132. Sekura RD, Jakoby WB. Phenol sulfotransferases. J Biol Chem 1979; 254:5658–5663.
133. Beckmann JD, Spurzem JR, Rennard SI. Phenol sulfotransferase expression in bovine airways: enzymological and immunohistochemical demonstration. Cell Tissue Res 1993; 274:475–485.
134. Walle T, Walle UK. Stereoselective sulfate conjugation of 4-hydroxypropranolol and terbutaline by the human liver phenolsulfotransferases. Drug Metab Dispos 1992; 20:333–336.
135. Farmer SG, Hay DWP. Airway epithelial modulation of smooth-muscle function. The evidence for epithelium-derived inhibitory factor. In: The Airway Epithelium. Farmer SG, Hay D, eds. New York, Marcel Dekker, 1991:437–483.
136. Stuart-Smith K, Vanhoutte PM. Interactions between epithelium and smooth muscle in canine airways. In: The Airway Epithelium. Farmer SG, Hay D, eds. New York, Marcel Dekker, 1991:485–503.
137. Gao Y, Vanhoutte PM. Attenuation of contractions to acetylcholine in canine bronchi by an endogenous nitric oxide-like substance. Br J Pharmacol 1993; 109:887–891.
138. Laitinen LA, Heino M, Laitinen A, Kava T, Haahtela T. Damage of the airway epithelium and bronchial reactivity in patients with asthma. Am Rev Respir Dis 1985; 131:599–606.
139. Frigas E, Loegering DA, Gleich GJ. Cytotoxic effects of the guinea pig eosinophil major basic protein on tracheal epithelium. Lab Invest 1980; 42:35–43.
140. Bousquet J, Chanez P, Lacoste JY, Barnéon G, Ghavanian N, Enander I, Venge P, Ahlstedt S, Simony-Lafontaine J, Godard P, Michel F-B. Eosinophilic inflammation in asthma. N Engl J Med 1990; 323:1033–1039.
141. Rickard KA, Taylor J, Rennard SI. Observations of development of resistance to detachment of cultured bovine bronchial epithelial cells in response to protease treatment. Am J Respir Cell Mol Biol 1992; 6:414–420.
142. Fick RB, Metzger WJ, Richerson HB, Zavala DC, Moseley PL, Schoderbek WE, Hunninghake GW. Increased bronchovascular permeability after allergen exposure in sensitive asthmatics. J Appl Physiol 1987; 63:1147–1155.
143. Kondo M, Finkbeiner WE, Widdicombe JH. Changes in permeability of dog tracheal epithelium in response to hydrostatic pressure. Am J Physiol 1992; 262(2 pt 1):L176–L182.
144. Lane BP, Gordon R. Regeneration of rat tracheal epithelium after mechanical injury. Proc Soc Exp Biol Med 1974; 145:1139–1144.

145. McDowell EM, Ben T, Newkirk C, Chang S, DeLuca LM. Differentiation of tracheal mucociliary epithelium in primary cell culture recapitulates normal fetal development and regeneration following injury in hamsters. Am J Pathol 1987; 129:511–522.

146. Rutten MJ, Ito S. Morphology and electrophysiology of guinea pig gastric mucosal repair in vitro. Am J Physiol 1983; 244:G171–182.

147. Moore R, Carlson S, Madara JL. Rapid barrier restitution in an in vitro model of intestinal epithelial injury. Lab Invest 1989; 60:237–244.

148. Odland G, Ross R. Human wound repair. I. Epidermal regeneration. J Cell Biol 1968; 39:135–157.

149. Keenan KP, Wilson TS, McDowell EM. Regeneration of hamster tracheal epithelium after mechanical injury. IV. Histochemical, immunocytochemical and ultrastructural studies. Virchows Arch Cell Pathol 1983; 43:213–240.

150. Clark RAF, Lanigan JM, DellaPelle P, Manseau E, Dvorak HF, Colvin RB. J Invest Dermatol 1982; 79:264–269.

151. Grinnell F, Billingham RE, Burgess L. Distribution of fibronectin during wound healing in vivo. J Invest Dermatol 1981; 76:181–189.

152. McGowan SE. Extracellular matrix and the regulation of lung development and repair. FASEB J 1992; 6:2895–2904.

153. Horiba K, Fukuda Y, Kanno S, Yamanaka N. Fibronectin receptor in epithelial and mesenchymal cells in wound healing of rat trachea (abstr). Am Rev Respir Dis 1993; 147:A47.

154. Romberger DJ, Beckmann JD, Claassen L, Ertl RF, Rennard SI. Modulation of fibronectin production of bovine bronchial epithelial cells by transforming growth factor-β. Am J Respir Cell Mol Biol 1992; 7:149–155.

155. Stoner GD, Katoh Y, Foidart JM, Trump BF, Steinert PM, Harris CC. Cultured human bronchial epithelial cells: blood group antigens, keratin, collagens, and fibronectin. In Vitro 1981; 17:577–587.

156. Morla A, Zhang Z, Ruoslahti E. Superfibronectin is a functionally distinct form of fibronectin. Nature 1994; 367:193–196.

157. Vollberg TM Sr, George MD, Jetten AM. Induction of extracellular matrix gene expression in normal human kertinocytes by transforming growth factor beta is altered by cellular differentiation. Exp Cell Res 1991; 193:93–100.

158. Goldstein RH, Polgar P. The effect and interaction of bradykinin and prostaglandins on protein and collagen production by lung fibroblasts. J Biol Chem 1982; 257:8630–8633.

159. Border WA, Ruoslahti E. Transforming growth factor-β in disease: the dark side of tissue repair. J Clin Invest 1992; 90:1–7.

160. Mustoe TA, Pierce GF, Thomason A, Gramates P, Sporn MB, Deuel TF. Accelerated healing of incisional wounds in rats induced by transforming growth factor-β. Science 1987; 237:1333–1336.

161. Kawamoto M, Romberger DJ, Nakamura Y, Tate L, Ertl RF, Spurzem JR, Rennard SI. Modulation of fibroblast type I collagen and fibronectin production by bovine bronchial epithelial cells. Submitted.

162. Rickard KA, Taylor J, Rennard SI, Spurzem JR. Migration of bovine bronchial epithelial cells to extracellular matrix components. Am J Respir Cell Mol Biol 1993; 8:63–68.

163. Kim JP, Zhang K, Kramer RH, Schall TJ, Woodley DT. Integrin receptors and RGD sequences in human keratinocyte migration: unique anti-migratory function of α3β1 epiligrin receptor. J Invest Dermatol 1992; 98:764–770.

164. Scharffetter-Kochanek K, Klein CE, Heinen G, Mauch C, Schaefer T, Adelmann-Grill BC, Goerz G, Fusenig NE, Krieg TM, Plewig G. Migration of a human keratinocyte cell line (HACAT) to interstitial collagen type IIs mediated by the α2β1-integrin receptor. J Invest Dermatol 1992; 98:3–11.

165. Nickoloff BJ, Mitra RS, Riser BL, Dixit VM, Varani J. Modulation of keratinocyte motility. Correlation with production of extracellular matrix molecules in response to growth promoting and antiproliferative factors. Am J Pathol 1988; 132:543–551.

166. Pilewski JM, Albelda SM. Adhesion molecules in the lung. Am Rev Respir Dis 1993; 148: S31–S37.

167. Sheppard D. Identification and characterization of novel airway epithelial integrins. Am Rev Respir Dis 1992; 148:S38–S42.
168. Albelda S. Endothelial and epithelial cell adhesion molecules. Am J Respir Cell Mol Biol 1991; 4:195–203.
169. Lark MW, Laterra J, Culp LA. Close and focal contact adhesions of fibroblasts to a fibronectin-containing matrix. Fed Proc 1985; 44:394–403.
170. Wang N, Butler JP, Ingber DE. Mechanotransduction across the cell surface and through the cytoskeleton. Science 1993; 260:1124–1127.
171. Ignotz RA, Heino J, Massaguè J. Regulation of cell adhesion receptors by transforming growth factor-β. J Biol Chem 1989; 264:389–392.
172. Sheppard D, Cohen DS, Wang A, Busk M. Transforming growth factor β differentially regulates expression of integrin subunits in guinea pig airway epithelial cells. J Biol Chem 1992; 267:17409–17414.
173. Spurzem JR, Sacco O, Rickard KA, Rennard SI. Transforming growth factor-β increases adhesion but not migration of bovine bronchial epithelial cells to matrix proteins. J Lab Clin Med 1993; 122:92–102.
174. DiMilla PA, Stone JA, Quinn JA, Albelda SM, Lauffenburger DA. Maximal migration of human smooth muscle cells on fibronectin and type IV collagen occurs at an intermediate attachment strength. J Cell Biol 1993; 122:729–737.
175. Postlethwaite AE, Keski-Oja J, Moses HL, Kang AH. Stimulation of the chemotactic migration of human fibroblasts by transforming growth factor β. J Exp Med 1987; 165:251–256.
176. Jetten AM, Shirley JE, Stoner G. Regulation of proliferation and differentiation of respiratory tract epithelial cells by TGF-β. Exp Cell Res 1986; 167:539–549.
177. Shoji S, Ertl RF, Linder J, Koizumi S, Duckworth WC, Rennard SI. Bronchial epithelial cells respond to insulin and insulin-like growth factor-I as a chemoattractant. Am J Respir Cell Mol Biol 1990; 2:553–557.
178. Zahm JM, Pierrot D, Puchele E. Fibronectin-mediated effect of epidermal growth factor in the wound healing of human respiratory epithelium in culture (abstr). Am Rev Respir Dis 1993; 147:A47.
179. Basson MD, Modlin IM, Madri JA. Human enterocyte (Caco-2) migration is modulated in vitro by extracellular matrix composition and epidermal growth factor. J Clin Invest 1992; 90:15–23.
180. Blay J, Brown KD. Epidermal growth factor promotes the chemotactic migration of cultured rat intestinal epithelial cells. J Cell Physiol 1985; 124:107–112.
181. Ohno I, Lea RG, Flanders KC, Clark DA, Banwatt D, Dolovich J, Denburg J, Harley CB, Gauldie J, Jordana M. Eosinophils in chronically inflamed human upper airway tissues express transforming growth factor β1 gene (TGFβ1). J Clin Invest 1992; 89:1662–1668.
182. Aderem AA. How cytokines signal messages within cells. J Infect Dis 1993; 167(suppl 1):S2–S7.
183. Stossel TP. On the crawling of animal cells. Science 1993; 260:1086–1094.
184. Ito H, Romberger DJ, Rennard SI, Spurzem JR. TNF-α enhances bronchial epithelial cell migration and attachment to fibronectin. Am Rev Respir Dis 1993; 147:A46.
185. Caterina MJ, Devreotes PN. Molecular insights into eukaryotic chemotaxis. FASEB J 1991; 5:3078–3085.
186. Rennard S, Thompson A, Daughton D, McKillip T, Orona C, Mueller M, Ertl R. Theophylline reduces neutrophil recruitment in vitro and lowers airway neutrophilia in chronic bronchitis in vivo. Eur Respir J 1990; 3:116S.
187. Ertl RF, Valenti V, Spurzem JR, Kawamoto M, Makamura Y, Veys T, Allegra L, Romberger DJ, Rennard SI. Prostaglandin E inhibits fibroblast recruitment (abstr). Am Rev Respir Dis 1992; 145:A19.
188. Nogami M, Romberger DJ, Rennard SI, Toews ML. Agonist-induced desensitization of beta adrenoceptors of bovine bronchial epithelial cells. Clin Sci 1993; 85:651–657.

13

Interleukin-1 and Tumor Necrosis Factor in Allergic Reactions

Edouard Vannier and Charles A. Dinarello
Tufts University School of Medicine and New England Medical Center,
Boston, Massachusetts

INTRODUCTION

An allergic reaction is initiated following the recognition of an antigen (allergen) by specific immunoglobulins (Ig) E that are bound to high-affinity IgE receptors expressed on the cell surface of mast cells and basophils. Cross-linking of IgE receptors activates mast cells and basophils to release their granule constituents and to synthesize arachidonate metabolites. These events initiate the development of the early phase of an allergic reaction. The early phase is essentially characterized by an intense vasodilation, accompanied by bronchoconstriction, when the lung is the target organ of the allergic reaction. Characteristically, the early phase occurs within the first 60 min, but is often followed a few hours later by a late-phase reaction. The late-phase reaction is associated with an accumulation of inflammatory cells at the site of allergen deposition. Release of granule constituents by activated eosinophils and basophils, as well as synthesis of arachidonate metabolites, leads to a further amplification of the local inflammatory response. In pulmonary allergic reactions, the late-phase response is associated with bronchial hyperreactivity. Chronic pulmonary inflammation and bronchial hyperreactivity are hallmarks of status asthmaticus. Thus, in the lung, the inflammatory nature of the late-phase reaction contrasts with the spasmogenic nature of the early-phase response. Although interleukin (IL)-1 and tumor necrosis factor (TNF)-α are unlikely to play a critical role in the development of an early-phase reaction, the inflammatory properties of IL-1 and TNF-α qualify them as potential mediators of the late-phase allergic response.

THE IL-1 NETWORK

Because activation of a cell by IL-1 requires few receptors, nature has developed a highly sophisticated network of regulations to control its activity (1). There are two agonist forms

309

of IL-1, namely, IL-1α and IL-1β, and at least three natural antagonisms to IL-1. The net effects of IL-1 ultimately reflect a balance between these agonists and antagonists. First, the naturally occurring IL-1 receptor antagonist (IL-1Ra) inhibits the binding of IL-1 to its receptors. Second, the IL-1 receptor type II (IL-1RII) is merely a binding protein (or decoy receptor) and diverts IL-1 away from the functional IL-1 receptor type I (IL-1RI), thus decreasing the cell sensitivity to IL-1. Third, soluble forms of the two IL-1 receptors bind IL-1 and prevent IL-1 from binding to its cell-bound receptors. The complexity and the specificity of the IL-1 network are presented in this section (Fig. 1).

The IL-1 Gene Family

The IL-1 gene family includes three members, two of which are agonists, the third member being an antagonist. IL-1α and IL-1β are structurally related proteins with nearly identical biological activities, as evidenced by their binding to the same receptors, although with different affinities. The IL-1 receptor antagonist (IL-1Ra) is structurally related to IL-1α and IL-1β, but does not display any biological activity when binding to the IL-1 receptors. Each of these proteins is encoded by separate genes.

IL-1α and IL-1β

The genes encoding for IL-1α and IL-1β have a similar structure; namely, they comprise seven exons and six introns (2,3). The IL-1α gene spans over a 10.5-kb region, whereas the IL-1β gene spans approximately 7.8 kb. Each gene encodes for a 31-kDa precursor polypeptide (4,5). These precursor forms of IL-1 do not contain the typical leader sequence that allows proteins to be incorporated into the endoplasmic reticulum (ER) and then processed through the Golgi apparatus toward the cell surface for secretion. Several alternative pathways have been proposed (6), but none has been fully elucidated. Although the precursor form of IL-1β contains several consensus sites for N-glycosylation (7,8), glycosylated forms of IL-1β have not been reported, supporting the hypothesis of an alternative pathway for secretion of IL-1β.

Interleukin-1β is localized mainly in the cytoplasmic ground substance, but is absent from the ER, the Golgi apparatus, and the plasma membrane of lipopolysaccharide (LPS)-stimulated human monocytes (9). Secretory proteins undergo three major modifications in the lumen of the ER and the Golgi apparatus: N-glycosylation, specific proteolytic cleavage, and formation of disulfide bonds. Disulfide-bonding between two cysteine residues occurs in the oxidizing milieu of the ER lumen and is a stabilizing force in the secondary structure of proteins. The mature form of IL-1α contains one cysteine residue (position 253) (8), whereas the mature form of IL-1β contains two cysteine residues (positions 124 and 187) (7). Accumulation of IL-1 precursor in the cytosol, a reducing milieu, may explain why thiol groups of cysteine residues are not engaged in a disulfide bond (10).

Mature forms of IL-1 have a molecular mass of 17.5 kDa and correspond to the COOH-terminus of their respective precursor forms (7,8). Interleukin-1β is generated by enzymatic cleavage of the precursor form by an intracellular cysteine protease, named IL-1β-converting enzyme (ICE) (11,12). The precursor form of IL-1β is as yet the only identified substrate for ICE, although other intracellular cysteine proteases recognize similar cleavage sites in other proteins. ICE cleaves between aspartic acid-116 and alanine-117. Mature IL-1α results from the enzymatic cleavage of its precursor form by calpains between positions 113 and 114 (13). Both mature forms of IL-1 are biologically active.

Both precursor forms of IL-1 are found in the cytosolic compartment. Mature forms are

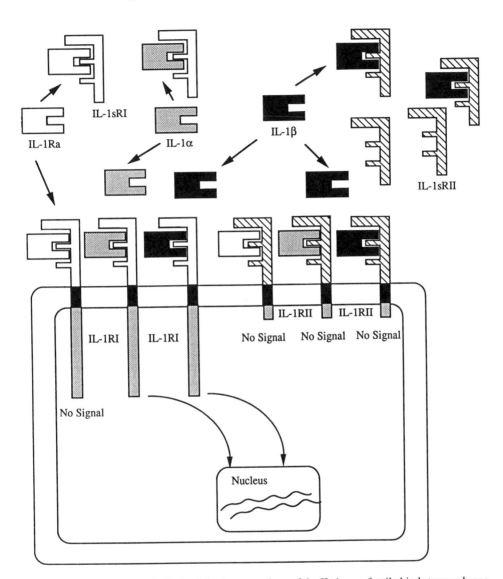

Figure 1   The IL-1 network: Each of the three members of the IL-1 gene family binds to membrane-bound IL-1 receptors. IL-1Ra and IL-1α have higher affinities for IL-1RI, whereas IL-1β has a higher affinity for IL-1RII. IL-1Ra inhibits IL-1 activities by blocking binding of IL-1α or IL-1β. Membrane-bound IL-1RI has a 213-residue cytoplasmic domain and initiates signal transduction for IL-1. In contrast, membrane-bound IL-1RII has a short cytoplasmic domain that comprises only 29 residues, does not trigger an intracellular signal, and serves as a decoy receptor. Soluble forms of each receptor are found in the extracellular milieu. IL-1sRI retains the ability to bind IL-1Ra, whereas IL-1sRII, preferentially and almost irreversibly, binds IL-1β.

found only in the extracellular environment, indicating that processing and secretion are two contemporary events (14). However, some precursor forms of IL-1 have been found extracellularly, suggesting that secretion does not require processing of its precursor form. Most of the mature IL-1α contingent stays in the cytosolic compartment, whereas mature IL-1β is secreted mainly in the extracellular milieu (15).

Recently, a high degree of homology between the human ICE gene product in mammalian cells and the *ced-3* gene described in *Caenorhabditis elegans* has suggested a possible role for ICE in programmed cell death, or apoptosis (16). In *C. elegans*, inhibition of *ced-3* prevents apoptosis. Such an inhibition can be achieved by activation of the *ced-9* gene. In *C. elegans*, programmed cell death would result from an imbalance between the *ced-3* and the *ced-9* gene products. In mammalian cells, overexpression of ICE induces programmed cell death (17). Reciprocally, inhibition of ICE activity by the viral *crm-A* gene product inhibits neuronal cell death (18). Cell death is also inhibited by *bcl-2*, the human homologue of *ced-9* (19). Thus, apoptosis in mammalian cells occurs when the expression of ICE predominates over that of *bcl-2*. Recently, a role for ICE in Fas-induced apoptosis has been established using thymocytes from ICE-deficient mice (20). However, lymphocytes from these ICE-deficient mice undergo normal programmed cell death when triggered by corticoids, supporting the concept of multiple pathways for apoptosis. Other intracellular cysteine proteases belonging to the ICE/*ced-3* family could be involved in programmed cell death. Such ICE-related proteins include Yama/CPP32 (21), Ich-1 (22), and the TX protein (23).

A role for ICE in apoptosis does not necessarily imply that IL-1β is a mediator of the apoptotic process. Although IL-1β is the only substrate yet described for ICE, ICE might use another substrate during apoptosis, since cell death has been observed in cells that do not express the IL-1β gene. In this circumstance, secretion of IL-1β in the extracellular environment would allow the surrounding cells to be affected by programmed cell death. Indirect apoptosis could occur through an IL-1-driven induction of nitric oxide (NO) synthesis. If IL-1β were not involved in apoptosis itself, the role of mature IL-1β could also be to initiate clearance of dead cells by neighboring cells.

Although mature IL-1 acts as a proinflammatory mediator, the role of the IL-1α precursor remains unclear. It is reasonable to speculate that the intracellular role of the IL-1α precursor may be more significant than that of the IL-1β precursor. First, the intracellular half-life of IL-1α is longer (15 h) than that of IL-1β (2.5 h) (14). Second, the IL-1α precursor is biologically active, whereas the IL-1β precursor is very weak (24,25). Third, the precursor form of IL-1α contains a nuclear-localization sequence, whereas the precursor form of IL-1β does not, suggesting that IL-1α could behave as a DNA-binding protein (26). These structural differences may account for the inhibitory effect of IL-1α mRNA antisense oligonucleotides on the senescence of endothelial cells (27).

IL-1 Receptor Antagonist

The third member of the IL-1 gene family was initially known as the IL-1 inhibitor (28). This IL-1 inhibitory activity was identified in the urine of febrile patients (29,30), or patients suffering from monocytic leukemia (31), and in the plasma of patients with juvenile rheumatoid arthritis (32). An IL-1 inhibitory activity was also reported in the supernatants of adherent monocytes cultured in IgG-coated plates (33). From a library of activated monocytes, Eisenberg and colleagues cloned, sequenced, and expressed a protein that displays the previously described IL-1 inhibitory activity (34,35). Because the IL-1 inhibitor binds to IL-1 receptors (35,36), does not induce any of the biological activities of IL-1

(37), and blocks the binding of IL-1 to its receptors (35,38), the IL-1 inhibitor behaved as a classic receptor antagonist and was renamed the IL-1 receptor antagonist (IL-1Ra).

The gene encoding for IL-1Ra is located on the long arm of human chromosome 2, in close proximity to the genes encoding for IL-1α and IL-1β, suggesting an early gene duplication (39). These three genes are thought to have evolved from a common ancestral gene some 350 million years ago. The IL-1Ra is believed to have diverged from this ancestral gene before the IL-1α gene diverged from the IL-1β gene (40). The IL-1Ra gene spans over 6.4 kb and is made of four exons and three introns. Two of the intron–exon junctions are conserved between the three IL-1 family member genes, further supporting the involvement of gene duplication in the creation of the IL-1 gene family.

The IL-1Ra gene encodes a 177-amino acid precursor polypeptide, the NH_2-terminus of which includes an hydrophobic stretch of amino acids typical of leader sequences required for secretion of proteins by the classical pathway (34,41). Incorporation of the precursor form of IL-1Ra into the endoplasmic reticulum is followed by cleavage of the first 25 amino acids located at its NH_2-terminus, thereby generating a 152-amino acid polypeptide. This mature form of IL-1Ra possesses multiple sites for *N*-glycosylation and is secreted as a glycoprotein with a molecular mass between 17 and 22 kDa. This form of IL-1Ra is known as the secretory IL-1Ra (sIL-1Ra).

Another form of IL-1Ra transcripts encodes for a 159-amino acid polypeptide, with no leader sequence (42). This form remains intracellular; hence, the designation intracellular IL-1Ra (icIL-1Ra). Differences between icIL-1Ra and the precursor form of IL-1Ra reside in their NH_2-terminus. The first three amino acids of icIL-1Ra are encoded by an alternative exon 1 located 9.6-kb upstream from the exon 1 used for the sIL-1Ra transcript. However, the four COOH-terminus amino acids of the leader sequence in the IL-1Ra precursor form are present in the same positions in icIL-1Ra. Furthermore, the 152 residues at the COOH-terminus of icIL-1Ra are those found in sIL-1Ra, thus conferring on icIL-1Ra the antagonistic activity of sIL-1Ra.

The IL-1 Receptors

Two distinct gene products have been identified, IL-1 receptor type I (IL-1RI) and IL-1 receptor type II (IL-1RII) (43–45). Both genes have been mapped to human chromosome 2 (45,46). IL-1RI is a 80-kDa protein, whereas IL-1RII is a 68-kDa protein. Originally, IL-1RI was thought to be present only on the surface of keratinocytes, endothelial cells, fibroblasts, hepatocytes, and T cells, whereas IL-1RII was thought to be the receptor expressed by B cells, monocytes, neutrophils, and bone marrow cells (47–49). However, it is now well accepted that every cell responsive to IL-1 expresses the IL-1RI (50,51). In contrast, IL-1RII does not transduce a signal and appears to serve the role of a decoy receptor (52,53). The paucity of IL-1RI receptors on some cells and the exquisite sensitivity of IL-1RI-bearing cells to IL-1 explain the previous simplistic classification based on the predominant IL-1R expression.

Both types of IL-1R belong to the immunoglobulin gene superfamily. Their extracellular domains contain three cysteine–cysteine bonds defining three loops and present a high degree of sequence homology. IL-1RI and IL-1RII differ mainly by the length of their cytoplasmic domains. The IL-1RI cytoplasmic domain is 213-amino acids long, whereas that of IL-1RII comprises only 29 amino acids. Because of such a short cytoplasmic domain, it was thought that IL-1RII would associate with an accessory protein or would dimerize with the functional type-I receptor. Both hypotheses are now excluded. IL-1RI and

IL-1RII display different affinities for each member of the IL-1 gene family (54). IL-1RI binds IL-1α and IL-1Ra with a greater affinity than it binds IL-1β. In contrast, IL-1RII binds IL-1β with higher affinity than it binds IL-1α and IL-1Ra. Binding of IL-1α or IL-1β to the IL-1RI chain allows the recruitment of an accessory chain to the IL-1–IL-1RI complexes (55). Such an event has not been observed with binding of IL-1Ra to IL-1RI. In contrast to IL-1RI, IL-1RII is unable to recruit the accessory chain upon binding of IL-1α, IL-1β, or IL-1Ra. Interestingly, this novel accessory chain does not bind any member of the IL-1 gene family in the absence of IL-1RI.

Soluble forms of each IL-1 receptor—namely, IL-1sRI and IL-1sRII—are found in the extracellular milieu. IL-1sRI retains the ability to bind IL-1Ra with an affinity comparable with cell-bound IL-1RI, but has a weaker affinity for IL-1α (56). IL-1sRI does not bind IL-1β. In contrast, IL-1sRII binds IL-1β with high affinity, but binds poorly to IL-1α and IL-1Ra (57,58). Interestingly, IL-1sRII also binds the IL-1β precursor, and it is speculated that this complex prevents processing of the IL-1β precursor into smaller forms (59). The selective loss of binding of some IL-1 gene family members to the soluble forms of IL-1 receptors likely results from the loss of specific binding sites following the shedding of membrane-bound IL-1 receptors. Because IL-1sRII binds almost exclusively IL-1β, constitutive shedding of the cell-bound IL-1RII likely represents a functional antagonism of IL-1 activity. On the other hand, the strong binding of IL-1Ra to IL-1sRI constitutes an impediment to the functional antagonism exerted by the inducible IL-1Ra.

BIOLOGICAL ACTIVITIES OF IL-1

A role for IL-1 in the development of an allergic reaction was first proposed when IL-1 was detected in blister fluids at sites of human skin allergic reactions (60). The bioactivity of IL-1 was observed during the cutaneous late-phase reaction, but was absent from the early-phase response. This bioactivity was mostly due to IL-1β, although IL-1α accounted for the remaining activity. Using radioimmunoassays, IL-1β was detected during the early phase. These findings indicated that IL-1β was secreted either as a biologically inactive form, such as the IL-1β precursor form, or the IL-1β bioactivity was hindered by IL-1 inhibitors, such as IL-1Ra or IL-1sRII. Although polyclonal antibodies raised against mature IL-1β recognize a significant percentage of IL-1β precursor molecules, one may question the former explanation, because a chymase released by dermal mast cells cleaves the IL-1β precursor into a biologically active mature fragment with an NH_2-terminus at 114 (61). The presence of IL-1 during allergic reactions was subsequently extended to the upper airways of allergic patients following antigenic challenge. IL-1 levels rose in nasal fluids during both the early and late phases of nasal allergic reactions (62). Interestingly, the IL-1 contingent of this early phase was biologically inactive. Increased IL-1α levels were also detected in nasal fluids during the early and late phases of an allergic reaction occurring in patients with allergic rhinitis (63). Taken together, these data suggested that IL-1 plays a role in the development of allergic reactions. Among the vast array of biological activities of IL-1, those that are relevant to allergy are discussed in the following sections (Fig. 2).

IL-1 and Histamine Release

Early studies suggested that recombinant IL-1β itself induced histamine release from human mast cells (64) and human basophils (65). These histamine-release assays were performed in the presence of deuterium oxide, a priming agent for degranulation of basophils and mast cells. A more detailed study revealed that IL-1 behaved as a histamine-releasing factor only in those basophil preparations that were sensitive themselves to deuterium oxide (66). Further studies clearly established that, in absence of deuterium oxide, IL-1 was not a histamine-releasing factor for either human basophils (67) or pulmonary mast cells (68).

Unlike IL-3, IL-5, and granulocyte–macrophage colony-stimulating factor (GM-CSF), IL-1 does not act as a priming agent for histamine release from basophils stimulated with IgE or the complement products C_{5a} and C_{3a} (67). However, IL-1 marginally enhances histamine release from basophils stimulated with platelet-activating factor (PAF) or IL-8 (67,69). In the light of the latter priming effect, it is important to consider the degree of contamination of the basophil preparations by monocytes as an explanation for the early claims that IL-1 itself was a histamine-releasing factor. In those basophil preparations, IL-1 may have acted as a priming agent for an IL-8-driven histamine release, for IL-1 is a potent inducer of IL-8 synthesis in monocytes.

In the chemokine gene family, the monocyte chemoattractant protein-1 (MCP-1) is of vital importance to this topic, as IL-1 induces the synthesis of MCP-1 by endothelial cells (70,71) and pulmonary epithelial cells (72). MCP-1 itself induces histamine release from basophils (73–75). The magnitude of MCP-1-induced degranulation is comparable with that induced by IL-8 in the presence of IL-3 (74). The potency of MCP-1 is further increased when basophils have been exposed to a priming agent, such as IL-3, IL-5, or GM-CSF. Thus, IL-1 may contribute indirectly to the degranulation of basophils by induction of MCP-1 synthesis.

IL-1 and Eosinophilic Infiltration

Recruitment of inflammatory cells at sites of allergic reactions results from a cascade of events taking place at the surface of an activated endothelium. The transendothelial migration of eosinophils is preceded by a two-step recognition of the endothelium by eosinophils; a rolling of eosinophils on activated endothelium, followed by their strong attachment to the endothelium. Eosinophils express the ligands for their counterreceptors present on the surface of activated endothelial cells. Interleukin-1 induces the surface expression of each of the three counterreceptors involved in the recruitment of eosinophils.

Rolling of Eosinophils on Activated Endothelium

Endothelial leukocyte adhesion molecule 1 (ELAM-1) is the counterreceptor for L-selectin, a glycoprotein constitutively expressed by eosinophils (76). Interleukin-1 induces the expression of ELAM-1 by endothelial cells (77,78). The recognition of L-selectin by ELAM-1 contributes to the adhesion process, as an anti-ELAM-1 partially reduces the adhesion of eosinophils to IL-1-activated endothelial cells (79). A role for IL-1 in the induction of ELAM-1 during late-phase cutaneous allergic reactions has also been confirmed in an in vitro model of human skin explants after exposure to the appropriate antigen (80). Rolling of eosinophils on the surface of activated endothelium is required for the exposure of eosinophils to inflammatory mediators released by activated endothelial cells or by the inflamed tissue.

Attachment of Eosinophils to Activated Endothelium

The initial rolling of eosinophils on the activated endothelium is followed by their tight attachment to the endothelium. Two distinct pathways have been identified, based on the interactions between the integrins expressed on the surface of eosinophils and the adhesion molecules expressed by activated endothelial cells. IL-1 induces the expression of intracellular adhesion molecule (ICAM)-1 and vascular cell adhesion molecule (VCAM-1) by

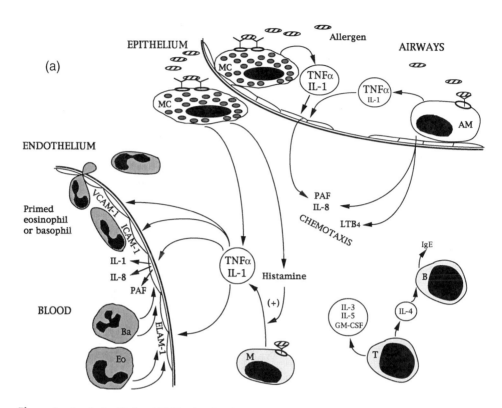

Figure 2 A role for IL-1 and TNF-α in allergic reactions. A schematic view of a pulmonary allergic reaction is presented in two parts. (a) Early-phase response: mast cells (MC) line the airway lumen as well as reside in the bronchial mucosa. Allergen deposition initiates the unfolding of the early-phase response. Cross-linking of the high-affinity receptors for IgE on mast cells induces the release of preformed mediators as well as the synthesis of arachidonate metabolites and various cytokines, including TNF-α and IL-1. Alveolar (AM) and tissue (M) macrophages also synthesize TNF-α and IL-1 after binding of immune complexes (allergen–antibody) to the low-affinity receptors for IgE. The reduced ability of alveolar macrophages to secrete IL-1 is indicated by the small type IL-1. Histamine released from mast cell granules may amplify the synthesis of TNF-α and IL-1. TNF-α and IL-1 initiate the onset of the late-phase response through a myriad of biological activities. These are also depicted. First, TNF-α and IL-1 stimulate bronchial epithelial cells to secrete PAF and IL-8, potent chemotactic factors for primed eosinophils (E_o). In addition to PAF and IL-8, alveolar macrophages secrete LTB_4, yet another chemotactic factor for primed eosinophils. Second, TNF-α and IL-1 induce surface expression of ELAM-1, ICAM-1, and VCAM-1 on endothelial cells. ELAM-1 is probably involved in the rolling of eosinophils and basophils (Ba) on the endothelium, whereas ICAM-1 and VCAM-1 mediate the strong attachment of primed eosinophils and basophils to activated endothelium. Third, TNF-α and IL-1 induce synthesis of PAF, IL-1, and IL-8 by endothelial cells. These mediators are potent activators of eosinophils and basophils. Activation is prerequisite step for the attachment of rolling cells to activated endothelium by β_1-integrins. After transendothelial migration, eosinophils and basophils move along a gradient of chemotactic factors toward sites of allergen deposition. In allergic asthma, allergen-specific CD4[+] T-cell clones (T) spontaneously secrete Th_2 lymphokines, including IL-3, IL-4, IL-5, and GM-CSF. IL-4, in conjunction with IL-13, maintains the synthesis of IgE by B cells (B).

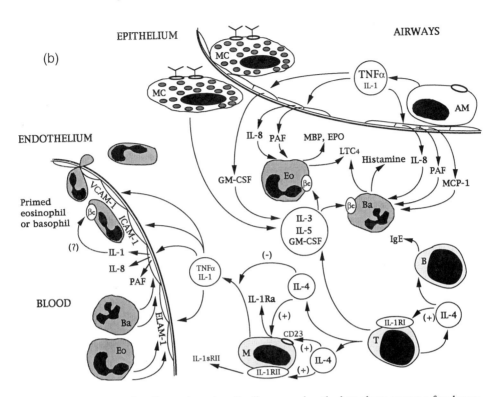

(b) Late-phase response: the allergen has virtually disappeared as the late phase occurs a few hours after mast cells have been activated. Alveolar macrophages still secrete TNF-α and IL-1. TNF-α and IL-1 induce synthesis of PAF, IL-8, and MCP-1 by bronchial epithelial cells. PAF and IL-8 induce synthesis of LTC$_4$ from primed basophils and eosinophils. Furthermore, PAF and IL-8 induce release of granule contents from these effector cells. Histamine increases the basal tonus of the bronchi, whereas MBP and EPO disrupt the epithelial barrier. MCP-1 is also a histamine-releasing factor for basophils. Priming of eosinophils and basophils results from an exposure to IL-3, IL-5, and GM-CSF. These Th$_2$ lymphokines are secreted by mast cells following exposure to the allergen and by allergen-specific CD4+ T-cell clones after antigen presentation. An indirect role for TNF-α and IL-1 in the priming event has been proposed because TNF-α and IL-1 up-regulate surface expression of the β-chain common (βc) to the receptors for IL-3, IL-5, and GM-CSF. Activated CD4+ T-cell clones also secrete IL-4. IL-4 displays anti-inflammatory effects on resident macrophages and infiltrated monocytes. IL-4 suppresses IL-1 and TNF-α production, but induces IL-1Ra synthesis. Furthermore, IL-4 increases surface expression for IL-1RII and its shedding as IL-1sRII. IL-4 induces surface expression of CD23 on monocytes and B cells. IL-4 up-regulates IL-1RI on T cells. The latter effect may compensate for the scarcity of IL-1 and, thus, may allow IL-1 to favor differentiation of uncommitted T cells toward a Th$_2$ profile.

endothelial cells (77,81). ICAM-1 is the counterreceptor for the β$_2$-integrins Mac-1 (82) and lymphocyte function-associated antigen (LFA)-1 (83), whereas VCAM-1 is the counter-receptor for the β$_1$-integrin very late activation antigen (VLA)-4 (84). The β$_2$-integrin pathway requires activated eosinophils, whereas constitutive expression of VLA-4 by resting eosinophils is sufficient for their adhesion to activated endothelial cells. Platelet-activating factor is a potent activator of eosinophils, and important sources of PAF are endothelial cells, monocytes, and alveolar macrophages after exposure to IL-1 (85–87). For the endothelial cells, most of the PAF remains cell-associated and, as such, is likely to be in the immediate vicinity of rolling eosinophils. A role for the β_2-integrins and ICAM-1 in the adhesion of activated eosinophils to IL-1-activated endothelial cells has been established in vitro by using specific antibodies directed either against each member of the β_2-integrin family or against ICAM-1 (79). In a similar fashion, the duo VLA-4–VCAM-1 has been reported to partly mediate the adhesion of eosinophils to IL-1-activated eosinophils (79).

Eosinophil Chemotaxis

Eosinophils cross the endothelial barrier and migrate within inflamed tissue toward sites of allergic reactions. This migration is thought to be driven by gradients of chemotactic factors, including PAF, leukotriene (LT) B_4, and IL-8. The role of IL-1 in eosinophil chemotaxis may be of considerable importance, since IL-1 induces the synthesis of these chemotactic factors. Interleukin-1 induces the release of PAF from alveolar macrophages (87) and monocytes (86). It is also a potent inducer of IL-8 synthesis by bronchial epithelial cells (88,89) and alveolar macrophages (90). A role for PAF and IL-8 in an IL-1-driven accumulation of eosinophils has recently been demonstrated in a rat model of cutaneous cellular infiltration (91). Importantly, the threshold for an eosinophil response to these chemotactic factors is greatly reduced when eosinophils have been exposed in vitro to IL-3, IL-5, or GM-CSF (92–94). These primed eosinophils are as responsive to PAF as their counterparts from patients with allergic asthma. Because IL-1 up-regulates gene and surface expression of β_c, the β-chain common to the receptors for IL-3, IL-5, and GM-CSF (95), another indirect role for IL-1 during a late-phase allergic reaction could consist in the amplification of the priming effects of IL-3 and IL-5 on eosinophils. However, it remains to be established whether IL-1 up-regulates β_c on eosinophils.

Because PAF and IL-8 are potent chemotactic factors for neutrophils, one wonders how eosinophils and basophils are selectively recruited at the sites of a late-phase allergic reaction (96). Interestingly, the IL-5 receptor is uniquely expressed by eosinophils and basophils (97,98). Furthermore, in contrast to eosinophils and basophils, neutrophils do not express the IL-3 receptor. Thus, the restricted expression of receptors for IL-3 and IL-5 is likely to be part of the molecular basis for selectivity in the recruitment of eosinophils and basophils. Although IL-1 is a weak activator of basophilic function, an IL-1-driven up-regulation of β_c expression on basophils cannot be excluded.

IL-1 and Eosinophil Survival

Circulating eosinophils are short-lived cells. Their accumulation within an inflamed tissue reflects the balance between infiltration and life span of these cells. Interestingly, IL-3, IL-5, and GM-CSF dramatically increase eosinophil survival in vitro (99–101). Whether IL-3, IL-5, and GM-CSF decrease enzymatic activities of ICE or related cysteine proteases remains unknown.

In bronchial inflammation, eosinophils accumulate in the vicinity of the epithelial layer. An indirect role for IL-1 in eosinophil survival has been suggested, for IL-1 induces the synthesis of GM-CSF by human bronchial epithelial cells (102), thereby prolonging the life span of eosinophils in vitro (103).

IL-1 and Activation of Effector Cells

Platelet-activating factor is a potent activator of primed eosinophils (104). Degranulation of activated eosinophils contributes to the development of bronchial hyperreactivity, an important feature of the late-phase response and also of status asthmaticus. Unique eosino-phil granule contents include cationic proteins, such as the major basic protein (MBP) and eosinophil peroxidase (EPO). Although MBP and EPO induce exfoliation and ciliostasis of epithelial cells in vitro, only MBP induces bronchial hyperreactivity in vivo (105). Both MBP and EPO induce bronchoconstriction. Activated eosinophils also synthesize LTC_4, which becomes converted into LTD_4 and LTE_4. These peptidoleukotrienes are broncho-constrictors and induce bronchial hyperreactivity. Because IL-1 is a potent inducer of PAF release, IL-1 could indirectly contribute to the activation of eosinophils. In a guinea pig model of pulmonary allergic reactions, blockade of IL-1 receptors has decreased the antigen-induced pulmonary recruitment of eosinophils and airway hyperreactivity (106).

Basophils could also contribute to the development of the late-phase reaction. Activated basophils degranulate and, in doing so, release histamine. Furthermore, primed basophils synthesize LTC_4 in response to PAF and, to a lesser extent, to IL-8 (67,69). IL-1 is a weak priming agent for histamine release from basophils stimulated with PAF or IL-8. However, IL-1 itself induces neither basophil degranulation nor LTC_4 synthesis. Furthermore, IL-1 does not prime basophils for LTC_4 synthesis induced by PAF or IL-8 (67,69). Thus, IL-1 is unlikely to be a major regulator of basophil function.

IL-1 and Differentiation of T-Helper Cells

Activated $CD4^+$ lymphocytes can be classified into two subsets, based on the profile of their cytokine production (107,108). Interferon-γ is the prototypic cytokine secreted by T-helper (Th_1) lymphocytes, whereas the secretion of IL-4 and IL-5 defines the Th_2 subset. Activated $CD4^+$ lymphocytes recruited at the sites of cutaneous late-phase reactions express the genes coding for IL-3, IL-4, IL-5, and GM-CSF but do not express the gene coding for IFN-γ (109). A similar Th_2 profile has been observed in T lymphocytes from bronchoalveolar lavage (BAL) of patients with allergic asthma (110). Although IL-1 fails to affect the differentiation of uncommitted human T-cell clones along the Th_1 pathway, IL-1 plays a significant role in the differentiation of these clones toward a Th_2 phenotype (111). In agreement with these observations, murine Th_2 clones established in the presence of antigens from the malaria parasite *Plasmodium chabaudi* express IL-1RI, whereas the Th_1 clones do not express detectable levels of IL-1RI (112). The importance of IL-1 in the differentiation of T cells along the Th_2 pathway in vivo remains uncertain, because IL-4 secreted by already committed Th_2 cells is likely to inhibit synthesis of IL-1 (see later discussion).

CELL SOURCES OF IL-1 IN ALLERGY

Detectable levels of IL-1 have been observed during the early and late phases of allergic reactions (60,62,63). What are the cell sources of IL-1?

Synthesis of IL-1 during the early-phase reactions is likely to be triggered by the allergen itself. Antigenic stimulation of murine mast cells induces the synthesis of IL-1 (113). Because IL-1 mRNA levels increase within the first 60 min after the exposure of mast cells to antigen, this rapid accumulation of IL-1 mRNA should take place during the develop-ment of the early-phase reaction. Alternatively, resident macrophages or freshly elicited monocytes could also be a source of IL-1. Indeed, an increased number of circulating monocytes and alveolar macrophages from patients with allergic asthma express the low-affinity receptor for IgE (FcϵRII) (114,115). Antigenic stimulation of monocytes from patients with asthma results in the synthesis of IL-1β (116); however, among the resident macrophages, alveolar macrophages are particularly poor producers of IL-1. Although alveolar macrophages from individuals with allergic asthma spontaneously secrete IL-1 (117), an antigenic stimulation does not further increase IL-1 secretion (118). These observations are not solely restricted to an antigenic challenge, for LPS is also a weak stimulus for the production of mature IL-1β in these cells (119). In fact, alveolar macrophages appear to be ill-suited for IL-1 secretion because they are inefficient at processing the precursor form of IL-1β into its mature form (120). These defects in cleavage and secretion of IL-1β likely reveal a limited ICE activity. The selectivity of these defects is best illustrated by the ability of alveolar macrophages to produce and secrete IL-1Ra (121).

The sources of IL-1 during the late-phase reactions probably include eosinophils, endothelial cells, and resident macrophages. Activated and primed eosinophils express the gene coding for IL-1α and produce IL-1α (122). Endothelial cells stimulated with TNF-α or IL-1 secrete IL-1β (123). It is also conceivable that resident macrophages and freshly elicited monocytes in the nasal mucosa or the dermal layer of the skin produce IL-1β after their exposure to TNF-α or IL-1.

MEDIATORS OF ALLERGY AND IL-1 ACTIVITY

Synthesis of IL-1 occurs in the midst of an intense inflammatory reaction. Mediators of the acute- and late-phase reactions are thus likely to regulate the synthesis of IL-1 as well as its activity.

Histamine

Early studies dealing with the regulation of IL-1 synthesis by histamine were performed with monocytes stimulated by LPS. Under these conditions, histamine marginally suppressed IL-1 synthesis (124). These immunomodulatory effects of histamine were mediated by activation of H_2 receptors. However, LPS as a stimulus is not relevant to an allergic reaction. In an attempt to better mimic the in vivo situation, IL-1 itself was used as a stimulus. Interestingly, histamine alone failed to induce IL-1β, but rather, enhanced gene expression and protein synthesis for IL-1β in IL-1α-stimulated peripheral blood mononuclear cells (125). This increase in self-induction of IL-1 was mediated by H_2 receptors. Activation of H_2 receptors leads to an increase in cAMP levels. Thus, it was not surprising to observe a similar effect in the presence of PGE_2, another activator of adenylate cyclase (125). In this in vitro model, histamine and PGE_2 also enhanced IL-8 synthesis (126). However, histamine did not affect the production of IL-1Ra induced by IL-1α (125). Thus, histamine release from mast cells and basophils may amplify the magnitude of the late-phase reactions by enhancing IL-1 synthesis and activities.

Lymphokines of the Th_2 Subset

Allergen-specific CD4[+] T-cell clones from allergic patients secrete a vast array of lymphokines that define the Th_2 profile in the murine system. These lymphokines include IL-4, IL-5, IL-10, and IL-13. However, human Th_2-like T-cell clones differ from their murine counterparts in that some of these lymphokines are also produced by human Th_1-like CD4[+] T-cell clones. Among those lymphokines are IL-10 (127) and IL-13 (128). Thus, secretion of IL-10 and IL-13 is not a characteristic feature of the Th_2 subset in humans. Nonetheless, these Th$_2$ lymphokines, as defined in the murine system, share the remarkable ability to inhibit IL-1 synthesis and activity.

IL-4

Interleukin-4 regulates IL-1 activity at multiple levels. It inhibits the synthesis of IL-1β in monocytes stimulated with IL-1α, but enhances the synthesis of IL-1Ra in the same cells (129). A similar regulation was observed when monocytes were stimulated with LPS (129–131). In addition, IL-4 itself induces the synthesis of IL-1Ra in resting monocytes (129,132). This inhibitory effect of IL-4 on IL-1 activity is further reinforced by its effect on IL-1RII. IL-4 enhances gene and surface expression of IL-1RII and increases the release of its soluble form in the extracellular milieu (53). Thus, the inhibitory effects of IL-4 on IL-1 activity are threefold: a decrease in the synthesis of the agonist IL-1, an induction of the synthesis of the naturally occurring antagonist IL-1Ra, and an increase in the surface expression of the decoy receptor IL-1RII, followed by the release of its soluble form IL-1sRII. Given this impressive triad of inhibitory effects, one might be puzzled by the increase in surface expression of IL-1RI upon exposure of murine Th$_2$ cells to IL-4 (133). If IL-1 is indeed an important mediator for the differentiation of T cells toward the Th$_2$ phenotype, the up-regulation of IL-1RI by IL-4 may compensate for the scarcity of IL-1 production under these conditions.

IL-5

The effect of IL-5 on the synthesis of IL-1 and IL-1Ra remains unknown. Although a weak inducer of IL-1 synthesis, GM-CSF is an excellent inducer of IL-1Ra synthesis by monocytes (134) and alveolar macrophages (135). Because receptors for IL-5 and GM-CSF share a common β-subunit involved in intracellular signaling (136), one should not rule out a possible effect of IL-5 on the synthesis of IL-1 by eosinophils. There is no report describing eosinophils as a source of IL-1Ra.

IL-10

The main effect of IL-10 on IL-1-related events resides in its ability to regulate IL-1β synthesis. Interleukin-10 dramatically suppressed IL-1β synthesis in human monocytes stimulated with LPS (137) and in human peripheral blood mononuclear cells stimulated with IL-1α (126a). Whether IL-10 is a major regulator of IL-1Ra production remains a controversial issue. Initial studies showed that IL-10 up-regulated IL-1Ra synthesis in LPS-stimulated monocytes (138). However, subsequent studies indicated that IL-10 marginally reduced LPS-induced IL-1Ra synthesis, despite a weak induction of IL-1Ra synthesis by IL-10 alone (139). Similar results were obtained when human peripheral blood mononuclear cells were stimulated with IL-1α (126a). These discrepancies could have arisen from the use of human serum in the initial studies, as human serum contains IgG subtypes, potent inducers of IL-1Ra synthesis (134,140). Taken together, these results could actually suggest that IL-10 possesses the ability to regulate IL-1Ra production induced by IgG. To our knowledge, there is no report documenting the effect of IL-10 on gene or surface expression for IL-1RI. In neutrophils, IL-10 does not affect surface expression of IL-1RII (141).

IL-13

Similar to IL-4, IL-13 regulates IL-1 activity. Alone, IL-13 induces IL-1Ra synthesis in resting monocytes (142), reduces IL-1β production in monocytes stimulated with LPS or IL-1α, and enhances IL-1Ra synthesis in these cells (126b,138). Furthermore, IL-13 increases surface expression of IL-1RII and induces the release of its soluble form, IL-1sRII

(143). The commonality between these activities of IL-4 and IL-13 results from the engagement of a common subunit of their heterodimeric receptors (144). This common subunit is thought to be the 130-kDa chain of the IL-4 receptor complex (145).

SPECIFIC BLOCKADE OF IL-1 IN ALLERGY

If one keeps in mind the vast array of biological activities of IL-1 relevant to allergic reactions, one might have anticipated the efficacy of a truncated, soluble form of the human IL-1RI in a recent clinical trial of cutaneous allergic reactions (146). This truncated form corresponds to the 313 residues located at the NH_2-terminus of IL-1RI and, hereafter, has been designated IL-1tRI. Intradermal injection of IL-1tRI was neither immunogenic nor toxic. Interleukin-1tRI remained without effect on the induration during the early phase of the cutaneous allergic reaction. Surprisingly, IL-1tRI marginally affected erythema formation, but dramatically reduced itching and discomfort sensation during the early phase. The latter parameter is essentially subjective, and one should not be left with the impression that IL-1 plays a critical role in the unfolding of the early phase. In contrast, IL-1tRI significantly reduced induration during the late-phase response. Furthermore, IL-1tRI reduced erythema and itching, although to a lesser extent. Indirect immunofluorescent staining of tissue biopsies for eosinophil granule MBP revealed a decrease, although not significant, in infiltrating eosinophils and in extracellular MBP deposition at sites treated with low doses of IL-1tRI, when compared with placebo sites. Thus, in this clinical trial, the improvement of clinical symptoms following administration of IL-1tRI likely results from a decreased activation of eosinophils and other effector cells, rather than from a reduced recruitment of these effector cells.

In this clinical trial, IL-1tRI was described as binding IL-1α and IL-1β, with affinities similar to those seen for membrane-bound IL-1RI (146). Although not mentioned, IL-1tRI conceivably binds IL-1Ra with an affinity similar to that seen with membrane-bound IL-1RI: it is tempting to propose that the use of IL-1sRII could have resulted in a greater suppression of the late-phase response. Unlike IL-1tRI, IL-1sRII preferentially binds IL-1β, but displays an extremely weak affinity for IL-1α or IL-1Ra. A clinical trial with human IL-1sRII could, in the future, strengthen the case for IL-1 in the development of allergic reactions.

ROLE OF TNF-α IN ALLERGIC REACTIONS

Interleukin-1 shares many of its biological activities with TNF-α (147). In most instances, IL-1 acts synergistically with TNF-α. In this section, we briefly describe the cell sources for TNF-α, the regulation of TNF-α synthesis, and the biological activities of TNF-α in the context of an allergic reaction.

Cell Sources of TNF-α

Synthesis of TNF-α during the early-phase reaction could occur in mast cells and resident macrophages. Early studies revealed that murine mast cells possess the unique ability to store TNF-α in their granules (148). This preformed TNF-α had a molecular mass of 50 kDa and was biologically active. Alternative mRNA splicing or degree of glycosylation could have accounted for the higher molecular mass of the preformed TNF-α, when compared with the precursor form (26 kDa) or the mature form (17 kDa) of TNF-α in human monocytes. The antigenic stimulation of murine mast cells resulted in the immediate release of preformed TNF-α, followed by a sustained release of newly synthesized TNF-α (149,150). The pool of preformed TNF-α accounted for only one-tenth of the whole amount of TNF-α released after antigenic stimulation of mast cells. It was later demonstrated in mice that mast cells contributed to the leukocyte recruitment during a cutaneous late-phase reaction by the release of TNF-α (151). The concept of preformed TNF-α has now been extended to human pulmonary (152) and dermal (153) mast cells. The preformed pool of human TNF-α is also biologically active, as evidenced in an in vitro model of human skin explants, in which preformed TNF-α was shown to be responsible for the expression of ELAM-1 by dermal endothelium after mast cell degranulation (153,154). A previous study indicated that resident cells from the skin of allergic patients were the probable source of TNF-α involved in the expression of ELAM-1 by dermal endothelium after an in vitro exposure of skin biopsies to the appropriate allergen (80). Thus, mast cells could orchestrate the recruitment of inflammatory cells at sites of allergen deposition. An immediate release of preformed TNF-α would trigger surface expression of adhesion molecules by a nearby endothelium. A second wave of newly synthesized TNF-α would allow, in conjunction with IL-1, a more sustained expression of these adhesion molecules. Basophils also express TNF-α (155), but whether preformed TNF-α is stored in their granules remains unknown.

Resident macrophages are also a likely source of TNF-α during the early-phase reaction. The differentiation of monocytes into macrophages is characterized by an increased capacity to produce TNF-α (156), and alveolar macrophages are no exception. Although alveolar macrophages are extremely poor producers of IL-1, secretion of TNF-α in response to LPS is enhanced severalfold in these cells, when compared with secretion of TNF-α by blood monocytes (157). This increase in TNF-α secretion is associated with an increase in TNF-α mRNA levels, indicating that increased TNF-α secretion does not result from a post-transcriptional modification. In allergic asthma, alveolar macrophages spontaneously secrete TNF-α (158). This spontaneous secretion is further increased by antigenic stimulation (158,159).

Among the likely sources of TNF-α during the late-phase reactions, one must mention alveolar macrophages (160), basophils, and eosinophils (161,162).

Regulation of TNF-α Synthesis

Histamine suppresses TNF-α synthesis in LPS-stimulated monocytes (163). However, a role for histamine in the regulation of TNF-α synthesis during allergic reactions remains speculative, as histamine fails to affect this synthesis when monocytes are stimulated with IL-1α, rather than LPS (164). On the other hand, IL-4 is a potent suppressor of TNF-α synthesis in monocytes stimulated with LPS (165). Similar results have been obtained with IL-10 (137) and IL-13 (138,166).

Biological Activities of TNF-α

An indirect role for TNF-α in the infiltration, activation, and survival of eosinophils has been suggested. TNF-α activates endothelial cells to express ELAM-1 (167), ICAM-1 (77), and VCAM-1 (81,168). The proteins ELAM-1, ICAM-1, and VCAM-1 contribute to the in vitro adhesion of eosinophils to TNF-α-treated endothelial cells (169,170). Furthermore, TNF-α induces the synthesis of PAF from endothelial cells (171) and macrophages (172). It also induces the synthesis of IL-8 by epithelial cells (88,89), alveolar macrophages (90), and endothelial cells (173). Moreover, TNF-α could increase the sensitivity of eosinophils to PAF and IL-8, because it up-regulates surface expression of the β-chain common to the receptors for IL-3, IL-5, and GM-CSF, priming agents for eosinophil activation (95). Each of these biological activities of TNF-α are shared with IL-1.

Unlike IL-1, TNF-α does not prime basophils to release histamine and synthesize LTC$_4$ in response to PAF (69). Nonetheless, TNF-α could play an indirect role in the degranulation of basophils, as it induces the synthesis of MCP-1 by bronchial epithelial cells (72) and endothelial cells (70,71). Unlike IL-1, TNF-α acts as a direct priming agent for eosinophils. For example, it primes eosinophils for LTC$_4$ synthesis (174).

CONCLUSION

One of the most striking differences between TNF-α and IL-1 in allergic reactions is that TNF-α, unlike IL-1, is stored within the granules of mast cells. TNF-α defines a new class of mast cell mediators that are both preformed and newly synthesized. This particular feature of TNF-α suggests that TNF-α precedes IL-1 in initiating the late-phase response. Soon after exposure to the allergen, resident macrophages join mast cells to increase the overall production of TNF-α and IL-1. Through myriad biological activities, TNF-α and IL-1 initiate and sustain the recruitment of eosinophils and other effector cells toward sites of allergen deposition. Moreover, TNF-α and IL-1 contribute indirectly to the activation of these effector cells, once they reach sites of allergic reaction. Mediators of the early phase, such as histamine, may magnify the importance of these cytokines by increasing their synthesis. However, the effects of TNF-α and IL-1 should eventually vanish as allergen-specific T-cell clones begin secreting a vast array of Th$_2$ lymphokines that share the ability to regulate synthesis and activities of both cytokines. Although useful in defining the possible molecular mechanisms of the allergic reactions, such a scenario is of only descriptive value. A role for IL-1 and TNF-α in the pathogenesis of allergic reactions can be established only by using specific inhibitors of each cytokine in vivo. A truncated form of IL-1RI has now been shown to limit the extent of a cutaneous late-phase response in humans, and IL-1Ra reduces pulmonary eosinophil accumulation and bronchial hyperreactivity in a guinea pig model of allergic reactions. There is as yet no report documenting a pharmacological approach specific for TNF-α in allergic reactions. Because IL-1 and TNF-α display similar activities, it would not be unexpected if a TNF "inhibitor" were to reduce the late-phase response of an allergic reaction.

ACKNOWLEDGMENTS

These studies are supported by National Institutes of Health grant AI-15614. The authors thank Dr. Giamila Fantuzzi for helpful comments during the preparation of the manuscript.

REFERENCES

1. Dinarello CA. The interleukin-1 family: 10 years of discovery. FASEB J 1994; 8:1314–1325.
2. Clark BD, Collins KL, Gandy MS, Webb AC, Auron PE. Genomic sequence for human prointerleukin 1 beta: possible evolution from a reverse transcribed prointerleukin 1 alpha gene. Nucleic Acids Res 1986; 14:7897–7914.
3. Furutani Y, Notake M, Fukui T, et al. Complete nucleotide sequence of the gene for human interleukin 1 alpha. Nucleic Acids Res 1986; 14:3167–3179.
4. Giri JG, Lomedico PT, Mizel SB. Studies on the synthesis and secretion of interleukin 1. I. A 33,000 molecular weight precursor for interleukin 1. J Immunol 1985; 134:343–349.

5. Limjuco G, Galuska S, Chin J, et al. Antibodies of predetermined specificity to the major charged species of human interleukin 1. Proc Natl Acad Sci USA 1986; 83:3972–3976.

6. Rubartelli A, Cozzolino F, Talio M, Sitia R. A novel secretory pathway for interleukin-1β, a protein lacking a signal sequence. EMBO J 1990; 9:1503–1510.

7. Auron PE, Webb AC, Rosenwasser LJ, et al. Nucleotide sequence of human monocyte interleukin 1 precursor cDNA. Proc Natl Acad Sci USA 1984; 81:7907–7911.

8. March CJ, Mosley B, Larsen A, et al. Cloning, sequence and expression of two distinct human interleukin-1 complementary DNAs. Nature 1985; 315:641–647.

9. Singer II, Scott S, Hall GL, et al. Interleukin 1β is localized in the cytoplasmic ground substance but is largely absent from the Golgi apparatus and plasma membranes of stimulated human monocytes. J Exp Med 1988; 167:389–407.

10. Priestle JP, Schär HP, Grütter MG. Crystal structure of the cytokine interleukin-1β. EMBO J 1988; 7:339–343.

11. Cerretti DP, Kozlosky CJ, Mosley B, et al. Molecular cloning of the interleukin-1β converting enzyme. Science 1992; 256:97–100.

12. Thornberry NA, Bull HG, Calaycay JR, et al. A novel heterodimeric cysteine protease is required for interleukin-1β processing in monocytes. Nature 1992; 356:768–774.

13. Kobayashi Y, Yamamoto K, Saido T, et al. Identification of calcium-activated neutral protease as a processing enzyme of human interleukin 1α. Proc Natl Acad Sci USA 1990; 87:5548–5552.

14. Hazuda DJ, Lee JC, Young PR. The kinetics of interleukin 1 secretion from activated monocytes. Differences between interleukin 1α and interleukin 1β. J Biol Chem 1988; 263:8473–8479.

15. Lonnemann G, Endres S, van der Meer JWM, et al. Differences in the synthesis and kinetics of release of interleukin 1α, interleukin 1β and tumor necrosis factor from human mononuclear cells. Eur J Immunol 1989; 19:1531–1536.

16. Yuan J, Shaham S, Ledoux S, Ellis HM, Horvitz HR. The C. elegans cell death gene ced-3 encodes a protein similar to mammalian interleukin-1β-converting enzyme. Cell 1993; 75:641–652.

17. Miura M, Zhu H, Rotello R, Hartwieg EA, Yuan J. Induction of apoptosis in fibroblasts by IL-1β-converting enzyme, a mammalian homolog of the C. elegans cell death gene ced-3. Cell 1993; 75:653–660.

18. Gagliardini V, Fernandez P-A, Lee RKK, et al. Prevention of vertebrate neuronal death by the crmA gene. Science 1994; 263:826–828.

19. Hengartner MO, Horvitz HR. C. elegans cell survival gene ced-9 encodes a functional homolog of the mammalian proto-oncogene bcl-2. Cell 1994; 76:665–676.

20. Kuida K, Lippke JA, Ku G, et al. Altered cytokine export and apoptosis in mice deficient in interleukin-1β converting enzyme. Science 1995; 267:2000–2003.

21. Tewari M, Quan LT, O'Rourke K, et al. Yama/CPP32β, a mammalian homolog of CED-3, is a CrmA-inhibitable protease that cleaves the death substrate poly(ADP-ribose) polymerase. Cell 1995; 81:801–809.

22. Wang L, Miura M, Bergeron L, Zhu H, Yuan J. Ich-1, an Ice/ced-3-related gene, encodes both positive and negative regulators of programmed cell death. Cell 1994; 78:739–750.

23. Faucheu C, Diu A, Chan AWE, et al. A novel human protease similar to the interleukin-1β converting enzyme induces apoptosis in transfected cells. EMBO J 1995; 14:1914–1922.

24. Mosley B, Urdal DL, Prickett KS, et al. The interleukin-1 receptor binds the human interleukin-1α precursor but not the interleukin-1β precursor. J Biol Chem 1987; 262:2941–2944.

25. Jobling SA, Auron PE, Gurka G, et al. Biological activity and receptor binding of human prointerleukin-1β and subpeptides. J Biol Chem 1988; 263:16372.

26. Wessendorf JHM, Garfinkel S, Zhan X, Brown S, Maciag T. Identification of a nuclear localization sequence within the structure of the human interleukin-1α precursor. J Biol Chem 1993; 268:22100–22104.

27. Maier JAM, Statuto M, Ragnotti G. Endogenous interleukin 1 alpha must be transported to the nucleus to exert its activity in human endothelial cells. Mol Cell Biol 1994; 14:1845–1851.

28. Arend WP. Interleukin-1 receptor antagonist. Adv Immunol 1993; 54:167–227.
29. Seckinger P, Lowenthal JW, Williamson K, Dayer J-M, MacDonald HR. A urine inhibitor of interleukin 1 activity that blocks ligand binding. J Immunol 1987; 139:1546–1549.
30. Seckinger P, Williamson K, Balavoine J-F, et al. A urine inhibitor of interleukin 1 activity affects both interleukin 1α and 1β but not tumor necrosis factor α. J Immunol 1987; 139:1541–1545.
31. Balavoine J-F, Galve de Rochemonteix B, Williamson K, et al. Prostaglandin E_2 and collagenase production by fibroblasts and synovial cells is regulated by urine-derived human interleukin 1 and inhibitor(s). J Clin Invest 1986; 78:1120–1124.
32. Prieur A-M, Kaufmann M-T, Griscelli C, Dayer J-M. Specific interleukin-1 inhibitor in serum and urine of children with systemic juvenile chronic arthritis. Lancet 1987; 2:1240–1242.
33. Arend WP, Joslin FG, Massoni RJ. Effects of immune complexes on production by human monocytes of interleukin 1 or an interleukin 1 inhibitor. J Immunol 1985; 134:3868–3875.
34. Eisenberg SP, Evans RJ, Arend WP, et al. Primary structure and functional expression from complementary DNA of a human interleukin-1 receptor antagonist. Nature 1990; 343:341–346.
35. Hannum CH, Wilcox CJ, Arend WP, et al. Interleukin-1 receptor antagonist activity of a human interleukin-1 inhibitor. Nature 1990; 343:336–340.
36. Dripps DJ, Verderber E, Ng RK, Thompson RC, Eisenberg SP. Interleukin-1 receptor antagonist binds to the type II interleukin-1 receptor on B cells and neutrophils. J Biol Chem 1991; 266:20311–20315.
37. Dripps DJ, Brandhuber BJ, Thompson RC, Eisenberg SP. Interleukin-1 (IL-1) receptor antagonist binds to the 80-kDa IL-1 receptor but does not initiate IL-1 signal transduction. J Biol Chem 1991; 266:10331–10336.
38. Granowitz EV, Clark BD, Mancilla J, Dinarello CA. Interleukin-1 receptor antagonist competitively inhibits the binding of interleukin-1 to the type II interleukin-1 receptor. J Biol Chem 1991; 266:14147–14150.
39. Steinkasserer A, Spurr NK, Cox S, Jeggo P, Sim RB. The human IL-1 receptor antagonist gene (IL1RN) maps to chromosome 2q14–21, in the region of the IL-1α and IL-1β loci. Genomics 1992; 13:654–657.
40. Eisenberg SP, Brewer MT, Verderber E, et al. Interleukin-1 receptor antagonist is a member of the interleukin-1 gene family: evolution of a cytokine control mechanism. Proc Natl Acad Sci USA 1991; 88:5232–5236.
41. Carter DB, Deibel MR, Dunn CJ, et al. Purification, cloning, expression and biological characterization of an interleukin-1 receptor antagonist protein. Nature 1990; 344:633–638.
42. Haskill S, Martin G, van Le L, et al. cDNA cloning of an intracellular form of the human interleukin 1 receptor antagonist associated with epithelium. Proc Natl Acad Sci USA 1991; 88:3681–3685.
43. Sims JE, March CJ, Cosman D, et al. cDNA expression cloning of the IL-1 receptor, a member of the immunoglobulin superfamily. Science 1988; 241:585–589.
44. Sims JE, Acres RB, Grubin CE, et al. Cloning the interleukin 1 receptor from human T cells. Proc Natl Acad Sci USA 1989; 86:8946–8950.
45. McMahan CJ, Slack JL, Mosley B, et al. A novel IL-1 receptor, cloned from B cells by mammalian expression, is expressed in many cell types. EMBO J 1991; 10:2821–2832.
46. Copeland NG, Silan CM, Kingsley DM, et al. Chromosomal location of murine and human IL-1 receptor genes. Genomics 1991; 9:44–50.
47. Bomsztyk K, Sims JE, Stanton TH, et al. Evidence for different interleukin 1 receptors in murine B- and T-cell lines. Proc Natl Acad Sci USA 1989; 86:8034–8038.
48. Chizzonite R, Truitt T, Kilian PL, et al. Two high-affinity interleukin 1 receptors represent separate gene products. Proc Natl Acad Sci USA 1989; 86:8029–8033.
49. Spriggs MK, Lioubin PJ, Slack J, et al. Induction of an interleukin-1 receptor (IL-1R) on monocytic cells: evidence that the receptor is not encoded by a T cell-type IL-1R mRNA. J Biol Chem 1990; 265:22499–22505.

50. McKean DJ, Podzorski RP, Bell MP, et al. Murine T helper cell-2 lymphocytes express type I and type II IL-1 receptors, but only the type I receptor mediates costimulatory activity. J Immunol 1993; 151:3500–3510.

51. Sims JE, Gayle MA, Slack JL, et al. Interleukin 1 signaling occurs exclusively via the type I receptor. Proc Natl Acad Sci USA 1993; 90:6155–6159.

52. Stylianou E, O'Neill LAJ, Rawlinson L, et al. Interleukin-1 induces NFκB through its type I but not type II receptor in lymphocytes. J Biol Chem 1992; 267:15836–15841.

53. Colotta F, Re F, Muzio M, et al. Interleukin-1 type II receptor: a decoy target for IL-1 that is regulated by IL-4. Science 1993; 261:472–475.

54. Dower SK, Fanslow W, Jacobs C, et al. Interleukin-1 antagonists. Ther Immunol 1994; 1: 113–122.

55. Greenfeder SA, Nunes P, Kwee L, et al. Molecular cloning and characterization of a second subunit of the interleukin 1 receptor complex. J Biol Chem 1995; 270:13757–13765.

56. Svenson M, Hansen MB, Heegaard P, Abell K, Bendtzen K. Specific binding of interleukin 1 (IL-1) β and IL-1 receptor antagonist (IL-1ra) to human serum. High-affinity binding of IL-1ra to soluble IL-1 receptor type I. Cytokine 1993; 5:427–435.

57. Symons JA, Eastgate JA, Duff GW. Purification and characterization of a novel soluble receptor for interleukin 1. J Exp Med 1991; 174:1251–1254.

58. Re F, Muzio M, De Rossi M, et al. The type II "receptor" as a decoy target for interleukin 1 in polymorphonuclear leukocytes: characterization of induction by dexamethasone and ligand binding properties of the released decoy receptor. J Exp Med 1994; 179:739–743.

59. Symons JA, Young PR, Duff GW. Soluble type II interleukin 1 (IL-1) receptor binds and blocks processing of IL-1β precursor and loses affinity for IL-1 receptor antagonist. Proc Natl Acad Sci USA 1995; 92:1714–1718.

60. Bochner BS, Charlesworth EN, Lichtenstein LM, et al. Interleukin-1 is released at sites of human cutaneous allergic reactions. J Allergy Clin Immunol 1990; 86:830–839.

61. Mizutani H, Schechter N, Lazarus G, Black RA, Kupper TS. Rapid and specific conversion of precursor interleukin 1β (IL-1β) to an active IL-1 species by human mast cell chymase. J Exp Med 1991; 174:821–825.

62. Sim TC, Grant JA, Hilsmeier KA, Fukuda Y, Alam R. Proinflammatory cytokines in nasal secretions of allergic subjects after antigen challenge. Am J Respir Crit Care Med 1994; 149:339–344.

63. Gosset P, Malaquin F, Delneste Y, et al. Interleukin-6 and interleukin-1α production is associated with antigen-induced late nasal response. J Allergy Clin Immunol 1993; 92:878–890.

64. Subramanian N, Bray MA. Interleukin 1 releases histamine from human basophils and mast cells in vitro. J Immunol 1987; 138:271–275.

65. Haak-Frendscho M, Dinarello C, Kaplan AP. Recombinant human interleukin-1 beta causes histamine release from human basophils. J Allergy Clin Immunol 1988; 82:218–223.

66. Massey WA, Randall TC, Kagey-Sobotka A, et al. Recombinant human IL-1α and -1β potentiate IgE-mediated histamine release from human basophils. J Immunol 1989; 143:1875–1880.

67. Bischoff SC, Brunner T, de Weck AL, Dahinden CA. Interleukin 5 modifies histamine release and leukotriene generation by human basophils in response to diverse agonists. J Exp Med 1990; 172:1577–1582.

68. Bischoff SC, Dahinden CA. c-kit ligand: a unique potentiator of mediator release by human lung mast cells. J Exp Med 1992; 175:237–244.

69. Brunner T, de Weck AL, Dahinden CA. Platelet-activating factor induces mediator release by human basophils primed with IL-3, granulocyte-macrophage colony-stimulating factor, or IL-5. J Immunol 1991; 147:237–242.

70. Rollins BJ, Yoshimura T, Leonard EJ, Pober JS. Cytokine-activated human endothelial cells synthesize and secrete a monocyte chemoattractant, MCP-1/JE. Am J Pathol 1990; 136:1229–1233.

71. Sica A, Wang JM, Colotta F, et al. Monocyte chemotactic and activating factor gene expression induced in endothelial cells by IL-1 and tumor necrosis factor. J Immunol 1990; 144:3034–3038.

72. Standiford TJ, Kunkel SL, Phan SH, Rollins BJ, Strieter RM. Alveolar macrophage-derived cytokines induce monocyte chemoattractant protein-1 expression from human pulmonary type II-like epithelial cells. J Biol Chem 1991; 266:9912–9918.

73. Alam R, Lett-Brown MA, Forsythe PA, et al. Monocyte chemotactic and activating factor is a potent histamine-releasing factor for basophils. J Clin Invest 1992; 89:723–728.

74. Bischoff SC, Krieger M, Brunner T, Dahinden CA. Monocyte chemotactic protein 1 is a potent activator of human basophils. J Exp Med 1992; 175:1271–1275.

75. Kuna P, Reddigari SR, Rucinski D, Oppenheim JJ, Kaplan AP. Monocyte chemotactic and activating factor is a potent histamine-releasing factor for human basophils. J Exp Med 1992; 175:489–493.

76. Griffin JD, Spertini O, Ernst TJ, et al. Granulocyte–macrophage colony-stimulating factor and other cytokines regulate surface expression of the leukocyte adhesion molecule-1 on human neutrophils, monocytes, and their precursors. J Immunol 1990; 145:576–584.

77. Pober JS, Gimbrone MA Jr, Lapierre LA, et al. Overlapping patterns of activation of human endothelial cells by interleukin 1, tumor necrosis factor, and immune interferon. J Immunol 1986; 137:1893–1896.

78. Bevilacqua MP, Pober JS, Mendrick DL, Cotran RS, Gimbrone MA Jr. Identification of an inducible endothelial–leukocyte adhesion molecule. Proc Natl Acad Sci USA 1987; 84:9238–9242.

79. Bochner BS, Luscinskas FW, Gimbrone MA Jr, et al. Adhesion of human basophils, eosino-phils, and neutrophils to interleukin-1-activated human vascular endothelial cells: contributions of endothelial cell adhesion molecules. J Exp Med 1991; 173:1553–1556.

80. Leung DYM, Pober JS, Cotran RS. Expression of endothelial–leukocyte adhesion molecule-1 in elicited late phase allergic reactions. J Clin Invest 1991; 87:1805–1809.

81. Wellicome SM, Thornhill MH, Pitzalis C, et al. A monoclonal antibody that detects a novel antigen on endothelial cells that is induced by tumor necrosis factor, IL-1, or lipopolysaccharide. J Immunol 1990; 144:2558–2565.

82. Diamond MS, Staunton DE, de Fougerolles AR, et al. ICAM-1 (CD54): a counter-receptor for Mac-1 (CD11b/CD18). J Cell Biol 1990; 111:3129–3139.

83. Marlin SD, Springer TA. Purified intercellular adhesion molecule-1 (ICAM-1) is a ligand for lymphocyte function-associated antigen 1 (LFA-1). Cell 1987; 51:813–819.

84. Elices MJ, Osborn L, Takada Y, et al. VCAM-1 on activated endothelium interacts with the leukocyte integrin VLA-4 at a site distinct from the VLA-4/fibronectin binding site. Cell 1990; 60:577–584.

85. Bussolino F, Breviario F, Tetta C, et al. Interleukin 1 stimulates platelet-activating factor production in cultured human endothelial cells. J Clin Invest 1986; 77:2027–2033.

86. Valone FH, Epstein LB. Biphasic platelet-activating factor synthesis by human monocytes stimulated with IL-1β, tumor necrosis factor, or IFN-γ. J Immunol 1988; 141:3945–3950.

87. Warren JS. Relationship between interleukin-1 beta and platelet-activating factor in the pathogenesis of acute immune complex alveolitis in the rat. Am J Pathol 1992; 141:551–560.

88. Standiford TJ, Kunkel SL, Basha MA, et al. Interleukin-8 gene expression by a pulmonary epithelial cell line. A model for cytokine networks in the lung. J Clin Invest 1990; 86:1945–1953.

89. Nakamura H, Yoshimura K, Jaffe HA, Crystal RG. Interleukin-8 gene expression in human bronchial epithelial cells. J Biol Chem 1991; 266:19611–19617.

90. Strieter RM, Chensue SW, Basha MA, et al. Human alveolar macrophage gene expression of interleukin-8 by tumor necrosis factor-α, lipopolysaccharide, and interleukin-1β. Am J Respir Cell Mol Biol 1990; 2:321–326.

91. Sanz M-J, Weg VB, Bolanowski MA, Nourshargh S. IL-1 is a potent inducer of eosinophil

accumulation in rat skin. Inhibition of response by a platelet-activating factor antagonist and an anti-human IL-8 antibody. J Immunol 1995; 154:1364–1373.

92. Warringa RAJ, Koenderman L, Kok PTM, Kreukniet J, Bruijnzeel PLB. Modulation and induction of eosinophil chemotaxis by granulocyte–macrophage colony-stimulating factor and interleukin-3. Blood 1991; 77:2694–2700.

93. Sehmi R, Wardlaw AJ, Cromwell O, et al. Interleukin-5 selectively enhances the chemotactic response of eosinophils obtained from normal but not eosinophilic subjects. Blood 1992; 79: 2952–2959.

94. Warringa RAJ, Mengelers HJJ, Kuijper PHM, et al. In vivo priming of platelet-activating factor-induced eosinophil chemotaxis in allergic asthmatic individuals. Blood 1992; 79:1836–1841.

95. Watanabe Y, Kitamura T, Hayashida K, Miyajima A. Monoclonal antibody against the common β subunit (βc) of the human interleukin-3 (IL-3), IL-5, and granulocyte–macrophage colony-stimulating factor receptors shows upregulation of βc by IL-1 and tumor necrosis factor-α. Blood 1992; 80:2215–2220.

96. Liu MC, Hubbard WC, Proud D, et al. Immediate and late inflammatory responses to ragweed antigen challenge of the peripheral airways in allergic asthmatics. Cellular, mediator, and permeability changes. Am Rev Respir Dis 1991; 144:51–58.

97. Lopez AF, Eglinton JM, Gillis D, et al. Reciprocal inhibition of binding between interleukin 3 and granulocyte–macrophage colony-stimulating factor to human eosinophils. Proc Natl Acad Sci USA 1989; 86:7022–7026.

98. Lopez AF, Vadas MA, Woodcock JM, et al. Interleukin-5, interleukin-3, and granulocyte–macrophage colony-stimulating factor cross-compete for binding to cell surface receptors on human eosinophils. J Biol Chem 1991; 266:24741–24747.

99. Owen WF Jr, Rothenberg ME, Silberstein DS, et al. Regulation of human eosinophil viability, density, and function by granulocyte/macrophage colony-stimulating factor in the presence of 3T3 fibroblasts. J Exp Med 1987; 166:129–141.

100. Rothenberg ME, Owen WF, Silberstein DS, et al. Human eosinophils have prolonged survival, enhanced functional properties, and become hypodense when exposed to human interleukin 3. J Clin Invest 1988; 81:1986–1992.

101. Rothenberg ME, Petersen J, Stevens RL, et al. IL-5-dependent conversion of normodense human eosinophils to the hypodense phenotype uses 3T3 fibroblasts for enhanced viability, accelerated hypodensity, and sustained antibody-dependent cytotoxicity. J Immunol 1989; 143: 2311–2316.

102. Marini M, Soloperto M, Mezzetti M, Fasoli A, Mattoli S. Interleukin-1 binds to specific receptors on human bronchial epithelial cells and upregulates granulocyte/macrophage colony-stimulating factor synthesis and release. Am J Respir Cell Mol Biol 1991; 4:519–524.

103. Cox G, Ohtoshi T, Vancheri C, et al. Promotion of eosinophil survival by human bronchial epithelial cells and its modulation by steroids. Am J Respir Cell Mol Biol 1991; 4:525–531.

104. Takafuji S, Bischoff SC, de Weck AL, Dahinden CA. IL-3 and IL-5 prime normal human eosinophils to produce leukotriene C_4 in response to soluble agonists. J Immunol 1991; 147: 3855–3861.

105. Gundel RH, Letts LG, Gleich GJ. Human eosinophil major basic protein induces airway constriction and airway hyperresponsiveness in primates. J Clin Invest 1991; 87:1470–1473.

106. Smith D, Watson ML, Bourne AD, Thompson RC, Westwick J. An interleukin-1 receptor antagonist inhibits antigen-induced eosinophil accumulation and bronchial hyperreactivity in guinea-pigs. Br J Pharmacol 1992; 105:128P.

107. Mosmann TR, Schumacher JH, Street NF, et al. Diversity of cytokine synthesis and function of mouse CD4+ T cells. Immunol Rev 1991; 123:209–229.

108. Romagnani S. Induction of Th_1 and Th_2 responses: a key role for the "natural" immune response? Immunol Today 1992; 13:379–381.

109. Kay AB, Ying S, Varney V, et al. Messenger RNA expression of the cytokine gene cluster, inter-

leukin 3 (IL-3), IL-4, IL-5, and granulocyte/macrophage colony-stimulating factor, in allergen-induced late-phase cutaneous reactions in atopic subjects. J Exp Med 1991; 173:775–778.

110. Robinson DS, Hamid Q, Ying S, et al. Predominant Th$_2$-like bronchoalveolar T-lymphocyte population in atopic asthma. N Engl J Med 1992; 326:298–304.
111. Manetti R, Barak V, Piccinni M-P, et al. Interleukin-1 favours the in vitro development of type 2 T helper (Th$_2$) human T-cell clones. Res Immunol 1994; 145:93–100.
112. Taylor-Robinson AW, Phillips RS. Expression of the IL-1 receptor discriminates Th$_2$ from Th$_1$ cloned CD4$^+$ T cells specific for *Plasmodium chabaudi*. Immunology 1994; 81:216–221.
113. Burd PR, Rogers HW, Gordon JR, et al. Interleukin 3-dependent and -independent mast cells stimulated with IgE and antigen express multiple cytokines. J Exp Med 1989; 170:245–257.
114. Melewicz FM, Zeiger RS, Mellon MH, O'Connor RD, Spiegelberg HL. Increased peripheral blood monocytes with Fc receptors for IgE in patients with severe allergic disorders. J Immunol 1981; 126:1592–1595.
115. Melewicz FM, Kline LE, Cohen AB, Spiegelberg HL. Characterization of Fc receptors for IgE on human alveolar macrophages. Clin Exp Immunol 1982; 49:364–370.
116. Borish L, Mascali JJ, Rosenwasser LJ. IgE-dependent cytokine production by human peripheral blood mononuclear phagocytes. J Immunol 1991; 146:63–67.
117. Pujol J-L, Cosso B, Daurès J-P, et al. Interleukin-1 release by alveolar macrophages in asthmatic patients and healthy subjects. Int Arch Allergy Appl Immunol 1990; 91:207–210.
118. Gosset P, Lassalle P, Tonnel AB, et al. Production of an interleukin-1 inhibitory factor by human alveolar macrophages from normals and allergic asthmatic patients. Am Rev Respir Dis 1988; 138:40–46.
119. Wewers MD, Herzyk DJ. Alveolar macrophages differ from blood monocytes in human IL-1β release. Quantitation by enzyme-linked immunoassay. J Immunol 1989; 143:1635–1641.
120. Herzyk DJ, Allen JN, Marsh CB, Wewers MD. Macrophage and monocyte IL-1β regulation differs at multiple sites. Messenger RNA expression, translation, and post-translational processing. J Immunol 1992; 149:3052–3058.
121. Galve de Rochemonteix B, Nicod LP, Junod AF, Dayer J-M. Characterization of a specific 20- to 25-kD interleukin-1 inhibitor from cultured human lung macrophages. Am J Respir Cell Mol Biol 1990; 3:355–361.
122. Weller PF, Rand TH, Barrett T, et al. Accessory cell function of human eosinophils. HLA-DR-dependent, MHC-restricted antigen-presentation and IL-1α expression. J Immunol 1993; 150:2554–2562.
123. Warner SJC, Auger KR, Libby P. Interleukin 1 induces interleukin 1. II. Recombinant human interleukin 1 induces interleukin 1 production by adult human vascular endothelial cells. J Immunol 1987; 139:1911–1917.
124. Dohlsten M, Kalland T, Sjögren HO, Carlsson R. Histamine inhibits interleukin-1 production by lipopolysaccharide-stimulated human peripheral blood monocytes. Scand J Immunol 1988; 27:527–532.
125. Vannier E, Dinarello CA. Histamine enhances interleukin (IL)-1-induced IL-1 gene expression and protein synthesis via H$_2$ receptors in peripheral blood mononuclear cells: comparison with IL-1 receptor antagonist. J Clin Invest 1993; 92:281–287.
126. Vannier E, Dinarello CA. Histamine enhances interleukin-1-induced interleukin-8 synthesis in peripheral blood mononuclear cells via H$_2$ receptors. Cytokine 1994; 6:551.
126a. Vannier E, Dinarello CA. Unpublished observations.
126b. Vannier E, de Waal Malefyt R, Salazar-Montes A, de Vries JE, Dinarello CA. Interleukin (IL)-13 induces IL-1 receptor antagonist gene expression and protein synthesis in peripheral blood mononuclear cells: inhibition by an IL-4 mutant protein. Blood 1996; in press.
127. del Prete G, de Carli M, Almerigogna F, et al. Human IL-10 is produced by both type 1 helper (Th$_1$) and type 2 helper (Th$_2$) T cell clones and inhibits their antigen-specific proliferation and cytokine production. J Immunol 1993; 150:353–360.

128. de Vries JE. Novel fundamental approaches to intervening in IgE-mediated allergic diseases. J Invest Dermatol 1994; 102:141–144.

129. Vannier E, Miller LC, Dinarello CA. Coordinated antiinflammatory effects of interleukin 4: interleukin 4 suppresses interleukin 1 production but up-regulates gene expression and synthesis of interleukin 1 receptor antagonist. Proc Natl Acad Sci USA 1992; 89:4076–4080.

130. Fenton MJ, Buras JA, Donnelly RP. IL-4 reciprocally regulates IL-1 and IL-1 receptor antagonist expression in human monocytes. J Immunol 1992; 149:1283–1288.

131. Orino E, Sone S, Nii A, Ogura T. IL-4 up-regulates IL-1 receptor antagonist gene expression and its production in human blood monocytes. J Immunol 1992; 149:925–931.

132. Wong HL, Costa GL, Lotze MT, Wahl SM. Interleukin (IL) 4 differentially regulates monocyte IL-1 family gene expression and synthesis in vitro and in vivo. J Exp Med 1993; 177:775–781.

133. Koch K-C, Ye K, Clark BD, Dinarello CA. Interleukin 4 (IL) 4 up-regulates gene and surface IL1 receptor type I in murine T helper type 2 cells. Eur J Immunol 1992; 22:153–157.

134. Poutsiaka DD, Clark BD, Vannier E, Dinarello CA. Production of interleukin-1 receptor antagonist and interleukin-1β by peripheral blood mononuclear cells is differentially regulated. Blood 1991; 78:1275–1281.

135. Janson RW, King JTE, Hance KR, Arend WP. Enhanced production of IL-1 receptor antagonist by alveolar macrophages from patients with interstitial lung disease. Am Rev Respir Dis 1993; 148:495–503.

136. Tavernier J, Devos R, Cornelis S, et al. A human high affinity interleukin-5 receptor (IL5R) is composed of an IL5-specific α chain and a β chain shared with the receptor for GM-CSF. Cell 1991; 66:1175–1184.

137. de Waal Malefyt R, Abrams J, Bennett B, Figdor CG, de Vries JE. Interleukin 10 (IL-10) inhibits cytokine synthesis by human monocytes: an autoregulatory role of IL-10 produced by monocytes. J Exp Med 1991; 174:1209–1220.

138. de Waal Malefyt R, Figdor CG, Huijbens R, et al. Effects of IL-13 on phenotype, cytokine production, and cytotoxic function of human monocytes. Comparison with IL-4 and modulation by IFN-γ or IL-10. J Immunol 1993; 151:6370–6381.

139. Jenkins JK, Malyak M, Arend WP. The effects of interleukin-10 on interleukin-1 receptor antagonist and interleukin-1β production in human monocytes and neutrophils. Lymphokine Cytokine Res 1994; 13:47–54.

140. Arend WP, Smith MF, Janson RW, Joslin FG. IL-1 receptor antagonist and IL-1β production in human monocytes are regulated differently. J Immunol 1991; 147:1530–1536.

141. Wells J, Giri J, Cousart S, McCall CE. Expression of the IL-1 type 2 receptor gene in normal and sepsis human neutrophils. Clin Res 1994; 42:153A.

142. Muzio M, Re F, Sironi M, et al. Interleukin-13 induces the production of interleukin-1 receptor antagonist (IL-1ra) and the expression of the mRNA for the intracellular (keratinocyte) form of IL-1ra in human myelomonocytic cells. Blood 1994; 83:1738–1743.

143. Colotta F, Re F, Muzio M, et al. Interleukin-13 induces expression and release of interleukin-1 decoy receptor in human polymorphonuclear cells. J Biol Chem 1994; 269:12403–12406.

144. Zurawski SM, Vega F Jr, Huyghe B, Zurawski G. Receptors for interleukin-13 and interleukin-4 are complex and share a novel component that functions in signal transduction. EMBO J 1993; 12:2663–2670.

145. Renard N, Duvert V, Banchereau J, Saeland S. Interleukin-13 inhibits the proliferation of normal and leukemic human B-cell precursors. Blood 1994; 84:2253–2260.

146. Mullarkey MF, Leiferman KM, Peters MS, et al. Human cutaneous allergic late-phase response is inhibited by soluble IL-1 receptor. J Immunol 1994; 152:2033–2041.

147. Dinarello CA. Interleukin-1 and interleukin-1 antagonism. Blood 1991; 77:1627–1652.

148. Young JD-E, Liu C-C, Butler G, Cohn ZA, Galli SJ. Identification, purification, and characterization of a mast cell-associated cytolytic factor related to tumor necrosis factor. Proc Natl Acad Sci USA 1987; 84:9175–9179.

149. Gordon JR, Galli SJ. Mast cells as a source of both preformed and immunologically inducible TNF-α/cachectin. Nature 1990; 346:274–276.

150. Gordon JR, Galli SJ. Release of both preformed and newly synthesized tumor necrosis factor α (TNF-α)/cachectin by mouse mast cells stimulated via the FcεRI. A mechanism for the sustained action of mast cell-derived TNF-α during IgE-dependent biological responses. J Exp Med 1991; 174:103–107.

151. Wershil BK, Wang Z-S, Gordon JR, Galli SJ. Recruitment of neutrophils during IgE-dependent cutaneous late phase reactions in the mouse is mast cell-dependent. Partial inhibition of the reaction with antiserum against tumor necrosis factor-alpha. J Clin Invest 1991; 87:446–453.

152. Gordon JR, Post T, Schulman ES, Galli SJ. Characterization of mouse mast cell TNF-α induction in vitro and in vivo, and demonstration that purified human lung mast cells contain TNF-α. FASEB J 1991; 5:A1009.

153. Walsh LJ, Trinchieri G, Waldorf HA, Whitaker D, Murphy GF. Human dermal mast cells contain and release tumor necrosis factor α, which induces endothelial leukocyte adhesion molecule 1. Proc Natl Acad Sci USA 1991; 88:4220–4224.

154. Klein LM, Lavker RM, Matis WL, Murphy GF. Degranulation of human mast cells induces an endothelial antigen central to leukocyte adhesion. Proc Natl Acad Sci USA 1989; 86:8972–8976.

155. Steffen M, Abboud M, Potter GK, Yung YP, Moore MAS. Presence of tumor necrosis factor or a related factor in human basophil/mast cells. Immunology 1989; 66:445–450.

156. Rich EA, Panuska JR, Wallis RS, et al. Dyscoordinate expression of tumor necrosis factor-alpha by human blood monocytes and alveolar macrophages. Am Rev Respir Dis 1989; 139:1010–1016.

157. Martinet Y, Yamauchi K, Crystal RG. Differential expression of the tumor necrosis factor/cachectin gene by blood and lung mononuclear phagocytes. Am Rev Respir Dis 1988; 138:659–665.

158. Gosset P, Tsicopoulos A, Wallaert B, et al. Tumor necrosis factor alpha and interleukin-6 production by human mononuclear phagocytes from allergic asthmatics after IgE-dependent stimulation. Am Rev Respir Dis 1992; 146:768–774.

159. Gosset P, Tsicopoulos A, Wallaert B, et al. Increased secretion of tumor necrosis factor α and interleukin-6 by alveolar macrophages consecutive to the development of the late asthmatic reaction. J Allergy Clin Immunol 1991; 88:561–571.

160. Lassalle P, Gosset P, Delneste Y, et al. Modulation of adhesion molecule expression on endothelial cells during the late asthmatic reaction: role of macrophage-derived tumour necrosis factor-alpha. Clin Exp Immunol 1993; 94:105–110.

161. Costa JJ, Matossian K, Resnick MB, et al. Human eosinophils can express the cytokines tumor necrosis factor-α and macrophage inflammatory protein-1α. J Clin Invest 1993; 91:2673–2684.

162. Finotto S, Ohno I, Marshall JS, et al. TNF-α production by eosinophils in upper airways inflammation (nasal polyposis). J Immunol 1994; 153:2278–2289.

163. Vannier E, Miller LC, Dinarello CA. Histamine suppresses gene expression and synthesis of tumor necrosis factor α via histamine H_2 receptors. J Exp Med 1991; 174:281–284.

164. Vannier E, Dinarello CA. Histamine enhances interleukin (IL)-1-induced IL-6 gene expression and protein synthesis via H_2 receptors in peripheral blood mononuclear cells. J Biol Chem 1994; 269:9952–9956.

165. Hart PH, Vitti GF, Burgess DR, et al. Potential antiinflammatory effects of interleukin 4: suppression of human monocyte tumor necrosis factor α, interleukin 1, and prostaglandin E_2. Proc Natl Acad Sci USA 1989; 86:3803–3807.

166. Minty A, Chalon P, Derocq J-M, et al. Interleukin-13 is a new human lymphokine regulating inflammatory and immune responses. Nature 1993; 362:248–250.

167. Bevilacqua MP, Stengelin S, Gimbrone MA, Seed B. Endothelial leukocyte adhesion molecule 1: an inducible receptor for neutrophils related to complement regulatory proteins and lectins. Science 1989; 243:1160–1165.

168. Osborn L, Hession C, Tizard R, et al. Direct expression cloning of vascular cell adhesion molecule 1, a cytokine-induced endothelial protein that binds to lymphocytes. Cell 1989; 59:1203–1211.

169. Kyan-Aung U, Haskard DO, Poston RN, Thornhill MH, Lee TH. Endothelial leukocyte adhesion molecule-1 and intercellular adhesion molecule-1 mediate the adhesion of eosinophils to endothelial cells in vitro and are expressed by endothelium in allergic cutaneous inflammation in vivo. J Immunol 1991; 146:521–528.

170. Weller PF, Rand TH, Goelz SE, Chi-Rosso G, Lobb RR. Human eosinophil adherence to vascular endothelium mediated by binding to vascular cell adhesion molecule 1 and endothelial leukocyte adhesion molecule 1. Proc Natl Acad Sci USA 1991; 88:7430–7433.

171. Bussolino F, Camussi G, Baglioni C. Synthesis and release of platelet-activating factor by human vascular endothelial cells treated with tumor necrosis factor or interleukin 1α. J Biol Chem 1988; 263:11856–11861.

172. Camussi G, Bussolino F, Salvidio G, Baglioni C. Tumor necrosis factor/cachectin stimulates peritoneal macrophages, polymorphonuclear neutrophils, and vascular endothelial cells to synthesize and release platelet-activating factor. J Exp Med 1987; 166:1390–1404.

173. Strieter RM, Kunkel SL, Showell HJ, et al. Endothelial cell gene expression of a neutrophil chemotactic factor by TNF-α, LPS, and IL-1β. Science 1989; 243:1467–1469.

174. Takafuji S, Bischoff SC, de Weck AL, Dahinden CA. Opposing effects of tumor necrosis factor-α and nerve growth factor upon leukotriene C_4 production by human eosinophils triggered with N-formyl-methionyl-leucyl-phenylalanine. Eur J Immunol 1992; 22:969–974.

14

Neuropeptides and Their Receptors in Allergic Airway Diseases

David A. Ingram, Sunil P. Sreedharan, Edward J. Goetzl, and Jeffrey L. Kishiyama
University of California, San Francisco, California

INTRODUCTION

Upper and lower respiratory airway structures, including smooth muscle, vasculature, and subepithelial glands, are densely innervated by an array of sensory, motor, and autonomic nerves, dedicated to regulation of airway tone, blood flow, and mucous secretion. Potent neuromediators, such as vasoactive intestinal peptide (VIP), peptide histidine methionine (PHM), calcitonin gene-related peptide (CGRP), somatostatin (SOM), neurokinin A (NKA), and substance P (SP), are detectable in tissues and fluids of airways affected by hypersensitivity diseases. Although the precise physiological roles of these neuropeptides have not been fully defined, their localization and functional effects have implied involvement in bidirectional interactions between the immune and neuroendocrine systems. The distinctive patterns of neuromediator release in allergic reactions and their ability to evoke tissue responses resembling immediate hypersensitivity reactions and acute inflammation suggest that neuropeptides contribute to the pathogenesis of human allergic airways disease.

INNERVATION OF THE RESPIRATORY TRACT

The respiratory tract contains autonomic pathways of the sympathetic (adrenergic) and parasympathetic (cholinergic) nervous system. A functionally distinct third system, which utilizes predominantly peptide neuromediators to modulate airway function, is termed the nonadrenergic, noncholinergic (NANC) pathway. The NANC components have been defined through responses to electrical field stimulation after pharmacological blockade of cholinergic and adrenergic pathways. Although both α- and β-adrenoceptors have been identified in bronchial tissue, there is little or no direct representation of sympathetic pathways in the airways. The NANC pathways, on the other hand, appear to be the major neural bronchodilating system in human airways (1). The NANC pathways may be inhibitory (bronchodilator) or excitatory (bronchoconstrictor) influences and exert their effects through released neuropeptides. Evidence suggests that probable mediators of inhibitory (bronchodilatory) NANC neurons include VIP and PHM. Likely mediators of excitatory (bronchoconstricting) NANC neurons include the tachykinins SP, NKA, NKB, and CGRP (2,3). The vasoactive and bronchoactive effects of VIP and SP, which are mediated by distinct cellular receptors, occur independently of cholinergic and adrenergic receptor activation.

Although neuropeptides such as VIP and SP (4,5) may be the primary neurotransmitters released by NANC neurons, they may also function as cotransmitters with classic neuromediators in other autonomic pathways. For instance, VIP is cosynthesized, colocalized, and coreleased with PHI–PHM. Vasoactive intestinal peptide may also be a cotransmitter in some neurons with the classic neurotransmitter acetylcholine, and be released in response to cholinergic stimuli. This mediator has also been demonstrated in the vagus nerve (6).

PRINCIPLES OF THE AXON REFLEX

Afferent fibers from the vagus nerve sense airway irritation (7). Protective reflexes trigger coughing and sneezing after inhalation of noxious chemicals or irritating particles (8). Local defense reactions, such as bronchoconstriction, vasodilation, and increased vascular permeability, can be initiated after stimulation of capsaicin-responsive sensory neurons (9–11). These sensory c-fibers transmit afferent signals from airway mucosa. Through antidromic mechanisms or "axon reflex," multiple neuropeptides are released from peripheral nerve terminals after sensory nerve stimulation.

The release of sensory neuropeptides has been described after electrical or physiological nerve stimulation (12). Initial airway stimuli may be physical or chemical irritation. Cigarette smoke, fumes, and particulate matter are common inhalant triggers of axon reflex. Airborne allergens, on the other hand, indirectly induce liberation of neuromediators through the effects of released histamine, serotonin, bradykinin, and prostaglandins (13,14).

The development of molecular probes and antibodies, useful for the detection of genetic messages (mRNA) and protein gene products, have become powerful tools for detection and localization of neuropeptides and their respective receptors. Takeda and colleagues used indirect immunofluorescent histochemistry and in situ hybridization with oligonucleotide probes for preprotachykinins to demonstrate the participation of SP and CGRP in guinea pig models of toluene diisocyanate (TDI)-induced allergic rhinitis (15). Substance P is an 11-amino acid neuropeptide belonging to the tachykinin family, along with NKA and NKB. All three of these tachykinins are generated from a single gene RNA transcript, preprotachykinin A mRNA, through alternative RNA splicing. Substance P elicits local tissue responses of inflammation, including protein extravasation, vasodilation, and glandular secretion. In Takeda's model of TDI-induced allergic rhinitis, repeated application of TDI to nasal mucosa causes increased expression of preprotachykinin mRNA in trigeminal ganglion neurons and increased immunoreactivity in nasal mucosa sensory nerve terminals. These findings are consistent with allergic disease-related increases in dorsal root ganglia synthesis, axonal transport, and antidromic release of tachykinins in nasal tissues (15).

Capsaicin, a neurotoxic agent extracted from red pepper, releases SP and CGRP from unmyelinated sensory nerve endings. Neurokinin A and possibly gastrin-releasing peptide (GRP) may also be localized within the same nociceptive neurons that innervate blood vessels, gland acini, and epithelium (16,17). Treatment with systemic and locally applied capsaicin has been used to deplete neuropeptides and inhibit hypersensitivity reactions such as TDI-induced nasal allergy reactions (18,19). Depletion of SP and other tachykinins by capsaicin has also been used to reduce the vasodilation and microvascular permeability induced by airway irritants, such as cigarette smoke (20). The physiological effects seen in animal models and the effects of capsaicin on allergen- and irritant-induced nasal reactions emphasize the neural contribution to nasal reactivity.

LOCALIZATION OF NEUROPEPTIDES AND RECEPTORS

Expression of peptide receptors, typical of the neuroendocrine system, has been demonstrated on immune and inflammatory cells, respiratory and gastrointestinal epithelium, and neural tissues. The G-protein–associated receptors for SP, NKA, NKB, and VIP have recently been cloned from immune cells.

Vasoactive Intestinal Peptide

Vasoactive intestinal peptide exerts potent, long-lasting bronchodilator activity on airway smooth muscle and vasodilator activity in nasal and bronchial vessels (Table 1). In vitro, the effects of VIP-induced bronchodilation are 50-fold greater than the effects of isoproterenol (3). Immunohistochemical staining demonstrates high concentrations of VIP-immunoreactive nerves in the upper and lower respiratory tract, around airways, mucous glands,

Table 1 Humoral Activities of Neuropeptides Implicated in Allergic Diseases

Neuropeptide	Activity
Substance P (SP)	Vasodilation
	Increased vascular permeability
	Secretion
	Bronchoconstriction, less potent than NKA
Neurokinin A (NKA)	Bronchoconstriction
	Vasodilation, less potent than SP
Vasoactive intestinal peptide (VIP)	Vasodilation
	Bronchodilation
	Secretion
Peptide histidine methionine (PHM)	Bronchodilation
	Secretion
	Vasodilation, less potent than VIP
Calcitonin gene-related peptide (CGRP)	Vasodilation
	Augments effects of SP
Gastrin-related peptide (GRP)	Bronchoconstriction
	Secretion

Source: Ref. 7.

and pulmonary vasculature. Immunoreactive staining of VIP and autoradiographic mapping of VIP-binding units demonstrate a high density of VIP-containing neurons and VIP receptors near the smooth-muscle layer of the trachea and main bronchi, but diminishing levels in the small airways (21).

The functional effects of VIP are mediated by specific, high-affinity receptors on target cells. The time-dependent, reversible, and saturable nature of the binding interaction suggests the presence of specific receptors for VIP. The VIP receptor possesses a seven-transmembrane segment structure functionally coupled to adenylate cyclase through regulatory G-proteins. The receptors on different cell types may vary in ligand affinity, size, and number of binding sites per cell. Initially described as a gut hormone, genetic message for high-affinity VIP receptors are found on a vast array of cell types, predominantly lung tissue, gastrointestinal epithelial cells, and subsets of lymphocytes, with weaker expression in brain, heart, kidney, liver, and placenta. Many lymphocytic cell lines including Molt 4b and other T lymphoblasts, Nalm 6 pre-B cells, and DAKIKI IgA-secreting B cells also express VIP receptors (22–26). The low-affinity VIP receptor, isolated from a line of pre-B lymphocytes demonstrates the highest degree of structural homology to receptors for peptide mediators of inflammation.

The bronchodilation and vasodilation induced by VIP are consistent with the physiological changes produced by electric field stimulation of inhibitory NANC neurons. Although most characterizations of NANC innervation have been done in animals, reflex neural bronchodilation of human airways from the trachea to the small airways appears to be mediated exclusively by NANC inhibitory nerves (27,28).

Tachykinins

Tachykinins cause vascular permeability and bronchoconstriction through specific membrane neuropeptide receptors. The diversity of tachykinin activities can be partly attributed to different classes of neurokinin receptors, with different tissue specificities and preferential binding affinities for variant forms of SP, NKA, and NKB (29–31). There are three distinct tachykinin receptor subtypes, NK_1, NK_2, and NK_3. Substance P binds with greatest affinity to the NK_1-type receptor, which is localized preferentially in the vasculature, although receptors are present in central and peripheral neurons, smooth muscle, endothelial cells, fibroblasts, and both T and B lymphocytes (32). The increased secretion of interferon (IFN)-γ by SP-treated, antigen-stimulated splenic and granuloma T cells is mediated by the NK_1-type tachykinin receptors (33).

As NKA, NKB, and SP represent different products from the same gene, significant homology exists, and each tachykinin demonstrates some binding to each of the tachykinin receptor subtypes. The rank order of tachykinin-binding affinities for the NK_1 receptor is SP > NKA > NKB. In comparison, the rank order of binding affinity for NK_2 receptors is NKA > NKB > SP. Although some binding cross-reactivity exists, the relative specificity of the receptor–ligand interaction can be demonstrated using specific receptor antagonists. The NK_1 receptor antagonists block the cellular effects of SP, whereas specific NK_2 receptor antagonists provide no inhibitory effects (33).

The clinical effects of these neuropeptides may be determined by the distribution of their high-affinity receptors. The NK_2-type receptors are found in very high concentrations in airway smooth muscle, compared with NK_1-type tachykinin receptors. Not surprisingly, infusion of NKA causes bronchoconstriction in asthmatic subjects, whereas infused SP causes primarily cardiovascular effects (34,35).

Calcitonin Gene-Related Peptide

The CGRP is a 37-amino acid peptide that contributes to nasal and bronchial congestion by increasing local blood flow, with potent and long-lasting direct airways effects and augmentation of mucosal edema through histamine and lipid mediators (20,36,37). CGRP may be stored together with SP in sensory nerve terminals, and CGRP receptors have been localized to bronchial vessels in airway mucosa.

IMMUNOMODULATION BY NEUROPEPTIDES

Immune organs, including the thymus, peripheral lymph nodes, Peyer's patches, and spleen, are extensively innervated with nerve terminals on or very near populations of lymphocytes, macrophages, and mast cells, allowing delivery of high concentrations of neuromediators in specific areas (38–40). Detection of immunoreactive nerve endings and shared neuromediator receptors on immune effector cells has led to the demonstration of neuropeptide modulation of immune systems. Ablational lesions in the central nervous system affects the number and function of lymphocytes and natural killer (NK) cells in the spleen, thymus, and systemic circulation (41).

The anatomical localization and elucidation of immunological modulatory effects of SP, SOM, and VIP have provided some insight into the normal immune role of neuromediators (Table 2). Neural influence on lymphoid distribution and thymic processing is evident during embryonic development (42). The VIP-immunoreactive nerve endings are concentrated in the internodular regions of the Peyer's patches and mesenteric lymph nodes and influence regional distribution and recycling of murine T cells, with greater effects on $CD4^+$ than $CD8^+$ subsets. To study the effects of VIP on lymphocyte trafficking, Ottaway and Greenberg down-regulated VIP receptor expression in cells obtained from rat Peyer's patches by incubation with VIP in vitro. The reinjected T lymphocytes demonstrated suppressed homing and reduced return to the gut-associated lymphoid tissues (43).

Table 2 Immunoregulatory and Immunopathogenetic Effects of Neuropeptides

Neuropeptide	Effects
SP	Increases production of IgA
	Enhances T-cell proliferation
	Elicits production of IL-1, IL-2, TNF-α, IL-6, IFN-γ
	Increases expression of IL-2 receptor
VIP	Decreases production of IgG and IgM
	Increases production of IgE
	Suppresses T-cell proliferation
	Inhibits synthesis of IL-2 and IL-4
	Increases IL-5 production
	Influences lymphocyte homing and distribution
SOM	Decreases production of IgM and IgA
	Suppresses T-cell proliferation
	Inhibits IgE-dependent mast cell/basophil mediator release

Source: Ref. 40.

Neuromediators may also affect development, functional priming of lymphocyte subsets, and other immunological responses.

Neuropeptides affect numerous immunological parameters, including lymphocyte proliferation, immunoglobulin production, leukocyte phagocytic function, and leukocyte chemotaxis. Specific, high-affinity neuropeptide receptors have been demonstrated on many immune effector cells. Significantly higher percentages of splenic lymphocytes express SP receptors compared with blood lymphocytes, quantified by flow cytometric analysis. Means of 53 and 34% of the T cells, and 65 and 47% of the B cells in Peyer's patches and spleen, respectively, bound SP. It has not been determined, whether SP-binding lymphocytes are attracted to and accumulate in these tissues, or whether they develop the receptors after tissue localization (44). In contrast, fewer than 20% of peripheral blood lymphocytes expressed receptors for SP (45). Payan and colleagues demonstrated specific binding of fluorescein-labeled SP to approximately 3–5% of normal peripheral blood T lymphocytes (46). Other members of the tachykinin family, NKA and NKB, have specific receptors of their own. At high concentrations, however, binding and stimulation of SP receptors can occur (47).

The studies of leukocyte immunomodulation have complemented the biochemical characterization of neuropeptide ligand–receptor binding and signal transduction. Vasoactive intestinal peptide significantly inhibits murine and human lymphocyte proliferation responses to mitogen (48,49). The proliferative responses of concanavalin A (Con-A)-stimulated lymphocytes can be inhibited by VIP, possibly through suppression of interleukin (IL)-2 production (50). The effects of VIP on immunoglobulin synthesis are tissue-specific, resulting in increased IgA synthesis by 30% in splenic lymphocytes, but decreased IgA synthesis by 70%, in Peyer's patch lymphocytes (51). The differential effects of VIP in different tissue compartments reflects the local nature of neuropeptide immunoregulation. The pattern of exposure to VIP may determine the effects of immunoglobulin production. Human blood mononuclear cells incubated with twice-daily additions of physiological concentrations of VIP demonstrated markedly suppressed IgG and IgM production by pokeweed mitogen (PWM), up to 90%. Secretion of IgE, induced by IL-4, was increased in the same system by three- to tenfold (52).

Somatostatin was initially described as a hypothalamic hormone, mediating the release of growth hormone in the central nervous system; however, SOM is also distributed widely in nonneural tissues and the peripheral nervous system (53). It is found in distinct dorsal root ganglia cells and transported to peripheral nerve terminals. The effects of SOM are mediated by stereospecific receptors and include suppression of lymphocyte proliferation and synthetic responses of splenic and Peyer's patches' lymphocytes, including IgA and IgM production (54). The separate role of SOM as a regulatory mediator is suggested by its late appearance after nasal challenge and its ability to inhibit IgE-mediated release of histamine, LTD_4, and LTE_4 from human basophils and some types of mast cells (55). Inhibitory effects of SOM on murine lymphocyte proliferation and inhibition of mitogen-induced leukocyte migration provide additional evidence of its immunomodulatory function (56,57).

Somatostatin and SP demonstrate opposing immunological effects analogous to their antagonistic actions in the nervous system. Substance P is a stimulatory neuromediator for several immune parameters, including lymphocyte proliferation and immunoglobulin production. Specific receptors have been documented on human lymphocytes that mediate SP's simulatory effect on proliferation and immunoglobulin synthesis (58); enhancement of mononcyte chemotaxis; macrophage oxidative burst; and release of arachidonic acid metabolites (59,60). Substance P increased the production of IgA in lymphocytes by 300% (61) and increased proliferation, as measured by [^{3}H]thymidine and [^{3}H]leucine uptake, by 60–70% in the presence or absence of mitogens (62).

NEUROPEPTIDE INTERACTIONS WITH MAST CELLS

In some tissues, over 85% of subepithelial mast cells are in contact with, or within 2 mm of, peptidergic nerve fibers containing SP and CGRP (63). In contrast to the inhibitory effects of SOM, high concentrations of SP degranulate mast cells and elicit release of preformed and newly generated mediators, by a mechanism that is independent of IgE (64,65). The demonstration of neuroimmunological effects on mast cell function is consistent with the close proximity of mast cell location to neuropeptide-containing nerve terminals. In rodent systems, approximately 65% of intestinal mucosal mast cells are in intimate contact with subepithelial peptidergic neurons (38). Pretreatment with capsaicin suppresses nasal allergy-like responses by depleting SP and CGRP from unmyelinated sensory nerves in guinea pig nasal mucosa (18). Skin itch and flare responses to injected SP resemble skin responses to histamine and are inhibited by antihistamines (66).

Numerous investigations have demonstrated neurogenic induction of mast cell degranulation and histamine release by direct electrical field stimulation of specific nerves (67–69). Leff et al. (66) extended the scope of these models to include neurogenic enhancement of antigen-induced hypersensitivity reactions during bronchial challenge with ascaris antigen. They were able to augment the lung histamine generation to antigen challenge by adding vagal nerve stimulation (66).

Several other features highlight the bidirectional communication between mast cells and peripheral nerves. Peptidergic neurons are not the only source of potent neuromediators, as mast cells and basophils generate authentic or variant forms of VIP; and eosinophils produce SP and VIP. The functional interaction between mast cells and peripheral nerves is reciprocal, as mast cell-derived histamine stimulates sensory nerves and facilitates neurotransmission in sympathetic ganglia by an H_1-predominant mechanism (70). In Bienenstock and co-workers' paradigm, mast cells are functional sensory receptors for the nervous system, capable of detecting antigens and informing the nervous system about environmental conditions (71).

Overall, the neuroendocrine–immune interactions seem to provide additional capacities to finely modify immune responses. Neuroimmune regulation affords broadened capacity for induction of immune reactivity, as both classic antigen presentation or physical nerve stimulation may generate an immune response. In addition to peripheral immune stimuli, the nervous system may trigger immune responses after central nervous or hormonal signals. The patterns of neural innervation allow generalization of responses over a larger area (72). Stimulation of respiratory epithelium at a single site may trigger a response throughout the entire airway. Alternatively, neuromodulation of immunity may localize the response to a given tissue compartment or focus. According to the view supported by Roche and colleagues (72,73), neuroimmune interactions are an adaptive feature of mucosal surfaces, which represent unique interfaces between tissue-bound immune cells and environmental or lumenal immunogenic substances. Such a system provides more rapid responses to mucosal stimuli, especially secondary responses with substantial upregulation of localized immunity.

THE EFFECTS OF NEUROPEPTIDES ON CYTOKINES

It has been hypothesized that neuropeptides may exert their modulatory effects on immune responses through regulation of cytokine production by target cells. Cytokines activate immune cells, regulate growth and differentiation, and affect immunoglobulin synthesis and class-switching. They are synthesized and released by inflammatory cells and modulate immune effector cells in an autocrine, paracrine, or hormonal fashion. Certain cytokine profiles have been identified in atopic disease and suggest a role in the pathogenesis of inflammatory diseases such as asthma and allergic rhinitis. Recent investigations have explored the effects of neuropeptides on cytokine production and have revealed this to be an important mechanism of neuroimmune modulation.

In purified human monocytes, Lotz et al. (74) observed SP and substance K (SK) induced production of IL-1, tissue necrosis factor (TNF)-α, and IL-6. A specific SP-antagonist, with D-isomeric substitutions of several amino acids, inhibited the increased IL-1 and TNF synthesis. As both IL-1 and TNF-α are proinflammatory mediators, initiating and maintaining humoral and cellular immune responses and contributing to tissue damage through induction of prostaglandin (PG)E$_2$ and collagenase secretion, the tachykinins were indirectly promoting inflammation.

Calvo and colleagues reported enhanced IL-2 secretion by peripheral blood T lymphocytes and Jurkat and HUT 78 T-cell lines after incubation with physiological concentrations of SP during phytohemagglutinin–phorbol myristate acetate (PHA/PMA) stimulation. Furthermore, expression of specific IL-2 mRNA was also increased by SP (75). The level of mRNA induced by SP with PMA is increased approximately fivefold over PMA alone in murine T-cell lines (76). Among the tachykinins tested, SP was the most potent inducer of IL-2 synthesis. In combination with Con-A or anti-CD3 antibody, SP stimulated IL-2 production in a dose-dependent manner, at four to five orders of magnitude lower concentrations than NKA, NKB, or physalaemin (76). Interleukin-2 is a major T-cell growth factor, secreted in autocrine and paracrine fashion by activated T lymphocytes, resulting in T-cell activation and clonal T-cell proliferation. By enhancing lymphocyte cytotoxicity, stimulating cytokine synthesis, and inducing antibody production, the primary immunological effects of IL-2 are stimulatory and production of inflammation.

Consistent with the pattern seen in most physiological regulatory networks, neuroendocrine modulation of immune responses and cytokine expression may be inhibitory, as well as stimulatory. In contrast to the stimulation of IL-2 by SP, moderate to high doses of VIP inhibit IL-2 synthesis by T cells activated by mitogen or through T-cell receptor (TCR) stimulation. In murine lymphocytes, very low concentrations of VIP can cause a marked increase in IL-2 secretion, followed by inhibition of both IL-2 and IL-4, in a dose-dependent fashion (98). Interestingly, the results published by Sun and Ganea (78) suggest that the molecular mechanisms responsible for the down-regulation of these two cytokines are distinct. The inhibition of IL-2 appears transcriptionally based, whereas down-regulation of IL-4 involves posttranscriptional mechanisms (63).

Neuropeptide-induced regulation of cytokine production is not limited to cells of lymphoid origin. Ansel et al. have demonstrated SP-induced synthesis of TNF-α in murine mast cells. Although mast cells may generate and secrete multiple cytokines, in addition to immediate hypersensitivity mediators such as histamine, proteoglycans, proteases, acid hydrolases, and eicosanoids, TNF-α production was selectively induced. There were no detectable changes in steady-state IL-1, IL-3, IL-4, IL-6, or GM-CSF in the murine mast cell line studied. The SP induction of TNF-α was also duplicated in freshly isolated murine peritoneal mast cells (79). Some investigators feel mast cell-derived TNF-α may contribute to IgE-mediated late-phase reactions by recruiting inflammatory leukocytes (80).

Neuroregulation of cytokine action may occur at multiple levels. Neurotensin enhances the functional effects of IL-1 through alteration of generation and release processes (75). Functional inhibition of IL-1 stimulation of thymocytes and fibroblasts can be selectively blocked by α-melanocyte-stimulating hormone (MSH) (81,82). Vasoactive intestinal peptide can rapidly increase IL-5 secretion from granuloma and splenic lymphocytes in a model of schistosomiasis-induced murine granulomas. Furthermore, Mathew et al. (83) postulate that VIP acts at some posttranscriptional level to stimulate IL-5 secretion, as IL-5 mRNA levels were not changed in VIP-stimulated lymphocytes, compared with Con-A-stimulated cells, which demonstrated increased gene expression (83).

INFLAMMATORY EFFECTS OF NEUROPEPTIDES

The release of neuropeptides has been demonstrated in models of inflammatory diseases such as asthma and rheumatoid arthritis (84). Local tissue reactions, resembling mast cell-dependent immediate hypersensitivity allergic reactions and acute inflammatory responses, can be generated neurogenically. The potential roles for neuropeptides in immediate hypersensitivity encompass direct tissue effects, recruitment of immune effector cells, and modulation of mediator release from basophils and mucosal mast cells (Table 3).

Several observations suggest that neuropeptide mediators may be involved in the pathogenesis of inflammation, or may provide an amplification loop for antigen-induced hypersensitivity reactions. The inflammation of rheumatoid arthritis is characterized by inflamed synovium, associated with increased numbers of T and B lymphocytes and plasma cells infiltrating the tissues and synovial fluid. Increased concentrations of SP and up-regulation of SP receptor expression in diseased joints, and demonstrable proinflammatory immunomodulatory functions, suggest SP plays a role in pathogenesis of synovitis (31). In experimental models of rheumatoid arthritis, SP enhances synovial inflammation, and capsaicin depletion of SP eliminates the inflammation (85). The effects of SP on blood flow and vascular permeability enhances the local delivery and accumulation of inflammatory cells. Substance P demonstrates potent stimulatory effects on neutrophil chemotactic and

Table 3 Inflammatory Effects of Neuropeptides in Allergy

Neuropeptide	Effects
SP	Stimulates degranulation of mast cell
	Increases mast cell production of TNF-α
	Augments monocyte and neutrophil chemotactic and phagocytic responses
	Evokes neutrophil and eosinophil accumulation in human skin
	Enhances macrophage oxidative burst and mediator release
VIP	Inhibits antigen-induced histamine release
	Induces neutrophil accumulation in human skin
	Enhances expression of surface LFA-1 adhesion molecules
SOM	Inhibits mast cell activation

Source: Ref. 117.

H_2O_2 responses to formyl–methionyl–leucyl–phenylalanine (FMLP) and C5a, increasing responses by 50–100% (86). Nevertheless, evidence suggests that cytokine production in rheumatoid arthritis may reflect direct stimulation of synoviocytes, rather than primary immune effector cell activation (87).

NEUROPEPTIDES IN UPPER AIRWAY HYPERSENSITIVITY RESPONSES

Walker et al. (88) performed nasal challenge with ryegrass antigen in a cohort of patients with a history of seasonal allergic rhinitis and positive skin test reactivity. Distinctive patterns of release of CGRP and SOM were detectable, with histamine in nasal lavage fluid (88). Whereas histamine concentrations reached peak levels at 15–60 min, SOM reached peak levels at 6 h after challenge, and CGRP continued to rise in some patients for up to 24 h. The late appearance of SOM, when the immediate hypersensitivity phase was subsiding, and the ability of SOM to suppress IgE-dependent mediator release from human basophils (89), suggested SOM's function may be physiologically inhibitory (88). In basophils and some types of mast cells, SOM has demonstrated inhibition of histamine, LTD_4, and LTE_4 release by up to 80% (89).

In contrast to the nasal allergen challenges by Walker and colleagues, Mosimann et al. (90) were able to detect SP and VIP in addition to CGRP in nasal secretions. The nasal lavage specimens were collected on ice, and a cocktail of protease inhibitors, including captopril, phosphoramidon, leupeptin, puromycin, and aprotinin, were added to restrict neuropeptide degradation before radioimmunoassay. Nasal challenges were performed with histamine, saline, and irrelevant allergen to serve as controls for challenge with relevant allergens. Rapid, brief, and dose-dependent increases in SP, CGRP, and VIP were seen in atopic subjects challenged with allergen, compared with nonatopic control subjects. The pattern was consistent with stimulation of sensory neural release of SP and CGRP by immediate hypersensitivity mediators, followed by reflexive liberation of VIP from para-sympathetic pathways. Interestingly, the histamine control challenge induced significant elevation in VIP concentrations, but not in SP or CGRP. This might represent preferential histamine stimulation of parasympathetic neurons over sensory nerves in human subjects. Alternatively, the dose delivered locally may have been too low to trigger axonal reflex by this stimulus (90).

Atopic patients with allergic rhinitis have upper airway hyperreactivity to cholinergic stimuli (91,92), as assessed objectively by measurements of symptom scores, secretion volumes, and nasal airway resistance after nasal provocation with methacholine. Nasal mucosal hyperreactivity may be due to hyperreactivity of effector organs (i.e., submucosal glands), or it may be secondary to hyperresponsiveness in the mucosal sensory system. Konno et al. (93,94) performed unilateral vidian neurectomies on seven subjects with perennial nasal allergic rhinitis to isolate and determine the contribution of the neural reflex in hyperrhinorrhea. With the unaffected side as a control, they were able to significantly blunt the nasal secretory responses by antigen or histamine. They concluded that direct effects of histamine on glandular secretion are insignificant compared with the reflex activation of sensory neurons by histamine (93,94).

The underlying molecular and cellular pathophysiological mechanisms of upper airway hyperreactivity have not been elucidated entirely, but may reflect increased expression of cell surface receptors, dampened inhibitory autonomic tone, or changes in airways degrada-tive enzymes, such as neutral endopeptidase. In guinea pig models of allergic rhinitis, increased numbers of muscarinic receptors were found in their nasal mucosa after sensitization with ovalbumin (79).

THE ROLE OF NEUROPEPTIDES IN ASTHMA

Many features of lower airway inflammation parallel those found in upper airways models. Glandular mucous secretions, bronchial blood flow, and microvascular permeability are increased, and there is an accumulation of inflammatory cells and mediators. Asthma is characterized by airways inflammation and bronchial hyperreactivity. A distinguishing feature of neurogenic inflammation in the lower airways is the effect of neuropeptides on airway smooth muscle. Numerous bronchoactive peptides have been identified, some with bronchoconstrictive effects: GRP, cholecystokinin, LTC_4, LTD_4, SP, NKA, CGRP; and some that relax airway smooth muscle: VIP, PHM–PHI, ANP, vasopressin, and oxytocin (96). Substance P and VIP are the neuropeptides present in the highest concentrations in the lung. The human bronchoconstrictive effects of NKA are more pronounced in small bronchi, compared with the effects of cholinergic stimuli, which cause obstruction in more proximal airways. These functional differences are consistent with the anatomical patterns of immunoreactivity seen with the various neuropeptides.

Neurogenic influences are hypothesized to worsen airway inflammation in asthma. The postulated sequence of events starts with bronchial inflammation, leading to epithelial shedding. The exposed airway sensory C-fibers potentiate antidromic release of neuropeptides by axon reflex. The liberated tachykinins have pronounced bronchoconstrictor effects and cause increased bronchial blood flow, increased microvascular permeability, and mucous secretions. They also promote immune cell activation, adherence, chemotaxis, and mediator release. This cascade continues to amplify inflammation by inducing cytokine expression, promoting mast cell degranulation, up-regulating gene expression, and potentiating neurotransmission.

Some researchers have theorized that a defect in VIP-induced bronchodilator influences contributes to the pathogenesis of asthma (97). In a study by Ollerenshaw et al. (98), lung tissues from five subjects with asthma and nine subjects without asthma were examined. At least 80 sections, including large and small airways, were examined from each specimen for presence of immunoreactivity to VIP. More than 92% of the sections from the lungs of patients without asthma demonstrated positive staining, but none of the sections from the asthmatic subjects showed immunoreactivity to VIP (98). Even in areas of intense inflammation, they found immunostaining for SP. Their study could not determine whether VIP synthesis was decreased, VIP degradation was increased, or there was a loss of neurons containing VIP. Nor could the study determine whether the lack of immunoreactive VIP was a primary abnormality or was secondary to the disease process.

Nevertheless, their findings sparked speculation that inflamed airways release enzymes, such as mast cell tryptase, that may rapidly degrade VIP, leading to exaggerated cholinergic tone or airway hyperresponsiveness. Four of the five asthmatic subjects included in Ollerenshaw's study, however, suffered from severe clinical disease. In fact, three lung tissue specimens were obtained postmortem. Doubt has arisen concerning the relevance of their findings to cases of reversible airways disease. In subsequent biopsies from patients with mild asthma, results of staining for VIP-immunoreactive nerves and VIP mRNA appear normal.

The potential pathogenic role of other peptidases has been examined in asthmatic subjects, as the activities of these enzymes may determine the effective potency and bio-specificity of the neuropeptide mediators. Neutral endopeptidase (NEP) causes rapid enzymatic degradation of neuropeptides in human airways, and inhibition of its activity pharmacologically or by cigarette smoke potentiates the effects of neurogenic inflammation (99). Nebulized thiorphan, an inhibitor of NEP, accentuates the bronchoconstrictor effects of inhaled TKA in normal and asthmatic subjects (100). In contrast, anti-inflammatory corticosteroids may up-regulate expression of NEP in human airways. Although it is tempting to speculate that NEP activity may be decreased in asthma, leading to exaggerated physiological effects of neuropeptides, immunohistochemical staining and in situ hybridization studies have failed to demonstrate disparate signals in the airways of asthmatic subjects compared with control groups (99–102).

IMPLICATIONS FOR THERAPY

Several levels of therapy may be potentially useful for pharmacological control of neuro-immunologically mediated allergic airways disease:

1. Modulation of mast cell activation by antigen or other stimuli
2. Blockade of ligand–receptor interaction of mast cell products, including histamine, platelet-activating factor, and arachidonic acid metabolites
3. Suppression of neurally sensitizing mediators, including histamine and diHETEs
4. Inhibition of release of proinflammatory neuropeptides
5. Antagonism of receptor-mediated effects of neuropeptides

Corticosteroids, allergen immunotherapy, and cromolyn sodium suppress mast cell responses to antigens and possibly other stimuli, thereby reducing release of mast cell mediators. Topical glucocorticoid therapy reduces the numbers of mucosal mast cells (103) and produces marked inhibition of in vitro basophil histamine and leukotriene release by IgE-dependent stimuli (104). Cromolyn sodium clearly suppresses human mast cell release in vitro (105) and exhibits dose–response inhibition of histamine release by antigen-stimulated rat peritoneal mast cells (106).

Prolonged treatment with topical steroids blunts both early and late pulmonary responses to antigen inhalation challenge (107) by various different mechanisms, including inhibition of mediators, such as cytokines, PAF, and eicosanoids. Steroid-induced decreases in hyperresponsiveness to nonspecific stimuli have also been demonstrated. Corticosteroids may also inhibit neurogenic inflammation, through modulation of interaction between neuropeptide and receptor. By reducing NK_1-receptor mRNA in asthmatic lungs, corticosteroids inhibit NK_1-receptor gene expression at the genetic level (108).

Antihistamines act through blockade of histamine receptors on end-organ tissues. Since histamine-facilitated neurotransmission is mediated through H_1-predominant mechanisms, antihistamines also suppress neurally mediated amplification of allergic responses. Newly developed agents are capable of competitively blocking the occupancy of receptors for PAF, LTD_4, and LTB_4. Cetirizine, a more potent nonsedating antihistamine, also inhibits cutaneous influx of eosinophils attracted by compound 48/80 and antigen in allergic subjects, but not in normal subjects nor in allergic patients challenged with histamine. These results suggest that mediator release or the effects of chemotactic factors are altered significantly by cetirizine (109).

Many first- and second-generation H_1-antagonists block mediator release as well as ligand–receptor interaction. Functional inhibition of histamine, eicosanoid, and other immediate hypersensitivity mediator release occurs in mast cells and basophils. The effect is seen with either antigen–IgE-dependent mast cell activation or degranulation by SP, compound 48/80, or calcium ionophore A23187 by undefined mechanisms (110–113).

8,15-Dihydroxy–eicosatetraenoic acid (8,15-di-HETE) is an arachidonic acid metabolite released by eosinophils, leukocytes, and epithelial cells. 8,15-di-HETE is a neuroactive eicosanoid that modulates the fundamental state of reactivity of nociceptive neurons to other stimuli. Potentially, agents that selectively inhibit the effects of neurally sensitizing 8,15-di-HETE could decrease neurogenic inflammation. Cytokines that possess neurotrophic effects include IL-1, and to a lesser extent, TNF. They may augment the production of nerve growth factor (NGF) and increase the intracellular content of SP in neural cells. Specific inhibitors of these cytokines may also suppress neurogenic inflammation.

Atropine and ipratropium bromide can be administered to the lungs by aerosol and have clinically significant anticholinergic activities. A reduction in airway obstruction through suppression of vagal tone might be anticipated with these therapies. Currently, these agents have limited usefulness for the treatment of asthma, possibly because of their nonspecific blockade of M_1, M_2, and M_3 muscarinic receptors. The M_1 and M_3 receptor subtypes are thought to mediate glandular secretion and bronchoconstriction, respectively, and blockade of these receptors may be beneficial. The M_2 receptors, however, are found on cholinergic nerves and autoinhibit release of acetylcholine from nerve terminals (114,115). Antagonism of M_2 receptor-mediated signals could promote inflammation by reducing physiological inhibition of cholinergic signals. Development of specific antagonists for M_1 and M_3 receptors, or agonists for M_2 receptors, however, could modulate the effects or release of neuropeptides.

Receptor-directed antagonists of neuropeptides exist and may modify allergic airways responses. Many of these therapies require refinement, however, as many are partial agonists, lack potency, or cannot be administered effectively, owing to proteolytic degradation or unacceptable systemic side effects. A common type of specific-binding antagonist are synthetic analogues, such as the VIP antagonist, 4-Cl-D-Phe-6,Leu-17VIP. Fragments of authentic neuropeptides may also demonstrate specific binding with partial agonist or competitive antagonistic activity.

The structurally diverse variants of VIP may be truncated forms of previously described VIP, or may represent forms derived by alternative splicing of mRNA (116). Immune cell-derived neuropeptide variants demonstrate different binding affinities and produce diverse responses, suggesting that each may have unique immunoregulatory roles (117). The primary mast cell-derived variants, VIP_{10-28} binds with one-tenth the affinity of authentic VIP (VIP_{1-28}) to lymphocyte receptors, and with $1/1000$ the affinity of VIP_{1-28} to rodent neural tissue receptors (118). The VIP fragment VIP_{10-28} is a naturally occurring VIP variant, the physiological role of which may be antagonism of VIP binding (119). The physiological effect of these neuropeptide variants may vary, reflecting different subtypes of receptors expressed by those target tissues. These agents are of interest for pharmacological study to characterize the physiology or biochemistry of neuropeptide receptors.

SUMMARY

Neuropeptides and other neural mediators influence allergic reactions by altering functions of lymphocytes, other leukocytes, and mast cells, as well as blood vessels, glandular elements, and smooth muscle. The further elucidation and characterization of the pathophysiological involvement of neuropeptides in upper and lower airway allergic diseases will lead to a better understanding of their separate and interactive roles. As we develop greater knowledge of the mechanisms of neurogenic inflammation and autonomic regulation of airway responses, distinctive therapies can be directed toward specific aspects of neuromediator structure and function in allergic rhinitis and asthma.

REFERENCES

1. Richardson JB. State of the art. Nerve supply to the lungs. Am Rev Respir Dis 1979; 19:785.
2. Andersson RG, Grundstrom N. The excitatory non-cholinergic, non-adrenergic nervous system of the guinea-pig airways. Eur J Respir Dis 1983; 64(suppl 121):141–157.
3. Barnes PJ. Neural control of human airways in health and disease. Am Rev Respir Dis 1986; 134:1289–1314.
4. Andersson RG, Grundstrom N. The excitatory non-cholinergic, non-adrenergic nervous system of the guinea-pig airways. Eur J Respir Dis 1983; 64:141–157.
5. Lundberg JM, Martling CR, Saria A. Substance P and capsaicin-induced contraction of human bronchi. Acta Physiol Scand 1983; 119:49–53.
6. Lundberg JM, Hokfelt T, Nilsson G, et al. Peptide neurons in the vagus, splanchnic and sciatic nerves. Acta Physiol Scand 1978; 34:50–62.
7. Goetzl EJ, Sreedharan SP. Mediators of communication and adaptation in the neuroendocrine and immune system. FASEB J 1992; 6:2646–2652.
8. Coleridge JCG, Coleridge HM. Afferent vagal C-fibre innervation of the lung and airways and its functional significance. Rev Physiol Biochem Pharmacol 1984; 99:1–110.
9. Lundberg JM, Saria A. Capsaicin-sensitive vagal neurons involved in control of vascular permeability in rat trachea. Acta Physiol Scand 1982; 116:473–476.
10. Hartung HP, Toyka KV. Activation of macrophages by substance P: induction of oxidative burst and thromboxane release. Eur J Pharmacol 1983; 89:301–305.
11. Lundblad L, Anggard A, Lundberg JM. Effects of antidromic trigeminal nerve stimulation in relation to parasympathetic vasodilatation in cat nasal mucosa. Acta Physiol Scand 1984; 119: 7–13.
12. Brimjoin S, Lundberg JM, Brodin E, Hokfelt T, Nilsson G. Axonal transport of substance P in the vagus and sciatic nerves of the guinea pig brain. Brain Res 1980; 191:443.
13. Saria A, Martling CR, Yan Z, Theodorsson-Norheim E, Gamse R, Lundberg JM. Release of multiple tachykinins from capsaicin-sensitive sensory nerves in the lung by bradykinin, histamine, dimethylphenyl piperazinium, and vagal nerve stimulation. Am Rev Respir Dis 1988; 137:1330–1335.
14. Baraniuk JN, Kaliner M. Neuropeptide and nasal secretion. J Allergy Clin Immunol 1990; 86: 620–627.
15. Tadeka N, Kalubi B, Abe Y, Irifune M, Ogino S, Matsunaga T. Neurogenic inflammation in nasal allergy: histochemical and pharmacological studies in guinea pigs. Acta Otolaryngol Suppl 1993; 501:21–24.
16. Baraniuk JN, Lundgren JD, Okayama M, Merida M, Kaliner M. Substance P and neurokinin A (NKA) in human nasal mucosa. Am J Respir Cell Mol Biol 1990; 3:165–173.
17. Baraniuk JN, Lundgren JD, Goff J, et al. Gastrin releasing peptide (GRP) in human nasal mucosa. J Clin Invest 1990; 85:998–1005.
18. Nagy JI. Capsaicin: a chemical probe for sensory neuron mechanisms. In: Iverson LL, Iverson SD, Snyder SH, eds. Handbook of Psychopharmacology. Vol 15. New York: Plenum Press, 1982:185–235.
19. Buck SH, Burks TF. The neuropharmacology of capsaicin: review of some recent observations. Pharmacol Rev 1986; 38:179–226.
20. Lundberg JM, Alving K, Karlsson JA, Matran R, Nilsson G. Sensory neuropeptide involvement

in animal models of airway irritation and of allergen-evoked asthma. Am Rev Respir Dis 1991; 143:1429–1431.

21. Dey RD, Shannon WA Jr, Said SI. Localization of VIP-immunoreactive nerves in airways and pulmonary vessels of dogs, cats and human submucosa. Cell Tissue Res 1981; 220:231–238.

22. Laburthe M, Breant B, Rouyer-Fessard C. Molecular identification of receptors for vasoactive intestinal peptide in rat intestinal epithelium by covalent cross-linking. Eur J Biochem 1984; 139:181–187.

23. McArthur KE, Wood CL, O'Dorisio MS, Zhou Z, Gardner JD, Jensen RT. Characterization of receptors for VIP on pancreatic acinar cell plasma membranes using covalent crosslinking. Am J Physiol 1987; 252:G404–G412.

24. Nguyen TD, Williams JA, Gray GM. Vasoactive intestinal peptide receptor on liver plasma membranes: characterization as a glycoprotein. Biochemistry 1986; 25:3361–3368.

25. Taylor DP, Pert CB. VIP: specific binding to rat brain membranes. Proc Natl Acad Sci USA 1979; 76:660–664.

26. Tseng J, O'Dorisio MS. Mechanism of vasoactive intestinal peptide (VIP)-mediated immuno-regulation. In: Goetzl AJ, Spector NH, eds. Neuroimmune Networks: Physiology and Diseases. New York: Alan R Liss, 1989:105–111.

27. Diamond L, O'Donnell M. A non-adrenergic vagal inhibitory pathway to feline airways. Science 1980; 208:185–185.

28. Irvin CG, Boileau R, Tremblay J, Martin RR, Macklem PT. Bronchodilatation: noncholinergic, nonadrenergic mediation demonstrated in vivo in the cat. Science 1980; 207:791–792.

29. Laufer R, Gilon C, Chorev M, Selinger Z. Characterization of neurokinin B receptor site in rat brain using a highly selective radioligand. J Biol Chem 1986; 261:10257–10263.

30. Bergstrom L, Beaujouan JC, Torrens Y, Saffroy M, Glowinski J, et al. Sulfhydryl reagents have different effects on substance P and neurokinin B binding sites in cortical synaptosomes in the rat. Mol Pharmacol 1987; 32:764–771.

31. Payan DG. Neuropeptides and inflammation: the role of substance P. Annu Rev Med 1989; 40: 341–352.

32. Goetzl EJ, Sreedharan SP. Mediators of communication and adaptation in the neuroendocrine and immune systems. FASEB J 1992; 6:2646.

33. Blum AM, Metwali A, Cook G, Mathew RC, Elliott D, Weinstock JV. Substance P modulates antigen-induced, IFN-γ production in murine schistosomiasis mansoni. J Immunol 1993; 151: 225–233.

34. Fuller RW, Maxwell DL, Dixon CMS, et al. The effects of substance P on cardiovascular and respiratory function in human subjects. J Appl Physiol 1987; 62:1473–1479.

35. Evans TW, Dixon CMS, Clarke B, Conradson TB, Barnes PJ. Comparison of NKA and SP on cardiovascular and airway function in man. Br J Clin Pharmacol 1988; 25:273–275.

36. Brain SD, Williams TJ, Tippins JR, Morris HR, MacIntyre I. Calcitonin gene-related peptide is a potent vasodilator. Nature 1985; 313:54–56.

37. Goodman EC, Iversen LL. Calcitonin gene-related peptide: novel neuropeptide. Life Sci 1986; 38:2169–2178.

38. Stead RH, Tomioka M, Quinonez G, Simon GT, Felten SY, Bienenstock J. Intestinal mucosal mast cells in normal and nematode-infected rat intestines are in intimate contact with pep-tidergic nerves. Proc Natl Acad Sci USA 1987; 84:2975–2979.

39. Lorton D, Bellinger DL, Felten SY, Felten DL. Substance P innervation of spleen in rats: nerve fibers associate with lymphocytes and macrophages in specific compartments of the spleen. Brain Behav Immun 1991; 5:29–40.

40. Goetzl EJ, Sreedharan SP. Mediators of communication and adaptation in the neuroendocrine and immune systems. FASEB J 1992; 6:2646–2652.

41. Cross RJ, Markesbery WR, Brooks WH, Roszman TL. Hypothalamic–immune interactions: neuromodulation of natural killer activity by lesioning of the anterior hypothalamus. Immunology 1984; 51:399–405.

42. Bulloch K, Tollefson L. Dual-label retrograde transport: CNS innervation of mouse thymus distinct from other mediastinum viscera. J Neurosci Res 1990; 25:20–28.

43. Ottaway CA, Greenberg GR. In vitro alteration of receptors for vasoactive intestinal peptide changes the in vivo localization of mouse T cells. J Exp Med 1984; 160:1054–1069.

44. Goetzl EJ, Adelman AC, Sreedharan SP. Neuroimmunology. Adv Immunol 1990; 48:161–190.

45. Stanisz A, Scicchitano R, Dazin P, Bienenstock J, Payan DG. Distribution of substance P receptors on murine spleen and Peyer's patch T and B cells J Immunol 1987; 139:749.

46. Payan DG, Brewster DR, Missirian-Bastian A, Goetzl EJ. Substance P recognition by a subset of human T lymphocytes. J Clin Invest 1984; 133:3260.

47. Cotrait M, Hospital M. Conformational behavior of some tachykinin C-terminal heptapeptides. Int J Peptide Protein Res 1986; 28:450–455.

48. Ottaway CA, Greenberg GR. Interaction of vasoactive intestinal peptide with mouse lymphocytes: specific binding and the modulation of mitogen responses. J Immunol 1984; 132:417–423.

49. Ottaway CA, Bernaerts C, Chan B, Greenberg GR. Specific binding of vasoactive intestinal peptide to human circulating mononuclear cells. J Physiol Pharmacol 1983; 61:664–671.

50. Ottaway CA. Selective effects of VIP on the mitogenic response of murine T cells. Immunology 1987; 62:291–297.

51. Hassner A, Lau MS, Goetzl EJ, Adelman DC. Isotype-specific regulation of human lymphocyte production of immunoglobulins by sustained exposure to vasoactive intestinal peptide (VIP). J Allergy Clin Immunol 1993; 92(6):891–901.

52. Elde R, Hokfelt T. Localization of hypophysiotropic peptides and other biologically active peptides within the brain. Annu Rev Physiol 1979; 41:587.

53. Stanisz AM, Befus D, Bienenstock J. Neuropeptides and immunity. J Immunol 1986; 136:152.

54. Goetzl EJ, Payan DG. Inhibition by somatostatin of release of mediators from human basophils and rat leukemic basophils. J Immunol 1984; 133:3255–3259.

55. Pawlikowski M, Stepien H, Kunert-Radek J, Zelazowski P, Schally AV. Immunomodulatory action of somatostatin. Ann NY Acad Sci 1986; 496:233–239.

56. Payan DG, Hess AC, Goetzl EJ. Inhibition by somatostatin of the proliferation of T-lymphocytes and Molt-4 lymphoblasts. Cell Immunol 1984; 84:433.

57. Schicchitano R, Bienenstock J, Stanisz AM. In vivo immunomodulation by the neuropeptide substance P. Immunology 1988; 63:733–736.

58. Hartung HP, Toyka KV. Activation of macrophages by substance P: induction of oxidative burst and thromboxane release. Eur J Pharmacol 1983; 89:301–305.

59. Hartung HP, Wolters K, Toyka KV. Substance P: binding properties and studies on cellular responses in guinea pig macrophages. J Immunol 1986; 136:3856–3863.

60. Stanisz AM, Befus D, Bienenstock J. Differential effects of vasoactive intestinal peptide, substance P and somatostatin on immunoglobulin synthesis and proliferation by lymphocytes from Peyer's patches, mesenteric lymph nodes, and spleen. J Immunol 1986; 136:152–156.

61. Payan DG, Brewster DR, Goetzl EJ. Specific stimulation of human T lymphocytes by substance P. J Immunol 1983; 131:1613–1615.

62. Stead RH, Tomioka M, Quinonez G, et al. Intestinal mucosal mast cells in normal and nematode-infected rat intestines are in intimate contact with peptidergic nerves. Proc Natl Acad Sci USA 1987; 84:2975–2979.

63. Erjavec F, Lembeck F, Florjanc-Irman T, Skofitsch G, Donnerer BJ, Saria A, Holzer P. Release of histamine by substance P. Naunyn Schmiedebergs Arch Pharmacol 1981; 317:67–70.

64. Foreman JC, Jordan CC, Oehme P, Renner H. Structure–activity relationships for some substance P-related peptides that cause wheal and flare reactions in human skin. J Physiol 1983; 335:49–65.

65. Hagermark O, Hokfelt T, Pernow B. Flare and itch induced by substance P in human skin. J Invest Dermatol 1978; 71:233–235.

66. Lundberg JM, Saria A. Capsaicin-sensitive vagal neurons involved in control of vascular permeability in rat trachea. Acta Physiol Scand 1982; 115:521–523.

67. Masini E, Rucci L, Cirri-Borghi MB, et al. Stimulation of resection of vidian nerve in patients with chronic hypertrophic non-allergic rhinitis. Agents Actions 1986; 18:251–253.

68. Leff AR, Stimler NP, Munoz NM, et al. Augmentation of respiratory mast cell secretion of histamine caused by vagus nerve stimulation during antigen challenge. J Immunol 1986; 136:1066–1073.

69. Undem BJ, Weinreich D. Functional interactions between mast cells and peripheral neurons. In: Goetzl EJ, Spector NH, eds. Neuroimmune Networks: Physiology and Diseases. New York: Alan R Liss, 1989:155–162.

70. Bienenstock J, Macqueen G, Sestini P, Marshall JS, Stead RH, Perdue MH. Inflammatory cell mechanisms: mast cell/nerve interactions in vitro and in vivo. Am Rev Respir Dis 1991; 143: S55–S58.

71. Nio DA, Moylan RN, Roche JK. Modulation of T lymphocyte function by neuropeptides. J Immunol 1993; 150:5281–5288.

72. Roche JK. Immunological mechanisms for chronic inflammatory diseases of mucosa. In: WS Lynn, ed. Inflammatory Cells and Lung Disease. New York: CRC Press, 1983:63–84.

73. Lotz M, Vaughan JH, Carson DA. Effect of neuropeptides on production of inflammatory cytokines by human monocytes. Science 1988; 241:1218.

74. Calvo CF, Chavanel G, Senik A. Substance P enhances IL-2 expression in activated human T cells. J Immunol 1992; 148:3498–3504.

75. Rameshwar P, Gascon P, Ganea D. Stimulation of IL-2 production in murine lymphocytes by substance P and related tachykinins. J Immunol 1993; 151:2484–2496.

76. Nio DA, Moylan RN, Roche JK. Modulation of T lymphocyte function by neuropeptides. J Immunol 1993; 150:5281–5288.

77. Sun L, Ganea D. Vasoactive intestinal peptide inhibits interleukin IL-2 and IL-4 production through different molecular mechanisms in T cells activated via the T cell receptor/CD3 complex. J Neuroimmunol 1993; 48:59–70.

78. Ansel JC, Brown JR, Payan DG, Brown MA. Substance P selectively activates TNF-α gene expression in murine mast cells. J Immunol 1993; 150:4478–4485.

79. Goeddel DV, Aggarwal BB, Gray PW, Leung DW, Nedwin GE, Palladio MA, Patton JS, Pennica D, Shepard HSM, Sugarman BJ, Wong G. Tumor necrosis factors: gene structure and biological activities. Cold Spring Harbor Symp Quant Biol 1986; 60:597.

80. Mason MJ, Van Epps D. Modulation of IL-1, tumor necrosis factor, and C5a-mediated murine neutrophil migration by alpha-melanocyte stimulating hormone. J Immunol 1989; 142:1646–1651.

81. Cannon JG, Tatro JB, Reichlin S, Dinarello CA. alpha Melanocyte stimulating hormone inhibits immunostimulatory and inflammatory actions of interleukin-1. J Immunol 1986; 137:2232–2236.

82. Mathew RC, Cook GA, Blum AM, Metwali A, Felman R, Weinstock JV. Vasoactive intestinal peptide stimulates T lymphocytes to release IL-5 in murine schistosomiasis mansoni infection. J Immunol 1992; 148:3572–3577.

83. Barnes PJ. Neural control of human airways in health and disease. Am Rev Respir Dis 1986; 134:1289–1314.

84. Levine JD, MA, Basbaum AI. The contribution of neurogenic inflammation in experimental arthritis. J Immunol 1985; 135:843s–846s.

85. Perianin A, Snyderman R, Malfroy B. Substance P primes neutrophil activation: a mechanism for neurological regulation of inflammation. Biochem Biophys Res Commun 1989; 161: 520–524.

86. Stanisz A, Agro A. Are lymphocytes a target for substance P modulation in arthritis? Arthritis Rheum 1992; 21:252–258.

87. Walker KB, Serwonska MH, Valone FH, Harkonen WS, Frick OL, Scriven KH, Ratnoff WD, Browning JG, Payan DG, Goetzl EJ. Distinctive patterns of release of neuroendocrine peptides after nasal challenge of allergic subjects with ryegrass antigen. J Clin Invest 1988; 8:108–113.
88. Goetzl EJ, Payan DG. Inhibition by somatostatin of the release of mediators from human basophils and rat leukemic basophils. J Immunol 1984; 133:3255–3259.
89. Mosimann BL, White MV, Hohman RJ, Boldrich MS, Kaulbach HC, Kaliner MA. Substance P, calcitonin gene-related peptide and vasoactive intestinal peptide increase in nasal secretions after allergen challenge in atopic patients. J Allergy Clin Immunol 1993; 92:95–104.
90. Borum P. Nasal methacholine challenge: a test for the measurement of nasal reactivity. J Allergy Clin Immunol 1979; 63:253.
91. Druce HM, Wright RH, Kossoff D, Kaliner MA. Cholinergic nasal hyperreactivity in atopic subjects. J Allergy Clin Immunol 1985; 76:445–452.
92. Konno A, Terada N, Okamoto Y, Togawa K. The role of chemical mediators and the mucosal hyperreactivity in nasal hypersecretion in nasal allergy. J Allergy Clin Immunol 1987; 79: 620–626.
93. Konno A, Togawa K. Vidian neurectomy for allergic rhinitis: evaluation of long-term results and some problems concerning operative therapy. Arch Otorhinolaryngol 1979; 225:67.
94. Konno A, Terada N. Participation of autonomic nervous system of the nasal mucosa in pathophysiology of nasal allergy. Otologia (Fukuoka) 1985; 31:1263.
95. Said SI. Influence of neuropeptides on airway smooth muscle. Am Rev Respir Dis 1987; 136:S52–S58.
96. Matsuzaki Y, Hamasaki Y, Said SI. Vasoactive intestinal peptide: possible transmitter of nonadrenergic relaxation of guinea pig airways. Science 1980; 210:1252–1253.
97. Ollerenshaw S, Jarvis D, Woolcock A, Sullivan C, Sheibner T. Absence of immunoreactive vasoactive intestinal polypeptide in tissue from the lungs of patients with asthma. N Engl J Med 1989; 320:1244–1248.
98. Nadel JA. Neutral endopeptidase modulates neurogenic inflammation. Eur Respir J 1991; 4: 745–754.
99. Cheung D, Bel EH, den Hartigh J, Kijkman JH, Sterk PJ. An effect of an inhaled neutral endopeptidase inhibitor, thiorphan, on airway responses to neurokinin A in normal humans in vivo. Am Rev Respir Dis 1992; 145:1275–1280.
100. Lazarus SC, Borson DB, Gold WM, Nadel JA. Inflammatory mediators, tachykinins and enkephalinase in airways. Int Arch Allergy Appl Immunol 1987; 82:372–373.
101. Stimler-Gerard NP. Neutral endopeptidase-like enzyme controls the contractile activity of substance P in guinea pig lung. J Clin Invest 1987; 79:1819–1825.
102. Pipkorn U. Effect of topical glucocorticoid treatment on nasal mucosal mast cells in allergic rhinitis. Allergy 1983; 38:125.
103. Schleimer RP, Lichtenstein LM, Gillespie E. Inhibition of basophil histamine release by anti-inflammatory steroids. Nature 1981; 292:454.
104. Assem ESK, Mongar JL. Inhibition of allergic reactions in man and other species by cromoglycate. Int Arch Allergy Appl Immunol 1970; 38:68.
105. Garland LG. Effect of cromoglycate on anaphylactic histamine release from rat peritoneal mast cells. Br J Pharmacol 1973; 49:128.
106. Dahl R, Johansson SA. Importance of duration of treatment with inhaled budesonide on the immediate and late bronchial reaction. Eur J Respir Dis 1982; 122:167.
107. Adcock IM, Peters M, Gelder C, Shirasaki H, Brown CR, Barnes PJ. Increased tachykinin receptor gene expression in asthmatic lung and its modulation by steroids. J Mol Endocrinol 1993; 11:1–7.
108. Fadel R, Richard N, Rihoux JP, Henocq E. Inhibitory effect of cetirizine 2HC1 on eosinophil migration in vivo. Clin Allergy 1987; 17:373–379.
109. Church MK, Gradidge CF. Inhibition of histamine release from human lung in vitro by antihistamines and related drugs. Br J Pharmacol 1980; 69:663.

110. Temple DM, McCluskey M. Loratadine, an antihistamine, blocks antigen- and ionophore-induced leukotriene release from human lung in vitro. Prostaglandins 1988; 35:549.
111. Little MM, Casale TB. Azelastine inhibits IgE-mediated human basophil histamine release. J Allergy Clin Immunol 1989; 83:862.
112. Radermecher M. Inhibition of allergen-mediated histamine release from human cells by keto-tifen and oxatomide. Respiration 1981; 41:45.
113. Barnes PJ. Muscarinic receptor subtypes: implications for lung disease. Thorax 1989; 44:161.
114. Mak JCW, Barnes PJ. Autoradiographic visualization of muscarinic receptor subtypes in human and guinea pig lung. Am Rev Respir Dis 1990; 141:1559.
115. Goetzl EJ, Sreedharan SP, Turck CW. Structurally distinct vasoactive intestinal peptide from rat basophilic leukemia cells. J Biol Chem 1988; 263:9083–9086.
116. Goetzl EJ, Turck CW, Peterson KE, Finch RJ, Kodama KT, Adelman DC, Sreedharan SP. Neuromediators of immunity and inflammation. In: Melchers F, ed. Progress in Immunology. Vol 7. Berlin: Springer-Verlag, 1989:772–779.
117. Finch RJ, Sreedharan SP, Goetzl EJ. High affinity receptors for vasoactive intestinal peptide on human myeloma cells. J Immunol 1989; 142:1977.
118. Rosselin G, Anteunis A, Astesano C, Boissard, Pali P, Hejblum G, Marie JC. Regulation of the vasoactive intestinal peptide receptor. Ann NY Acad Sci 1988; 527:220–237.
119. O'Dorisio MS, Wood CL, O'Dorisio TM. Vasoactive intestinal peptide and neuropeptides modify the immune response. J Immunol 1985; 135:792s.

15

Histamine-Releasing Factors and Inhibitors: Relationship to the Chemokines

Rafeul Alam and J. Andrew Grant

The University of Texas Medical Branch, Galveston, Texas

INTRODUCTION

The granules of mast cells and basophils contain a myriad of mediators that have potent inflammatory activity. These mediators include histamine, leukotrienes, prostaglandins, platelet-activating factor, tryptase, kininogenase, and other proteolytic enzymes (1). Recent studies suggest that these cells are the source of some important cytokines. Mast cells produce interleukin (IL)-4, IL-5, IL-6, tumor necrosis factor (TNF), and other cytokines (2,3). Basophils produce IL-4 (4,5) and macrophage inflammatory protein (MIP)-1α (Li H, Alam R, unpublished data). By virtue of IL-4 production and the expression of CD40 on their surface, basophils can drive IgE production by B cells in the absence of T cells (6). The presence of IL-4 is sine qua non for the differentiation of T_{H2} cells (7). Since T_{H0} cells are poor producers of IL-4, basophils and mast cells are thought to be the initial source of IL-4. The release of IL-4 from these cells leads to the generation of T_{H2} cells. However, how these cells are activated in the absence of IgE in a primary immune response is unknown. Basophils are activated in the late-phase allergic reaction that occurs 4–6 h after the initial exposure to the allergens (8). The mechanism of their activation in the late-phase reaction is also unknown. Thus, basophil or mast cell activation occurs in various conditions wherein the nature of the secretagogue(s) remains undefined. Cytokines are one group of molecules that activate a variety of cells. For this reason we focused our attention on cytokine-dependent activation of basophils and mast cells.

HISTAMINE-RELEASING FACTOR

Thueson et al. initially described a group of cytokines, called histamine-releasing factor (HRF) that activate basophils (9) and some subtypes of mast cells (reviewed in Refs. 1 and 10). Histamine-releasing factor induced typical immediate-type degranulation of basophils, as judged by electron microscopy (11). It caused the synthesis of leukotrienes from lung mast cells (12). Furthermore, partially purified HRF had chemotactic activity for basophils and monocytes. It is produced by mononuclear cells (MNC), T cells and B cells (13), monocyte–macrophages (14,15), platelets (16), and neutrophils (17).

HRF and Clinical Correlates

The synthesis of HRF is stimulated by specific allergens in sensitive patients (18). The production of HRF by MNC from asthmatic patients has been correlated with bronchial hyperreactivity (19) and symptoms of asthma (20). Immunotherapy reduced the production of HRF by MNC in patients with asthma (20) and allergic rhinitis (21). The MNC cells from patients with atopic dermatitis who had concurrent food allergy spontaneously produced high amounts of HRF that reverted to normal levels after 2 years of elimination therapy (22). Basophils from these patients spontaneously released a large percentage of intracellular histamine, which was also reduced after the elimination therapy. HRF-like activity was recovered from cutaneous blister fluid obtained during the late-phase allergic reaction (23). Furthermore, lesional blister fluid from patients with chronic idiopathic urticaria had higher levels of HRF than nonlesional blister fluid (24). HRF-like activity was also recovered from nasal washings (25) and bronchoalveolar lavage fluid (26).

IgE-Dependent and IgE-Independent HRF

One species of HRF induced histamine release from basophils obtained from select basophil donors only (27). Basophils stripped of the surface IgE lost sensitivity to the HRF, which was restored by sensitization with IgE obtained from the responder donors, but not from nonresponder donors or myeloma IgE. The most allergic and symptomatic patients had the most responsive basophils. On the basis of these experiments, the Johns Hopkins group hypothesized that patients whose basophils respond to this species of HRF have a special type of IgE, so-called IgE$^+$ (28). According to this hypothesis, one species of HRF binds to the IgE$^+$ on the surface of basophils and induces histamine release. The IgE from less severe atopic patients and nonallergic individuals (IgE$^-$) lacks this HRF-binding property. The molecular identity of IgE$^+$ and of the HRF species are currently being investigated. Many species of MNC-derived HRF act in an IgE-independent manner and cause histamine release from basophils obtained from allergic as well as from nonallergic normal subjects.

The molecular identity of various species of HRF was studied by protein purification of cell culture supernatants. Several species of HRF, with various molecular weights, were identified in different laboratories (29,30). Direct sequencing was hampered by low amounts of purified materials and by the blocked NH_2-terminal. Simultaneously, we studied histamine-releasing activity of newly cloned interleukins and cytokines. Among the cytokines identified first, none had any detectable histamine-releasing activity except IL-3 and granulocyte–macrophage colony-stimulating factor (GM-CSF) (31,32). The latter two cytokines released small amounts of histamine from basophils obtained from some select allergic donors.

THE CHEMOKINES, A UNIQUE FAMILY OF CYTOKINES

Chemokines represent a new family of relative low molecular mass (8–10 kDa) cytokines that are predominantly chemotactic for inflammatory cells (Table 1). This family is divided

Table 1 Chemokines

CXC chemokines	C–C chemokines
Interleukin-8 (NAP-1)	MCP-1 (MCAF)
Gro-α (MGSA, MIP-2)	MCP-2 (HC-14)
Gro-β	MCP-3 (FIC, MARC)
Gro-γ	MIP-1α (LD78, AT464, GOS19)
ENA-78	MIP-1β (Act-2, AT744, G-26)
GCP-2	RANTES
IP-10	I-309
PF-4	
PBP and its truncated fragments:	
CTAP III	
NAP-2	
Genomic structure:	
4 exons/3 introns except for PF-4 and PBP 3 exons/2 introns	3 exons/2 introns
Chromosomal location:	
Chromosome 4, q12–21	Chromosome 17, q11–21

into two subfamilies: the CXC subfamily is characterized by the presence of two cysteines separated by a single amino acid of various types (reviewed in Refs. 33, 34). The members of the CXC family include IL-8, Gro(α, β, γ)–melanocyte growth-stimulating activity (MGSA)–macrophage inflammatory protein-2 (MIP-2), neutrophil-activating protein-2, connective tissue-activating protein III (CTAP III), β-thromboglobulin, platelet factor-4 (PF-4), and inducible protein-10 (IP-10). The C–C subfamily contains two adjacent cysteines in its sequence. The members of the C–C subfamily include monocyte chemotactic protein-1 (MCP-1/MCAF), MCP-2, MCP-3, macrophage inflammatory protein-1α (MIP-α)/LD78, MIP-1β/Act-2, RANTES, and I-309. Both subfamilies have a similar organization of exons and introns, suggesting that they might have emerged from a single gene by duplication. The genes for these families in humans are located on chromosomes 4 and 17, respectively (34).

The C–C chemokines are produced by a variety of cells (Table 2). MCP-1 was initially isolated from mononuclear cells, but later studies demonstrated that mast cells, fibroblasts, airway epithelial cells, synovial cells, and various tumor cells can produce this chemokine. Interleukin-1, TNF, GM-CSF, and interferon (IFN)-γ are potent stimuli for the synthesis of MCP-1. RANTES was initially cloned from T cells. The production of RANTES by T cells is stimulated by specific antigens or mitogens. Subsequently, platelets were shown to contain RANTES, and release the chemokine after stimulation with thrombin (35) and PAF (36). MIP-1α is produced by monocytes, T cells, B cells, neutrophils, and airway epithelial cells. The production of RANTES and MIP-1α by T cells can be specifically stimulated by allergens in sensitive patients (36).

HRF and the C–C Chemokines

Recent studies from our laboratory and from two other groups have demonstrated that most species of HRF belong to the C–C chemokine family. We first evaluated monocyte chemotactic peptide–monocyte chemotactic and activating factor (MCP-1/MCAF) and demonstrated that MCP-1 was one of the most potent secretagogues for basophils (37). It

Table 2 Cellular Source of the C–C Chemokines

Chemokine	Source
MCP-1	Monocytes, macrophages
	Endothelial cells
	Epithelial cells
	Fibroblasts
	Keratinocytes
	Mesangial cells
	Synoviocytes
	Smooth muscle
	Tumor cells
MCP-2 (HC14) and MCP-3	Monocytes
	Osteosarcoma cells
MIP-1α and MIP-1β	T cells
	B cells
	Fibroblasts
	U937, HL-60
RANTES	T cells
	Platelets
I-309	T cells

induced histamine release from basophils obtained from allergic and from normal subjects in an IgE-independent manner. The quantity of histamine released by MCP-1 was correlated with the cellular response to crude HRF, but not with anti-IgE. Anti-MCP-1 antibody removed more than 50% of the histamine-releasing activity of crude HRF produced by blood mononuclear cells (MNC). Kuna et al. (38) and Bischoff et al. (39) confirmed these effects.

Subsequently, we and others demonstrated that MIP-1α (40) and RANTES (41) also had histamine-releasing activity, although these chemokines are significantly weaker secretagogues than MCP-1. Moreover, basophils from only some select donors responded to MIP-1α and RANTES. Recently, we reported that MCP-2, MCP-3, and FIC/MARC (homologous to human MCP-3) also had histamine-releasing activity (42). Similar to MCP-1, MCP-3 was active on basophils obtained from allergic and from nonallergic subjects. In a comparative study, we have observed that the order of histamine-releasing potency of all C–C chemokines is as follows: MCP-1 > MCP-3 > FIC > MIP-1 = RANTES > MCP-2 (Table 3). Finally we found that all C–C chemokines had an additive effect on allergen-induced histamine release.

The C–C chemokines are chemotactic for a variety of cells, both in vitro and in vivo. MCP-1, MCP-2, and MCP-3 cause chemotaxis of monocytes (43); RANTES induces directed migration of eosinophils (44), CD4, CD45 RO$^+$ T cells, and monocytes (45). MIP-1α attracts T cells (46), neutrophils (47), and basophils (40). MCP-3 has recently been shown to induce chemotaxis of eosinophils (48). Thus, the C–C chemokines attract cells that play a dominant role in the pathogenesis of allergic inflammation. MIP-1β, a T-cell chemotactic factor, has been expressed by endothelial cells of the small vessels (49), suggesting that this chemokine may directly promote cellular adhesion to the endothelium and, thereby, facilitate emigration. Whether other C–C chemokines are similarly involved in cell adhesion and migration is currently unknown.

Table 3 List of Cytokines with Histamine-Releasing Activity

Cytokine	Basophil		Mast cell direct release
	Direct release	Augmentation	
MCP-1	+++	−	−
MCP-3	+++	−	?
FIC/MARC	++	−	?
RANTES	++[a]	−	−
MIP-1α	++[a]	−	+
MCP-2	+[a]	−	?
IL-3	+[a]	+	−
GM-CSF	+[a]	+	−
Il-8	+[a]	−	−
CTAP-III/NAP-2	+[a]	−	−
c-*kit* ligand	−	+	+

[a]Select donors only.

C–C Chemokines and Basophil Cytokine Synthesis

Mast cells produce several cytokines that have potent immunoregulatory properties. We and others reported that basophils produce IL-4 after stimulation with anti-IgE (4,5). The effect of MCP-1 on basophil IL-4 synthesis was investigated by reverse-transcription polymerase chain reaction (PCR), which showed that MCP-1 induced the synthesis of mRNA for IL-4 in purified basophils. This observation is important from the standpoint that T_{H0} cells are poor producers of IL-4. MCP-1-dependent secretion of IL-4 by basophils could foster the generation of T_{H2} cells in a primary immune response. The T_{H2} cells, differentiated in this manner, could initiate and sustain the production of IgE by B cells.

C–C Chemokines and Mast Cell Activation

Crude and partially purified HRF was previously shown to degranulate lung cells (12). We studied MCP-1, RANTES, and MIP-1α for mast cell histamine release. Initially, murine peritoneal mast cells were used for this purpose. Only MIP-1α showed histamine-releasing activity when evaluated with peritoneal mast cells obtained from certain species of mice (40). Subsequently, chopped human lung tissue and dispersed lung cells were examined. Once again, MIP-1α was the only chemokine that induced histamine release from human lung mast cells (unpublished observation). Lung mast cells usually respond poorly to many known secretagogues compared with cutaneous and mucosal mast cells of the gastrointestinal tract. Therefore, it is possible that MCP-1 and RANTES may activate cutaneous or mucosal mast cells.

Production and Recovery of the C–C Chemokines from Tissue Effluents

The production of chemokines by human bronchoalveolar cells was investigated in allergic asthmatic patients and in normal controls by reverse-transcription PCR. We found that mRNAs for MCP-1, MCP-3, RANTES, and MIP-1α were produced by bronchoalveolar lavage (BAL) cells from all asthmatic and normal subjects (50). Interleukin-8 was synthesized by BAL cells from all asthmatic patients and by those from 50% of the normal subjects. The secretion of RANTES and MIP-1α was examined by enzyme-linked immunosorbent assay (ELISA). The mean levels of MCP-1, RANTES, MIP-1α, and IL-8 were 284 ± 84, 429 ± 91, 62 ± 35, and 2270 ± 521 pg/ml in the asthmatic group, and 100 ± 16, 178 ± 81, 6 ± 2.5, and 1460 ± 509 pg/ml in the healthy control group, respectively. The difference in the production of MCP-1, RANTES, and MIP-1α between the two groups were significant ($p < 0.05$). Thus, we have shown that chemokines are produced by BAL cells, and that increased production of MCP-1, RANTES, and MIP-1α is observed in patients with asthma.

The effect of nasal allergen challenge on the chemokine production was studied in allergic patients (51). Small amounts of MIP-1α were recovered during the immediate-phase, which increased considerably during the late-phase reaction. RANTES was detected in the late-phase nasal reaction. The detection of MIP-1α in the early-phase reaction may suggest a mast cell or macrophage origin. Treatment of the patients with a topical steroid improved symptom scores and significantly reduced the recovery of the C–C chemokines.

C–C Chemokines and Eosinophils

We studied the effect of MCP-1, MIP-1α, and RANTES on eosinophil chemotaxis. MIP-1α had modest chemotactic activity, but RANTES was strongly chemotactic for eosinophils (44). Furthermore, RANTES activated eosinophils and induced the secretion of ECP. Eosinophils became hypodense after incubation with RANTES. The latter observation suggests that RANTES induces a generalized state of activation of eosinophils. More recently, we found that eosinophils produce RANTES (Alam R, et al., submitted). Thus, RANTES could induce a self-sustained inflammatory response.

Activity of the C–C Chemokines In Vivo

Partially purified HRF induces immediate cutaneous and bronchial responses in humans (52). To determine the in vivo activity of the C–C chemokines, we used the mouse footpad-swelling reaction as the model for inflammation. The injection of MCP-1 and MIP-1α into the mouse footpad induced an immediate swelling response, beginning at 30 min, that evolved into a sustained late-phase reaction lasting 6 h (53). Similar to the human cutaneous immediate- and late-allergic reactions, the footpad-swelling reaction was not biphasic, and the immediate phase evolved into the late phase. Light microscopic examination of the footpad obtained at 2 h showed that MIP-1α induced an intense inflammatory reaction consisting of neutrophils and mononuclear cells. MCP-1 induced only minor soft-tissue swelling, but no cellular infiltrates. Electron microscopy demonstrated that MIP-1α induced intense degranulation of the majority of the mast cells, whereas MCP-1 only modestly caused mast cell activation. Thus, we demonstrated that both MIP-1α and MCP-1 were active in vivo. RANTES has also induced a cutaneous eosinophilic inflammation when injected in dogs (54).

Interleukin-8 and MIP-1α are chemotactic for neutrophils, whereas RANTES attracts and activates eosinophils. We and others detected increased concentrations of IL-8 in the BAL fluid from asthmatic patients; however, eosinophils, not neutrophils, are characteristics of allergic inflammation. To understand this paradox, we recently investigated chemokine levels in tissue effluents from sites of neutrophil-rich inflammation. We studied synovial fluids obtained from patients with rheumatoid arthritis (55); the ratios of RANTES/MIP-1α/IL-8 in the synovial fluid from patients with rheumatoid arthritis and osteoarthritis were 4:6:80 and 1:0.2:13, respectively. Thus, there were 4-, 30-, and 6-fold increase in RANTES, MIP-1α, and IL-8, respectively, in rheumatoid arthritis, compared with osteoarthritis. The ratios of RANTES/MIP-1α/IL-8 in the BAL fluid were 4:0.6:22 in asthmatic patients, and 1:0.06:11 in healthy controls. The increase in RANTES, MIP-1α, and IL-8 were four-, ten-, and two-fold higher, respectively, in asthmatics compared with the controls. We believe that the ratio of RANTES to MIP-1α and IL-8 favors eosinophilic inflammation in bronchial asthma, whereas it favors neutrophilic inflammation in rheumatoid arthritis. Also, the production sequence of the chemokines may be of importance. Some of the receptors for chemokines are promiscuous (56), and there is significant cross-desensitization among the members of the chemokine family. Thus, the chemokine that is produced first may desensitize cells to the effect of other chemokines.

HISTAMINE-RELEASE INHIBITORY FACTOR

We described a histamine-release inhibitory factor produced by human mononuclear cells (57,58). This inhibitory factor blocked activation of basophils by histamine-releasing factors, but not by other secretagogues, such as anti-IgE, C5a, and formyl-methionyl-leucyl-phenylalanine (FMLP). After high-performance liquid chromatographic (HPLC) purification and sodium dodecyl sulfate–polyacrylamide gel electrophoresis (SDS–PAGE) analysis, HRIF had two prominent forms, 8–12 kDa and 41 kDa in apparent size. Our subsequent studies showed that the smaller HRIF could probably be attributed to IL-8 (59). Both IL-8 and HRIF had a similar molecular size, and had an identical retention time on C4 reverse-phase HPLC. Interleukin-8 inhibited histamine release induced with MNC-derived HRF and defined cytokines such as MCP-1, but did not inhibit C5a and anti-IgE. The molecular basis of this inhibition can be explained by the existence of promiscuous receptors for these chemokines on cell surfaces. It is likely that the binding of one chemokine to the receptor desensitizes the cell to the other chemokines (homologous desensitization). Inhibition of cytokine-induced basophil histamine release was observed with other chemokines that had lower intrinsic activity.

CONCLUDING REMARKS

The identification of the majority of HRF with the C–C chemokines underscores the importance and potential pathogenetic implications of these cytokines. The hallmark of allergic inflammation is infiltration with eosinophils, mast cells, basophils, and T cells (60). The C–C chemokines may play a crucial role in the chemotaxis of these effector cells to the site of allergic inflammation. Furthermore, some of the C–C chemokines activate basophils, eosinophils, and mast cells. The activation of basophils and mast cells by the C–C chemokines in a primary immune response may result in the production of IL-4, thereby setting the stage for the generation of T_{H2} cells and IgE production. Eosinophil-derived toxic proteins, such as major basic protein (MBP) and cationic protein (ECP), are frequently detected in the sputum and BAL fluids from asthmatic patients (61). RANTES may play an important role in the activation of eosinophils in this condition. Thus, regulation of the C–C chemokines may hold the key to our success in combating allergic disease.

REFERENCES

1. Alam R, Grant JA. Basophils: biology and function in airway disease. In: Busse W, Holgate ST, eds. Asthma and Rhinitis. Cambridge: Blackwell Scientific, 1994.
2. Plaut M, Pierce JH, Watson CJ, Hanley-Hyde J, Nordan RP, Paul WE. Mast cell lines produce

lymphokines in response to cross-linkage of FcεRI or to calcium ionophores. Nature 1989; 339: 64–67.

3. Gordon JR, Burd PR, Galli SJ. Mast cells as a source of multifunctional cytokines. Immunol Today 1990; 11:458–464.

4. Brunner T, Heusser CH, Dahinden CA. Human peripheral blood basophils primed by IL-3 produce IL-4 in response to immunoglobulin E receptor stimulation. J Exp Med 1993; 177: 605–611.

5. Lett-Brown MA, Li H, Stafford S, Hilsmeier K, Sim T, Grant JA, Alam R. Human basophils produce IL-4 in response to anti-IgE (abstr). J Allergy Clin Immunol 1993; 91:257.

6. Gauchat J-F, Henchoz S, Mazzel G, Aubry J-P, Brunner T, Blasey H, Life P, Talabot D, Flores-Remo L, Thompson J, Kishi K, Butterfield J, Dahinden C, Bonnefoy JY. Induction of human IgE synthesis in B cells by mast cells and basophils. Nature 1993; 365:340–343.

7. Mosmann TR, Cherwinski H, Bond MW, Gieldin MA, Coffman RL. Two types of murine helper T cell clone: I. Definition according to profiles of lymphokine activities and secreted proteins. J Immunol 1986; 136:2348–2357.

8. Gao CB, Liu MC, Galli SJ, Kagey-Sobotka A, Lichtenstein LM. The histamine containing cells in the late phase response in the lung are basophils (abstr). J Allergy Clin Immunol 1990; 85:172.

9. Thueson DO, Speck LS, Lett-Brown MA, Grant JA. Histamine-releasing activity (HRA). I. Production by mitogen- or antigen-stimulated human mononuclear cells. J Immunol 1979; 123: 626–632.

10. Grant JA, Alam R, Lett-Brown MA. Histamine-releasing factors and inhibitors: historical perspectives and possible implications in human illness. J Allergy Clin Immunol 1991; 88:683–693.

11. Dvorak AM, Lett-Brown MA, Thueson DO, Pyne K, Raghuprasad PK, Galli SJ, Grant JA. Histamine releasing activity (HRA) III. HRA induces human basophil histamine release by provoking noncytotoxic granule exocytosis. Clin Immunol Immunopathol 1984; 32:142–150.

12. Ezeamuzie IC, Assem ES. A study of histamine release from basophils by products of lymphocyte stimulation. Agents Actions 1985; 13:222–230.

13. Alam R, Forsythe PA, Lett-Brown MA, Grant JA. Cellular origin of histamine releasing factor produced by peripheral blood mononuclear cells. J Immunol 1989; 142:3951–3956.

14. Liu MC, Proud D, Lichtenstein LM, et al. Human lung macrophage-derived histamine-releasing activity is due to IgE-dependent factors. J Immunol 1986; 136:2588–2595.

15. Schulman ES, McGettigan MC, Post TJ, Vigderman RJ, Shapiro SS. Human monocytes generate basophil histamine releasing activities. J Immunol 1988; 7:2369–2375.

16. Orchard MA, Kagey-Sobotka A, Proud D, Lichtenstein LM. Basophil histamine release induced by a substance from stimulated human platelets. J Immunol 1986; 136:2240–2244.

17. White MV, Kaplan AP, Haak-Frendscho M, Kaliner MA. Neutrophils and mast cells: comparison of neutrophil-derived histamine-releasing activity with other histamine-releasing factors. J Immunol 1988; 141:3575–3583.

18. Alam R, Rozniecki J, Selmaj K. A mononuclear cell-derived histamine releasing factor (HRF) in asthmatic patients. Histamine release from basophils in vitro. Ann Allergy 1984; 53:66–69.

19. Alam R, Kuna P, Rozniecki J, Kuzminska B. The magnitude of the spontaneous production of histamine releasing factor (HRF) by lymphocytes in vitro correlates with the state of bronchial hyperreactivity in asthmatic patients. J Allergy Clin Immunol 1987; 79:103–108.

20. Kuna P, Alam R, Kuzminska B, Rozniecki J. The effect of preseasonal immunotherapy on the production of histamine-releasing factor (HRF) by mononuclear cells from patients with seasonal asthma: results of a double-blind, placebo-controlled, randomized study. J Allergy Clin Immunol 1989; 83:816–824.

21. Brunet C, Bedard PM, Lavoie A, Jobin M, Hebert J. Allergic rhinitis to ragweed pollen. II. Modulation of histamine-releasing factor production by specific immunotherapy. J Allergy Clin Immunol 1992; 89:87–94.

22. Sampson HA, Broabent KR, Bernhisel-Broadbent J. Spontaneous basophil histamine release and histamine releasing factor in patients with atopic dermatitis and food hypersensitivity. N Engl J Med 1989; 321:228–232.

23. Warner JA, Pienkowski MM, Plaut M, Norman PS, Lichtenstein LM. Identification of a histamine-releasing factor in the late phase of cutaneous IgE-mediated reactions. J Immunol 1986; 136:2583–2587.

24. Jacques P, Lavoie A, Bedard P-M, Brunet C, Hebert J. Chronic idiopathic urticaria: profiles of skin mast cell histamine release during active disease and remission. J Allergy Clin Immunol 1982; 89:1139–1143.

25. Sim TC, Alam R, Forsythe PA, Welter JB, Lett-Brown MA, Grant JA. Measurement of histamine-releasing a factor activity in individual nasal washings: relationship with atopy, basophil response and membrane-bound IgE. J Allergy Clin Immunol 1992; 89:1157–1165.

26. Alam R, Welter J, Forsythe PA, Lett-Brown MA, Rankin JA, Boyars M, Grant JA. Detection of histamine release inhibitory factor- and histamine releasing factor-like activities in broncho-alveolar lavage fluids. Am Rev Respir Dis 1990; 141:666–671.

27. MacDonald SM, Lichtenstein LM, Proud D, Plaut M, Naclerio RM, MacGlashan DW, Kagey-Sobotka A. Studies of IgE-dependent histamine releasing factors: heterogeneity of IgE. J Immunol 1987; 139:506–512.

28. Lichtenstein LM. Histamine releasing factor and IgE heterogeneity. J Allergy Clin Immunol 1988; 81:814–820.

29. Lett-Brown MA, Thueson DO, Plank DE, Duffy LK, Grant JA. Histamine releasing activity (HRA). V. Characterization and purification using high performance liquid chromatography. Cell Immunol 1984; 87:445–451.

30. Baeza ML, Reddigari S, Haak-Frendscho M, Kaplan AP. Purification and further characterization of human mononuclear cell histamine-releasing factor. J Clin Invest 1989; 83:1204–1210.

31. Haak-Frendscho M, Arai N, Arai K-I, Baeza ML, Finn A, Kaplan AP. Human recombinant granulocyte–macrophage colony stimulating factor and interleukin 3 cause basophil histamine release. J Clin Invest 1988; 82:17–22.

32. Alam R, Welter JB, Forsythe PA, Lett-Brown MA, Grant JA. Comparative effect of recombinant IL-1, -2, -3, -4, and -6, IFN-γ, granulocyte–macrophage colony-stimulating factor, tumor necrosis factor-α, and histamine-releasing factors on the secretion of histamine from basophils. J Immunol 1989; 142:3431.

33. Baggiolini M, Dewald B, Moser B. Interleukin-8 and chemotactic cytokines—CXC and CC chemokines. Adv Immunol 1993; 55:97–179.

34. Baggiolini M, Dahinden CA. CC chemokines in allergic inflammation. Immunol Today 1994; 15:127–133.

35. Kameyoshi Y, Doorschner A, Mallet AI, Christophers E, Schroder J-M. Cytokine RANTES released by thrombin-stimulated platelets is a potent attractant for human eosinophils. J Exp Med 1992; 176:587–592.

36. Forsythe P, Alam R, Nevils Y. Characterization of RANTES secretion by mononuclear cells and platelets: differential stimulation of secretion by allergens, PAF, Con A and thrombin. FASEB J 1994; 8:A764.

37. Alam R, Lett-Brown MA, Forsythe PA, Anderson-Walters D, Kenamore C, Kormos C, Grant JA. Monocyte chemotactic and activating factor is a potent histamine-releasing factor for basophils. J Clin Invest 1992; 89:723–728.

38. Kuna P, Reddigari SR, Rucinski D, Oppenheim JJ, Kaplan AP. Monocyte chemotactic and activating factor is a potent histamine-releasing factor for human basophils. J Exp Med 1992; 175:489–493.

39. Bischoff SC, Krieger M, Brunner T, Dahinden CA. Monocyte chemotactic protein 1 is a potent activator of human basophils. J Exp Med 1992; 175:1271–1275.

40. Alam R, Forsythe P, Lett-Brown MA, Grant JA. Macrophage inflammatory protein-1α is an activator of basophils and mast cells. J Exp Med 1992; 176:781–786.

41. Kuna P, Reddigari SR, Schall TJ, Rucinski D, Viksman MY, Kaplan AP. RANTES, a monocyte and T lymphocyte chemotactic cytokine releases histamine from human basophils. J Immunol 1992; 149:636–642.

42. Alam R, Forsythe P, Stafford S, Heinrich J, Bravo R, Proost P, Van Damme J. Monocyte

chemotactic protein-2 (MCP-2), monocyte chemotactic protein-3 (MCP-3), and fibroblast-induced cytokine, three novel chemokines, induce histamine release from basophils. J Immunol (in press).

43. Opdenakker G, Froyen G, Fiten P, Proost P, Van Damme J. Human monocyte chemotactic protein-3 (MCP-3): molecular cloning of the cDNA and comparison with other cytokines. Biophys Biochem Res Commun 1993; 191:535–542.

44. Alam R, Stafford S, Forsythe P, Grant JA. RANTES is a chemotactic and activating factor for eosinophils. J Immunol 1993; 150:3442–3447.

45. Schall TJ, Bacon K, Toy KJ, Goeddel DV. Selective attraction of monocytes and T lymphocytes of the memory phenotype by cytokine RANTES. Nature 1990; 347:669–671.

46. Taub DD, Conlon K, Lloyd AR, Oppenheim JJ, Kelvin DJ. Preferential migration of activated $CD4^+$ and $CD8^+$ T cells in response to MIP-1α and MIP-1β. Science 1993; 260:355–358.

47. Wolpe SD, Cerami A. Macrophage inflammatory proteins 1 and 2: members of a novel superfamily of cytokines. FASEB J 1989; 3:2565–2571.

48. Dahinden CA, Geiser T, Brunner T, Von Tscharner V, Caput D, Ferrara P, Minty A, Baggiolini M. Monocyte chemotactic protein 3 is a most effective basophil- and eosinophil-activating chemokine. J Exp Med 1994; 179:751–756.

49. Tanaka Y, Adams DH, Hubscher S, Hirano H, Siebenlist U, Shaw S. T cell adhesion induced by proteoglycan-immobilized cytokine MIP-1β. Nature 1993; 361:79–82.

50. Alam R, York J, Boyars M, Grant JA, Stafford S, Forsythe P, Lee J, Weido A. The involvement of chemokines in bronchial asthma. The detection of the mRNA for MCP-1, MCP-3, RANTES, MIP-1α, and IL-8 in bronchoalveolar lavage cells and the measurement of RANTES and MIP-1α in the lavage fluid. Am Rev Respir Crit Care Med 1994; 149:A951.

51. Bitticks L, Hilsmeier K, Schreiber D, Sim T. Secretion profile of IL-1β, GM-CSF, and chemokines (IL-8, MIP-1α, and RANTES) in allergen-induced nasal responses: inhibition by topical steroids. J Allergy Clin Immunol 1994; 93:270.

52. Alam R, Rozniecki J. A mononuclear cell-derived histamine-releasing factor in asthmatic patients. Activity in vivo. Allergy 1985; 40:124–129.

53. Alam R, Kumar D, Anderson-Walters D, Forsythe PA. Macrophage inflammatory protein-1α and monocyte chemoattractant protein-1 elicit immediate and late cutaneous reactions and activate mast cells in vivo. J Immunol 1994; 152:1298–1303.

54. Meurer R, Van Riper G, Feeney W, Cunningham P, Hora D Jr, Springer MS, MacIntyre DE, Rosen H. Formation of eosinophilic and monocytic intradermal inflammatory sites in the dog by injection of human RANTES, but not human MCP-1, MIP-1α, or human IL-8. J Exp Med 1993; 178:1913–1921.

55. Baethge B, Forsythe P, Lisse JR, Alam R. Macrophage inflammatory protein-1α, RANTES and IL-8 in synovial fluids. FASEB J 1994; 8:A760.

56. Neote K, DiGregorio D, Mak JY, Horuk R, Schall TJ. Molecular cloning, functional expression, and signaling characteristics of a C–C chemokine receptor. Cell 1993; 72:425–425.

57. Alam R, Lewis DM, Olenchock. Identification of a histamine release inhibitory factor (HRIF) and an inhibitor of histamine releasing factor (HRF) synthesis (IHS) produced simultaneously by guinea-pig lymphoid cells. Cell Immunol 1988; 115:447–459.

58. Alam R, Grant JA, Lett-Brown MA. Identification of a histamine release inhibitory factor (HRIF) produced by human mononuclear cells in vitro. J Clin Invest 1988; 82:2056–2062.

59. Alam R, Forsythe PA, Lett-Brown MA, Grant JA. Interleukin 8 and RANTES inhibit basophil histamine release induced with monocyte chemotactic and activating factor and histamine-releasing factor. Am J Respir Cell Mol Biol 1992; 7:427–433.

60. Djukanovic R, Roche WR, Wilson JW, Beasley CRW, Twentyman OP, Howard PW, Holgate ST. Mucosal inflammation in asthma. Am Rev Respir Dis 1990; 142:434–457.

61. Frigas E, Gleich GJ. The eosinophil and the pathophysiology of asthma. J Allergy Clin Invest 1986; 77:527–537.

16

IL-2, IL-4, IL-6, IL-10, IFN-γ, Their Receptors, Modulation of Their Actions, and Role in Allergic Responses

Toshio Tanaka, Yoshinori Katada, Hiroshi Ochi, Masaki Suemura, and Tadamitsu Kishimoto
Osaka University Medical School, Osaka, Japan

INTRODUCTION

Cytokines are a set of molecules that communicate between cells in immune and hemato-poietic systems. These proteins exert their biological functions through their binding to specific receptors and by inducing biochemical signals on target cells. Recent progress in the cytokine research over the last 5 years has revealed that most cytokines and their receptors have been identified at the molecular level and that cytokines have important functions in many physiological responses and in the pathophysiology of many diseases (1,2).

The type 1 (immediate) allergic response is characterized by a hyperproduction of specific immunoglobulin (Ig)E in response to environmental allergens, such as house dust mite, pollen, animal dander, and others, and the interaction of allergen with specific IgE on the Fcε receptor I (FcεRI)-expressing cells induces the activation and infiltration of inflammatory cells (3). In this process cytokines also play a major role by regulating IgE synthesis and inflammatory cell function. In this chapter we will review cytokines—especially interleukin (IL)-2, IL-4, IL-6, IL-10, and interferon (IFN)-γ—their receptors, and their roles in allergic responses.

CYTOKINES, THEIR RECEPTORS, AND SIGNAL TRANSDUCTION

Cytokines (IL-2, IL-4, IL-6, IL-10, and IFN-γ)

With cloning of cytokine genes, utilization of recombinant cytokines, neutralizing anti-bodies, and the technology of the transgenic or knockout mouse, in which the target gene (of cytokine or its receptor) is overexpressed or disrupted, reveal its biological functions not only in vitro but also in vivo. Table 1 lists the property of five of these molecules and their major functions (of considerable importance is the functions of these cytokines on the

Table 1 Properties of IL-2, IL-4, IL-6, IL-10, and IFN-γ

Cytokine	Cell source	Molecular mass	Biological function
IL-2	T cells (naive and T_H1)	14–16 kDa	Stimulates T-, B-, and NK-cell growth and differentiation
IL-4	T_H2 cells, basophils, mast cells	20 kDa	Stimulates T-cell growth, induces T_H2 differentiation, promotes B-cell activation, isotype-switching for IgG4 and IgE; induces CD23 expression, enhances class II MHC antigen expression
IL-6	Ubiquitous; mainly macrophages, T_H2 cells	22–29 kDa	Induces B-cell differentiation, and growth of plasma cells, induces acute-phase proteins, promotes megakaryocyte maturation
IL-10	T_H2 cells, B cells	20 kDa	Induces B-cell growth and differentiation, inhibits monokine and IFN-γ synthesis
IFN-γ	T cells (T_H1), NK cells	20–25 kDa	Inhibits viral replication, activates macrophages

process of the allergic responses, which will be discussed). It should be pointed out that each cytokine as shown in the table shows a variety of actions on different target cells and also on the same cells (pleiotropy) and a different cytokine exerts the same action on the responding cells (redundancy); for instance not only IL-2, but also IL-4 induces T-cell growth. These cytokines are briefly reviewed in the following.

IL-2

Interleukin-2 was originally defined as a T-cell growth factor produced by lymphocytes in response to antigen or mitogen stimulation (4). It is synthesized mainly by T cells and natural killer (NK) cells. Among cytokines, it shows a comparatively limited range of activity in lymphoid cells: thymocyte, T, B, and NK cell growth and differentiation and in activation of monocytes (5). Clinical trials of IL-2 have been in progress, with an expectation of its anti-tumor effect mediated by activation of NK—lymphokine-activated killer (LAK)—cells. Therapy with IL-2 results in 10–20% objective responses in patients with metastatic renal cell carcinoma or malignant melanoma (6).

IL-4

Interleukin-4 was initially described as a T-cell-derived costimulation factor that augmented proliferation of murine B cells stimulated by submitogenic doses of anti-IgM antibody (7). It is produced by helper T cells (T_H2 cells) and IgE Fc-receptor type 1 ($Fc_\varepsilon RI$)-positive cells such as mast cells and basophils (8–10). IL-4 shows a wide range of functions on responding cell populations (11); induction of T-cell growth, promoting differentiation of naive T cells into T_H2 cells, inhibiting IL-2-induced IFN-γ production by NK cells, activation of resting B cells, enhancement of expression of major histocompatibility complex (MHC) class II and CD23 expression, induction of class-switching for IgE and IgG4(human) or IgG1(mouse), modulating colony formation by hematopoietic precursor cells, and induction of vascular cell adhesion molecule (VCAM) and suppressing intracellular adhesion molecule (ICAM)-1 expression by endothelial cells (12). IL-4 is also involved in the induction of cytotoxic T cells and NK cells. IL-4, IL-13, IL-5, granulocyte–macrophage colony-stimulating factor (GM-CSF), and IL-3 are very closely related molecules, based on the several types of evidence (13). The genes for these cytokines are located on human chromosome 5q23–31 and mouse chromosome 11. The exon structure of their genes is very similar, and homology of primary sequences has been demonstrated. These cytokines are produced by similar cell types. Recently, Marsh et al. (14) have shown that there is a close linkage of this region (chromosome 5q23–31) with an elevated level of IgE in atopic patients.

So far, clinical phase II study of IL-4 in patients with malignant tumors, including multiple myeloma, showed no objective response (15). Biological responses of IL-4 treatment include a striking increase of IL-1R antagonist and soluble CD23.

IL-6

Interleukin-6 was originally identified as a B-cell differentiation factor that induces the final maturation of B cells into antibody-producing cells (16). However, a series of subsequent studies have revealed that this cytokine functions not only in the immune system, but also in the hematopoietic, endocrine, hepatic, and even neural systems (17,18). It promotes proliferation of many cells, including myeloma/hybridoma/plasmacytomas, T cells, Epstein–Barr virus (EBV)-transformed B cells, mesangial cells, keratinocytes, and hematopoietic cells. It inhibits growth of myeloid leukemic cell lines and breast carcinoma cell lines. IL-6 induces neural differentiation of PC12 cells, cytotoxic T-cell differentiation, megakaryocyte maturation, macrophage differentiation of myeloid leukemic cell lines, immunoglobulin production by activated B cells, and production of acute-phase proteins in hepatocytes. It is also associated with osteoporosis by activating osteoclasts. IL-6 is synthesized by a wide variety of cells, including lymphocytes, monocytes, fibroblasts, bone marrow stromal cells, mesangial cells, keratinocytes and endothelial cells. Its overproduction is reported to be associated with pathogenesis of a variety of diseases, such as cardiac myxoma, rheumatoid arthritis, Castleman's disease, multiple myeloma, Lennert's T-cell lymphoma, mesangial proliferative glomerulonephritis, and development of acquired immunodeficiency syndrome (AIDS) Kaposi's sarcoma.

The inhibitory effect of tumor growth in some malignant neoplasms and its hematopoietic effect of IL-6 provided a rationale for clinical testing of this cytokine. The main hematological effect of IL-6 in vivo is a significant increase (200%) in platelet counts; but as yet no objective antitumor response has been achieved in a phase I trial (15).

IL-10

Interleukin-10 was originally described as a T_H2 cell-derived factor that inhibits cytokine synthesis by T_H1 cells (19). It is now known to be produced by T_H2 cells, monocytes, activated B cells, mast cells, and basophils (20). IL-10 inhibits production of monokines and IFN-γ. It inhibits or augments expression of MHC class II molecules by monocytes or B cells, respectively. IL-10 enhances activated B cell growth and immunoglobulin production. It acts on mast cells, leading to its prolonged survival.

IFN-γ

The IFNs were initially shown to have antiviral activities (21). IFN-γ is synthesized by T cells and NK cells. In addition to its antiviral activity, it shows multiple functions: antiproliferative activity on tumor cells, induction of MHC class I or II molecules, activation of monocytes and NK cells, and inhibition of osteoclast activation (22). It inhibits IL-4-induced CD23 expression and IgE synthesis by B cells. Thus, in many aspects IFN-γ counteracts functions of IL-4.

Treatment with IFN-γ has been effective in many forms of neoplasia, infectious diseases, and chronic granulomatous diseases. Its clinical trials in allergic diseases will be discussed later.

The Cytokine Receptor and Its Signal Transduction

Recent progress of molecular cloning of cytokine receptors, their associated molecules, and their signal transducers, and the analyses of signaling pathways revealed a molecular basis for the characteristic feature of cytokines: pleiotropy and redundancy (23).

Cytokine receptors now fall into several families, based on their structure (Fig. 1) (1,2). Most of the cytokine receptors, including IL-2Rβ, IL-2Rγ (γc), IL-4R, IL-6R, and its signal transducer, gp130, fall into the type 1 cytokine receptor family, the extracellular domain of which contains two fibronectin type 3 domains, with a set of four spaced cysteines and a WSXWS motif in the membrane-distal and membrane-proximal domain. The type 2 cytokine receptor family includes IL-10 and interferon receptors and has one or two similar domains at the extracellular portion, with a set of spaced cysteines, but without a WSXWS motif.

Functional IL-2R exists at two forms (24): the high-affinity form of IL-2R(K_d = 10–50 pM) is made up of an α-chain (Tac antigen, 55 kDa) (25), a β-chain (70–75 kDa) (26), and a γ-chain (65 kDa) (27). In some cells, such as NK cells or resting T cells, intermediate-

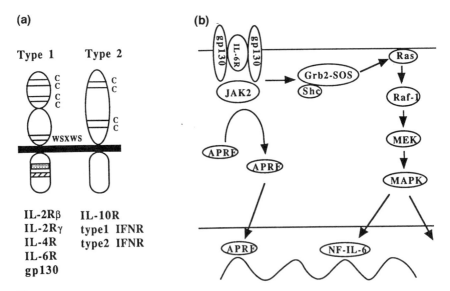

Figure 1 Cytokine receptor and its signal transduction: (a) Cytokine receptors fall into several families; IL-2R β- and γ-chain, IL-4R, IL-6R, and its signal transducer, gp130 belong to the type 1 family. The type 2 family includes IL-10R and IFNRs. (b) Signaling pathway through the cytokine receptor; as with IL-6 signal transduction, two major pathways have been demonstrated. Stimulation of JAK2 leads to an activation of APRF (STAT3) or other transcriptional regulators, including NF-IL-6 through a phosphorylation cascade.

affinity form of IL-2R (K_d = 1–5 nM), consisting of a β- and a γ-chain appears to be expressed. In T cells antigen or mitogen stimulation induces a dramatic expression of the α-chain, leading to an increased number of high-affinity IL-2R.

IL-4R is 140-kDa molecule with a K_d of 20–300 pM (28). It forms a complex with IL-2Rγ (γc) chain to provide its signaling (29).

IL-6R is an 80-kDa molecule and exists at two forms on responding cells: high-affinity (K_d = 10 pM) and low-affinity (700 pM) (30). IL-6 can exert its function by binding to membrane IL-6R as well as to the soluble form of IL-6R, leading to the homodimerization of gp130 (31).

In the IL-10 receptor system, one chain (α-chain) has been recently cloned (32), but it has been postulated that an uncloned associated molecule is required for the formation of a high-affinity receptor to IL-10 by forming the complex with cloned IL-10R.

IFN-γR (type 2 IFN-R) (33) is a 90-kDa molecule, with a K_d of 0.1–1 nM, but it seems that an accessory molecule is also required for its functional receptor.

The redundancy of cytokine function is now explained by the existence of a common signal transducer, such as gp130, βc, and γc (2,34). The gp130 molecule was first demonstrated as a signal transducer that is commonly used for IL-6R, oncostatin-MR, leukemia inhibitory factor (LIF)R, ciliary neurotrophic factor (CNTF)R, and, perhaps, IL-11R. Similarly, βc is shared with IL-3R, IL-5R, and GM-CSFR; and IL-2, IL-4, IL-7, and perhaps, IL-9 also use common γc in association with its unique receptor for its signaling. Mutations or deletions of γc genes are primary causes of X-linked severe combined immunodeficiency in patients whose maturation of T cells is defective (35). In the IL-6 and CNTF system, the complex of ligand and soluble form of its receptor is also capable of inducing signaling, but in many other systems, it seems that soluble forms of receptors inhibit signal transduction by inhibiting ligand binding to the membrane receptor, thus indicating that transmembrane and intracytoplasmic domains of both IL-6R and CNTFR are not required for transmitting their signals, and these complexes, even in the soluble form, are believed to trigger the formation of homo- or heterodimers of gp130 (36). In contrast, in other cytokine receptors the cytoplasmic portion is certainly essential for the signal transduction as well as the existence of a common signal transducer, such as βc or γc.

The characteristic pleiotropy of cytokines may also be explained by the recent discovery of (at least) two signaling pathways of cytokine receptors (37). Figure 1 shows the IL-6 signaling pathway as one representative.

The binding of a growth factor induces receptor oligomerization and activation of the Janus kinase (JAK) family of cytoplasmic tyrosine kinases. The activated JAKs phosphorylate the receptor as well as cytoplasmic proteins belonging to a family of transcription factors, called the signal transducer and activators of transcription (STATs; in the IL-6 system, APRF or STAT3; 38), leading to the activation of the target gene(s). The second pathway is mediated by the stimulation of Ras-dependent mitogen-activated protein (MAP) kinase cascade, initiated by the interaction of phosphorylated Shc with Grb2. Grb2, in turn, is shown to bind tightly to Sos through SH3 domain, and then the complex can activate Ras, leading to the activation of a serine–threonine–tyrosine phosphorylation cascade in which Raf, MAPK/ERK, and MAP kinases are sequentially phosphorylated. This second pathway finally leads to the stimulation of the transcription factor(s), such as NF-IL-6 in the IL-6 signaling pathway (39). These activated transcriptional factors then stimulate or inhibit targeted gene activation.

For IL-2 and IL-4 signaling, JAK3 kinase is perhaps a mediator and IL-4 STAT has been recently cloned (40). The binding of IFN-γ to its receptor induces activation of JAK1 and

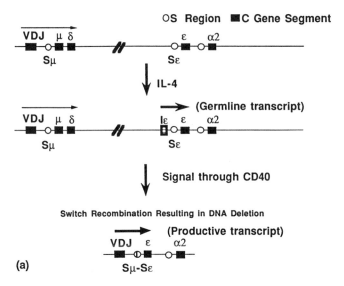

Figure 2 Mechanisms regulating IgE synthesis: (a) Molecular basis of class-switching to the ε gene. The immunoglobulin heavy chain gene of resting mature B cells is made up of rearranged VDJ and unrearranged C_H region. IL-4, by acting on B cells, induces expression of germline transcript of Cε gene, consisting of Iε and Cε. The signal through CD40 activates the mechanisms for switching recombination, leading to Sμ–Sε recombination and then productive transcript of the Cε gene, consisting of VDJ, and Cε is expressed. (b) A variety of cytokines modulate IgE synthesis: TNF-α, IL-5, IL-6, IL-9, and the soluble form of CD23 up-regulate IgE production, whereas IFN-α, IFN-γ, IL-8, IL-12, and TGF-β inhibit its synthesis.

JAK2 (41,42), leading to the stimulation of STAT1 (43). However, IL-10-mediated signaling still remains to be determined.

ALLERGIC RESPONSES

The principal characteristic feature of allergic individuals is the capacity to produce IgE response to environmental allergens, which is usually accompanied by an elevated total serum IgE level (3). Predisposition to allergy appears to result from interaction of genetic factors with environmental ones. In allergic patients, this overproduced IgE is captured by mast cells, basophils, or other cells expressing FcεRI. Allergen then activates these cells by cross-linking of FcεRI by an allergen-specific IgE, leading to the release of chemical mediators, such as histamines, leukotrienes, chemotactic factors, and cytokines. Thus, allergic reaction can be divided into two phases: IgE production phase (afferent phase) and inflammatory phase (effector phase). The functional roles of cytokines in this process will be discussed next.

Immunoglobulin E Synthesis and Cytokines

Induction of IgE synthesis by purified B cells requires two stimulants: a class-switching factor IL-4 and an activator for the switching recombination mechanisms at the DNA level (Fig. 2A; 44). Interleukin-4, when acting on B cells, induces expression of germline

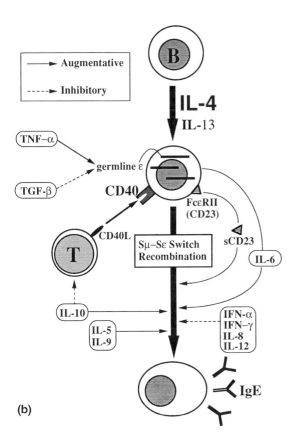

(b)

transcript of Cε gene, made up of an intervening exon (Iε) and Cε, perhaps by activation of IL-4 STAT (45). In general, this transcript is not translated into protein, thus it is also called a sterile transcript. Although the exact role of this transcript in the switching process remains to be determined, it is believed that its appearance is essential for the following S–S recombination, since the disruption of I exon (Iγ1) causes failure of class-switching to γ1 (46). The second signal has been generated by LPS (47), EBV infection (48), or activated T cells (49) and, recently, it has become clear that the physiological responsive molecule for generating the second signal is CD40 (50), which belongs to a family of tumor necrosis factor–nerve growth factor receptor (TNF, NGFR) (51). The signals through CD40 lead to actual recombination of the switching regions between μ and ε, after which a productive transcript of Cε, consisting of VDJ and Cε, is expressed. However, the precise mechanisms of signal transduction by CD40 that lead to S–S recombination are not yet clarified. The molecule that physiologically interacts and activates CD40 expressed on B cells is the recently cloned CD40 ligand (CD40L), or gp39 (52,53). Mutations or deletions of CD40L genes are primary causes for X-linked hyper-IgM immunodeficiency in patients whose serum levels of IgG, IgA, and IgE are decreased or lacked (54–58).

In this IgE-inducing system, other cytokines have also been demonstrated to modulate its synthesis (see Fig. 2B). IFN-α, IFN-γ, TGF-β, IL-8, and IL-12 inhibit its production, whereas TNF-α, IL-5, IL-6, IL-9 and soluble products of CD23 (FcεRII) enhance IgE synthesis by peripheral blood mononuclear cells stimulated by IL-4 or B cells with anti-

CD40 antibody plus IL-4 (59–66). The mechanisms through which these cytokines affect IgE production are unclear, but transforming growth factor (TGF)-β or TNF-α inhibit or enhance IgE secretion by down-regulating or up-regulating, respectively, expression of a germline transcript of the Cε gene. IFN-γ in mouse counteracts IL-4 in the induction of Cε germline transcript (67), but in humans the acting point of IFN-γ on the inhibition of IgE production remains unknown. IL-10 augments IgE synthesis independently of IL-6 by B cells incubated with anti-CD40 plus IL-4, whereas it is reported to inhibit IL-4-induced IgE secretion by peripheral mononuclear cells (68). Interleukin-6, which is endogenously produced by stimulated B cells is capable of enhancing expression of productive transcript without affecting Cε germline expression, thereby acting as a B-cell differentiation factor. In the mouse, IL-2 inhibits IL-4 plus LPS-induced IgE secretion (69), but the inhibitory effect of IL-2 in human IgE synthesis is less clear. In the human system, IL-13 is also capable of inducing expression of a germline transcript of Cε by B cells in the absence of IL-4 (70), but it seems that it does not function in the mouse system.

In addition to regulation of IgE synthesis by cytokines, adhesion molecules also affect its synthesis by B cells stimulated with anti-CD40 plus IL-4 (71,72). The incubation of purified resting B cells with these reagents causes a strong B-cell aggregation, associated with an increase of expression of ICAM-1, CD43, and CD23, with and avidity change of the LFA-1 molecule. The addition of anti-ICAM-1 antibody enhances IgE production by such stimulated B cells by augmenting expression of a germline transcript of Cε gene, suggesting that B cell–B cell interaction through ICAM-1 also modulates IgE synthesis.

IL-4 Producers: T$_H$2 Cells and FcεRI-Positive Cells

In 1986, Mosmann et al. described two distinct types of cloned mouse T-cell lines, based on the profile of secreting cytokines: T$_H$1, but not T$_H$2, cells produce IL-2, IFN-γ, and TNF-β, whereas T$_H$2 cells secrete IL-4, IL-5, IL-6, and IL-10. Interleukin-3 and GM-CSF are secreted by both types (73). Since IFN-γ is a strong activator for monocytes and macrophages, the primary function of T$_H$1 cells is involved in mediating the delayed-type hypersensitivity (DTH) response. The T$_H$2 cells can produce IL-4, a class-switching factor for IgE, IL-5, IL-6, and IL-10, which enhances IgE secretion, whereas, the T$_H$1 product IFN-γ is capable of inhibiting its synthesis. Thus, selective expansion of T$_H$2 cells is considered to be associated with overproduction of IgE.

The mechanism that regulates the differentiation of naive T cells into T$_H$1 or T$_H$2 cells has been explored in the mouse. A variety of in vitro and in vivo experiments support the idea that cytokines themselves are major determinants for this differentiation of T cells (74,75). Figure 3 shows such a model. When naive T cells are activated by antigen stimulation in the presence of antigen-presenting cells (APC), the presence of IL-4 preferentially induces its differentiation into T$_H$2 cells and inhibits that into T$_H$1 cells. In contrast, the presence of IL-12 or IFN-γ directs naive T cells to T$_H$1 cells. In humans, although not so dramatically demonstrated, this process mode is thought to be regulated similarly. The cell source of IL-12 is macrophages or B cells, whereas the origin of IL-4 acting on naive T cells remains to be determined. One of the candidates is FcεRI-positive cells (and already differentiated effector T$_H$2 cells). Brown et al. (76) and Plaut et al. (8) first demonstrated that mouse mast cell lines can produce IL-4 in response to cross-linking FcεRI or ionomycin. The following studies revealed that mast cells or basophils in humans can also produce T$_H$2 type cytokines (9,10), including IL-4, IL-5, IL-6, and IL-10. Because these activated cells also express CD40L, they provide two signals for B cells to differentiate into

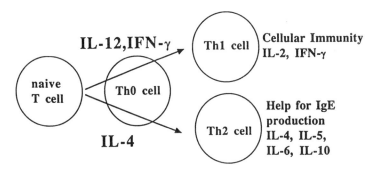

Figure 3 Cytokines determines naive T-cell differentiation: IL-4 is a major determinant for naive T cells to differentiate into T_H2 cells, whereas IL-12 or IFN-γ preferentially induces its differentiation into T_H1 cells.

IgE-secreting cells (77), although whether IL-4 derived directly from these cells determines the direction of differentiation of T cells is still unknown.

Relevance of T_H1 and T_H2 Cells in Human Allergic Diseases

Whether or not overproduction of specific IgE into allergen, which is characteristic for allergic patients, is mediated by the generation of T_H2 cells for allergen has been examined. In situ hybridization techniques revealed that infiltrating T cells in allergic inflammation, such as allergen-induced late-phase reactions in the atopic subjects, or bronchoalveolar lavage fluids from asthmatic patients, expressed IL-3, IL-4, IL-5, GM-CSF, but not IFN-γ, suggesting that T_H2-like cells play a role in the inflammation, although whether or not these cells are specific for allergen is not clarified (78,79). The study by Wierenga et al. demonstrated that most T-cell clones for allergen from the patients secrete high levels of IL-4 and IL-5, but little IFN-γ in response to allergen stimulation (80). In contrast, T-cell clones for bacterial antigens, from the same patients, produce IL-2 and IFN-γ, indicating a preferential expansion of T_H2 cells for allergen in the patients. We also examined whether or not allergen (house dust mite)-specific IL-4-producing T cells might be preferentially generated in allergic patients in vivo, by using a highly sensitive bioassay with IL-4-responsive T-cell line huCT.4S (81). Although IL-4 synthesis by peripheral blood lymphocytes (PBL) in response to polyclonal T-cell stimulants did not significantly differ between the control and allergic subjects, it was clear that the allergen induced IL-4 synthesis by PBL from the patients with elevated radioallergosorbent test (RAST) score, but not from the controls, and we found a good correlation between IL-4 production and RAST score among allergic patients, except for the patients in whom serum level of IgE was extremely elevated. These results directly indicate that, indeed, in the allergic patients, allergen-specific T_H2 cells are more highly generated in vivo.

In the allergic patients with markedly elevated serum IgE levels, spontaneous IgE secretion by PBL and overexpression of CD23 on B cells and monocytes that have elevated soluble CD23 in the serum have been demonstrated (82). Since IL-4 plays an important role on the induction of CD23 expression as well as IgE synthesis, and IFN-γ counteracts IL-4's functions, these observations suggest that imbalance of IL-4 and IFN-γ may account for immunological features of the patients with highly elevated IgE polyclonally. Indeed, the capacity of T cells to produce IL-4 or IFN-γ from such patients was reported to be dysregulated in response to polyclonal stimulation (83,84).

These reports thus indicate that, in allergic patients, polyclonally or monoclonally T cells are preferentially differentiated into T_H2 type cells, but the reason for this skewed differentiation of naive T cells in allergic patients is still unknown. To determine whether or not an intrinsic dysfunction of T cells from allergic patients with a markedly elevated IgE might account for their preferential differentiation into T_H2 cells, we examined the capacity of CD45RA-positive (naive) T cells to secrete IL-4 after being stimulated with anti-CD3 in the presence of IL-4 or anti-IL-4 (85). In controls, the addition of IL-4 at the priming caused a striking enhancement of IL-4 synthesis by T cells when restimulated with anti-CD3. In contrast, the enhancing effect of IL-4 on IL-4 production by the patients' T cells was small, suggesting that rather than a spontaneous differentiation of naive T cells into T_H2 cells, the in vitro differentiation seems to be suppressed.

Cytokines in Allergic Inflammation

Allergen-induced reactions are clinically characterized by a biphasic response. Exposure to allergen induces release of chemical mediators, chemotactic factors, and cytokines by mast cells in the tissue. An immediate response is usually observed within 15 min and subsides 30–90 min later. Frequently, after the immediate response ceases (3–7 h later, the onset of an inflammatory response, called the late-phase reaction (LPR), begins (86). This response is associated with cellular infiltration of eosinophils, neutrophils, and mononuclear cells, and these cells are thought to play a role in chronic allergic inflammation. The targeting of eosinophils to sites of allergic reaction depends on generation of adhesive molecules by endothelial cells. Locally produced IL-1, TNF-α, and IFN-γ induce expression of ICAM-1 on endothelial cells (87,88), but regulation of VCAM expression seems to depend on IL-4 (12,89). VLA-4, a counterreceptor for VCAM, is expressed on eosinophils, but not on neutrophils, and so eosinophil infiltration into the local allergic inflammatory sites strongly depends on the VCAM–VLA-4 interaction. Thus, locally produced IL-4 plays a role in the infiltration of eosinophils.

Moreover, cytokines, such as IL-5, IL-3, and GM-CSF, produced by FcεRI-positive cells and T cells, regulate eosinophil survival, proliferation, and activation, leading to the formation of chronic allergic inflammation (90).

MODULATION OF CYTOKINES' ACTIONS ON THE ALLERGIC RESPONSE TO THERAPY

The actions of five cytokines, IL-2, IL-4, IL-6, IL-10, and IFN-γ, on the allergic responses are summarized as follows. Generally, T_H2 cells and FcεRI-positive cell-derived products—IL-4, IL-6, and IL-10—play a positive role on the induction of allergic responses. Of particular importance is IL-4, which is a class-switching factor for IgE and a differentiation factor for conversion of naive T cells into T_H2 cells, and it also has a substantial effect on infiltration of eosinophils by up-regulating expression of VCAM on endothelial cells. Interleukin-6 and IL-10 are B-cell differentiation factors that up-regulate IgE synthesis, and IL-10 also inhibits IFN-γ synthesis by the macrophage-dependent system. In contrast, IL-2 and IFN-γ, T_H1 cell products, have an important influence on inhibition of allergic responses by suppressing IgE synthesis, and IFN-γ inhibits T-cell differentiation into T_H2 cells. Indeed, in allergic patients, allergen-specific or polyclonal generation of T_H2 cells was demonstrated.

The clinical efficiency of glucocorticoids in allergic diseases is widely accepted (91). Although clinically, in allergic responses, this drug seems to be more effective in LPR than in IPR, it has been postulated that it modulates afferent and effector phases of allergic reactions. Glucocorticoids inhibit mediator release by triggering production of lipocortin, which inhibits phospholipase A_2 and, thereby, prevents release of arachidonic acid, leading to an inhibition of leukotrienes and prostaglandins. They also suppress induction of adhesion molecules' expression and of cytokine gene activation by their binding to AP-1 (93,94).

Cyclosporine (cyclosporin-A; Cy-A), an immunosuppressive drug, inhibits cytokine gene activation by inhibiting activation of the NF-AT transcriptional factor, through inactivation of calcineurin (95,96). Moreover, it also suppresses degranulation of chemical mediators and CD40L expression. Indeed the administration of Cy-A in the allergic patients is reported to decrease clinical symptoms (97,98), although this reagent cannot specifically inhibit IL-4 synthesis or the function of T_H2 cells.

There has been much interest in the development of therapy modifying imbalance of cytokines involved in the allergic responses (99,100). Several approaches are considered to suppress the allergic response, and some of them are now in progress. Theoretically, various means are possible to neutralize actions of cytokines: for IL-4, monoclonal antibodies to IL-4, IL-4 receptor, soluble IL-4R that inhibit the binding of IL-4 to IL-4R; inhibitors for IL-4 gene activation, release of IL-4, and signal transduction by IL-4R; and inhibition of IL-4-induced target gene expression. Among them, some experimental modulators have already been studied in clinical trials. For example Leung et al. (101) showed that thymopentin, a synthetic pentapeptide, that induces IL-2 and IFN-γ production by thymocytes and T cells, produced significant relief of atopic dermatitis in a double-blind, placebo-controlled study.

A new compound, IPD-1151T, is an inhibitor of IL-4 synthesis of a cloned T-cell line and inhibits IgE synthesis, without affecting IgM nor IgG production. Moreover, it inhibits antigen-induced histamine release from mast cells. Clinical trials of efficacy of IPD-1151T are underway with allergic patients, and it has produced a good response (102).

The in vivo effect of IFN-γ for hyper-IgE syndrome and atopic dermatitis patients has been examined and has shown a marked reduction in clinical symptoms, without serious side effects (103). Interestingly, it is reported that the injection of IFN-γ in the atopic dermatitis patients caused a significant reduction in the number of circulating eosinophils (104), raising a possibility that the administration of IFN-γ in vivo may act by inhibiting T_H2 cell expansion and, thereby, in a decrease of IgE synthesis and eosinophil differentiation by inhibiting IL-4 and IL-5 production, although further studies are required for this hypothesis.

Ideally, in the allergic patients who are sensitive to a limited number of allergens, if we could manipulate in vivo differentiation of allergen-specific T cells into T_H1 cells, or could induce an unresponsive state of allergen-specific T cells, it would be a most beneficial therapy, without any side effect. Perhaps the in vivo experiment of mice infected with the parasite, *Leishmania major* gives us such a good model (105). In Balb/c mice when infected with *L. major*, IL-4-producing T_H2 cells dominate, whereas in many other mice expanded T cells can produce mainly IFN-γ. However, Balb/c mice, treated with anti-IL-4 antibodies, IFN-γ, or IL-12 at the time of priming, developed an immune response in which T_H1 cells dominated, and they cleared the parasites, rather than developing a progressive infection. The reverse is also true; when other mice were treated with anti-IFN-γ antibodies or IL-4 at the priming, they died with an expansion of T_H2 cells. This experiment indicates that in vivo artificially injected cytokine or anti-cytokine antibodies can alter the direction of naive

T cells into T_H1 or T_H2 cells, irrespective of the genetic factor that appears to determine the in vivo response. In humans specific-allergen immunotherapy has proved effective, to some extent, in the treatment of some allergic patients. As one of the mechanisms of this therapy, a recent report showed that allergen-specific IL-4 production (but not IFN-γ) by T cells is decreased in the effective allergic patients (106). Although whether this effect is mediated by action on memory T_H2 cells or inhibition of the differentiation of naive T cells into T_H2 cells is not yet clarified. It is possible that the administration of these cytokines (IFN-γ or IL-12) or anti-IL-4 antibodies with allergen could develop allergen-specific T_H1 cells in a manner similar to vaccination.

REFERENCES

1. Taga T, Kishimoto T. Cytokine receptors and signal transduction. FASEB J 1993; 7:3387–3396.
2. Kishimoto T, Taga T, Akira S. Cytokine signal transduction. Cell 1994; 76:253–262.
3. Ishizaka K, Ishizaka T. Allergy. In: Paul WE, ed. Fundamental Immunology II. New York: Raven Press, 1989:867–888.
4. Morgan DA, Ruscetti FW, Gallo RG. Selective in vitro growth of T-lymphocytes from normal human bone marrows. Science 1976; 193:1007–1008.
5. Smith KA. The interleukin-2 receptor. Adv Immunol 1988; 42:165–179.
6. Whittington R, Faulds D. Interleukin-2: a review of its pharmacological properties and therapeutic use in patients with cancer. Drugs 1993; 46:446–514.
7. Howard M, Farrar J, Hilfier M, Johnson B, Takatsu K, Hamaoka T, Paul WE. Identification of a T cell-derived B cell growth factor distinct from interleukin-2. J Exp Med 1982; 155:914–923.
8. Plaut M, Pierce JH, Watson CJ, Hanley-Hyde J, Nordan RP, Paul WE. Mast cell lines produce lymphokines in response to cross-linkage of FcεRI or to calcium ionophores. Nature 1989; 339:64–68.
9. Paul WE, Seder RA, Plaut M. Lymphokine and cytokine production by FcεRI$^+$ cells. Adv Immunol 1992; 53:1–29.
10. Piccini M-P, Macchia P, Parronnchi P, Gindizi MG, Bellesi G, Grossi A, Maggi E, Romagnani S. Human bone marrow non-B, non-T cells produce IL-4 in response to cross-linkage of Fcε and Fcγ receptors. Proc Natl Acad Sci USA 1991; 88:8656–8660.
11. Paul WE. Interleukin-4: a prototypic immunoregulatory lymphokine. Blood 1991; 77:1859–1870.
12. Schleimer RP, Sterbinsky SA, Kaiser J, Bickel CA, Klunk DA, Tomioka K, Newman W, Luscinskas FW, Gimbrone MA Jr, McIntyre BW, Bochner BS. IL-4 induces adherence of human eosinophils and basophils but neutrophils to endothelium: association with expression of VCAM-1. J Immunol 1992; 148:1086–1092.
13. Boulay J-L, Paul WE. The interleukin-4-related lymphokines and their binding to hematopoietin receptors. J Biol Chem 1992; 267:20525–20528.
14. Marsh DG, Neely JD, Breazeale DR, Ghosh B, Freidhoff LR, Ehrlich-Kautzky E, Schou C, Krishnaswamy G, Beaty TH. Linkage analysis of IL-4 and other chromosome 5q31.1 markers and total serum immunoglobulin E concentrations. Science 1994; 264:1152–1156.
15. Aulitzky WE, Schuler M, Peschel C, Huber C. Interleukins; clinical pharmacology and therapeutic use. Drugs 1994; 48:667–677.
16. Muraguchi A, Kishimoto T, Miki Y, Kuritani T, Kaieda T, Yoshizaki K, Yamamura Y. T cell-replacing factor (TRF)-induced IgG secretion in human B blastoid cell line and demonstration of acceptors for TRF. J Immunol 1981; 127:412–416.
17. Kishimoto T. The biology of interleukin-6. Blood 1989; 74:1–10.
18. Kishimoto T, Akira S, Taga T. Interleukin-6 and its receptor: a paradigm for cytokines. Science 1992; 258:593–597.

19. Fiorentino D, Bond M, Mosmann T. Two types of mouse helper T cells. IV Th2 clones secrete a factor that inhibits cytokine production by Th1 clones. J Exp Med 1989; 170:2081–2095.

20. Moore KW, O'Garra A, Malefyt R de W, Viera P, Mosmann TR. Interleukin-10. Annu Rev Immunol 1993; 11:165–190.

21. Sen GC, Lengyel P. The interferon system. J Biol Chem 1992; 267:5017–5020.

22. Gray PW, Goeddel PV. Molecular biology of interferon-gamma. Lymphokines 1987;13: 151–162.

23. Paul WE. Pleiotropy and redundancy; T cell-derived lymphokines in the immune response. Cell 1989; 57:521–526.

24. Minami Y, Kono T, Miyazaki T, Taniguchi T. The IL-2 receptor complex; its structure, function, and target genes. Annu Rev Immunol 1993; 11:245–267.

25. Nikaido T, Shimizu A, Ishida N, Sabe H, Teshigawara K, Maeda M, Uchiyama T, Yodoi J, Honjo T. Molecular cloning of cDNA encoding human interleukin-2 receptor. Nature 1984; 311:631–635.

26. Hatakeyama M, Tsudo M, Minamoto S, Kono T, Doi T, Miyata T, Miyasaka M, Taniguchi T. Interleukin-2 receptor beta chain gene: generation of three receptor forms by cloned human alpha and beta chain cDNAs. Science 1989; 244:551–556.

27. Takeshita T, Asao H, Ohtani K, Ishii N, Kumaki S, Tanaka N, Munakata H, Nakamura M, Sugamura K. Cloning of the γ chain of the human IL-2 receptor. Science 1992; 257:379–382.

28. Idzerda RL, March CJ, Mosley B, Lyman SD, Vanded Bos T. Human interleukin 4 receptor confers biological responsiveness and defines a novel receptor family. J Exp Med 1990; 171:861–873.

29. Russel SM, Keegan AD, Harada N, Nakamura Y, Noguchi M, Leland P, Friedmann MC, Miyajima A, Puri RK, Paul WE, Leonard WJ. Interleukin-2 receptor γ chain: a functional component of interleukin-4 receptor. Science 1993; 262:1880–1883.

30. Yamasaki K, Taga T, Hirata Y, Yawata H, Kawanishi Y, Seed B, Taniguchi T, Hirano T, Kishimoto T. Cloning and expression of the human interleukin-6 (BSF-2/IFNb) receptor. Science 1988; 241:825–828.

31. Hibi M, Murakami M, Saito M, Hirano T, Taga T, Kishimoto T. Molecular cloning and expression of an IL-6 signal transducer, gp130. Cell 1990; 63:1149–1157.

32. Ho A, Liu Y, Khan TA, Hsu D-W, Bazan JF, Moore KW. A receptor for interleukin-10 is related to interferon receptors. Proc Natl Acad Sci USA 1993; 90:11267–11271.

33. Aguet M, Dembic Z, Merlin G. Molecular cloning and expression of the human interferon-γ receptor. Cell 1988; 55:273–280.

34. Miyajima A, Kitamura T, Harada N, Yokota T, Arai K. Cytokine receptors and signal transduction. Annu Rev Immunol 1992; 10:295–331.

35. Noguchi M, Yi H, Rosenblatt HM, Filipovich AH, Adelstein S, Modi WS, McBridge OW, Leonard WJ. Interleukin-2 receptor γ chain mutation results in X-linked severe combined immunodeficiency in humans. Cell 1993; 73:147–157.

36. Murakami M, Hibi M, Nakagawa N, Nakagawa T, Yasukawa K, Yamanishi K, Taga T, Kishimoto T. IL-6-induced homodimerization of gp130 and associated activation of a tyrosine kinase. Science 1993; 260:1808–1810.

37. Ihle JN, Witthuhn BA, Quelle FW, Yamamoto K, Thierfelder WE, Kreider B, Silvennoinen O. Signaling by the cytokine receptor superfamily: Jaks and STATS. Trends Biochem Sci 1994; 19:222–227.

38. Akira S, Nishio Y, Inoue M, Wang X-J, Wei S, Matsusaka T, Yoshida K, Sudo T, Naruto M, Kishimoto T. Molecular cloning of APRF, a novel IFN-stimulated gene factor 3 p91-related transcription factor involved in the gp130-mediated signaling pathway. Cell 1994; 77:63–71.

39. Akira S, Isshiki H, Sugita T, Tanabe O, Kinoshita S, Nishio Y, Nakajima T, Hirano T, Kishimoto T. A nuclear factor for IL-6 expression (NF-IL-6) is a member of a C/EBP family. EMBO J 1990; 9:1897–1906.

40. Hou J, Schindler U, Henzel WJ, Ho TC, Brasseur M, McKnight SL. An interleukin-4-induced transcription factor: IL-4 STAT. Science 1994; 265:1701–1706.
41. Muller M, Briscoe J, Laxton C, Guschin D, Ziemiecki A, Silvennoinen O, Harpur A-G, Bargeri G, Witthuhn BA, Schindler C, Pellegrimi S, Wilks AF, Ihre JN, Stark GR, Kerr IM. The protein tyrosine kinase JAK1 components defects in interferon-α/β and -γ signal transduction. Nature 1993; 366:129–135.
42. Watling P, Guschin D, Muller M, Silvennoinen O, Witthuhn BA, Quelle FW, Rogers NC, Schindler C, Stark GR, Ihle JN, Kerr IM. Complementation by the protein tyrosine kinase JAK2 of a mutant cell line defective in the interferon-γ signal transduction pathway. Nature 1993; 366:166–170.
43. Shuai K, Stark GR, Ker IM, Darnell JE Jr. Activation of transcription by IFN-γ: tyrosine phosphorylation of a 91 kD DNA binding protein. Science 1992; 258:1808–1812.
44. Purkerson J, Isakson P. A two signal model for regulation of immunoglobulin isotype switching. FASEB J 1992; 6:3245–3250.
45. Gauchat J-F, Lebman DA, Coffman RL, Gascan H, de Vries JE. Structure and expression of germline ε transcripts in human B cells induced by interleukin 4 to switch to IgE production. J Exp Med 1990; 172:463–474.
46. Jung S, Rajewsky K, Radbruch A. Shutdown of class switch recombination by deletion of a switch region control element. Science 1993; 259:984–987.
47. Coffman RL, Ohara J, Bond MH, Carty J, Zlotnik A, Paul WE. B cell stimulatory factor-1 enhances IgE response of lipopolysaccharide-activated B cells. J Immunol 1986; 136:4538–4544.
48. Thyphronitis G, Tsokos GC, June CH, Levine AD, Finkelman AD. IgE secretion by Epstein–Barr virus-infected purified human B lymphocytes is stimulated by interleukin-4 and suppressed by interferon-γ. Proc Natl Acad Sci USA 1989; 86:5580–5584.
49. Lebman DA, Coffman RL. Interleukin-4 causes isotype switching to IgE in T cell-stimulated clonal B cell cultures. J Exp Med 1988; 168:853–862.
50. Jabara HH, Fu SM, Geha RS, Vercelli D. CD40 and IgE: synergism between anti-CD40 MAb and IL-4 in the induction of IgE synthesis by highly purified B cells. J Exp Med 1990; 172:1861–1864.
51. Stamenkovic I, Clark EA, Seed B. A B-lymphocyte activation molecule related to the nerve growth factor receptor and induced by cytokines in carcinomas. EMBO J 1989; 8:1403–1410.
52. Armitage RJ, Fanslow WC, Strockbine L, Sato TA, Clifford KN, Macduff BM, Anderson DM, Gimpel SD, Davis-Smith T, Maliszewski C, Clark EA, Smith CA, Grabstein KH, Cosman D, Spriggs MK. Molecular cloning and biological characterization of a murine ligand for CD40. Nature 1992; 357:80–82.
53. Gauchat J-F, Aubry J-P, Mazzei G, Life P, Jomotte T, Elson G, Bonnefoy J-Y. Human CD40-ligand: molecular cloning, cellular distribution and regulation of expression by factors controlling IgE production. FEBS Lett. 1993; 315:259–266.
54. Korthauer U, Graf D, Mages HW, Briere F, Padayachee M, Malcolm S, Ugazio AG, Notarangelo LD, Levinsky RJ, Kroczek RA. Defective expression of T-cell CD40 ligand causes X-linked immunodeficiency with hyper-IgM. Nature 1993; 361:539–541.
55. DiSanto JP, Bonnefoy JY, Gauchat JF, Fischer A, de Saint Basile G. CD40 ligand mutations in X-linked immunodeficiency with hyper-IgM. Nature 1993; 361:541–543.
56. Allen RC, Armitage RJ, Conley ME, Rosenblatt H, Jenkins NA, Copeland NG, Bedell MA, Edelhoff S, Disteche CM, Simoneaux DK, Fanslow WC, Belmont FJ, Spriggs MK. CD40 ligand gene defects responsible for X-linked hyper-IgM syndrome. Science 1993; 259:990–993.
57. Aruffo A, Farrington M, Hollenbaugh D, Li X, Milatovich A, Nonoyama S, Bajorath J, Grosmaire LS, Stenkamp R, Neubauer M, Roberts RL, Noelle RJ, Ledbetter JA, Francke U, Ochs HD. The CD40 ligand, gp39, is defective in activated T cells from patients with X-linked hyper-IgM syndrome. Cell 1993; 72:291–300.

58. Fuleihan R, Ramesh N, Loh R, Jabara H, Rosen RS, Chatila T, Fu SM, Stamenkovic I, Geha RS. Defective expression of the CD40 ligand in X chromosome-linked immunoglobulin deficiency with normal or elevated IgM. Proc Natl Acad Sci USA 1993; 90:2170–2173.

59. Pene J, Rousset F, Briere F, Chretien I, Paliard X, Banchereau J, Spits H, de Vries JE. IgE production by normal human lymphocytes is induced by interleukin 4 and suppressed by interferon-γ and -α and prostaglandin E_2. Proc Natl Acad Sci USA 1988; 85:6880–6884.

60. Gauchat JF, Aversa G, Gascan H, de Vries JE. Modulation of IL-4 induced germline ε RNA synthesis in human B cells by tumor necrosis factor-α, anti-CD40 monoclonal antibodies or transforming growth factor-β correlates with levels of IgE production. Int Immunol 1992; 4: 397–406.

61. Kimata H, Yoshida A, Ishioka C, Lindley I, Mikawa H. Interleukin 8 (IL-8) selectively inhibits immunoglobulin E production induced by IL-4 in human B cells. J Exp Med 1992; 176:1227–1231.

62. Kiniwa M, Gately M, Gubler U, Chizzonite R, Fargeas C, Delespesse G. Recombinant interleukin-12 suppresses the synthesis of immunoglobulin E by interleukin-4 stimulated human lymphocytes. J Clin Invest 1992; 90:262–266.

63. Pène J, Rousset F, Brière F, Chrètien I, Wideman J, Bonnefoy JY, de Vries JE. Interleukin 5 enhances interleukin 4-induced IgE production by normal human B cells. The role of soluble CD23 antigen. Eur J Immunol 1988; 18:929–935.

64. Dugas B, Renauld JC, Pène J, Bonnefoy JY, Peti-Frère C, Braquet P, Bousquet J, Van SJ, Mencia HJ. Interleukin-9 potentiates the interleukin-4-induced immunoglobulin (IgG, IgM and IgE) production by normal human B lymphocytes. Eur J Immunol 1993; 23:1687–1692.

65. Vercelli D, Jabara HH, Arai K, Yokota T, Geha RS. Endogenous IL-6 plays an obligatory role in IL-4 induced human IgE synthesis. Eur J Immunol 1989; 19:1419–1425.

66. Sarfati M, Rector E, Wong K, Rubio-Trujillo M, Sehon AH, Delespesse G. In vitro synthesis of IgE by human lymphocytes; II. Enhancement of the spontaneous IgE synthesis by IgE-binding factors secreted by RPMI 8866 lymphoblastoid B cells. Immunology 1984; 53:197–205.

67. Rothman P, Chen Y-Y, Lutzker S, Li SC, Stewart V, Coffman R, Alt FW. Structure and expression of germline immunoglobulin heavy-chain ε transcripts: interleukin-4 plus lipopolysaccharide-directed switching to Cε. Mol Cell Biol 1990; 10:1672–1680.

68. Punnonen J, Malefyt R de W, Vlasselaer PV, Gauchat J-F, Vries JE. IL-10 and viral IL-10 prevent IL-4-induced IgE synthesis by inhibiting the accessory function of monocytes. J Immunol 1993; 151:1280–1289.

69. Nakanishi K, et al. Personal communication.

70. Punnonen J, Aversa G, Cocks BG, McKenzie ANJ, Menon S, Zurawski G, Malefyt RDW, de Vries JE. Interleukin 13 induces interleukin 4-independent IgG4 and IgE synthesis and CD23 expression by human B cells. Proc Natl Acad Sci USA 1993; 90:3730–3734.

71. Thoma S, Hirohata S, Lipsky PE. The role of CD11a/CD18–CD54 interactions in human T cell-dependent B cell activation. J Immunol 1993; 146:492–499.

72. Katada Y, Tanaka T, Ochi H, Aitani M, Yokota A, Kikutani H, Suemura M, Kishimoto T. B cell–B cell interaction through intercellular adhesion molecule 1 and lymphocyte functional antigen I regulates immunoglobulin E synthesis by B cells stimulated with interleukin-4 and anti-CD40 antibody. Eur J Immunol 1996 (in press).

73. Mosmann TR, Cherwinski H, Bond MW, Giedlin MA, Coffman RL. Two types of murine helper T ell clone. I. Definition according to profiles of lymphokine activities and secreted proteins. J Immunol 1986; 136:2348–2357.

74. Paul WE, Seder RA. Lymphocyte responses and cytokines. Cell 1994; 76:241–251.

75. Seder RA, Paul WE. Acquisition of lymphokine-producing phenotype by CD4$^+$ T cells. Annu Rev Immunol 1994; 12:635–674.

76. Brown MA, Pierce JH, Watson CJ, Falco J, Ihle JN, Paul WE. B cell stimulatory factor-1/interleukin-4 mRNA is expressed by normal and transformed mast cells. Cell 1989; 50: 809–816.

77. Gauchat JF, Henchoz S, Mazzei G, Aubry JP, Brunner T, Blasey H, Life P, Talabot D, Flores RL, Thompson J, Kishi K, Butterfield J, Dahinden C, Bonnefoy J-Y. Induction of human IgE synthesis in B cells by mast cells and basophils. Nature 1993; 365:340–343.

78. Kay AB, Ying S, Varney V, Gaga M, Durham SR, Moqbel R, Wardlaw AJ, Hamid Q. Messenger RNA expression of the cytokine gene cluster, interleukin 3 (IL-3), IL-4, IL-5 and granulocyte/ macrophage colony-stimulating factor, in allergen-induced late phase cutaneous reactions in atopic subjects. J Exp Med 1991; 173:775–778.

79. Robinson DS, Qutayba H, Ying S, Tsicopoulos A, Barkans J, Bentley AM, Conigan C, Durham S, Kay AB. Predominant Th2-like bronchoalveolar T-lymphocyte population in atopic asthma. N Engl J Med 1992; 326:298–304.

80. Wierenga EA, Snoek M, deGroot C, Chreitien I, Bos JD, Jansen HM, Kapsenberg ML. Evidence for compartmentalization of functional subsets of CD4$^+$ T-lymphocytes in atopic patients. J Immunol 1990; 144:4651–4656.

81. Ochi H, et al. Submitted.

82. Suemura M, Kikutani H, Barsumian EL, Kishimoto T. IL-4 and Fcε receptor II in allergy. Cytokines 1989; 2:18–36.

83. Vollenweider S, Saurat J-H, Rocken M, Hauser C. Evidence suggesting involvement of inter-leukin-4 (IL-4) production in spontaneous in vitro IgE synthesis in patients with atopic der-matitis. J Allergy Clin Immunol 1991; 87:1088–1095.

84. Rousset F, Robert J, Andary M, Bonnin J-P, Souillet G, Chretien I, Briere F, Pene J, de Vries JE. Shifts in interleukin-4 and interferon-γ production by T cells of patients with elevated serum IgE levels and the modulatory effects of these lymphokines on spontaneous IgE synthesis. J Allergy Clin Immunol 1991; 87:58–69.

85. Ochi H, Tanaka T, Katada Y, Naka T, Aitani M, Hashimoto S, Maeda K, Toyoshima K, Igarashi T, Suemura M, Kishimoto T. Functional disturbance of naive T lymphocytes in very high IgE producers: Depletion of interleukin-4-induced interleukin-4-producing cells. Int Arch Allergy Immunol 1996 (in press).

86. Dolovich J, Hargreave FE, Chalmers R, Shier KJ, Gauldie J, Bienenstock J. Late cutaneous allergic responses in isolated IgE-dependent reactions. J Allergy Clin Immunol 1973; 52:38–46.

87. Prober JS, Gimbrone MA Jr, Lappierre LA, Mendrick DL, Fiers W, Rothlein R, Springer TA. Overlapping patterns of activation of human endothelial cells by interleukin-1, tumor necrosis factor, and immune interferon. J Immunol 1986; 137:1893–1896.

88. Renkonen R, Mattila P, Majuri ML, Paavonen T, Silvennoinen O. IL-4 decreases IFN-gamma-induced endothelial ICAM-1 expression by a transcriptional mechanism. Scand J Immunol 1992; 35:525–530.

89. Thornhill MA, Haskard DO. IL-4 regulates endothelial cell activation by IL-1, tumor necrosis factor, or IFN-γ. J Immunol 1990; 145:865–872.

90. Coffman RL, Seymour BW, Hudak S, Jackson J, Rennick D. Antibody to interleukin-5 inhibits helminth-induced eosinophilia in mice. Science 1989; 245:308–310.

91. Schleimer RP. Effects of glucocorticoids on inflammatory cells relevant to their therapeutic applications in asthma. Am Rev Respir Dis 1990; 141:S59–S69.

92. McFadden ER Jr. Evolving concepts with pathogenesis and management of asthma. Adv Intern Med 1994; 39:357–394.

93. Schule R, Rangarajan P, Kliewer S, Ransome LJ, Bolado J, Yang N, Verma IM, Evans RM. Functional antagonism between oncoprotein c-*jun* and the glucocorticoid receptor. Cell 1990; 62:1217–1226.

94. Yang-Yen H-F, Chambard J-C, Sun Y-L, Smeal T, Schmidt TJ, Drouin J, Karin M. Transcrip-tional interference between c-*jun* and the glucocorticoid receptor: mutual inhibition of DNA binding due to direct protein–protein interaction. Cell 1990; 62:1205–1215.

95. Sigal NH, Dumont FJ. Cyclosporin A, FK-506, and rapamycin, pharmacologic probes of lymphocyte signal transduction. Annu Rev Immunol 1992; 10:519–560.

96. Liu J, Farmer JD Jr, Lane WS, Friedman J, Weissman I, Schreiber SL. Calcineurin is a common target of cyclophilin–cyclosporin A and FKBP-FK506 complexes. Cell 1991; 66:807–815.
97. Alexander A, Barnes NC, Kay AB. Cyclosporin A (CyA) in chronic severe asthma: a double-blind, placebo-controlled trial. Am Rev Respir Dis 1991; 143:A633.
98. Van Joost T, Stolz E, Heule F. Efficacy of low-dose cyclosporine A in severe atopic skin disease. Arch Dermatol 1987; 97:166–167.
99. Hetzel C, Lamb JR. CD4+ T cell-targeted immunomodulation and the therapy of allergic disease. Clin Immunol Immunopathol 1994; 73:1–10.
100. Katz MF, Beer DJ. T lymphocytes and cytokine networks in asthma: clinical and therapeutic implications. Adv Intern Med 1993; 38:189–222.
101. Leung DYM, Hirsch RL, Schneider L, Moody C, Takaoka R, Li SH, Meyerson LA, Mariam SG, Goldstein G, Hanifin JM. Thymopentin therapy reduces the clinical severity of atopic dermatitis. J Allergy Clin Immunol 1990; 85:927–934.
102. Koda A, Yanagihara Y, Matsuura N. Modulation of IgE synthesis by a new drug, IPD-1151T. Prog Allergy Clin Immunol 1992; 2:41–45.
103. King CL, Gallin JI, Malech HL, Abramson SL, Nutman TB. Regulation of immunoglobulin production in hyperimmunoglobulin E recurrent-infection syndrome by interferon-γ. Proc Natl Acad Sci USA 1989; 86:1085–1089.
104. Boguniewicz M, Jaffe HS, Izu A, Sullivan MJ, York D, Geha RS, Leung DYM. Recombinant gamma interferon in treatment of patients with atopic dermatitis and elevated IgE levels. Am J Med 1990; 88:365–370.
105. Sher A, Coffman RL. Regulation of immunity to parasites by T cells and T cell-derived cytokines. Annu Rev Immunol 1992; 10:385–409.
106. Secrist H, Chelen CJ, Wen Y, Marshall JD, Uematsu DT. Allergen immunotherapy decreases interleukin 4 production in CD4+ T cells from allergic individuals. J Exp Med 1993; 178:2123–2130.

17

Interleukin-3, Granulocyte–Macrophage Colony-Stimulating Factor, Interleukin-5, and Their Receptors

Joshua A. Boyce and William F. Owen, Jr.
Harvard Medical School and Brigham and Women's Hospital, Boston, Massachusetts

INTRODUCTION

Cytokine-mediated intercellular signaling appears to control many facets of inflammation, including the development of hematopoietic cells in the bone marrow, the recruitment of these cells to foci of inflammation, and regulation of the function of these scells (1–20). In the study of allergic inflammation, the hematopoietic cytokines interleukin-3 (IL-3), granulocyte–macrophage colony-stimulating factor (GM-CSF), and interleukin-5 (IL-5) are of particular interest for several reasons. First, these cytokines regulate the proliferation and maturation of granulocytes (1,2,3). Second, they arise from a cluster of closely related genes (21). Despite little homology at the amino acid level, they share structural features critical for function. Third, there is considerable functional overlap among these three cytokines, and each can serve to functionally up-regulate the granulocytes involved in allergic inflammation, such as the eosinophil (6,9,12,17,18). Lastly, the receptors for these cytokines share common subunits (22), and the study of these molecules has contributed greatly to the emerging body of knowledge on signal transduction mechanisms and regulation of cellular function.

This chapter deals with the structure and function of IL-3, GM-CSF, IL-5, and their receptors. The specific bioactivities of these molecules as they apply to hematopoiesis and inflammation will be reviewed. The molecular cloning of the receptors and their biology will be summarized as it applies to the overlapping functions of the three cytokines.

MOLECULAR CLONING AND BIOACTIVITY OF IL-3, GM-CSF, AND IL-5

IL-3

Of the hematopoietic cytokines under discussion, IL-3 is the least lineage-specific in its bioactivity. Murine IL-3 was initially identified as a mast cell growth factor, found in media conditioned by the myelomonocytic leukemia cell line WEHI-3 (23). The cloned cDNA encoded a protein of 166 amino acids, including a leader sequence (5,23,24). The mature glycosylated species has a molecular mass of 28-kDa. Cloning of the human homologue was accomplished following the expression cloning of gibbon IL-3, which cross-hybridized with the human sequence (5,25,26). The coding regions of the murine and primate molecules were divergent, accounting for the initial difficulty in cross-hybridization. However, there was strong conservation of specific A- and T-rich domains in the 3'-noncoding region. This made the cloning of a human cDNA encoding IL-3 from a library derived from stimulated lymphocytes possible using a murine cDNA probe (26). Human IL-3 has a predicted length of 133 amino acids and a deduced molecular mass of 15,091 Da. The recombinant proteins resulting from expression of both the human and the gibbon cDNAs produced hematopoietic bioactivity similar to that of the murine product, confirming the evolutionary relation among them (25,26).

Activated T lymphocytes are thought to be the predominant source of IL-3 in vivo. It is also elaborated by activated monocytes and natural killer (NK) cells (27,28). Interleukin-3 has widespread bioactivity on hematopoietic cells at all stages of differentiation. In picomolar concentrations, it supports the formation of multilineage [colony-forming unit (CFU)-GEMM], granulocyte–macrophage (CFU-GM), granulocyte (CFU-G), macrophage (CFU-M), megakaryocyte (CFU-MEG), eosinophil (CFU-EO), and basophil (CFU-B) colonies in cells from human bone marrow in vitro (4). It acts synergistically with erythropoietin in stimulating the formation of both early and late erythroid colonies. Interleukin-3 is also unique among the hematopoietic cytokines in its ability to promote the growth of the most primitive known bone marrow progenitors, CFU-blast (1,2,4,5). This broad specificity prompted the name "multi-CSF."

The bioactivities of IL-3 overlap considerably with those of GM-CSF for in vitro models of hematopoiesis. However, IL-3 is considerably less potent in supporting granulocyte colony formation than is GM-CSF, suggesting that at least some granulocyte colonies lose their responsiveness to IL-3 during development, particularly neutrophils (29). These observations support the hypothesis that IL-3 is an important early-acting cytokine in hematopoiesis, whereas GM-CSF acts later (1). However, this view is countered by a school of thought that IL-3 does not act constitutively in hematopoiesis. Proponents of the latter view point to the restricted cell expression of IL-3, and the finding that murine stromal cell lines capable of supporting in vitro hematopoiesis do not elaborate IL-3 (30). Instead, IL-3 may be elaborated in response to inflammation or systemic illness for the purpose of accelerating hematopoiesis (28,31). Similar to GM-CSF, the hematopoietic effects of IL-3 have prompted interest in its use in the treatment of hematological disorders, such as myelodysplastic syndromes, aplastic anemia, acquired immunodeficiency syndrome (AIDS), and in salvage therapy following bone marrow transplantation (32–38). Thus, IL-3 is a hematopoietic cytokine capable of stimulating the proliferation and differentiation of multiple hematopoietic cell lineages, both in vitro and in vivo.

Dysregulated production of IL-3 may be involved in the pathogenesis of some myeloproliferative disorders. For example, a t(5;14)(q31;q32) translocation is described in association with B-cell acute lymphoblastic leukemia, resulting in a fusion of the IgH and IL-3 genes with detectable serum IL-3 levels. These patients develop eosinophilia and granulocytosis (39). Similarly, lethally irradiated mice, receiving syngeneic transplants of bone marrow cells transfected with a cDNA encoding IL-3, develop a myeloproliferative syndrome with multiorgan leukocytic infiltration (40). Thus, the overproduction of IL-3 in vivo may result in myeloproliferative disease.

In addition to its hematopoietic effects, IL-3 has proinflammatory effects on mature granulocytes in vitro. For example, human monocytes exposed to picomolar concentrations of IL-3 in vitro show increased surface expression of CD11b and exhibit a biphasic adhesion to both plastic surfaces and to cultured human umbilical vein endothelial cells (HUVEC) (41). Picomolar doses of IL-3 also augment the tumoricidal activity of monocytes in vitro by their increased synthesis of tumor necrosis factor (TNF)-α (42), and prolong the survival of monocytes in culture (8). Eosinophils exposed continuously to picomolar concentrations of IL-3 have prolonged survival in vitro, for as long as 21 days, by inhibition of programmed cell death (apoptosis) (6,43). Continuous exposure to IL-3 prevents the time-dependent internucleosomal DNA degradation that is characteristic of the programmed cell death of eosinophils (43). During the period of exposure in vitro, eosinophils undergo a decrement in their relative centrifugation density ("hypodense" eosinophils). Hypodense eosinophils become primed for augmented antibody-dependent cellular cytotoxicity (ADCC), superoxide production, and leukotriene (LT)C_4 synthesis (6), similar to the effects of IL-5 or GM-CSF on eosinophils (9,12,18,43,44). Interleukin-3 also promotes the release of histamine by mature basophils (histamine-releasing factor; HRF) (7). Thus, IL-3 is capable of regulating many phases of the inflammatory response, including increased myelopoiesis, adhesion of granulocytes to vascular endothelium, maintenance of granulocyte viability, and enhancement of selected functions of eosinophils, basophils, and monocytes. Neutrophils, which lose the capacity to respond to IL-3 during hematopoiesis, do not respond to IL-3 (29).

GM-CSF

Similarly to IL-3, the discovery of GM-CSF arose from the study of hematopoiesis in vitro. Myelopoiesis experiments with hematopoietic bone marrow-derived progenitors revealed a dependency on exogenous T-cell–derived factors for the growth and differentiation of granulocytes (45–47). Both human T-cell lines and unfractionated human lymphocytes, stimulated with phytohemagglutinin (PHA), elaborate colony-stimulating activity in vitro (46,47), suggesting that the colony-stimulating factors were at least partly T-cell-derived. Murine GM-CSF was the first of the hematopoietic cytokines to be characterized, following its initial isolation and purification from a mouse lung-conditioned medium (48). Subsequently, neuraminidase treatment of GM-CSF yielded sufficient quantities of murine asialo-GM-CSF to obtain NH_2-terminal sequence data (49). This sequence was used to construct the probe with which the murine cDNA was cloned (50).

Human GM-CSF was originally purified from media conditioned by the HTLV-II-infected lymphoblastic cell line, Mo-1 (46,51). This cell line was also used to prepare a cDNA library. Following transfection in COS African green monkey kidney cells, GM-CSF was cloned by expression from this library (52).

Human and murine GM-CSF are 144 and 118 amino acids in length, respectively (50,52). They are 60% homologous at the nucleotide level, and 54% at the amino acid level (52). The two proteins share some highly conserved features. Both have 17-amino acid leader sequences that are glycosylated, and removal of these leader sequences by enzymatic deglycosylation results in molecules with enhanced bioactivity (53). Two intrachain disulfide bonds are present that are essential to bioactivity, and amino acid residues 21–31 and 78–94 are essential for bioactivity on hematopoietic cells (54,55). The expression of GM-CSF is less lineage-restricted than that of IL-3. GM-CSF is elaborated by several cell types, including activated T lymphocytes, macrophages, eosinophils, and mast cells (55). Both endothelium and fibroblasts release GM-CSF following stimulation with IL-1 and tumor necrosis factor (TNF)-α or TNF-β (43,55–58).

There is some overlap in the hematopoietic functions of GM-CSF and IL-3. Similar to IL-3, GM-CSF acts as a growth factor, stimulating proliferation and maturation of myeloid progenitor cells in vitro (59). The culture of normal hematopoietic progenitors from human bone marrow with GM-CSF in vitro results in the development of eosinophil, monocyte, and neutrophil colonies (59,60). Unlike IL-3, GM-CSF does not promote colony formation of the earliest hematopoietic progenitors (CFU-BLAST), prompting speculation that GM-CSF acts somewhat later than IL-3 in hematopoiesis in vivo (61). In conjunction with erythropoietin, GM-CSF also stimulates proliferation of erythroid burst-forming units from peripheral blood-derived erythroid progenitors in vitro (62) (Table 1). Recombinant human GM-CSF administered intravenously to primates results in reticulocytosis and a dramatic leukocytosis (63). GM-CSF and IL-3 have synergistic effects on hematopoiesis in vitro and in vivo. Interleukin-3 and GM-CSF together promote the formation of a greater number of colonies than either one alone in bone marrow proliferation assays in vitro. Sequential subcutaneous administration of IL-3 and GM-CSF in cancer patients with normal hemato-poietic potential results in greater increases in circulating neutrophils and eosinophils, as well as circulating hematopoietic progenitors (38). GM-CSF has also been used in the treatment of chemotherapeutically induced myelosuppression, myelodysplastic syndromes, AIDS, bone marrow transplantation, and other disorders involving disordered myelo-poiesis. The reader is referred to recent excellent reviews for further discussion of these clinical applications (64,65). The clinical use of recombinant GM-CSF primarily results in increased granulopoiesis, monocytosis, and, to a lesser extent, eosinophilia (32).

As with IL-3, GM-CSF is expressed constitutively in some cases of leukemia (66). Furthermore, lethally irradiated mice, receiving syngeneic transplants of bone marrow cells transfected with a GM-CSF cDNA, develop a lethal myeloproliferative syndrome, much like the aforementioned mice receiving IL-3-expressing transplants (67). Thus, aberrant production of GM-CSF, as with IL-3, is a cause of abnormal myeloproliferation.

Analogous with IL-3, GM-CSF is a potent functional agonist of mature granulocytes in vitro. For example, picomolar doses of GM-CSF cause a biphasic adherence of human monocytes to plastic surfaces and to HUVEC in vitro (13,41), prolongs the viability of cultured monocytes (8), and stimulates their tumoricidal capability by augmenting their generation of TNF-α (42). These effects are shared with IL-3. With eosinophils, the effects of GM-CSF are also similar to those of IL-3 (6,9,10,43,68–70). For example, eosinophils primed in vitro with GM-CSF show increased expression of surface HLA-DR and the leukocyte integrin CR3 (CD11b) (15). GM-CSF in picomolar doses converts eosinophils to the functionally primed hypodense phenotype in vitro (12,70). Eosinophils primed in vitro by GM-CSF exhibit augmented cytotoxicity to antibody-coated schistosomes and generate increased quantities of LTC_4 in response to calcium ionophore (9,12). Furthermore, the priming of eosinophils by GM-CSF in vitro in the presence of 3T3 fibroblasts results in an augmented respiratory burst and production of LTC_4 in response to the bacterial peptide N-formyl-L-methionyl-L-leucyl-L-phenylalanine (FMLP) (69), whereas nonprimed eosino-phils do not respond to FMLP alone. GM-CSF-primed eosinophils exhibit enhanced phagocytosis of opsonized yeast (71). The synthesis and size of eosinophil cell-associated proteoglycans is increased by the culture of eosinophils with GM-CSF (68). In mature basophils, GM-CSF alone causes histamine release, an effect shared with IL-3 (7). Thus, similar to IL-3, GM-CSF is a functional agonist of monocytes, eosinophils, and basophils, and is capable of regulating the expression of adhesion molecules and stimulating the effector functions of these mature granulocytes.

Table 1 Bioactivities of IL-3, GM-CSF, and IL-5 In Vitro

Cytokine	Chromosomal location	Cells of origin	Hematopoietic activity	Activity on mature cells
IL-3	Same	CD4 T cells, monocytes, NK cells, eosinophils	Colony-forming-unit (CFU)-blast, monocytes, neutrophils, eosinophils, basophils, megakaryocytes, erythrocytes (synergy with erythropoietin for erythrocytes)	*Eosinophils*: conversion to hypodense phenotype, enhanced viability, increased CR3 and HLA-DR expression, augmented cytotoxicity, increased LTC_4 generation, increased superoxide production *Basophils*: histamine-releasing factor *Monocytes*: enhanced viability, enhanced adhesion to endothelial cells, increased expression of CD18, augmented cytotoxicity
GM-CSF	5q23–31 (human) 11 (mouse)	CD4 T cells, fibroblasts, macrophage/monocytes, endothelial cells, neutrophils, eosinophils	Eosinophils, monocytes, neutrophils, erythrocytes (synergy with erythropoietin for erythrocytes)	*Eosinophils*: conversion to hypodense phenotype, enhanced viability, increased CR3 and HLA-DR expression, augmented cytotoxicity, increased LTC_4 generation, increased superoxide production *Neutrophils*: increased surface Mo-1 and pl50,95, increased number of affinity of FMLP receptors, enhanced superoxide production, augmented production of 20-OH and 20-COOH LTB_4, increased degranulation, augmented cytotoxicity and phagocytosis, inhibition of chemotaxis *Basophils*: histamine-releasing factor *Monocytes*: enhanced viability, increased expression of CD18, adhesion to endothelium, augmented cytotoxicity
IL-5	Same	CD4 T cells, eosinophils, mast cells, macrophages	Eosinophils	*Eosinophils*: Conversion to hypodense phenotype, enhanced viability, increased CR3 and HLA-DR expression, increased ICAM-1 expression, enhanced chemotactic response, augmented cytotoxicity, increased LTC_4 generation, increased superoxide production, augmented degranulation *Basophils*: histamine-releasing factor *B cells (murine)*: proliferation and differentiation, IgE and IgG_1 class switch

Unlike IL-3, GM-CSF is also a potent stimulator of mature neutrophil function. For example, neutrophils exposed in vitro to 500 pM GM-CSF exhibited increased surface expression of the adhesion molecules Mo-1 and LeuM5 (pl50,95) (72). GM-CSF also inhibits the chemotaxis of neutrophils in vitro and primes them for augmented oxidative metabolism in response to physiological chemoattractants, such as FMLP, C5a, and LTB$_4$ (51,71,73,74). Neutrophils primed by GM-CSF in vitro demonstrate augmented synthesis of platelet-activating factor (PAF), a chemoattractant and functional agonist for neutrophils and eosinophils (14). As with eosinophils, the culture neutrophils in the presence of picomolar doses of GM-CSF primes them for augmented functional responses to FMLP (75,76). These primed neutrophils, which have an increased number and affinity of FMLP receptors (75), exhibit augmented superoxide production (74) and biosynthesis of LTB$_4$, 20-hydroxy-LTB$_4$, and 20-carboxy-LTB$_4$ in response to either FMLP or the complement fragment C5a (76). GM-CSF induces degranulation of neutrophils in vitro by a pertussis toxin-sensitive mechanism, both alone and in response to FMLP, PAF, or calcium ionophore (77,78). Other proinflammatory effects of GM-CSF on neutrophil function include stimulation of phagocytosis of opsonized yeast or *Staphylococcus aureus* (10,79); an increase in their cytotoxic capacity in vitro against antibody-coated targets, such as human promyelocytic leukemia cells and malignant B cell lines (11); and prolongation of their survival in culture by several hours (71). Thus, GM-CSF is a potent priming stimulus for mature neutrophils and, therefore, has more widespread bioactivity in the myeloid cell series than IL-3 does.

The bioactivity of GM-CSF in vitro is not confined to cells of hematopoietic origin. Small-cell lung cancer lines express a high-affinity receptor for GM-CSF, and both GM-CSF and interferon-γ (IFN-γ) inhibit the growth of these cell lines in vitro (80,81). GM-CSF receptors also have been identified in an simian virus (SV) 40-transformed marrow stromal cell line (82), colonic adenocarcinoma cells (83), melanoma cells (84), and other malignant cells and lines. Endothelial cells, which both produce GM-CSF (43) and express receptors for GM-CSF (85), exhibit migratory and proliferative responses to GM-CSF (86). Therefore, the bioactivity of GM-CSF in vivo may not be limited to its hematopoietic and proinflammatory effects alone.

IL-5

Interleukin-5 is unique among the hematopoeitins by its restricted eosinophil lineage-specific effects in humans. The bioactivities of IL-5 were originally described as T-cell-replacing factor, B-cell growth factor II, and eosinophil-activating factor (87,88). The activity of IL-5 was originally recognized in mouse spleen-conditioned media that exhibited eosinophil colony-stimulating activity on marrow cells (89). The development of a lipid media assay for eosinophil peroxidase activity and a liquid medium system for in vitro eosinophilopoiesis ultimately led to the discovery and isolation of IL-5 (90–93). Subsequently, the murine IL-5 cDNA was cloned, followed shortly by the human homologue (93).

Unlike IL-3 and GM-CSF, the nucleotide and amino acid sequences and bioactivities of IL-5 are highly conserved between the species (93). The human and murine molecules are 70% homologous at the amino acid level, and there is cross-species bioactivity (92,93). The IL-5 protein is a 115-amino acid homodimer. The monomer has a molecular mass of 12 kDa. Subsequent glycosylation results in a mature glycoprotein of 40–45 kDA, although as with GM-CSF, glycosylation is not necessary for bioactivity (94). The dimer is arranged in an antiparallel configuration, and there are probably two receptor-binding sites per molecule (95–97). However, IL-5 binds to its receptor in a 1:1 molar ratio (98).

Interleukin-5 is the most lineage-specific of the hematopoietic cytokines, and it is potentially involved at all stages of eosinophil-associated disease, including eosinophilopoiesis, maintenance of cellular viability, chemotaxis, adhesion, and activation of eosinophils. In humans, the hematopoietic bioactivity of IL-5 and the effects of IL-5 on mature granulocytes are confined to eosinophils and basophils (99,100). Interleukin-5 appears to be the major cytokine involved in the selective production of eosinophilia, as well as the functional activation and maintenance of eosinophil viability at sites of inflammation (100,101). The existence of a hematopoietic growth factor with specificity for eosinophils was first suspected based on the observation that T-cell function was necessary for mice to develop eosinophilia in response to a helminthic infection. This observation prompted speculation that a T-cell–derived factor was necessary for eosinophil development (102–104). Subsequently, the T_H2 class of helper T cells were shown to be the primary source of IL-5 (100,105). This cytokine may also be produced by mast cells (106), by macrophages (100), and by eosinophils themselves (100,107). The latter finding has potential significance for IL-5 as an effector for the autoregulatory capacity of eosinophils.

The hematopoietic function of IL-5 has been compared with that of IL-3 and GM-CSF in both liquid and semisolid culture media using progenitors from peripheral blood, umbilical cord blood, and bone marrow (90,108–116). Although IL-5, GM-CSF, and IL-3, all support the formation of eosinophil colonies, only IL-5 does so in a selective fashion (3,108, 112,114,116). Furthermore, the concentration of IL-3 or GM-CSF required to support eosinophil colonies is roughly tenfold greater than that required of IL-5 (109–112). Interleukin-5 acts synergistically with IL-3 and GM-CSF in semisolid hematopoietic culture systems and appears to function as a terminal differentiation factor for eosinophil progenitors, whereas IL-3 and GM-CSF promote the development of early eosinophil precursors (109–114). Compared with IL-5 alone, IL-3 plus IL-5, GM-CSF plus IL-5, or all three cytokines together, produce a greater number of eosinophil progenitors (112,115). Thus, a network of cytokines may act in concert to produce eosinophils in vitro, with IL-5 being the terminal element of this network.

Despite evidence that IL-5 acts in concert with IL-3 and GM-CSF during eosinophilopoiesis in vitro, IL-5 may act alone in the production of eosinophilia in vivo. Transgenic mice constitutively expressing IL-5 develop eosinophilia in the absence of neutrophilia or monocytosis (116–118). Passive immunization with anti-IL-5 monoclonal antibody blocks this eosinophilia (119) and also prevents the increase in eosinophilia following experimental helminth infection (120). In contrast to lethally irradiated mice receiving syngeneic bone marrow transplants that constitutively produce IL-3 or GM-CSF (40,67), the IL-5 transgenic mice remain healthy, despite striking peripheral blood eosinophilia (118). Furthermore, patients treated with intravenous infusions of IL-3 or GM-CSF typically develop only modest eosinophilia compared with increases in other cell lines (32–38). Alternatively, IL-5 detectable in the serum is associated with selective eosinophilia, as is seen in the tryptophan-associated eosinophilia–myalgia syndrome, the idiopathic hypereosinophilic syndrome, or episodic angioedema with eosinophilia (121–123). Furthermore, the local production of IL-5 in diseases, such as asthma, Hodgkin's disease, and eosinophilic pneumonia, is associated with peripheral blood and tissue eosinophilia (105,124,125). Thus, in vivo, IL-5 alone may be capable of supporting eosinophilopoiesis, and the production of IL-5 is associated with certain human diseases characterized by selective eosinophilia.

Similar to IL-3 and GM-CSF, IL-5 influences the function of mature eosinophils and basophils. Eosinophils cultured in the presence of IL-5 for 7 days are converted to the hypodense phenotype (44). IL-5 inhibits the programmed cell death of eosinophils in vitro, enhancing their survival and inducing resistance to the cytotoxic effects of corticosteroids

(43,126). It also has chemotactic and chemokinetic activity for eosinophils (17). It primes them for augmented chemotactic responses to PAF, LTB_4, and FMLP (127), as well as to the chemotactic cytokines RANTES, IL-8, and MIP-1α (128). IL-5 induces eosinophils to express intercellular adhesion molecule (ICAM)-1 (129), thereby priming them for augmented adhesion. It enhances the adhesion of peripheral blood eosinophils to human umbilical vein endothelial cells (HUVEC) by increasing the numbers of surface complement receptor 3 (CR3) (130,131). Furthermore, the affinity of eosinophil surface CR3 for opsonized zymosan particles is increased by the exposure of peripheral blood eosinophils to picomolar concentrations of IL-5 in vitro (132). However, both IL-3 and GM-CSF are more potent at inducing CR3 expression than IL-5 (130). Thus, the recruitment of eosinophils to inflammatory foci in vivo may be enhanced by prior priming with IL-5, IL-3, or GM-CSF. By augmenting the chemotactic response to selected stimuli, and by up-regulating the number or affinity of CR3, eosinophil adhesion to vascular endothelium may be augmented. IL-5 acts synergistically with corticosteroids to induce the expression of the major histocompatibility complex (MHC) class II antigens, HLA-DR and HLA-DQ, on mature eosinophils in vitro (133). Therefore, IL-5 might promote the antigen-presenting function of eosinophils. For basophils, IL-5, at doses of 0.1–10 ng/ml, increases histamine release and their generation of LTC_4 in response to C5a, neutrophil-activating peptide 1, and C3a (134). Thus, the behavior of eosinophils and basophils at inflammatory foci may be selectively up-regulated by IL-5.

Interleukin-5 effects the differentiation of murine B cells, but analogous bioactivity has not been identified in human cells. A population of mouse B cells possess IL-5 receptors (135). Murine B cells develop IL-5 receptors when their antigen receptor is engaged, and they are subsequently stimulated with a polyclonal activation signal such as lipopolysaccharide (LPS), dextran sulfate (136), or anti-Ig–dextran conjugates (138): this proliferation and immunoglobulin secretion in response to IL-5 may be indicative of the functionality of IL-5 receptors on B cells (137). In murine B cells, IL-5 acts synergistically with IL-4 to induce a class switch from IgM to IgE or IgG subclass 1 (138,139). Furthermore, TGF-β acts synergistically with IL-5 to promote IgA production in murine B cells (140). In contrast, IL-5 has no activity in standard B-cell proliferation assays using human B cells (141), and likely has no significant effects on human B cells in vivo. However, human B cells transformed by the Epstein–Barr virus (EBV) in vitro produce IL-5 and proliferate in response to IL-5 (142,143). Under these conditions, IL-5 may be an autocrine growth factor for EBV-transformed human B cells.

Under certain culture conditions, IL-5 may be bioactive on human T cells. T cells cultured for 24 h in the presence of IL-2, and subsequently cultured with IL-5, show increased synthesis of both IL-2 receptor subunits. No change occurred after the T cells were cultured with IL-5 alone. Therefore, the possibility exists that IL-2 induces IL-5 responsiveness in T cells (144).

The Cytokine Gene Cluster and Common Structural Features of IL-3, GM-CSF, and IL-5

Despite significant overlap in hematopoietic and proinflammatory function, there is little homology among the primary amino acid sequences of IL-3, IL-5, and GM-CSF. Nonetheless, these molecules may have arisen from a common evolutionary antecedent. The genes encoding IL-3, IL-5, and GM-CSF all map to a region on the long arm of human chromosome 5 (21,145) and murine chromosome 11 (146). This region also contains multiple other genes encoding cytokines and cytokine receptors (147). Deletions in the long arm of chromosome 5 are often associated with myelodysplastic syndromes and acute leukemias. One such disorder, the 5q$^-$ syndrome, is characterized by a refractory microcytic anemia and deletion of region 5q23-q31, which includes the genes encoding GM-CSF, IL-5, and IL-3 (148–151). In both mouse and human, each of the genes is a single copy composed of four exons and three introns, except the IL-3 gene, which contains an extra exon (152). The 5′-flanking regions of the IL-3, IL-5, and GM-CSF genes contain putative promotor sequences, with strongly conserved elements across the cytokine genes and across species; included is a highly conserved GC-rich region (152).

Critical functional domains of the hematopoietic cytokines have been identified utilizing site-directed mutagenesis and construction of hybrid cytokines. Interleukin-3, IL-5, and GM-CSF, all possess an unusual NH$_2$-terminal α-helical bundle fold consisting of four α-helices (153,154). These helices have positionally conserved adjacent lysine and glutamic acid residues. A hybrid cytokine containing the NH$_2$-terminal region of GM-CSF and the remainder of the molecule from IL-5 can bind to the IL-5 receptor. Despite little homology between their primary amino acid sequences, the features responsible for receptor binding are conserved between IL-5 and GM-CSF (153). In particular, hydrophilic amino acid residues in the NH$_2$-terminal α-helices of IL-3, IL-5, and GM-CSF are critical in governing bioactivity and receptor binding of these cytokines (153–157).

CHARACTERIZATION AND CLONING OF THE RECEPTORS FOR IL-3, GM-CSF, AND IL-5

The molecular cloning and characterization of the cytokine receptors elegantly explains the overlapping biological activities of IL-3, IL-5, and GM-CSF. This functional overlap was recognized shortly following the cloning of these cytokines and the availability of their recombinant products (25,50,93). IL-3, IL-5, and GM-CSF had similar bioactivities on cells possessing receptors for more than one cytokine, such as monocytes (IL-3, GM-CSF receptors; 158), eosinophils (IL-3, IL-5, GM-CSF; 159,160), and basophils (IL-3, IL-5, GM-CSF; 161). Furthermore, the hematopoietic functions of IL-3 and GM-CSF were similar (34,36,37,60,63).

Early studies of the receptors for IL-3, IL-5, and GM-CSF revealed two classes of cytokine binding, high and low affinity. High- and low-affinity binding of GM-CSF has been demonstrated on KG-1 cells (162). Because IL-3 specifically competes for high- but not low-affinity binding of GM-CSF, a shared receptor subunit was suggested (163). Cross-competition between IL-3 and GM-CSF does not occur in the human histiocytic lymphoma cell line U937, nor the gastric carcinoma cell line Kato-3, which lack IL-3 receptors. This finding suggests that cross-competition between IL-3 and GM-CSF is not based on competitive inhibition by one cytokine on the binding of the other, and that IL-3 and GM-CSF receptors might share a common subunit (163). Similar cross-competition has subsequently been demonstrated on basophils, for IL-3, GM-CSF, and IL-5 (161); on eosinophils, for IL-3, GM-CSF, and IL-5 (159,160); and on monocytes, for GM-CSF and IL-3 (158). Therefore, cross-competition between GM-CSF, IL-3, and IL-5 occurs on cells that are known to bind more than one of the three cytokines. Thus, human neutrophils, which express only receptors for GM-CSF, exhibit no cross-competition, whereas eosinophils, which bind all three, do show cross-competition (159,160).

Cross-competition of binding between IL-3, GM-CSF, and IL5, as well as their overlapping hematopoietic and proinflammatory bioactivities, has been explained since the receptors for IL-3, GM-CSF, and IL-5 have been cloned. Each of these receptors is composed of two subunits: a subunit responsible for recognition and binding of the cytokine (α-subunit), and a subunit essential for signal transduction (β-subunit). Whereas the α-subunits of the receptors for IL-3, IL-5, and GM-CSF are distinct molecules that are entirely specific to the respective cytokines, the β-subunit is shared among the three receptors (22). This shared β-subunit accounts for the overlap in bioactivity observed for IL-3, IL-5, and GM-CSF. It also helps explain cross-competition of binding.

IL-3 Receptor

The IL-3 receptor was characterized initially by cross-linking studies using radiolabeled ligand in equilibrium binding assays and Scatchard plot analysis. These studies showed that IL-3 bioactivity is mediated by a low-abundance, high-affinity receptor on murine and human cells. Affinity studies suggested that the murine IL-3 receptor bound IL-3 with a K_d of 100–300 pM, and approximately 100–5000 receptors per cell (164,165). The observation of a bimodal distribution of ligand binding on some cell types suggested two populations of receptors, a high-affinity receptor (K_d 100–300 pM) and a low-affinity receptor (K_d 10 nM) with the capacity for rapid dissociation from the ligand (166). Cross-linking and affinity isolation of the murine IL-3 receptors using specific antibodies indicated that it was a molecule of 60–75 kDa (167–169). Subsequent studies indicated that the high-affinity IL-3 receptor was composed of multiple subunits. Proteins of 140, 120, and 70 kDa were described in a high-affinity receptor complex (170,171), and 140 kDa alone for the low-affinity receptor (166). Thus, early evidence suggested a multisubunit high-affinity receptor.

The subunits of the murine IL-3 receptor were cloned and used to reconstitute the functional high- and low-affinity receptors. A murine cDNA encoding an IL-3-binding protein, designated A1C2A, was cloned and expressed in COS African green monkey cells (172). A1C2A encoded a mature glycoprotein of 110–120 kDa, a size in keeping with one of the subunits previously revealed by cross-linking experiments (163,172). The deduced peptide was 856 amino acids in length, with a putative extracellular domain of 417 amino acids, containing two homologous sequences of 200 amino acids. There was a single, short transmembrane domain and a serine- and proline-rich cytoplasmic domain, similar to that found in the IL-4, IL-2, G-CSF, and EPO receptors (173). The expressed molecule bound murine IL-3 with low affinity (K_d 10 nM), supporting the hypothesis that other subunits composed the high-affinity IL-3 receptor. Experiments with A1C2A affinity columns confirmed that the high-affinity IL-3 receptor included this subunit (174).

A second murine cDNA, similar to A1C2A, designated A1C2B, was cloned (175). This molecule was 91% homologous to A1C2A at the primary amino acid sequence level, and was 896 amino acids in length. Comparable with A1C2A, A1C2B contained a pair of homologous 200-amino acid motifs in the extracellular domain (175), and also had a single transmembrane domain and a serine- and proline-rich cytoplasmic domain. However, unlike A1C2A, the protein encoded by A1C2B showed no cytokine-binding capability by itself. A1C2B encoded a receptor subunit that was shared by the receptor complexes for murine GM-CSF and IL-5 (β-subunit) (176,177), whereas A1C2A proved to encode a unique ligand-specific β-subunit utilized only by the murine IL-3 receptor (174). Thus, in the murine system, there are two β-subunits: one entirely specific to the IL-3 receptor heterodimer and one shared with the IL-5 and GM-CSF receptors.

The cDNA encoding the ligand-specific α-subunit of the murine IL-3 receptor was cloned (173). The predicted encoded protein was 396 amino acids and included an extra-cellular domain with two motifs similar to those of A1C2A and A1C2B, and a single transmembrane domain. In contrast with the two murine β-subunits, the murine IL-3 receptor α-subunit had an extremely short cytoplasmic tail. The mature glycosylated product was 70 kDa. Although cells transfected with this cDNA had low-affinity (K_d 300 pM) binding of murine IL-3, cotransfection with A1C2A resulted in a reconstitution of high-affinity binding. In keeping with the native receptor, cross-linking of this reconstituted receptor for murine IL-3 yielded three proteins of 140, 120, and 70 kDa. High-affinity binding of IL-3 could also be reconstituted by cotransfection with the cloned α-subunit and A1C2B, indicating that the murine IL-3 receptor was capable of utilizing either of these closely related β-subunits (178). Thus, the murine receptor for IL-3 is composed of at least two subunits. No explanation is yet available for the third cross-linked protein of 120 kDa.

Characterization of the human IL-3 receptor was initially carried out using the human IL-3-dependent cell line TF-1. The high-affinity receptor consisted of two cross-linked proteins of 135 and 70 kDa, with a K_d of 170 pM (179). Therefore, both the human and murine IL-3 receptors were apparently composed of multiple subunits. The cDNA encoding the human homologue of A1C2B, the common β-subunit of the human IL-3, IL-5, and GM-CSF receptors, was cloned using the cDNA for the β-subunit of the murine IL-3 receptor as a probe (180). The encoded human β-subunit has 56 and 55% identity with A1C2A and A1C2B at the amino acid level, respectively. Much like the murine homologues, the encoded protein has a 440-amino acid extracellular domain, with two conserved motifs, a single transmembrane domain, and a 411-amino acid cytoplasmic tail. Similar to A1C2B, human cells transfected with this cDNA alone do not bind IL-3. A human cDNA encoding an IL-3-binding protein, the IL-3 receptor α-subunit, was cloned using an expression strategy (181). When this cDNA was coexpressed with the human homologue of A1C2B (β-subunit) on CTLL-2 cells, a proliferative response to IL-3 was exhibited (182). The α-subunit of the human IL-3 receptor is a 70-kDa protein with structural features shared with the murine α-subunit: an extracellular domain containing two motifs of the cytokine receptor superfamily, a single transmembrane domain, and a short cytoplasmic domain. Transfection with the α-subunit alone results in low-affinity binding only (181). Like the murine IL-3 receptor, the human IL-3 receptor is composed of two subunits: a ligand-specific α-subunit that, by itself, confers only low-affinity binding for IL-3, and a β-subunit that is mandatory for high-affinity binding and for signal transduction. However, unlike the mouse IL-3 receptor, only a single β-subunit of the IL-3 receptor has been identified.

The gene encoding the ligand-specific α-subunit of the IL-3 receptor is mapped to the pseudoautosomal region of the sex chromosomes, in close proximity to the gene encoding the GM-CSF receptor α-subunit (183,184). The β-subunit, shared by the IL-3, IL-5, and GM-CSF receptors, maps to the long arm of human chromosome 22 (184) (Table 2).

GM-CSF Receptor

Similar to the receptor for IL-3, the murine GM-CSF receptor was initially characterized by binding studies using radioiodinated GM-CSF on cells of the myelomonocytic lineage (185,186). Scatchard analyses revealed the presence of two populations of receptors, both low (K_d 1 nM) and high (K_d 20 pM) affinity (186). Analogous to the IL-3 receptor, low-affinity binding is attributed to an α-subunit specific for the GM-CSF receptor, whereas high-affinity binding occurs as a result of the presence of both α- and β-subunits, the latter

Table 2 Biochemical Features of the Receptor Subunits for IL-3, GM-CSF, and IL-5

Receptor subunit	Human chromosome	WSXWS motifs	High-affinity binding	Low-affinity binding	Signal transduction	Soluble isoform
IL-3α	X-Y pseudoautosomal	1	No	Yes	No	Unknown
GM-CSFα	X-Y pseudoautosomal	1	No	Yes	No	Yes
Il-5α	3p24-26	1	No	Yes	No	Yes
Common β (human)	22q12.2-q13.1	2	No	No	Yes	No
Common β (mouse)		2	No	Yes (A1C2A for IL-3)	Yes	No

shared with the IL-3 and IL-5 receptors (A1C2B). The cDNA encoding the murine GM-CSF receptor α-subunit was cloned by direct expression (187). Coexpression in COS-7 cells of the murine GM-CSF receptor α-subunit, with the β-subunit cDNA, A1C2B, results in a reconstituted high-affinity murine GM-CSF receptor. This reconstitution indicated that A1C2B is a subunit of the murine GM-CSF receptor and is analogous to the human β-subunit (187).

Similar to the murine GM-CSF receptor, the human GM-CSF receptor is composed of multiple subunits. Cross-linkage studies using specific antibodies initially suggested a predominant protein of 97 kDa, or three cross-linked species of masses 150, 115, and 95 kDa (185,188–191). Scatchard analysis of human myelopoietic cells revealed discordant binding affinities. For example, mature neutrophils possess a single population of high-affinity (K_d 50 pM) receptors, and only 1000 receptors per cell (189,191). However, in hematopoietic cell lines possessing GM-CSF receptors, including HL-60, TF-1, and U937, and in mature human monocytes (193), both low- and high-affinity binding of GM-CSF was identified (192,193). Furthermore, two distinct patterns of high-affinity binding of GM-CSF are present in the human system (194), designated as class I and class II binding. Class I binding is found on mature neutrophils and exhibits down-regulation by GM-CSF, PMA, and calcium ionophore A23187. This pattern of high-affinity binding is not competed for by IL-3. Class II binding exhibits cross-competition with IL-3 and is seen on leukemic blasts (194,195). Both classes of high-affinity binding for GM-CSF are found on normal bone marrow progenitors and mature monocytes. Thus class II high-affinity binding may be confined to hematopoietic cells exhibiting cytological immaturity (194). The functional significance and structural correlate(s) of this dichotomy of GM-CSF binding are unknown.

Two subunits compose the high-affinity receptor for human GM-CSF, and they have been cloned and expressed. The ligand-specific α-subunit was cloned from a placental cDNA library by expression cloning (196). The predicted protein was 44 kDa, with subsequent glycosylation, resulting in an 85-kDa molecule. The cDNA encoded an open-reading frame of 400 amino acids that included a 22-amino acid signal peptide. Similar to other cytokine receptors, the human GM-CSF α-subunit has four positionally conserved cysteines and a region immediately extracellular of the transmembrane domain with a WSXWS motif. This motif is identical with that found in IL-3 and IL-5 receptors (see following discussion). Similar to the α-subunit of the IL-3 receptor, the GM-CSF receptor α-subunit has a single hydrophobic transmembrane domain and a short cytoplasmic tail. Transfection of this cDNA into COS cells resulted in low-affinity binding (K_d 2–8 nM) for ^{125}I-GM-CSF, indicating that the α-subunit by itself could reconstitute only a low-affinity receptor for GM-CSF (196). Overexpression of this receptor in a murine IL-3–GM-CSF-dependent cell line resulted in a proliferative response to high doses of human GM-CSF at concentrations consistent with the dissociation constant of the receptor (1–10 nM). Therefore, the cloned low-affinity receptor was functional (197).

Subsequently, the IL-3 and GM-CSF receptors were found to share a common β-subunit (181). Reconstitution of the high-affinity human GM-CSF and IL-3 receptors was accomplished by cotransfection of the cDNA species encoding the common β-subunit and the respective α-subunits of the IL-3 and GM-CSF receptors (181,182). These reconstituted receptors bound both IL-3 and GM-CSF with high affinity. Furthermore, cross-competition between IL-3 and GM-CSF was demonstrated in transfected cells expressing both α-subunits and the common β-subunit (182), and cross-linking of the reconstituted receptors revealed patterns similar to those for the native receptors (181,198,199). Thus, it was demonstrated that the human receptors for IL-3 and GM-CSF share the common β-subunit.

A second isoform of the human GM-CSF receptor α-subunit has subsequently been identified, arising through an alternative splicing event (200). This molecule encodes a predicted protein of 410 amino acids that possesses a short, serine-rich cytoplasmic domain and retains the functional capabilities of the first α-subunit. Only one GM-CSF receptor α-subunit has been identified thus far in the mouse.

In addition to the membrane-bound GM-CSF receptor α-subunit, a soluble isoform of the GM-CSF receptor α-subunit has been identified (201). When compared with the membrane-bound GM-CSF receptor α-subunit, the soluble isoform contains an internal deletion of 97 nucleotides. The encoded protein, which retains its capacity to bind GM-CSF, lacks the 84 COOH-terminal amino acids. The deleted COOH-terminal region of the GM-CSF receptor includes the transmembrane and cytoplasmic domains. The functional significance of the soluble GM-CSF receptor in vivo is unknown.

Similar to the α-subunit of the IL-3 receptor, the human gene for the GM-CSF receptor α-subunit has recently been mapped to the pseudoautosomal region of the sex chromosomes (183,184,202; see Table 2).

IL-5 Receptor

As with the IL-3 and GM-CSF receptors, the IL-5 receptor was initially characterized by cross-linking and Scatchard analysis studies. On murine IL-5-dependent cells, low (K_d 1 nM) and high (K_d 40 pM) binding sites were identified, and cross-linkage studies revealed two proteins with molecular masses of 60 and 130 kDa, respectively (203). A library was prepared from an IL-5-dependent pre-B-cell line, and the murine cDNA encoding the 60-kDa subunit of the murine IL-5 receptor was cloned (204). The encoded product was a glycoprotein of 415 amino acids, containing a hydrophobic NH_2-terminal region of 17 amino acids, a transmembrane domain of 22 amino acids, a cytoplasmic domain of 54 amino acids, and a glycosylated extracellular domain. Transfection of this cDNA into COS cells yielded a protein that bound murine IL-5 with low affinity (K_d 2–10 nM). However, when FDC-P1 cells, which constitutively express A1C2B (β-subunit), were transfected with the 60-kDa IL-5 receptor subunit, both low-affinity and high-affinity bindings were seen. The cells had acquired a proliferative response to IL-5 (177). The monoclonal antibody R52.120 inhibited the binding of both IL-3 and IL-5 and precipitated a doublet of 120 kDa. This doublet was composed of the proteins encoded by A1C2A and A1C2B. Cotransfection revealed that A1C2B, but not A1C2A, encoded the second subunit of the murine IL-5 receptor (177,205). Thus, A1C2B is shared among the murine IL-3, GM-CSF, and IL-5 receptors.

The human IL-5 receptor was characterized initially on the promyelocytic leukemia cell line HL-60, that exhibited both high- and low-affinity binding of IL-5. After stimulation with butyrate, all IL-5 binding was converted to high-affinity binding (K_d 40 pM) (206). Cross-linking revealed two proteins, similar in size to the murine homologues. A cDNA encoding an IL-5-binding protein was cloned from an HL-60 cDNA library. The reading frame encoded a predicted protein of 335 amino acids that was 71% homologous with the α-subunit of the murine IL-5 receptor. However, it lacked the putative cytoplasmic and transmembrane domains because of a TAA stop codon upstream from these coding regions in the murine homologue. Therefore, this cDNA clone apparently encoded a soluble isoform of the human IL-5 receptor (207). Furthermore, this soluble isoform was inhibitory in an eosinophil differentiation assay, suggesting it may serve a counterregulatory function for the eosinophilopoietic effect of IL-5 (207). However, the role of the soluble IL-5 receptor in vivo has yet to be determined.

Use of RNA blot analysis of HL-60 cells and eosinophils revealed a predominant 1.4-kb transcript, consistent with the size of the cloned cDNA encoding the soluble IL-5 receptor, and two more minor bands of 2.0 and 4.4 kb. Subsequently, a full-length cDNA encoding the membrane-bound isoform of the human IL-5 receptor α-subunit was cloned from a library derived from TF-1, a human erythroleukemic cell line (208). The sequence was identical with the previously cloned soluble IL-5 receptor isoform, except that this cDNA contained coding regions for a 21-amino acid transmembrane domain and an extremely short cytoplasmic tail of 55 amino acids. The open-reading frame encoded a 400-amino acid receptor, with an extracellular domain including two pairs of cysteines and a WSXWS motif, similar to the IL-3 and GM-CSF receptors (181,195,196). Furthermore, an amino acid sequence similar to the type-3 fibronectin (FBN-III) molecule was near the NH_2-terminus. This region, which is potentially important in governing interactions with other receptor subunits or with IL-5 itself (207,208), is conserved among other growth factor receptors, including the growth hormone and prolactin receptors (209,210), the G-CSF receptor (211), the erythropoietin and IL-2 receptors (212), and the IL-6 receptor (213). The expressed IL-5 receptor protein was 55–60 kDa, identical with the size noted on normal human eosinophils. Because of its short cytoplasmic tail, the authors concluded that the molecule was probably incapable of signal transduction of its own accord and concurred that a second subunit would likely be necessary for signal transduction (208).

The fact that the human IL-5 receptor shared a β-subunit with the IL-3 and GM-CSF receptors was proved in studies utilizing a chimeric receptor. The chimeric receptor included transmembrane and cytoplasmic domains from the mouse IL-5 receptor homologue (α-subunit) and the extracellular domain of the soluble human IL-5 receptor (α-subunit) that lacked a cytoplasmic or transmembrane domain (207). When the chimeric cDNA was cotransfected with the human homologue of A1C2B (β-subunit), high-affinity binding of IL-5 was reconstituted. Furthermore, cotransfection of COS 1 cells with the GM-CSF α-subunit, the IL-5 receptor α-subunit, and the common β-subunit, resulted in cross-competition in binding by GM-CSF and IL-5. These studies provided evidence that the human IL-5 receptor was composed of two subunits: a ligand-specific α-subunit, and a β-subunit that was shared among human IL-3, IL-5, and GM-CSF receptors. The commonality of subunits explained the similarity in patterns of cross-linking in studies of the three cytokine receptors, and also likely accounted for overlap in the bioactivities of IL-3, GM-CSF, and IL-5. Furthermore, these experiments suggested that the critical structural elements that governed the interaction between the α- and β-subunits of the IL-5 receptor were conserved across species.

The gene encoding the IL-5 receptor α-subunit is located on chromosome 3 (3p26) (214,215), unlike the genes encoding the human GM-CSF and IL-3 α-subunits, which map to the pseudoautosomal region of the sex chromosomes (183,184). The functional domains of the IL-5 receptor α-subunit are encoded by separate exons. Two separate exons encode three fibronectin type-III-like modules and a signal peptide; the membrane anchor and the cytoplasmic tail are encoded by two exons, the first of which contains a proline cluster region (214). Five prime upstream of the membrane anchor domain is an exon containing a TAA stop codon, followed by a polyadenylation signal. Therefore, normal RNA splicing results in a soluble isoform of the IL-5 receptor, whereas alternative splicing results in an isoform that contains the membrane anchoring region.

As noted earlier, HL-60 cells possess both low- and high-affinity binding sites for IL-5 that are converted exclusively to high-affinity binding by butyrate treatment of the cells (206). On normal human eosinophils, there are also both low- and high-affinity binding sites (K_d 2.6 nM and 518 pM, respectively). Overnight incubation in the presence of picomolar concentrations of GM-CSF increases specific binding of IL-5 and converts all binding sites to high-affinity (216). Other studies have observed that eosinophils may have only high-affinity binding sites for IL-5 (217,218). These discrepancies may be explained by differences in the state of activation in vivo of the eosinophils in question. Hypodense eosinophils, that are functionally primed, and normodense eosinophils have IL-5 receptors with different binding constants (217).

FUNCTIONAL SIGNIFICANCE OF HETERODIMERIC RECEPTORS AND CONSERVED FEATURES OF THE CYTOKINE RECEPTOR SUPERFAMILY

In all studies to date of the IL-3, IL-5 and GM-CSF receptors, the presence of the common β-subunit appears essential for high-affinity binding to occur in response to GM-CSF, IL-3, or IL-5 (176,177,180,181,195,205). Most of these studies suggest that the β-subunit is essential for signal transduction as well. With the exception of the murine IL-3 receptor β-subunit A1C2A, which binds IL-3 with low affinity, the high-affinity binding of IL-3, IL5, and GM-CSF requires interactions between the α-subunit, β-subunit, and specific residues of the NH_2-terminal α-helix of IL-3, IL-5, and GM-CSF, particularly a glutamic acid residue at position 21 (153–157). Mutagenesis that results in an alanine substitution at residue 21 abrogates high-affinity binding of GM-CSF, but low-affinity binding is unaffected (155,157). Site-directed mutagenesis and binding studies revealed that amino acid residues Tyr-365, His-367, and Ile-368 of the common human β-subunit are essential for the high-affinity binding of GM-CSF and IL-5, but not IL-3, to occur (219). This region of the β-subunit apparently binds residue 21 of the NH_2-terminal α-helix of GM-CSF and IL-5. Therefore, ligand binding to the common β-subunit of the receptors may involve different NH_2-terminal residues in IL-3 than in IL-5 or GM-CSF (219).

It is apparent that the α- and β-subunits of the receptors for IL-3, IL-5, and GM-CSF associate with one another and with the ligand in a ternary complex (220). According to this model, the two subunits are loosely associated at the cell membrane before ligand binding. Subsequent binding of the ligand results in stabilization of this complex (220). Radiolabled GM-CSF associates with its receptor in stoichiometric fashion at a concentration sufficient to saturate high-affinity binding sites (220). Unless prior ligand binding occurs, solubilization of the cell membrane results in dissociation of the two receptor subunits. It is likely that the physical association of α- and β-receptor subunits creates a new binding site that allows the activation of signaling molecules and signal transduction (185).

Although there is little homology between the respective murine and human receptor homologues, there is likely preservation of residues critical for the interaction between α- and β-receptor subunits and between the β-subunit and IL-3, IL-5, or GM-CSF. For example, in the murine GM-CSF responsive cell line, FDC-P1, which possesses functional high-affinity GM-CSF receptors, expression of the human GM-CSF receptor α-subunit results in low- but not high-affinity binding to human GM-CSF (197). Nevertheless, a growth signal was transduced at high concentrations of GM-CSF (10 nM). Therefore, signal transduction may occur in response to the human α- and the murine β-subunits, becoming associated in a ternary complex with GM-CSF. Furthermore, when the human GM-CSF receptor α-subunit is expressed in the murine T-cell line, CTLL, that lacks endogenous β-subunits, no growth signal is obtained in response to human GM-CSF. When CTLL cells are cotransfected with both human α- and β-subunits, these cells become responsive to human GM-CSF (176). Finally, cotransfection of the human GM-CSF receptor α-subunit and the murine β-subunit (A1C2B) results in transduction of a growth signal despite suboptimal binding. These findings confirm that the presence of the GM-CSF receptor β-subunit is necessary for signal transduction to occur, and that residues governing the interaction between α- and β-subunits, and possibly between the β-subunits and IL-3, IL-5, and GM-CSF may be conserved across species.

Studies of site-directed mutagenesis of the common IL-3, IL-5, and GM-CSF β-subunit have been employed to define the domains of the β-subunit that are critical to its function. The murine IL-3-dependent pre-B-cell line BaF3 was cotransfected with a series of mutant β-subunits and with the α-subunit of the murine GM-CSF receptor. Two domains were identified that were critical to the preservation of proliferation signals. Arg-456–Phe-487 was essential for proliferation, whereas Val-518–Asp-544, which was nonessential, enhanced proliferation in response to GM-CSF. Mutants lacking Val-518–Leu-626 were incapable of mediating tyrosine phosphorylation of 60- and 95-kDa proteins. However, mutants lacking residues downstream from Val-518 were able to transmit an herbimycin-sensitive growth signal, suggesting that tyrosine kinase activity was preserved. By contrast, mutations of the ligand-specific α-subunit influenced signal transduction to a smaller degree (221).

The ligand-specific α-subunits of the IL-3, GM-CSF, and IL-5 receptors contain positionally conserved amino acid residues, with specific functional significance. Each murine α-subunit has tryptophan residues at positions 137 and 238 (207,222). In the human IL-5 receptor, a proline cluster spans residues Leu-371–Asp-384, which is shared with the receptors for GM-CSF, growth hormone, and prolactin (177,207). Four cysteine residues are highly conserved that define one or more immunoglobulin-like domains, and disulfide bonds have been demonstrated between these adjacent residues. This arrangement is similar to the growth hormone receptor (223). As noted previously for the IL-5 receptor, there is also homology between the receptors for IL-3 and GM-CSF with the type III fibronectin structure (FBN-III) (207,208). Modeling of the secondary structure of FBN-III predicts that this molecule is composed of seven conserved blocks and that the molecule forms antiparallel β-strands similar to the extracellular domains of the cytokine receptors (224).

Although the intracytoplasmic domains of murine and human receptors for IL-3, IL-5, and GM-CSF show greater divergence than their extracellular domains, there are some conserved features. All three α-subunits have very short cytoplasmic tails, which are felt to participate only minimally in signal transduction (22,207,208). Each has a conserved FPPVPAPK sequence just distal to the transmembrane domains that may participate in the interaction with the common β-subunit (177,185). Like many of the cytokine receptor superfamily members, the β-subunit has a large proportion of proline–serine and proline–threonine residues in its intracytoplasmic domain. These residues are recognition sites for a class of serine–threonine kinases (225), which are potentially important in signal transduction.

The receptors for GM-CSF, IL-3, and IL-5 belong to a superfamily of cytokine receptors that includes the receptors for erythropoietin, IL-4, G-CSF, and IL-7 (209–213,224). Despite little homology in primary sequence, these receptors share common features. This receptor superfamily has conserved WSXWS motifs in their extracellular domains (222). In the β-subunit of the IL-3, IL-5, and GM-CSF receptors, two WSXWS motifs are present, and each α-subunit has one. The nucleotide sequence encoding the WSXWS motif is also highly conserved. A hinge region exists in the β-subunits of these receptors that is between the two WSXWS motifs. This structure permits their participation in ligand binding (224).

The WSXWS motif may be involved in the physical interactions between receptor sub-units (188).

REGULATION OF RECEPTOR EXPRESSION

Expression of the receptors for IL-3, IL-5, and GM-CSF may be subject to autocrine or paracrine control mechanisms. High-affinity GM-CSF receptor expression is increased markedly in mouse peritoneal macrophages in response to picomolar concentrations of GM-CSF or IL-3 (226). Interferon-γ increases steady-state transcript levels encoding the common β-subunit in human monocytes by increasing mRNA synthesis and attenuating its degradation (227). Tissue necrosis factor-α increases high-affinity receptors for IL-3 and GM-CSF on human AML blasts, but not in normal neutrophils (228). In the human erythroleukemic cell line TF-1, which expresses receptors for all three cytokines, exposure in vitro to IL-1 or TNF-α increases expression of the common β-subunit protein (229). However, IL-1 was the sole cytokine that augmented proliferative responses to IL-3, IL-5, and GM-CSF. These findings indicate that high-affinity binding alone is insufficient to bring about increased proliferative responses in TF-1.

Another potential mechanism for regulation of cytokine-induced responses is the biosynthesis of soluble receptor isoforms that are inhibitory of hematopoietic or proinflammatory bioactivity. Soluble IL-5 receptors and GM-CSF receptors have been described in vitro (207,208,230–232). The mRNAs that encode these soluble isoforms arise from normal splicing events. In the IL-5 receptor, in all cells studied, the transcript encoding the soluble receptor is more abundant than the membrane-bound isoform, including TF-1, HL-60 cells, and human eosinophils (207,208). The soluble IL-5 receptor inhibited IL-5-induced eosinophil differentiation in vitro (207). Thus, soluble cytokine receptors may function in an autoregulatory "negative-feedback" loop, preventing overstimulation of mature cells or controlling eosinophilopoiesis. The biological function in vivo of soluble receptors is unproved.

CONCLUSION

In summary, IL-3, IL-5, and GM-CSF are hematopoietic cytokines with stimulatory effects on the function of mature granulocytes. Each cytokine arises from a cluster of closely related genes, and shares common structural features, despite little amino acid sequence homology. The receptors for IL-3, IL-5, and GM-CSF exist as heterodimers, having a shared β-subunit that is responsible for signal transduction. This feature of their receptors likely accounts for the overlapping biological functions of IL-3, IL-5, and GM-CSF. The bioactivity of each cytokine is implicated in the control of the cells that participate in the effector limb of adaptive immunity.

It may be possible to employ the interaction between the cytokines and their receptors as a therapeutic target for patients with inflammatory disease. For instance, it may be possible to control diseases associated with the overproduction of IL-5, such as the idiopathic hypereosinophilic syndrome (121), by using specific IL-5 receptor antagonists or by administering blocking antibodies directed against IL-5. Anti-IL-5 antibodies have already been employed in IL-5 transgenic mice and result in reversal of the animals' eosinophilia (119). Soluble isoforms of the IL-5 receptor have been cloned and expressed (98). The capacity of soluble cytokine receptors to compete for ligand binding may provide a more efficacious means of attenuating the biological response. Alternatively, cytokine–toxin conjugates, similar to that generated for IL-2 and diphtheria toxin (233), may offer a means of selectively eliminating the allergic effector cell.

REFERENCES

1. Clark SC, Kamen R. The human hematopoietic colony-stimulating factors. Science 1987; 236:1229–1237.
2. Rennick DM, Lee FD, Yokota T, Arai KI, Cantor H, Nabel GJ. A cloned MCGF cDNA encodes a multilineage hematopoietic growth factor: multiple activities of interleukin 3. J Immunol 1985; 134:910–914.
3. Saito H, Hatake K, Dvorak AM, Leiferman KM, Donnenberg AD, Arai N, Ishizaka K, Ishizaka T. Selective differentiation and proliferation of hematopoietic cells induced by recombinant human interleukins. Proc Natl Acad Sci USA 1988; 85:2288–2295.
4. Ihle JN, Keler J, Oroszlan S, Henderson LE, Copeland TD, Fitch F, Prystowski MB, Goldwasser E, Schrader JW, Palaszynski E, Dy M, Lebel B. Biologic properties of homogeneous interleukin 3. I. Demonstration of WEHI-3 growth factor activity, mast cell growth factor activity, colony-stimulating factor activity, and histamine-producing cell-stimulating activity. J Immunol 1983; 131:282–287.
5. Yang Y-C, Clark SC. Interleukin-3: molecular biology and biologic activities. Hematol Oncol Clin North Am 1989; 3:441–452.
6. Rothenberg ME, Owen WF, Siberstein DS, Woods J, Soberman RJ, Austen KF, Stevens RL. Human eosinophils have prolonged survival, enhanced function and become hypodense when exposed to human interleukin 3. J Clin Invest 1988; 81:1986–1992.
7. Haak-Frendscho M, Arai N, Arai K, Baeza ML, Finn A, Kaplan AP. Human recombinant granulocyte–macrophage colony-stimulating factor and interleukin 3 cause basophil histamine release. J Clin Invest 1988; 82:17–20.
8. Elliot MJ, Vadas MA, Eglinton JM, Park LS, To LB, Cleland LG, Clark SC, Lopez AF. Recombinant human interleukin-3 and granulocyte–macrophage colony-stimulating factor show many common biological effects and binding characteristics on human monocytes. Blood 1989; 74:2349–2359.
9. Silberstein DS, Owen WF, Gasson JC, DiPersio JF, Golde DW, Bina JC, Soberman R, Austen KF, David JR. Enhancement of human eosinophil cytotoxicity and leukotriene synthesis by biosynthetic (recombinant) granulocyte–macrophage colony-stimulating factor. J Immunol 1986; 137:3290–3294.
10. Fleishmann J, Golde DW, Weisbart RH, Gasson JC. Granulocyte–macrophage colony-stimulating factor enhances phagocytosis of bacteria by human neutrophils. Blood 1986; 68: 708–711.
11. Fabian I, Baldwin GC, Golde DW. Biosynthetic granulocyte–macrophage colony-stimulating factor enhances neutrophil cytotoxicity toward human leukemia cells. Leukemia 1987; 1:613–617.
12. Owen WF, Rothenberg ME, Silberstein DS, Gasson JC, Stevens RL, Austen KF, Soberman RJ. Regulation of human eosinophil viability, density and function by granulocyte/macrophage colony-stimulating factor in the presence of 3T3 fibroblasts. J Exp Med 1987; 166:129–141.
13. Gamble JR, Elliot MJ, Jaipargas E, Lopez AF, Vadas MA. Regulation of human monocyte adherence by granulocyte–macrophage colony-stimulating factor. Proc Natl Acad Sci USA 1989; 86:7169–7173.
14. DeNichilo MO, Stewart AG, Vadas MA, Lopez AF. Granulocyte–macrophage colony-stimulating factor is a stimulant of platelet-activating factor and superoxide generation by human neutrophils. J Biol Chem 1991; 266:4896–4902.
15. Koenderman L, Hermans SW, Capel PJ, van de Winkel JG. Granulocyte-macrophage colony-stimulating factor induces sequential activation and deactivation of binding via a low-affinity IgG Fc receptor, hFc gamma RII, on human eosinophils. Blood 1993; 81:2413–2419.
16. Sanderson CJ, Warren DJ, Strath M. Identification of a lymphokine that stimulates eosinophil

differentiation in vitro. Its relationship to interleukin 3, and functional properties of eosinophils produced in culture. J Exp Med 1985; 162:60–74.

17. Yamaguchi Y, Hayashi Y, Sumaga Y, Miura Y, Kasahara T, Kitamura S, Torishu M, Mita S, Tominaga A, Takatsu K. Highly purified murine interleukin 5 (IL-5) stimulates eosinophil function and prolongs in vitro survival. IL-5 as an eosinophil chemotactic factor. J Exp Med 1988; 167:43–56.

18. Lopez AF, Sanderson CJ, Gamble JR, Campbell HD, Young IG, Vadas MA. Recombinant human interleukin 5 is a selective activator of human eosinophil function. J Exp Med 1988; 167:219–224.

19. Walsh GM, Wardlaw AJ, Hartnell A, Sanderson CJ, Kay AB. Interleukin-5 enhances the in vitro adhesion of human eosinophils, but not neutrophils, in a leukocyte integrin (CD11/18)-dependent manner. Int Arch Appl Immunol 1991; 94:174–178.

20. Hansel TT, De Vries IJ, Carballido JM, Braun RK, Carballido-Perrig N, Rihs S, Blaser K, Walker C. Induction and function of eosinophil intercellular adhesion molecule-1 and HLA-DR. J Immunol 1992; 149:2130–2136.

21. Van-Leeuwen BH, Martinson ME, Webb GC, Young IG: Molecular organization of the cytokine gene cluster, involving the human IL-3, IL-4, IL-5 and GM-CSF genes, on human chromosome 5. Blood 1989; 73:1142–1148.

22. Nicola NA, Metcalf D. Subunit promiscuity among hematopoietic growth factor receptors. Cell 1991; 67:1–4.

23. Fung MC, Hapel AJ, Ymer S, Cohen DR, Johnson RM, Campbell HD, Young IG. Molecular cloning of cDNA for murine interleukin 3. Nature 1984; 307:233–237.

24. Yokota T, Lee F, Rennick D, Hall C, Arai N, Mosmann T, Nabel G, Cantor H, Arai K. Isolation and characterization of a mouse cDNA clone that expresses mast-cell growth factor activity in monkey cells. Proc Natl Acad Sci USA 1984; 81:1070–1074.

25. Yang YC, Ciarletta AB, Temple PA, et al. Identification by expression cloning of a novel hematopoietic growth factor related to murine IL-3. Cell 1986; 47:3–10.

26. Dorssers L, Burger H, Bot F, Delwel R, Geurts van Kessel AHM, Lowenberg B, Wagemaker G. Characterization of a human multilineage colony-stimulating factor identified by a conserved noncoding sequence in mouse interleukin-3. Gene 1987; 55:115–124.

27. Wimperis JZ, Niemeyer CM, Sieff CA, Mathey-Prevot B, Nathan DG, Arceci RJ. Granulocyte–macrophage colony-stimulating factor and interleukin-3 mRNAs are produced by a small fraction of blood mononuclear cells. Blood 1989; 74:1525–1530.

28. Otsuka T, Miyajima A, Brown N, et al. Isolation and characterization of an expressible cDNA encoding human IL-3. Induction of IL-3 mRNA in human T cell clones. J Immunol 1988; 140:2288–2295.

29. Lopez AF, Dyson PG, To LB, Elliot MJ, Milton SE, Russell JA, Juttner CA, Yang YC, Clark SC, Vadas MA. Recombinant human interleukin-3 stimulation of hematopoiesis in humans: loss of responsiveness with differentiation in the neutrophilic myeloid series. Blood 1988; 72:1797–1804.

30. Li CL, Johnson GR. Stimulation of multipotential, erythroid, and other murine haemopoietic progenitor cells by adherent cell lines in the absence of detectable multi-CSF (IL-3). Nature 1985; 31:633–636.

31. Schrader JW. The panspecific hematopoietin of activated T lymphocytes (interleukin-3). Annu Rev Immunol 1986; 4:205–230.

32. Vadhan-Raj S, Keating M, LeMaistre A. Effects of recombinant human granulocyte-macrophage colony-stimulating factor in aplastic anemia and myelodysplastic syndromes. N Engl J Med 1987; 317:1545–1552.

33. Ganser A, Lindemann A, Seipelt G, Ottmann OG, Herrmann F, Eder M, Frisch J, Schulz G, Mertelsmann R, Hoelzer D. Effects of recombinant human interleukin-3 in patients with bone marrow failure. Blood 1990; 76:666–676.

34. Ottmann OG, Ganser A, Seipelt G, Eder M, Schulz G, Hoelzer D. Effects of recombinant human interleukin-3 on human hematopoietic progenitor and precursor cells in vivo. Blood 1990; 76:1494–1502.
35. Vadhan-Raj S, Buescher S, Broxmeyer HE, et al. Stimulation of myelopoiesis in patients with aplastic anemia by recombinant human granulocyte–macrophage colony-stimulating factor. N Engl J Med 1988; 319:1628–1634.
36. Ganser A, Volkers B, Greher J, Ottmann OG, Walther F, Becher R, Bergmann L, Schulz G, Hoelzer D. Recombinant human granulocyte–macrophage colony-stimulating factor in patients with myelodysplastic syndromes—a phase I/II trial. Blood 1989; 73:31–37.
37. Ganser A, Seipelt G, Lindemann A, et al. Effects of recombinant human interleukin-3 in patients with myelodysplastic syndromes. Blood 1990; 76:455–462.
38. Ganser A, Lindemann A, Ottmann OG, et al. Sequential in vivo treatment with two recombinant human hematopoietic growth factors (interleukin-3 and granulocyte–macrophage colony-stimulating factor) as a new therapeutic modality to stimulate hematopoiesis: results of a phase I study. Blood 1992; 79:2583–2591.
39. Meeker TC, Hardy D, Willman C, Hogan T, Abrams J. Activation of the interleukin-3 gene by chromosome translocation in acute lymphocytic leukemia with eosinophilia. Blood 1990; 76:285–289.
40. Chang JM, Metcalf D, Lang RA, Gonda TJ, Johnson GR. Nonneoplastic hematopoietic myelo-proliferative syndrome induced by dysregulated multi-CSF (IL-3) expression. Blood 1989; 73:1487–1497.
41. Elliot MJ, Vadas MA, Cleland LG, Gamble JR, Lopez AF. IL-3 and granulocyte–macrophage colony-stimulating factor stimulate two distinct phases of adhesion in human monocytes. J Immunol 1990; 145:167–176.
42. Cannistra SA, Vennenga E, Groshek P, Rambaldi A, Griffin JD. Human granulocyte–macrophage colony-stimulating factor and interleukin-3 stimulate monocyte cytotoxicity through a tumor necrosis factor-dependent mechanism. Blood 1988; 71:672–676.
43. Her E, Frazer J, Austen KF, Owen WF. Eosinophil hematopoietins antagonize the programmed cell death of eosinophils: cytokine and glucocorticoid effects on eosinophils maintained by endothelial cell conditioned medium. J Clin Invest 1992; 88:1982–1987.
44. Rothenberg ME, Petersen J, Stevens RL, Silberstein DS, McKenzie DT, Austen KF, Owen WF. IL-5-dependent conversion of normodense eosinophils to the hypodense phenotype uses 3T3 fibroblasts for enhanced viability, accelerated hypodensity, and sustained antibody-dependent cytotoxicity. J Immunol 1989; 143:2311–2316.
45. Bradley TR, Metcalf D. The growth of mouse bone marrow cells in vitro. Aust J Exp Biol Med Sci 1966; 44:287–299.
46. Golde DW, Quan SG, Cline MJ. Human T lymphocyte cell line producing colony-stimulating activity. Blood 1978; 52:1068–1072.
47. Cline MJ, Golde DW. Production of colony-stimulating activity by human lymphocytes. Nature 1974; 248:703–704.
48. Burgess AW, Camakaris J, Metcalf D. Purification and properties of colony-stimulating factor from mouse lung-conditioned medium. J Biol Chem 1977; 252:1998–2003.
49. Sparrow LG, Metcalf D, Humkapiller MW, Hood LE, Burgess AW. Purification and partial amino acid sequence of asialo murine granulocyte-macrophage colony-stimulating factor. Proc Natl Acad Sci USA 1985; 82:292–296.
50. Gough NM, Gough J, Metcalf D, Kelso A, Grail D, Nicola NA, Burgess AW, Dunn AR. Molecular cloning of a cDNA encoding a murine hematopoietic growth regulator, granulocyte–macrophage colony-stimulating factor. Nature 1984; 309:763–767.
51. Gasson JC, Weisbart RH, Kaufman SE, Clark SC, Hewick RM, Wong GG, Golde DW. Purified human granulocyte–macrophage colony-stimulating factor: direct action on neutrophils. Science 1984; 226:1339–1342.

52. Wong GG, Witeck JS, Temple PA, Wilkens KM, Leary AC, Luxenburg DP, Jones SS, Brown EL, Kay RM, Orr EC, Shoemaker C, Golde DW, Kaufman RJ, Hewick RM, Wang EA, Clark SC. Human GM-CSF: molecular cloning of the complementary DNA and purification of the natural and recombinant proteins. Science 1985; 228:810–815.

53. Moonen P, Mermod J-J, Ernst JF, Hirschi M, Delamarter JF. Increased biological activity of deglycosylated recombinant human granulocyte–macrophage colony-stimulating factor produced by yeast or animal cells. Proc Natl Acad Sci USA 1987; 84:4428–4431.

54. Kaushanski K, Shoemaker SG, Alfaro S, Brown C. Hematopoietic activity of granulocyte/macrophage colony-stimulating factor is dependent upon two distinct regions of the molecule: functional analysis based upon the activities of interspecies hybrid growth factors. Proc Natl Acad Sci USA 1989; 86:1213–1217.

55. Gasson JC. Molecular physiology of granulocyte–macrophage colony-stimulating factor. Blood 1991; 77:1131–1145.

56. Broudy VC, Kaushansky K, Harlan JM, Adamson JW. Interleukin 1 stimulates human endothelial cells to produce granulocyte/macrophage colony-stimulating factor. J Immunol 1987; 129:464–468.

57. Seiff CA, Tsai S, Faller DV. Interleukin 1 induces cultured endothelial cell production of granulocyte–macrophage colony-stimulating factor. J Clin Invest 1987; 79:48–51.

58. Zucali JR, Dinarello CA, Oblon DJ, Gross MA, Anderson L, Weiner RS. Interleukin 1 stimulates fibroblasts to produce granulocyte–macrophage colony-stimulating activity and prostaglandin E_2. J Clin Invest 1986; 77:1857–1863.

59. Seiff CA, Emerson SG, Donahue RE, Nathan DG, Wang EA, Wong GG, Clark SC. Human recombinant granulocyte–macrophage colony-stimulating factor: a multilineage hematopoietin. Science 1985; 230:1171–1173.

60. Tomonaga M, Golde DW, Gasson JC. Biosynthetic (recombinant) human granulocyte–macrophage colony-stimulating factor: effect on normal bone marrow and leukemia cell lines. Blood 1986; 67:31–36.

61. Miyajima A. Molecular structure of the IL-3, GM-CSF and IL-5 receptors. Int J Cell Cloning 1992; 10:126–134.

62. Donahue RE, Emerson SG, Wang EA, Wong GG, Clark SC, Nathan DG. Demonstration of burst-promoting activity of recombinant human GM-CSF on circulating erythroid progenitors using an assay involving the delayed addition of erythropoietin. Blood 1985; 86:1479–1481.

63. Donahue RE, Wang EA, Stone DK, Kamen R, Wong GG, Sehgal PK, Nathan DG, Clark SC. Stimulation of haematopoiesis in primates by continuous infusion of recombinant human GM-CSF. Nature 1986; 321:872–875.

64. Lieschke GJ, Burgess AW. Granulocyte colony-stimulating factor and granulocyte–macrophage colony-stimulating factor (part 1 of 2). N Engl J Med 1992; 327:28–35.

65. Lieschke GJ, Burgess AW. Granulocyte colony-stimulating factor and granulocyte–macrophage colony-stimulating factor (part 2 of 2). N Engl J Med 1992; 327:991–996.

66. Schreurs J, Gorman DM, Miyajima A. Cytokine receptors: a new superfamily of receptors. Int Rev Cytol 1992; 137B:121–155.

67. Johnson GR, Gonda TJ, Metcalf D, Hariharan IK, Cory S. A lethal myeloproliferative syndrome in mice transplanted with bone marrow cells infected with a retrovirus expressing granulocyte–macrophage colony-stimulating factor. EMBO J 1989; 8:441–448.

68. Rothenberg ME, Pomerantz JL, Owen WF, Avraham S, Soberman RJ, Austen KF, Stevens RL. Characterization of a human eosinophil proteoglycan and augmentation of its biosynthesis and size by interleukin 3, interleukin 5, and granulocyte/macrophage colony-stimulating factor. J Biol Chem 1988; 263:13901–13908.

69. Owen WF, Petersen J, Austen KF. Eosinophils altered phenotypically and primed by culture with granulocyte/macrophage colony-stimulating factor and 3T3 fibroblasts generate leukotriene C_4 in response to fMLP. J Clin Invest 1991; 87:1958–1963.

70. Tomioka K, MacGlashan DW Jr, Lichtenstein LM, Bochner BS, Schleimer RP. GM-CSF regulates human eosinophil responses to f-Met peptide and platelet activating factor. J Immunol 1993; 151:4989–4997.

71. Lopez AF, Williamson DJ, Gamble JR, Begley CG, Harlan JM, Klebanoff SJ, Waltersdorph A, Wong G, Clark SC, Vadas MA. Recombinant human granulocyte–macrophage colony-stimulating factor stimulates in vitro mature human neutrophil and eosinophil function, surface receptor expression, and survival. J Clin Invest 1986; 78:1220–1228.

72. Arnaout MA, Wang EA, Clark SC, Sieff CA. Human recombinant granulocyte–macrophage colony-stimulating factor increases cell-to-cell adhesion and surface expression of adhesion-promoting surface glycoproteins on mature granulocytes. J Clin Invest 1986; 78:597–601.

73. Weisbart RH, Golde DW, Clark SC, Wong GG, Gasson JC. Human granulocyte–macrophage colony-stimulating factor is a neutrophil activator. Nature 1985; 314:361–363.

74. Weisbart RH, Kwan L, Golde DW, Gasson JC. Human GM-CSF primes neutrophils for enhanced oxidative metabolism in response to the major physiological chemoattractants. Blood 1987; 69:18–21.

75. Weisbart RH, Golde DW, Gasson JC. Biosynthetic human GM-CSF modulates the number and affinity of neutrophil f-Met-Leu-Phe receptors. J Immunol 1986; 137:3584–3587.

76. Dehinden CA, Zingg J, Maly FE, de Weck AL. Leukotriene production in human neutrophils primed by recombinant human granulocyte/macrophage colony-stimulating factor and stimulated with the complement component C5a and fMLP as second signals. J Exp Med 1988; 167: 1281–1295.

77. Richter J, Andersson T, Olsson I. Effect of tumor necrosis factor and granulocyte–macrophage colony-stimulating factor on neutrophil degranulation. J Immunol 1989; 142:3199–3205.

78. Kaufman S, Dipersio JF, Gasson JC. Effects of human GM-CSF on neutrophil degranulation in vitro. Exp Hematol 1989; 17:800–804.

79. Metcalf D, Begley CG, Johnson GR, Nicola NA, Vadas MA, Lopez AF, Williamson DJ, Wong GG, Clark SC, Wang EA. Biologic properties in vitro of a recombinant human granulocyte–macrophage colony-stimulating factor. Blood 1986; 67:37–45.

80. Ruff MR, Farrar WL, Pert CB. Interferon γ and granulocyte–macrophage colony-stimulating factor inhibit growth and induce antigens characteristic of myeloid differentiation in small-cell lung cancer cell lines. Proc Natl Acad Sci USA 1986; 83:6–7.

81. Baldwin GC, Gasson JC, Kaufman SE, Quan SG, Williams RE, Avalos BR, Gazdar AF, Golde DW, DiPersio JF. Nonhematopoietic tumor cells express functional GM-CSF receptors. Blood 1989; 73:1033–1037.

82. Dedhar S, Gaboury L, Galloway P, Eaves C. Human granulocyte–macrophage colony-stimulating factor is a growth factor active on a variety of cell types of non hematopoietic origin. Proc Natl Acad Sci USA 1988; 85:9253–9257.

83. Berdel WE, Danhauser-Riedl S, Steinhauser G, Winton EF. Various human hematopoietic growth factors (interleukin 3, GM-CSF, G-CSF) stimulate clonal growth of nonhematopoietic tumor cells. Blood 1989; 73:80–83.

84. Baldwin GC, Golde DW, Widhopf GF, Economou J, Gasson JC. Identification and characterization of a low-affinity granulocyte–macrophage colony-stimulating factor receptor on primary and cultured human melanoma cells. Blood 1991; 78:609–615.

85. Colotta F, Bussolino F, Polentarutti N, Guglielmetti A, Sironi M, Bocchietto E, De Rossi M, Mantovani A. Differential expression of the common β and specific α-chains of the receptors for GM-CSF, IL-3 and IL-5 in endothelial cells. Exp Cell Res 1993; 206:311–317.

86. Bussolino F, Wang JM, Defillipi P, Turrini F, Sanavio F, Edgell CJ, Aglietta M, Arese P, Mantovani A. Granulocyte–macrophage colony-stimulating factors induce human endothelial cells to migrate and proliferate. Nature 1989; 337:471–473.

87. Takatsu K, Tominaga A, Harada N, Mita S, Matsumoto M, Takahashi T, Kikuchi Y, Yamaguchi N. T cell-replacing factor (TRF)/interleukin 5 (IL-5): molecular and functional properties. Immunol Rev 1988; 102:107–135.

88. Yokota T, Arai N, De Vries J, Spits H, Bachereau J, Zlotnick A, Rennick D, Howard M, Takebe Y, Miyatake S, Lee F, Arai K. Molecular biology of interleukin 4 and interleukin-5 genes and biology of their products that stimulate B cells, T cells and hemopoietic cells. Immunol Rev 1988; 102:137–187.

89. Metcalf D, Parker JW, Chester HM, Kincade PW. Formation of eosinophil-like granulocyte colonies by mouse bone marrow cells in vitro. J Cell Physiol 1974; 84:275–289.

90. Strath M, Warren DJ, Sanderson CJ. Detection of eosinophils using an eosinophil peroxidase assay. Its use as an assay for eosinophil differentiation factors. J Immunol Methods 1985; 83: 209–215.

91. Ruscetti FW, Cypress RH, Chervenick PA. Specific release of neutrophilic- and eosinophilic-stimulating factors from sensitized lymphocytes. Blood 1976; 47:757–765.

92. Lopez AF, Begley CG, Williamson DJ, Warren DJ, Vadas MA, Sanderson CJ. Murine eosinophil differentiation factor: an eosinophil-specific colony-stimulating factor with activity on human cells. J Exp Med 1986; 163:1085–1099.

93. Azuma C, Tanabe T, Konishi M, Kinashi T, Noma T, Matsuda F, Yaoita Y, Takatsu K, Hammarstrom L, Smith CIE, Severinson E, Honjo T. Cloning of cDNA for human T-cell replacing factor (interleukin-5) and comparison with the murine homologue. Nucleic Acids Res 1986; 14:9149–9158.

94. Tominaga A, Takahashi T, Kikuchi Y, Mita S, Noami S, Harada N, Yamaguchi N, Takatsu K. Role of carbohydrate moiety of IL-5: effect of tunicamycin on the glycosylation of IL-5 and the biologic activity of deglycosylated IL-5. J Immunol 1990; 144:1345–1352.

95. McKenzie ANJ, Ely B, Sanderson CJ. Mutated interleukin-5 monomers are biologically inactive. Mol Immunol 1991; 28:155–158.

96. Minamitake Y, Kodama S, Katayama T, Adachi H, Tanaka S, Tsujimoto M. Structure of recombinant human interleukin 5 produced by Chinese hamster ovary cells. J Biochem (Tokyo) 1990; 107:292–297.

97. Proudfoot AE, Davies JG, Turcatti G, Wingfield PT. Human interleukin-5 expressed in *Escherichia coli*: assignment of the disulfide bridges of the purified unglycosylated protein. FEBS Lett 1991; 283:61–64.

98. Devos R, Guisez Y, Cornelis S, Verhee A, Van der Heyden J, Maaeberg M, Lahm HW, Fiers W, Tavernier J, Plaetinck G. Recombinant soluble human interleukin-5 (hIL-5) receptor molecules. Cross-linking and stoichiometry of binding to IL-5. J Biol Chem 1993; 268:6581–6587.

99. Denburg JA. Basophil and mast cell lineages in vitro and in vivo. Blood 1992; 79:846–860.

100. Sanderson CJ. Interleukin-5, eosinophils, and disease. Blood 1992; 79:3101–3109.

101. Ohnishi T, Kita H, Weiler D, Sur S, Sedgwick JB, Calhoun WJ, Busse WW, Abrams JS, Gleich GJ. IL-5 is the predominant eosinophil-active cytokine in the antigen-induced pulmonary late-phase reaction. Am Rev Respir Dis 1993; 147:901–907.

102. Basten A, Beeson PB. Mechanism of eosinophilia. II. Role of the lymphocyte. J Exp Med 1970; 131:1288–1305.

103. Nielsen K, Fogh L, Andersen S. Eosinophil response to migrating *Ascaris suum* larvae in normal and congenitally thymus-less mice. Acta Pathol Microbiol Immunol Scand 1974; 82:919–920.

104. Hz CK, Hz SH, Whitney RA, Hansen CT. Immunopathology of schistosomiasis in athymic mice. Nature 1976; 262:397–399.

105. Walker C, Virchow J-C, Bruijnzeel PLB, Blaser K. T cell subsets and their products regulate eosinophilia in allergic and nonallergic asthma. J Immunol 1991; 146:1829–1835.

106. Bradding P, Feather IH, Wilson S, Bardin PG, Heusser CH, Holgate ST, Howarth PH. Immuno-localization of cytokines in the nasal mucosa of normal and perennial rhinitic subjects. The mast cell as a source of IL-4, IL-5, and IL-6 in human allergic mucosal inflammation. J Immunol 1993; 151:3853–3865.

107. Broide DH, Paine MM, Firestein GS. Eosinophils express interleukin 5 and granulocyte–macrophage colony-stimulating factor mRNA at sites of allergic inflammation in asthmatics. J Clin Invest 1992; 90:1414–1424.

108. Clutterbuck EJ, Sanderson CJ. Human eosinophil hematopoiesis studied in vitro by means of murine eosinophil differentiation factor (IL-5): production of functionally active eosinophils from normal human bone marrow. Blood 1988; 71:6346.
109. Campbell HD, Sanderson CJ, Wang Y, Hort Y, Martinson ME, Tucker WQ, Stellwagen A, Strath M, Young IG. Isolation, structure and expression of cDNA and genomic clones for murine eosinophil differentiation factor. Comparison with other eosinophilopoietic lymphokines and identity with interleukin-5. Eur J Biochem 1988; 174:345–352.
110. Sanderson CJ. Control of eosinophilia. Int Arch Allergy Appl Immunol 1991; 94:122–126.
111. Yamaguchi Y, Suda T, Suda J, Eguchi NM, Miura Y, Harasda N, Tominaga A, Takatsu K. Purified interleukin 5 supports the terminal differentiation and proliferation of murine eosinophilic precursors. J Exp Med 1988; 167:43–56.
112. Clutterbuck EJ, Sanderson CJ. The regulation of human eosinophil precursor production by cytokines: a comparison of rhIL-1, rhIL-3, rhIL-4, rhIL-6, and rh granulocyte–macrophage colony-stimulating factor. Blood 1990; 75:1774–1779.
113. Warren DJ, Moore MA. Synergism among interleukin 1, interleukin 3, and interleukin 5 in the production of eosinophils from primitive hemopoietic stem cells. J Immunol 1988; 140:94–99.
114. Lu L, Lin ZH, Shen RN, Warren DJ, Leemhuis T, Broxmeyer HE. Influence of interleukins 3, 5 and 6 on the growth of eosinophil progenitors in highly enriched human bone marrow in the absence of serum. Exp Hematol 1990; 18:1180–1186.
115. Ema H, Suda T, Nagayoshi K, Miura Y, Civin CI, Nakauchi H. Target cells for granulocyte colony-stimulating factor, interleukin-3 and interleukin-5 in differentiation pathways of neutrophils and eosinophils. Blood 1990; 76:1956–1961.
116. Sonoda Y. Humoral regulation of eosinophilopoiesis by interleukin-3, granulocyte–macrophage colony-stimulating factor (GM-CSF) and interleukin-5. Nippon Rinsho 1993; 51:565–570.
117. Vaux DL, Lalor PA, Cory S, Johnson GR. In vivo expression of interleukin 5 induces an eosinophilia and expanded Ly-1B lineage populations. Int Immunol 1990; 2:965–971.
118. Dent LA, Strath M, Mellor AL, Sanderson CJ. Eosinophilia in transgenic mice expressing IL-5. J Exp Med 1990; 172:1425–1431.
119. Hitoshi Y, Yamaguchi N, Korenaga M, Mita S, Tominaga A, Takatsu K. In vivo administration of antibody to murine IL-5 receptor inhibits eosinophilia of transgenic mice. Int Immunol 1991; 3:135–139.
120. Coffman RL, Seymour BW, Hudak S, Jackson J, Rennick D. Antibody to interleukin-5 inhibits helminth-induced eosinophilia in mice. Science 1989; 245:308–310.
121. Owen WF, Rothenberg ME, Petersen J, Weller PF, Silberstein DS, Sheffer A, Stevens RL, Soberman RJ, Austen KF. Interleukin 5 and phenotypically altered eosinophils in the blood of patients with the idiopathic hypereosinophilic syndrome. J Exp Med 1989; 170:343–348.
122. Owen WF, Petersen J, Sheff DM, Folkerth RD, Anderson RJ, Corson JM, Sheffer AL, Austen KF. Hypodense eosinophils and interleukin 5 activity in the blood of patients with the eosinophilia–myalgia syndrome. Proc Natl Acad Sci USA 1990; 87:8647–8651.
123. Butterfield JH, Leiferman KM, Abrams J, Silver JE, Bower J, Gonchoroff N, Gleich GJ. Elevated serum levels of interleukin-5 in patients with the syndrome of episodic angioedema and eosinophilia. Blood 1992; 79:688–692.
124. Samoszuk M, Nansen L. Detection of interleukin-5 messenger RNA in Reed-Sternberg cells of Hodgkin's disease with eosinophilia. Blood 1990; 75:13–16.
125. Matsumoto R, Ando M, Kohrogi H, Araki S, Takatsu K. Interleukin-05 levels of pleural fluid and serum samples in a patient with PIE syndrome. Chest 1992; 102:1296–1297.
126. Yamaguchi Y, Suda T, Ohta S, Tomonaga K, Miura Y, Kasahara T. Analysis of the survival of mature human eosinophils: interleukin-5 prevents apoptosis in mature human eosinophils. Blood 1991; 78:2542–2547.
127. Sehmi R, Wardlaw AJ, Cromwell O, Kurihara K, Waltmann P, Kay AB. Interleukin-5 selectively enhances the chemotactic response of eosinophils obtained from normal but not eosinophilic subjects. Blood 1992; 79:2952–2959.

128. Schweizer RC, Welmers BA, Raaijmakers JA, Zanen P, Lammer JW, Koenderman L. RANTES- and interleukin-8-induced responses in normal human eosinophils: effects of priming with interleukin-5. Blood 1994; 83:3697–3704.

129. Hansel TT, De Vries IJ, Carballido JM, Braun RK, Carballido-Perrig N, Rihs S, Blaser K, Walker C. Induction and function of eosinophil intercellular adhesion molecule-1 and HLA-DR. J Immunol 1992; 149:2130–2136.

130. Hartnell A, Kay AB, Wardlaw AJ. Interleukin-3-induced up-regulation of CR3 expression on human eosinophils is inhibited by dexamethasone. Immunology 1992; 77:488–493.

131. Walsh GM, Wardlaw AJ, Hartnell A, Sanderson CJ, Kay AB. Interleukin-5 enhances the in vitro adhesion of human eosinophils, but not neutrophils, in a leukocyte integrin (CD11/18)-dependent manner. Int Arch Allergy Appl Immunol 1991; 94:174–178.

132. Blom M, Tool AT, Kok PT, Koenderman L, Roos D, Verhoeven AJ. Granulocyte–macrophage colony-stimulating factor, interleukin-3 (IL-3), and IL-5 greatly enhance the interaction of human eosinophils with opsonized particles by changing the affinity of complement receptor type 3. Blood 1994; 83:2978–2984.

133. Guida L, O'Hehir RE, Hawrylowicz CM. Synergy between dexamethasone and interleukin-5 for the induction of major histocompatibility complex class II expression by human peripheral blood eosinophils. Blood 1994; 84:2733–2740.

134. Bischoff SC, Brunner T, De Weck AL, Dahinden CA. Interleukin 5 modifies histamine release and leukotriene generation by human basophils in response to diverse agonists. J Exp Med 1990; 172:1577–1582.

135. Hitoshi Y, Yamaguchi N, Mita S, Sonoda E, Takaki S, Tominaga A, Takatsu K. Distribution of IL-5 receptor-positive B cells. Expression of IL-5 receptor on Ly-1 (CD5)+ B cells. J Immunol 1990; 144:4218–4225.

136. Wetzel GD. Induction of interleukin 5 responsiveness in resting B cells by engagement of the antigen receptor and perception of a second polyclonal activation signal. Cell Immunol 1991; 137:358–366.

137. Allison KC, Strober W, Harriman GR. Induction of IL-5 receptors in normal B cells by cross-linking surface Ig with anti-Ig-dextran. J Immunol 1991; 146:4197–4203.

138. Purkeson JM, Isakson PC. Interleukin 5 (IL-5) provides a signal that is required in addition to IL-4 for isotype switching to immunoglobulin (Ig) G1 and IgE. J Exp Med 1992; 175:973–982.

139. Purkeson J, Isakson P. A two-signal model for regulation of immunoglobulin isotype switching. FASEB J 1992; 6:3245–3252.

140. Sonoda E, Hitoshi Y, Yamaguchi N, Ishii T, Tominaga A, Araki S, Takatsu K. Differential regulation of IgA production by TGF-beta and IL-5: TGF-beta induces surface IgA-positive cells bearing IL-5 receptor, whereas IL-5 promotes their survival and maturation into IgA-secreting cells. Cell Immunol 1992; 140:158–172.

141. Clutterbunk E, Shields JG, Gordon J, Smith SH, Boyd A, Callard RE, Campbell HD, Young IG, Sanderson CJ. Recombinant human interleukin 5 is an eosinophil differentiation factor but has no activity in standard human B cell growth factor assays. Eur J Immunol 1987; 17:1743–1750.

142. Baumann MA, Paul CC. Interleukin-5 is an autocrine growth factor for Epstein–Barr virus-transformed B lymphocytes. Blood 1992; 79:1763–1767.

143. Paul CC, Keller JR, Armpriester JM, Baumann MA. Epstein–Barr virus transformed B lympho-cytes produce interleukin-5. Blood 1990; 75:1400–1403.

144. Hara M, Kitani A, Harigai M, Hirose T, Suzuki K, Kawakami M, Ishizaka T, Kawaguchi Y, Hidaka T, Kawagoe M, et al. Interleukin 5 up-regulates high-affinity interleukin 2 receptor expression by human resting peripheral T cells: a comparison with the effect of interleukin 4 on B cells. Cytokine 1991; 3:584–592.

145. Chandrasekharappa SC, Rebelsky MS, Firak TA, Le Beau MM, Westbrook CA. A long-range restriction map of the interleukin-4 and interleukin-5 group on chromosome 5. Genomics 1990; 6:94–99.

146. Lee JS, Campbell HD, Kozak CA, Young IG. The IL-4 and IL-5 genes are closely linked and are part of a cytokine gene cluster on mouse chromosome 11. Somat Cell Mol Genet 1989; 15: 143–152.

147. Westbrook CA, Neuman WL, Hewitt J, Kidd KK, Le Beau MM, Williamson R. Report of the chromosome 5 workshop. Genomics 1991; 10:1105–1109.

148. Le Beau MM, Pettenati MJ, Lemons RS, Diaz MO, Westbrook CA, Larson PA, Sherr CJ, Rowley JD. Assignment of the GM-CSF, CSF-1 and FMS genes to human chromosome 5 provides evidence for linkage of a family of genes regulating hematopoiesis and for their involvement in the deletion (5q) in myeloid disorders. Cold Spring Harbor Symp Quant Biol 1986; 51:899–909.

149. Sutherland GR, Baker E, Callen DF, Campbell HD, Young IG, Sanderson CJ, Garson OM, Lopez AF, Vadas MA. Interleukin-5 is at 5q31 and is deleted in the 5q- syndrome. Blood 1988; 71:1150–1152.

150. Le Beau MM, Westbrok CA, Diaz MO, Larson RA, Rowley JD, Gasson JC, Golde DW, Scherr CJ. Evidence for the involvement of GM-CSF and FMS in the deletion (5q) in myeloid disorders. Science 1986; 231:984–987.

151. Huebner K, Isobe M, Croce CM, Golde DW, Kaufman SE, Gasson JC. The human gene encoding GM-CSF is at 5q21-q32, the chromosome region deleted in the 5q− anomaly. Science 1985; 230:1282–1285.

152. Muto A, Yokota T. IL-3 gene, receptor and signal transduction. Nippon Rinsho 1992; 50:1781–1786.

153. Shanafelt AB, Miyajima A, Kitamura T, Kastelein RA. The amino-terminal helix of GM-CSF and IL-5 governs high-affinity binding to their receptors. EMBO J 1991; 10:4105–4112.

154. Shanafelt AB, Kastelein RA. High affinity ligand binding is not essential for granulocyte–macrophage colony-stimulating factor receptor activation. J Biol Chem 1992; 267:25466–25472.

155. Meropol N, Altmann SW, Shanafelt AB, Kastelein RA, Prystowski M. The requirement of hydrophilic amino-terminal residues for granulocyte–macrophage colony-stimulating factor bioactivity and receptor binding. J Biol Chem 1992; 267:14266–14269.

156. Lopez AF, Shannon MF, Hercus T, Nicola NA, Canberi B, Dottore M, Layton MJ, Eglinton L, Vadas MA. Residue 21 of human granulocyte–macrophage colony-stimulating factor is critical for biological activity and for high but not low-affinity binding. EMBO J 1992; 11:909–916.

157. Diedrichs K, Boone T, Karplus PA. Novel fold and putative receptor binding site of granulocyte–macrophage colony-stimulating factor. Science 1991; 254:1779–1782.

158. Park LS, Friend D, Price V, Anderson D, Singer J, Prickett KS, Urdal DL. Heterogeneity in human interleukin-3 receptors. A subclass that binds human granulocyte-macrophage colony-stimulating factor. J Biol Chem 1989; 264:5420–5427.

159. Lopez AF, Eglinton JM, Gillis D, Park LS, Clark S, Vadas MA. Reciprocal inhibition of binding between interleukin 3 and granulocyte–macrophage colony-stimulating factor to human eosinophils. Proc Natl Acad Sci USA 1989; 86:7022–7026.

160. Lopez AF, Vadas MV, Woodcock JM, Milton SE, Lewis A, Elliot MJ, Gillis D, Ireland REO, Park LS. Interleukin-5, interleukin-3 and granulocyte–macrophage colony-stimulating factor cross-compete for binding to cell surface receptors on human eosinophils. J Biol Chem 1991; 266:24741–24747.

161. Lopez AF, Eglinton JM, Tapley PM, To LB, Parl LS, Clark SC, Vadas MA. Human interleukin-3 inhibits the binding of granulocyte–macrophage colony-stimulating factor and interleukin-5 to basophils and strongly enhances their functional activity. J Cell Physiol 1990; 145:69–77.

162. Gesner TG, Mufson RA, Norton CR, Turner KJ, Yang YC, Clark SC. Specific binding, internalization, and degradation of human recombinant interleukin-3 by cells of the acute myelogenous leukemia line, KG-1. J Cell Physiol 1988; 136:493–499.

163. Taketazu F, Chiba S, Shibuya K, Kuwaki T, Tsumura H, Miyazono K, Miyagawa K, Takaku F.

IL-3 specifically inhibits GM-CSF binding to the higher-affinity receptor. J Cell Physiol 1991; 146:251–257.

164. Park LS, Friend D, Gillis S, Urdal D. Characterization of the cell surface receptor for a multi-lineage colony-stimulating factor (CSF-2 alpha). J Biol Chem 1986; 261:205–210.

165. Nicola NA, Metcalf D. Binding of iodinated multipotential colony-stimulating factor (interleukin-3) to murine bone marrow cells. J Cell Physiol 1986; 128:180–188.

166. Schreuers J, Arai K, Miyajima A. Evidence for a low-affinity interleukin-3 receptor. Growth Factors 1990; 2:221–234.

167. Nicola NA, Peterson L. Identification of distinct receptors for two hematopoietic growth factors (granulocyte colony-stimulating factor and multipotential colony-stimulating factor) by chemical cross-linking. J Biol Chem 1986; 261:12384–12389.

168. May S, Ihle JN. Affinity isolation of the interleukin-3 surface receptor. Biochem Biophys Res Commun 1986; 135:870–879.

169. Sorensen P, Farber NM, Krystal G. Identification of the interleukin-3 receptor using an iodinatable, cleavable photoreactive cross-linking agent. J Biol Chem 1986; 261:9094–9097.

170. Schreuers J, Sugawara M, Arai K, Ohta Y, Miyajima A. A monoclonal antibody with IL-3-like activity blocks IL-3 binding and stimulates tyrosine phosphorylation. J Immunol 1989; 142: 819–825.

171. Isfort RJ, Stevens D, May WS, Ihle JN. Interleukin 3 binds to a 140-kDa phosphotyrosine-containing cell surface protein. Proc Natl Acad Sci USA 1988; 85:7982–7986.

172. Yonehara S, Ishii A, Yonehara M, Koyasu S, Miyajima A, Schreurs J, Arai K, Yahara I. Identification of a cell surface 105 kD protein (A1C-2 antigen) which binds interleukin-3. Int Immunol 1990; 2:143–150.

173. Itoh N, Yonehara S, Schreuers J, Gorman DM, Maruyama K, Ishii A, Yahara I, Arai KI, Miyajima A. Cloning of an interleukin-3 receptor gene: a member of a distinct receptor gene family. Science 1990; 247:324–327.

174. Schreuers J, Hung P, May WS, Arai K, Miyajima A. A1C2A is a component of the purified high affinity mouse IL-3 receptor: temperature-dependent modulation of A1C2A structure. Int Immunol 1991; 3:1231–1242.

175. Gorman DM, Itoh N, Kitamura T, Schreuers J, Yonehara S, Yahara I, Arai K, Miyajima A. Cloning and expression of a gene encoding an interleukin 3 receptor-like protein: identification of another member of the cytokine receptor gene family. Proc Natl Acad Sci USA 1990; 87: 5459–5463.

176. Kitamura T, Hayashida K, Sakamaki K, Yokota T, Arai K, Miyajima A. Reconstitution of a functional human granulocyte–macrophage colony-stimulating factor (GM-CSF) receptor: evidence that A1C2B is a subunit of murine GM-CSF receptor. Proc Natl Acad Sci USA 1991; 88: 5082–5086.

177. Takaki S, Mita S, Kitamura T, Yonehara S, Yagamuchi N, Tominaga A, Miyajima A, Takatsu K. Identification of the second subunit of the murine interleukin-5 receptor: interleukin-3 receptor-like protein, AIC2B is a component of the high affinity interleukin-5 receptor. EMBO J 1991; 10:2833–2838.

178. Hara T, Miyajima A. Two distinct functional high affinity receptors for mouse interleukin-3 (IL-3). EMBO J 1992; 11:1875–1884.

179. Kuwaki T, Kitamura T, Tojo A, Matsuki S, Tamai Y, Miyazono K, Takaku F. Characterization of human interleukin-3 receptors on a multi-factor-dependent cell line. Biochem Biophys Res Commun 1989; 161:16–22.

180. Hayashida K, Kitamura T, Gorman DM, Arai K, Yokota T, Miyajima A. Molecular cloning of a second subunit of the human GM-CSF receptor. Proc Natl Acad Sci USA 1990; 87:9655–9659.

181. Kitamura T, Sato N, Arai K, Miyajima A. Expression cloning of the human IL-3 receptor cDNA reveals a shared subunit for the human IL-3 and GM-CSF receptors. Cell 1991; 66:1165–1174.

182. Miyajima A, Kitamura T. Functional reconstruction of the human IL-3 receptor. Blood 1992; 80:84–90.

183. Kremer E, Baker E, D' Andrea RJ, et al. A cytokine receptor gene cluster in the X-Y pseudo-autosomal region? Blood 1993; 82:22–28.
184. Shen Y, Baker E, Callen DF, Sutherland GR, Wilson TA, Rakar S, Gough NM. Localization of the human GM-CSF receptor beta chain (CSF2RB) to chromosome 22q12.2→q13.1. Cytogenet Cell Genet 1992; 61:175–177.
185. Kastelein RA, Shanafelt AB. GM-CSF receptor. Interactions and activation. Oncogene 1993; 8:231–236.
186. Walker F, Burgess AW. Specific binding of radioiodinated granulocyte-macrophage colony-stimulating factor to hematopoietic cells. EMBO J 1985; 4:933–939.
187. Park LS, Martin U, Sorensen R, Luhr S, Morrisey PJ, Cosman D, Larsen A. Cloning of the low-affinity murine granulocyte–macrophage colony-stimulating factor receptor and reconstitution of a high-affinity receptor complex. Proc Natl Acad Sci USA 1992; 89:4295–4299.
188. Park LS, Friend D, Gillis S, Urdal DL. Characterization of the cell surface receptor for human granulocyte/macrophage colony-stimulating factor. J Exp Med 1986; 164:251–262.
189. Gasson JC, Kaufman SE, Weisbart RH, Tomonaga M, Golde DW. High-affinity binding of granulocyte–macrophage colony-stimulating factor to normal and leukemic myeloid cells. Proc Natl Acad Sci USA 1986; 83:669–673.
190. Baldwin GC, Gasson JC, Kaufman SE, Quan SG, Williams RE, Avalos BR, Gazdar AF, Golde DW, DiPersio JF. Nonhematopoietic tumor cells express functional GM-CSF receptors. Blood 1989; 73:1033–1037.
191. DiPersio J, Billing P, Kaufman S, Eghtesady P, Williams RE, Gasson JC. Characterization of the human granulocyte–macrophage colony-stimulating factor receptor. 1988; 263:1834–1841.
192. Chiba S, Tojo A, Kitamura T, Urabe A, Miyazono K, Takaku F. Characterization and molecular features of the cell surface receptor for human granulocyte–macrophage colony-stimulating factor. Leukemia 1990; 4:29–36.
193. Park LS, Waldron PE, Friend D, Sassenfeld HM, Prie V, Anderson D, Cosman D, Andrews RG, Berstein ID, Urdal DL. Interleukin-3, GM-CSF and G-CSF receptor on cell lines and primary leukemia cells: receptor heterogeneity and relationship to growth factor responsiveness. Blood 1989; 74:56–65.
194. Cannistra SA, Koenigsmann M, DiCarlo J, Groshek P, Griffin JD. Differentiation-associated expression of two functionally distinct classes of granulocyte–macrophage colony-stimulating factor receptors by human myeloid cells. 1990; 265:12656–12663.
195. Rapoport AP, Abboud CN, DiPersio JF. Granulocyte–macrophage colony-stimulating factor (GM-CSF) and granulocyte colony-stimulating factor (G-CSF): receptor biology, signal transduction, and neutrophil activation. Blood Rev 1992; 6:43–57.
196. Gearing DP, King JA, Gough NM, Nicola NA. Expression cloning of a receptor for human granulocyte macrophage colony-stimulating factor. EMBO J 1989; 8:3667–3776.
197. Metcalf D, Nicola NA, Gearing DP, Gough NM. Low-affinity placenta-derived receptors for human granulocyte–macrophage colony-stimulating factor can deliver a proliferative signal to murine hematopoietic cells. Proc Natl Acad Sci USA 1990; 87:4670–4674.
198. Park LS, Friend D, Gillis S, Urdal DL. Characterization of the cell surface receptor for granulocyte–macrophage colony-stimulating factor. J Biol Chem 1986; 261:4177–4183.
199. Gesner TG, Mufson RA, Turner KJ, Clark SC. Identification through chemical cross-linking of distinct granulocyte–macrophage colony-stimulating factor and interleukin-3 receptors on myeloid leukemic cells, KG-1. Blood 1989; 2652–2656.
200. Crosier KE, Wong GG, Mathey-Prevot B, Nathan DG, Sieff CA. A functional isoform of the human granulocyte/macrophage colony-stimulating factor receptor has an unusual cytoplasmic domain. Proc Natl Acad Sci USA 1991; 88:7744–7748.
201. Raines MA, Liu L, Quan SG, Joe V, DiPersio JF, Golde DW. Identification and molecular cloning of a soluble human granulocyte–macrophage colony-stimulating factor receptor. Proc Natl Acad Sci USA 1991; 88:8203–8207.
202. Gough NM, Gearing DP, Nicola NA, Baker E, Pritchard M, Callen DF, Sutherland GR.

Localization of the human GM-CSF receptor gene to the X-Y pseudoautosomal region. Nature 1990; 345:734–736.

203. Mita S, Tominaga A, Hitoshi Y, Sakamoto K, Honjo T, Akagi M, Kikuchi Y, Yamaguchi N, Takatsu K. Characterization of high-affinity receptors for interleukin-5 on interleukin 5-dependent cell lines. Proc Natl Acad Sci USA 1989; 86:2311–2315.

204. Takaki S, Tominaga A, Hitoshi Y, Mita S, Sonoda E, Yagamuchi N, Takatsu K. Molecular cloning and expression of the murine interleukin-5 receptor. EMBO J 1990; 9:4367–4374.

205. Devos R, Plaetinck G, Van der Heyden J, Cornelis S, Vanderckhove J, Fiers W, Tavernier J. Molecular basis of a high-affinity murine interleukin-5 receptor. EMBO J 1991; 10:2133–2137.

206. Plaetinck G, Van der Heyden J, Tavernier J, Fache I, Tuypens T, Fischkoff S, Fiers W, Devos R. Characterization of interleukin 5 receptors on eosinophilic sublines from human promyelocytic leukemia (HL-60) cells. J Exp Med 1990; 172:683–691.

207. Tavernier J, Devos R, Cornelis S, Tuypens T, Van der Heyden J, Fiers W, Plaetinck G. A high affinity interleukin-5 receptor (IL-5R) is composed of an IL-5 specific alpha chain and a beta chain shared with the receptor for GM-CSF. Cell 1991; 66:1175–1184.

208. Murata Y, Takaki S, Migita M, Kikuchi Y, Tominaga A, Takatsu K. Molecular cloning and expression of the human interleukin-5 receptor. J Exp Med 1992; 175:341–351.

209. Bazan JF. A novel family of growth factor receptors: a common binding domain in the growth hormone, prolactin, erythropoietin and IL-6 receptors, and the p75 IL-2 receptor beta chain. Biochem Biophys Res Commun 1989; 164:788–795.

210. Patthy L. Homology of a domain of the growth hormone/prolactin receptor family with type III modules of fibronectin. Cell 1990; 61:13–14.

211. Larsen A, Davis T, Curtis BM, Gimpel S, Sims JE, Cosman D, Park L, Sorensen E, March CJ, Smith CA. Expression cloning of a human granulocyte colony-stimulating factor: a structural mosaic of hematopoietin receptor, immunoglobulin, and fibronectin domains. J Exp Med 1990; 172:1559–1570.

212. D'Andrea AD, Fasman GD, Lodish HF. Erythropoietin and interleukin-2 receptor beta chain: a new receptor family. Cell 1989; 58:1023–1024.

213. Hibi M, Murakami M, Saito M, Hirano T, Taga T, Kishimoto T. Molecular cloning and expression of an IL-6 signal transducer, gp130. Cell 1990; 63:1149–1157.

214. Tuypens T, Plaetinck G, Baker E, Sutherland G, Brusselle G, Fiers W, Devos R, Tavernier J. Organization and chromosomal location of the human interleukin 5 receptor gene. Eur Cytokine Network 1992; 3:451–459.

215. Isobe M, Kumura Y, Murata Y, Takaki S, Tominaga A, Takatsu K, Ogita Z. Localization of the gene encoding the alpha subunit of the human interleukin-5 receptor (IL-5R-α) to chromosome region 3p24-3p26. Genomics 1992; 14:755–758.

216. Chihara J, Plumas J, Gruart V, Tavernier J, Prin L, Capron A, Capron M. Characterization of a receptor for interleukin 5 on human eosinophils: variable expression and induction by human granulocyte/macrophage colony-stimulating factor. J Exp Med 1990; 172:1347–1351.

217. Migita M, Yamaguchi N, Mita S, Higuchi S, Hitoshi Y, Yoshida Y, Tominaga M, Matsuda F, Tominaga A, Takatsu K. Characterization of the human IL-5 receptors on human eosinophils. Cell Immunol 1991; 133:484–497.

218. Ingley E, Young IG. Characterization of a receptor for interleukin-5 on human eosinophils and the myeloid leukemia line HL-60. Blood 1991; 78:339–344.

219. Woodcock JM, Zacharakis B, Plaetinck G, Bagley CJ, Qiyu S, Hercus TR, Tavernier J, Lopez AF. Three residues in the common beta chain of the human GM-CSF, IL-3 and IL-5 receptors are essential for GM-CSF and Il-5 but not IL-3 high affinity binding and interact with Glu 21 of GM-CSF. EMBO J 1994; 13:5176–5185.

220. Hoang T, De Lean A, Haman A, Beauchemin V, Kitamura T, Clark SC. The structure and dynamics of the granulocyte macrophage colony-stimulating factor receptor defined by the ternary complex model. J Biol Chem 1993; 268:11881–11887.

221. Shakamaki K, Miyajima I, Kitamura T, Miyajima A. Critical cytoplasmic domains of the

common beta subunit of the human GM-CSF, IL-3 and IL-5 receptors for growth signal transduction and tyrosine phosphorylation. EMBO J 1992; 11:3541–3549.

222. Wang H-M, Ogorochi T, Arai K, Miyajima A. Structure of mouse interleukin 3 (IL-3) binding protein (A1C2A): amino acid residues critical for IL-3 binding. J Biol Chem 1992; 267:979–983.

223. Fuh G, Mulkerrin MG, Bass S, McFarland N, Brochier M, Bourell JH, Light DR, Wells JA. The human growth hormone receptor. Secretion from *Escherichia coli* and disulfide bonding pattern of the extracellular binding domain. J Biol Chem 1990; 265:3111–3115.

224. Bazan JF. Structural design and molecular evolution of a cytokine receptor superfamily. Proc Natl Acad Sci USA 1990; 87:6934–6938.

225. Maller JL. Xenopus oocytes and the biochemistry of cell division. Biochemistry 1990; 29:3157–3166.

226. Fan K, Ruan Q, Sensenbrenner L, Chen BD. Up-regulation of granulocyte–macrophage colony-stimulating factor (GM-CSF) receptors in murine peritoneal exudate macrophages by both GM-CSF and IL-3. J Immunol 1992; 149:96–102.

227. Hallek M, Lepisto EM, Slattery KE, Griffin JD, Ernst TJ. Interferon-gamma increases the expression of the gene encoding the beta subunit of the granulocyte–macrophage colony-stimulating factor receptor. Blood 1992; 80:1736–1742.

228. Elbaz O, Budel LM, Hoogerbrugge H, Touw IP, Delwel R, Mahmoud LA, Lowenberg B. Tumor necrosis factor regulates the expression of granulocyte–macrophage colony-stimulating factor (GM-CSF) and interleukin-3 (IL-3)-receptors on human acute myeloid leukemia cells. Blood 1991; 77:989–995.

229. Wantanabe Y, Kitamura T, Hayashida K, Miyajima A. Monoclonal antibody against the common beta subunit (beta c) of the human interleukin-3(IL-3), IL-5 and granulocyte–macrophage colony-stimulating factor receptors shows upregulation of beta c by IL-1 and tumor necrosis factor alpha. Blood 1992; 80:2215–2220.

230. Ashworth A, Kraft A. Cloning of a potentially soluble receptor for human GM-CSF. Nucleic Acids Res 1990; 18:7178.

231. DiPersio JF, Hedvat C, Ford CF, Golde DW, Gasson JC. Characterization of the soluble human granulocyte–macrophage colony-stimulating factor receptor complex. J Biol Chem 1991; 266:279–286.

232. Tavernier J, Tuypens T, Plaetinck G, Verhee A, Fiers W, Devos R. Molecular basis of the membrane-anchored and two soluble isoforms of the human interleukin 5 receptor alpha subunit. Proc Natl Acad Sci USA 1992; 89:7041–7045.

233. Finberg RW, Wahl SM, Allen JB, Saman G, Strom TB, Murphy JR, Nichols JC. Selective elimination of HIV-1-infected cells with an interleukin-2 receptor-specific cytotoxin. Science 1991; 252:1703–1705.

18

Nitric Oxide

Richard A. Robbins and Joseph H. Sisson
University of Nebraska Medical Center, Omaha, Nebraska

INTRODUCTION

The attention given to nitric oxide (NO) in the past 7 years has been remarkable. Attesting to the interest generated, NO was named "The Molecule of the Year" by the editors of *Science* in 1992, and it has now estimated that over 10% of all manuscripts submitted to biomedical research journals deal with some aspect of NO (1). Much of the resultant information explosion has emphasized that NO is involved in a vast number of diverse physiological and pathophysiological processes (1,2). Proposed roles for NO include regulation of smooth-muscle tone, neurotransmission, host defense, and cytotoxicity. Many of these suggested functions implicate NO in basic allergic mechanisms and disorders. It is the intent of this chapter to review the recent advances in the understanding of NO, emphasizing those most relevant to the pathophysiology of allergic diseases.

The capacity of the endothelium to dilate blood vessels by releasing activity that decreases the tone of the underlying vascular smooth muscle has been recognized for several years (3). However, the identity of this endothelial-derived relaxing factor (EDRF) remained baffling because of its exceedingly short half-life, until two groups independently reported that EDRF was analogous with NO (4,5). At about the same time, two groups investigating the mechanisms of macrophage-mediated cytotoxicity described that one mechanism could be accounted for by a molecule resembling NO (6,7). Taken together these initial investigations have laid the foundation on which many of the more recent advances have occurred.

FORMATION OF NITRIC OXIDE

Nitric oxide is formed when the guanido group of the essential amino acid L-arginine is cleaved, forming NO and L-citrulline (Fig. 1) (1,2). The reaction is catalyzed by nitric oxide

415

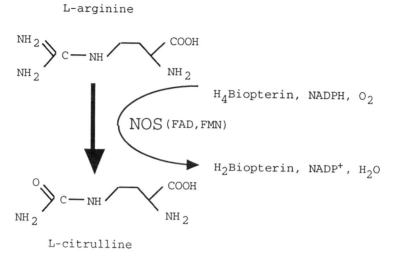

L-arginine

Figure 1 Diagrammatic representation of the L-arginine–nitric oxide pathway. The guanido group of L-arginine is cleaved, generating nitric oxide (NO) and L-citrulline. The reaction is catalyzed by nitric oxide synthase (NOS) and several cofactors, including NADPH, tetrahydrobiopterin (H_4 biopterin), and the flavones (FAD, FMN).

synthase (NOS) and several cofactors. The reaction is stereospecific (i.e., only L-arginine is cleaved by NOS to form L-citrulline); D-arginine does not interact with NOS.

Nitric oxide synthase exists in several forms (Table 1; 8). Although arginine transport into the cell is probably necessary for continued NO production, NOS activity appears to be the major rate-limiting step of NO formation in vivo (2). In the vasculature, a constitutive NOS (cNOS) exists, which is a constitutively expressed, calcium-dependent enzyme (9,10). The enzyme migrates as a monomer of 135 kDa on gel electrophoresis, and it is homologous with cytochrome P-450 reductase (11,12). Constitutive NOS accounts for the baseline production of small, picomolar amounts of NO from endothelial cells, but has also been identified in a variety of nonendothelial cells (see Table 1; 13–22).

Brain NOS (bNOS, also called neural NOS or nNOS) is another constitutively expressed NOS and similar in many aspects to cNOS (8,23). Both are calcium-dependent and produce picomolar amounts of NO. The similarity is not surprising, since the enzymes are about 60% homologous (8–11,23).

An inducible form of NOS (iNOS) has been detected in a variety of tissues and organs in addition to vascular endothelium (see Table 1; 6,7,18,22,24–29). Inducible NOS appears to be approximately 50% homologous with cNOS or bNOS (26,30,31). However, in contrast with cNOS or bNOS, iNOS is not usually expressed in most tissues, but is induced by lipopolysaccharide (LPS) or cytokines (2,8). Induction of iNOS can result in the formation of much larger, nanomolar amounts of NO than the picomolar amounts that result from cNOS or bNOS (2).

The NOSs have several cofactors, including flavones (FAD, FMN), tetrahydrobiopterin, and NADPH (2,8,32). Brain NOS colocalizes with NADPH diaphorase, and it now appears that bNOS and NADPH diaphorase are, in fact, the same enzyme (33). This activity is

Table 1 Comparison of the Different Forms of Nitric Oxide Synthase

	cNOS	bNOS	iNOS
Location	Endothelium Neutrophils Platelets Mast cells Renal glomeruli and tubules Myocardium Gastric mucosa	Nervous system Lung epithelium	Endothelium Macrophages Fibroblasts Smooth muscle Hepatocytes Neutrophils Lung epithelium Myocardium Pancreatic islets Chrondocytes
Amount of NO produced	Picomolar	Picomolar	Nanomolar
Calcium-dependent	Yes	Yes	No or partially
Increases activity	Sheer stress Calcium Calmodulin	Appropriate receptor stimulation Calcium Calmodulin	TNF-α IL-1β IFN-γ LPS
Decreases activity	Hypoxia NO LPS TNF-α	Protein kinase C	Corticosteroids Transforming growth factor-β IL-10 Monocyte chemotactic protein-1 IL-4

useful in that nitroblue tetrazolium can be used to localize bNOS activity (34). Presumably, other NOS activities could also be localized with nitroblue tetrazolium (22).

Both cNOS and bNOS are clearly calcium-dependent enzymes and are activated by Ca^{2+} or calmodulin (2,8). Thus, stimuli that increase intracellular calcium also increase cNOS or bNOS activity, resulting in a rise of NOS activity in a matter of a few seconds (34). In the endothelium, sheer stress over 24 h increases cNOS mRNA and protein (36). Recent studies have determined that hypoxia down-regulates cNOS in pulmonary endothelium, presumably as a mechanism to shunt blood to better-ventilated areas (37–39). Nitric oxide also appears to be capable of decreasing cNOS activity, thereby providing a negative-feedback loop that prevents overproduction of NO (40). Interestingly, in contrast with iNOS (see later), tumor necrosis factor-α (TNF-α) and LPS actually decrease cNOS (36,41).

Brain NOS appears to be regulated in a manner similar to cNOS, predominantly through Ca^{2+} and calmodulin (2,8,23). Brain bNOS transfected into kidney 293 cells is phosphory-lated and, consequently, inhibited by protein kinase C (PKC; 42). However, both cNOS and bNOS have an AMP-dependent protein kinase phosphorylation site, but phosphorylation of bNOS by this kinase has no effect on catalytic activity (35). Therefore, the significance of such phosphorylation is unclear.

In contrast with cNOS and bNOS, iNOS is thought to be calcium-independent, although recent studies using hepatocyte iNOS, cloned into human embryonic kidney cells, suggest a partial calcium dependence (26). The major regulator of iNOS activity appears to be transcriptional regulation of iNOS mRNA. Stimuli, such as LPS, or cytokines, such as (TNF), interleukin-1β (IL-1), or interferon (IFN)-γ, increase iNOS mRNA, which correlates with iNOS protein expression and function (25,43). In pulmonary endothelial cells and lung epithelial cell lines, combinations of cytokines with or without LPS appear to be more potent in augmenting iNOS mRNA than individual cytokines or LPS alone (25,43). In vitro it takes several hours to increase iNOS mRNA and, once induced, the RNA has a half-life of several hours (43). Corticosteroids, transforming growth factor β (TGF-β), IL-10 monocyte chemotactic protein (MCP)-1, IL-4, and a cigarette smoke extract have recently been reported to inhibit cytokine- or LPS-induced increases in iNOS (43–54).

METABOLISM OF NITRIC OXIDE

Nitric oxide is a highly reactive radical (most correctly represented by $NO^{\cdot}$) and has an estimated half-life of seconds in biological tissues (55). Nitric oxide reacts rapidly with O_2^{-} to form peroxynitrite (OONO$^-$; 56–58):

$$NO^{\cdot} + O_2^{-} \rightarrow OONO^{\cdot} + H^{+} \rightarrow OONOH \rightarrow OH^{\cdot} + NO_2$$

Peroxynitrite is a strong, oxidizing agent that spontaneously forms nitrite (NO_2^{-}) and hydroxyl (OH^{-}) anions (59,60). Both of the latter facilitate lipid peroxidation; therefore, they could be important in both host defense or tissue damage resulting from NO formation (56,59,60). Nitrite is stable for several hours in water and plasma, but is rapidly converted to nitrate in whole blood (2,61).

There are also several pathways other than by reacting with oxygen by which NO can be metabolized. It reacts with a variety of heme and non–heme-containing metalloproteins (55,62,63). Binding of NO to the porphyrin ring of guanylate cyclase results in activation of the enzyme, leading to formation of GMP (64). The increase in cGMP leads to relaxation of vascular smooth muscle, accounting for the reduction in blood pressure induced by NO (2,64). In addition, NO can react with various other proteins, including hemoglobin, myoglobin, cytochrome c, catalase, succinate dehydrogenase, lipoxygenase, ascorbate oxidase, ceruloplasmin, and tyrosinase and, in some instances, modifies the function of these proteins (65).

Sulfur-containing compounds can react with NO, forming S-nitrosothiols (RS-NO; 55). This may be one mechanism that attenuates the toxicity of NO and its formation of peroxynitrite (55,66). A variety of nitrosothiols have been found under physiological conditions, including S-nitrosoalbumin, S-nitrosoglutathione, S-nitrosocysteine, and S-nitroso-homocysteine (67–72). However, the formations of these compounds are reversible reactions, and NO can be released with a change in redox state, pH, or thiol content (73). Therefore, these reactions might be thought of as an NO repository (74).

Nitric oxide can also react with DNA (75,76). In vitro, NO can deaminate deoxynucleosides, deoxynucleotides, and intact DNA (75). These reactions result in the formation of C→T transitions in bacteria in vivo, with resultant mutagenesis (75). Presumably, the same type of reactions could occur in humans. Furthermore, similar reactions might occur in the primary amines of amino acids, resulting in alteration of protein structure and sequence (75).

In summary, the oxidant chemistry of NO metabolism may be extremely complex. There are several demonstrated or potential reactions by which NO might chemically alter the basic composition of cellular lipids, proteins, and DNA. Therefore, the potential for NO to alter cellular function is extensive and, only recently, has this potential become appreciated.

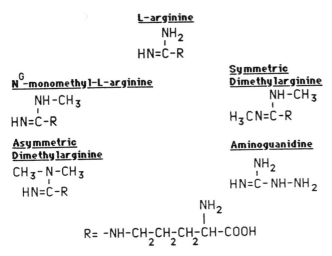

Figure 2 Structures of L-arginine, N^G-monomethyl-L-arginine (L-NMMA), asymmetric dimethyl-arginine, symmetric dimethylarginine, and aminoguanidine. L-NMMA, asymmetric dimethyl-arginine, and symmetric dimethylarginine have been identified in human urine and plasma. L-NMMA and asymmetric dimethylarginine are competitive NOS inhibitors, but symmetric is the inactive isomer of asymmetric dimethylarginine. Aminoguanidine is a competitive NOS inhibitor.

PHARMACOLOGY OF NITRIC OXIDE

A variety of synthetic and naturally occurring inhibitors of NOS have been described (Fig. 2). Most of these inhibitors have substitutions made in the guanido group of arginine and compete with arginine for the active site on NOS (2). As with arginine, only the L-forms are active (2). Asymmetric dimethylarginine and N^G-monomethyl-L-arginine (L-NMMA), inhibitors of NOS, and symmetric dimethylarginine, an inactive isomer of asymmetric dimethylarginine, are present in plasma and urine and, therefore, are naturally occurring inhibitors (2,77). These compounds accumulate in renal failure and have been hypothesized to lead to the hypertension seen in this disorder (2,77).

Several other NOS inhibitors have been commonly used to block the action of cNOS, bNOS, and iNOS in the laboratory. These include not only the naturally occurring L-NMMA, but also L-N^G-nitroarginine methyl ester (L-NAME), N^G-nitro-L-arginine (L-NOARG), N^G-iminoethyl-L-ornithine (L-NIO), L-N^G-nitroarginine-p-nitroanilide (L-NAPNA), L-canavanine, hydroxycobalamin, and aminoguanidine (78). Both L-NMMA and L-NIO inhibit arginine transport into the cell, suggesting an additional mechanism for inhibition of NO production other than competitive NOS inhibition (79). Hydroxy-cobalamin appears to be a more selective inhibitor of endothelial cNOS than bNOS (80), and conversely, L-NAPNA appears to be more selective for bNOS than endothelial cNOS (81). Aminoguanidine has been reported to have 10- to 100-fold greater inhibitory activity for iNOS than for cNOS, suggesting that it might have potential therapeutic use in those situations when selective inhibition of iNOS is desirable (82).

Glucocorticoids inhibit induction of iNOS, but do not cNOS (43–45). The action appears to be by reduction of iNOS mRNA transcription and not by a direct effect on the enzyme (43–45).

In addition to inhibitors of NOS that decrease NO, a variety of NO generators are known that release NO. Two of the more common are nitroglycerin and sodium nitroprusside, and current thought is that both drugs exert their effects predominantly by release of NO (83). In addition, various synthetic donors, including S-nitroso-N-acetylpenicillamine (SNAP) and spermine-NO (SPERNO) have been synthesized for use in laboratory investigations (75,84).

PHYSIOLOGY OF NITRIC OXIDE

Vasodilation

Vasodilation of the microcirculation is a key component of the inflammatory reaction and influences edema formation and leukocyte accumulation. Nitric oxide has a well-established role in the endothelial-dependent control of blood pressure (2). In addition, there is evidence to suggest that NO-mediated vasodilation may potentiate edema. Nitric oxide appears to mediate the edema response to substance P, LPS, and ultraviolet light irradiation in rat skin (85–87). An attractive hypothesis is that the initial edema formation during allergen skin tests might involve a local increase in cNOS activity, caused by release of bradykinin, acetylcholine, substance P, thrombin, or adenine nucleotides, with a resultant increase in local intracellular calcium concentrations. Later, an increase in local cytokine production results in stimulation of iNOS, leading to edema formation during the late allergic skin reaction. Although such a hypothesis would conform to current thoughts on NO production and edema formation, it is untested.

Nitric oxide might be involved in neural stimulation of vascular relaxation (2,35). In addition to its direct vasodilatory properties, NO can also mediate endothelium-independent vascular smooth-muscle relaxation in cerebral and other arteries, as well as the penile corpus cavernosum (88–90). These responses are sensitive to tetrodotoxin, which blocks the voltage-dependent Na^+ channels responsible for propagation of action potentials in nerves. Depolarization of nerves, resulting in an increased cytosolic Ca^{2+} concentration, stimulates bNOS in nerve terminals which, in turn, results in production of NO and stimulation of guanylate cyclase in vascular smooth muscle, causing relaxation (35).

Inflammation

The role of NO in an inflammatory response is unclear and, at times, contradictory. It is either endogenously released from neutrophils or monocytes or, when exogenously added, it appears to enhance chemotaxis of these cells by a cGMP-dependent mechanism (Fig. 3; 91–93). However, NO appears to inhibit adhesion of leukocytes to vascular endothelium and bronchial epithelium (94,95).

Nitric oxide has been hypothesized to mediate both acute and chronic inflammatory reactions. Inhibitors of NOS attenuate the degree of acute inflammation in rats with adjuvant arthritis and immune–complex-mediated lung and dermal injury (96–98). Inhibitors of NOS also inhibit experimental models of ileitis (99). In support of the role of NO participation in inflammatory responses, nitrite is increased in joint fluid aspirated from patients with rheumatoid arthritis (100).

However, other experimental evidence has led to the hypothesis that NO suppresses inflammation. Lymphocytes can release NO, and murine macrophage release of NO can

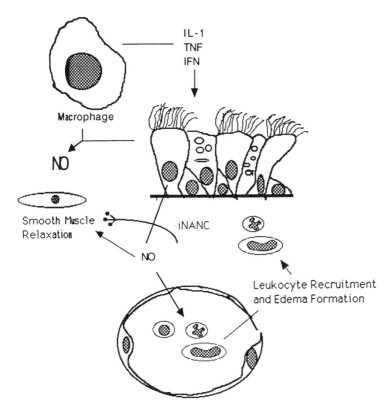

Figure 3 Schematic representation of possible roles for NO in the lung. Stimulation of alveolar macrophages results in release of cytokines and NO. The cytokines estimate bronchial epithelium, causing additional NO production. The NO can be released into the airway and detected in the exhaled air, or can interact with smooth muscle or blood vessels. The NO together with the NO-dependent inhibitory nonadrenergic, noncholinergic (iNANC) pathway results in bronchodilatation. NO interaction with blood vessels and leukocytes may result in edema formation and enhanced recruitment of inflammatory cells.

reduce lymphocyte activation (101–105). These observations have led to the hypothesis that local NO production plays a suppressor role in allograph rejection (104,105).

Taken together, these varied observations suggest a potential role for NO in inflammation and specific immunity. However, as evidenced by the opposing experimental results and hypotheses, a precise role for NO remains to be defined.

Bronchodilatation

Nitric oxide appears to be capable of mediating bronchodilatation by several mechanisms (see Fig. 3). It has long been known that NO donors, such as nitroglycerin or sodium nitroprusside, can relax airway smooth muscle in vitro (106,107). Nitric oxide gas also relaxes tracheal muscle and reduces methacholine-induced bronchoconstriction (84, 108,109). Interestingly, these effects appear to be more marked in denuded epithelium strips, suggesting that the epithelium may serve as a barrier, preventing access of NO to the bronchial smooth muscle (110). In support of the capacity for NO to relax smooth muscle, it has recently been demonstrated that NO reduces methacholine-induced bronchoconstriction in patients with asthma (110). However, NO does not alter bronchial tone in normal volunteers (112).

There is increasing evidence that NO may function as the neurotransmitter of the inhibitory nonadrenergic, noncholinergic (iNANC) bronchodilator response (see Fig. 3). Brain NOS has been localized to airway nerves in the guinea pig, ferret, and human airways that innervate airway vessels, smooth muscle, and submucosal glands, and also has been detected in the parasympathetic, sympathetic, and sensory ganglia supplying the airways (112–115). Nitric oxide appears to account for a portion of iNANC response in pig, guinea pig, cat, and horse airways (116–121). Recent evidence suggests that NO neurotransmission accounts for nearly all the human iNANC response (122–125). This may have functional significance, because NANC nerves are the only known neural bronchodilator mechanism in human airways (126).

In contrast with its bronchodilatatory role by neurotransmission or direct action on smooth muscle, the potential exists for NO to potentiate bronchial narrowing (see Fig. 3). Nitric oxide is a potent bronchial vasodilator in animal airways (127). It is feasible that NO-mediated dilation of bronchial blood vessels could at least partly account for the edema seen in narrowing of the airway in conditions such as asthma. In support of this concept, NO inhibitors reduce neurogenic plasma exudation in guinea pig airway (128).

Host Defense

Murine macrophages produce antimicrobial activity that is L-arginine-dependent through production of NO (6,7,129). In addition, NO may also be cytotoxic for tumor cells (130,131). These effects appear to be dependent on the combination of NO with enzymes of the respiratory cycle and on DNA synthesis in the target cells (75,131–133). These data suggest that NO production by macrophages may be an important mechanism in host defense against microorganisms and tumor cells. Neutrophils also produce NO, suggesting that these cells may also participate in host defenses by a similar mechanism (14).

Nitric oxide is also generated by respiratory tract epithelial cells (21,22,43,134). Although it is controversial whether iNOS is constitutively expressed by these cells or must be induced (22,134), cytokines released by macrophages can increase iNOS mRNA transcription, producing a marked increase in NO production (43,134). This suggests that not only may macrophages directly participate in host defenses by releasing NO, but may also indirectly participate by releasing cytokines that stimulate resident epithelial cells to release NO.

Removing particulate matter and microorganisms by modulating the mucociliary escalator represents another mechanism by which NO may enhance host defense: NO increases ciliary beat frequency above baseline (135). Isoproterenol increases ciliary beat frequency within minutes, and NOS inhibitors attenuate this increase (135). The cytokines TNF and IL-1 also increase ciliary beat frequency, although it takes several hours to note the increase (136); NOS inhibitors also decrease this later cytokine-mediated increase. These observations would be consistent with the early effect being mainly through a cNOS mechanism, and the later cytokine-mediated response being through an iNOS mechanism, although this remains unproved. The later cytokine-mediated increase provides further evidence that macrophage release of cytokines may enhance NO production by bronchial epithelial cells.

NITRIC OXIDE IN HUMAN DISEASE

Asthma

Nitric oxide has been detected in the exhaled air of normal humans and animals (137,138). Asthma is a bronchospastic disorder characterized by a bronchitis, consisting of eosinophils, neutrophils, macrophages, and lymphocytes (139). Macrophages obtained from asthmatic subjects release increased amounts of cytokines (140,141). Therefore, it does not seem surprising that exhaled NO levels are increased in asthmatic subjects (Fig. 4) (142–144). Furthermore, inhaled corticosteroids decreased the exhaled NO levels, consistent with their in vitro inhibitory effects on iNOS mRNA transcription (43, 142). The cellular source of the increase in exhaled NO is unclear, but bronchial epithelial cells obtained from asthmatics have increased expression of iNOS, suggesting that this is one potential source (134).

The role that increased NO might be playing in the lower respiratory tract of asthmatics is unclear. It could be argued that low amounts of NO released from epithelial cells or macrophages might be beneficial in relaxing airway smooth muscle. However, NO might represent a double-edged sword, and high amounts could potentially contribute to airway hyperemia, resulting in airway narrowing, or epithelial cytotoxicity and shedding.

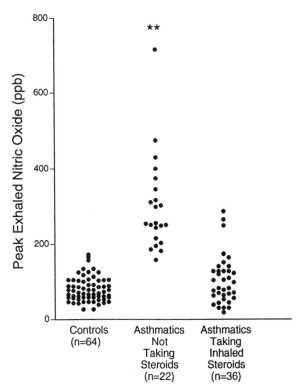

Figure 4   Peak exhaled nitric oxide levels in normal nonasthmatic, nonsmoking controls, subjects with asthma not taking corticosteroids, and subjects with asthma taking inhaled corticosteroids. **p < 0.01 compared with controls and asthmatic subjects receiving corticosteroids. (Data from Ref. 54.)

Hypertension and Hypotension

Endothelial cell production of NO has a fairly well-established role in the regulation of blood pressure (2). Several lines of evidence suggest that NO at least partly contributes to essential hypertension. Endothelial-dependent vasodilation is decreased in patients with essential hypertension, and the response to L-NMMA is reduced in these patients (145,146). In addition, arginine infusion into human with or without hypertension produces a reduction in blood pressure (147,148).

It is thought that NO plays an important role in shock. The NOS inhibitors can prevent the hypotension in animals produced by anaphylaxis, LPS, TNF, or hemorrhage (149). Initial studies demonstrated that NOS inhibitors improved blood pressure in some patients with septic shock (150); however, more recent data have been disappointing (151). Perhaps the degree of NO inhibition may be crucial for the outcome of treatment (152). Excessive inhibition of NO might lead to severe vasoconstriction, with resultant end-organ damage. This has led to the concept that selective inhibition of iNOS or inhibition of endogenous NO, while administering small amounts of a nitrovasodilator, may lead to an improved outcome.

Adult Respiratory Distress Syndrome

Recent data have demonstrated that inhalation of NO might be beneficial to patients with the adult respiratory distress syndrome (ARDS). Nitric oxide is a known pulmonary vasodilator, leading to the concept that inhalation of NO would improve ventilation–perfusion matching by selectively vasodilating those areas of the lung that are well ventilated. Rossaint and co-workers (153) administered low doses (18–36 ppm) through the ventilator of patients with ARDS and found an improvement in ventilation–perfusion matching. Interestingly, administration of NO for 7 days resulted in improvement in lung function, which did not appear to be totally explained by pulmonary vasodilation. This improvement suggests that NO might produce a beneficial effect by other mechanisms, such as reducing lung inflammation, or by improving lung healing.

Cigarette Smoking

Cigarette smoking has many adverse health consequences, including increased incidences of hypertension, heart disease, and lower respiratory tract infection (154–156). The potential exists for NO to play a role in each of these disorders. Recent data have demonstrated that exhaled NO is reduced in cigarette smokers, compared with those who do not smoke, suggesting that smoke may inhibit NOS (54,144). Nitric oxide is contained in high levels in cigarette smoke, and NO can inhibit its own production by inhibiting NOS (40,157). However, this did not appear to be the mechanism, because inhalation of NO in amounts approximating the levels in cigarette smoke did not reduce exhaled NO levels (54).

REFERENCES

1. Culotta E, Koshland DE, NO news is good news. Science 1992; 258:1862–1863.
2. Moncada S, Higgs A. The L-arginine–nitric oxide pathway. N Engl J Med 1993; 329:2002–2012.
3. Furchgott RF, Zawadski JV. The obligatory role of endothelial cells in the relaxation of arterial smooth muscle by acetylcholine. Nature 1980; 288:373–376.

4. Palmer RMJ, Ferrige AG, Moncada S. Nitric oxide release accounts for the biological activity of endothelium-derived relaxing factor. Nature 1987; 327:524–526.

5. Ignarro LJ, Buga CM, Wood KS, Byrns RE, Chaudhuri G. Endothelium derived relaxing factor produced and released from artery and vein is nitric oxide. Proc Natl Acad Sci USA 1987; 84:9265–9269.

6. Hibbs JB, Taintor RR, Vaurin Z. Macrophage cytotoxicity: role of L-arginine deaminase activity and imino nitrogen oxidation to nitrite. Science 1987; 235:473–476.

7. Iyenger R, Stuehr DJ, Marletta MA. Macrophage synthesis of nitrite, nitrate, and N-nitrosamines; precursors and role of the respiratory burst. Proc Natl Acad Sci USA 1987; 84:6369–6373.

8. Förstermann U, Schmidt HHHW, Pollock JS, Sheng H, Mitchell JA, Warner TD, Masaki N, Murad F. Isoforms of nitric oxide synthase: characterization and purification from different cell types. Biochem Pharmacol 1991; 10:1849–1857.

9. Lamas S, Marsden PA, Li GK, Tempst P, Michel T. Endothelial nitric oxide synthase: molecular cloning and characterization of a distinct constitutive enzyme isoform. Proc Natl Acad Sci USA 1992; 89:6348–6352.

10. Janssens SP, Shimouchi A, Quertermous T, Bloch DB, Block KD. Cloning and expression of a cDNA encoding human endothelium-derived relaxing factor/nitric oxide synthase. J Biol Chem 1992; 267:14519–14522.

11. Pollock JS, Förstermann U, Mitchell JA, Warner TD, Schmidt HHHW, Nakane M, Murad F. Purification and characterization of particulate endothelium-derived relaxing factor synthase from cultured and native bovine aortic endothelial cells. Proc Natl Acad Sci USA 1991; 88:10480–10484.

12. Bredt DS, Hwang PM, Glatt CE, Lowenstein C, Reed RR, Snyder SH. Cloned and expressed nitric oxide synthase structurally resembles cytochrome P-450 reductase. Nature 1991; 351:714–718.

13. Salvemini D, Masini C, Anggard E, Mannaioni PF, Vane J. Synthesis of nitric oxide-like factor from L-arginine by rat serosal mast cells: stimulation of guanylate cyclase and inhibition of platelet aggregation. Biochem Biophys Res Commun 1990; 169:596–601.

14. Yui Y, Hattori R, Kosuga K, Eizawa H, Hiki K, Ohkawa S, Ohnishi K, Terao S, Kawai C. Calmodulin-independent nitric oxide synthase from rat polymorphonuclear neutrophils. J Biol Chem 1991; 266:3369–3371.

15. Hiki K, Yui Y, Hattori R, Eizawa H, Kosuga K, Kawai C. Three regulation mechanisms of nitric oxide synthase. Eur J Pharmacol 1991; 206:163–164.

16. Radomski NW, Moncada S. Biological role of nitric oxide in platelet function. In: Moncada S, Higgs EA, Berrazueta JR, eds. Clinical Relevance of Nitric Oxide in the Cardiovascular System. Madrid: Edicomplet, 1991:45–56.

17. Smith JA, Shah AM, Lewis MJ. Factors released from endocardium of the ferret and pig modulate myocardial contraction. J Physiol 1991; 439:1–14.

18. DeBelder AJ, Radomski MW, Why HJF, Richardson PJ, Bucknall CA, Salas E, Martin JF, Moncada S. Nitric oxide synthase activities in human myocardium. Lancet 1993; 341:84–85.

19. Terada Y, Tomita K, Nonoguchi H, Marumo F. Polymerase chain reaction localization of constitutive nitric oxide synthase and soluble guanylate cyclase messenger RNAs in microdissected rat nephron segments. J Clin Invest 1992; 90:659–665.

20. Brown JF, Tepperman BL, Hanson PJ, Whittle BJR, Moncada S. Differential distribution of nitric oxide synthase between cell fractions isolated from the rat gastric mucosa. Biochem Biophys Res Commun 1992; 184:680–685.

21. Robbins RA, Hamel FG, Floreani AA, Gossman GL, Nelson KJ, Belenky S, Rubinstein I. Bovine bronchial epithelial cells metabolize L-arginine to L-citrulline: possible role of nitric oxide synthase. Life Sci 1993; 52:709–716.

22. Kobzik L, Bredt DS, Lowenstein CJ, Drazen J, Gaston B, Sugarbaker D, Stamler JS. Nitric

oxide synthase in human and rat lung: immunochemical and histochemical localization. Am J Respir Cell Mol Biol 1993; 9:371–377.

23. Bredt DS, Snyder SH. Isolation of nitric oxide synthetase, a calmodulin-requiring enzyme. Proc Natl Acad Sci USA 1990; 87:682–685.

24. Jorens PG, van Overveld FJ, Vermeire PA, Bult H, Herman AG. Synergism between inter-leukin-1β and the nitric oxide synthase inducer interferon-γ in rat lung fibroblasts. Eur J Pharmacol 1992; 224:7–12.

25. Nakayama DR, Geller DA, Lowenstein CJ, Davies P, Pitt BR, Simmons RL, et al. Cytokines and lipopolysaccharides induce nitric oxide synthase in cultured rat pulmonary artery smooth muscle. Am J Respir Cell Mol Biol 1992; 7:471–476.

26. Geller DA, Lowenstein CJ, Shapiro RA, et al. Molecular cloning and expression of inducible nitric oxide synthase from human hepatocytes. Proc Natl Acad Sci USA 1992; 90:3491–3495.

27. McCall TB, Broughton-Smith NK, Palmer RMJ, Whittle BJR, Moncada S. Synthesis of nitric oxide from L-arginine by neutrophils. Release and interaction with superoxide anions. Biochem J 1989; 169:596–601.

28. Eizirik DL, Björklund A, Welsh N. Interleukin-1-induced expression of nitric oxide synthase in insulin-producing cells is preceded by c-*fos* induction and depends on gene transcription and protein synthesis. FEBS Lett 1993; 317:62–66.

29. Stadler J, Stefanovic-Racic M, Billiar TR, Curran RD, McIntyre LA, Georgescu HI, Simmons RL, Evans CH. Articular chondrocytes synthesize nitric oxide in response to cytokines and lipopolysaccharide. J Immunol 1991; 147:3915–3920.

30. Xie Q-W, Cho HJ, Claycay J, et al. Cloning and characterization of inducible nitric oxide synthase from mouse macrophages. Science 1992; 256:225–228.

31. Lyons CR, Orloff GJ, Cunningham JM. Molecular cloning and functional expression of an inducible nitric oxide synthase from a murine macrophage cell line. J Biol Chem 1992; 172:1246–1252.

32. Kwon NS, Nathan CF, Stueh DS. Reduced biopterin as a cofactor in the generation of nitrogen oxides by murine macrophages. J Biol Chem 1989; 264:20496–20501.

33. Hope BT, Michael GJ, Knige KM, Vincent SR. Neuronal NADPH-diaphorase is a nitric oxide synthase. Proc Natl Acad Sci USA 1991; 88:2811–2814.

34. Hope BT, Vincent SR. Histochemical characterisation of neuronal NADPH-diaphorase. J Histochem Cytochem 1989; 37:653–661.

35. Knowles RG, Moncada S. Nitric oxide as a signal in blood vessels. Trend Biol Sci 1992; 17:399–402.

36. Nishida K, Harrison DG, Navas JP, Fisher AA, Dockery SP, Uematsu M, Nerem RM, Alexander RW, Murphy TJ. Molecular cloning and characterization of the constitutive bovine aortic endothelial cell nitric oxide synthase. J Clin Invest 1992; 90:2092–2101.

37. Liu SF, Crawley DE, Barnes PJ, Evans TW. Endothelium-derived nitric oxide inhibits pulmon-ary vasoconstriction in isolated blood perfused rat lungs. Am Rev Respir Dis 1991; 143:32–37.

38. Persson MG, Gustafsson LE, Wiklund NP, Moncada S, Hedqvist P. Endogenous nitric oxide as a probable modulator of pulmonary circulation and hypoxic pressor response in vivo. Acta Physiol Scand 1990; 140:449–457.

39. Adnos S, Raffestin B, Eddamibi S, Braquet P, Chabrier PE. Loss of endothelium-dependent relaxant activity in the pulmonary circulation of rats exposed to chronic hypoxia. J Clin Invest 1991; 87:155–162.

40. Buga GM, Griscavage JM, Rogers NE, Ignarro LJ. Negative feedback regulation of endothelial cell function by nitric oxide. Circ Res 1993; 73:808–812.

41. Myers PR, Wright TF, Tanner MA, Adams HR. EDRF and nitric oxide production in cultured endothelial cells: direct inhibition by *E. coli* endotoxin. Am J Physiol 1992; 262:H710–H718.

42. Bredt DS, Ferris CD, Snyder SH. Nitric oxide synthase sites. Phosphorylation by cyclic AMP-dependent protein kinase, protein kinase C, and calcium/calmodulin protein kinase; identifica-tion of flavin and calmodulin binding sites. J Biol Chem 1992; 267:10976–10981.

43. Robbins RA, Springall DR, Warren JB, Kwon OJ, Buttery LDK, Wilson AJ, Adcock IM, Rivers-Moreno V, Moncada S, Polak J, Barnes PJ. Inducible nitric oxide synthase is increased in murine lung epithelial cells by cytokine stimulation. Biochem Biophys Res Commun 1994; 198:835–843.

44. DiRosa M, Radomski M, Carnuccio R, Moncada S. Glucocorticoids inhibit the induction of nitric oxide synthase in macrophages. Biochem Biophys Res Commun 1990; 172:1246–1252.

45. Radomski MW, Palmer RMJ, Moncada S. Glucocorticoids inhibit the expression of an inducible, but not the constitutive nitric oxide synthase in vascular endothelial cells. Proc Natl Acad Sci USA 1990; 87:10043–10049.

46. Junquero DC, Schini VB, Scott-Burden TS, Vanhoutte PM. Transforming growth factor-β_1 inhibits L-arginine-derived relaxing factor(s) from smooth muscle cells. Am J Physiol 1992; 262:H1788–H1795.

47. Ding A, Nathan CF, Graycar J, Derynck R, Steuhr DJ, Srimal S. Macrophage deactivating factor and transforming growth factors β-1, β-2 and β-3 inhibit induction of macrophage nitrogen oxide synthase by interferon-gamma. J Immunol 1990; 145:940–944.

48. Pfeilschifter J, Vosbeck K. Transforming growth factor β_2 inhibits interleukin 1β- and tumour necrosis factor α-induction of nitric oxide synthase in rat renal mesangial cells. Biochem Biophys Res Commun 1991; 175:372–379.

49. Liew FY, Li Y, Severn A, Millot S, Schmidt J, Salter M, Moncada S. A possible novel pathway of regulation of murine T helper type-22 (Th2) cells of a Th1 cell activity via the modulation of the induction of nitric oxide synthase on macrophages. Eur J Immunol 1991; 21:2489–2494.

50. Cunha FQ, Moncada S, Liew FY. Interleukin-10 (IL-10) inhibits the induction of nitric oxide synthase by interferon-γ in murine macrophages. Biochem Biophys Res Commun 1992; 182:1155–1159.

51. Heck DE, Laskin DL, Gardner RC, Laskin DJ. Epidermal growth factor suppresses nitric oxide and hydrogen peroxide production by keratinocytes: potential role for nitric oxide in the regulation of wound healing. J Biol Chem 1992; 267:21277–21280.

52. McCall TB, Palmer RMJ, Moncada S. Interleukin-8 inhibits the induction of nitric oxide synthase in rat peritoneal macrophages. Biochem Biophys Res Commun 1992; 186:680–685.

53. Rojas A, Delgado R, Claria L, Palacios M. Monocyte chemotactic protein-1 inhibits the induction of nitric oxide synthase in J774 cells. Biochem Biophys Res Commun 1993; 196:274–279.

54. Kharitonov SA, Yates DJ, Robbins RA, Keatings VM, Robichaud A, Barnes PJ. Cigarette smoking decreases exhaled nitric oxide. Am J Respir Crit Care Med 1994; 149:A199.

55. Stamler JS, Singel DJ, Loscalzo J. Biochemistry of nitric oxide and its redox-activated forms. Science 1992; 258:1898–1902.

56. Beckman JS, Beckman TW, Chen J, Marshall PA, Freeman BA. Apparent hydroxyl radical production by peroxynitrite: implications for endothelial injury from nitric oxide and superoxide. Proc Natl Acad Sci USA 1990; 87:1620–1624.

57. Blough NV, Zafiriou OC. Reaction of superoxide with nitric oxide to form peroxynitrite in alkaline aqueous solution. Inorg Chem 1985; 24:3502–3504.

58. Saran M, Michel C, Bors W. Reaction of NO with $O_2{}^-$: implications for the action of endothelium-derived relaxing factor (EDRF). Free Radic Res Commun 1990; 10:221–226.

59. Radi R, Beckman JS, Bush KM, Freeman BA. Peroxynitrite-induced membrane lipid peroxidation: the cytotoxic potential of superoxide and nitric oxide. Arch Biochem Biophys 1991; 288:481–487.

60. Radi R, Beckman JS, Bush KM, Freeman BA. Peroxynitrite oxidation of sulfhydryls: the cytotoxic potential of superoxide and nitric oxide. J Biol Chem 1991; 266:4244–4250.

61. Kelm M, Feelisch M, Grude R, Motz W, Strauer BE. Metabolism of endothelium-derived nitric oxide in human blood. In: Mocada S, Marletta MA, Hibbs JB Jr, Higgs EA, eds. The Biology of Nitric Oxide. Vol. 1. London: Portland Press, 1992:319–322.

62. Marletta MA, Tayeh MA, Hevel JM. Unraveling the biological significance of nitric oxide. Biofactors 1990; 2:219–225.

63. McCleverty JA. Reactions of nitric oxide coordinated to transition metal. Chem Rev 1979; 79:53–76.

64. Waldman SA, Murad F. Biochemical mechanisms underlying vascular smooth muscle relaxation: the guanylate cyclase–cyclic GMP system. J Cardiovasc Pharmacol 1988; 12 (suppl 5): S115–S118.

65. Henry Y, Ducrocq C, Drapier J-C, Servent D, Pellat C, Guissani A. Nitric oxide: a biological effector: electron paramagnetic resonance detection of nitrosyl–iron–protein complexes in whole cells. Eur Biophys J 1991; 20:1–15.

66. Kanner J, Harel S, Granit R. Nitric oxide as an antioxidant. Arch Biochem Biophys 1991; 289:130–136.

67. Stamler JS, Jaraki O, Osborne J, Simon D, Keaney J, Vita J, Singel D, Valeri CR, Loscalzo J. Nitric oxide circulates in mammalian plasma primarily as an *S*-nitroso adduct of serum albumin. Proc Natl Acad Sci USA 1992; 89:7674–7677.

68. Stamler JS, Simon DI, Osborne JA, Mulline ME, Jaraki O, Michel T, Singel DJ, Loscalzo J. *S*-Nitrosylation of proteins with nitric oxide; synthesis and characterization of biologically active compounds. Proc Natl Acad Sci USA 1992; 89:444–448.

69. Lascalzo J. *N*-Acetylcysteine potentiates inhibition of platelet aggregation by nitroglycerine. J Clin Invest 1985; 76:703–708.

70. Wei EP, Kontos HA. H_2O_2 and endothelium-dependent cerebral arteriolar dilation. Hypertension 1990; 16:162–169.

71. Myers PR, Minor RL, Guerra R, Bates JN, Harrison DG. Vasorelaxant properties of the endothelium-derived relaxing factor more closely resemble *S*-nitrosocysteine than nitric oxide. Nature 1990; 345:161–163.

72. Stamler JS, Simon DI, Jaraki O, Osborne JA, Francis S, Mullins M, Singel D, Loscalzo J. *S*-Nitrosylation of tissue-type plasminogen activator confers vasodilatory and antiplatelet properties of the enzyme. Proc Natl Acad Sci USA 1992; 89:8087–8091.

73. Mirvish S. Formation of *N*-nitroso compounds; chemistry, kinetics and in vivo occurrence. Toxicol Appl Pharmacol 1975; 31:325–351.

74. Gaston B, Drazen JM, Loscalzo J, Stamler JS. The biology of nitrogen oxides in the airways. Am J Respir Crit Care Med 1994; 149:538–551.

75. Wink DA, Kasprzak KS, Maragos CM, et al. DNA deaminating ability and genotoxicity of nitric oxide and its progenitors. Science 1991; 254:1001–1003.

76. Nguyen T, Brunson D, Crespi CL, Penman BW, Wishok JS, Tannenbaum SR. DNA damage and mutation in human cells exposed to nitric oxide in vitro. Proc Natl Acad Sci USA 1992; 89: 3030–3034.

77. Vallance P, Leone A, Calver A, Collier J, Moncada S. Accumulation of an endogenous inhibitor of nitric oxide synthesis in chronic renal failure. Lancet 1992; 339:572–575.

78. Rees DD, Palmer RMJ, Schulz R, Hodson MF, Moncada S. Characterization of three inhibitors of endothelial nitric oxide synthase in vitro and in vivo. Br J Pharmacol 1990; 101:746–752.

79. Bogle RG, Moncada S, Pearson JD, Mann GE. Identification of inhibitors of nitric oxide synthase that do not interact with the endothelial cell L-arginine transporter. Br J Pharmacol 1992; 105:768–770.

80. Rajanayagam MAS, Li C-G, Rand MJ. Differential effects of hydroxycobalamin on NO-mediated relaxations in rat aorta and ancoccygeus muscle. Br J Pharmacol 1993; 108:3–5.

81. Baddedge RC, Moore PK, Gathen Z, Hart SL. L-N^G-nitroarginine-*p*-nitroanilide (L-NAPNA): a selective inhibitor of nitric oxide synthase in the brain. Br J Pharmacol 1993; 107:194P.

82. Misko TP, Moore WM, Kasten TP, et al. Selective inhibition of inducible nitric oxide synthase by aminoguanidine. Eur J Pharmacol 1993; 233:119–125.

83. Feelisch M. The biochemical pathways of nitric oxide formation from nitrovasodilators; appro-

priate choice of exogenous NO donors and aspects of preparation and handling of aqueous NO solutions. J Cardiovasc Pharmacol 1991; 17(suppl 3):S25–S33.

84. Dupuy G, Shore SA, Drazen JM, Frostell C, Hill WA, Zapol WM. Bronchodilator action of inhaled nitric oxide in guinea pigs. J Clin Invest 1992; 90:421–428.

85. Hughes SR, Williams TJ, Brain SD. Evidence that endogenous nitric oxide modulated oedema formation induced by substance P. Eur J Pharmacol 1990; 191:481–484.

86. Pons F, Williams TJ, Warren JB. Nitric oxide, but not interleukin-1, mediates the local blood flow response to lipopolysaccharide in rabbit skin. Eur J Pharmacol 1993; 239:23–30.

87. Warren JB, Loi RK, Couglan ML. Involvement of nitric oxide synthase in the delayed vasodilator response to ultraviolet light irradiation of rat skin in vivo. Br J Pharmacol 1993; 109: 802–806.

88. Toda N, Okamura T. Modification by L-N^G-monomethyl-arginine (L-NMMA) of the response to nerve stimulation in isolated dog mesenteric and cerebral arteries. Jpn J Pharmacol 1990; 52:170–173.

89. Gaw AJ, Aberdeen J, Humphrey PPA, Wadsworth RM, Burnstock G. Relaxation of sheep cerebral arteries by vasoactive intestinal polypeptide and neurogenic stimulation: inhibition by L-N^G-monomethyl-arginine in endothelium-denuded vessels. Br J Pharmacol 1991; 102: 567–572.

90. Rajfer J, Aronson WJ, Bush PA, Dorey FJ, Ignarro LJ. Nitric oxide as a mediator of relaxation of the corpus cavernosum in response to nonadrenergic, noncholinergic neurotransmission. N Engl J Med 1992; 326:90–94.

91. Kaplan SS, Billiar T, Curran RD, Zdziarski UE, Simmons RL, Basford RE. Attenuation of chemotaxis with N^G-monomethyl-L-arginine: a role for cyclic GMP. Blood 1989; 74:1885–1887.

92. Belenky SN, Robbins RA, Rennard SI, Gossman GL, Nelson KJ, Rubinstein I. Inhibitors of nitric oxide synthase attenuate neutrophil chemotaxis in vitro. J Lab Clin Med 1993; 122: 388–394.

93. Belenky SN, Robbins RA, Rubinstein I. Nitric oxide synthase inhibitors attenuate human monocyte chemotaxis in vitro. J Leukoc Biol 1993; 53:498–503.

94. Kubes P, Suzuki M, Granger DN. Nitric oxide: an endogenous modulator of leukocyte adhesion. Proc Natl Acad Sci USA 1991; 88:289–292.

95. Robbins RA, Nelson KJ, Gossman GL, Spurzem JM, Sisson JH, Romberger DJ, Rennard SI, Rubinstein I. Modulation of neutrophil adhesion to bronchial epithelial cells by nitric oxide. Am Rev Respir Dis 1993; 147:A435.

96. Isalenti A, Ianaro A, Moncada S, Di Rosa M. Modulation of acute inflammation by endogenous nitric oxide. Eur J Pharmacol 1992; 211:177–182.

97. Ialenti A, Moncada S, Di Rosa M. Modulation of adjuvant arthritis by endogenous nitric oxide. Br J Pharmacol 1993; 110:701–706.

98. Mulligan MS, Hevel JM, Marletta MA, Ward PA. Tissue injury caused by deposition of immune complexes is L-arginine dependent. Proc Natl Acad Sci USA 1991; 88:6338–6342.

99. Miller MJS, Sadowska-Krowicka H, Chotinauruemol S, Kakkis JL, Clark DA. Amelioration of chronic ileitis by nitric oxide synthase inhibition. J Pharmacol Exp Ther 1993; 264:11–16.

100. Farrell AJ, Blake DR, Palmer RMJ, Moncada S. Increased concentrations of nitrite in synovial fluid and serum samples suggest increased nitric oxide synthesis in rheumatic diseases. Ann Rheum Dis 1992; 51:1219–1222.

101. Kirk SJ, Regan MC, Barbul A. Cloned murine T lymphocytes synthesize a molecule with biological characteristics of nitric oxide. Biochem Biophys Res Commun 1990; 173:660–665.

102. Hoffman RA, Lanrehr JM, Billiar TR, Curran RD, Simmons RL. Alloantigen-induced activation of rat splenocytes is regulated by the oxidative metabolism of L-arginine. J Immunol 1990; 145:2220–2226.

103. Albina JE, Abate JA, Henry WL Jr. Nitric oxide production is required for murine resident

peritoneal macrophages to suppress mitogen-stimulated T cell proliferation; role of IFN-γ in the induction of the nitric oxide-synthesizing pathway. J Immunol 1991; 147:144–148.

104. Langrehr JM, Hoffman RA, Billiar TR, Lee KKW, Schraut WH, Simmons RL. Nitric oxide synthesis in the in vivo allograft response; a possible regulatory mechanism. Surgery 1991; 110:335–342.

105. Mills CD. Molecular basis of "suppressor" macrophages; arginine metabolism via the nitric oxide synthetase pathway. J Immunol 1991; 146:2719–2723.

106. Gruetter CA, Childers CC, Bosserman MK, Lemke SM, Ball JG, Valentovic MA. Comparison of relaxation induced by glyceryl trinitrate, isosobide dinitrate and sodium nitroprusside in bovine airways. Am Rev Respir Dis 1989; 139:1192–1197.

107. Kishen R, Bleuvry BJ. Some actions of sodium nitroprusside and glyceryl trinitrate on guinea pig isolated trachealis muscle. J Pharm Pharacol 1985; 37:502–504.

108. Masaki Y, Munakata M, Ukita H, Houma Y, Kawakami Y. Nitric oxide (NO) can relax canine airway smooth muscle. Am Rev Respir Dis 1989; 139:A350.

109. Högman M, Frostell C, Arnberg H, Hedenstierna G. Inhalation of nitric oxide modulates methacholine-induced bronchoconstriction in the rabbit. Eur Respir J 1993; 6:177–180.

110. Munakata M, Masaki Y, Saxuma I, et al. Pharmacological differentiation of epithelium-derived relaxing factor from nitric oxide. J Appl Physiol 1990; 69:665–670.

111. Högman M, Frostell CG, Hedenström H, Hedenstierna G. Inhalation of nitric oxide modulates adult human bronchial tone. Am Rev Respir Dis 1993; 148:1474–1478.

112. Hulks G, Warren PM, Douglas NJ. The effect of inhaled nitric oxide on bronchomotor tone in the normal human airway. Am Rev Respir Dis 1993; 147:A515.

113. Fischer A, Mundel P, Mayer B, Preissler U, Philippin B, Dummer W. Nitric oxide synthase in guinea-pig lower airway innervation. Neurosci Lett 1993; 149:157–160.

114. Dey RD, Dalal G, Pinkstaff CA, Mayer B, Kummer W, Said SI. Nitric oxide synthase and vasoactive intestinal peptide are colocalized in neurons of the ferret tracheal plexus. Am Rev Respir Dis 1993; 147:A288.

115. Fischer A, Hoffman B, Hauser-Kronberger C, Mayer B, Kummer W. Nitric oxide synthase in the innervation of the human respiratory tract. Am Rev Respir Dis 1993; 147:A662.

116. Tucker JF, Brane SR, Charalambons L, Hobbs AJ, Gibson A. L-N^G-Nitroarginine inhibits non-adrenergic, non-cholinergic relaxations of guinea pig trachea. Br J Pharmacol 1990; 100: 663–664.

117. Li CG, Rand MJ. Evidence that part of the NANC relaxant response of guinea-pig trachea to electrical field stimulation is mediated by nitric oxide. Br J Pharmacol 1991; 102:91–94.

118. Kannan MS, Johnson DE. Functional innervation of pig tracheal smooth muscle: neural and non-neural mechanisms of relaxation. J Pharmacol Exp Ther 1992; 260:1180–1184.

119. Kannan MS, Johnson DE. Nitric oxide mediates the neural nonadrenergic, noncholinergic relaxation of pig tracheal smooth muscle. Am J Physiol 1993; 262:L511–L514.

120. Fischer JT, Anderson JW, Waldron MA. Nonadrenergic noncholinergic neurotransmission of feline trachealis: VIP or nitric oxide? J Appl Physiol 1993; 74:31–39.

121. Yu M, Robinson E, Wang Z. Regional distribution of nitroxidergic and adrenergic nerves in equine airway smooth muscle. Am Rev Respir Dis 1993; 147:A286.

122. Belvisi MG, Stretton CD, Barnes PJ. Nitric oxide is the endogenous neurotransmitter of bronchodilator nerves in human airways. Eur J Pharmacol 1992; 210:221–222.

123. Belvisi MG, Stretton CD, Miura M, et al. Inhibitory NANC nerves in human tracheal smooth muscle: a quest for the neurotransmitter. J Appl Physiol 1992; 73:2505–2510.

124. Ellis JL, Undem BJ. Inhibition by L-N^G-nitro-L-arginine of nonadrenergic noncholinergic mediated relaxations of human isolated central and peripheral airways. Am Rev Respir Dis 1992; 146:1543–1547.

125. Bai TR, Bramley AM. Effect of an inhibitor of nitric oxide synthase on neural relaxation in human bronchi. Am J Physiol 1993; 8:425–430.

126. Lammers JWJ, Barnes PJ, Chung KF. Non-adrenergic, non-cholinergic airway inhibitory nerves. Eur Respir J 1992; 5:239–246.

127. Alving K, Fornhem C, Wietzberg E, Lundber JM. Nitric oxide mediates cigarette–smoke-induced vasodilatory responses in the lung. Acta Physiol Scand 1992; 146:407–408.

128. Kuo H-P, Liu S, Barnes PJ. The effect of endogenous nitric oxide on neurogenic plasma exudation in guinea pig airways. Eur J Pharmacol 1992; 221:177–182.

129. Marletta MA, Yoon PS, Iyengar R, Leaf CD, Wishnok JS. Macrophage oxidation of L-arginine to nitrite and nitrate; nitric oxide is an intermediate. Biochemistry 1988; 27:8706–8611.

130. Fast DJ, Shannon JB, Herriott MJ, Kennedy MJ, Rummage JA, Leu RW. Staphylococcal exotoxins stimulate nitric oxide-dependent murine macrophage tumoricidal activity. Infect Immun 1991; 59:2987–2993.

131. Hibbs JB Jr, Taintor RR, Vavrin Z, et al. Synthesis of nitric oxide from a terminal guanidino nitrogen atom of L-arginine: a molecular mechanism regulating cellular proliferation that targets intracellular iron. In: Moncada S, Higgs EA, eds. Nitric Oxide from L-Arginine: A Bioregulatory System. Amsterdam: Excerpta Medica, 1990:189–223.

132. Ignarro LJ. Heme-dependent activation of guanylate cyclase by nitric oxide: a novel signal transduction mechanism. Blood Vessels 1991; 28:67–73.

133. Lepoivre M, Flaman J-M, Henry Y. Early loss of the tyrosyl radical ribonucleotide reductase of adenocarcinoma cells producing nitric oxide. J Biol Chem 1992; 267:22994–223000.

134. Hamid Q, Springall DR, Riveros-Moreno V, et al. Induction of nitric oxide synthase in asthma. Lancet 1993; 342:1510–1513.

135. Jain B, Rubinstein I, Robbins RA, Leise KL, Sisson JH. Modulation of airway epithelial cell ciliary beat frequency by nitric oxide. Biochem Biophys Res Commun 1993; 191:83–88.

136. Jain B, Robbins RA, Rubinstein I, Sisson JH, TNFα and IL-1β modulate airway epithelial ciliary activity by a nitric oxide-dependent mechanism. Clin Res 1994; 42:115A.

137. Gustafsson LE, Leone AM, Persson MG, Wiklund NP, Moncada S. Endogenous nitric oxide is present in the exhaled air of rabbits, guinea pigs and humans. Biochem Biophys Res Commun 1991; 181:852–857.

138. Borland C, Cox Y, Higenbottam T. Measurement of exhaled nitric oxide in man. Thorax 1993; 48:1160–1162.

139. Barnes PJ. New concepts in the pathogenesis of bronchial hyperresponsiveness and asthma. J Allergy Clin Immunol 1989; 83:1013–1026.

140. Ohna I, Ohkawara Y, Yamauchi K, Tanno Y, Takishima T. Production of tumor necrosis factor with IgE receptor triggering from sensitized lung tissue. Am J Respir Cell Mol Biol 1990; 3:285–289.

141. Borish L, Mascali JJ, Dishuck J, Beam WR, Martin RJ, Rosenwasser LJ. Detection of alveolar macrophage-derived IL-1β in asthma: inhibition with corticosteroids. J Immunol 1992; 149:3078–3082.

142. Kharitonov SA, Yates D, Robbins RA, Logan-Sinclair R, Shinebourne EA, Barnes PJ. Increased nitric oxide in exhaled air of asthmatic patients. Lancet 1994; 343:133–135.

143. Alving K, Wietzberg E, Lundberg JM. Increased amount of nitric oxide in exhaled air of asthmatics. Eur Respir J 1993; 6:1368–1370.

144. Persson MG, Zetterström O, Agrenius V, Ihre E, Gustafsson LE. Single-breath nitric oxide measurements in asthmatic patients and smokers. Lancet 1994; 343:146–147.

145. Panza JA, Quyyumi AA, Brush JE Jr, Epstein SE. Abnormal endothelium-dependent vascular relaxation in patients with essential hypertension. N Engl J Med 1990; 323:22–27.

146. Calver A, Collier J, Moncada S, Vallance P. Effect of local intra-arterial N^G-monomethyl-L-arginine in patients with hypertension: the nitric oxide dilator mechanism appears abnormal. J Hypertens 1992; 10:1025–1031.

147. Nakaki T, Hishikawa K, Suzuki H, Saruta T, Kato R. L-Arginine-induced hypotension. Lancet 1990; 336:696.

148. Petros AJ, Hewlett AM, Bogle RG, Pearson JD. L-Arginine-induced hypotension. Lancet 1991; 337:1044–1045.
149. Moncada S. The L-arginine:nitric oxide pathway. Acta Physiol Scand 1992; 145:201–227.
150. Petros A, Bennett D, Vallance P. Effect of nitric oxide synthase inhibitors on hypotension in patients with septic shock. Lancet 1991; 181:852–857.
151. Petros A, Lamb G, Leone A, Moncada S, Bennett D, Vallance P. Effects of a nitric oxide synthase inhibitor in humans with septic shock. Cardiovasc Res 1994; 28:34–39.
152. Wright CD, Rees DD, Moncada S. Protective and pathological roles of nitric oxide in endotoxin shock. Cardiovasc Res 1992; 26:48–57.
153. Rossaint R, Falke KJ, López F, Slama K, Pison U, Zapol WM. Inhaled nitric oxide for the adult respiratory distress syndrome. N Engl J Med 1993; 328:399–405.
154. Bartecchi CE, MacKenzie TD, Schrier RW. The human cost of tobacco use. N Engl J Med 1994; 330:907–912, 975–980.
155. Monto AS, Ross H. Acute respiratory illness in the community: effect of family composition, smoking and chronic symptoms. Br J Prev Soc Med 1977; 31:101–108.
156. Aronson MD, Weiss ST, Ben RL, Komaroff AL. Association between cigarette smoking and acute respiratory tract illness in young adults. JAMA 1982; 248:181–183.
157. Norman V, Keith CM. Nitrogen oxides in tobacco smoke. Nature 1965; 205:915–916.

19

Leukotrienes: Their Receptors, Antagonists, and Synthesis Inhibitors

I. Caroline Crocker and Robert G. Townley
Creighton University School of Medicine, Omaha, Nebraska

INTRODUCTION

Leukotrienes, arachidonic acid metabolites synthesized by leukocytes, are important mediators in the pathophysiology of allergic diseases. Increased production of leukotrienes has been observed in atopic asthmatic patients, both when their condition is stable and during exacerbations (1). Similarly, elevated leukotriene levels can be detected in nasal lavage from persons with allergic rhinitis (2). Because bronchial or nasal challenge with leukotrienes precipitates many of the pathological changes observed in asthma or allergic rhinitis, considerable effort has been devoted to the development of pharmaceutical agents that, being effective against leukotrienes, could have potential in the treatment of atopic disease. The synthesis and effects of leukotrienes, their receptors, antagonists, and synthesis inhibitors, with particular reference to asthma and allergic rhinitis, is reviewed in this chapter.

HISTORICAL PERSPECTIVES

Leukotrienes (LT) were initially described as the slow-reacting substance of anaphylaxis (SRS-A) when investigators noticed that a perfusate of guinea pig lung tissue that had been treated with cobra venom caused contraction of smooth-muscle tissue (3). Although this group suggested a role for SRS-A in asthma in 1940 (4), leukotrienes were not identified as arachidonic acid metabolites and inflammatory mediators until the late 1970s. Indeed, that LTC_4, LTD_4, and LTE_4, together are the SRS-A was only established in 1983 (5). After characterization of the individual leukotrienes (6,7), the biochemical pathways involved in their synthesis and metabolism were elucidated (8).

SYNTHESIS AND METABOLISM

Leukotrienes are synthesized from arachidonic acid (5,8,11,14-eicosatetraenoic acid)—which is found as a normal part of the phospholipid bilayer of many biological membranes—through a complex and highly regulated cascade (Fig. 1). After stimulation of the cell by receptor activation, antigen–antibody interactions, cold, or an altered ionic environment, phospholipase A_2 (PLA_2) liberates arachidonic acid from the cell membrane (9). 5-Lipoxygenase (5-LO), an iron-containing enzyme (10), translocates from the euchromatin region of the nucleus to the nuclear membrane (11–17) where, in intact cells, the involvement of an 18 kDa 5-lipoxygenase-activating protein (FLAP) becomes necessary for the cascade to continue (18,19). 5-Lipoxygenase then catalyzes the oxygenation of arachidonic acid at C-5 to form 5(S)-hydroperoxy-6,8,11,14-eicosatetraenoic acid (5-HPETE) (20), which is quickly dehydrated by 5-LO to form LTA_4 (11,18,19,21). This unstable epoxide is the first compound in the cascade that has the conjugated triene sequence that gives the leukotrienes their chromophore properties (three ultraviolet-absorbing peaks). The name of these inflammatory mediators *leukotrienes* reflects both their origin and this property (10).

After formation, LTA_4 is released into the cell cytosol and quickly undergoes further metabolism, either within that cell or after transport to another cell (22; Fig. 2). The nature of the next step is determined by the cell type. First, LTA_4 may be hydrolyzed by a cytosolic

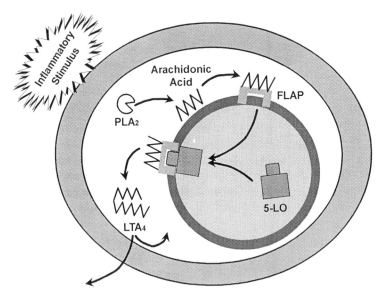

Figure 1 The formation of leukotriene A_4 from arachidonic acid that results from cell stimulation. Stimulation of the cell by an inflammatory stimulus, such as receptor activation, antigen–antibody interactions, cold, or an altered ionic environment, causes phospholipase A_2 (PLA_2) to cleave arachidonic acid from the membrane. 5-Lipoxygenase (5-LO) translocates from the euchromatin of the nucleus to the nuclear membrane where it interacts with 5-lipoxygenase-activating protein (FLAP). The arachidonic acid is then oxygenated and, subsequently, dehydrated to form leukotriene A_4 (LTA_4). This is then metabolized further either within the cell, or after transport to another cell. (Courtesy of MK Church.)

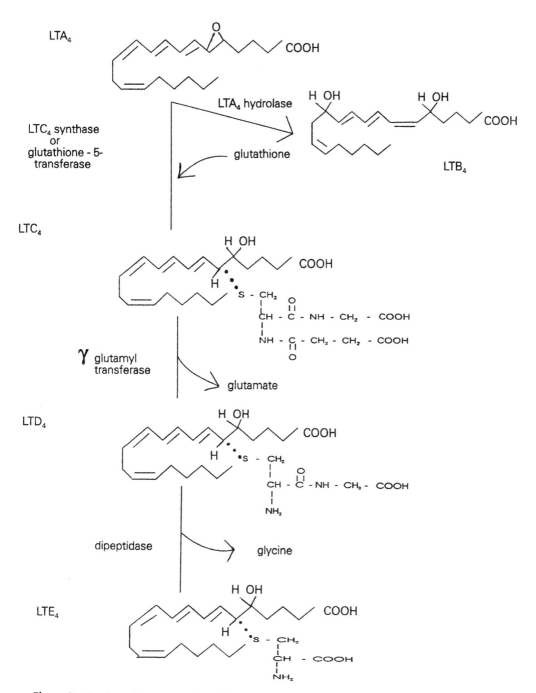

Figure 2 A schematic representation of the metabolism of leukotriene A_4 into either leukotriene B_4 or the sulfidopeptide leukotrienes.

zinc-containing metalloenzyme, LTA_4 hydrolase, to form a dihydroxy acid LTB_4 (21,23), which is eventually metabolized by ω-oxidation at C-20 to a less-active form (24).

Alternatively, glutathione-S-transferase (LTC_4 synthase) may catalyze the stereospecific conjugation of LTA_4 and glutathione to form a sulfidoleukotriene, LTC_4 (25). The enzyme γ-glutamyl transpeptidase removes the glutamic acid to yield LTD_4 (24), and then another peptidase cleaves the glycine residue leaving LTE_4 (20). In the human lung, this metabolism from LTC_4 to LTE_4 is complete within 10 min (26). LTE_4 and its β and ω-oxidation products are then excreted into the bile (~85%) and urine (~15%) (27). Locally, LTE_4 may eventually be degraded by reactive oxygen species that are generated by activated leukocytes to biologically inactive sulfoxides (28,29).

Control of leukotriene biosynthesis is achieved by three main mechanisms. The liberation of arachidonic acid is critical to the activity of 5-LO in cells that have been exposed to receptor-mediated stimuli (30). Indeed, although formyl-methiomyl-leucyl-phenylalanine (FMLP), the complement component C5a, platelet-activating factor (PAF), and LTB_4 are poor activators of 5-LO in neutrophils (31–33), enzyme activity and LT synthesis is greatly enhanced by the addition of arachidonic acid to the culture medium (22,31,34). In addition, preincubation of the cells with granulocyte–macrophage colony-stimulating factor (GM-CSF), tumor necrosis factor (TNF)-α, lipopolysaccharides (LPS), or PAF before stimulation will also increase LT synthesis by neutrophils. This priming effect is not due to up-regulation of 5-LO activity, but to increased release of arachidonic acid from the cell membrane (35–40). Cytokines [interleukin (IL)-3, IL-5, and GM-CSF] also increase LTC_4 release after stimulation by a second agonist in basophils (41), eosinophils (42), and neutrophils (41). Clearly, any modulation of the secretion of these cytokines will also regulate leukotriene formation.

Second, formation of leukotrienes is controlled by the state of activation of 5-LO. A membrane-bound protein, FLAP, is necessary for 5-LO activity in cells (18,19). The 5-LO activity is also influenced by cellular redox states (22), requires the presence of ATP (43), and is dependent on transforming growth factor (TGF)-β found in serum (22).

Finally, transcellular biosynthesis may play an important role in regulation of leukotriene biosynthesis (Table 1). For example, many cell types that contain 5-LO do not

Table 1 Cell Types Capable of Synthesizing Leukotrienes

Cell type	Substrate[a]	Product	Refs.
Macrophage	AA	LTB_4, LTC_4	45
Monocyte	AA	LTB_4, LTC_4	220, 221
Mast cell	AA	LTB_4, LTC_4	222
Neutrophil	AA	LTB_4	6
Eosinophil	AA	LTC_4	57
Basophil	AA	LTC_4	223
Platelet	LTA_4	LTC_4	224
Lymphocyte	LTA_4	LTB_4	52
Erythrocyte	LTA_4	LTB_4	46

[a]AA, arachidonic acid.
Source: Modified from Ref. 225.

express LTA_4 hydrolase, whereas others have LTC_4 synthase, but not 5-LO (43). 5-Lipoxygenase protein expression and activity is mainly found in myeloid cells: granulocytes, monocytes, macrophages, mast cells, and B lymphocytes (6,7,44–47). The lung also stains positively for 5-LO by immunohistochemistry, but this may be due to the presence of macrophages and granulocytes (48). Leukotriene-B_4 is the major product of alveolar macrophages (45,49) and neutrophils (28), both of which contain LTA_4 hydrolase. The LTA_4 hydrolase activity is also found in lymphocytes, erythrocytes, endothelial cells, epithelial cells, and fibroblasts (46,50–53). Although these cells may not contain 5-LO, they can synthesize LTB_4 in the presence of LTA_4 release by other cells. Similarly, the sulfidopeptide or cysteinyl LT (LTC_4, LTD_4, and LTE_4) are produced by eosinophils (54–58), macrophages, monocytes (59), basophils (60), and mast cells (61,62). Platelets, which do not express 5-LO, also secrete LTC_4 if exposed to LTA_4 (64). In conclusion, control of the liberation of arachidonic acid, activation of 5-LO, and transcellular biosynthesis allows the leukotriene response to be amplified and regulated by the cellular microenvironment.

BIOLOGICAL ACTIVITY OF LEUKOTRIENES

The two leukotriene classes (LTB_4 and the sulfidopeptide leukotrienes, *S*LT) have very dissimilar active profiles, separate cell surface receptors, and act on different types of cells. Therefore, the actions and receptors of LTB_4 and the *S*LT will be considered separately.

Since LTB_4's main target is the leukocyte, stimulation with LTB_4 evinces considerable evidence that leukocytes have been activated. Leukotriene-B_4 is a potent neutrophil chemoattractant (64–66) and also has some chemotactic properties for eosinophils (67). For example, in vivo treatment of human lung segments with LTB_4 versus saline results in a 17-fold higher concentration of neutrophils than in the segments exposed to LTD_4 (68). However, the importance of neutrophils in asthma is uncertain (67). Although the chronic inflammatory nature of asthma suggests that chemotaxis of cells from the circulation to the site of inflammation is important, other mediators may be more potent for eosinophils than LTB_4 (9,69), possibly indicating that LTB_4 plays only a minor role in asthma and allergic rhinitis. Other actions of LTB_4 include neutrophil aggregation, adherence to endothelial vessel walls, extravasation, degranulation, calcium mobilization, and superoxide generation (64,70–73). One group of investigators found that LTB_4 suppresses T-lymphocyte function, enhances natural killer (NK) cell activity, and stimulates keratinocyte proliferation (59), whereas another group reported LTB_4 up-regulation of T-cell proliferation (74) and IL-6 secretion by monocytes (75,76) (see Ref. 77 for a review of the biological activity of LTB_4).

Although its cell activation mechanisms have not been completely elucidated, LTB_4 appears to act through either two receptors (78–80), or two affinity states of one receptor (81). This latter idea is supported by the observation that LTB_4 antagonists show no selectivity for the functional responses requiring a low dose of LTB_4 (chemotaxis, chemokinesis, adherence) than those needing a higher dose (80,82), although results are sometimes complicated by the antagonist's partial agonist activity. However, the G-coupled receptor is a member of the rhodopsin-like superfamily (78,79), and the stereospecific LTB_4 binding requires the (5*S*,12*R*)-hydroxyl groups, a *cis* double bond at C-6, and an intact eicosanoid backbone (83–85).

The *S*LTs, which generally act on contractile cells (10), are important mediators of airway obstruction in asthma (1). In addition to causing fibroblast (86) and epithelial cell

(87) proliferation, SLTs are known to mediate bronchoconstriction (88–90), hyperreactivity, mucous secretion, vascular permeability, and plasma exudation (91).

The number and specificity of the SLT receptors in humans is controversial. Although an LTC_4 receptor has been described on the lungs of guinea pigs (92–94) and rats (95), it has not been found in humans; LTE_4 appears to bind at a similar receptor site (96,97). The LTD_4 receptor that has been reported in human lung parenchyma, similar to the LTB_4 receptor, is known to be a member of the rhodopsin-like superfamily, but further molecular characterization has not yet been possible (98). There is evidence that LTC_4 probably interacts at the same site as LTD_4, in that a selective LTD_4 receptor antagonist prevents contraction after treatment with either LTC_4 or LTD_4 (99–101). Indeed, LTE_4 is also a partial agonist at this site (102). The use of only one receptor may explain the relatively delayed bronchoconstriction potentiated by LTC_4 (10–20 min) in comparison with LTD_4 and LTE_4 (4–6 min). It is possible that LTC_4 undergoes further metabolism before attaching to the receptor (103). Once attached, the SLTs precipitate many of the pathophysiological characteristics of atopic disease.

Several studies, both in vivo and in vitro, have demonstrated that the SLTs mediate bronchoconstriction. In human and animal preparations of explanted bronchial segments, LTC_4 and LTD_4 are 100-fold more potent than histamine (60). The relative potency of LTE_4 is still controversial (104,105). In vivo exposure of the bronchial passages to an SLT by inhalation also causes constriction of the airways, both in asthmatic (91,106) and in normal subjects (90,107), although the response is amplified in the former. In this system, LTC_4 and LTD_4 are equipotent (108). Leukotriene E_4 is 30–100 times less potent, but causes longer-lasting contractions (108).

Besides mediating airway obstruction, sulfidoleukotrienes also appear to contribute to the nonspecific hyperresponsiveness observed after allergen challenge (10). Studies with receptor antagonists have shown that long-term treatment results in amelioration of airway hyperreactivity, indicating that these mediators play an important causative role in this area. Some of these studies will be described in the following.

The SLTs are also 100–1000 times more potent than histamine in causing microvascular leak in the guinea pig airways (109). Topical application of a leukotriene caused extravasation in guinea pig and hamster cheek pouches and throughout the bronchial tree (69). In addition, in humans, intradermal application of the SLTs produces a weal-and-flare reaction within minutes (110). The leukotrienes cause endothelial gaps to be formed in the postcapillary venules, allowing the escape of macromolecules first and then of water, leading to edema and further obstruction (1).

A major pathological feature of asthma is the increased production of mucus that plays a part in airway obstruction and, in severe cases, mucous plugging (1). Although many mediators may be involved in this process (histamine, prostaglandins, thromboxane A_2, or PAF), in vitro the SLTs are some of the most potent mucous secretagogues studied (111,112). Indeed, it has been demonstrated that LTC_4 up-regulated mucous secretion from the tracheal submucosal glands of dogs and that the SLTs are ten times more potent than methacholine in causing mucous secretion in human airways (112).

Because leukotrienes can mediate many of the pathological changes detected in atopic disease, it would be of interest to verify whether increased leukotriene production is indeed a characteristic feature of asthma and allergic rhinitis. The release of SRS-A from human lung tissue was first documented in 1960 (113). More recently, ex vivo studies have demonstrated that mixed leukocytes from atopic asthmatic and allergic rhinitis patients make three to five times more LTB_4 and LTC_4 than cells from normal controls (114,115).

Several research groups have shown LTE_4 release into the urine after allergen challenge (116–120) or exacerbations (121) in atopic asthmatics. Aspirin challenge of aspirin-sensitive asthmatics (120,122) and nocturnal asthma (123) also results in increased urinary LTE_4. Finally, increased levels of LTC_4 and LTD_4 have been detected in the plasma and bronchoalveolar lavage (BAL) fluid of persons with stable asthma (124,125), suggesting that the decreased FEV_1 of these persons may be due to "leukotriene tone."

The role of leukotrienes in asthma that is induced by indirect stimuli, such as exercise or cold, dry air, remains controversial. Indeed, at least two groups have failed to detect elevated levels of leukotrienes in BAL fluid obtained immediately after exercise from patients with exercise-induced asthma (126,127). In addition, these stimuli also do not induce elevated levels of urinary LTE_4 excretion (118). Although direct evidence for LT involvement in exercise asthma is lacking, there are some other indications that they are implicated. For example, both a LTD_4 antagonist and a 5-LO inhibitor protect against asthma induced by exercise or hyperventilation of cold, dry air (128,129). As even small quantities of these potent mediators released in situ can have great effects (primed basophils produce LT after hyperosmotic stimuli; 130), it would appear that LTs may even have a role in bronchoconstriction caused by indirect stimuli. In conclusion, because the SLTs have many proinflammatory properties and elevated levels are present in the biological fluids of asthmatics when compared with normal subjects, it is probable that they are instrumental in the pathogenesis of both chronic and acute asthma.

Leukotrienes also appear to be implicated in the disease mechanisms of allergic rhinitis. Although LTE_4 is undetectable in the urine of allergic rhinitis patients (116), both individuals with symptomatic allergic perennial rhinitis (131) and those with seasonal allergic rhinitis (132) have elevated levels of LTC_4 in their nasal lavage fluid in comparison with normal controls. Nasal lavage from patients undergoing allergen challenge also contain increased LTC_4 levels compared with normal controls within between 5 and 30 min of challenge (133–135). Similarly, nasal cold air challenge of cold-sensitive individuals and ocular allergen challenge of atopic patients resulted in significantly higher amounts of LTE_4 in nasal lavage (136) and tear fluid (137) in comparison with normals and the unchallenged eye, respectively. Direct nasal challenge with either LTC_4 (133) or LTD_4 (138) produced congestion and increased resistance, as measured by rhinomanometry, but no sneezing or pruritus.

ANTILEUKOTRIENE CHEMOTHERAPY

Pharmacological control of leukotriene synthesis is accomplished either by antagonism of the specific leukotriene receptor or by inhibition of 5-LO or FLAP, preventing the formation of LTs. Antagonists have been developed around the acetophenone structure, by synthetically altering the LT functional groups or, as with ICI 198,615, by a combination of the two approaches (139). Inhibition of 5-LO can be achieved with (1) substrate analogues, such as eicosatetraenoic acid or prostaglandin (PG) I_2 analogues; (2) hydroxyurea derivatives, such as zileuton; (3) iron-chelators, such as the acetohydroxamic acids; and (4) antioxidants, such as flavonoids, nafazatrom (BAY-G576), retinol (vitamin A); or naphthalene derivatives [lonapalene (RS-43,179) Wy-47,288] (140–142). In comparison, both indole derivatives, such as MK-886, and quinoline–indole hybrids, such as MK-0591, inhibit FLAP (19,141,142).

In addition to those drugs that specifically inhibit leukotrienes, other drugs that are commonly used to treat asthma may also modulate the LT system. It has been postulated that corticosteroids induce production of lipocortin, an intracellular messenger which, in turn, may inhibit phospholipase A_2, preventing the liberation of arachidonic acid that occurs with cell activation (143). However, as aspirin-sensitive asthmatics receiving fairly high doses of inhaled budesonide still secrete significant quantities of LTE_4 into the urine, the importance of this mode of action is questionable (10). Alternatively, corticosteroids may make the effector cells unresponsive to stimulation by LT; this has been suggested by the increased vascular permeability engendered by these inflammatory mediators (144).

Anti-inflammatory agents, such as nedocromil sodium and cromolyn, are often effective in the treatment of asthma. Although these drugs are perceived to operate primarily by preventing mast cell mediator release, in airways and other systems, they have a direct antiexudative effect, as well. Indeed, nedocromil sodium inhibits LTB_4-induced chemotaxis (145).

B_2-Adrenergic agonists, particularly the new long-acting drugs, may functionally antagonize leukotrienes both at the synthesis level and at the level of the target cells. Both formoterol and salmeterol inhibit LTB_4-induced plasma extravasation in guinea pig airways and hamster cheek pouches, respectively (146,147). There is also evidence that β-adrenoceptor agonists partially inhibit leukotriene release from inflammatory cells, such as eosinophils (148,149).

Terfenadine, a histamine receptor antagonist, can have some inhibitory effects on leukotriene production by anti–IgE-stimulated eosinophils from atopic asthma patients (150). Leukotriene-C_4 levels in the supernatant of cells were reduced by 59.8% after treatment with 20 μM terfenadine, possibly owing to an increase in intracellular calcium (Fig. 3). When the effect of 10 μM ketotifen, another antiallergy drug, on eosinophil LTC_4 production was studied in the same system, similar results were obtained with an inhibition of release of 23% (151).

Leukotriene D_4 Receptor Antagonists

Leukotriene antagonists are one of the most interesting classes of antiasthma drugs because they are the first mediator antagonists to be demonstrated as effective in the treatment of

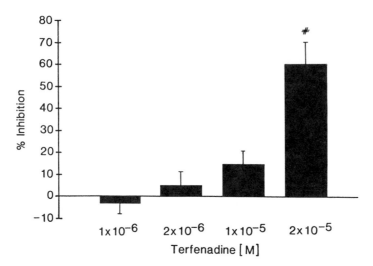

Figure 3   The inhibitory effect of terfenadine on calcium ionophore-induced LTC_4 production by eosinophils. # Indicated $p < 0.05$ compared with buffer. (Data from Ref. 150.)

Table 2 Leukotriene D_4 Receptor Antagonists

Antagonist	Common name	Refs.
FPL-55712		153–155
LY-171883	Tomelukast	102, 152, 157
SK&F-104,353	Pobilukast	102, 158–159, 226
ICI-204,219	Accolate, zafirlukast	102, 157, 161–173, 188
ONO-1078	Pranulast	174–180, 227
MK-571		102, 181–186, 228
MK-679	Verlukast	1, 187–189, 229
L-648,051		182
L-649,923		156
ONO-RS-411		43
Wy-48,252		43
AS-35		230, 231
DS-4574		232, 233
ICI-198,615		160, 161

clinical asthma (Table 2). Although the early studies, which evaluated only the effect of one dose or a short period of treatment on asthma, were discouraging, further work revealed that the effects of receptor antagonists are cumulative (152). Indeed, recent work has shown that the more potent antagonists are very effective against both bronchoconstriction and non-specific bronchial hyperreactivity engendered by allergen exposure. The major leukotriene antagonists are reviewed in this section.

FPL-55712 was one of the first and least effective leukotriene antagonists developed (153). In vitro pretreatment of guinea pig trachea and human bronchi with FPL-55712 inhibits antigen-induced smooth-muscle contraction and, in fact, reverses established contraction (153). In contrast, improvement was noted in only two of four patients with chronic asthma given nebulized FPL-55712 in a study that could not be blinded because of the taste of FPL-55712 and the transient discomfort it produces in the throat after inhalation (154). The previous findings that this compound has a short half-life and poor bioavailability may explain these results (155). More recent drugs are often more than 1000 times as potent as FLP-55712.

Tomelukast or LY-171883 is an early leukotriene antagonist that produces a three- to fourfold shift to the right in the inhaled LTD_4 dose–response curve (102). A single dose of 400 mg had a small, but significant, protective effect on the early allergic reaction (EAR) after allergen challenge. No effect on the late allergic reaction (LAR) was observed (156). This is probably because maximum efficacy of these drugs is often reached only after extended periods of treatment. In a double-blind, placebo-controlled study by Cloud et al. (152), 138 mild, chronic asthmatics were treated with 600 mg of LY-171883 per day for 6 weeks. Although there were no differences between those receiving drug and those being given placebo in diurnal peak flow rates and frequency of attacks, there was a steady improvement in the forced expiratory volume in 1 second (FEV_1), which reached 7% by 6 weeks ($p = 0.003$; Fig. 4). In addition, by 6 weeks, the need for rescue medication by those receiving tomelukast had significantly decreased in comparison with those patients taking placebo. Another study in 19 asthmatic patients indicated that tomelukast may also be of slight benefit in the prevention of bronchoconstriction caused by hyperventilation of cold, dry air (157).

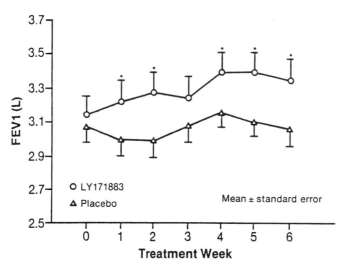

Figure 4 Improvement in the mean weekly FEV_1 after treatment with LY171883 compared with placebo. *Indicates $p < 0.05$ compared with placebo. (Data from Ref. 152.)

Pobilukast edamine (SK&F-104,353) is a leukotriene antagonist that is designed to be administered by inhalation. It has a potency three to four times as great as tomelukast, as measured by the prevention of a drop in FEV_1 engendered by inhalation of LTD_4 by normal and asthmatic individuals (102). Furthermore, a randomized, double-blind, crossover, placebo-controlled study in aspirin-sensitive asthmatics revealed that pobilukast partially inhibits aspirin-induced bronchoconstriction, preventing the drop in FEV_1 by 47% (158). Finally, it has been observed in another placebo-controlled, randomized, crossover study that exercise-induced asthma can also be attenuated with this drug (159). It would seem that pobilukast may be effective against bronchoconstriction induced by direct challenge with SLT, pseudoallergies (i.e., aspirin sensitivity), or indirect challenges.

One of the more potent leukotriene antagonists (zafirlukast accolate; ICI-204,219), is also one of the most extensively studied. Accolate is a structural analogue of ICI-198,615, an antagonist without enough bioavailability to be studied in humans (160,161). It is known that ICI-204,219 inhibits PAF-induced bronchoconstriction in normal males (162). Two groups have demonstrated attenuation of an inhaled LTD_4-induced fall in FEV_1 by a single dose of zafirlukast (102,163). This agent is approximately 100 times as potent at tomelukast in preventing LTD_4-induced bronchoconstriction (102). In comparison, Drazen and group (102) also showed that a 40-mg dose of zafirlukast inhibits allergen-induced bronchoconstriction with a potency 30 times that of tomelukast. These apparently differing results may be the consequence of diverse methods of administration, particle size, and so forth. In another study, the effect of a single 40-mg dose of this oral leukotriene antagonist on bronchial response to standardized cat allergen was investigated. Each of the 13 patients in this placebo-controlled, double-blinded, randomized, crossover study underwent bronchoprovocation with cat dander until a 20% fall in FEV_1 was observed. The concentration of allergen required to cause this drop was increased tenfold after zafirlukast administration, in comparison with placebo, showing that 40 mg of oral ICI-204,219 antagonizes both inhaled cat allergen-induced early and late bronchoconstriction (164). The area under the curve (AUC) for percentage change in FEV_1 from baseline to 5 h was improved from -69.6 to -9.7%. When this study was repeated with ten patients and inhaled zafirlukast (total dose 1600 µg), no effect on the late phase was observed ($p = 0.17$), whereas the early response was inhibited $p = 0.007$. This could possibly be due to a pharmacokinetic effect (165).

The effects of zafirlukast on bronchoconstriction after cumulative bronchial challenge were investigated in a randomized, placebo-controlled, double-blind, crossover study (166). Ten mildly asthmatic atopic men were challenged with specific allergen before and 2 h after either placebo or 20 mg of this agent. Results showed that zafirlukast significantly increased (5.5 times) the median allergen dose necessary to provoke a fall in FEV_1 of 20%, whereas the average PD_{20} was elevated 2.5 times.

Finnerty (167) also found that a 20-mg dose of oral zafirlukast, administered 2 h before challenge, is effective against exercise-induced asthma. The FEV_1 was assessed over a 30-min period subsequent to challenge with dry air while on a treadmill. The mean maximum fall in FEV_1 in the group receiving either the drug or placebo was 21.6 and 36.0%, respectively ($p < 0.01$). These results were confirmed in a randomized, double-blind, placebo-controlled, crossover study with nine mild to moderate asthmatic subjects (168). Again, 400 µg of zafirlukast given 30 min before challenge significantly attenuated the exercise-provoked bronchoconstriction from 30.2% to 14.5% ($p = 0.043$) and reduced recovery time from 60 to 20 min (median; $p = 0.018$).

In addition to ameliorating the response to challenges, zafirlukast appears to reverse the leukotriene tone observed in chronic, unchallenged asthmatics. Hui and Barnes conducted a placebo-controlled study in ten chronic asthmatic patients in whom 40 mg of oral ICI-204,219 caused a significant 8% (2–14%) improvement in FEV_1 that was sustained for 4 h posttreatment (169). Spector et al. (170) conducted a 6-week, multicenter, placebo-controlled, randomized, double-blind parallel study in 266 mild to moderate asthma outpatients. Patients received either placebo or 10, 20, or 40 mg of zafirlukast daily. The group treated with the highest dosage showed significant improvement in evening peak expiratory flow rate (11%), nighttime awakenings (46%), morning inhaler use (37%), and asthma symptom scores (27%), in comparison with the group given placebo (170). These results have been confirmed in a currently ongoing multicenter study (Table 3; 171).

The efficacy of zafirlukast in preventing the EAR and LAR after bronchial allergen challenge was evaluated in a double-blind, placebo-controlled crossover study (172). A single oral 40-mg dose of zafirlukast not only prevented early and late bronchoconstriction, but it also suppressed the nonspecific bronchial hyperreactivity to histamine that occurs after allergen exposure ($p < 0.01$).

The potential of zafirlukast against allergic rhinitis has also been studied. In a double-blind, placebo-controlled, parallel group study, 164 ragweed-sensitive patients were equally divided into four groups and given 10, 20, 40, or 100 mg of zafirlukast each morning for 2 consecutive days (173). The remainder of each day (9 h) was spent in a local park. On both day 1 and 2 the 20-, 40-, and 100-mg groups had less nasal congestion than the placebo group, whereas rhinorrhea was significantly attenuated in only the 20- and 40-mg groups. Frequency of sneezing was not affected on day 1, but was significantly lower than placebo on day 2 in the 10-, 20-, and 40-mg groups. This could be because leukotrienes do not directly cause sneezing, but their inhibition may prevent the release of substances that do.

Pranulast (ONO-1078) is an oral LTD_4 antagonist that has been effective in the attenuation of chronic asthma (174), allergen-induced EAR and LAR in asthmatics (175), and aspirin-induced asthma (176). Pranulast is active in inhibiting the decline in FEV_1 induced

Table 3 The Mean Difference Between Zafirlukast (Accolate) and Placebo at Endpoint

Assessment	Accolate Versus Placebo		
	Week 2 (5 mg)	Week 4 (20 mg)	Week 6 (40 mg)
Asthma symptom score	−0.25*	−0.13*	−0.16
Awakenings	−1.11*	−0.67	−0.92*
Morning with asthma	−1.22**	−0.48	−1.04*
β-Agonist use (puffs/day)	−0.61*	−0.24	−0.58
AM perfusion (L/min)	16.23*	19.23*	24.23**
PM perfusion (L/min)	20.94**	6.61	9.49
FEV$_1$	0.20*	0.14*	0.16*
% of predicted FEV$_1$	4.89*	3.17	3.64

*$p < 0.05$; **$p < 0.01$.
Source: Ref. 171.

by inhalation of LTD_4 by normal subjects and asthmatics (177). Guinea pig lung studies have shown that pranulast preferentially binds to the LTD_4 and LTE_4 receptor with a potency 2000–3000 times greater than FPL-55712 (178). Although, as with all leukotriene antagonists, it has no effect on histamine-induced contraction, pranulast reverses both LTD_4 and allergen-induced contraction of the guinea pig trachea (178).

Two short-term, double-blind, placebo-controlled, crossover studies have shown that therapy with pranulast causes a small, but significant, improvement in bronchoconstriction and hyperreactivity in mild to moderate asthmatics (178,180). A 24-week study in 11 patients, treated with 450 mg twice a day, demonstrated a reduction in asthma severity symptoms after 2 weeks and continued improvement in FEV_1 and PC_{20} at 12 and 24 weeks (174). This shows that the efficacy of LT antagonists is cumulative over time.

MK-571, another leukotriene antagonist, can be given either orally or by intravenous infusion. It inhibits allergen-induced pulmonary eosinophilia in guinea pigs (181), albumin-induced dyspnea in sensitized rats (182), and is 30- to 40-fold more potent that tomelukast at preventing bronchoconstriction after inhalation of LTD_4 by humans (102).

Infusion of MK-571 inhibited both the immediate (0–3 h) and late (3–10 h) asthmatic response to allergen in a double-blind, placebo-controlled, crossover study by Rasmussen and colleagues (183). The high (450-mg) dose resulted in a prevention of inhibition of 62% for the EAR and 50% for the LAR. As would be expected, allergen challenge increased mean LTE_4 excretion whether or not the LTD_4 receptor antagonist was administered in the early phase, but in the later phase, the levels of excreted LTE_4 fell. In a randomized, placebo-controlled study with 43 patients with mild to moderate asthma, administration of 75 mg tid for 2 weeks and 150 mg tid for 4 weeks resulted in significant overall clinical improvement (184). Similarly, another study (4 weeks with moderate to severe asthmatics) showed that baseline FEV_1 improved by 15% and the need for rescue medication decreased by 30% (184). Again, this significant elevation of baseline airway caliber points to the possibility of the existence of leukotriene tone (185). As with several of the other antagonists, it has been demonstrated that MK-571 also significantly attenuates the decrease in FEV_1 (65%) and recovery time (8.4 min as compared with 33.4 min) after exercise (186).

Verlukast (MK-0679), a potent and specific investigational LTD_4 receptor antagonist, causes rapid bronchodilation after intravenous infusion (187). Single doses of MK-0679 (125 or 500 mg) or placebo were administered to nine patients with moderate but stable asthma on individual study days in a three-period, double-blind, randomized, crossover study. Fifteen minutes after the end of infusion there was an improvement in FEV_1 of 15.8 and 7.8% with the 500- and 125-mg doses, respectively. In comparison, FEV_1 decreased 2.6% with placebo. In another study, treatment of asthma patients for 6 weeks with oral verlukast resulted in an 18% increase in FEV_1 and a 30% decrease in the use of β-adreno-ceptor agonists (188). These results were confirmed by Hutchinson et al. in a 4-week study (1). Finally, verlukast has also proved effective in the inhibition of aspirin-induced airway obstruction (189).

Finally, preliminary studies have shown that leukotriene antagonists may have potential in preventing airway hyperreactivity (180,183). Nine days of treatment with L-648,051 not only attenuated the EAR and LAR to inhaled allergen, but also improved reactivity to methacholine by 1.5-doubling dilutions (183), a degree of improvement similar to that seen after use of inhaled corticosteroids for 2 weeks or more.

Leukotriene B_4 Receptor Antagonists

A few specific LTB_4 receptor antagonists have recently become available, but they have low potencies and considerable partial agonist activity, complicating the interpretation of data (10). Nonetheless, as two have been evaluated in guinea pigs, it is of use to mention them at this point. The first, NZ-107 was studied for its effect on airway inflammation caused by intratracheal injection of LTB_4 or IL-5, or by inhalation of PAF, and by cell activation (190). Analysis of the BAL fluid revealed that both LTB_4-induced eosinophilia and neutrophilia were suppressed. Surprisingly, although PAF and superoxide generation were inhibited in macrophages and eosinophils, NZ-107 had no effect on neutrophil activation. The second, U-75302 was similarly studied in guinea pigs and inhibited LTB_4-induced chemotaxis of eosinophils in vitro and antigen-induced lung eosinophilia in vivo (191).

5-Lipoxygenase-Activating Protein Inhibitors

Because both FLAP and 5-LO are vital to in vivo leukotriene synthesis, inhibition of either will prevent both LTB_4 and SLT formation. Specific FLAP inhibitors have only recently been developed and, as such, extensive data are not available. Summaries of the available data on major compounds are presented in this section (Table 4).

Sulfido-LT production by mixed leukocytes from atopic volunteers was dramatically depressed after treatment with BAYX-1005 whether the cells were stimulated with anti-IgE or allergen (192). The effect of BAYX-1005, a FLAP inhibitor, has also been evaluated in a guinea pig model (193). Allergen challenge of the lung parenchyma caused a biphasic

Table 4 5-Lipoxygenase-Activating
Protein (FLAP) Inhibitors

FLAP inhibitor	Refs.
BAYX1005	192–194
MK-0591	195, 234, 235
MK-886	142, 192, 194, 198–200

response (immediate, then plateau). Interestingly, BAYX-1005 depressed only the plateau phase; however, a combination of the FLAP inhibitor and an antihistamine depressed both phases of the response (194). A similar experiment with ICI-198,615, anti-IgE, and human bronchi yielded very similar results. That is, the response of the human bronchi to anti-IgE was completely abolished by the FLAP inhibitor in concert with an antihistamine. ICI-198,615 by itself merely rendered the bronchi insensitive to exogenous leukotrienes and ablated the plateau phase of bronchoconstriction (194).

MK-0591 is a quinoline–indole hybrid that is administered orally. Diamant et al. (195) evaluated the effects of this drug on the EAR and LAR after challenge with dust mite extract in eight allergic men with mild to moderate asthma (195). Three doses of 250 mg each were given 24, 12, and 1.5 h before allergen challenge. The results were impressive, showing that LTB_4 production after ex vivo calcium ionophore activation of whole blood and excretion of urinary LTE_4 was reduced by 99 and 87%, respectively. Similarly, the EAR drop in FEV_1 was decreased by 79% and the LAR by 39%.

MK-0591 was also evaluated in a multicenter, parallel group, double-blind study with 239 patients with mild to moderate asthma (196). Patients either received placebo or one of four doses of oral MK-1591 for 6 weeks after a 3-week run-in period with placebo. The results demonstrated that treatment with MK-0951 decreased asthma symptoms and the need for β-adrenoceptor agonists. In comparison, peak flow rates and pulmonary function were improved. The decrease in urinary LTE_4 levels that were found indicates that MK-0591 was acting by blocking the formation of SLT.

MK-886, another FLAP inhibitor, is an indole derivative that attenuates both the EAR and LAR after allergen inhalation and prevents ex vivo LTB_4 production by whole blood (142). Results obtained in guinea pig lung parenchyma and in mixed leukocytes were similar to those with BAYX1005 (192,193); that is, both phases of the constriction response to allergen could be ameliorated with the inhibitor and an antihistamine. Another group confirmed that MK-886 inhibits allergen-induced bronchoconstriction in guinea pigs, but could find no effect against airway eosinophilia (197). MK-886 was also evaluated in the human bronchi experiment conducted with ICI 198,615, an LTD_4 receptor antagonist and, again, combination with an antihistamine completely abolished contraction after anti-IgE exposure (194).

Finally, MK-886 was studied in a two-point, double-blind, crossover study in eight atopic men (198). All received doses of 800 and 250 mg 1 h before and 2 h after allergen inhalation, respectively. The results showed that ex vivo LTB_4 production by whole blood after stimulation with calcium ionophore was reduced by 54% for 6 h after the allergen challenge. The urinary LTE_4 concentration was similarly decreased: 51 and 80% in the EAR and LAR, respectively (196). In another study in human subjects, it was demonstrated that, unlike LTD_4 antagonists, MK-886 does not protect against airway hyperresponsiveness (199), but this could be a function of the length of the study.

5-Lipoxygenase Inhibitors

Studies in chronically bronchoconstricted asthmatics, laboratory-induced bronchoconstriction, and allergic rhinitis indicate that pharmacological manipulation of the 5-LO enzyme may be useful in the treatment of asthma. In this section a few of the major 5-LO inhibitors will be reviewed (Table 5).

The 5-LO inhibitor, docebenone (AA-681) was evaluated for efficacy in prevention of allergic rhinitis during allergy season by Ancill et al. (200). Patients (123) were enrolled in a

Table 5 Five Lipoxygenase (5-LO) Inhibitors

5-LO Inhibitor	Common name	Refs.
AA-681	Docebenone	182, 201, 236
A-64077	Zileuton	202–207, 237, 238
ICI-D2138		208–210
U-60257	Piriprost	239
FR-110,302		240
B1-6-239		241
A-78773		242

10-week placebo-controlled, parallel group, double-blind study and given either 75 mg bid of AA-861 or placebo. Although ocular symptoms and mean daily use of terfenadine were unaffected by this regimen, total nasal symptoms reported were significantly lower in the group receiving docebenone than in those receiving placebo in an evaluation at weeks 5 and 8.

Zileuton (A-64077) is a hydroxyurea derivative with chelating activity that inhibits the active site iron of 5-LO (201). This drug has also been evaluated in allergic rhinitis. Eight patients were given a nasal allergen challenge 3 h after a single dose of 800 mg of zileuton or placebo. Both LTB_4 levels in nasal washings and ex vivo LTB_4 synthesis were much lower in the zileuton-treated group than in those who had received placebo. In addition, nasal congestion was significantly reduced by zileuton, although, as seen with zafirlukast, frequency of sneezing and histamine release was not attenuated by one dose of the inhibitor (202).

Treatment with zileuton also improves airway function in patients with asthma, as shown in a randomized, placebo-controlled, double-blind study on 139 persons (baseline FEV_1, 40–75%; 15% reversibility; 1). The first dose (600 mg) was administered in the hospital and produced a 14.6% increase in FEV_1 in 1 h. After 4 weeks of use (2.4 or 1.6 g/day), the higher dosage reduced the symptom scores, frequency of β-adrenergic agonist usage, and mean urinary LTE_4 levels. The mean FEV_1 and FVC were increased by 13.4 and 14.6%, respectively. As the peak expiratory flow rate continued to improve and β-agonist use continued to drop until the end of the trial, the maximum efficacy of the drug may not have been reached.

The same group have demonstrated that zileuton (one 800-mg dose) also significantly attenuated the asthmatic response to cold, dry air in 13 asthmatic patients in a double-blind, placebo-controlled, randomized trial (203). In addition to inhibiting LTB_4 production by whole blood by 74% after challenge with calcium ionophore, zileuton propagated a 47% increase in the quantity of air needed to cause the FEV_1 to drop by 10%. Similarly, zileuton reduces the decrease in FEV_1 experienced by aspirin-sensitive asthmatics after aspirin challenge. In this system, the concomitant angioedema, gastrointestinal symptoms, and nasal congestion were also alleviated by zileuton (204). Finally, zileuton, which has now been examined in over 800 individuals, has also been reported to be beneficial in ulcerative colitis, rheumatoid arthritis, and asthmatic challenge studies (182,203,205,206).

The effect of a nonredox 5-LO inhibitor ICI-D2138 was examined in a double-blind, randomized, placebo-controlled study with seven aspirin-sensitive asthmatics with baseline FEV_1 of more than 67% (207). Challenge with aspirin 4 h after one dose of 350 mg ICI-D2138 compared with placebo resulted in a fall of FEV_1 of 4.9 versus 20.3%, respectively.

In addition, there was a 72% inhibition of LTB_4 generation in whole blood and the increase in urinary LTB_4 was depressed by 74%.

ICI-D2138 is the most potent and selective 5-LO inhibitor yet reported. Unlike zileuton, it does not operate by a redox or iron chelation mechanism, but by an enantioselective mechanism (10). The short-term efficacy and safety of ICI-D2138 was tested in a 10-day, placebo-controlled, double-blind study in rheumatoid arthritis patients (206). Prevention of the flare after nonsteroidal anti-inflammatory drug withdrawal was demonstrated, showing that ICI-D2138 has anti-inflammatory properties.

This agent has also been tested in patients with mild asthma in two double-blind allergen challenge studies (208). However, after either a single 350-mg dose or ten daily doses of 37.5, 125, or 350 mg, no blocking of allergen-induced bronchoconstriction could be observed. This is in contrast to a study by McMillan et al. (209) in which ICI-D2138 potently inhibited bronchoconstriction in guinea pigs that were pretreated with pyrilamine, indomethacin, and propranolol (209). Therefore, these results do not exclude the possibility that ICI-D2138 may be an effective drug in the treatment of asthma, but may indicate that the allergen challenge model may not be a positive indicator of the efficacy of antiasthmatic agents (10). Clearly, further work is required.

ADVERSE EFFECTS

Most studies now completed report that the leukotriene antagonists and synthesis inhibitors are well-tolerated, with few adverse effects. The early antagonist FPL-55712 has an unpleasant taste, and patients complain of discomfort in the throat after inhalation, but it is not serious (154). However, several of the earlier compounds (MK-886, LY-171,883, MK-571) were withdrawn from further clinical trials because of changes in hepatic enzymes. Other complaints have included mild adverse effects, such as gastrointestinal disturbances and headaches. For example, tomelukast (600 mg bid) caused mild diarrhea in 4 of 138 patients (156), and 6 of 139 patients receiving zileuton experienced mild dyspepsia (154). Single doses of MK-679 (187), ICI-D2138 (208), and zafirlukast (154) caused no significant adverse effects. Although several patients receiving zileuton, tomelukast, or zafirlukast reported headaches, the frequency was the same as in those receiving placebo (1).

CONCLUSION

There is much evidence that leukotrienes are critical mediators in asthma and allergic disease (43). First, LTB_4 and the sulfidoleukotrienes are potent biological mediators of bronchoconstriction, hypersensitivity, and plasma exudation (88,210). Second, leukotrienes can be detected in the blood, urine, and BAL fluid of asthmatics both after allergen challenge and during an exacerbation (211,212). Patients with psoriasis and those with allergic rhinitis also have increased levels of leukotrienes in the urine and nasal lavage, respectively (131,213). Third, leukotrienes are produced by the cells that mediate inflammation in asthma. In fact, in the EAR, most cells, which are stimulated by anti-IgE, degranulate, releasing LTC_4, histamine, and possibly, prostanoids (214–217). Then, during the LAR, there is an influx of neutrophils and eosinophils (218), both of which release SLT and PAF.

Finally, it has been amply demonstrated that pharmacological agents that modulate leukotrienes attenuate both asthma and allergic rhinitis symptoms. This is of interest because other mediator antagonists do not have these beneficial effects in asthma. Antihistamines do not influence asthma symptoms, and PAF antagonists have no significant effects on the EAR or LAR, nor do they exhibit any anti-inflammatory effects (219). Leukotriene antagonists, on the other hand, have a cumulative effect, and their full potential may not yet have been seen. The effects of leukotriene antagonists are additive to those of β-adrenergic agonists and reduce the need for steroids. This suggests that leukotriene antagonists have anti-inflammatory actions as well as bronchodilatory effects. In the future it will be important to test the newer, more potent drugs, vary the dosages and methods of delivery, increase the treatment periods, and try the drugs in combination with other classes of antiallergy drugs. Further results are eagerly awaited.

REFERENCES

1. Chanarin N, Johnston SL. Leukotrienes as a target in asthma therapy. Drugs 1994; 47:12–24.
2. Naclerio RM, Baroody FM. Observations on the response of the nasal mucosa to allergens. Otolaryngol Med Neck Surg 1994; 111:355–363.
3. Feldberg W, Kellaway CH. Liberation of histamine and formation of lysolethicin like substances by cobra venom. J Physiol 1938; 94:187–226.
4. Kellaway CH, Threthewie RE. The liberation of a slow reacting smooth muscle stimulating substance of anaphylaxis. J Exp Physiol 1940; 30:121–145.
5. Samuelsson B. Leukotrienes: mediators of immediate hypersensitivity reactions and inflammation. Science 1983; 220:568–575.
6. Borgeat P, Samuelsson B. Transformation of arachidonic acid by rabbit polymorphonuclear leukocytes. Formation of a novel dihydroxy eicosanoic acid. J Biol Chem 1979; 254:2643–2646.
7. Murphy RC, Hammarstrom S, Samuelsson B. Leukotriene C: a slow reacting substance from murine mastocytoma cells. Proc Natl Acad Sci USA 1979; 76:4275–4279.
8. Holtzman MJ. Arachidonic acid metabolism. Am Rev Respir Dis 1991; 143:188–203.
9. Drazen JM, Austen KF. Leukotrienes and airway responses. Am Rev Respir Dis 1987; 136: 985–998.
10. Hedqvist P, Raud J, Palmertz U, Kumlin M, Dahlen SE. Eicosanoids as mediators and modulators of inflammation. Adv Prostaglandin Thromboxane Leukot Res 1991; 21B:537–543.
11. Rouzer CA, Kargman S. Translocation of 5-lipoxygenase to the membrane in human leukocytes challenged with ionophore A23187. J Biol Chem 1988; 263:10980–10988.
12. Wong A, Cook MN, Hwang SM, Sarau HM, Foley JJ, Crooke ST. Stimulation of leukotriene production and membrane translocation of 5-lipoxygenase by cross-linking of the IgE receptors in RBL-2H3 cells. Biochemistry 1992; 31:4046–4053.
13. Kargman S, Prasit P, Evans JF. Translocation of HL-60 cell 5-lipoxygenase—inhibition of A23187 or N-formyl-methionyl-leucyl-phenylalanine-induced translocation by indole and quinolone leukotriene synthesis inhibitors. J Biol Chem 1991; 266:23745–23752.
14. Malaviya R, Malaviya R, Jakschik BA. Reversible translocation of 5-lipoxygenase in mast cells upon IgE/antigen stimulation. J Biol Chem 1993; 268:4939–4944.
15. Peters-Golden M, McNish RW. Redistribution of 5-lipoxygenase and cytosolic phospholipase-A_2 to the nuclear fraction upon macrophage activation. Biochem Biophys Res Commun 1993; 196:147–153.
16. Woods JW, Evans JF, Ethier D, Scott S, Vickers PJ, Hearn L, Heibein JA, Charleson S, Singer II. 5-Lipoxygenase and 5-lipoxygenase activating protein are localized in the nuclear envelope of activated human leukocytes. J Exp Med 1994; 178:1935–1946.
17. Woods JW, Coffey MJ, Brock TG, Singer II, Peters-Golden M. 5-Lipoxygenase is located in the euchromatin of the nucleus in resting human alveolar macrophages and translocates to the nuclear envelope upon cell activation. J Clin Invest 1995; 95:2035–2046.

18. Dixon RAF, Diehl RE, Opas E, Rands E, Vickers PJ, Evans JF, Gillard JW, Miller DK. Requirement of a 5-lipoxygenase-activating protein for leukotriene synthesis. Nature 1990; 343: 282–284.

19. Miller DK, Gillard JW, Vickers PJ, Sadowski S, Leveille C, Mancini JA, Charleson P, Dixon RAF, Ford-Hutchinson AW, Fortin R, Gauthier JY, Rodkey J, Rosen R, Rouzer C, Sigal IS, Strader CD, Evans JF. Identification and isolation of a membrane protein necessary for leukotriene production. Nature 1990; 343:278–281.

20. Samuelsson B, Dahlen SE, Lindgren JA, Rouzer CA, Serhan CN. Leukotrienes and lipoxins: structures, biosynthesis, and biological effects. Science 1987; 237:1171–1176.

21. Samuelsson B, Funk CD. Enzymes involved in the biosynthesis of leukotriene B_4. J Biol Chem 1989; 264:19469–19472.

22. Steinhilber D. 5-Lipoxygenase: enzyme expression and regulation of activity. Pharm Acta Helv 1994; 69:3–14.

23. Minami M, Ohno S, Kawasaki H, Radmark O, Samuelsson B, Jornvall H, Shimizu T, Seyama Y, Suzuki K. Molecular cloning of a cDNA coding for human leukotriene A_4 hydrolase. Complete primary structure of an enzyme involved in eicosanoid synthesis. J Biol Chem 1987; 262: 13873–13876.

24. Henderson WR Jr. Eicosanoids and platelet-activating factor in allergic respiratory diseases. Am Rev Respir Dis 1991; 143:S86–90.

25. Penrose JF, Gagnon L, Goppelt-Struebe M, Myers P, Lam BK, Jack RM, Austen KF, Soberman RJ. Purification of human leukotriene C_4 synthase. Proc Natl Acad Sci USA 1992; 89:11603–11606.

26. Kumlin M, Dahlen SE. Characteristics of formation and further metabolism of leukotrienes in the chopped human lung. Biochim Biophys Acta 1990; 1044:201–210.

27. Keppler D, Guhlman A, Oberdorfer F, Kraus K, Muller J, Ostertag H, Huber M. Generation and metabolism of cysteinyl leukotrienes in vivo. Ann NY Acad Sci 1991; 629:100–104.

28. Henderson WR, Klebanoff SJ. Leukotriene production and inactivation by normal, chronic granulomatous disease and myeloperoxidase-deficient neutrophils. J Biol Chem 1983; 258: 13522–13527.

29. Henderson WR. Formation and oxidative degradation of leukotrienes by eosinophils and neutrophils. In: Samuelsson B, Berti F, Folco GC, et al. Drugs Affecting Leukotrienes and Other Eicosanoid Pathways. New York: Plenum Press, 1985:339–349.

30. Haines KA, Giedd KN, Rich AM, Korchak HM, Weissmann G. The leukotriene B_4 paradox: neutrophils can, but will not, respond to ligand–receptor interactions by forming leukotriene B_4 or its omega-metabolites. Biochemistry 1987; 241:55–62.

31. Clancy RM, Dahinden CA, Hugli TE. Arachidonate metabolism by human polymorphonuclear leukocytes stimulated by N-formyl-Met-Leu-Phe or complement component C5a is independent of phospholipase activation. Proc Natl Acad Sci USA 1983; 80:7200–7204.

32. McDonald PP, McColl S, Naccache PH, Brogeat P. Studies on the activation of human neutrophil 5-lipoxygenase by natural agonists and Ca^{2+}-ionophore A23187. Biochem J 1991; 280: 379–385.

33. Sellmayer A, Strasser T, Weber PC. Differences in arachidonic acid release, metabolism and leukotriene B_4 synthesis in human polymorphonuclear leukocytes activated by different stimuli. Biochim Biophys Acta 1987; 927:417–422.

34. Mahadevappa VG, Powell WS. The metabolism of arachidonic and eicosapentaenoic acids in human neutrophils stimulated by A23187 and FMLP. J Cell Biochem 1989; 40:341–352.

35. DiPersio JF, Naccache PH, Borgeat P, Gasson JC, Nguyen M, McColl S. Characterization of the priming effects of human granulocyte–macrophage colony stimulating factor on human neutrophil leukotriene synthesis. Prostaglandins 1988; 36:673–691.

36. Doerfler ME, Danner RL, Shelhamer JH, Parrillo JE. Bacterial lipopolysaccharides prime human neutrophils for enhanced production of leukotriene B_4. J Clin Invest 1989; 83:970–977.

37. Hatzelmann A, Haurand M, Ullrich V. Involvement of calcium in the thiomersal-stimulated formation of leukotrienes by FMLP in human polymorphonuclear leukocytes. Biochem Pharmacol 1990; 39:559–567.

38. Roubin R, Elsas PP, Fiers W, Dessein AJ. Recombinant human tumor necrosis factor (rTNF) enhances leukotriene biosynthesis in neutrophils and eosinophils stimulated with the Ca-ionophore A23187. Clin Exp Immunol 1987; 70:484–490.

39. Wirthmueller U, Baggiolini M, De Weck AL, Dahinden CA. Receptor-operated activation of polymorphonuclear leukocytes—different effects of NAP-1/IL-8 and fMet-Leu-Phe or C5a. Biochem Biophys Res Commun 1991; 176:972–978.

40. Dahinden CA, Zingg J, Maly FE, DeWeck AL. Leukotriene production in human neutrophils primed by recombinant human granulocyte–macrophage colony stimulating factor and stimulated with complement component C5a and FMLP as second signals. J Exp Med 1988; 167:1281–1295.

41. Bischoff SC, Brunner T, de Weck AL, Dahinden CA. Interleukin 5 modifies histamine release and leukotriene generation by human basophils in response to diverse agonists. J Exp Med 1990; 172:1577–1582.

42. Takafuji S, Bischoff SC, de Weck AL, Dahinden CA. Interleukin 3 and interleukin 5 prime human eosinophils in produce leukotriene C_4 in response to soluble agonists. J Immunol 1991; 147:3855.

43. Henderson WR. The role of leukotrienes in inflammation. Ann Intern Med 1994; 121:684–697.

44. Claesson H-E, Haeggstrom J. Human endothelial cells stimulate leukotriene synthesis and convert granulocyte released leukotriene A_4 into leukotrienes B_4, C_4, and E_4. J Lipid Mediat 1988; 173:93–100.

45. Fels AOS, Pawlowski NA, Cramer EB, King TKC, Cohn ZA, Scott WA. Human alveolar macrophages produce leukotriene B_4. Proc Natl Acad Sci USA 1983; 80:5425–5429.

46. Fitzpatrick FA, Ligget W, McGee J, Bunting S, Morton D, Samuelsson B. Metabolism of leukotriene A_4 by human erythrocytes. J Biol Chem 1984; 259:11403–11407.

47. Jakobsson PJ, Steinhilber D, Odlander B, Radmark O, Claesson HE, Samuelsson B. On the expression and regulation of 5-lipoxygenase in human lymphocytes. Proc Natl Acad Sci USA 1992; 89:3521–3525.

48. Yamamoto S. Mammalian lipoxygenases: molecular structures and function. Biochim Biophys Acta 1992; 1128:117–131.

49. Martin TR, Altman LC, Albert RK, Henderson WR. Leukotriene B_4 production by human alveolar macrophages: a potential mechanism for amplifying inflammation in the lung. Am Rev Respir Dis 1984; 129:106–111.

50. Radmark O, Shimizu T, Jornvall H, Samuelsson B. Leukotriene A_4 hydrolase in human leukocytes: purification and properties. J Biol Chem 1984; 259:12339–12345.

51. Feinmark SJ, Cannon PJ. Endothelial cell leukotriene C_4 synthesis results from intracellular transfer of leukotriene A_4 synthesized by polymorphonuclear leukocytes. J Biol Chem 1986; 261:16466–16472.

52. Odlander B, Jakobsson P-J, Rosen A, Claesson H-E. Human B and T lymphocytes convert leukotriene A_4 into leukotriene B_4. Biochem Biophys Res Commun 1988; 153:203–208.

53. Bigby TD, Lee DM, Meslier N, Gruenert DC. Leukotriene A_4 hydrolase activity of human airway epithelial cells. Biochem Biophys Res Commun 1989; 164:1–7.

54. Sur S, Adolphson CR, Gleich GJ. Eosinophils: biochemical and cellular aspects. In: Middleton E, Reed CE, Ellis EF, Adkinson NF, Yunginger JW, Busse WW, eds. Allergy: Principles and Practice. St. Louis: CV Mosby, 1993:169–200.

55. Jorg A, Henderson WR, Murphy RC, Klebanoff SJ. Leukotriene generation by eosinophils. J Exp Med 1982; 155:390–402.

56. Owen WF Jr, Soberman RJ, Yoshimoto T, Sheffer AL, Lewis RA, Austen KF. Synthesis and release of leukotriene C_4 by human eosinophils. J Immunol 1987; 138:532–538.

57. Weller PK, Lee AV, Foster DW, Corey EJ, Austen KF, Lewis RA. Generation and metabolism of 5-lipoxygenase pathway leukotrienes by human eosinophils: predominant production of leukotriene C_4. Proc Natl Acad Sci USA 1983; 80:7626–7630.

58. Tamura N, Agrawal DK, Townley RG. Leukotriene C_4 production from human eosinophils in vitro: role of eosinophil chemotactic factors on eosinophil activation. J Immunol 1988; 141: 4291–4297.

59. Valone FH, Boggs JM, Goetzl EJ. Lipid mediators of hypersensitivity and inflammation. In: Middleton E, Reed CE, Ellis EF, Adkinson NF, Yungiger JW, Busse WW, eds. Allergy: Principles and Practice. St. Louis: CV Mosby, 1993:302–319.

60. MacGlashan DW Jr, Schleimer RP, Peters SP, Schulman ES, Adams GK, Sobotka AK, Newball HH, Lichtenstein LM. Comparative studies of human basophils and mast cells. Fed Proc 1983; 42:2504–2509.

61. Schleimer RP, MacGlashan DW Jr, Peters SP, Pinckard RN, Adkinson NF Jr, Lichtenstein LM. Characterization of inflammatory mediator release from purified human lung mast cells. Am Rev Respir Dis 1986; 133:614–617.

62. Samuelsson B. Leukotrienes: mediators of immediate hypersensitivity reactions and inflammation. Science 1983; 220:568–575.

63. Maclouf JA, Murphy RC. Transcellular metabolism of neutrophil-derived leukotriene A_4 human platelets. A potential cellular source of leukotriene C_4. J Biol Chem 1988; 263:174–181.

64. Ford-Hutchinson AW, Bray WM, Doig MV, Shipley ME, Smith MJH. Leukotriene B_4, a potent chemokinetic and aggregating substance released from PMN leucocytes. Nature 1980; 286: 263–264.

65. Nagy L, Lee TH, Goetzl EJ, Pickett WC, Kay AB. Complement receptor enhancement and chemotaxis of human neutrophils and eosinophils by leukotrienes and other lipoxygenase products. Clin Exp Immunol 1983; 71:394–398.

66. Erger RA, Casale TB. Comparative studies indicate that platelet-activating factor is a relatively weak eosinophilotactic mediator. Am J Respir Cell Mol Biol 1995; 12:65–70.

67. Djukanovic R, Roche WR, Wilson JW, Beasley CRW, Twentyman OP. Mucosal inflammation in asthma. Am Rev Respir Dis 1990; 142:434–457.

68. Martin TR, Pistorese BP, Chi EY, Goodman RB, Matthay MA. Effects of leukotriene B_4 in the human lung. Recruitment of neutrophils into the alveolar spaces without a change in protein permeability. J Clin Invest 1989; 84:1609–1619.

69. Piacentini GL, Kaliner MA. The potential roles of leukotrienes in bronchial asthma. Am Rev Respir Dis 1991; 143:S96–99.

70. Feinmark SJ, Lindgren JA, Claesson H-E, Malmsten C, Samuelsson B. Stimulation of human leukocyte degranulation by leukotriene B_4 and its ω-oxidized metabolites. FEBS Lett 1981; 136: 141–144.

71. Bjork J, Arfors K-E, Hedqvist P, Dahlen S-E, Lingren JA. Leukotriene B_4 causes leukocyte emigration from postcapillary venules in the hamster cheek pouch. Microcirculation 1982; 2:271.

72. Palmblad J, Malmsten CL, Uden A-M, Radmark O, Engstedt L, Samuelsson B. Leukotriene B_4 is a potent and stereospecific stimulator of neutrophil chemotaxis and adherence. Blood 1981; 58:658–661.

73. Serhan CN, Fridovich J, Goetzl EJ, Dunham PB, Weissman G. Leukotriene B_4 and phosphatidic acid are calcium ionophores: studies employing arsenazo III in liposomes. J Biol Chem 1982; 257:4746–4752.

74. Rola-Pleszczynski M, Chavaillaz PA, Lemaire I. Stimulation of interleukin-w and interferon gamma production by leukotriene B_4 in human lymphocyte cultures. Prostaglandins Leukot Med 1986; 23:207–210.

75. Rola-Pleszczynski M, Stankova J, Leukotriene B_4 enhances interleukin-6 (IL-6) production and IL-6 messenger RNA accumulation in human monocytes in vitro: transcriptional and posttranscriptional mechanisms. Blood 1992; 80:1004–1011.

76. Brach MA, de Vos S, Arnold C, Gruss HJ, Mertselmann R, Hermann F. Leukotriene B_4 transcriptionally activates interleukin-6 expression involving NK-$_\kappa$B and NF-IL6. Eur J Immunol 1992; 22:2705–2711.

77. Wasserman MA, Smith EF, Underwood DC, Barnetts MA. Pharmacology and pathophysiology of 5-lipoxygenase products. In: Crooke ST, Wong A, eds. Lipoxygenases and Their Products. San Diego: Academic Press, 1991:1–50.

78. Goldman DW, Goetzl EJ. Specific binding of leukotriene B_4 to receptors on human polymorphonuclear leukocytes. J Immunol 1982; 129:1600–1604.

79. Lin AH, Ruppel PL, Gorman RR. Leukotriene B_4 binding to human neutrophils. Prostaglandins 1984; 28:837–849.

80. Goldman DW, Goetzl EJ. Heterogeneity of human polymorphonuclear leukocyte receptors for leukotriene B_4. Identification of a subset of high affinity receptors that transduce the chemotactic response. J Exp Med 1984; 159:1027–1041.

81. Votta B, Mong S. Transition of affinity states for leukotriene B_4 receptors in sheep lung membranes. J Pharmacol Exp Ther 1990; 265:841–847.

82. Johnson HM, Russel JK, Torres BA. Second messenger role of arachidonic acid and its metabolites in interferon gamma production. J Immunol 1991; 347:3053–3056.

83. Ng CF, Sun FF, Taylor BM, Wolin MS, Wong PY. Functional properties of guinea pig eosinophil leukotriene B_4 receptor. J Immunol 1991; 147:3096–103.

84. Bomalski JS, Mong S. Binding of leukotriene B_4 and its analogues to human polymorphonuclear leukocyte membrane receptors. Prostaglandins 1987; 33:855–867.

85. LeBlanc Y, Fitzsimmons BJ, Charleson S, Alexander P, Evans JF, Rokach J. Analogues of leukotriene B_4: effects of modification of the hydroxyl groups on leukocyte aggregation and binding to leukocyte leukotriene B_4 receptors. Prostaglandins 1987; 33:617–625.

86. Baud L, Perez J, Denis M, Ardaillou R. Modulation of fibroblast proliferation by sulfidopeptide leukotrienes; effect of indomethacin. J Immunol 1987; 138:1190–1195.

87. Leikauf G, Claesson H-E, Doupnik C, Hybbinette S, Grafstrom R. Cysteinyl leukotrienes enhance growth in human airway epithelial cells. Am J Physiol 1989; 259:L255–L261.

88. Dahlen S-E, Hedqvist P, Hammarstrom S, Samuelsson B. Leukotrienes are potent constrictors of human bronchi. Nature 1980; 288:484–486.

89. Hanna CJ, Bach MK, Pare PD, Schellenberg RR. Slow reacting substances (leukotrienes) contract human airway and pulmonary vascular smooth muscle. Nature 1981; 290:343–344.

90. Holroyde MC, Altounyan REC, Cole M, Dixon M, Elliott EV. Bronchoconstriction produced in man by leukotrienes C and D. Lancet 1981; 6:17–18.

91. Griffin M, Weiss JW, Leitch AG, McFadden ER Jr, Corey EJ, Austen KF, Drazen JM. Effects of leukotriene D on the airways in asthma. N Engl J Med 1983; 308:436–439.

92. Hogaboom GK, Mong S, Wu HL, Crooke ST. Peptidoleukotrienes: distinct receptors for leukotriene C_4 and D_4 in the guinea-pig lung. Biochem Biophys Res Commun 1983; 116:1136–1143.

93. Cheng JB, Lang D, Bewtra AK, Townley RG. Tissue distribution and functional correlation of [^{3}H]leukotriene C_4 and [^{3}H]leukotriene D_4 binding sites in guinea-pig uterus and lung preparations. J Pharmacol Exp Ther 1985; 232:80–87.

94. Cheng JB, Townley RG. Identification of leukotriene D_4 receptor binding sites in guinea pig lung homogenates using [^{3}H]leukotriene D_4. Biochem Biophys Res Commun 1984; 118: 20–26.

95. Pong SS, DeHaven RN, Kuehl FA Jr, Egan RW. Leukotriene C_4 binding to rat lung membranes. J Biol Chem 1983; 116:1136–1143.

96. Cheng JB, Townley RG. Evidence for a similar receptor site for binding of [^{3}H]leukotriene E_4 and [^{3}H]leukotriene D_4 to the guinea-pig crude lung membrane. Biochem Biophys Res Commun 1984; 122:949–954.

97. Cheng JB, Townley RG. Effect of the serine–borate complex on the relative ability of leukotriene C_4, D_4, and E_4 to inhibit lung and brain [^{3}H]leukotriene D_4 and [^{3}H]leukotriene C_4

binding: demonstration of the agonists' potency order for the leukotriene D_4 and leukotriene C_4 receptors. Biochem Biophys Res Commun 1984; 119:612–617.

98. Rovati GE, Giovanazzi S, Mezzetti M, Nicosia S. Heterogeneity of binding sites for ICI 198,615 in human lung parenchyma. Biochem Pharmacol 1992; 44:1411–1415.

99. Buckner CK, Krell RD, Laravuso RB, Coursin DB, Berstein PR, Will JA. Pharmacological evidence that human intralobar airways do not contain different receptors that mediate contractions to leukotriene C_4 and leukotriene D_4. J Pharmacol Exp Ther 1986; 237:558–562.

100. Buckner CK, Saban R, Castleman WL, Will JA. Analysis of leukotriene receptor antagonists on isolated human intralobar airways. Ann NY Acad Sci 1988; 524:181–186.

101. Aharony D, Falcone RC. Binding of tritiated LTD-4 and the peptide leukotriene antagonist tritiated ILI-198615 to receptors on human lung membranes. In: Zor U, Naor Z, Danon A, eds. New Trends in Lipid Mediators Research. Basel: S Karger, 1989:67–71.

102. Drazen JM. Leukotrienes in asthma and rhinitis. In: Busse W, Holgate S, eds. Asthma and Rhinitis. Oxford: Blackwells, 1994.

103. Drazen JM. Comparative contractile responses to sulfidopeptide leukotrienes in normal and asthmatic human subjects. Ann NY Acad Sci 1988; 524:289–297.

104. Jones TR, Davis C, Daniel EE. Pharmacological study of the contractile activity of leukotriene C_4 and D_4 on isolated human airway smooth muscle. Can J Physiol Pharmacol 1982; 60: 638–843.

105. Samhoun MN, Conroy DM, Piper PJ. Pharmacological profile of leukotrienes E_4, N-acetyl$_4$ and four of their novel omega and beta oxidative metabolites in airways of guinea pig and men in vitro. Br J Pharmacol 1989; 98:1406–1412.

106. Adelroth E, Morris MM, Hargreave FE, O'Bryne PM. Airway responsiveness to LTC_4 and D_4 and to methacholine in patients with asthma and normal controls. N Engl J Med 1986; 315: 480–484.

107. Barnes NC, Piper PJ, Costello JF. Comparative effects of inhaled leukotriene C_4, leukotriene D_4, and histamine in normal human subjects. Thorax 1984; 39:500–504.

108. Davidson AE, Lee TH, Scanlon PD, Solaway J, McFadden R. Bronchoconstrictor effects of LTE_4 in normal and asthmatic subjects. Am Rev Respir Dis 1987; 135:333–337.

109. Woodward DF, Weichman BM, Gill CA, Wasserman MA. The effect of synthetic leukotrienes on tracheal microvascular permeability. Prostaglandins 1983; 25:131–142.

110. Camp RDR, Coutts AA, Greaves MW, Kay AB, Walport. Responses of human skin to intradermal injection of leukotrienes C_4, D_4, and B_4. Br J Pharmacol 1983; 80:497–502.

111. Coles ST, Neill KH, Reid LM, Auten KF, Nii Y. Effects of leukotrienes C_4 and D_4 on glycoproteins and lysozyme secretion by human bronchial mucosa. Prostaglandins 1983; 25: 155–170.

112. Marom Z, Shelhamer JH, Bach MK, Morton DR, Kaliner MA. Slow reacting substances, leukotrienes C_4 and D_4 increase the release of mucus from human airways in vitro. Am Rev Respir Dis 1982; 126:449–451.

113. Brocklehurst WE. The release of histamine and formation of a new slow reacting substance (SRS-A) during anaphylactic shock. J Physiol 1960; 151:416–435.

114. Sampson AP, Thomas RU, Costello JF, Piper PJ. Enhanced leukotriene synthesis in leukotrienes of atopic and asthmatic subjects. Br J Pharmacol 1989; 98:1406–1412.

115. Kohi F, Miyagawa H, Agrawal DK, Bewtra AK, Townley RG. Generation of leukotriene B_4 and C_4 from granulocytes of normal controls, allergic rhinitis, and asthmatic subjects. Ann Allergy 1990; 65:228–232.

116. Taylor GW, Taylor I, Black P, Maltby NH, Turner N, Fuller RW, Dollery CT. Urinary leukotriene E_4 after antigen challenge and in acute asthma and allergic rhinitis. Lancet 1989; 1:584–587.

117. Manning PJ, Rokash J, Malo J-L, Ethier D, Cartier A, Girard Y, Charleson S, O'Byrne PM. Urinary leukotriene E_4 levels during early and late asthmatic responses. J Allergy Clin Immunol 1990; 86:211–220.

118. Tagari P, Rasmussen JB, Delorme D, Girard Y, Eriksson L-O, Charleson S, Ford-Hutchinson AW. Comparison of urinary leukotriene E_4 and 16-carboxytetranordihydroleukotriene E_4 excretion in allergic asthmatics after inhaled allergen. Eicosanoids 1990; 3:75–80.

119. Westcott JY, Smith HR, Wenzel SE, Larsen GL, Thomas RB, Felsien D, Voelkel NF. Urinary leukotriene E_4 in patients with asthma. Am Rev Respir Dis 1991; 143:1322–1238.

120. Kumlin M, Dahlen B, Bjorck T, Zetterstrom O, Granstrom E, Dahlen S-E. Urinary excretion of leukotriene E_4 and 11-dehydro-thromboxane B_2 in response to bronchial provocations with allergen, aspirin, leukotriene D_4 and histamine in asthmatics. Am Rev Respir Dis 1992; 145: 1087–1091.

121. Drazen JM, O'Brien J, Sparrow D, Weiss ST, Matins MA. Recovery of leukotriene D_4 from the urine of patients with airway obstruction. Am Rev Respir Dis 1992; 146:104–108.

122. Sladek K, Szczeklik A. Cysteinyl leukotrienes overproduction and mast cell activation in aspirin-provoked bronchospasm in asthma. Eur Respir J 1993; 6:391–399.

123. Bellia V, Cuttitta G, Mirabella A, Profita M, Bonanno A, Catania G, Bonsignore G. Urinary leukotriene E_4 as a marker of nocturnal asthma. Am Rev Respir Dis 1992; 145:A16.

124. Lam S, Chan H, LeRiche JC, Chan-Yeung M, Salari H. Release of leukotrienes in patients with bronchial asthma. J Allergy Clin Immunol 1988; 81:711–717.

125. Wardlaw AJ, Hay H, Cromwell O, Collins JW, Kay AB. Leukotrienes LTC_4 and LTB_4 in bronchoalveolar lavage in bronchial asthma and other respiratory diseases. J Allergy Clin Immunol 1989; 84:19–26.

126. Broide DH, Lotz M, Cuomo AJ, Coburn DA, Federman EC, Wasserman SI. Cytokines in symptomatic asthma airways. J Allergy Clin Immunol 1992; 89:958–967.

127. Busse W. Exercise-induced asthma: a role for the eosinophil? J Allergy Clin Immunol 1991; 88: 695–698.

128. Manning PJ, Watson RM, O'Byrne PM. Exercise-induced refractoriness in asthmatic subjects involves leukotriene and prostaglandin interdependent mechanisms. Am Rev Respir Dis 1993; 148:950–954.

129. Israel E, Dermarkarian R, Rosenberg M, Sperling R, Taylor G, Rubin P, Drazen JM. The effects of a 5-lipoxygenase inhibitor on asthma induced by cold, dry air. N Engl J Med 1990; 323:1769–1770.

130. Eggleston PA, Kagey-Sobotka A, Proud D, Adkinson NF Jr, Lichtenstein LM. Disassociation of the release of histamine and arachidonic acid metabolites from osmotically activated basophils and human lung mast cells. Am Rev Respir Dis 1990; 141:960–964.

131. Knani J, Campbell A, Enander I, Peterson CGB, Michel F, Bousquet J. Indirect evidence of nasal inflammation assessed by titration of inflammatory mediators and enumeration of cells in nasal secretions of patients with chronic rhinitis. J Allergy Clin Immunol 1992; 90:880–889.

132. Skoner DP, Lee L, Doyle WJ, Boehm S, Fireman P. Nasal physiology and inflammatory mediators during natural pollen exposure. Ann Allergy 1990; 65:206–210.

133. Miadonna A, Tedeschi A, Leggieri E, Lorini M, Folco G, Sala A, Qualizza R, Froldi M, Zanussi C. Behavioral and clinical relevance of histamine and leukotrienes C_4 and B_4 in grass–pollen-induced rhinitis. Am Rev Respir Dis 1987; 136:357–362.

134. Georgitis JW, Stone BD, Gottschlich G. Nasal inflammatory mediator release in ragweed allergen patients: correlation with cellular influx into nasal secretions. Int Arch Allergy Appl Immunol 1991; 96:231–237.

135. Ramis I, Catafau JR, Serra J, Bulbena O, Picada C, Gelpi E. In vivo release of 15-HETE and other arachidonic acid metabolites in nasal secretions during early allergenic reactions. Prostaglandins 1991; 42:411–420.

136. Togias AG, Naclerio RM, Peters SP, Nimmagadda I, Proud D, Kagey-Sobotka A, Adkinson F, Norman PS, Lichtenstein LM. Local generation of sulfidopeptide leukotrienes upon nasal provocation with cold, dry air. Am Rev Respir Dis 1986; 133:1133–1137.

137. Bisgaard H, Ford-Hutchinson AW, Charleson S, Taudorf E. Detection of leukotriene C_4-like

immunoreactivity in tear fluid from subjects challenged with specific allergen. Prostaglandins 1984; 27:369–374.

138. Okuda M, Watase T, Mezawa A, Liu C. The role of leukotriene D_4 in allergic rhinitis. Ann Allergy 1988; 60:537–540.

139. Snyder DW, Giles RE, Keith RA, Yee YK, Krell RD. The in vitro pharmacology if ICI 198,615: a novel, potent and selective peptide leukotriene antagonist. J Pharmacol Exp Ther 1987; 243: 548–556.

140. Snyder DW, Fleisch JH. Leukotriene receptor antagonists as potential therapeutic agents. Annu Rev Pharmacol Toxicol 1989; 29:123–143.

141. Salmon JA, Garland LG. Leukotriene antagonists and inhibitors of leukotriene biosynthesis as potential therapeutic agents. Prog Drug Res 1991; 37:9–90.

142. Ford Hutchinson AW. Leukotriene antagonists and inhibitors as modulators of IgE-mediated reactions. Springer Semin Immunopathol 1993; 15:37–50.

143. Davidson FF, Dennis EA. Biological relevance of lipocortins and related proteins as inhibitors of phospholipase A_2. Biochem Pharmacol 1989; 38:3645–3651.

144. Tsurufuji S, Sugio K, Takemasa F. The role of glucocorticoid receptor and gene expression in the antiinflammatory action of dexamethasone. Nature 1979; 280:408–410.

145. Dahlen S-E, Bjorck T, Kumlin M, Sydbom A, Raud J, Palmertz U, Franzen L, Gronneberg R, Hedqvist P. Dual inhibitory action of nedocromil sodium on antigen-induced inflammation. Drugs 1989; 37(suppl 1):63–68.

146. Erjefalt I, Persson CG. Pharmacologic control of plasma exudation into tracheobronchial airways. Am Rev Respir Dis 1991; 143:1008–1014.

147. Raud J, Palmertz U, Hedqvist P, Dahlen S-E. Salmeterol inhibits plasma exudation and leukocyte emigration induced by leukotriene B_4 in the hamster cheek pouch. Am Rev Respir Dis 1992; 145:A741.

148. Howarth PH, Durham SR, Lee TH, Kay AB, Church MK, Holgate ST. Influence of albuterol, cromolyn sodium and ipratropium bromide on the airway and circulating mediator responses to allergen bronchial provocation in asthma. Am Rev Respir Dis 1985; 132:986–992.

149. Eda R, Sugiyama H, Hopp RJ, Okada C, Bewtra AK, Townley RG. Inhibitory effects of formoterol on platelet-activating factor induced eosinophil chemotaxis and degranulation. Int Arch Allergy Immunol 1993; 102:391–398.

150. Nabe M, Agrawal DK, Sarmiento EU, Townley RG. Inhibitory effect of terfenadine on mediator release from human blood basophils and eosinophils. Clin Exp Allergy 1989; 19:515–520.

151. Nabe M, Miyagawa H, Agrawal DK, Sugiyama H, Townley RG. The effect of ketotifen on eosinophils as measured at LTC_4 release and by chemotaxis. Allergy Proc 1991; 12:267–271.

152. Cloud ML, Enas GC, Kemp J, Platt-Mills T, Altman LC, Townley RG, Tinkelman D, King T Jr, Middleton E, Shefer AL, McFadden R Jr, Farlow DS. A specific LTD_4/LTE_4-receptor antagonist improves pulmonary function in patients with chronic, mild asthma. Am Rev Respir Dis 1989; 140:1336–1339.

153. Adams GK, Lichtenstein LM. Antagonism of antigen induced contraction of guinea pig and human airways. Nature 1977; 270:255–257.

154. Lee TH, Walport MJ, Wilkinson AH, Turner-Warwick M, Kay AB. Slow reacting substances of anaphylaxis antagonist FPL55712 in chronic asthma. Lancet 1981; 2:304–305.

155. Augstein J, Farmer JB, Lee TB, Sheard P, Tattersall ML. Selective inhibitor of slow reacting substance of anaphylaxis. Nature 1973; 245:215–217.

156. Fuller RW, Black PN, Dollery CT. Effect of the oral leukotriene D_4 antagonist LY171883 on inhaled and intradermal challenge with antigen and LTD_4 in atopic subjects. J Allergy Clin Immunol 1989; 83:939–944.

157. Israel E, Juniper EF, Callaghan JT, Mathur PN, Morris MM, Dowell AR, Enas GG, Hargreave FE, Drazen JM. Effect of a leukotriene antagonist, LY171883, on cold air-induced broncho-constriction in asthmatics. Am Rev Respir Dis 1989; 140:1458–1453.

158. Christie PE, Smith CM, Lee TH. The potent and selective sulfidoleukotriene antagonist, SK&F 104353, inhibits aspirin-induced asthma. Am Rev Respir Dis 1991; 144:957–958.

159. Robuschi M, Riva E, Fucella LM, Vida E, Rossi BM, Gambara G, Spagnotto S, Bianco S. Prevention of exercise-induced bronchoconstriction by a new leukotriene antagonist (SK&F 104353). A double-blind study versus disodium cromoglycate and placebo. Am Rev Respir Dis 1992; 145:1285–1288.

160. Bernstein PR. Accolate. Drugs Future 1994; 19:217–220.

161. Krell RD. The emergence of potent and selective peptide leukotriene receptor antagonists. Pulm Pharmacol 1989; 2:27–31.

162. Kidney JC, Ridge SM, Chung KF, Barnes PJ. Inhibition of platelet-activating factor-induced bronchoconstriction by the leukotriene D_4 receptor antagonist ICI-204,219. Am Rev Respir Dis 1993; 147:215–217.

163. Smith LJ, Geller S, Ebright L, Glass M, Thyrum PT. Inhibition of leukotriene D_4-induced bronchoconstriction in normal subjects by the oral LTD_4 receptor antagonist ICI 204,219. Am Rev Respir Dis 1990; 141:988–992.

164. Findlay SR, Barden JM, Easley CB, Glass M. Effect of the oral leukotriene antagonist, ICI 204,219, on antigen-induced bronchoconstriction in subjects with asthma. J Allergy Clin Immunol 1992; 89:1040–1045.

165. O'Shaughnessy KM, Taylor IK, O'Connor B, O'Connell F, Thomson H, Dollery CT. Potent leukotriene D_4 receptor antagonist ICI 204,219 given by the inhaled route inhibits the early but not the late phase of allergen-induced bronchoconstriction. Am Rev Respir Dis 1993; 147:1431–1435.

166. Dahlen B, Zetterstrom O, Bjorck T, Dahlen S-E. The leukotriene-antagonist ICI-204,219 inhibits the early airway reaction to cumulative bronchial challenge with allergen in atopic asthmatics. Eur Respir J 1994; 7:324–331.

167. Finnerty JP, Wood-Baker R, Thomson H, Holgate ST. Role of leukotrienes in exercise-induced asthma. Inhibitory effect of ICI 204219, a potent leukotriene D_4 receptor antagonist. Am Rev Respir Dis 1992; 145:746–749.

168. Makker HK, Lau LC, Thomson HW, Binks SM, Holgate ST. The protective effect of inhaled leukotriene D_4 receptor antagonist ICI 204,219 against exercise-induced asthma. Am Rev Respir Dis 1993; 147:1413–1418.

169. Hui KP, Barnes NC. Lung function improvement in asthma with a cysteinyl leukotriene receptor antagonist. Lancet 1991; 337:1062–1063.

170. Spector SL, Smith LJ, Glass M. The Accolate (ICI 204,219). Clin Res 1993; 41:199A.

171. Townley RG, Glass M, Minkwitz MC. Six-week, dose-escalation study with Accolate (zafirlukast) in patients with mild to moderate asthma. Am J Respir Crit Care Med 1995; 151:A379.

172. Taylor IK, O'Shaughnessy KM, Fuller RW, Dollery CT. Effect of cysteinyl-leukotriene receptor antagonist ICI 204,219 on allergen-induced bronchoconstriction and airway hyperreactivity in atopic subjects. Lancet 1991; 337:690–694.

173. Donnelly A, Glass M, Muller B, Smart S, Hutson J, Minkwitz M, Casale TB. Leukotriene D_4 (LTD_4) antagonist ICI 204,219 relieves ragweed allergic rhinitis symptoms. J Allergy Clin Immunol 1993; 91:997–1004.

174. Taki F, Suzuki R, Torii K, Matsumoto S, Taniguchi H, Takagi K. Reduction of the severity of bronchial hyperresponsiveness by the novel leukotriene antagonist 4-oxo-8-[4-phenyl-butoxy)benzoylamino]-2-(tetrazol-5-yl)4*H*-1-benzopyran hemihydrate. Arzneimittelforschung 1994; 44:330–333.

175. Yamai T, Watanabe S, Motojima S, Fukada T, Makino S. The significance of leukotriene in antigen-induced late asthmatic response. Am Rev Respir Dis 1989; 139:A462.

176. Yamamoto H, Nagata M, Kuramitu K, Kiuchi H, Sakamoto Y, Yamamoto K, Doi Y. J Clin Med Ther 1993; 9(suppl 1):229–232.

177. Nakagawa T, Mizushima Y, Ishii A, Nambu F, Motoishi M, Yui Y, Shida T, Miyamoto T. Effect of leukotriene antagonist on experimental and clinical bronchial asthma. Adv Prostaglandins Thromboxane Leukotriene Res 1990; 21:465–468.
178. Obata T, Okada Y, Motoishi M, Nakagawa N, Terawaki T, Aishita H. In vitro antagonism of ONO-1078, a newly developed anti-asthma agent, against peptide leukotrienes in isolated guinea pig tissues. Jpn J Pharmacol 1992; 60:227–237.
179. Miyamoto T, Takishima T, Makino S, Shida T, Nakashima M, Hanaoka K. J Clin Therap Med 1993; 9(suppl 1):71–107.
180. Fujimura M, Sakahoto S, Kamis Y, Matsuda T. Effect of a leukotriene antagonist ONO 1978 on bronchial hyperresponsiveness in patients with asthma. Respir Med 1993; 87:133–138.
181. Foster A, Chan CG. Peptide leukotriene involvement in pulmonary eosinophil migration upon antigen challenge in the actively sensitized guinea pig. Int Arch Allergy Appl Immunol 1991; 96:279–284.
182. Jones TR, Zamboni R, Belley M, Champion E, Charette L, Ford-Hutchinson AW, Frantte R, Gauthier J-Y, Leger S, Masson P, MacFarlane CS, Piechuta H, Rokach J, Williams H, Young RN. Pharmacology of L-660,711 (MK-571): a novel potent and selective leukotriene D_4 receptor antagonist. Can J Physiol Pharmacol 1989; 67:17–28.
183. Rasmussen JB, Eriksson L-O, Margolskee DJ, Tagari P, Williams VC, Anderson K-E. Leukotriene D_4 receptor blockade inhibits the immediate and late bronchoconstrictor responses to inhaled antigen in patients with asthma. J Allergy Clin Immunol 1992; 90:193–201.
184. Margolskee D, Bodman S, Dockhorn R, Israel E, Kemp J, Mansmann H, Minotti DA, Spector S, Stricker W, Tinkelman D, Townley RG, Winder J, Williams V. The therapeutic effects of MK-571, a potent and selective leukotriene (LT)D_4 receptor antagonist, in patients with chronic asthma. J Allergy Clin Immunol 1991; 87:309.
185. Kips JC, Joos GF, Lepeleire I, Margolskee DJ, Buntinx A, Pauwels RA, Van der Straeten ME. MK-571, a potent antagonist of leukotriene D_4-induced bronchoconstriction in the human. Am Rev Respir Dis 1991; 144:617–621.
186. Manning PJ, Watson RM, Margolskee DJ, Williams VC, Schwartz JI, O'Byrne PM. Inhibition of exercise-induced bronchoconstriction by MK-571, a potent leukotriene D_4-receptor antagonist. N Engl J Med 1990; 323:1736–1739.
187. Impens N, Reiss TF, Teahan JA, Desmet M, Rossing TH, Shingo S, Zhang J, Schandevyl W, Verbesselt R, Dupont AG. Acute bronchodilation with an intravenously administered leukotriene D_4 antagonist, MK-679. Am Rev Respir Dis 1993; 147:1442–1446.
188. Margolskee D, Friedman B, Williams V, et al. The therapeutic effects of MK-0679, a selective leukotriene D_4 receptor antagonist, in patients with chronic asthma. Eighth International Conference on Prostaglandins and Related Compounds, July 1992:163.
189. Dahlen B, Kumlin M, Margolskee DJ, Larsson C, Blomqvist H, Williams VC, Zetterstrom O, Dahlen SE. The leukotriene-receptor antagonist MK-0679 blocks airway obstruction induced by inhaled lysine–aspirin in aspirin-sensitive asthmatics. Eur Respir J 1993; 6:1018–1026.
190. Iwama T, Nagai H, Koda A. Effects of NZ-107 on airway inflammation and cell activation in guinea-pigs. J Pharm Pharmacol 1993; 45:286–291.
191. Richards IM, Griffin RL, Oostveen JA, Morris J, Wishka DG, Dunn CJ. Effect of the selective leukotriene B_4 antagonist U-75302 on antigen-induced bronchopulmonary eosinophilia in sensitized guinea pigs. Am Rev Respir Dis 1989; 140:1712–1716.
192. Crocker IC, Tanimoto Y, Maruo H, Zhou C-Y, Romero F, Townley RG. Evaluation of a cellular antigen stimulation test (CAST) ELISA system. Asthma: Theory to Treatment 1995:27.
193. Jonsson EWE, Dahlen S-E. Interactions between leukotriene and histamine in the anaphylactic contraction of guinea pig lung parenchyma. J Pharmacol Exp Ther 1994; 271–615–623.
194. Bjorck T, Dahlen S-E. Leukotrienes and histamine mediate IgE-dependent contractions of human bronchi: pharmacological evidence obtained with tissues from asthmatic and non-asthmatic subjects. Pulm Pharmacol 1993; 6:87–96.
195. Diamant Z, Timmers MC, van der Veen H, Friedman BS, De Smet M, Depre M, Hilliard D, Bel

EH, Sterk PJ. The effect of MK-0591, a novel 5-lipoxygenase activating protein inhibitor on leukotriene biosynthesis and allergen-induced airway responses in asthmatic subjects in vivo. J Allergy Clin Immunol 1995; 95:42–51.

196. Storms W, Friedman B, Zhang J, et al. Treating asthma by blocking the lipoxygenase pathway. Am Rev Respir Dis 1995; In press.

197. Ishida K, Thomson RJ, Schellenberg RR. Role of leukotrienes in airway hyperresponsiveness in guinea pigs. Br J Pharmacol 1993; 108:700–704.

198. Friedman BS, Bel EH, Buntinx A, Tanaka W, Han YH, Shingo S, Spector R, Sterk P. Oral leukotriene inhibitor (MK-886) blocks allergen-induced airway responses. Am Rev Respir Dis 1993; 147:839–844.

199. Bel EH, Timmers MC, Hermans J, Dijkman JH, Sterk PJ. The long-term effects of nedocromil sodium and beclomethasone diproprionate on bronchial responsiveness to methocholine in nonatopic asthmatic subjects. Am Rev Respir Dis 1990; 141:21–28.

200. Ancill RJ, Takahashi Y, Kibune Y, Campbell R, Smith JR. Randomized double-blind, placebo-controlled clinical trial of a selective 5-lipoxygenase inhibitor (AA-861) for the prevention of seasonal allergic rhinitis. J Int Med Res 1990; 18:75–88.

201. Carter GW, Young PR, Albert DH, et al. 5-Lipoxygenase inhibitory activity of zileuton. J Pharmacol Exp Ther 1991; 256:929–937.

202. Knapp HR. Reduced allergen-induced nasal symptoms and leukotriene synthesis with an orally active 5-lipoxygenase inhibitor. N Engl J Med 1990; 323:1745–1748.

203. Israel E, Dermarkarian R, Rosenberg M, Sperling R, Taylor G, Rubin P, Drazen JM. The effects of a 5-lipoxygenase inhibitor on asthma induced by cold, dry air. N Engl J Med 1990; 323:1740–1744.

204. Israel E, Fischer AR, Rosenberg MA, Lilly CM, Callery JC, Shapiro J, Cohn J, Rubin P, Drazen JM. The pivotal role of 5-lipoxygenase products in the reaction of aspirin-sensitive asthmatics to aspirin. Am Rev Respir Dis 1993; 148:1447–1451.

205. Collawn C, Rubin P, Perez N, Bobadilla J, Cabrera G, Reyes E, Borovoy J, Kershenobich D. Phase II study of the safety and efficacy of a 5-lipoxygenase inhibitor in patients with ulcerative colitis. Am J Gastroenterol 1992; 87:342–346.

206. Sperling RI, Coblyn JS, Larkin JK, Benincaso AI, Austen KF, Weinblatt ME. Inhibition of leukotriene B_4 synthesis in neutrophils from patients with rheumatoid arthritis by a single oral dose of methotrexate. Arthritis Rheum 1990; 33:1149–1155.

207. Nasser SM, Bell GS, Foster S, Spruce KE, MacMillan R, Williams AJ, Lee TH, Arm JP. Effect of the 5-lipoxygenase inhibitor ZD2138 on aspirin-induced asthma. Thorax 1994; 49:749–756.

208. Hui KP, Taylor GW, Rubin P, Kesterson J, Barnes NC, Barnes PJ. Effect of a 5-lipoxygenase inhibitor on leukotriene generation and airway responsiveness after allergen challenge in asthmatic patients. Thorax 1991; 46:184–189.

209. McMillan RM, Spruce KE, Crawley GC, Walker ERH, Foster SJ. Pre-clinical pharmacology of ICI D2138, a potent orally-active non-redox inhibitor of 5-lipoxygenase. Br J Pharmacol 1992; 107:1042–1047.

210. Dahlen SE, Bjork J, Hedqvist P, Arfors K-E, Hammarstrom S, Lindgren JA, Samuelsson B. Leukotrienes promote plasma leakage and leukocyte adhesion in postcapillary venules: in vivo effects with relevance to the acute inflammatory response. Proc Natl Acad Sci USA 1981; 78:3887–3891.

211. Denzlinger C, Rapp S, Hagmann W, Keppler D. Leukotrienes as mediators in tissue trauma. Science 1985; 230:330–332.

212. Hagmann W, Denzlinger C, Keppler D. Production of peptide leukotrienes in endotoxin shock. FEBS Lett 1985; 180:309–313.

213. Brain SD, Camp RDR, Kobza Black A, Dowd PM, Greaves MW, Ford-Hutchinson AW, Charleson S. Leukotrienes C_4 and D_4 in psoriatic skin lesions. Prostaglandins 1985; 29:611–619.

214. Wenzel SE, Larsen GL, Johnston K, Voekel NF, Westcott JY. Elevated levels of leukotriene C_4 in

bronchoalveolar lavage fluid from atopic asthmatics after endobronchial challenge. Am Rev Respir Dis 1990; 142:112–119.

215. Wenzel SE, Westcott JY, Larsen GL. Bronchoalveolar lavage fluid mediator levels 5 minutes after allergen challenge in atopic subjects with asthma: relationship to the development of late asthmatic responses. J Allergy Clin Immunol 1991; 87:540–548.

216. Liu MC, Bleeker R, Lichtenstein LM, Kagey-Sobotka A, Niv Y, McLemore TL, Permutt S, Proud D, Hubbard WC. Evidence for elevated histamine, prostaglandin D_2 and other bronchoconstricting prostaglandins in the airway of subjects with mild asthma. Am Rev Respir Dis 1990; 142:126–132.

217. Sladek K, Dworski R, Fitzgerald GA, Buitkus KL, Block FJ, Marney SR Jr, Sheller JR. Allergen-stimulated release of thromboxane A_2 and leukotriene E_4 in humans. Effect of indomethacin. Am Rev Respir Dis 1990; 141:1441–1445.

218. Larsen GL. The pulmonary late-phase response. Hosp Prac 1987; 22:155–169.

219. Lee TH, Horton CE, Kyan-Aung U, Haskard D, Crea AE, Spur BW. Lipoxin A_4 and B_4 inhibit chemotactic responses of human neutrophils stimulated by leukotriene B_4 and N-formyl-L-methionyl-L-leucyl-L-phenylalanine. Clin Sci 1989; 77:195–203.

220. Goldyne ME, Burrish GF, Poubelle P, Borgeat P. Arachidonic acid metabolism among human mononuclear leukocytes: lipoxygenase-related pathways. J Biol Chem 1984; 259:8815–8819.

221. Williams JD, Czop JK, Austen KF. Release of leukotrienes by human monocytes on stimulation of the phagocytic receptor for particulate activators. J Immunol 1984; 132:3034–3040.

222. Freeland HS, Schleimer RP, Schulman ES, Lichtenstein LM, Peters SP. Generation of leukotriene B_4 by lung fragments and purified human lung mast cells. Am Rev Respir Dis 1988; 138:389–394.

223. Warner JA, Peters SP, Lichtenstein LM, Hubbard W, Yancey KB, Stevenson HC, Miller PJ, MacGlashan JDW. Differential release of mediators from human basophils: differences in arachidonic acid metabolism following activation by unrelated stimuli. J Leukoc Biol 1989; 45:558–571.

224. Edenius C, Heidvall K, Lindgren JA. Novel transcellular interaction: conversion of granulocyte-derived LTA_4 into cysteinyl-containing leukotrienes by human platelets. Eur J Biochem 1988; 178:81–86.

225. Stenke L, Reizenstein P, Lindgren JA. Leukotrienes and lipoxins—new potential performers in the regulation of human myelopoiesis. Leukot Res 1994; 18:727–732.

226. Evans JM, Barnes NC, Zakrzewski JT, Sciberras DG, Stahl EG, Piper PJ, Costello JF. L-648,051, a novel cysteinyl-leukotriene antagonist is active by the inhaled route in man. Br J Clin Pharmacol 1989; 28:125–135.

227. Krell RD, Aharony D, Buckner CK, et al. The preclinical pharmacology of ICI 204,219. A peptide leukotriene antagonist. Am Rev Respir Dis 1990; 141:978–987.

228. Gaddy JN, Margolskee DJ, Bush RK, Williams VC, Busse WW. Bronchodilation with a potent and selective leukotriene D_4 (LTD_4) receptor antagonist (MK-571) in patients with asthma. Am Rev Respir Dis 1992; 146:358–363.

229. Dahlen B, Kumlin M, Margolskee DJ, Larsson C, Blomqvist H, Williams VC, Zetterstrom O, Dahlen SE. Leukotriene receptor antagonist MK-0679 blocks airway obstruction induced by inhaled lysin-aspirin in aspirin-sensitive asthmatics. Eur Respir J 1993; 6:1018–1026.

230. Bando T, Fujimura M, Shintani H, Saito M, Kurashima K, Nishi K, Matsuda T. Inhibitory effect of aerosol administration of a sulfidopeptide leukotriene antagonist on bronchoconstriction induced by antigen inhalation in guinea pigs. Arzneimittelforschung 1994; 44:754–757.

231. Saito M, Fujimura M, Ogawa H, Matsuda T. Role of leukotrienes and platelet activating factor in allergic bronchoconstriction and their interactions in guinea pig airways in vivo. Prostaglandins Leukot Essent Fatty Acids 1993; 49:579–585.

232. Aibara S, Mori M, Tsukada W. Inhibitory effect of DS-4574 on leukotriene- or antigen-induced bronchoconstriction in guinea pigs. Int Arch Allergy Immunol 1993; 100:268–273.

233. Tabuchi Y, Kurebayashi Y. Effect of DS-4574, a novel peptidoleukotriene antagonist with mast

cell stabilizing action, on acute gastric lesions and gastric secretion in rats. Jpn J Pharmacol 1992; 60:335–340.

234. Prasit P, Belley M, Blouin M, et al. A new class of leukotriene biosynthesis inhibitor: the development of MK-0591. J Lipid Mediat 1993; 6:239–244.

235. Brideau C, Chan C, Charleson S, et al. Pharmacology of MK 0591, a potent orally active leukotriene biosynthesis inhibitor. Can J Physiol Pharmacol 1994. In press.

236. Fujimura M, Sasaki F, Nakatsumi Y, Takakashi M, Hifumi S, Taga K, Mifune J, Tanaka T, Matsuda T. Effects of a thromboxane synthetase inhibitor (OKY-046) and a lipoxygenase inhibitor (AA 861) on bronchial responsiveness to acetylcholine in asthmatic subjects. Thorax 1986; 41:955–959.

237. Israel E, Rubin P, Kemp JP, et al. The effect of inhibition of 5-lipoxygenase by zileuton in mild-to-moderate asthma. Ann Intern Med 1993; 119:1059–1066.

238. Abraham WM, Ahmed A, Cortes A, Sielczak MW, Hinz W, Bouska J, Lanni C, Bell RL. The 5-lipoxygenase inhibitor zileuton blocks antigen-induced late airway responses, inflammation and airway hyperresponsiveness in allergic sheep. Eur J Pharmacol 1992; 217:119–126.

239. Mann JS, Robinson C, Sheridan AQ, Clement P, Bach MK, Holgate ST. Effect of inhaled piriprost (U60,257) a novel leukotriene inhibitor, on allergen and exercise induced bronchoconstriction in asthma. Thorax 1986; 41:746–752.

240. Asano M, Inamura N, Nakahara K, Nagayoshi T, Isono T, Hamada K, Oku T, Notau Y, Kohsaka M, Ono T. A 5-lipoxygenase inhibitor FR110302, suppresses hyperresponsiveness and lung eosinophilia induced by Sephadex particles in rats. Agents Actions 1992; 36:215–221.

241. Wegner CD, Gundel RH, Abraham WM, et al. The role of 5-lipoxygenase products in preclinical models of asthma. J Allergy Clin Immunol 1993; 91:917–929.

242. Howarth PH, Harrison K, Lau L, Dube L, Cohn J. The influence of the 5-lipoxygenase inhibitor A-78773 on the nasal response to allergen in rhinitis. J Allergy Clin Immunol 1994; 93:297.

20

Platelet-Activating Factor and Its Antagonists in Allergic and Inflammatory Disorders

Matyas Koltai and David Hosford
Institut Henri Beaufour, Le Plessis Robinson, France

Pierre G. Braquet
Bio-Inova, Plaisir, France

INTRODUCTION

Platelet-activating factor (PAF), identified as 1-*O*-alkyl-2-acetyl-*sn*-glyceryl-3-phosphoryl-choline [1] (1), a potent phospholipid autacoid, is rapidly generated by an acyltransferase

$$\begin{array}{c} H_2C-O-(CH_2)_n-CH_3 \\ | \\ \overset{O}{\underset{\|}{}} \\ CH_3-C-O-CH \\ | \quad\quad O \\ CH_2-O-\overset{\|}{P}-O-CH_2-CH_2-\overset{+}{N}(CH_3)_3 \\ | \\ {}_-O \end{array}$$

[1]   PAF: n = 15 or 17

from its inactive precursor lyso-PAF and released from the cells. A considerable part, however, remains cell-associated, indicating that this phospholipid induces fundamental intracellular changes (2). As reviewed recently, PAF has been implicated as mediator in inflammation, ischemic disorders, and shock conditions, such as traumatic shock and gram-negative septic shock (3,4). Furthermore, it is produced by a great variety of cells, including endothelial cells, polymorphonuclear leukocytes, platelets, monocytes, basophils, eosino-phils, mast cells, and lymphocytes (5–7).

Transduction of important signals brought about by endogenous mediators and agonists from cell membrane receptors to the activation site has a pivotal role in cellular function. Several of these pathways, for example, signal transduction through inositol phosphates and cAMP, have now been well defined (8). Phosphoinositides play an important role in the release of intracellular calcium $[Ca^{2+}]_i$, which appears to be involved in a great variety of cellular responses (9). Early studies clearly showed that PAF affects cellular phospho-inositide metabolism in platelets of various species. This effect has been characterized as an early rapid and transient decrease in phosphatidylinositol 4,5-biphosphate in washed rabbit platelets labeled with [³H]inositol when stimulated with low concentrations of PAF (10). Lyso-PAF has no such an effect, and the response, which is clearly observed within 5 s after addition of PAF, is concentration-dependent. Interestingly, within 15 s an increase in [³H]lysophosphatidylinositol was also seen, pointing to a close relationship between PAF release and changes of phosphoinositide metabolism. The stimulation by PAF of phospho-inositide metabolism was first suggested to be linked to the mobilization of membrane-bound $[Ca^{2+}]_i$ horse platelets (11). Alternatively, trifluoperazine and N-(6-aminohexyl)-5-chloro-l-naphthalene sulfonamide, two calmodulin antagonists, inhibited PAF biosynthesis in neutrophil leukocytes stimulated by the Ca^{2+} ionophore A23187 (12). Later on, when the fluorescent probe fura-2 became available and frequently used, PAF-induced release of $[Ca^{2+}]_i$ was confirmed by exact measurements in U937 human monocytic cell line. This response was antagonized by various specific PAF receptor antagonists, again emphasizing the role of PAF in $[Ca^{2+}]_i$ signaling (13). This signal transduction involves activation of GTPase (14,15), it is linked to G-protein–coupled receptors (16–19), and directly affects membrane ion pumps (20). There is also convincing evidence that through activation of phospholipase A_2 (PLA_2), PAF releases arachidonic acid (AA), resulting in eicosanoid formation both on the cyclooxygenase and lipoxygenase pathways (2,5).

The present chapter is designed first to overview the most important PAF receptor antagonists that have been developed, then to summarize functional changes induced by PAF in pathophysiological conditions, such as immediate-type hypersensitivity, in particular bronchial asthma, and acute or chronic inflammatory responses of allergic or nonallergic origin in various tissues. Finally, the effect of PAF receptor antagonists under these conditions is also reviewed.

SPECIFIC PAF RECEPTOR ANTAGONISTS

The PAF antagonists selectively bind PAF receptors, and since these drugs possess an affinity for these binding sites greater than that of PAF, they concentration-dependently inhibit the effect of the lipid mediator. There is an indication that molecular changes of PAF receptors exist in various tissue; therefore, some PAF receptor antagonists may exhibit tissue specificity.

The chemical structures of the most important PAF receptor antagonists reviewed in this chapter are shown by bold numbers in brackets. Fundamentally, two groups of PAF antagonists may be distinguished: synthetic and natural compounds. Synthetic and natural PAF antagonists have a great variability in their chemical structure that might have importance in their different pharmacological profile. Most of these drugs are under development; however, several have recently undergone clinical trials.

Natural Compounds

The most widely examined natural PAF antagonists are the ginkgolides [2] (21–24), in particular, ginkgolide B (BN 52021), which exhibits the highest potency among these agents. The first total synthesis of ginkgolides was performed by Corey and Gavai (25) and Corey et al. (26) and has been considered to be a great success for a computed synthetic process, since these compounds have a complicated secondary structure. Kadsurenone [3],

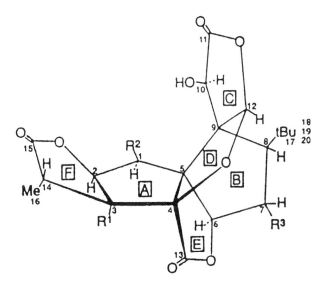

Ginkgolide	Nomenclature	R¹	R²	R³
A	BN 52020	OH	H	H
B	BN 52021	OH	OH	H
C	BN 52022	OH	OH	OH
J	BN 52024	OH	H	OH
M	BN 52023	H	OH	OH
synthetic	BN 50580	OH	OMe	H
synthetic	BN 50585	OH	OEt	H

[2]   Ginkgolides

[3]   Kadsurenone

a benzofuranoid neolignan, isolated from *Piper futokadsurae* by the Merck group (27) was the first natural PAF receptor antagonist and has greatly facilitated the molecular modeling of the PAF receptor and has led to the development of potent synthetic PAF antagonists.

Two moderately active marine natural products, chantancin and phomactin A, have been processed by Sankyo (28,29). Swietemohonin A, a tetranortriterpenoid, is a very weak PAF antagonist (30). Futoxide and prehispanolone are derived from Chinese medicinal herbs, whereas LC 5504, a compound that is more stable and active than the natural drug, is obtained by hydrogenating the dihydrofuran ring and replacing the keto group of prehispanolone with a hydroxyl group (31). Tetrahydrocannabinol-7-oic acid, the major cannabis metabolite, has also reduced PAF-induced paw edema and lethality in mice (32). More recently, it has been reported that aglafoline from *Aglaia elliptifolia* Merr. exhibits PAF antagonist effect (33).

Synthetic Derivatives Derived from Natural Compounds

Fujisawa has developed a series of diketopiperazine compounds of microbial origin (e.g., FR 76600) that inhibit PAF-induced hypotension (34). From this series, FR 900,452 has been isolated from the culture broth of *Streptomyces phaeofaciens* (35). PCA 4248 belongs to the PAF antagonists have a dihydropyridine framework. This compound inhibits plasma extravasation induced by immunoglobulin G (IgG) aggregates and endotoxin (36). Sch 37370 is a dual antihistamine and PAF antagonist (37) that attenuates PAF- and histamine-induced bronchoconstriction in the guinea pig. The metabolite of the compound exhibits only antihistaminic but not PAF antagonist property.

Synthetic Compounds

In the last couple of years, a great variety of synthetic compounds with specific PAF receptor antagonist effects have been developed. Most of them have been extensively studied in animal experiments, whereas relatively few have been evaluated in clinical trials.

Quaternary Nitrogen PAF Antagonists

These compounds have structural resemblance to PAF. The earliest drugs in this group, synthesized by Takeda, were CV-3988 [4] and CV-6209 [5] that show clear structural

$$CH_2OCONHC_{18}H_{37}$$

$$MeOCH$$

$$CH_2OPO(CH_2)_2 - N$$

[4]   CV-3988

analogy to PAF (38,39). More recent compounds in this group, SRI 63-072 [6] and SRI 63-441, developed by Sandoz, with a *cis*-2,5-substituted tetrahydrofuran framework, exhibit less similarity to PAF, but they still have quaternary nitrogen in their structure (40). Uriach has evaluated 2-alkoxytetrahydrofuran PAF antagonists, such as UR-10324 and UR-11353, that inhibit PLA_2 and also PLC activity (41). Furthermore, E-5880 [7] elabo-

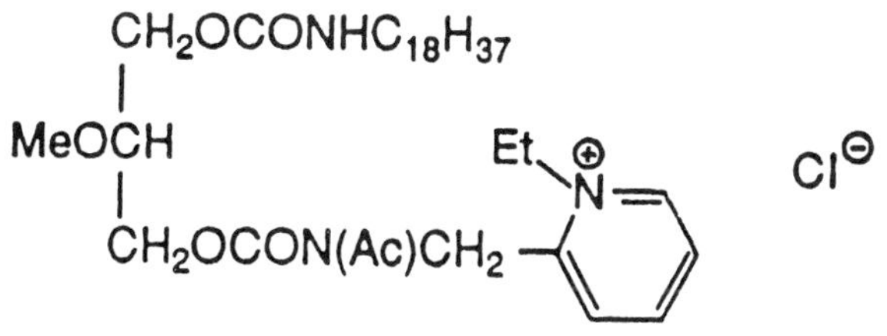

$$CH_2OCONHC_{18}H_{37}$$
$$|$$
$$MeOCH$$
$$|$$
$$CH_2OCON(Ac)CH_2$$

[5]   CV-6209

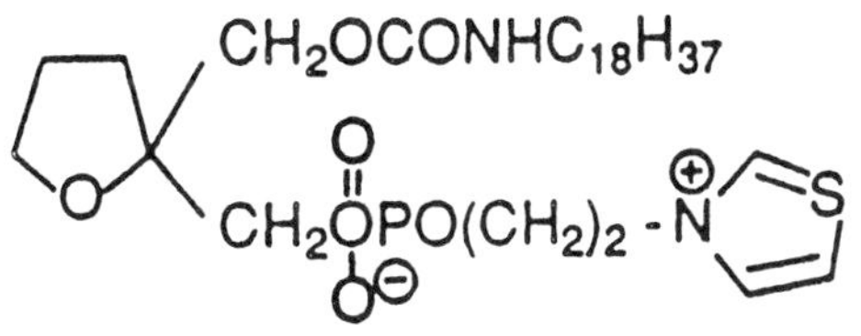

$$CH_2OCONHC_{18}H_{37}$$

$$CH_2OPO(CH_2)_2$$

[6]   SRI 63-072

OCH₃
CO
OCH₃
NHC₁₈H₃₇
Cl⁻ C₂H₅

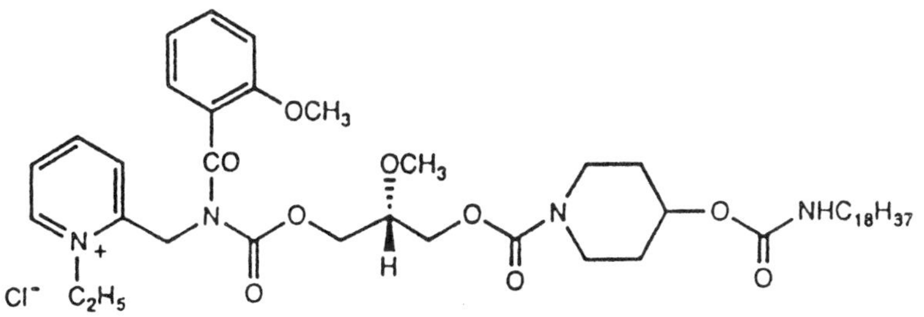

[7]   E-5880

rated by Eisai, is the lead compound in a series of potent quaternary nitrogen PAF antagonists that have a 4-substituted piperidinocarbamate moiety between the glycerol spacer and the lipophilic group (42). American Cyanamid patented quaternary nitrogen compounds that also feature alkoxyaryl lipophilic moiety, such as CL 184,005 [8], that have been claimed to prevent endotoxin-induced lethality in mice when combined with a Celltech murine tumor necrosis factor-α (TNF-α) monoclonal antibody. Recently, the synthesis of a series of aryl phosphoglyceride or bisaryl phosphate (43) and bisaryl amide or bisaryl urea compounds (44) have been reported. TCV-309 [9] with a 50% effective dose peroral (ED$_{50}$) value of 1 mg/kg, that provides 69% inhibition of PAF-induced hypotension in the rat for longer than 8 h, belongs to this group (45,46). In contrast to CV-3988 and CV-6209, TCV-309 does not induce hemolysis in whole blood because of its lack of detergent-like action (38).

[8]   CL 184005

[9]   TCV-309

Heterocyclic sp² Nitrogen PAF Antagonists

In this class of compounds a heterocyclic sp² nitrogen atom, which is able to interact with the receptor as a hydrogen bond acceptor, is a crucial requirement for the PAF antagonist activity. Other structural features in this group are a sulfur atom and a carbonyl moiety that carry specific, potent ability to bind the receptors. Among others, this pyridyl carboxamide group is represented by Ro-74,719, introduced by Hoffmann-La Roche, that inhibits PAF binding at a concentration of 900 nM (47).

Hetrazepine Derivatives Boehringer-Ingelheim discovered the first hetrazepine-type PAF receptor antagonist, WEB 2086 [10] (apafant), the development of which was followed by the synthesis of WEB 2170 [11] (bepafant) and WEB 2347 (48,49). All these drugs exhibit potent in vitro effect and excellent peroral bioavailability, with a long-lasting pharmacological effect. WEB 2170 inhibits active anaphylaxis in guinea pigs or mice when given perorally at doses of 0.04 and 3 mg/kg or 1 and 10 mg/kg, along with low doses of mepyramine to minimize the effect of anaphylactic histamine release (50,51). Systemic administration of WEB 2086 is highly effective in horses and has been proposed for veterinary use (52). Novel compounds in this series exemplified by WEB 2315 exhibit receptor binding properties at subnanomolar concentrations.

From the hetrazepine group, Yoshitomi has chosen to develop Y-24180, which possesses a 6-methyl group and a lipophilic 4-isobutylphenylethyl thiopentene substituent (53,54), whereas Eisai has synthesized a molecule named E-6123 in which the tetrahydropyridyl ring is modified. E-6123 shows a potent PAF receptor antagonistic property (55,56).

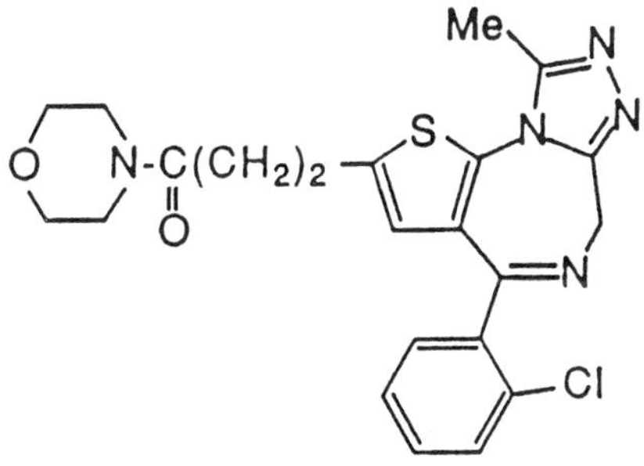

[10]   WEB 2086, apafant

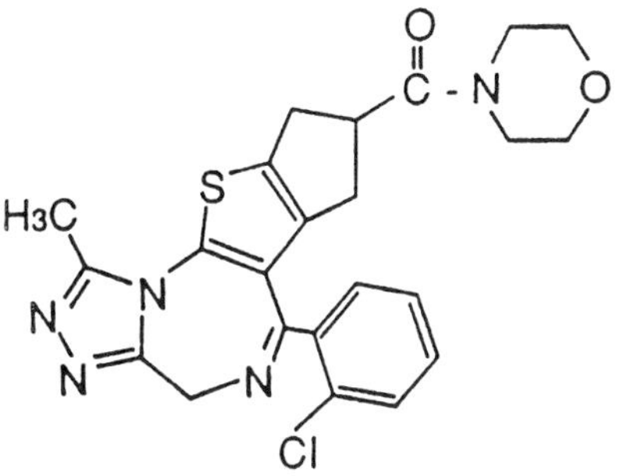

[11]   WEB 2170, bepafant

Interestingly, the PAF antagonistic properties of these compounds are related to the *S*-enantiomers, showing 40 times higher activity than the *R*-enantiomer (51).

The IPSEN-Beaufour group has developed a new series of compounds with hetrazepine framework: BN 50726, BN 50727, BN 50730, and BN 40739 [12] (57–59). These com-

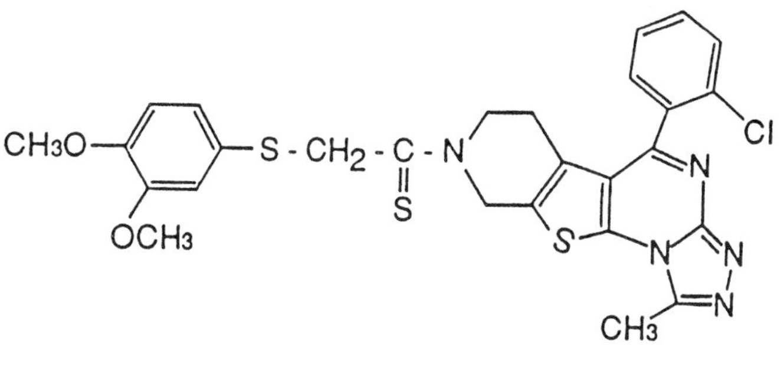

[12]   BN 50739

pounds have undergone pharmacological trials, and exert high potency after parenteral administration, and their effect lasts longer than 8 h after a single injection. BN 50739 is particularly effective in endotoxic and traumatic shock (63). Furthermore, it protects against stroke in animal models (64), whereas BN 50730 exhibits potency against PAF- and antigen-induced bronchoconstriction (65). Hoffmann-La Roche has synthesized Ro-24-4736, which has been selected for clinical trials in asthma and septic shock (66).

3-Pyridyl Derivatives   Several PAF receptor antagonists have a 3-pyridyl group as heterocyclic nitrogen constituent. The lead compound from Hoffmann-La Roche is Ro 24-0238 [13], which exhibits moderate potency (47). Replacement of the 3-pyridyl group

[13]   Ro 24-0238

with a 2-pyridyl or 4-pyridyl group greatly reduces activity, supporting the concept that the sp^2 nitrogen is an acceptor of a hydrogen bond from the receptor.

Rhône-Poulenc Rorer has also developed compounds with this framework. The original lead compound RP 48740 has low potency; however, its substitution resulted in RP 59227 [14] (tulopafant) and RP 66681 [15], showing high potency in vitro and good peroral

[14]   RP 59227, tulopafant

activity in vivo (67–69). RP 59227, being a competitive inhibitor, exhibits different affinities for macrophage membrane PAF receptors when compared with WEB 2986, which has been classified as a noncompetitive inhibitor (70). Several analogues of these compounds have been prepared by Yamanouchi, and YM 264 is effective at a peroral dose of 0.19 mg/kg against PAF-induced death in mice (71) and puromycin-induced nephropathy in rats (72). Another compound of this series, with a highly selective PAF antagonist effect, YM 461 (73) prevents PAF-induced death in mice with a peroral ED$_{50}$ of 0.35 mg/kg and dose-dependently inhibits PAF-induced hypotension in rats, with an IV ED$_{50}$ of 0.3 mg/kg, and a peroral dose of 3 mg/kg protects conscious guinea pigs against antigen-induced anaphylactic challenge for more than 6 h. Abbott has identified a class of *N*-substituted

[15]   RP 66681

tetrahydrobenzopyrano(3,4-c)pyridine PAF antagonists that exhibit K_i values ranging between 131 and 167 nM in a [^{3}H]PAF-binding assay (74).

Sumitomo has synthesized a *cis*-diastereomer compound named SM-10661 that is more
active than the *trans*-diastereomer (75). When the methyl group in the *trans*-diastereomer is
replaced by a longer substituent, the compound acquires higher potency. Accordingly, the
2R,5S-(+)-enantiomer of SM-10661 is 150 times more active than the 2S,5R-(4−)-
enantiomer (76). Several analogues have also been identified, among them a compound that
is orally active (77) and protective against airway hypersensitivity in passively sensitized
guinea pigs, against leukocyte infiltration in actively sensitized animals, as well as against
experimental disseminated intravascular coagulation (78). Sanofi developed SR 27417 [16],

[16]   SR 27417

a highly potent, orally active compound of this series (79). SR 27417 inhibits lethal
anaphylactic and endotoxic shock, with peroral ED_{50} values of 1.25 mg/kg and 0.15 mg/kg,
respectively (80). Studies on the effect of SR 27417 on ex vivo rabbit platelet aggregation
yielded ED_{50} values of 80, 35, 50, and 1250 μg/kg at 1, 3, 24, and 72 h after peroral
administration, and [^{3}H]PAF binding to washed platelets revealed a competitive-type
inhibition.

Imidazolyl Derivatives   The imidazo[4,5-c]pyridyl moiety is a particularly favored
heterocycle, substituted either at position-1 or position-5. A series of compounds of this

type have been patented by Searle, whereas Pfizer has developed PAF antagonists with a dihydropyridine framework. UK-74,505 [17] (modipafant) inhibits PAF-induced lethality

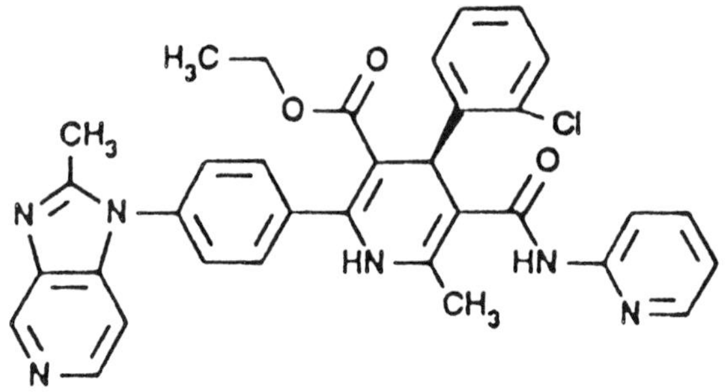

[17]   UK-74,505, modipafant

in mice, with a peroral ED_{50} of 110 μg/kg, and ex vivo platelet aggregation in dog with 75 μg/kg for 8 h after administration (81). For this compound, the group used for substitution at position-2 of the imidazo[4,5-c]pyridyl is similar to that substituted at position-9 of the hetrazepine series of PAF antagonists (82). Pfizer has also disclosed compounds in which the dihydropyridine structure is replaced by a benzodiazepine, benzazepine, or a wide variety of other lipophilic moieties, and explores the relationship between their series of compounds and hetrazipines. Starting from UK-74,505, British Biotechnology has performed molecular modeling and found that the methyl group is the optimal substituent at position-2 of the benzimidazole heterocycle, as was previously shown in UK-74,505 and at position-9 in WEB-2086 (83). This program has resulted in BB-182, an early lead benzimidazole derivative, and modification of the lipophilic group in BB-823 [18] considerably

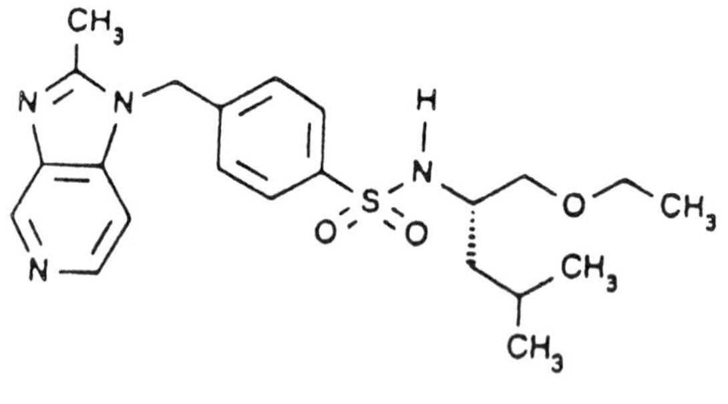

[18]   BB-823

enhanced activity. BB-823 inhibits PAF- and endotoxin-induced hypotension in the rat with an IV ED_{50} of 0.7 and 5.5 mg/kg, respectively, and offers maximal inhibition of ex vivo PAF-induced [³H]serotonin release from rabbit platelets. BB-654, a 2-methylimidazo-[4,5-c]pyridine heterocycle, with an aryl 3-pyridyl lipophilic moiety, inhibits PAF-induced hypotension in rats, with an IV ED_{50} of μg/kg.

    SDZ 64-412 [19] and SDZ 65-123 [20], developed by Sandoz, inhibit PAF-induced bronchoconstriction at a peroral ED_{50} of 1 mg/kg (40). Schering and Wellcome have

[19]   SDZ 64-412

[20]   SDZ 65-123

patented similar imidazolyl derivatives that also possess antiviral activity and are orally active in the rat adjuvant arthritis model. The imidazo[1,2-*b*]pyridazine heterocycle has been synthesized by Takeda in a series of perorally active PAF antagonists.

Diaryl PAF Antagonists: Tetrahydrofuran Derivatives   Merck has identified L-652,731 as a key lead compound, with a tetrahydrofuran spacer, being one of many moderately active lignan PAF antagonists that are rapidly metabolized in the organism (84). On the basis of electrostatic potential maps, L-652,731 was used to develop the "ear muff" and multipolarized cyclinder models for the PAF receptors (85,86). Differential substitution of aryl groups yielded a compound L-659,898 [21] with enhanced in vitro potency and an im-

[21]   L-659,898

proved in vivo profile (87). The *trans*-diastereomers of both compounds possess considerably greater potency for the PAF receptors than the *cis*-diastereomers. Of the two enantiomers of L-659,898, the $S,5S$-(−)-enantiomer is the most potent in vitro (88). Further identification of L-659,898 led to the synthesis of MK 287, showing improved metabolic stability and pharmacokinetics. Surprisingly, MK 287 exhibits gender-dependent oral activity being less potent in male animals than in females. Therefore, Merck conducted further research that has resulted in the synthesis of L-671,284 [22], which is devoid of

[22]   L-671,284

gender-dependent peroral activity (89). Further research in Merck has elaborated a racemic sulfonated 2,5-diaryltetrahydrofuran, L-668,750, a potent, specific, orally active PAF receptor antagonist, the negative enantiomer, of which L-680,573, a −-*trans*-(2S,5S)-2-[3-(2-oxopropyl)sulfonyl]-4-*n*-propoxy-[5-(3-hydroxy-propoxy) phenyl]-5-tri-(3,4,5-methoxy-phenyl)tetrahydrofuran is more effective than the positive enantiomer L-680,574 (90). The two compounds could successfully be separated in rat plasma using a chiral a 1-acid glycoprotein high-performance liquid chromatography (HPLC) (91). L-680,573 is one of the most potent PAF receptor antagonists, with ED_{50} values of 60 μg/kg orally, or 4μg/kg IV, respectively, as measured in PAF-induced plasma extravasation and elevated *N*-acetyl-β-D-glucoronamidase levels in male rats (90). Several water-soluble prodrugs and metabolites that are equally potent PAF antagonists, when applied through a duodenal catheter, have also been described. A series of 4-substituted 2-alkoxytetrahydrofuran derivatives featuring an acetal group has high activity and long-lasting action (92). The lead compound of UR-11353 protects against PAF-induced death and hypotension at a dose of 1 μg/kg as long as 10 h after IV administration. The chemical and biochemical characterization of lignan analogues has been reviewed (84).

Tetrahydronaphthalene Derivative   The in vitro and in vivo PAF antagonist effects of CIS-19, a *cis*-2-(3,4-dimethoxyphenyl)-6-isopropoxy-7-methoxyl-1-(*N*-methylform-amido)-1,2,3,4-tetrahydronaphthalene), was recently described (93). CIS-19, in a selective and concentration-dependent manner, inhibited the aggregation and ATP release reaction of rabbit platelets induced by PAF. The concentration−effect curves of PAF-induced aggregation were shifted to the right with pA_2 and pA_{10} values of 7.1 and 6.1, respectively. CIS-19 does not influence thromboxane (TX)B_2 formation induced by AA, collagen, or thrombin of washed platelets below a concentration of 4000 nM; however, it completely blocks PAF-induced, but not collagen- or thrombin-induced [³H]IP$_1$ formation of washed platelets at a concentration of 250 nM. When injected IV, doses of 2.5 and 5 mg/kg. CIS-19 do not change blood pressure; however, they inhibit PAF-induced, but not AA-induced, hypotensive shock either preventively or curatively. These doses also inhibit PAF- but not AA-induced bronchoconstriction in guinea pigs.

Piperazinyl Derivatives   IPSEN-Beaufour developed a series of piperazinyl derivatives in which the most effective compound carries substituent at position-2 (86). One of these compounds consists of a propylphenyl group and exhibits potent in vitro activity. Takeda has patented related compounds in which one of the aryl groups is fused with a cyclopentano ring. Among these, one compound inhibits PAF-induced hypotension at a peroral dose of 3 μg/kg for 4 h after dosing. A Sankyo compound has an IV antihypotensive ED_{50} of 6.7 μg/kg. A series of (pyridylcyanomethyl)piperazines has recently been prepared and evaluated for PAF antagonist activity (92). Activity was found mainly in four skeletons: 1-acyl-4-(3-pyridylcyanomethyl)piperazine, 1-acyl-4-(4-pyridylcyanomethyl)piperazine, 1-acyl-4-(3-pyridylcyanomethyl)piperidine, and 1-acyl-4-cyano-4-(3-pyridylamino)-piperazine. The acyl substituents, diphenylacetyl and 3,3-diphenylpropionyl, provided the most active compounds, and the introduction of an amine or hydroxy group in the 3,3-diphenylpropionyl substituent, developed by Uriach, further improved peroral activity.

THE EFFECT OF PAF AND ITS ANTAGONISTS IN ALLERGIC DISEASES

PAF and Airway Hyperresponsiveness

Platelet-activating factor induces bronchoconstriction, an effect that can be selectively blocked by PAF receptor antagonists. This has been confirmed by BN 50730, a new hetrazepine PAF antagonists in the cat (65). Inhaled lyso-PAF increased airway microvascular leakage in the guinea pig, presumably after conversion to active PAF, since WEB 2086 prevented the response (94). PAF has also induced bronchoconstriction in asthmatic human volunteers (95,96), which was inhibited by WEB 2086 (97). Increased plasma PAF levels were detected in children with acute asthmatic attacks, and after immunotherapy, decreased in vivo and in vitro PAF production was detectable, suggesting the involvement of PAF in the pathogenesis of bronchial asthma (98).

The interaction of PAF with bronchial smooth muscle and the attenuation by specific PAF receptor antagonists of allergic bronchoconstriction have raised the concept that PAF may be involved in the pathomechanism of allergic airway hyperresponsiveness; consequently, PAF receptor antagonists may be useful in the treatment of human asthma. This concept is supported by the close relation between airway hyperresponsiveness and platelet activation (99,100) as well as eosinophil accumulation (95,101). Eosinophil activation and function are modulated by the cytokines granulocyte–macrophage colony-stimulating factor (GM-CSF), interleukin (IL)-3, and IL-5. Eosinophils derived from asthmatic patients exhibited a primed phenotype, as deduced from enhanced responses toward formyl-methionyl-leucyl-phenylalanine (FMLP) and PAF (102). Allergic challenge in asthmatic patients increased the effect of these stimulants. Indeed, eosinophils isolated 3 h after antigen challenge exhibited a more pronounced primed phenotype, which was reflected by an induction of responsiveness toward IL-8. Eosinophil responses induced by PAF, FMLP, complement fragment C5a, IL-3, IL-5, and GM-CSF were significantly altered after antigen challenge. These data have provided evidence that eosinophils are already primed in the peripheral blood of individuals with allergic asthma, most likely owing to the presence of circulating lymphokines. This in vivo priming results in selective up-regulation and down-regulation of responses toward various chemotaxins, which may be released in the lung during allergic inflammation.

Reactivity of Anaphylactic Bronchoconstriction to PAF Receptor Antagonists

BN 52021 and other PAF antagonists are effective inhibitors of anaphylactic bronchoconstriction in guinea pigs sensitized by homologous (103) or heterologous antiovalbumin (OA) serum (104). The potency of BN 52021 was lower in actively sensitized than in passively sensitized animals. Combined treatment with SDZ 264-412 or WEB 2086 with an H_1-receptor antagonist in a guinea pig model of IgE-induced airway hypersensitivity triggered by aerosol allergen (105), or in IgE-induced systemic anaphylaxis in the rabbit (106), respectively, is even more potent.

Booster Injection and Sensitivity of Allergic Bronchoconstriction to PAF Antagonists

In a model of anaphylactic bronchoconstriction evoked by intratracheal administration of OA after booster injections, regardless of the interval between repeated OA applications, the efficacy of BN 52021 to block anaphylactic bronchoconstriction is completely abolished (107). Furthermore, the PAF antagonist became ineffective not only against the antigen-induced smooth-muscle contraction, but also in blocking TXB_2 release. It was suggested previously that WEB 2086, which has a framework unrelated to that of BN 52021, also lost its effect against anaphylactic bronchoconstriction in guinea pigs actively sensitized and then boosted (108), whereas WEB 2086 was effective when used up to 4 days after booster injection (109). These observations indicate that repeated intake of allergen modifies airway responsiveness within a few days.

Pretolani et al. (110) have recently described that human recombinant IL-5 (rhIL-5) increased bronchoconstriction and TXA_2 release when applied intra-arterially subsequent to PAF administration in perfused lungs isolated from actively sensitized guinea pigs. This synergistic effect was also seen after booster application, but was not present in lungs derived from passively sensitized animals. Apparently, an active immune response is required for priming the effect of PAF by rhIL-5. Since the recruitment of eosinophils into the airways and the development of hyperresponsiveness to PAF are concomitant, eosinophils are suggested as target cells for interaction between rhIL-5 and PAF.

In a recent paper by Rabinovici et al. (111), IL-2 induced acute lung injury, characterized by elevated water content, myeloperoxidase activity, and serum TXB_2 in the rat, which was attenuated by BN 50739, suggesting the involvement of PAF in lung inflammation. Ongoing studies are exploring the chronic inflammatory changes in the lung under hypersensitivity states and after chronic PAF administration: infusion of PAF by Alzet osmotic mini-pump induces morphological changes in the lung (112). In clinical patients with bronchial asthma, the relation between heightened locomotor reactions and mediator release from activated inflammatory cells to the bronchoalveolar lumen has been explored (113).

Booster Injection and Sensitivity of Allergic Inflammation to PAF Antagonists

Another important aspect of altered tissue sensitivity to PAF antagonists during active immunization has been recognized in studies of local inflammatory response induced by allergen injection in mice actively sensitized 21 days earlier (114). The interference of WEB 2170 with OA-induced paw edema is markedly changed in boosted or unboosted sensitized mice. The intensity of the inflammatory edema induced by OA or PAF was the same in either group; however, IP treatment with WEB 2170 1 h before challenge dose-dependently reduced the edema in boosted mice, but did not modify the response in unboosted ones.

WEB 2170 was more effective against PAF-induced paw edema in boosted than in un-boosted mice. Furthermore, topical and selective desensitization to PAF inhibited the edema evoked by antigen only in boosted animals. Therefore, it appears likely that, in contrast with anaphylactic bronchoconstriction in guinea pigs, the booster injection during immunization process shifts the anaphylactic paw edema from a PAF-independent to a PAF-dependent reaction.

The negative results with PAF antagonists in antigen-induced bronchoconstriction of the guinea pig after booster injection and the ineffectiveness of UK-74,505 on early and late asthmatic responses induced by repeated administration of the specific allergen in humans suggest that administration of PAF receptor antagonists in this disease has no beneficial effect. Further research on the mechanism of allergic response caused by continuous exposure to allergen in clinical patients or in guinea pigs after booster injections may shed more light on the presently obscure role of PAF in allergic bronchoconstriction and inflammation. Alterations in the allergic inflammatory response in boosted mice (114) point to the possible significance of inflammatory cell recruitment developing during immediate hypersensitivity, the mechanism of which remains to be elucidated.

Recent immunopathological studies have revealed that isolated lungs from guinea pigs actively sensitized by ovalbumin and booster 2 weeks thereafter display an enhanced bronchoconstriction and release a larger amount of secondary mediators compared with lungs from nonimmunized animals when stimulated by PAF or other agonists (115). Seven days after booster administration lungs were resected and frozen, and cryostat sections were stained by monoclonal antibodies that recognize T cells, T-cell subsets, or other relevant epitopes. Cyanide-resistant peroxidase activity was used to identify eosinophils. A large number of T cells, mainly of the CD4$^+$ subset, and eosinophils were recruited into the bronchi, compared with nonimmunized or nonboosted animals. In antigen-challenged animals, the number of T cells did not change, but the number of eosinophils was further increased at the 24-h time point. Also at this time point, a population of cells with a dendritic appearance was seen in the bronchial wall that did not express macrophage markers, but was strongly class II-positive. Class II positivity was also noted in the bronchial epithelium and on many cells infiltrating the mucosa. These findings suggest that activated T cells or their products may play an important role in the immunopathology associated with the development of bronchial hyperreactivity. These alterations between healthy, actively sensitized, and boosted animals may, at least partly, be responsible for the loss of bronchodilator effect of PAF antagonists after booster application (116).

From these results the following conclusions can be drawn: (1) conventionally used animal models are insufficient to provide relevant results on whether an effective antagonist of PAF will be useful in clinical trials; (2) all PAF antagonists selected for development as a potential treatment of bronchial asthma should be reexamined using the protocol of boosterization; (3) finally, new trends in searching for PAF antagonists that are able to influence the fundamental alterations that develop in drug responsiveness during human allergic disorders should be carefully taken into account.

Clinical Findings with WEB 2086 in Bronchial Asthma

WEB 2086, produced by Boeringher-Ingelheim, was the first specific PAF receptor antago-nist selected for development as a therapeutic agent in human bronchial asthma. The clinical evaluation of the drug has recently been finished, and a part of the multicenter, randomized, double-blind, placebo-controlled phase III trials, including eight atopic, mildly asthmatic subjects, has recently been published (117). The purpose of the study was to evaluate the effects of WEB 2086, given in a dose of 100 mg three times a day for 1 week, which treatment of human subjects has antagonized the effects of inhaled PAF on allergen-induced early and late asthmatic responses and on airway hyperresponsiveness. Neither early nor late asthmatic responses induced by inhalation of the specific antigen changed. These results, consistent with those found in animal studies after booster administration, suggest that the PAF antagonist WEB 2086 does not attenuate allergen-induced early and late responses of airway hyperresponsiveness in clinical patients.

PAF in the Inflammatory Response

Inflammation is an important, natural defense mechanism, and PAF mimics the symptoms of the acute inflammatory response. PAF activates various inflammatory cells and interacts with various cytokines, which has led to the concept of a PAF-induced, autogenerated, regulatory feedback network of inflammatory mediator release (118–120). Overactivation of this mechanisms leads to priming (i.e., amplification of inflammatory mediator release with consecutive disease states), whereas PAF may down-regulate mediator production through formation of eicosanoids and activation of adenylate cyclase (121,122).

Skin and Mucosal Inflammation

When injected locally, PAF induces an inflammatory response characterized by increased blood flow, extravasation of plasma proteins, and transient intravascular cellular accumulation, followed by perivascular, mixed cellular infiltration. PAF antagonists, such as UR-10324, UR-11353, CV-6209, and WEB 2086, all are able to reduce the acute non-immune inflammatory response induced by several irritants in the mouse ear (Merlos et al., 1991). SR 27417 has been claimed to be 660 times more potent than WEB 2086 in inhibiting PAF-induced edema formation in the rabbit skin and, when mixed with the antigen, it inhibited allergen-induced plasma extravasation (80), indicating the PAF may play a major role in cutaneous anaphylaxis.

As measured by accumulation of radiolabeled platelets and edema formation in the rabbit skin challenged by zymosan; or from a reverse, passive Arthus reaction, UK 74-505, a novel long-acting PAF antagonist markedly moderated the inflammatory response (123).

The role of PAF in mucosal hypersensitivity to topical histamine challenge was studied in guinea pig models of nasal allergy (124). Histamine sensitivity was significantly increased by nasal allergen challenge in actively sensitized animals. Histamine hypersensitivity was inhibited by an anti-PAF agent SM 10661, and PAF also increased histamine hypersensitivity of the nasal mucosa.

Arthritis

Recent emerging evidence indicates that the inflammatory response causing rheumatoid arthritis may be associated with various mediators released by inflammatory cells: PAF stimulates inflammation in animal models used for mimicking human rheumatoid arthritis (125).

This pathophysiological entity may involve an increased production and release of nonpancreatic, extracellular PLA_2 (126). When rabbit platelet PLA_2 activity was measured, Ro 19-3704, a PAF antagonist (127), inhibited the enzyme activity, in validation of the concept that PAF antagonists may have beneficial supplementary effects through which the inflammatory response may be attenuated. In an in vitro system in which rate basophilic leukemia cells, passively sensitized by exposure to monoclonal antitrinitrophenol mouse IgE and triggered with suboptimal concentration of trinitrophenol OA conjugate, Ro

19-3704 and Ro 19-1400, two structural analogues of PAF, potently inhibited histamine and LT release (128). These effects may not be related to the PAF receptor antagonistic properties of these compounds, since WEB 2086 and BN 52021, two structurally distinct PAF antagonists, were relatively ineffective.

PAF aggravates the early phase of tissue damage in antigen-induced arthritis in healthy rabbits, and TNF can amplify the inflammatory response induced by PAF (129). In this model, BN 50726 attenuated inflammatory synovial fluid formation, leukocyte accumulation, PGE_2 release, and preserved proteoglycan content.

PAF in the Generalized Inflammatory Response

To develop a more uniform set of definitions, it has recently been proposed that sepsis and similar disorders may be called *systemic inflammatory response syndrome* (SIRS; 130). As reviewed recently, there is circumstantial evidence that PAF is involved in the pathogenesis of SIRS (3,131); however, this is beyond the scope of this review.

Crohn's Disease and Ulcerative Colitis

The mediator role of PAF in intestinal inflammation and ulceration has been proposed (131). In the gastrointestinal tract, some regional differences have been shown in response to PAF. PAF increases ion transport and epithelial permeability in the distal colon, but not in the caecum (132); also induces bowel necrosis (133).

PAF content and acetylhydrolase activity in the stool of patients with Crohn's disease are higher than in patients with irritable bowel syndrome and diarrhea, or with diarrhea and malabsorption (134). Alternatively, the PAF content in the stool has been claimed to be a sensitive marker of the severity of the disease (135).

Both Crohn's disease and ulcerative colitis appear to have immune etiological factors. This is mainly based on the effectiveness of therapeutic interventions. Crohn's disease is responsive to prednisolone and azathioprine, whereas ulcerative colitis can be treated with corticosteroids and sulfasalazine. In both diseases, an increased formation of PAF has been demonstrated (136–138).

More recently, an increased generation of PAF by intestinal mucosal epithelial cells and lamina propria mononuclear cells isolated from surgical specimen of patients with ulcerative colitis has been described when compared with that of control patients (139). Resting and A23187 ionophore-stimulated PAF levels in these highly purified cells were also increased in patients with bowel disease when compared with controls. The difference was especially expressed in epithelial cells, suggesting their pivotal role in the pathogenesis of ulcerative colitis.

Systemic Lupus Erythematosus

Platelet activating factor has recently been suggested to play an important role in immune glomerulonephritis, favoring the formation of immune deposits in glomeruli and contributing to the local inflammatory reaction. Morigi et al. (140) have studied urinary PAF excretion in New Zealand black × New Zealand white mice, representing a model of genetically determined immune complex diseases that mimic human systemic lupus. Long-term treatment with L-659,989 delayed the onset of proteinuria and prolonged survival. Similar findings have recently been obtained in patients with immune-mediated glomerulonephritis (141). Increased urinary PAF excretion was not due to increased acetylhydrolase activity, which remained comparable with controls. These results suggest that signs of renal disease activity in human membranous nephropathy are associated with an excessive synthesis of PAF. Interestingly enough, augmented PAF production by polymorphonuclear cells isolated from immune-mediated glomerulonephritis was comparable with controls, pointing to the potential significance of humoral and tissue components. The condition of 16-week-old MRL/MpJ-++(/+) mice having a lupus-like severe glomerulonephritis, with proteinuria and reduction of kidney function, treatment with the PAF antagonist L659,989 for 4 weeks provided significant improvement of functional renal parameters (142).

Recently, a diet supplemented with flaxseed, rich in α-linoleic acid and plant lignans, with potent PAF receptor antagonist properties, was given to MRL/lpr mice, representing a murine model of lupus nephritis (143). The diet considerably improved all kidney parameters measured and significantly increased survival rate.

Insulitis

The BB rat spontaneously develops insulin-dependent diabetes mellitus (IDDM) in association with marked "insulitis" in the islet of Langerhans. Diabetes-prone BB/W or rats were treated daily from weaning at 25 days until 105 days of age with BN 52021 and the effect of the PAF antagonist were compared with rats given an appropriate placebo (144). The overall incidence of IDDM was unaffected by treatment; however, quantitative analysis of the insulin-producing area showed a dose-dependent protection of β-cells by the PAF receptor antagonist. At the same time, the glucagon/insulin ratio was also improved. Severe insulitis decreased from 84 to 59% in comparison with the inflammatory response in the saline-treated rats. The preservation of pancreatic β-cells by BN 52021 may suggest a role for PAF in this pathophysiological condition and the benefit of PAF antagonists as immunomodulators in IDDM.

Allergic Encephalomyelitis and Multiple Sclerosis

In rats developing experimental allergic encephalomyelitis, IV PAF aggravated the disease when injected 5, 6, and 7 days after adjuvant injection, and PAF antagonists markedly attenuated the development of symptoms (145). In the guinea pig, normal vascular endothelial cells do not express major histocompatibility complex (MHC) class II antigens. In the acute phase of relapsing experimental allergic encephalomyelitis, these cells exhibited MHC class II antigens, as measured by monoclonal antibodies HLA-DR, 27E7, and MSgp8 (146,147). This suggests that these cells may be the target for the development of allergic encephalomyelitis.

Since local allergic inflammatory responses can frequently be reduced by PAF antagonists, these findings prompted the Beaufour group to begin a pilot study in patients with multiple sclerosis. Ten patients with relapsing, remitting multiple sclerosis in acute relapse were treated with a 5-day course of intravenous BN 52021, a specific PAF receptor inhibitor, and eight of them showed improved neurological course, beginning 2–6 days after the initiation of the therapy. The improvement was sustained in five and transient in three patients. Two out of the three patients with secondary failure and of the two who did not respond to ginkgolide B therapy, received IV methylprednisolone. Three patients experienced mild side effects under ginkgolide therapy, but none of them had any serious adverse effects. A controlled randomized study is underway to confirm these results and to test higher doses and more-prolonged administration of BN 52021 (148).

CONCLUDING REMARKS

The data summarized in this review clearly show that PAF is an important phospholipid mediator that plays a regulatory role in the function of inflammatory, endothelial, and smooth-muscle cells (5–7). It triggers the release of $[Ca^{2+}]_i$ through stimulating phosphoinosotide metabolism that results in IP_3 formation and activation of PLA_2, leading to increased eicosanoid generation and interaction with various cytokines (118,119), thereby fundamentally affecting inflammatory cellular function. The discovery of PAF, as well as its numerous, structurally different natural and synthetic antagonists, has initiated intensive research to clarify the complex role of this phospholipid mediator in various pathophysiological conditions and diseases, as well as the eventual benefit of PAF antagonists in clinical disorders.

Recent experimental and clinical results have shed more light on the mechanism of action of PAF in the allergic and inflammatory responses. From the first experimental findings showing that PAF is a potent bronchoconstricting agent, it was hypothesized that PAF antagonists might be useful in the treatment of human bronchial asthma. A careful analysis of the role of PAF in the pathomechanism of airway hypersensitivity observed in passive and active anaphylaxis and after booster administration has revealed, that PAF antagonists exhibit different abilities to inhibit bronchoconstriction induced by various challenges (107–109). These agents profoundly inhibit PAF-induced and passive anaphylactic challenge-induced bronchoconstriction; however, these drugs are less active in actively sensitized animals, and they become entirely ineffective after booster injection (107,109). In accord with the recognition that boosterization is the best experimental animal model of human bronchial asthma, clinical trials conducted by Boeringher-Ingelheim have proved that WEB 2086 is ineffective in asthmatic patients (117).

Further research has shown that cellular responses to various cytokines, especially to IL-5, are fundamentally altered after booster injection, which may be responsible for the ineffectiveness of PAF antagonists under these conditions (108).

PAF triggers inflammatory response when injected locally, and its effect is blocked by PAF receptor antagonists. The conventionally used animal models of acute and chronic inflammatory responses, however, exhibit low sensitivity to the antagonists of PAF. In contrast to airway hypersensitivity, booster injection increases PAF production in allergic inflammatory responses (114,115,123,128), and this is accompanied by an augmented potency of PAF antagonists under these pathophysiological conditions. There is recent experimental and clinical evidence that PAF production is increased in inflammatory diseases (138,139). PAF antagonists improve allergic inflammatory responses in the gastrointestinal tract, especially in bowel diseases, and in arthritis. There is indication that these drugs may exert beneficial effects in animal models of Crohn's disease (134,135,138) and ulcerative colitis (136,139) as well as arthritis (125,129). Animal studies have proved that allergic nephropathies that mimic the symptoms of systemic lupus erythematosus are markedly improved after treatment with PAF antagonists (140–143). Insulitis in BB rats also appears sensitive to PAF antagonists (144), as has been demonstrated in experimental allergic encephalomyelitis in the rat (145). A recent clinical trial has shown a beneficial effect of BN 52021 in patients with remittent multiple sclerosis (144).

The future trends of research, therefore, should be devoted to clarify the cellular background of these fundamental alterations that occur during the development of airway hypersensitivity and allergic inflammatory responses. This process may clarify clinical indications, other than bronchial asthma, for specific PAF receptor antagonists.

REFERENCES

1. Hanahan DJ, Demopoulos CA, Liehr J, Pinckard RN. Identification of platelet-activating factor isolated from rabbit. J Biol Chem 1980; 255:5514–5516.

2. Prescott SM, Zimmerman GA, McIntyre TM. Platelet-activating factor. J Biol Chem 1990; 265:1781–1784.

3. Koltai M, Hosford D, Braquet PG. Platelet-activating factor in septic shock. New Horizons 1993; 1:87–95.

4. Koltai M, Tosaki A, Guillon J-M, Hosford D, Braquet P. PAF antagonists as potential therapeutic agents in cardiac anaphylaxis and myocardial ischemia. Cardiovasc Drug Rev 1989; 7:177–198.

5. Braquet P, Touqui L, Shen TS, Vargaftig BB. Perspectives in platelet-activating factor research. Pharmacol Rev 1987; 39:97–145.

6. Koltai M, Hosford D, Guinot P, Esanu A, Braquet P. Platelet-activating factor (PAF): a review of its effects, antagonists and possible future clinical applications. Drugs 1991; 42(part 1):9–29.

7. Koltai M, Hosford D, Guinot P, Esanu A, Braquet P. Platelet-activating factor (PAF): a review of its effects, antagonists and possible future clinical applications. Drugs 1991; 42(part 2): 174–204.

8. Hall IP. Inositol phosphates, cyclic AMP and signal transduction. DNP 1993; 6:5–11.

9. Berridge MJ. Inositol triphosphate and calcium signalling. Nature 1993; 361:315–325.

10. Shukla SD, Hanahan DJ. An early decrease in phosphatidylinositol 4,5-biphosphate upon stimulation of rabbit platelets with acetylglycerylether phosphorylcholine (platelet activating factor). Arch Biochem Biophys 1983; 227:626–629.

11. Billah M, Lapetina G. Platelet activating factor stimulates metabolism of phosphoinositides in horse platelets: possible relationship to Ca^{2+} mobilization during stimulation. Proc Natl Acad Sci USA 1983; 80:965–968.

12. Billah M, Siegel MI. Calmodulin antagonists inhibit formation of platelet activating factor in stimulated human neutrophils. Biochem Biophys Res Commun 1984; 118:629–635.

13. Weber C, Aepfelbacher M, Lux I, Zimmer B, Weber PC. Docosahexaenoic acid inhibits PAF and LTD4 stimulated (Ca^{2+})i increase in differentiated monocytic U937 cells. Biochim Biophys Acta 1991; 1133:38–45.

14. Shukla SD. Platelet activating factor receptor and signal transduction mechanisms. FASEB J 1992; 6:2296–2301.

15. Avdonin PV, Svitina Ulitina IV, Tkachuk VA. Selective inactivation by endogenous protein kinase C of human platelet high affinity GTPase coupled with PAF receptors. J Mol Cell Cardiol 1989; 21:139–143.

16. Mori M, Bito H, Sakanaka C, Honda Z, Kume K, Izumi T, Shimizu T. Activation of mitogen activated protein kinase and arachidonate release via two G protein coupled receptors expressed in the rat hippocampus. Ann NY Acad Sci 1994; 744:107–125.

17. Braquet P, Hosford D,Koltz P, Guilbaud J, Paubert-Braquet M. Effect of platelet-activating factor on tumor necrosis factor-induced superoxide generation from human neutrophils: possible involvement of G proteins. Lipids 1991; 26:1071–1075.

18. Honda Z, Nakamura M, Miki I, Minami M, Watanabe T, Seyama Y, Okado H, Toh H, Ito K, Miyamoto T. Cloning by functional expression of platelet activating factor receptor from guinea pig lung. Nature 1991; 349:342–346.

19. Hwang SB. Specific receptors of platelet activating factor, receptor heterogeneity, and signal transduction mechanisms. J Lipid Mediat 1990; 2:123–158.

20. Pedemonte CH. Structure–function relationship of membrane ion pumps. DNP 1993; 6: 498–507.

21. Braquet P, Hosford D. Ethnopharmacology and the development of natural PAF antagonists as therapeutic agents. J Ethnopharmacol 1991; 32:135–139.

22. Braquet P, Esanu A, Busine E, Hosford D, Broquet C, Koltai M. Recent progress in ginkgolide research. Med Res Rev 1991; 11:295–355.

23. Braquet P, Spinnewyn B, Braquet M, Bourgain RH, Taylor JE, Etienne A, Drieu K. BN 52021 and related compounds: a new series of highly specific PAF-acether antagonists isolated from *Ginkgo biloba*. Blood Vessels 1985; 16:559–572.

24. Huxtable JR. The pharmacology of extinction. J Ethnopharmacol 1992; 37:1–11.

25. Corey EJ, Gavai AV. Enantioselective route to a key intermediate in the total synthesis of ginkgolide B. Tetrahedron Lett 1988; 29:3201–3204.

26. Corey EJ, Rao KS. Enantioselective total synthesis of ginkgolide derivatives lacking the *tert*-butyl group, an essential structural subunit for antagonism of platelet activating factor. Tetrahedron Lett 1991; 32:4623–4626.

27. Shen TY, Hwang SB, Chang MN, Doebber TW, Lam MH, Wu MS, Wang X, Han GQ, Li RZ. Characterization of a platelet-activating factor antagonist isolated from haifenteng (*Piper futokadsura*): specific inhibition of in vitro and in vivo platelet-activating factor-induced effects. Proc Natl Acad Sci USA 1985; 82:672–676.

28. Sugano M, Shindo T, Sato A, Iijima Y, Oshima T, Furuya K, Kuwano H, Hata T, Hanzawa H. Phomactin A: a novel PAF antagonist from marine fungus *Phoma* sp. J Am Chem Soc 1991; 113:5463–5464.

29. Sugano M, Shindo T, Sato A, Iijima Y, Oshima T, Kuwano H, Hata T. Chantancin, a PAF antagonist from soft coral, *Sacrophyton* sp. J Org Chem 1990; 55:5802–5805.

30. Ekimoto H, Irie Y, Araki Y, Han G-Q, Kadota S, Kikutchi T. Platelet aggregation inhibitors from the seeds of *Swietenia mahagoni*: inhibition of in vitro and in vivo platelet-activating factor-induced effects of tetranortriterpenoids related to swietenine and swietenolide. Planta Med 1991; 57:56–58.

31. Lee CM, Jiang LM, Shang HS, Hon PM, He Y, Wong HN. Prehispanolone, a novel platelet activating factor receptor antagonist from *Leourus heterophyllus*. Br J Pharmacol 1991; 103:1719–1724.

32. Burstein SH, Audette CA, Doyle SA, Hull K, Hunter SA, Latham V. Antagonism to the actions of platelet activating factor by a nonpsychoactive cannabinoid. J Pharmacol Exp Ther 1989; 251:531–535.

33. Ko FN, Wu TS, Liou MJ, Huang TF, Teng CM. PAF antagonism in vitro and in vivo by aglafoline from *Aglaia elliptifolia* Merr. Eur J Pharmacol 1992; 218:129–135.

34. Hemmi K, Shimazaki N, Shima I, Okamoto M, Yoshida K, Hashimoto M. PAF antagonists from microbial origin: structure-activity relationships of diketopiperazine derivatives. In: Braquet P, ed. Handbook of PAF and PAF Antagonists. Boca Raton: CRC Press, 1991:71–79.

35. Shimazaki N, Shima I, Okamoto M, Yoshida K, Hemmi K, Hashimoto M. PAF inhibitory activity of diketopiperazines: structure–activity relationships. Lipids 1991; 26:1175–1178.

36. Fernandez-Gallardo S, Ortega MP, Priego JG, de Casa Juana MF, Sunkel C, Sanchez-Crespo M. Pharmacological actions of PCA 4248, a new platelet-activating factor receptor antagonist: in vivo studies. J Pharmacol Exp Ther 1990; 255:34–39.

37. Billah MM, Chapman RM, Egan RW, Gilchrest H, Piwinski JJ, Sherwood J, Siegel M, West RE Jr, Kreutner W. SCS 324, a potent, orally active, dual antagonist of platelet-activating factor and histamine. J Pharmacol Exp Ther 1990; 252:1090–1096.

38. Takatani M, Tsushima S. Structure activity relationship in CV-3988 and CV-6209 PAF antagonist series. In: Braquet P, ed. Handbook of PAF and PAF Antagonists. Boca Raton: CRC Press, 1991:97–118.

39. Terashita ZI, Kawamura M, Takatani M, Tsushima S, Imura Y, Nishikawa K. Beneficial effects of TCV-309, a novel potent and selective platelet activating factor antagonist in endotoxin and anaphylactic shock in rodents. J Pharmacol Exp Ther 1992; 260:748–755.

40. Terashita ZI, Imura Y, Takatani M, Tsushima S, Nishikawa K. CV-6209, a highly potent antagonist of platelet activating factor in vitro and in vivo. J Pharmacol Exp Ther 1987; 242:263–268.

41. Terashita ZI, Takatani M, Nishikawa K. Pharmacological profile of TCV-309—a potent PAF antagonist. J Lipid Mediat 1992; 5:183–185.

42. Houlihan WJ. Structure activity relationship in cyclic analogs of PAF with PAF antagonist properties. In: Braquet P, ed. Handbook of PAF and PAF Antagonists. Boca Raton: CRC Press, 1991:157–170.

43. Merlos M, Gomez M, Giral M, Vericat ML, Garcia-Rafanell J, Forn J. Effects of PAF-

antagonists in mouse ear oedema induced by several inflammatory agents. Br J Pharmacol 1991; 104:990–994.

44. Nagaoka J, Harada K, Kimura A, Kobayashi S, Murakami M, M, Yoshimura T, Yamada K, Asano O, Katayama K, Yamatsu I. Inhibitory effects of the novel platelet activating factor receptor antagonist, 1-ethyl-2-[N-(2-methoxy)benzoyl-N-[(2R)-2-methoxy-3-(4-octadecyl-carbamoyloxy)piperidino carbonyloxypropyloxy] carbonylaminomethyl pyridinium chloride, in several experimentally induced shock models. Arzneimittelforschung 1991; 41:719–724.

45. Wissner A, Carroll ML, Green KE, Kerwar SS, Pickett WC, Schaub RE, Torley LW, Wrenn, S, Kohler CA. Analogues of platelet activating factor. 6. Mono- and bis-aryl phosphate antagonists of platelet-activating factor. J Med Chem 1992; 35:1650–1662.

46. Wissner A, Carroll ML, Johnson BD, Kerwar SS, Pickett WC, Schaub E, Torley LW, Trova MP, Kohler CA. Analogues of platelet activating factor. 7. Bis-aryl amide and bis-aryl urea receptor antagonists of platelet-activating factor. J Med Chem 1992; 35:4779–4789.

47. Tilley JW, O'Donnell M. N-[ω-(Heteroalkyl)alkyl]carboxamide derivatives as platelet activating factor antagonists: structure–activity relationships, and biological data. In: Braquet P, ed. Handbook of PAF and PAF Antagonists. Boca Raton: CRC Press, 1991:229–258.

48. Casals-Stenzel J. Thieno-triazolo-1,4-diazepines as antagonists of platelet-activating factor: present status. Lipids 1991; 26:1157–1161.

49. Heuer HO. Pharmacology of a new very potent and long acting hetrazepinoic PAF-antagonist and its action in repeatedly sensitized guinea-pigs. J Lipid Mediat 1991; 4:39–44.

50. Heuer HO. Inhibition of active anaphylaxis in mice and guinea pigs by the new hetrazepinoic PAF antagonist bepafant (WEB 2170). Eur J Pharmacol 1991; 199:157–163.

51. Heuer HO, Keller B, Urich K. Action of the racemate and the isomers of the platelet-activating factor antagonist bepafant (WEB 2170) after oral administration to guinea-pigs and rats. Naunyn Schmiedebergs Arch Pharmacol 1991; 343:546–550.

52. Foster AP, Lees P, Andrews MJ, Cunningham FM. Effects of WEB 2086, an antagonist to the receptor for platelet-activating factor (PAF), on PAF-induced responses in the horse. Equine Vet J 1992; 24:203–207.

53. Terasawa M, Aratani H, Setoguchi M, Tahara T. Pharmacological actions of Y-24180: I. A potent and specific antagonist of platelet activating factor. Prostaglandins 1990; 40:571–579.

54. Takehara S, Mikashima H, Setoguchi M, Tahara T. Pharmacological actions of Y-24180, a new specific antagonist of platelet activating factor (PAF): II. Interactions with PAF and benzo-diazepine receptors. Prostaglandins 1990; 40:553–583.

55. Karasawa A, Rochester JA, Lefer AM. Beneficial actions of BN 50739, a new PAF antagonist, in murine traumatic shock. Methods Find Exp Clin Pharmacol 1990; 12:231–237.

56. Sakuma Y, Muramoto K, Harada K, Katayama S, Tsunoda H, Katayama K. Inhibitory effect of a novel PAF antagonist E6123 on anaphylactic responses in passively and actively sensitized guinea pigs and passively sensitized mice. Prostaglandins 1991; 42:541–555.

57. Tsunoda H, Sakuma Y, Shirato M, Obaishi H, Harada K, Yamada K, Shimomura N, Machida Y, Yamatsu I, Katayama K. Activity of a novel thienodiazepine derivative as a platelet-activating factor antagonist in guinea pig lungs. Arzneimittelforschung 1991; 41:224–227.

58. Braquet P, Esanu A. New trends in PAF antagonist research: a new series of potent hetrazepine-derived PAF antagonists. Agents Actions 1991; 32:34–36.

59. Braquet P, Laurent B, Rolland A, Martin C, Pommier J, Hosford D, Esanu A. From ginkgolides to N-substituted piperidinothieno-diazepines, a new series of highly potent dual antagonists. Adv Prostaglandins Tromboxane Leukot Res 1990; 21:929–937.

60. Castaner J, Koltai M, Spinnewyn B, Duverger D, Pirotzky E, Esanu A, Braquet P. BN 50739. Drugs Future 1990; 16:413–419.

61. Yue T-L, Rabinovici R, Farhat M, Feuerstein G. Pharmacological profile of BN 50739, a new PAF antagonist in vitro and in vivo. Prostaglandins 1990; 39:469–480.

62. Yue T-L, Rabinovici R, Farhat M, Feuerstein G. Inhibitory effect of new PAF antagonists on PAF-induced rabbit platelet aggregation in vitro and in vivo. J Lipid Mediat 1991; 3:13–26.

63. Rabinovici R, Yue TL, Farhat M, Smith EF III, Esser KM, Slivjak M, Feuerstein G. Platelet activating factor (PAF) and tumor necrosis factor-α (TNFα) interactions in endotoxemic shock: studies with BN 50739, a novel PAF antagonist. J Pharmacol Exp Ther 1990; 255:256–263.

64. Lindsberg PJ, Hallenbeck JM, Feuerstein G. Platelet-activating factor in stroke and brain injury. Ann Neurol 1991; 30:117–129.

65. Dyson MC, Bellan JA, Minkes RK, Beckerman RC, Wegman MJ, Braquet P, McNamara DB, Kadowitz PJ. Influence of SK&F 95587 and BN 50730 on bronchoconstrictor responses in the cat. J Pharmacol Exp Ther 1990; 255:1320–1327.

66. Crowley HJ, Yaremo B, Selig WM, Janero DR, Burghardt C, Welton A, O'Donnell M. Pharmacology of a potent platelet-activating factor antagonist: Ro 24-4736. J Pharmacol Exp Ther 1991; 259:78–85.

67. Lavé D. Structure–activity relationships in pyrrolo[1,2-c]thiazoles PAF receptor antagonists. In: Braquet P, ed. Handbook of PAF and PAF Antagonists. Boca Raton: CRC Press, 1991:203–228.

68. Floch A, Bousseau A, Hetier E, Floch F, Bost PE, Cavero I. RP 55778, a PAF receptor antagonist, prevents and reserves LPS-induced hemoconcentration and TNF release. J Lipid Mediat 1989; 1:349–360.

69. Floch A, Tahraoui L, Sedivy P, Cavero I. The platelet activating factor receptor antagonist, RP 59227, blocks platelets activating factor receptors mediating liberation of reactive oxygen species in guinea pig macrophages and human polynuclear leukocytes. J Pharmacol Exp Ther 1991; 258:567–575.

70. Underwood SL, Lewis SA, Raeburn D. RP 59227, a novel PAF receptor antagonist: effects in guinea pig models of airway hyperreactivity. Eur J Pharmacol 1992; 210:97–102.

71. Yamada T, Tomioka K, Horie M, Sakurai Y, Nagaoka H, Mase T. Effects of YM264, a novel PAF antagonist, on puromycin aminonucleoside-induced nephropathy in the rat. Biochem Biophys Res Commun 1991; 176:781–785.

72. Yamada T, Tomioka K, Saito M, Horie M, Mase T, Nagaoka H. Pharmacological properties of YM264, a potent and orally active antagonist of platelet-activating factor. Arch Int Pharmacodyn 1990; 308:23–136.

73. Yamada T, Saito M, Mase T, Hara H, Nagaoka H, Murase K, Tomioka K. Pharmacological properties of YM461, a new orally active platelet-activating factor antagonist. Lipids 1991; 26:1179–1183.

74. Guinn DE, Summers JB, Heyman HR, Conway RG, Rhein DA, Albert DH, Magoc T, Carter GW. Synthesis and structure–activity relationships of a series of novel benzopyran-containing platelet-activating factor antagonists. J Med Chem 1992; 35:2055–2061.

75. Tanabe Y, Suzukamo G, Komuro Y, Imanishi N, Morooka S, Enomoto M, Kojima A, Sanemitsu Y, Mizutani M. Structure–activity relationship of optically active 2-(3-pyridyl)thiazolidin-4-ones as a PAF antagonist. Tetrahedron Lett 1991; 32:379–382.

76. Komuro Y, Imanishi N, Uchida M, Morooka S. Biological effects of orally active platelet-activating factor receptor antagonist SM-10661. Mol Pharmacol 1990; 38:378–384.

77. Sugasawa T, Imanishi N, Morooka S. Effect of the selective PAF antagonist SM-10661 in an asthmatic model. 2. The effect of antigen-induced dual asthmatic response and infiltration of leukocytes into airways in actively sensitized conscious guinea pigs. Lipids 1991; 26:1305–1309.

78. Imanishi N, Komuro Y, Morooka S. Effect of a selective PAF antagonist SM-10661 (($\pm$)-cis-3,5,dimethyl-2-(3-pyridyl)thiazolidin-4-one HCl) on experimental disseminated intravascular coagulation (DIC). Lipids 1991; 26:1391–1395.

79. Herbert JM, Bernat A, Valette G, Gigo V., Lale A, Laplace MC, Lespy L. Maffrand JP, Le Fur G. Biochemical and pharmacological activities of SR 27417, a highly potent, long-acting platelet-activating factor receptor antagonist. J Pharmacol Exp Ther 1991; 259:44–51.

80. Herbert JM, Laplace MC, Bernat A, Salel V, Maffrand JP. Effect of SR 27417 on oedema formation induced in rabbit skin by platelet-activating factor or antigen. Eur J Pharmacol 1992; 216:175–181.

81. Alabaster VA, Keir RF, Parry MJ, de Souza RN. UK-74,505, a novel and selective PAF antagonist, exhibits potent and long lasting activity in vivo. Agents Actions 1991; 34(suppl):221–227.

82. Weber KH, Heuer HO. Hetrazepines as antagonists of platelet activating factor. Med Res Rev 1989; 9:181–218.

83. Hodgkin EE, Miller A, Whittaker M. A partial pharmacophore for the platelet activating factor (PAF) receptor. Bioorg Med Chem Lett 1992; 2:597–602.

84. Shen TY. Chemical and biochemical characterization of lignan analogs as novel PAF receptor antagonists. Lipids 1991; 26:1154–1156.

85. Dive G, Godfroid JJ, Lamotte-Brasseur J, Batt JP, Heymans F, Dupont L, Braquet P. PAF-receptor. 1. "Cache-oreilles" effect of selected high-potency platelet-activating factor (PAF) antagonists. J Lipid Mediat 1989; 1:201–215.

86. Batt J-P, Lamouri A, Tavet F, Heymans F, Dive G, Godfroid JJ. New hypothesis on the conformation of the PAF receptor from studies on the geometry of selected platelet-activating factor antagonists. J Lipid Mediat 1991; 4:343–346.

87. Ponpipom MM, Bugianesi RL, Chabala JC. Enantioselective cyclization of chiral butane-1,4-diols to chiral tetrahydrofurans: synthesis of chiral *trans*-2-(3-methoxy-5-methylsulfonyl-4-propoxyphenyl)-5-(3,4,5-methylsulfonyl-4-propoxyphenyl)-5-(3,4,5-trimethoxyphenyl)tetrahydrofuran, a potent PAF-receptor antagonist. Tetrahedron Lett 1988; 29:6211–6214.

88. Ponpipom MM, Hwang S-B, Doebber TW, Acton JJ, Alberts AW, Bitfu T, Brooker DR, Bugianesi RL, Chabala JC, Gamble NL, Graham DW, Lam M-H, Wu MS. *trans*-2-(3-Methoxy-5-methylsulfonyl-4-propoxyphenyl)-5-(3,4,5-trimethoxyphenyl)tetrahydrofuran (L-659,989), a novel, potent PAF-receptor antagonist. Biochem Biophys Res Commun 1988; 150:1213–1220.

89. Bugianesi RL, Ponpipom MM, Parsons WH, Hwang SB, Doebber TW, Lam M-H, Wu MS, Alberts AW, Chabala JC. Synthesis and biological activity of the platelet-activating factor antagonist (±)-*trans*-2-(3-methoxy-4-phenylsulfonyl-ethoxy-5-*n*-propylsulfonylphenyl)-5-(3,4,5-trimethoxyphenyl)tetrahydrofuran (L-671,284) and its analogs. Bioorg Med Chem Lett 1992; 2:181–184.

90. Girotra NN, Biftu T, Ponpipom MM, Acton JJ, Alberts AW, Bach TN, Ball RG, Bugianesi RL, Parsons WH, Chabala JC. Development, synthesis, and biological evaluation of (−)-*trans*-(2S,5S)-2-(3-((2-oxopropyl)sulfonyl)-4-*n*-propoxy-5-(3-hydroxypropoxy)-phenyl)-5-(3,4,5-trimethoxyphenyl)tetrahydrofuran, a potent orally active platelet-activating factor (PAF) antagonist and its water soluble prodrug phosphate ester. J Med Chem 1992; 35:3474–3482.

91. Alvaro RF, Rosegay A, Chiu SH. Determination of enantiomeric concentrations of a 2,5-diaryltetrahydrofuran (L-668,750), a platelet-activating factor antagonist, in the rat plasma using a chiral alpha 1-acid glycoprotein high-performance liquid chromatography column. J Chromatogr 1992; 24:327–332.

92. Carceller E, Merlos M, Bartroli J, Garcia-Rafanell J, Forn J. (Pyridylcyanomethyl)piperazines as orally active PAF antagonists. J Med Chem 1992; 35:676–683.

93. Ko FN, Yu SM, Chen IS, Ishii H, Chang YL, Huang TF, Teng CM. CIS-19, a novel platelet activating factor receptor antagonist: in vitro and in vivo studies. Biochim Biophys Acta 1993; 1175:225–231.

94. Sakamoto T, Elwood W, Barnes PJ, Chung KF. Effect of inhaled lyso-platelet-activating factor on airway vascular leakage in the guinea pig. J Appl Physiol 1993; 74:1117–1122.

95. Barnes PJ. PAF, eosinophils and asthma. J Lipid Mediat 1992; 5:155–158.

96. Chung KF, Barnes PJ. Effect of platelet activating factor on airway calibre, airway responsivenss, and circulating cells in asthmatic subjects. Thorax 1989; 44:108–115.

97. Adamus WS, Heuer HO, Meade CJ, Schilling JC. Inhibitory effects of the new PAF-acether antagonist WEB 2086 on pharmacologic changes induced by PAF inhalation in human beings. Clin Pharmacol Ther 1990; 47:456–462.

98. Hsieh KH, Ng CK. Increased plasma platelet-activating factor in children with acute asthmatic attacks and decreased in vivo and in vitro production of platelet-activating factor after immunotherapy. J Allergy Clin Immunol 1993; 91:650–657.

99. Gresele P, Dottorini M, Selli ML, Innacci L, Canino S, Todisco T, Romano S, Crook P, Page CP, Nenci GG. Altered platelet function associated with the bronchial hyperresponsiveness accompanying nocturnal asthma. J Allergy Clin Immunol 1993; 91:894–902.

100. Taylor ML, Stewart GA, Thompson PJ. The differential effect of aspirin on human platelet activation in aspirin-sensitive asthmatics and normal subjects. Br J Clin Pharmacol 1993; 35: 227–234.

101. Cheng JB, Pillar JS, Shirley JT, Showell HJ, Watson JW, Cohan VL. Antigen-mediated pulmonary eosinophilia in immunoglobulin G_1-sensitized guinea pigs: eosinophil peroxidase as a simple specific marker for detecting eosinophils in bronchoalveolar lavage fluids. J Pharmacol Exp Ther 1993; 264:922–929.

102. Warringa RA, Mengelers HJ, Raaijmakers JA, Bruijnzeel PL. Koenderman L. Upregulation of formyl-peptide and interleukin-8-induced eosinophil chemotaxis in patients with allergic asthma. J Allergy Clin Immunol 1993; 91:1198–1205.

103. Lagente V, Touvay C, Randon J, Desquand S, Cirino M, Vilain B, Lefort J, Braquet P, Vargaftig BB. Interference of the PAF-acether antagonist BN 52021 with passive anaphylaxis in the guinea-pig. Prostaglandins 1987; 33:265–274.

104. Desquand S, Vargaftig BB. Interference of the PAF-acether antagonist BN 52021 with bronchopulmonary anaphylaxis. Can a case be made for PAF-acether in bronchopulmonary anaphylaxis in the guinea-pig? In: Braquet P, ed. Ginkgolides Chemistry, Biology, Pharmacology and Clinical Perspectives. No. 1. Barcelona: Prous Sciences Publishers, 1988:171–181.

105. Handley DA, LeLeo JJ, Havill AM. Induction by aerosol allergen of sustained and nonspecific IgE-mediated airway hyperreactivity in the guinea pig. Agents Actions 1992; 37:201–203.

106. Lohman IC, Halonen M. The effects of combined histamine and platelet-activating factor antagonism on systemic anaphylaxis induced by immunoglobulin E in the rabbit. Am J Respir Dis 1993; 147:1223–1228.

107. Desquand S, Lefort J, Dumarey C, Vargaftig BB. Interference of BN 52021, an antagonist of PAF, with different forms of active anaphylaxis in the guinea-pig: importance of the booster injection. Br J Pharmacol 1991; 102:687–695.

108. Pretolani M, Lefort J, Leduc D, Vargaftig BB. Effect of human recombinant interleukin-5 on in vitro responsiveness of PAF of lung from actively sensitized guinea-pigs. Br J Pharmacol 1992; 106:677–684.

109. Desquand S, Lefort J, Dumarey C, Vargaftig BB. The booster injection of antigen during active sensitization modifies the anti-anaphylactic activity of the PAF antagonist WEB 2086. Br J Pharmacol 1990; 100:217–222.

110. Pretolani M, Lefort J, Malenchère E, Vargaftig BB. Interference of the novel PAF-acether antagonist WEB 2086 with the bronchopulmonary responses to PAF-acether and to active and passive shock in the guinea-pig. Eur J Pharmacol 1987, 140:311–321.

111. Rabinovici R, Yeh CG, Hillegas LM, Griswold DE, Dimartino MJ, Vernick J, Fong KL, Feuerstein G. Role of complement in endotoxin/platelet-activating factor-induced lung injury. J Immunol 1992; 149:1744–1750.

112. Touvay C, Pfister A, Vilain B, Page CP, Lelleouch-Tubiana A, Pignol B, Mencia-Huerta JM, Braquet P. Effect of long-term infusion of platelet-activating factor on pulmonary responsiveness and morphology in the guinea-pig. Pulm Pharmacol 1991; 4:43–51.

113. Rabier M, Damon M, Chanez P, Mencia-Huerta JM, Braquet, P, Bousquet J, Godard P. Neutrophil chemotactic activity of PAF, histamine and neuromediators in bronchial asthma. J Lipid Mediat 1991; 4:265–275.

114. Amorin CZ, Martins MA, Cordeiro RBS, Vargaftig BB. Differential inhibition by the PAF antagonist, WEB 2170, of allergic inflammation in single sensitized and boosted mice. Eur J Pharmacol 1992; 211:29–33.

115. Lapa e Silva JR, Bachelet CM, Pretolani M, Baker D, Scheper RJ, Vargaftig BB. Immunopathologic alterations in the bronchi of immunized guinea pigs. Am J Respir Cell Mol Biol 1993; 9:44–53.

116. Pretolani M, Vargaftig BB. From lung hypersensitivity to bronchial hyperreactivity. What can we learn from studies on animal models? Biochem Pharmacol 1993; 45:791–800.

117. Freitag A, Watson RM, Matsos G, Eastwood C, O'Byrne PM. Effect of a platelet activating factor antagonist, WEB 2086, on allergen induced asthmatic responses. Thorax 1993; 48:594–598.

118. Braquet P, Paubert-Braquet M, Bourgain R, Bussolino F, Hosford D. PAF/cytokine autogenerated feedback networks in microvascular immune injury: consequences in shock, ischemia and graft rejection. J Lipid Mediat 1989; 1:75–112.

119. Braquet P, Paubert-Braquet M, Koltai M, Bourgain R, Bussolino F, Hosford D. Is there a case for PAF antagonists in the treatment of ischemic states? Trends Pharmacol Sci 1989; 10:23–30.

120. Gatti S, Faggioni R, Echtenacher B, Ghezzi P. Role of tumour necrosis factor and reactive oxygen intermediates in lipopolysaccharide-induced pulmonary oedema and lethality. Clin Exp Immunol 1993; 91:456–461.

121. Heller R, Bussolino F, Ghido D, Garbarino G, Schroeder H, Pescarmona G, Till U, Bosia A. Protein kinase C and cyclic AMP modulate thrombin-induced platelet-activating factor synthesis in human endothelial cells. Biochim Biophys Acta 1991; 1093:55–64.

122. Zimmerman GA, McIntyre TM, Prescott SM. Production of platelet-activating factor by human vascular endothelial cells: evidence for a requirement for specific agonists and modulation by prostacyclin. Circulation 1985; 72:718–727.

123. Pons F, Rossi AG, Norman KE, Williams TJ, Nourshargh S. Role of platelet-activating factor (PAF) in platelet accumulation in rabbit skin: effect of the novel longlasting PAF antagonist, UK 74-505. Br J Pharmacol 1993; 109:234–242.

124. Narita S, Asakura K. The role of platelet-activating factor on histamine hypersensitivity in nasal allergy in guinea pig models. Int Arch Allergy Appl Immunol 1993; 100:373–377.

125. Sharma JN. Pro-inflammatory actions of the platelet activating factor: relevance to rheumatoid arthritis. Exp Pathol 1992; 43:47–50.

126. Vadas P, Browning J, Edelson J, Pruzanski W. Extracellular phospholipase A_2 expression and inflammation. The relationship with associated disease states. J Lipid Mediat 1993; 8:1–30.

127. Mounier C, Hatmi M, Faili A, Bon C, Vargaftig BB. Competitive inhibition of phospholipase A_2 activity by the platelet-activating factor antagonist Ro 19-3704 and evidence for a novel suppressive effect of platelet activation. J Pharmacol Exp Ther 1993; 264:1460–1467.

128. Gilfillan AM, Wiggan GA, Hoppe WC, Patel BJ, Welton AF. Ro 19-3704 directly inhibits immunoglobulin E-dependent mediator release by a mechanism independent of its platelet-activating factor antagonist properties. Eur J Pharmacol 1990; 176:255–262.

129. Zarco P, Maestre C, Herrero-Beaumont G, Gonzales E, Garcia-Hoyo. Involvement of platelet-activating factor and tumour necrosis factor in the pathogenesis of joint inflammation in rabbits. Clin Exp Immunol 1992; 88:318–323.

130. Koltai M, Hosford D, Braquet P. PAF-induced amplification of mediator release in septic shock: prevention of down-regulation by PAF antagonists. J Lipid Mediat 1993; 6:183–198.

131. Wallace JL, Whittle BJR. Profile of gastrointestinal damage induced by platelet-activating factor. Prostaglandins 1988; 12:137–141.

132. Travers SPL, Jewell DP. Regional differences in the response to platelet-activating factor in rabbit colon. Clin Sci 1992; 82:673–680.

133. Zhwang C, Hsueh W. PAF-induced bowel necrosis: effect of vasodilators. Dig Dis Sci 1991; 36:634–640.

134. Denizot Y, Chaussade S, Nathan N, Colombel JF, Bossant MJ, Cherouki N, Benveniste J, Couturier D. PAF-acether and acetylhydrolase activity in stool of patients with Crohn's diseases. Dig Dis Sci 1992; 37:432–437.

135. Chaussade S, Denizot Y, Colombel JF, Benveniste J, Couturier D. PAF-acether in stool as a marker of intestinal inflammation. Lancet 1992; 339:739.

136. Eliakim R, Karmeli F, Razim E, Rachmilewitz. Role of platelet-activating factor in ulcerative colitis: enhanced production during active disease and inhibition by sulfasalazine and prednisolone. Gastroenterology 1988; 95:1167–1172.

137. Jewell DP, Campieri M, Jarnerot G, Modigliani R, Rask-Madsen J. New therapeutic modalities for inflammatory bowel disease. Gastroenterol Int 1993; 6:1–12.
138. Kald B, Olaison G, Sjodahl R, Tagesson C. Novel aspect of Crohn's disease: increased content of platelet-activating factor in ileal and colonic mucosa. Digestion 1990; 46:199–204.
139. Ferraris L, Karmeli F, Eliakim R, Klein J, Fiocchi C, Rachmilevitz D. Intestinal cells contribute to the enhanced generation of platelet activating factor in ulcerative colitis. Gut 1993; 34: 665–668.
140. Morigi M, Macconi D, Riccardi E, Boccarfo P, Zilio P, Bertani T, Remuzzi R. Platelet-activating factor receptor blocking reduces proteinuria and improves survival in lupus autoimmune mice. J Pharmacol Exp Ther 1991; 258:601–606.
141. Norris M, Benigni A, Boccardo P, Gotti E, Benfenati E, Aiello S, Todeschini M, Remuzzi G. Urinary excretion of platelet activating factor in patients with immune-mediated glomerulonephritis. Kidney Int 1993; 43:426–429.
142. Baldi E, Emanccipator SN, Hassan MO, Dunn MJ. Platelet activating factor receptor blockade ameliorates murine systemic lupus erythematosus. Kidney Int 1990; 38:1030–1038.
143. Hall AV, Parbtani A, Clark WF, Spanner E, Keeney M, Chin-Yee I, Philbrick DJ, Holub BJ. Abrogation of MRL:lpr lupus nephritis by dietary flaxseed. Am J Kidney Dis 1993; 22: 326–332.
144. Beck JC, Goodner CJ, Wilson D, Glidden D, Baskin DG, Lernmark A, Braquet P. Effects of ginkgolide B, a platelet-activating factor inhibitor on "insulitis" in spontaneously diabetic BB rats. Autoimmunology 1991; 9:225–235.
145. Howat DW, Chand N, Braquet P, Willoughby DA. An investigation into the possible involvement of platelet activating factor in experimental allergic encephalomyelitis in rats. Agents Actions 1989; 27:473–476.
146. Wilcox CE, Baker D, Butter C, Willoughby DA, Turk JL. Differential expression of guinea pig class II major histocompatibility complex antigens on vascular endothelial cells in vitro in experimental allergic encephalomyelitis. Cell Immunol 1989; 120:82–91.
147. Wilcox CE, Healey DG, Butter C, Willoughby DA, Turk JL. Presentation of myelin basic protein by normal guinea pig brain endothelial cells and its relevance to experimental allergic encephalomyelitis. Immunology 1989; 67:435–440.
148. Brochet B, Orgogozo M, Guinot P, Dartigues JF, Henry P, Loisseau F. Etude pilott d'un inhibiteur du PAF-acether, le ginkgolide B dans le traitement des pousses aigues de sclerose en plaques [Pilot study of ginkgolide B, a PAF-acether specific inhibitor in the treatment of acute outbreaks of multiple sclerosis]. Rev Neurol (Paris) 1992; 148:299–301.

21

Adrenergic Receptors, Mechanisms, and the Late Allergic Reaction: Therapeutic Role of the New Long-Acting β-Agonists

Robert G. Townley
Creighton University School of Medicine, Omaha, Nebraska

STRUCTURE AND FUNCTION OF ADRENERGIC RECEPTORS

New insights into receptor structure and function and the cloning of many receptors have provided a whole new approach to study receptor regulation in inflammatory cells in lung disease. The genes for cytokines, neurotransmitters, and the various adrenergic receptors have now been cloned and expressed. This has made it possible to study the pharmacology of the receptors in a cultured cell line. This has also led to an understanding of the parts of the protein structure involved in ligand binding, signal transduction, and receptor regulation. It has also been possible to delete specific nucleotide sequences in the receptor gene and produce mutant receptors by a process called deletion mutagenesis. The cloning of mutant receptors has contributed to the understanding of the function of various parts of the receptor molecule. The discovery of related subtypes of receptors, such as the three subtypes of β- and seven subtypes of α-adrenergic receptors has come about partly as a result of receptor cloning and the development of selective antagonists.

Adrenergic agonists elicit changes in the target organs of asthma and allergic response by interaction with cell membrane receptors that are coupled to intracellular guanine nucleotide-binding regulatory proteins, designated G-proteins. These G-proteins mediate the signal transduction generated from the effect of adrenergic agents on their specific receptors (Fig. 1). G-proteins are composed of α-, β- and γ-subunits and have been extensively reviewed (1,2). G-protein–coupled receptors are changed in their conformation following β-adrenergic agonist binding, and GTP replaces GDP within the α-subunit on the G-protein. This results in a dissociation of the α-subunits from the β- and γ-subunits and, ultimately, is responsible for relaying the activity of the various effector systems. These effector systems include not only effects on adenylate cyclase and cAMP, but also several other systems, including effects on cyclic-GMP (cGMP) phosphodiesterase, ion channels,

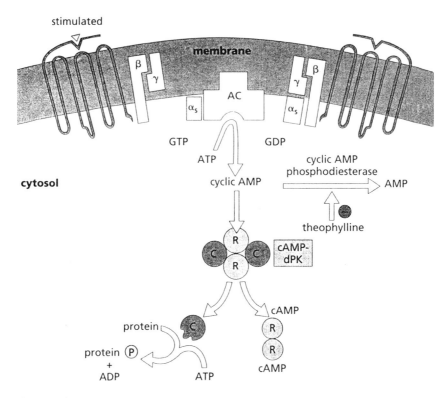

Figure 1 Activation of adenylate cyclase and protein kinases. The diagram shows two β-adrenergic receptor molecules, each of which is composed of three transmembrane loops. Stimulation of the receptor (left) causes its activation in which the α_s-unit of the heterotrimeric G_s-protein binds GTP and dissociates from the complex to the adenylate cyclase (AC) catalytic unit. Activated AC catalyzes the formation of cyclic AMP (cAMP), which binds to the regulatory units (R) of cAMP-dependent protein kinases (cAMP dPK), thus freeing the catalytic units (C) to phosphorylate specific proteins. The activated state exists only transiently, ATP hydrolysis to ADP leads to reassociation of the $\alpha_s\beta\gamma$-complex of G_s, inactivation of AC, receptor regeneration, and the breakdown of AMP by phosphodiesterases. (From Ref. 168.)

and phospholipases. These various changes result in various metabolic and ion changes within the cell or on the cell surface, which will have a variety of physiological consequences not only on airway smooth muscle, but also on the wide array of cells in the airway and the inflammatory cells associated with the allergic response (Table 1).

Molecular biology studies with molecular cloning and sequence analysis of genes encoding these G-proteins and the various subtypes of receptors, including β_1, β_2, β_3-adrenergic receptors, as well as α_{1A}, α_{1B}, α_{1C}, α_{2A}, α_{2B}, α_{2C}, and α_{2D}-adrenergic receptors, provide a much greater complexity, as well as a greater understanding, of the functional interaction among the various G-proteins and the various adrenergic receptors (Table 2).

These various adrenergic receptors all have in common seven membrane-spanning amino acid sequences. There is a high degree of homology among the various adrenergic receptor subtypes in terms of the amino acid sequences that span the transmembrane

Table 1 Cellular Effects of β_2-Adrenergic Receptor Stimulation

Cell	Response
Airway smooth muscle	Bronchodilation
Mast cells	Inhibition of mediator release
Eosinophils	Inhibition of mediator release and chemotaxis
Lymphocytes	Inhibition of activation
Skeletal muscle	Tremor
Metabolic	Hypokalemia, hyperglycemia
Mucous glands	Increased water content of mucus
Epithelial cells	Increased ciliary activity
Vascular endothelium	Decreased microvascular leakage
Alveolar type II cells	Increased surfactant secretion

domain in the seven α-helices of the receptors. The adrenergic receptors are, for the most part, glycoproteins.

The β_1-adrenergic receptors have a rank order of agonist potency of isoproterenol > epinephrine $\geq$ norepinephrine. The gene encoding the β_1-adrenergic receptor has been mapped to human chromosome 10q24–26 which happens to be the same region where the α_{2A}-adrenergic receptor gene is located. Interestingly, this enables one to test the hypothesis of cross-talk or interaction between the β_1-receptor that on stimulation increases adenylate cyclase, and the α_2-adrenergic receptor that would decrease adenylate cyclase.

The gene for the β_2-adrenergic receptor has been localized to human chromosome 5q31–32, which is the same region as that for the α_{1B}-receptor. This could result in physiological antagonism if there were some genetic defect in asthma at the respective chromosomal sites. Thus, the interesting hypothesis that there could be an imbalance between the α- and β-adrenergic receptor functions in asthma may now be testable at the molecular and genetic level. Much less is known about the β_3-adrenergic receptor other than it has a much lower

Table 2 Pharmacological Properties and Tissue Distribution of Cloned Adrenergic Receptors

Receptor subtype	Tissue distribution	Agonists	Antagonists
α_{1A}-Adrenergic	Brain, vas deferens, heart, spleen	NE>Epi>PE	Praz>WB-4101
α_{1B}-Adrenergic	Lung, brain, heart, liver, kidney, spleen	Oxy>Epi>NE	Praz>WB-4101
α_{1C}-Adrenergic	Dentate gyrus	Oxy>Epi>NE	Praz$\geq$WB-4101
α_{2A}-Adrenergic	Brain, platelets	p-AC>UK[>]t Epi	Yoh>Praz
α_{2B}-Adrenergic	Kidney, neonatal lung	Clon>NE>Oxy	Yoh>Praz
α_{2C}-Adrenergic	Kidney	Oxy>NE	Ida>Praz
α_{2D}-Adrenergic	Brain, kidney, salivary gland	Oxy>Epi>NE	Ida>Phent
β_1-Adrenergic	Brain, heart, pineal gland	Iso>Epi$\geq$NE	Betax>ICI 118,551
β_2-Adrenergic	Lung, prostate	Iso>Epi>NE	ICI 118,551>Betax
β_3-Adrenergic known	Adipose tissue	BRL37344>Iso	No high-affinity antagonists

Source: Ref. 2.
NE, norepinephrine; Epi, epinephrine; PE, phenylephrine; Oxy, oxymetazoline; p-AC, paraaminoclonidine, Clon; clonidine; Praz, prazosin; Yoh, yohimbine; Phent, phentolamine; Betax, betaxolol.

affinity for β-adrenergic antagonists and for catecholamine agonists and appears to play a functional role in tissues, such as muscle and adipocytes, with a particular distribution to brown and white adipose tissue. It now appears that once the adrenergic receptor has been activated, then several effector mechanisms can be activated, in contrast with previously held views in which a single receptor was thought to activate a single pathway, such as stimulation of adenylate cyclase. This results in a much greater fine-tuning of the autonomic responses and a greater complexity of the physiological events that can occur.

REGULATION OF ADRENERGIC RECEPTORS

It has long been recognized that glucocorticoids produce a marked increase in the β-adrenergic receptor density in lung cells (3,4). It is now recognized that this increase in β-receptors by corticosteroids is due to an increase in the level of a receptor-specific mRNA, and the genes for the β-adrenergic receptors contain DNA-binding sites for glucocorticoid receptors (5). The effect of β-adrenergic agents on β-receptors and the desensitization of the receptors that occurs have important implications in the therapy of asthma, particularly in the use of potent long-acting β-agonists. This effect is very germane to the controversy of the regular use of β-agonists versus an intermittent or demand basis. This prolonged exposure of β-receptors results in receptor phosphorylation and is associated with impaired receptor–G protein coupling (6). Lefkowitz's group (6) have also reported that phosphorylation of β-receptors by prolonged exposure to β-agonist may increase their internalization from the cell surface and, therefore, make them unavailable for activation by β-adrenergic agonists.

The identification of a cAMP-independent, β-adrenergic receptor kinase has been identified (βARK) (7). This βARK results in agonist-specific or homologous desensitization of the receptor. The activation of protein kinases A and C (PKA and PKC) provide feedback mechanisms of desensitization following activation of adenylate cyclase, by a variety of mechanisms, including histamine acting through H_2-receptors or prostaglandin (PG)E with stimulation of adenylate cyclase and protein kinase. This type of regulation, known as heterologous desensitization, may be an important mechanism in the decreased cAMP response that occurs in the lymphocytes of asthmatics following allergen challenge and the associated late reaction with airway hyperresponsiveness, as reported by Meurs and Kauffman (8). At the cellular level, this heterologous desensitization has been demonstrated in various in vitro preparations (9,10). The tremendous advance in understanding the various diverse types of adrenergic receptors at their genetic and molecular biological level provides important opportunities to bring these advances into the clinic in terms of autonomic deregulation in asthma and the interaction of the inflammatory response as a result of the allergic reaction.

INTERACTION OF α- AND β-ADRENERGIC MECHANISMS

Further studies involving the autonomous imbalance in asthma can address the controversy over the role of adrenergic receptors in this disorder. The administration of an α-agonist, such as methoxamine, provokes airway narrowing (11,12). α-Adrenergic responsiveness, following administration of phenylephrine, was increased only in asthmatic patients compared with normal subjects and allergic rhinitis subjects (13). Studies of the skin, pupil, and blood pressure by several investigators (13–16) provide evidence of increased α- and decreased β-adrenergic function in asthmatic subjects. Although α-adrenergic-blocking agents have not shown clinical efficacy in the treatment of asthma, they have shown some protection against exercise-induced asthma, as well as cold air challenges, but have no effect on the airway response to inhaled histamine or ragweed (17).

The presence of α-adrenergic receptors on human airways has been tested in the presence of β-adrenergic-blocking agents to avoid the contribution of β-receptor stimulation that could have a counterregulatory effect. In testing human trachea in vitro, the human tracheal smooth muscle was contracted by epinephrine in the presence of propranolol. (18) (Fig. 2). In the presence of hydrocortisone or the α-adrenergic blockers, phentolamine and phenoxybenzamine, the contracting effect of epinephrine was reduced or abolished (18). In patients with chronic obstructive lung disease (COPD), airway smooth muscle shows a greater direct responsiveness to α-agonist than airways from normal individuals (19). Normal individuals showed only α-adrenergic contraction of the smooth muscle when the smooth muscle was already partially depolarized by histamine or potassium chloride. Thus, it appears that if the airway smooth muscle is partially depolarized, the effect of an α-agonist on contraction is enhanced.

The well-known observation that β-adrenergic-blocking agents adversely affect asthmatic subjects could be related to an increased α-adrenergic responsiveness, as a result of airway inflammation (19). The potential cross-talk between α- and β-adrenergic receptors may also exist between α- and muscarinic receptors. Thus, methoxamine-induced bronchoconstriction is inhibited by ipratropium bromide and by cromolyn, which suggests involvement of cholinergic neurotransmission in bronchoconstriction induced by the α-agonist, methoxamine (12).

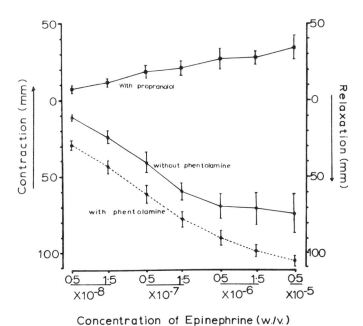

Figure 2   Effect of epinephrine on human tracheal relaxation response. Relaxation was expressed as response to epinephrine alone and to epinephrine in the presence of the α-adrenergic-blocking agent phentolamine. When propranolol was added to the bath, the response to epinephrine resulted in contraction. The vertical lines represent the standard errors of the mean.

α_2-Adrenergic receptors are present in human airways and may mediate an inhibition of cholinergic neurotransmission at the parasympathetic ganglia or on postganglionic parasympathetic nerve endings. Clonidine, which is an α_2-adrenergic agonist, when inhaled, will inhibit allergen-induced bronchoconstriction in patients with allergic asthma. This effect has been interpreted to be related to the α_2-adrenergic receptor regulation of vagal excitatory nerve activity (20).

Several investigators have shown that antigen challenge in sensitized guinea pigs results in a diminution of the β_2-receptor and an increase in the α_1-receptor in lungs of animals exposed to a specific antigen (21,22). Additional studies, done in sheep sensitized and challenged with a specific antigen, demonstrate an alteration of the pharmacological response in the airway smooth muscle. The relaxation induced by isoproterenol was reduced, and the normal relaxing response of epinephrine was converted to contraction in airways of sensitized animals (23,24). Thus, the possibility exists that in the asthmatic patients, following repeated exposure to allergens, the inflammatory response that occurs may be associated with an increased α- and decreased β-receptor activity. The observation that α-antagonists, phentolamine and thymoxamine, restore the capacity of leukocytes from asthmatics to synthesize cAMP in response to a β-receptor agonist is consistent with this hypothesis (25,26) The use of newer antihypertensive agents, such as celiprolol, which has β_1-receptor blocking activity, as well as α_2-receptor antagonist properties, did not cause airway obstruction in asthmatics, nor did it block the bronchodilating action of terbutaline. In contrast, propranolol caused bronchoconstriction and blocked the bronchodilating effect of terbutaline in these same subjects (27).

SITE-DIRECTED MUTAGENESIS

The technique of site-directed mutagenesis has been valuable in understanding the structure and function of receptors. One example is replacement of cystine residues at the positions 106 and 184 in the second and third extracellular domains in the hamster lung β_2-receptor. Impairment of the β-receptor ligand-binding affinity occurs with substitution of either of these cystine residues with isoleucine (28). A marked reduction in the binding affinity and coupling to adenylate cyclase occurs with substitution of either of the adjacent cystine residues at positions 190 and 191 on the third cytoplasmic loop of the human β_2-receptor (29). Site-directed mutagenesis can affect agonist-binding affinity but not G_s activation. Deletion mutagenesis studies in which stretches of the amino acid sequence are removed indicate that the third intracellular loop is critical for interaction between β_2-adrenergic receptors (β_2-ARs) and G_s (30).

Recent studies show that there are at least six different polymorphic forms of β_2-ARs. Although these mutations are not the primary cause of asthma, they may account for some of the clinical heterogeneity among patients with asthma. Mutations of small regions, or even single amino acids, of the β_2-AR can affect receptor function. Liggett and associates recently attempted to determine whether such mutations occur and might be important in the pathogenesis of asthma or its response to therapy (31,32).

Reihaus et al. (31) developed a method of studying β_2-AR mutations. This method involved identifying a single amino acid deviation from the wild-type β_2-AR–coding sequence, using temperature gradient gel electrophoresis (31). The lymphocytes of 56 healthy persons and 51 patients with moderately severe asthma were used to isolate the genomic DNA.

The distribution of β_2-AR mutations in the two populations studied is shown in Figure 3 (32). Darkened residues indicate the nine regions of DNA mutations, there were no changes

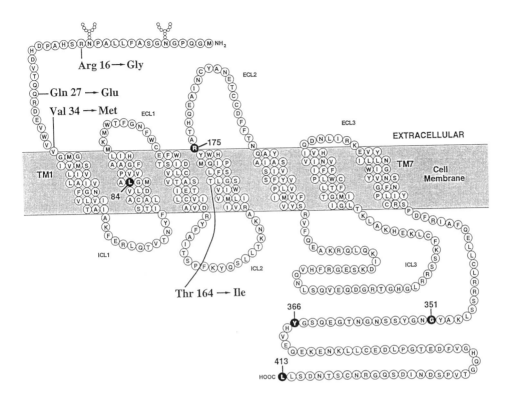

Figure 3 Adrenergic receptor mutations found in patients with and without asthma are illustrated. The darkened circles indicate where nucleic acid changes were detected. Regions of amino acid change ("missense mutations") are indicated by the amino acid substitutions (for example, Ag-16 → Gly). Of the nine mutations found, five resulted in no amino acid changes, whereas four resulted in changes in the encoded residues indicated at amino acid positions 16, 27, 34, and 164. ECL1–ECL3 denote extracellular loops 1–3, and ICL1–ICL3 denote intracellular loops. TM1 and TM7 denote transmembrane segments 1 and 7. (From Ref. 32.)

in the encoded amino acids at five of these codons. However, four mutations did cause changes in the encoded residues. These mutations are indicated at amino acid positions 16, 27, 34, and 164. There was no difference between patients with asthma and the controls in the distribution frequency of both homozygous and heterozygous polymorphisms in this group. Liggett and colleagues did notice, however, a clustering of patients with ARG-16 to Gly polymorphism in 75% of patients who were corticosteroid-dependent—defined as the need for prednisone 20 mg/day for more than 6 months. These authors then compared this mutated receptor with the wild-type β_2-AR and found several abnormalities (33).

One such abnormality of this Gly-16 polymorphism of the β_2-AR mutation that results in enhanced down-regulation of receptor number, is its overrepresentation in patients with nocturnal asthma (34). This frequency of the Gly-16 allele was 80.4% in the nocturnal group as compared with 52.2% in the nonnocturnal asthma group ($p = 0.007$).

Liggett and colleagues, in a study of 65 patients with asthma (35), also reported an association of Glu-27 β_2-adrenergic receptor polymorphism, with a fourfold lower airway reactivity to methacholine compared with the wild-type Gln-27 genotype.

In a study of 17 normal and 47 asthmatic subjects, Turki and Liggett (36) found β_2-AR autoantibodies in 5% of normal subjects and about 40% of asthmatic subjects. Although these authors have not reported an association of these autoantibodies with genetic polymorphism of the β_2-receptor, they did observe a 40% inhibition of binding to β_2-receptor and a 50% attenuation of isoproterenol-stimulated cAMP production by these β_2-AR antibodies. Because only 40% of asthmatic subjects had antibodies to the β_2-AR, they felt that it was unlikely that such antibodies played a causal role in asthma. However, the therapeutic response in such persons to β_2 agonists might be reduced.

The Thr-164 to Ile-164 mutation resulted in receptor-bound agonists that had hydroxyl groups on their β-carbons and had affinities for β-agonists about four times lower than that of the wild-type. This decreased binding of catecholamines resulted in significant impairment of agonist-promoted signal transduction. The effect of epinephrine on the stimulation of adenylate cyclase was decreased about 50% in the Thr-164 to Ile-164 polymorphism.

The foregoing data suggest that several different forms of β_2-AR are found in persons with and without asthma, and that mutation of β_2-AR are not the primary cause of asthma. However, it is conceivable that the severity of asthma or its response to therapy may differ according to the β_2-AR genotype, as evidenced by the differences in agonist binding, agonist activation of the receptor, or agonist-mediated regulation of the receptor.

Corticosteroids prevent the desensitization and down-regulation of β-receptors on human leukocytes (37). Corticosteroids increase the level of β_2-receptor mRNA in cultured hamster smooth-muscle cells, which suggests that steroids increase β-receptor density by increasing the rate of gene transcription (38).

There is evidence that β-receptors may be abnormal or have decreased function in the airways of patients with asthma, and this may be due to uncoupling of receptors owing to phosphorylation by activation of protein kinase C that is stimulated through inflammatory-mediated receptors (39,40). The understanding of the structure and function of receptors in the lungs of asthmatic subjects will most likely be markedly improved through the results of new developments in molecular biology. The further understanding of receptor function and structure will be important in the development of new drugs that interact with the transcriptional or posttranslational formation of receptors.

THE ROLE OF COUPLING β-RECEPTORS TO ION CHANNELS AND RELAXATION OF AIRWAY SMOOTH MUSCLE

It is not commonly appreciated by most physicians that stimulation of β_2-adrenergic receptors causes hyperpolarization of airway smooth muscle and inhibits tension (41). β-Agonist bronchodilators increase membrane conductance of potassium, as evidenced by the observation that potassium channel blockers inhibit the hyperpolarization (42). The application of β-agonist to tracheal smooth-muscle cells results in the stimulation of calcium-activated potassium channels (43). Stimulation of β-adrenergic receptors activates K_{Ca} channels by a second messenger, which results in phosphorylation of the channel protein and the opening of the potassium channel (44). The K_{Ca} channels are an important mechanism by which β-adrenergic receptors relax airway smooth muscles (45; see Chap. 23).

β-Adrenergic receptors are also directly coupled to K_{Ca} channels through the guanine–nucleotide-binding protein. It is important to remember that this is only one of several mechanisms involved in adrenergic inhibition of contracted airway smooth muscle. Other mechanisms include inhibition of inositol triphosphate (IP$_3$) formation and calcium release. Similarly the inhibition of membrane voltage-dependent calcium channels may be an additional regulatory mechanism.

THE ACTION OF G-PROTEINS IN AIRWAY SMOOTH MUSCLE AND ASTHMA

The G-proteins are composed of three subunits: α-, β-, and a γ-subunit. The structure and functional diversity of G-protein α-subunits is illustrated in Table 3. The G-protein $\beta\gamma$-subunits appear to play a role in attaching G-proteins to the plasma membrane. However, the $\beta\gamma$-subunits also appear to be involved with effector activity, including adenylate cyclase and phospholipase A$_2$ (PLA$_2$) (46). One example is the effect of allergic inflammation or production of cytokines interleukin (IL)-1β or tumor necrosis factor (TNF)-α on decreased responses to isoproterenol in association with increased production of G$_i$ protein. The guanine regulatory protein G$_i$ inhibits adenylate cyclase.

One hypothesis for the increased sensitivity of airway smooth muscle to contractile agonist could be the reduced sensitivity of β-adrenergic-receptor-induced excitation–contraction uncoupling in the airway of asthmatic subjects. This could be a consequence of aberrant G-protein regulation of adenylate cyclase (47). These authors have postulated that G$_s$ is a substrate for phosphorylation by protein kinase C, and this phosphorylation is likely to elicit a profound inhibitory effect on subsequent GTP-stimulated adenylate cyclase activity. Because of the increased number and activity of inflammatory cells in airways of asthmatics, this could result in releasing mediators capable of activating protein kinase C which, in turn, would phosphorylate G$_s$ and, subsequently, alter agonist-stimulated adenylate cyclase (see Fig. 4; 47). These authors hypothesized that, in asthmatic airways, there could be a decreased expression of G$_s$ because of its down-regulation, and there would be less G$_s$ available to couple to receptors. An analogous situation could exist in cardiac muscle for which prolonged treatment of heart myocytes with a β-agonist leads to down-regulation of G$_s$ caused by inhibition of mRNA translation in the protein and a coincident upregulation of G$_i$ (48). Thus, a possible mechanism for a decreased activity of β-agonist following prolonged use can be due to down-regulation of G-protein in cells. Thus, the introduction of a long-acting β_2-receptor agonist in the treatment of asthma could lead to homologous down-regulation by such agonists. Similarly, the heterologous down-regulation of G$_s$ in response to a variety of biological mediators as a result of the allergic

Table 3 Structural and Functional Diversity of G-Protein α-Subunits

G-protein type	Forms	Function
G$_s$ (45/52 kDa)	4 forms	Stimulates adenylate cyclase, activates Ca^{2+} channels
G$_i$ (41 kDa)	3 forms	Inhibits adenylate cyclase, activates K$^+$ channels, activates phospholipase C
G$_o$ (39 kDa)	2 forms	Regulates Ca^{2+} channels
G$_q$ (43 kDa)	6 forms	Activates phospholipase C
G$_z$ (42 kDa)	1 form	Unknown function
G$_t$ (39 kDa)	2 forms	Activates cGMP phosphodiesterase
G$_s$ olf (45 kDa)	1 form	Activates olfactory adenylate cyclase

Source: Ref. 47.

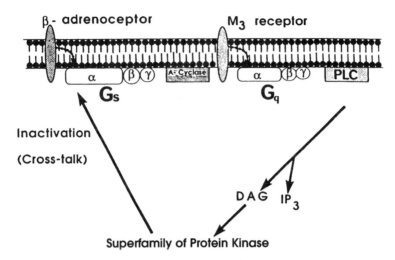

Figure 4 Schematic representation of the molecular cross-talk between cAMP and PtdIns(4,5)P$_2$ signal cascades; leading to protein kinase C activation and phosphorylation of G$_{s\alpha}$. In asthma, such an event may lead to reduced β-adrenergic receptor sensitivity in airway smooth muscle. DAG, diacylglycerol; IP$_3$, inositol triphosphate. (From Ref. 47.)

inflammatory process could result in a decreased response to bronchodilators. Support for involvement of G-protein studies in asthma comes from the work of Meurs et al. (49). These investigators evaluated the regulation of the β-receptor–adenylate cyclase system in lymphocytes of allergic patients with asthma and the possible role of protein kinase C in allergen-induced nonspecific refractoriness of adenylate cyclase. Thus, lymphocytes of allergic individuals, obtained after a late reaction induced with an allergen challenge, showed a decreased adenylate cyclase activity, as well as G_s-protein responses to β-agonist, prostaglandin E, and GTP analogues.

At least three mechanisms may be involved in relaxation of airway smooth muscle. One is mediated by elevation of tissue cAMP content either by β-receptor activation or prostaglandin E stimulation of adenylate cyclase or by inhibiting the breakdown of cAMP with phosphodiesterase inhibitors. The second mechanism is the elevation of tissue cGMP by agents, such as nitric oxide or atrial natriuretic peptide. The third mechanism of relaxation is mediated by direct action of drugs on ion channels, including voltage-operated calcium channel antagonists, which have a relatively weak effect, and potassium channel activators. It has also become apparent that there is significant cross-talk between second-messenger pathways involving relaxation through the adenylate cyclase path and inositol phospholipid as a result of its formation in airway inflammatory cells and airway smooth muscle. An example of this interrelation is the report that histamine-induced inositol phosphate formation could be inhibited by β$_2$-adrenoceptor agonist in tracheal smooth muscle of animals (50). Since patients with asthma are very sensitive to inhalation of histamine and since histamine is increased in the airway of asthmatics and contributes to increased airway tone, it would seem potentially beneficial to inhibit its formation with long-acting β$_2$-agonists.

Potential mechanisms mediating cAMP-induced airway smooth-muscle relaxation directly or indirectly involve and result from a reduction in intracellular calcium. The clinical effect of continuous use of β-adrenergic agents and their mechanisms involved in airway smooth-muscle relaxation are the source of controversy. Since β-adrenergic-blocking agents, including inhalation of propranolol, cause bronchoconstriction in asthmatics, but not in normal subjects, and since β-agonists have a striking effect in relieving asthmatic bronchoconstriction, it has been suggested that there might be a defect in the β-adrenergic receptor function in asthma (51). Several possible abnormalities involving adrenergic control have been proposed by Barnes et al. (52). Human airways apparently do not show functional adrenergic nerves to control airways smooth muscle; however, adrenergic nerves do influence cholinergic neurotransmission by prejunctional β-receptors (53,54). Adrenergic nerves do not directly control human airway smooth muscle; therefore, it seems probable that circulating catecholamines would have a primary role in regulating bronchomotor tone. However, even during acute exacerbations of asthma, there does not appear to be elevation of plasma epinephrine. Since several studies have demonstrated that airways from asthmatic patients fail to relax normally to isoproterenol, this suggests a possible defect in β-receptor function in airway smooth muscle (39,40,55). Still to be resolved is whether this is due to a quantitative or qualitative abnormality in β-receptors, or to some abnormality in receptor coupling or in the biochemical pathways leading to relaxation (56). In a study by Bai et al. (40), the density of β-receptors of airways smooth muscle from asthmatic subjects was normal, thereby suggesting that a defect in the coupling of the β-receptors is a more likely mechanism.

FUNCTION AND LOCATION OF β-ADRENERGIC RECEPTOR IN THE TARGET TISSUE OF ASTHMA

It is conceivable that the synthesis and release of platelet-activating factor (PAF) and certain cytokines as a result of the allergic response could cause a further derangement of autonomic function by decreasing the β-adrenergic and increasing the cholinergic response in the airways (57).

The bronchodilating β-adrenergic receptor activity is determined by the β-adrenergic-receptor function and circulating catecholamines. Szentivanyi (51) postulated that bronchial asthma might be partly due to impaired β-adrenergic-receptor function. A decrease in such receptor function can result either from exogenously administered β-antagonist or from exposure to allergens, resulting in a late bronchial reaction. In a guinea pig model of asthma, several investigators have observed down-regulation of β-adrenergic receptors and an up-regulation of α-receptors (21,22,58). In patients with bronchial asthma, the lymphocyte β-adrenergic-receptor density was reduced after an allergen-induced asthmatic reaction (8,59,60). Relaxation of human central and peripheral airways is mediated by the β_2-adrenergic receptors (61,62). The density of these receptors progressively increases from the trachea to the terminal bronchials, as demonstrated by autoradiography (63). Distribution of the subtypes of β-adrenergic receptors in the airway is consistent with the hypothesis that the β_2-receptors are regulated by circulating epinephrine and the β_1-receptors by sympathetic nerves.

Density, as well as the affinity, of β-receptors was significantly higher in bovine epithelial membranes than in bovine tracheal smooth muscle (64). If the airway epithelium is damaged, this results in increased bronchial reactivity. This is consistent with the finding that isoproterenol is a more potent relaxant in the presence of intact airway epithelium and less potent when the epithelium has been damaged, for example, by eosinophils, as occurs in clinical asthma or in the late reaction (65). Damage or partial denudation of the airway epithelium results in a loss of epithelial-derived relaxant factor (EDRF) (66). As stated, the loss of epithelium also results in the loss of β_2-adrenergic receptors and is consistent with the decreased response to β_2-agonists in inflamed airway mucosa, as occurs in the late reaction. With intact airway epithelium the β-adrenergic receptors maintain the integrity of tight junctions and thereby regulate the ion and fluid transport across epithelial cells. β_2-adrenergic receptors increase cAMP levels, and cAMP regulates the permeability of epithelial tight junctions.

Autoradiographic studies show a high density of β-adrenergic receptors in airway glands, and the submucosal glands were primarily of the β_2-subtype. Stimulating β_2-adrenergic receptors increases mucociliary clearance and increases the beat frequency of the respiratory tract ciliated cells (67).

Human alveolar macrophages obtained by bronchial alveolar lavage (BAL) contain about 5600 β_2-adrenergic receptors, with a K_D of about 29 pM (68). Stimulation of these β_2-receptors with isoproterenol results in a sixfold increase in cAMP production. The effect of β_2-adrenergic-receptor agonist in asthma may also be related to their effect on alveolar macrophages, since macrophages contain several mediators, including leukotriene (LT) B_4, LTC_4, platelet-activating factor (PAF), interleukin (IL)-1, tumor necrosis factor (TNF), and superoxide anions, as well as hydrogen peroxide. All of these mediators, as well as fibronectin-mediated phagocytosis and phagocytosis of immune complexes, can be modulated by cAMP. An increase in cAMP through activation of the β_2-receptors may inhibit migration and release of lysosomal enzymes and mediators from alveolar macrophages (69,70).

In addition to their potent effects on airway smooth muscle, β-adrenergic agonists regulate many aspects of lung function. These effects include inhibition of mast cell degranulation, regulation of fluid and ion transport across epithelial cells, and inhibition of microvascular permeability (71; see Table 1).

In the late-phase reaction of bronchial asthma, the recruitment of inflammatory cells to the airways could be influenced by β-adrenergic agonists. Margination and the appearance of neutrophils can be attenuated by β-adrenergic agents in vitro. The inflammatory process with the release of oxygen radicals and lytic enzymes from neutrophils and eosinophils, as well as alveolar macrophages, may be under β-adrenergic control. Recently, Okada et al. (72) observed that in the late-phase reaction, formoterol was very effective not only in inhibiting the number of eosinophils and macrophages, but in inhibiting the production of superoxide from eosinophils. The production of superoxide was markedly enhanced in eosinophils and macrophages in BAL cells 24 h after antigen challenge. Stimulation of these cells obtained by BAL with phorbol myristate acetate (PMA) or PAF was inhibited by pretreatment with formoterol, but not with isoproterenol. These changes are consistent with the therapeutic and anti-inflammatory effects of corticosteroids in leukocytes (73) and in the airways, where corticosteroids increase β-adrenergic responses (74) and decrease α-adrenergic responses (18).

THE EFFECT OF β-ADRENERGIC-BLOCKING AGENTS, DIMINISHED cAMP RESPONSE, AND AUTONOMIC DYSREGULATION

Two characteristic features of asthma are the known contraindications for the use of β-adrenergic-blocking agents and the diminished cAMP response to β-adrenergic agonists. It has long been recognized that β-adrenergic blockade accentuates the immediate response to an allergen, as well as to mediators that act directly on smooth muscle, such as histamine, methacholine, and serotonin (75). The effect of these agents on the late reaction has not been studied. Townley et al. (75) reported that β-adrenergic blockade increased the sensitivity to histamine, methacholine, and serotonin in guinea pigs and mice. However, in this same study β-adrenergic blockade had a much greater effect on the sensitivity to an antigen. This may be because β-adrenergic receptors are located on a wide variety of the target tissues of asthma and not just the airway smooth muscle.

β-Adrenergic hyporesponsiveness and cholinergic and α-adrenergic hyperresponsiveness have been implicated in the etiology and pathogenesis of asthma (71). However, other investigators interpret these changes as being secondary to the disease process, rather than to a primary determinant (76).

In asthmatic subjects, pretreatment with propranolol potentiates the bronchoconstriction caused by histamine (77), methacholine (78), acetylcholine (79), and cigarette smoke (80). However, in normal subjects, the bronchomotor response to methacholine (81) or to histamine (82) was not increased by pretreatment by propranolol. In contrast, subjects with allergic rhinitis, who were insensitive to methacholine, developed a transient sensitivity to methacholine and symptoms of asthma after propranolol inhalation (81). Inhalation of β-blockers alone has been used as a bronchoconstrictor challenge test in suspected asthmatic subjects. In propranolol-induced bronchoconstriction, it is believed that unopposed parasympathetic tone may be involved in propranolol bronchoconstriction, since atropine prevents and partially reverses this effect in patients with mild asthma (83).

EFFECT OF THE ALLERGIC REACTION AND PAF ON β-ADRENERGIC RESPONSES

Although β_2-agonists are by far the most potent agents in inhibiting and preventing the immediate allergic reaction, including mast cell mediator release, there is increasing evidence that mediators from eosinophils, macrophages, and lymphocytes, which are of primary importance in the late bronchial reaction, are also modulated by β_2-adrenergic receptors (84). It is, therefore, possible that an abnormality in β-adrenergic receptor function or of circulating catecholamines could contribute to airway hyperresponsiveness and perhaps contribute to the late bronchial reaction. The question of whether or not a defect in airway β-receptor function is present in bronchial asthma has not been answered conclusively (85). The effects of anaphylactic challenge on the sensitized guinea pig tracheal smooth muscle; the diminished relaxing effects of isoproterenol, prostaglandin E_2, and forskolin; but not of aminophylline, have been reported (85). These results suggest an impairment in the adenylate cyclase system in the airways after the anaphylactic reaction. These findings are also consistent with the results of Meurs et al. (59,60) in studying human peripheral blood lymphocytes 24 h after an antigen challenge and a late reaction. These investigators showed decreased cAMP response not only to β-agonist, but to nondegradable GTP analogues. Thus several independent laboratories provide evidence suggesting a decrease in the adenylate cyclase response and cAMP production following antigen challenge. Although several groups of investigators report altered adrenergic responsiveness and decreased number of β-adrenergic receptors in asthmatics (86–89), the evidence would indicate a defect beyond the β-receptor itself.

Several possible mechanisms for this decrease response as a result of antigen challenge can be postulated. The release of circulating catecholamines as a result of antigen challenge could conceivably result in a homologous down-regulation of β-adrenergic receptors. Alternatively, the synthesis of certain cytokines and mediators following the allergic reaction, including platelet-activating factor, could have an effect on β-adrenergic receptor function in the airways. Other investigators have also demonstrated that antigen challenge of sensitized guinea pigs in vivo resulted in diminished in vitro β-adrenergic receptor-mediated relaxation of airway smooth muscle (90). These investigators then studied the effect of proinflammatory cytokines TNF-α, IL-1β, or IL-2. None of these cytokines affected the contractile response of tracheas to carbamylcholine; however, the relaxation response to isoproterenol was significantly reduced by TNF-α and IL-1β, but not by IL-2. These observations led these authors to conclude that proinflammatory cytokines are able to result in diminished β-adrenergic receptor function, as seen in the antigen-challenged guinea pig model (Figs. 5 and 6; 90).

Two possible mechanisms include the induction of G_i-coupling protein or the induction of phospholipase A_2 (PLA_2). In endothelial cells IL-1β is able to produce increased mRNA levels for G_i proteins (91). The induction of G_i protein synthesis could cause a decreased β-adrenergic response by inhibiting adenylate cyclase. Alternatively, IL-1β and TNF-α are able to induce PLA_2 and increase production of lipid mediators, including PAF and leukotrienes. Phospholipase A_2 has been reported to reduce β-adrenergic responsiveness in experimental asthma (90).

Interleukin-1 causes the synthesis of PAF by vascular endothelial cells (92). Platelet-activating factor can cause bronchoconstriction, inflammation and edema, and chemotaxis of inflammatory cells, especially of eosinophils (57). Furthermore, PAF can activate eosinophils to release superoxide and leukotrienes, as well as activate basophils to release histamine and leukotrienes. In vivo incubation of human lung tissue with PAF decreases density of β-adrenergic receptors in human lung membranes (92,93). It has also been reported to induce a decrease in the density of β-receptors in other tissues (94). In functional studies of isolated trachea and lung parenchyma of guinea pig or human, PAF significantly reduced the potency of isoproterenol to reverse methacholine- or histamine-induced contraction. These changes were protected against by a specific PAF receptor antagonist BN52021 (92,93).

In our in vivo studies in guinea pigs, PAF aerosol potentiated the increase in specific airway resistance produced by methacholine. In contrast, the reversal of this airway obstruction by isoproterenol or prostaglandin E_2 was diminished (95). This decreased response to bronchodilators could lead to increase nonspecific airway hyperresponsiveness. However, PAF has been reported to activate PLA_2, and the PAF-induced desensitization of β-adrenergic receptor responses may also be due to an increase in PLA_2 activity (92).

Although these animal studies of PAF-induced airway hyperresponsiveness and decreased β-adrenergic responses suggest a possible role for PAF in asthma, recent studies in humans do not support this. A potent PAF antagonist WEB-2086 failed to protect against the antigen-induced late bronchial reaction in humans (96). This failure of the PAF antagonist to prevent the late reaction, in spite of other effects of the PAF antagonist WEB-2086 to inhibit platelet aggregation in these same subjects, provides strong evidence against the primary role of PAF in the late reaction.

Nevertheless, PAF, by decreasing the β-adrenergic receptor responsiveness in human airways, could contribute to the adrenergic imbalance, which could deprive the bronchial tissue of its normal counterregulatory bronchodilating effect. Sensitivity to antigen has been reported to be markedly increased in a variety of animal studies, as well as human studies, when the β-adrenergic receptors are blocked (51,75,78,82,97). Therefore, when histamine, leukotrienes, and other mediators are released as a result of the allergic reaction,

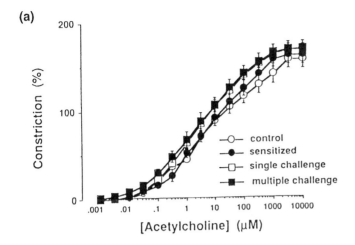

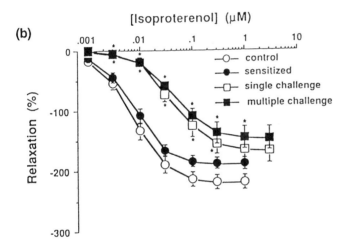

Figure 5 Constriction–relaxation responses of tracheas isolated from guinea pigs sensitized with ovalbumin. The constrictor response (a) to acetylcholine and (b) the relaxant response to isoproterenol after preconstruction with 0.1 μM ET-1 were isometrically measured using tracheas isolated from various animals: control (open circles), sensitized (closed circles), single-challenged (open squares), and multichallenged (closed squares) guinea pigs, according to the method described in the text. Relaxation was expressed as percentage of the constriction produced by 50 mM KCl, a nonreceptor-mediated constriction. (From Ref. 90.)

they are able to cause bronchoconstriction that may be at least partly unopposed by the usually intact β-receptors that normally serve to maintain bronchodilation.

β-Adrenergic receptor agonists and PAF can induce β-adrenergic receptor kinase (βARK) translocation in blood lymphocytes and suggests a functional role for the βARK mechanism of homologous receptor desensitization in immune cells (98). More recently these same investigators have demonstrated the expression of βARK and several G-protein–coupled receptor kinases that are actively and selectively modulated according to the functionary state of T lymphocytes and result in β-adrenergic homologous desensitization (99).

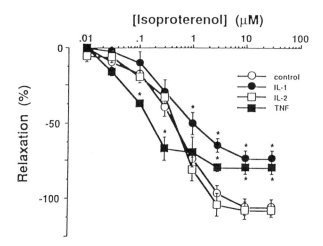

Figure 6 Effects of proinflammatory cytokines on isoproterenol-induced relaxation of cultured tracheas. Relaxation was expressed as percentage of the maximal contraction to carbamylcholine. Isoproterenol responses were studied after no exposure to cytokines (open circles $n = 12$) and incubation with IL-1β (4 ng/ml; closed circles, $n = 4$), IL-2 (0.2 μg/ml; open squares, $n = 4$), and TNF-α (0.1 μg/ml; closed squares, $n = 4$). Data were the means ± SEM. *The values marked were significantly different from the control value as determined by ANOVA ($p \leq 0.05$). (From Ref. 90.)

HOMOLOGOUS AND HETEROLOGOUS DOWN-REGULATION OF β-ADRENERGIC RESPONSIVENESS

The correlation between decreased β-adrenergic receptor function and disease severity (100,101) might be caused by repeated and prolonged release of endogenous catechol-amines, or by exogenous administration, resulting in a homologous down-regulation of β-adrenergic responsiveness. Alternatively, it could be a result of heterologous β-adrenergic down-regulation and hyporesponsiveness. Clearly, repeated and prolonged β-agonist treatment results in a marked decrease not only in the density of β-receptors, but also in the cAMP response (86,87,102). Nevertheless some investigators report decreased lymphocyte β-receptor density, as well as decreased β-adrenergic cAMP responsiveness of lympho-cytes in asthmatics who have not been taking a β2-agonist for at least 2 weeks (89,103).

Lymphocytes, particularly helper-type 2 T cells, play a primary role in orchestrating the immune response in the airways, including production of various lymphokines, such as interleukins 3, 4, and 5, which are very important in mast cell, basophil, and eosinophil growth and differentiation. Future studies comparing physiological effects of β-agonists on the release of these lymphokines, as well as the effect of IL-1 and TNF-α on β-adrenergic receptors could be very important in understanding the interaction of β-receptors with cytokines.

DESENSITIZATION OF β-ADRENERGIC RECEPTORS

Desensitization of β-adrenergic receptors can result from (1) loss of β-receptors (104), (2) loss of high-affinity receptors (105), or (3) loss of physiological response, without loss of β-receptors. Uncoupling or reduction in density of β-receptors after catecholamine exposure in human neutrophils has been reported by Davies and Lefkowitz (106). Uncoupling of β-receptors in lymphocytes without down-regulation, caused by the change of posture from supine to ambulation, has been demonstrated by Feldman et al. (107). More recently, Collins and Lefkowitz reported that mutation of human β-adrenergic receptors results in marked uncoupling of the β-receptor with the G-protein and decreased adenylate cyclase responsiveness (108). In patients with atopic dermatitis, desensitization of the cAMP system in lymphocytes has been reported (109), as well as heterologous desensitization in granulocytes of patients with bronchial asthma (110). Alternatively, a decreased cAMP response could result from elevated phosphodiesterase activity (111,112). The role of the various subtypes of phosphodiesterase and their inhibitors, particularly in inflammatory cells, such as the eosinophil and alveolar macrophage in asthma, has been recently reviewed (113,114). The development of specific phosphodiesterase IV inhibitors potentially has very significant therapeutic advantages over theophylline (115; see Chap. 22).

THE EFFECT OF CORTICOSTEROIDS ON β-ADRENERGIC RESPONSES

The effect of glucocorticoids on pulmonary β-adrenergic receptors and responses suggests an important role for glucocorticoids to increase β-adrenergic receptors and responsiveness (4). This is in addition to the anti-inflammatory effects of corticosteroids. Glucocorticoids lower the threshold of relaxation response of β-adrenergic receptors and inhibit the α-adrenergic contractile response to catecholamines in isolated tracheas from humans and guinea pigs (18,74). The homologous down-regulation and decreased responsiveness to β-adrenergic agonist induced by prolonged treatment with β-agonist drugs can be reversed by glucocorticoid hormones in airways of normal (116) and asthmatic subjects (117). Glucocorticoids also potentiate the stimulation of adenylate cyclase by β-adrenergic agonists in human leukocytes (118) and canine tracheal smooth muscle (119). We observed that oral prednisone, 15 mg tid for 5 days, showed a significant increase in the density of leukocyte β-receptors beginning on day 2, without a significant change in the dissociation constant. Pulmonary function improved, granulocyte cAMP doubled, and the increased neutrophil and decreased eosinophil and lymphocyte count changed as expected (120). Furthermore, in animal studies, the density of β-receptors in the lung increased by 70% after prolonged administration of hydrocortisone (4). Adrenalectomy produced the opposite effect, with a 29% fall in the density of β-receptors, without altering the affinity for β-receptors. These findings suggest that glucocorticoids potentiate β-adrenergic receptor stimulation at lest partly by increasing β-receptor density. Glucocorticoids also increase adrenergic responsiveness (121) and the density of β-receptors (122) in human lung cells in culture.

THE CONTROVERSY OVER CONTINUOUS USE OF β-ADRENERGIC AGONISTS

The current and recurrent controversy of the use of inhaled self-administered high doses of β-agonist drugs by patients with asthma before they are admitted to the hospital or die, underlines the basis for some degree of confusion in the minds of the public, as well as of physicians, whether the fatal or near fatal attacks are due to undertreatment or to overtreatment (123–129). A report in the lay press, including the *New York Times*, August 11, 1991, stated that patients dying from bronchial asthma were using up to twice the recommended number of inhalations per month of the inhaled β-agonist before death. This has led to confusion among physicians and patients about whether they should use their β-agonist in times of severe asthma.

The question of increased mortality from asthma as a result of undertreatment versus overtreatment is particularly important, because of the recent availability of powerful new long-acting inhaled β-agonists. Although there has been extensive investigation into the recent increase in asthma deaths in the United States (130), as well as in the United Kingdom and in New Zealand (125, 131), the cause of the increasing number of deaths caused by asthma is still undetermined. It has been argued that the overuse of β-agonist drugs may lead to temporary relief of symptoms, without treating the underlying inflammatory process, and may result in the delayed administration of oxygen and lifesaving anti-inflammatory corticosteroids (129,132,133).

The observation that regular treatment with isoproterenol (134) and fenoterol (135) is associated with worsening of asthma and a predisposition to increased risk of life-threatening attack led these authors to suggest that overtreatment with these agents is detrimental.

The role of cardiotoxicity, particularly in the presence of hypoxemia, although demonstrated in animals (136), has been difficult to assess in patients presenting themselves with life-threatening attacks of asthma. The study by Molfino et al. (123) attempts to address this question. These authors evaluated ten asthmatic patients with respiratory arrest and analyzed their clinical and laboratory characteristics. They concluded that undertreatment, evidenced by severe asphyxia and hypoxia, rather than overtreatment, is one of the major factors involved in the increased number of deaths from asthma. Molfino et al. suggest that asphyxia, rather than cardiac complication of bronchodilator therapy, is the cause for the overwhelming majority of deaths secondary to bronchial asthma in young and middle-aged patients.

The debate of the beneficial versus detrimental effects of the powerful new long-acting β_2-agonists has received considerable attention since the report of worsening of asthma from regular use of β_2-agonists by Sears et al. (135). These investigators reported that on-demand inhaled bronchodilator therapy was more effective than regular use of inhaled bronchodilator therapy. Fenoterol 0.2 mg/dose or a matched placebo was inhaled four times daily for 24 weeks. Of the 64 patients who completed the trial, the results favored regular use of placebo over regular use of fenoterol. The placebo-treated group showed a higher percentage of subjects who were able to reduce the need for oral prednisone, had lower bronchial reactivity, reported fewer nocturnal or daytime symptoms, had higher morning peak flow recordings, and had better overall control. Five of the six sever exacerbations requiring hospitalization occurred in the group on regular fenoterol. In the overall study, 17 had better control while on fenoterol four times a day, whereas 40 patients showed better control of asthma during placebo treatment.

The mechanism behind why regular use of β-agonist could worsen asthma is unknown; however, Sears and colleagues speculate that patients protected by regular use of β_2-agonist may tolerate higher exposure to allergens and thus early allergic response may be blunted, but not the late response.

It has long been recognized that the severity of asthma is associated with the degree of airway reactivity (137). It is the late response that is associated with increased airway reactivity. This association has been recently emphasized (138).

The regular use of inhaled β-agonist has been reported (139) to result in a mild increase in airway reactivity. However, the clinical relevance of this has been questioned. In fact, the new long-acting β_2-agonist salmeterol actually decreased airway reactivity and completely protected against the late bronchial reaction (140). The argument has not yet been settled, and the current availability of long-acting β_2-agonists has served to heighten the controversy.

TOLERANCE AND CONTINUOUS USE OF β-ADRENERGIC AGONISTS

The homologous down-regulation of β-adrenergic responses in leukocytes with continued use of β_2-agonists raises the question of whether the long-acting β_2-agonist will only further down-regulate these β-adrenergic responses. Whether these agents will be beneficial or detrimental will ultimately be assessed at the clinical level. However, prolonged administration of β_2-agonists in asthmatic subjects usually results in no diminution of the peak bronchodilating effect. More apparent is a shortening of the duration of the bronchodilation (141,142). There is no indication that long-term treatment with salmeterol or formoterol results in tolerance to their bronchodilating effect in asthma. Of some concern, however, is the finding that regular treatment with salmeterol for 4 and 8 weeks resulted in significant tolerance to its protective effect against the bronchoconstrictor stimulus of methacholine (143). This occurred without any evidence of tolerance to its bronchodilating effect. The authors suggest that the reduced protection against methacholine might be caused by tolerance to the functional antagonism by salmeterol. The clinical implication is that patients receiving regular monotherapy with a β_2-agonist may become more susceptible to an acute bronchoconstricting stimulus. Consequently, it has been advocated to use inhaled corticosteroids to prevent this tolerance to the protective effect of a long-acting β_2-agonist.

Tolerance to the protective effect of inhaled terbutaline against the bronchoconstrictive effect of AMP was even greater than for methacholine (144). Because allergens and AMP act on mast cells to release mediators, whereas methacholine acts directly on airway smooth muscle, these authors (144) concluded that regular use of β_2-agonists may result in increased acute bronchoconstriction from inhaled allergens. Nelson and colleagues (145) discussed whether regular use of inhaled fenoterol has a greater potential to down-regulate the number of β-adrenergic receptors than other commonly used β_2-agonists. These authors argue that Sears and colleagues (135) studied only fenoterol, and their report failed to provide any quantitative data in terms of the percentage of patients showing better control during administration of fenoterol by demand, rather than on a regular basis. Nevertheless, Sears et al. reported that of the 26 patients who developed a significant increase in bronchial responsiveness to methacholine 22 were more responsive with regular use of fenoterol (135).

The fact that nocturnal asthma was worse in the subjects receiving continuous fenoterol is consistent with other findings (146): patients with nocturnal asthma, as opposed to asthmatics without nocturnal asthma, had a decrease in their leukocyte β-adrenergic receptor density at 4:00 A.M., and this was accompanied by an impaired response to β-adrenergic stimulation (146).

In contrast with the work of Sears et al. (135), Sheppard and co-workers (147) found that the use of albuterol, two puffs four times a day, was clearly better than treatment with placebo. Similarly, the mean daily peak flow rates, as well as morning peak flows, were better in the albuterol treatment phase (147). In another study (148), subjects treated with albuterol, two puffs four times a day, had more symptoms during the night, particularly 4 h after the last inhalation of albuterol, than did patients treated with long-acting theophylline alone or a combination of long-acting theophylline and albuterol four times a day. Other studies (149,150) have reported results opposite those of Sears and colleagues. The patients studied by VanderWalker (150) were maintained on theophylline throughout the study; however, for the 2-week period that they received inhaled terbutaline, they did better than when taking a matching placebo in terms of all major variables, such as asthma control, use of as-needed inhaled bronchodilator, and both AM and PM peak flow rates. These results argue that long-acting theophylline may protect the patients against early-morning exacerbations. Whether theophylline plays a role in preventing subsensitivity to β_2-agonists need to be evaluated. Agents that increase cAMP, such as β-adrenergic agents, result in increased phosphodiesterase IV and the resultant increased metabolism of cAMP (115). If this proves to be true for airway tissue, it would provide a rational basis for using phosphodiesterase inhibitors in combination with β_2-agonists (see Chap. 22).

REAPPRAISAL OF ASTHMA MANAGEMENT: SALMETEROL AND FORMOTEROL—POSSIBLE ANTI-INFLAMMATORY ACTIVITY AND EFFECTS ON LATE REACTION AND AIRWAY RESPONSIVENESS

Both salmeterol and formoterol are potent, selective long-acting β_2-agonists, with sustained effects for at least 12 and up to 20 h. A reappraisal of the role of β_2-agonists in asthma is indicated because both of these new agents appear to have a marked inhibitory effect on the late reaction, which is in contrast with existing dogma of β_2-agonists. Furthermore, there is preliminary evidence that both of these agents may exert some degree of anti-inflammatory activity.

Salmeterol

Twentyman et al. (140) studied the effect of salmeterol on the early- and late-phase airway responses provoked by inhaled allergen. They observed that salmeterol, 50 μg inhaled before allergen challenge, prevented both the early- and late-phase bronchoconstriction. In this placebo-controlled study, salmeterol also completely inhibited the allergen-induced increase in nonspecific bronchial responsiveness over a 24-h period. These effects were unrelated to prolonged bronchodilatation or functional antagonism. These authors concluded that these actions extended beyond the protective action on airway smooth muscle and suggest novel actions for this long-acting β_2-agonist in asthma. In this study, following placebo, allergen caused a mean 30 and 20% fall in FEV_1 at 20 min and 7.5 h, respectively. Salmeterol inhibited both the immediate- and late-phase bronchoconstriction with 3.4 and 6.4% increases in FEV_1 at the same time points. In addition, there was a twofold doubling-dilution decrease in the PC_{20} to histamine with placebo administration, in contrast to a 1.55-fold increase with salmeterol 7.5 h after allergen challenge.

An unusual feature of salmeterol is that its sustained effects are reversed with a β-adrenergic blocker, but are reasserted when the β-blocker is removed. Radioligand-binding studies indicate that salmeterol has a high affinity ($K_i = 33$ nM). It appears to have little or no dissociation from its receptor. Salmeterol also exhibits anti-inflammatory activity in that it inhibits mediator release in human lung for up to 20 h, whereas the other β_2-agonists commonly used are ineffective after 4 h. Inhaled salmeterol attenuates the extravasation of plasma protein and inflammatory cell infiltration in the lung for 6–8 h.

The bronchoalveolar lavage (BAL) cells and the mediators' composition in BAL fluid content of markers of eosinophil, neutrophil, macrophage, and mast cell activity was decreased following salmeterol administration (151). Furthermore, the decrease in the chemotactic and phagocytic responsiveness may be interpreted as a dampening of these cellular changes and mediators following administration of salmeterol or placebo to 12 young asthmatics after 4 weeks of treatment in a double-blind manner. Stimulation with zymosan showed that alveolar macrophages' chemiluminescence was decreased with salmeterol. Similarly the eosinophil cationic protein was decreased in the BAL after salmeterol administration. In addition, the pulmonary function was increased and the histamine sensitivity was decreased (151).

In another study (152) of the anti-inflammatory effects of salmeterol, 10^{-5}M of salmeterol caused significant inhibition of thromboxane B_2 release from alveolar macrophages, which was not altered by propranolol. Salmeterol did inhibit alveolar macrophage function, whereas isoproterenol and albuterol (salbutamol) failed to do so in these same subjects.

Salmeterol, 50 µg by inhalation (153), protected against methacholine challenge for 12 h, whereas albuterol, 200 µg by inhalation, protected at 1 h, but not at 4 h. Salmeterol, 50 µg twice daily, in a controlled study significantly decreased nocturnal asthma, as well as improved morning and daytime symptoms, and peak expiratory flow rate. As part of a multicenter, double-blind parallel study of 667 mild to moderate asthmatics (154), salmeterol had a greater effect on the morning peak expiratory flow, evening peak expiratory flow, a decrease in nocturnal asthma, and a decrease in requirement for additional albuterol. In this large multicenter study, salmeterol, 50 µg twice a day, was more effective in each of the foregoing parameters than albuterol, 200 µg four times a day. A similar study in the United States resulted in improvement in these same parameters (155).

However, it is essential that patients receiving salmeterol also carry with them another β_2-agonist inhaler with a quicker onset of action. In spite of this warning in the package insert, a series of 20 deaths and respiratory arrests were reported in late 1994 as a result of patients using salmeterol for acute asthma attacks. This was considered to be related to the slow onset of action of salmeterol and to patients not having or not using a β_2-agonist with quicker onset of bronchodilation.

Formoterol

Formoterol (156) is a second new long-acting β_2-adrenergic agent. Formoterol fumarate is a catecholamine derivative with a formylamino-substituted catecholamine. It was originally developed in Japan and has been marketed there as an oral formulation since 1986. Formoterol for inhalation has been developed by Ciba Geigy Pharmaceuticals for use as a metered-dose inhaler. Inhalation of 12–24 µg of formoterol suspension showed near maximal bronchodilator effect within 5 min and a duration of action up to 12 h. In several comparative trials, formoterol solution aerosol at a dose of 12 µg twice daily showed greater bronchodilator effects than fenoterol (200 µg tid), albuterol (200 µg qid), and terbutaline (250 µg qid). The side effects observed after inhalation of formoterol were similar in frequency and type to those observed with the other β_2-adrenergic drugs studied. Because of its rapid onset of action, patients using formoterol, in contrast with salmeterol, should not need to carry a second β_2-agonist inhaler to obtain quick relief (156).

Formoterol is not structurally related to fenoterol and is two orders of magnitude more potent than albuterol or isoproterenol (156). Formoterol is only slowly washed out from tissues, and is lipophilic, but not as lipophilic as salmeterol. Its anti-inflammatory effects are suggested by its ability to inhibit histamine release, with an ED_{50} of 10^{-11} M. Tokuyama et al. (157) reported that inhaled formoterol inhibits histamine-induced airflow obstruction and airway microvascular leakage. They observed that formoterol is approximately 35 times more potent than albuterol in inhibiting both microvascular leakage and airflow obstruction induced by histamine aerosol. This finding is consistent with a report by Lofdahl and Svedmyr (158) that inhaled formoterol is approximately 40 times more potent than albuterol. Although formoterol and albuterol were both effective in inhibiting histamine-induced microvascular leak, albuterol has no inhibitory effect against plasma leakage induced by IV platelet-activating factor in animals (159). We are not aware of any data determining whether formoterol is able to protect against platelet-activating factor-induced microvascular leakage in humans.

THE EFFECT OF β-AGONISTS ON THE LATE ALLERGIC REACTION AND AIRWAY HYPERRESPONSIVENESS

The microvascular leakage in small airways results in mucosal thickening that could have a profound influence on the tendency of small airways to close. The relative ability of formoterol to protect against the microvascular leak and the potential related inflammatory response could exert an important beneficial role in the late bronchial reaction for which the usual β_2-agonists are thought to be relatively ineffective.

Conventional β_2-agonists inhibit the immediate allergic response by inhibiting the effect on mast cell mediator release, in addition to their direct bronchodilating effects. By contrast, conventional β_2-agonists do not inhibit the late allergic reaction (LAR) after antigen challenge or the accompanying rise in nonspecific bronchial responsiveness (160,161). Previous studies suggest that the late allergic response and the associated increase in bronchial hyperresponsiveness are the clinical manifestations of airway inflammation caused by mediators released as a consequence of inhaled antigens (162,163). β-Agonists have been thought to treat only the symptoms of asthma, without affecting the underlying inflammatory processes.

We, therefore, studied the effect of formoterol on the late asthmatic response and the airway inflammation in guinea pigs (164). After antigen challenge under cover of an H_1-receptor antagonist, specific airway conductance (SGaw) was measured using a two-chambered whole-body plethysmograph. Formoterol (10 μg/ml), isoproterenol (1 mg/ml), or saline was inhaled 15 min before challenge. Bronchoalveolar lavage was performed 24 h after challenge. The provocative concentrations of histamine required to decrease SGaw by 50% (SGaw-PC_{50}) were obtained before challenge, at 24 h, and at 72 h after challenge. The LAR (52.7 ± 7.7% of the baseline, $p < 0.02$) was observed 6–8 h after antigen challenge. An increased cellular influx in BAL (especially eosinophils and macrophages) and an increased bronchial responsiveness to histamine occurred 24 h after antigen challenge. Formoterol completely inhibited the LAR and the cellular increase in BAL, although isoproterenol failed to prevent them. Formoterol also decreased the antigen-induced increase in bronchial reactivity. These findings suggest that formoterol has novel actions on the underlying inflammatory processes in asthma other than by its prolonged bronchodilation.

In the foregoing study (164), formoterol completely suppressed the appearance of the LAR and the antigen-induced airway inflammation, whereas isoproterenol, a conventional short-acting β_2-agonist, failed to inhibit LAR and the increased airway inflammation. Formoterol also decreased the antigen-induced bronchial responsiveness to histamine. In asthmatic children, formoterol has been reported to decrease airway responsiveness to methacholine, even at 12 h after inhalation (165). Formoterol has also been reported to improve bronchial hyperresponsiveness to histamine and cold air after long-term adminis-tration. Both formoterol and salmeterol, given before antigen challenge, attenuate the LAR in asthmatics (140,166,167).

Thus, these new long-acting β_2-agonists such as formoterol and salmeterol, but not short-acting β_2-agonists, apparently are able to inhibit the LAR and the accompanying rise in bronchial responsiveness. Whether these inhibitory effects of formoterol and salmeterol on the LAR and the airway inflammation are due to the long persisting action of β_2-receptor stimulation or to some additional anti-inflammatory mechanism is yet to be determined. Further studies are needed to determine the effect of inhaled corticosteroids alone and in combination with long-acting β_2-antagonists on the clinical response, the LAR, the BAL inflammatory response, and the airway hyperresponsiveness in asthmatic subjects.

REFERENCES

1. Gilman AG. G proteins: transducers of receptor-generated signals. Annu Rev Biochem 1987; 56:615–649.
2. Fraser CM. Adrenergic agents. In: Middleton E Jr, Reed CE, Ellis EF, et al. Allergy Principles and Practice. St Louis: CV Mosby, 1993:778–815.
3. Fraser CM, Venter JC. The synthesis of β-adrenergic receptors in cultured human lung cells: induction by glucocorticoids. Biochem Biophys Res Commun 1980; 94:390–397.
4. Mano K, Akbarzadeh A, Townley RG. Effect of hydrocortisone on beta-adrenergic receptors in lung membranes. Life Sci 1979; 25:195.
5. Malbon CC, Hadcock JR. Evidence that glucocorticoid response elements in the 5-noncoding region of the hamster β-adrenergic receptor gene are obligate for glucocorticoid regulation of receptor mRNA levels. Biochem Biophys Res Commun 1988; 154:676–681.
6. Sibley DR, Lefkowitz RJ. Molecular mechanisms of receptor desensitization using the β-adren-ergic receptor-coupled adenylate cyclase systems as a model. Nature 1985; 317:124–129.
7. Benovic JL, Strasser RH, Caron MG, et al. β-Adrenergic receptor kinase: identification of a novel protein kinase that phosphorylates the agonist-occupied form of the receptor. Proc Natl Acad Sci USA 1986; 83:2797.
8. Meurs H, Kauffman HF, Timmermans A, de Monchy JAR, Koeter GH, de Vries K. Specific immunological modulation of lymphocyte adenylate cyclase in asthmatic patients after aller-genic bronchial provocation. Int Arch Allergy Appl Immunol 1986; 81:224.
9. Morris GM, Hadcock JR, Malbon CC. Cross-regulation between G-protein–coupled receptors. J Biol Chem 1991; 266:2233.
10. Lee NH, Fraser CM. Regulation and cross-talk of the cloned M_1 muscarinic and β-adrenergic receptors co-expressed in CHO cells. FASEB J 1991; 5:A1254.
11. Black JL, Salome C, Yan K, Shaw J. The action of prazosin and propylene glycol on methoxamine-induced bronchoconstriction in asthmatic subjects. Br J Clin Pharmacol 1984; 18: 349–353.
12. Black J, Vincene L, Salome C. Inhibition of methoxamine-induced bronchoconstriction by ipratropium bromide and disodium cromoglycate in asthmatic subjects. Br J Clin Pharmacol 1985; 20:41.
13. Henderson WR, Shelhamer JH, Reingold DG, Smith LS, Evans R, Kaliner M. α-Adrenergic hyperresponsiveness in asthma: analysis of vascular and pupillary responses. N Engl J Med 1979; 300:642–647.
14. Sanstron T, Henriksson R, Hornvist R, et al. Increased peripheral α-adrenoceptor responses in allergic asthmatics. Allergy 1988; 43:49.
15. Davis PB, Paget GL, Turi V. alpha-Adrenergic responses in asthma. J Lab Clin Med 1985; 105: 164–169.
16. Davis PB. Pupillary responses and airway reactivity in asthma. J Allergy Clin Immunol 1986; 77:667–673.

17. Blecker ER, Chahal KS, Mason P, et al. The effect of alpha-adrenergic blockade in nonspecific airways reactivity and exercised induced asthma. Eur J Respir Dis 1983; 64(suppl):258.

18. Townley RG, Honrath T, Guirgis HM. The inhibitory effect of hydrocortisone on the alpha-adrenergic responses of human and guinea pig isolated respiratory smooth muscle. J Allergy Clin Immunol 1972; 49:88.

19. Kneussel MP, Richardson JB. alpha-Adrenergic receptors in human canine tracheal and bronchial smooth muscle. J Appl Physiol 1978; 45:307–311.

20. Lindgren BRE, Elström T, Anderson RGG. The effect of inhaled clonidine in patients with asthma. Am Rev Respir Dis 1986; 134:266–269.

21. Barnes PJ, Dollery CT, Macdermot J. Increased pulmonary alpha-adrenergic and reduced beta-adrenergic receptors in experimental asthma. Nature 1990; 285:569.

22. Takeyama HF, Jedruska-Witt S, Takeyama FM, Bewtra A, Townley RG. Adrenergic receptors in guinea pig experimental asthma. Am Rev Respir Dis 1984; 73:128.

23. Mirbahar KB, Eyre P. Autonomic and autocoid activity in antigen-sensitized and control ovine pulmonary vein and artery. J Vet Pharmacol Ther 1982; 5:137–144.

24. Mirbahar KB, Eyre P. Autocoid and autonomic reactivity of bovine and ovine bronchus: modifications by antigenic sensitization. Arch Int Pharmacodyn Ther 1982; 5:60–70.

25. Logsdon PJ, Carnright DV, Middleton E Jr, Coffey RG. The effect of phentolamine on adenylate cyclase and on isoproterenol stimulation in leukocytes for asthmatics and nonasthmatic subjects. J Allergy Clin Immunol 1973; 52:148.

26. Alston WC, Patel KR, Kerr JW. Response of leukocyte adenyl cyclase to isoprenaline and effect of alpha-blocking drugs in extrinsic bronchial asthma. Br Med J 1974; 1:90–93.

27. Matthys H, Doshan HD, Ruhle KH, Braig H, Pohl M, Applin WS, Caruso FS, Neiss ES. The broncho-sparing effect of celiprolol, a new $beta_1$–$alpha_2$-receptor antagonist on pulmonary function of propranolol-sensitive asthmatics. J Clin Pharmacol 1985; 25:354–359.

28. Strader CD, Sigal IS, Candelore MR, Rands E, Hill WS, Dixon RAF. Conserved aspartic acid residues 79 and 113 of the β-adrenergic receptor have different roles in receptor function. J Biol Chem 1988; 263:10267–10271.

29. Fraser CM, Chung FZ, Wang CD, Venter JC. Site-directed mutagenesis of human β-adrenergic receptors: substitution of aspartic acid-130 by asparagine produces a receptor with high-affinity agonist binding that is uncoupled for adenylate cyclase. Proc Natl Acad Sci USA 1988; 85: 5478–5482.

30. O'Dowd BF, Hantowich M, Regan JW, Leader WM, Caron MG, Lefkowitz RJ. Site-directed mutagenesis of the cytoplasmic domains of the human β-adrenergic receptor. J Biol Chem 1988; 263:15985–15992.

31. Reihsaus E, Innis M, MacIntyre N, Liggett SB. Mutations in the gene encoding for the β-adrenergic receptor in normal and asthmatic subjects. Am J Respir Cell Mol Biol 1993; 8: 334–339.

32. Liggett SB. β-Adrenergic receptor structure and function. J Respir Dis 1994; 15:28–38.

33. Green SA, Cole G, Jacinto M, et al. A polymorphism of the human β-adrenergic receptor within the fourth transmembrane domain alters ligand binding and functional properties of the receptor. J Biol Chem 1993; 268:23116–23121.

34. Turki J, Pak J, Green SA, Martin RJ, Liggett SB. Genetic polymorphisms of the β-adrenergic receptor in nocturnal and nonnocturnal asthma. J Clin Invest 1995; 95:1635–1641.

35. Hall IP, Wheatley A, Wilding P, Liggett SB. Association of Glu 27 $beta_2$-adrenoceptor polymorphism with lower airway reactivity in asthmatic subjects. Lancet 1995; 345:1213–1214.

36. Turki J, Liggett SB. Receptor-specific functional properties of β-adrenergic receptor autoantibodies in asthma. Am J Respir Cell Mol Biol 1995; 12:531–539.

37. Davis AO, Lefkowitz RJ. Regulation of β-adrenergic receptors by steroid hormones. Annu Rev Physiol 1984; 46:119–130.

38. Collins S, Caron MG, Lefkowitz RJ. beta-Adrenergic receptors in hamster smooth muscle cells are transcriptionally regulated by glucocorticoids. J Biol Chem 1988; 263:9067–9070.

39. Goldie RG, Spina D, Hery PJ, Lulich KM, Paterson JW. In vitro responsiveness of human asthmatic bronchus to carbachol, histamine, β-adrenoceptor agonists and theophylline. Br J Clin Pharmacol 1986; 22:669–676.

40. Bai TR, Mak JCW, Barnes PJ. A comparison of β-adrenergic receptors and in vitro relaxant responses to isoproterenol in asthmatic airway smooth muscle. Am J Respir Cell Mol Biol 1992; 6:647–651.

41. Boyle JP, Davies JM, Gosling JA, Small RC. Pharmacological, electrophysiological, and immunocytochemical studies of VIP in guinea pig isolated trachea. Pflugers Arch 1988; 411:R201.

42. Allen SL, Beech DJ, Foster RW, Morgan GP, Small RC. Electrophysiological and other aspects of the relaxant action of isoprenaline in guinea-pig isolated trachealis. Br J Pharmacol 1985; 86:843–854.

43. Kume H, Takai A, Tokuno H, Tomita T. Regulation of Ca^{2+}-dependent K^+-channel activity in tracheal myocytes by phosphorylation. Nature 1989; 341:152–154.

44. Ewald DA, Williams A, Levitan IB. Modulation of single Ca^{2+}-dependent K^+-channel activity by protein phosphorylation. Nature 1985; 315:503–506.

45. Jones TR, Charette L, Garcia ML, Kaczorowski GJ. Selective inhibition of relaxation of guinea-pig trachea by charybdotoxin, a potent Ca^{2+} activated K^+-channel inhibitor. J Pharmacol Exp Ther 1990; 255:697–706.

46. Jelsema CL, Axelrod J. Stimulation of phospholipase A_2 activity in bovine rod outer segments by the βγ subunits of transducin and the inhibition by the α subunit. Proc Natl Acad Sci USA 1987; 84:3623–3627.

47. Pyne NJ, Rodger IW. Guanine nucleotide binding regulatory protein and receptor-mediated actions. In: Chung KF, Barnes PI, eds. Pharmacology of the Respiratory Tract. New York: Marcel Dekker, 1993:49–61.

48. Hadcock JR, Ros M, Watkins DC, Malbon CC. Cross-regulation between G-protein mediated pathways. Stimulation of adenylyl cyclase increases expression of the inhibitory G-protein. Gix II. J Biol Chem 1990; 265:14784–14790.

49. Meurs H, Kauffman HF, Koeter GH, Timmermans A, de Vries K. Regulation of β-receptor adenylate cyclase system in lymphocytes of allergic patients with asthma: possible role for protein kinase C in allergen-induced non-specific refractoriness of adenylate cyclase. J Allergy Clin Immunol 1987; 80:326–339.

50. Hall IP, Hill SJ. $beta_2$-Adrenoceptor stimulation inhibits histamine-stimulation inositol phospholipid hydrolysis in bovine tracheal smooth muscle. Br J Pharmacol 1988; 95:1204–1212.

51. Szentivanyi A. The beta adrenergic theory of the atopic abnormality in bronchial asthma. J Allergy 1968; 42:203–232.

52. Barnes PJ. Adrenergic regulation of airway function. In: Kaliner MA, Barnes PJ, eds. The Airway Neural Control in Health and Disease. New York: Marcel Dekker, 1988:57–85.

53. Barnes PJ. Neural control of human airways in health and disease. Am Rev Respir Dis 1986; 134:1289–1314.

54. Hall IP, Tattersfield AE. beta Agonists. In: Clark TJ, Godfrey S, Lee T, eds. Asthma. London: Chapman & Hall, 1992:341–365.

55. Cerrina J, Ladurie MIR, Labat C, Raffestin B, Bayol A, Brink C. Comparison of human bronchial muscle responses to histamine in vivo with histamine and isoproterenol agonists in vitro. Am Rev Respir Dis 1986; 134:57–61.

56. Bai TR. Abnormalities in airway smooth muscle in fatal asthma: a comparison between trachea and bronchus. Am Rev Respir Dis 1991; 143:441–443.

57. Townley RG, Hopp RJ, Agrawal DK, Bewtra AK. Platelet-activating factor and airway reactivity. J Allergy Clin Immunol 1989; 83:997–1010.

58. Gatto C, Green TP, Johnson MG, Marchessault RP, Seybold V, Johnson DE. Localization of quantitative changes in pulmonary beta-receptors in ovalbumin-sensitized guinea pigs. Am Rev Respir Dis 1987; 136:150–154.

59. Meurs H, Koeter GH, DeVries K, Kauffman HF. The beta-adrenergic system and allergic bronchial asthma: changes in lymphocyte beta adrenergic receptor number and adenylate cyclase activity after an allergen-induced asthmatic attack. J Allergy Clin Immunol 1982; 70:272.

60. Meurs H, Zaagsma J. Pharmacological and biochemical changes in airway smooth muscle in relation to bronchial hyperresponsiveness. In: Agrawal DK, Townley RG, eds. Pharmacology and Toxicology: Inflammatory Cells and Mediators in Bronchial Asthma. Boca Raton, FL: CRC Press, 1991:1–38.

61. Zaagsma J, van der Heijden PMCM, van der Schaar MWG, Bank CMC. Comparison of functional beta-adrenoceptor heterogeneity in central and peripheral airway smooth muscle of guinea pig and man. J Recep Res 1983; 3:89

62. Goldie RG, Paterson JW, Spira D, Wale JL. Classification of beta-adrenoceptors in human and porcine bronchus. Br J Pharmacol 1984; 81:611.

63. Barnes PJ, Basbaum BJ, Nadel JA. Autoradiography localization of autonomic receptors in airway smooth muscle. Marked differences between large and small airways. Am Rev Respir Dis 1983; 127:758.

64. Agrawal DK, Schugel JW, Townley RG. Comparison of beta adrenoceptors in bovine airway epithelium and smooth muscle cells. Biochem Biophys Res Commun 1987; 148:178–183.

65. Partanen M, Laitinen A, Hervonen A, Toivanen M, Laitinen LA. Catecholamine and acetylcholinesterase containing nerves in human lower respiratory tract. Histochemistry 1982; 76:175.

66. Vanhoutte PM. Epithelium-derived relaxing factor(s) and bronchial reactivity. Am Rev Respir Dis 1988; 138:S24–30.

67. Sanderson MJ, Dirksen ER. Mechano-sensitive and beta-adrenergic control of the ciliary beat frequency of mammalian respiratory tract cells in culture. Am Rev Respir Dis 1989; 139: 432–440.

68. Liggett SB. Identification and characterization of a homogeneous population of $beta_2$-adrenergic receptors on human alveolar macrophages. Am Rev Respir Dis 1989; 139:552–555.

69. Pick E. Cyclic AMP affects macrophage migration. Nature 1972; 238:176–177.

70. Rankin JA. Macrophages and their potential role in hyperreactive airways disease. In: Agrawal DK, Townley RG, eds. Pharmacology and Toxicology: Inflammatory Cells and Mediators in Bronchial Asthma. Boca Raton, FL: CRC Press, 1990:89–106.

71. Kaliner M, Shelhamer JH, Davis EB, Smith LJ, Venter JC. NIH Conference: Autonomic nervous system abnormalities and allergy. Ann Intern Med 1982; 96:349.

72. Okada C, Sugiyama H, Eda R, et al. The effect of formoterol on superoxide anion generation from bronchoalveolar lavage cells after antigen challenge in guinea pigs. Am J Respir Cell Mol Biol 1993; 8:509–517.

73. Sano Y, Begley M, Watt G, Townley R. Corticosteroid increases leukocyte beta-adrenergic receptors in vivo. J Allergy Clin Immunol 1980; 65:233.

74. Townley RG, Reeb R, Fitzgibbons T, Adolphson RL. The effect of corticosteroids on the beta-adrenergic receptors in bronchial smooth muscle. J Allergy 1970; 45:118.

75. Townley RG, Trapani IL, Szentivanyi A. Sensitization to anaphylaxis and to some of its pharmacological mediators by blockage of the beta adrenergic receptors. J Allergy 1967; 39: 177–197.

76. Leff AR. Role of the adrenergic nervous system in asthma. In: Kaliner MA, Barnes PJ, Persson CG, eds. Asthmatic Pathology and Treatment. New York: Marcel Dekker, 1992:357–374.

77. Ploy-Song-Sand Y, Corbin RP, Engel LA. Effects of intravenous histamine on lung mechanics in man after beta-blockade. J Appl Physiol 1978; 44:690–695.

78. Ryo UY, Townley RG. Comparison of respiratory and cardiovascular effects of isoproterenol, propranolol, and practolol in asthmatic and normal subjects. J Allergy Clin Immunol 1976; 57: 12–24.

79. Orehek J, Gayrard P, Grimaud C, Charpin J. Effect of maximal respiratory manoeuvres on bronchial sensitivity of asthmatic patients as compared to normal people. Br Med J 1975; 1: 123–125.

80. Zuskin E, Mitchell CA, Bouhuys A. Interaction between effects of beta blockade and cigarette smoke on airways. J Appl Physiol 1974; 36:449–452.

81. Townley RG, McGeady S, Bewtra A. The effect of beta adrenergic blockade on bronchial sensitivity to acetyl-beta-methacholine in normal and allergic rhinitis subjects. J Allergy Clin Immunol 1976; 57:358–366.

82. Zaid G, Beall GN. Bronchial response to beta-adrenergic blockade. N Engl J Med 1966; 275: 580–584.

83. Grieco MH, Pierson RN Jr. Mechanism of bronchoconstriction due to beta-adrenergic blockade. J Allergy 1971; 48:143–152.

84. Townley RG, Agrawal DK. Adrenergic and cholinergic receptors and airway responsiveness. In: Agrawal DK, Townley RG, eds. Airway Smooth Muscle: Modulation of Receptors and Responses. Boca Raton, FL: CRC Press, 1990:229–257.

85. Yukawa T, Makino S, Fukuda T, Kamikawa Y. Experimental model of anaphylaxis-induced beta-adrenergic blockade in the airways. Ann Allergy 1986; 57:219.

86. Conolly ME, Greenacre JK. The lymphocyte beta-adrenoceptor in normal subjects and patients with bronchial asthma. J Clin Invest 1976; 58:1307–1316.

87. Morris HG, Rusnake SA, Selner JC, Barzens K, Barnes J. Adrenergic desensitization in leukocytes of normal and asthmatic subjects. J Cyclic Nucleotide Res 1977; 3:439–446.

88. Tashkin DP, Conolly ME, Deutsch RI, Hui KK, Littner M, Scarpace P, Abrass I. Subsensitization of beta-adrenoceptors in airways and lymphocytes of healthy and asthmatic subjects. Am Rev Respir Dis 1982; 125:185.

89. Sano Y, Watt G, Townley RG. Decreased mononuclear cell beta-adrenergic receptors in bronchial asthma: parallel studies of lymphocyte and granulocyte desensitization. J Allergy Clin Immunol 1983; 72:495–503.

90. Wills-Karp, Uchida Y, Lee JY, Jinot J, Hirata A, Hirata F. Organ culture with proinflammatory cytokines reproduces impairment of the β-adrenoceptor mediated relaxation in tracheas of a guinea pig antigen model. Am J Respir Cell Mol Biol 1993; 8:153–159.

91. Lee RT, Brock TA, Tolman C, et al. Subtype-specific increase in G protein α subunit mRNA by interleukin-1β. FEBS Lett 1989; 249:139–142.

92. Agrawal DK, Townley RG. PAF, human lung beta-adrenoceptors and ginkgolide B (BN 52021). In: Braquet P, ed. Ginkgolides—Chemistry, Biology, Pharmacology, and Clinical Perspectives. Barcelona: JR Prous Science Publishers, 1988:355–364.

93. Agrawal DK, Townley RG. Effect of platelet-activating on beta-adrenoceptors in human lung. Biochem Biophys Res Commun 1987; 143:1–6.

94. Braquet P, Etienne A, Clostre F. Down-regulation of beta$_2$ adrenergic receptors by PAF-acether and its inhibition by the PAF-acether antagonist BN 52021. Prostaglandins 1985; 30:721.

95. Agrawal DK, Bergren DR, Byorth PJ, Townley RG. Platelet-activating factor induces nonspecific desensitization to bronchodilators in guinea pigs. J Pharmacol Exp Ther 1991; 259:1–7.

96. Freitag A, Watson RM, Matsos G, Eastwood, O'Byrne PM. The effect of treatment with an oral platelet activating factor antagonist (WEB 2086) on allergen induced asthmatic responses in human subjects. Am Rev Respir Dis 1991; 143:A157.

97. Lang DM, Alpern MB, Visintainer PF, Smith ST. Increased risk for anaphylactoid reaction from contrast media in patients on beta-adrenergic blockers with asthma. Ann Intern Med 1991; 115: 270–276.

98. Chuang TT, Sallese M, Ambrosini G, Parruti G, DeBlasi A. High expression of β-adrenergic receptor kinase in human peripheral blood leukocytes. Isoproterenol and platelet activating factor can induce kinase translocation. J Biol Chem 1992; 267:6886–6892.

99. DeBlasi A, Parruti G, Sallese M. Regulation of G protein coupled receptor kinase subtypes in

activated T-lymphocytes. Selective increase of β-adrenergic receptor kinase 1 and 2. J Clin Invest 1995; 95:203–210.

100. Apold J, Aksenes L. Correlation between increased bronchial responsiveness to histamine and diminished plasma cyclic adenosine monophosphate response after epinephrine in asthmatic children. J Allergy Clin Immunol 1977; 59:343–347.

101. Makino S, Ikemori K, Kashima T, Fukuda T. Comparison of cyclic adenosine monophosphate response of lymphocytes in normal and asthmatic subjects to norepinephrine and salbutamol. J Allergy Clin Immunol 1977; 59:348–352.

102. Morris HG, Rusnak SA, Barzens K. Leukocyte cyclic adenosine monophosphate in asthmatic children: effect of adrenergic therapy. Clin Pharmacol Ther 1977; 22:352–357.

103. Sato T, Bewtra AK, Hopp RJ, Townley RG. Alpha and beta adrenergic receptor systems in bronchial asthma and non-asthmatic subjects: reduced mononuclear cell beta receptors in bronchial asthma. J Allergy Clin Immunol 1990; 86:839–850.

104. Johnson GL, Wolfe BB, Harden TK, Molinoff PB, Perkins JP. Role of beta adrenergic receptors in catecholamine-induced desensitization of adenylate cyclase in human astrocytoma cells. J Bio Chem 1978; 253:1472–1480.

105. Wessels MR, Mullikin D, Lefkowitz RJ. Selective alteration in high affinity agonist bindings: a mechanism of beta adrenergic receptor desensitization. Mol Pharmacol 1979; 16:10–20.

106. Davies AO, Lefkowitz RJ. In vitro desensitization of beta adrenergic receptors in human neutrophils. J Clin Invest 1983; 71:565–571.

107. Feldman RD, Limbird LE, Nadeau J, Fitzgerald GA, Robertson D, Wood AJJ. Dynamic regulation of leukocyte beta adrenergic receptor-agonist interactions by physiological changes in circulating catecholamines. J Clin Invest 1983; 72:164–170.

108. Collins S, Altsehmeid J, Herbsman O, Caron MG, Mellon PI, Lefkowitz RJ. A cAMP response element in the beta$_2$-adrenergic receptor gene confers transcriptional autoregulation by cAMP. J Biol Chem 1990; 265:19330–19335.

109. Safko MJ, Chan SC, Cooper KD, Hanifin JM. Heterologous desensitization of leukocytes: a possible mechanism of beta-adrenergic blockade in atopic dermatitis. J Allergy Clin Immunol 1981; 68:218–225.

110. Busse WW, Sosman J. Decreased H$_2$ histamine response of granulocytes of asthmatic patients. J Clin Invest 1977; 59:1080–1087.

111. Grewe SR, Chan SC, Hanifin JM. Elevated leukocyte cyclic AMP–phosphodiesterase in atopic disease: a possible mechanism for cyclic AMP–agonist hyporesponsiveness. J Allergy Clin Immunol 1982; 70:452–457.

112. Butler JM, Chan SC, Stevens S, Hanifin JM. Inceased leukocyte histamine release with elevated cyclic AMP–phosphodiesterase activity in atopic dermatitis. J Allergy Clin Immunol 1983; 74: 490–497.

113. Torphy T, Undem B. Phosphodiestrase inhibitors: new opportunities for the treatment of asthma. Thorax 1991; 46:512–523.

114. Townley RG. Elevated cAMP-phosphodiesterase in atopic disease: cause or effect? (Editorial). J Lab Clin Med 1993; 121:15–17.

115. Torphy TJ, Zhou HL, Cieslinski LB. Stimulation of beta adrenoceptors in a human monocyte cell line (u937) upregulates cyclic AMP-specific phosphodiesterase. J Pharmacol Exp Ther 1992; 263:1195–1205.

116. Holgate ST, Baldwin CJ, Tattersfield AE. beta-Adrenergic agonist resistance in normal human airways. Lancet 1977; 2:375–377.

117. Ellul-Micallef R, Fenech FF. Effect of intravenous prednisolone in asthmatics with diminished adrenergic responsiveness. Lancet 1975; 2:1269–1273.

118. Coffey RG, Logsdon PJ, Middleton E Jr. Effects of glucocorticoids on leukocyte adenyl cyclase and ATPase of asthmatic and normal children. J Allergy Clin Immunol 1972; 49:87.

119. Rinand GA. Effects of hydrocortisone and isoproterenol on cyclic AMP formation and relaxation in canine trachea smooth muscle. Fed Proc 1979; 38:1082.

120. Sano Y, Begley M, Watt G, Townley RG. Corticosteroid increases leukocyte beta-adrenergic receptors in vivo. J Allergy Clin Immunol 1980; 65:223.

121. Smith BT. Cell line A 549: a model system for the study of alveolar type II cell function. Am Rev Respir Dis 1977; 115:285–293.

122. Fraser CM, Venter JC. The synthesis of β-adrenergic receptors in cultured human lung cells: induction by glucocorticoids. Biochem Biophys Res Commun 1980; 94:390–397.

123. Molfino NA, Nannini LJ, Martelli AN, Slutky AS. Respiratory arrest in near fatal asthma. N Engl J Med 1991; 324:285–288.

124. Windom HH, Burgess CD, Crane J, Pearce N, Dwong T, Beasley R. The self-administration of inhaled beta agonist drugs during severe asthma. NZ Med J 1990; 103:205–207.

125. Sears MR, Rea HH. Patients at risk for dying of asthma: New Zealand experience. J Allergy Clin Immunol 1987; 80:477–481.

126. Fraser PM, Speizer FE, Waters SD, Doll R, Mann NM. The circumstances preceding death from asthma in young people in 1968 to 1969. Br J Dis Chest 1971; 65:71–84.

127. Speizer FE, Doll R. A century of asthma deaths in young people. Br Med J 1968; 3:245–246.

128. Sears MR, Beaglehole R. Asthma mortality and morbidity: New Zealand. J Allergy Clin Immunol 1987; 80:383–388.

129. Jackson R. Undertreatment and asthma deaths. Lancet 1985; 2:500.

130. Barger LW, Vollmer WM, Felt RW, Buist AS. Further investigation into the recent increase in asthma death rates: a review of 41 asthma deaths in Oregon in 1982. Ann Allergy 1988; 60:31–39.

131. Johnson AJ, Nunn AJ, Somner AR, Stableforth DE, Stewart CJ. Circumstances of death from asthma. Br Med J 1984; 288:1870–1872.

132. Stolley PD. Asthma mortality; why the United States was spared an epidemic of deaths due to asthma. Am Rev Respir Dis 1972; 105:883–890.

133. Crane J, Pearce N, Flatt A, et al. Prescribed fenoterol and death from asthma in New Zealand, 1981–83: case-control study. Lancet 1989; 1:917–922.

134. Van Metre TE Jr. Adverse effects of inhalation of excessive amounts of nebulized isoproterenol in status asthmaticus. J Allergy 1969; 43:101.

135. Sears MR, Taylor DR, Print CG, et al. Regular inhaled beta-agonist treatment in bronchial asthma. Lancet 1990; 336:1391.

136. Collins JM, McDevitt DG, Shanks RG, Swanton JG. The cardio-toxicity of isoprenaline during hypoxia. Br J Pharmacol 1969; 36:35–45.

137. Ryo Y, Townley RG, Kolotkin BM, Kang B. Bronchial sensitivity to methacholine in current and former asthmatics and allergic rhinitis and control subjects. J Allergy Clin Immunol 1975; 56:429–442.

138. O'Hollaren MT, Yunginger JW, Offord KP, et al. Exposure to an aeroallergen as a possible precipitating factor in respiratory arrest in young patients with asthma. N Engl J Med 1991; 324:359–363.

139. Britton J, Hanley SP, Garrett HV, Hadfield JW, Tattersfield AE. Dose-related effects of salbutamol and ipratropium bromide on airway caliber and reactivity in subjects with asthma. Thorax 1988; 43:300–305.

140. Twentyman OP, Finnerty JP, Harris A, Palmer J, Holgate ST. Protection against allergen-induced asthma by salmeterol. Lancet 1990; 336:1338.

141. Weber RW, Smith JA, Nelson HS. Aerosolized terbutaline in asthmatics: development of subsensitivity with long-term administration. J Allergy Clin Immunol 1982; 70:417–422.

142. Repsher LH, Anderson JA, Bush RW, et al. Assessment of tachyphylaxis following prolonged therapy of asthma with inhaled albuterol aerosol. Chest 1984; 85:34.

143. Cheng D, Timmers MC, Zwinderman AH, et al. Long term effects of a long-acting $beta_2$-adrenoreceptor agonist, salmeterol, on airway hyperresponsiveness in patients with mild asthma. N Engl J Med 1992; 327:1198–1203.

144. O'Connor BJ, Aikman SL, Barnes PJ. Tolerance to the nonbronchodilator effects of inhaled β_2-agonists in asthma. N Engl J Med 1992; 327:1204–1208.

145. Nelson HS, Szefler, Martin RJ. Regular inhaled beta-adrenergic agonists in the treatment of bronchial asthma: beneficial or detrimental? (Editorial). Am Rev Respir Dis 1991; 144: 249–250.

146. Szefler SJ, Ando R, Cicutto LC, Surs W, Hill MR, Martin RJ. Plasma histamine, epinephrine, cortisol, and leukocyte beta-adrenergic receptors in nocturnal asthma. Clin Pharmacol Ther 1991; 49:59–68.

147. Shepherd GL, Hetzel MR, Clark TJH. Regular versus symptomatic aerosol bronchodilator treatment of asthma. Br J Dis Chest 1981; 75:215–217.

148. Joad JP, Ahrens RC, Lindgren SD, Weinberger MM. Relative efficacy of maintenance therapy with theophylline, inhaled albuterol and the combination for chronic asthma. J Allergy Clin Immunol 1987; 79:78–85.

149. Smith JA, Weber RW, Nelson HS. Theophylline and aerosolized terbutaline in the treatment of bronchial asthma: double-blind comparison of optimal doses. Chest 1980; 78:816–818.

150. VandeWalker ML, Kray KT, Weber RW, Nelson HS. Addition of terbutaline to optimal theophylline therapy: double-blind crossover study in asthmatic patients. Chest 1986; 90:198–203.

151. Dahl R, Pedersen B. Society of European Pulmonary Disease (SEP-SEPCR) Special Symposium: A Reappraisal of Asthma Management. London, September 12, 1990.

152. Fuller RW, Baker AJ. Society of European Pulmonary Disease (SEP-SEPCR) Special Symposium: A Reappraisal of Asthma Management. London, September 12, 1990.

153. Pauwels R, Derom E, VanDerStraten N. Society of European Pulmonary Disease (SEP-SEPCR) Special Symposium: A Reappraisal of Asthma Management. London, September 12, 1990.

154. Britton MG. Salmeterol and salbutamol: large multicenter studies. Eur Respir Rev 1991; 1: 288–292.

155. Pearlman DS, Chervinsky P, LaForce C, et al. A comparison of salmeterol with albuterol in the treatment of mild-to-moderate asthma. N Engl J Med 1992; 327:1420–1425.

156. Anderson GP. Formoterol: pharmacology, molecular basis of agonism and mechanism of long duration of a highly potent and selective β_2-adrenoceptor agonist bronchodilator. Life Sci 1993; 52:2145–2160.

157. Tokuyama K, Lotvall JO, Lofdahl CG, Barnes PJ, Chung KF. Inhaled formoterol inhibits histamine-induced airflow obstruction and airway microvascular leakage. Eur J Pharmacol 1991; 193:35–39.

158. Arvidsson P, Larsson S, Lofdahl CG, Melander B, Wahlander L, Svedmyr N. Formoterol, a new long-acting bronchodilator for inhalation. Eur Respir J 1989; 2:325–330.

159. Boschetto P, Roberts RN, Rogers DF, Barnes PJ. Effect of antiasthma drugs on microvascular leakage in guinea pig airways. Am Rev Respir Dis 1989; 139:416–421.

160. Cockcroft DW, Murdock KY. Comparative effects of inhaled salbutamol, sodium cromoglycate, and beclomethasone diproprionate on allergen-induced early asthmatic responses, late asthmatic responses, and increased bronchial responsiveness to histamine. J Allergy Clin Immunol 1987; 79:734–740.

161. Hutson PA, Holgate ST, Churck MK. The effect of cromolyn sodium and albuterol on early and late phase bronchoconstriction and airway leukocyte infiltration after allergen challenge of nonanesthetized guinea pigs. Am Rev Respir Dis 1988; 138:1157–1163.

162. De Monchy JG, Kauffman HF, Venge P, Koeter GH, Jansen HM, Sluiter HJ, de Vries K. Bronchoalveolar eosinophilia during allergen-induced late asthmatic reactions. Am Rev Respir Dis 1985; 131:373–376.

163. Metzger WJ, Richerson HB, Worden K, Monick M, Hunninghake GW. Bronchoalveolar lavage of allergic asthmatic patients following allergen bronchoprovocation. Chest 1986; 89:477–483.

164. Sugiyama H, Okada C, Bewtra AK, Hopp RJ, Townley RG. The effect of formoterol on the late asthmatic response in guinea pigs. J Allergy Clin Immunol 1992; 89:858–866.

165. Becker AB, Simons FER. Formoterol, a new long acting selective beta$_2$-adrenergic receptor agonist: double blind comparison with salbutamol and placebo in children with asthma. J Allergy Clin Immunol 1989; 84:891–895.

166. VonBerg A, Berdel D. Efficacy of formoterol metered aerosol in children. Lung 1990; 168(S): 90–98.

167. Palmqvist M, Balder B, Lowhagen O, Melander B, Svedmyr N, Wahlander L. Late asthmatic reaction prevented by inhaled salbutamol and formoterol. J Allergy Clin Immunol 1989; 83:244.

168. Holgate ST, Church MK. Allergy. London: Gower Medical Publishing, 1993.

22

Phosphodiesterase IV Inhibitors as Potential Therapeutic Agents in Allergic Disease

Mark A. Giembycz
Royal Brompton National Heart and Lung Institute,
London, England

John E. Souness
Rhône-Poulenc Rorer, Ltd., Essex, England

INTRODUCTION

Allergy originally encompassed all aspects of immunology, but now refers specifically to the tissue-damaging or irritant effects to the host of immunological reactions. Allergic diseases, including asthma, atopic and contact dermatitis, rhinitis, sinusitis, hypersensitivity pneumonitis, extrinsic alveolitis, angioedema and anaphylaxis, urticaria, eczema, and certain forms of migraine and gastrointestinal disorders, affect 20% of the population and represent a highly significant cause of morbidity and mortality. If allergic asthma is taken as a specific example, recent epidemiological studies indicate that the prevalence and severity of this disease is increasing (1) together with the number of reported cases of fatal asthma (2,3). These are particularly alarming statistics given the marked increase in the prescribing of various antiasthma therapies (4,5). According to a recent review, the cost associated with the diagnosis and treatment of allergic diseases as a whole is immense (6). In the United States, for example, it has been estimated that money spent on over-the-counter antihistamines far exceeds the entire annual budget for the National Institutes of Health (6).

The etiology of allergy is incompletely understood, although the last 5 years have seen significant advances in our understanding of the pathogenesis of many allergic disorders. In particular, the likely participation of immunoglobulin (Ig)E-driven mechanisms in many allergic diseases, including all of those just cited, has been identified and recognized by the World Health Organization (7). It is only too clear, given the enormity of the problem, which has now reached epidemic proportions, that drugs that can prevent the overt and covert manifestations of allergic reactions and, ideally, suppress or even prevent the process of host sensitization could have a profound effect (both clinical and economic) in the control of these diseases. Although glucocorticosteroids are probably the most effective antiallergic–anti-inflammatory drugs currently available, they are nonselective in action

523

and not without side effects that may preclude their routine use, especially in children. New drugs with enhanced selectivity and improved side effect profiles are clearly required. One group of drugs that may exhibit powerful anti-inflammatory and immunomodulatory activity comprises the cyclic nucleotide phosphodiesterase (PDE) inhibitors (8–12). Although theophylline, a drug that nonselectively inhibits all cyclic nucleotide PDEs, has been used in the treatment of allergic asthma for many years, its main beneficial activity has been generally attributed to its weak bronchodilator action. The last decade, however, has seen a most remarkable resurgence of interest in PDE inhibitors, not only as smooth-muscle relaxants, but also as potential antiallergic–anti-inflammatory agents. This stems primarily from the realization that PDEs represent a highly heterogeneous group of enzymes (seven families have now been clearly defined; see section on properties and classification) that are differentially expressed in cells. The obvious ramification of these findings is the potential for drugs that act selectively on a particular PDE isoenzyme. This could theoretically permit the discrete and selective manipulation of cell types that express this PDE variant. The clinical (and economic) potential of these compounds is so great that most of the world's major pharmaceutical companies have an active PDE research program and have developed potent and highly selective PDE inhibitors, many of which are currently undergoing clinical evaluation (Table 1; Fig. 1).

The purpose of this chapter is fourfold: to briefly describe the cellular and molecular mechanisms that are currently believed to underlie the genesis of allergic disease and, this foundation having been laid, to describe (1) the multiplicity and tissue distribution of PDE isoenzymes in cells that participate in allergic reactions, (2) the differences in the complement of PDEs expressed by normal versus allergic proinflammatory cells, and (3) the potential sites at which selective PDE inhibitors could act to alleviate the acute and chronic manifestations of allergic disease. Since inhibitors of the AMP-specific PDE (see later section on PDE IV) show the most promising pharmacology for the suppression of mediator release from a variety of proinflammatory–immunocompetent cells, and many functional and biochemical indices of chronic allergic inflammation (see Refs. 8–12, and following discussion), the PDE IV isoenzyme family will form the basis of this review.

ROLE OF IgE IN ALLERGIC DISEASES

How are susceptible individuals rendered sensitized to foreign substances (i.e., allergens or antigens)? Although a complete understanding of this phenomenon is lacking, the generation of IgE by B lymphocytes is believed to play a central role in this process.

In many allergic diseases in which IgE-dependent mechanisms are implicated, exposure of susceptible individuals to allergen, whether it be by inhalation or through the skin, usually results in opsonization of the allergen (i.e., the deposition of complement fragment C3b or antibody on the foreign protein), followed by ingestion of the opsonized particles by so-called antigen-presenting cells (APC). Several cells can act as APC, including alveolar and tissue macrophages, B lymphocytes, dendritic cells, Langerhans cells, and possibly epithelial cells. Once inside an APC the allergen is *processed* and then *presented* to CD4$^+$ T lymphocytes (i.e., T cells that express the receptor for major histocompatibility complex [MHC] class II molecules) in a way that is recognized as being foreign. This sequence of events is necessary because T lymphocytes do not recognize native (unprocessed) antigen (Fig. 2).

Over the last 10 years, evidence has emerged for at least two CD4$^+$ T-lymphocyte subsets, denoted T_H1 and T_H2 that are formed by an ill-defined process from putative T_H0 cells. This taxonomy is based on the profile of cytokines that T cells release (13,14). Thus,

Table 1 Representative Cyclic AMP Phosphodiesterase Inhibitors for Allergic Diseases

Company[a]	Drug	Isoenzyme selectivity	Indication	Development stage
Rhône-Poulenc Rorer	RP 73401	IV	Asthma	Phase II
Sandoz	STZ MKS 492	IV	Asthma	Preclinical
Troponwerke	Nitraquazone	IV	Inflammation	Discontinued
Almirall	LAS 31025	IV	Asthma	Phase III
Eli-Lilly	Tibenelast	IV	Asthma	Phase III
Organon	Org 20241	III/IV	Asthma	Phase I
Byk-Gulden	B-9004-070	IV	Asthma	Preclinical
Wyeth-Ayerst	WAY PDE 641	IV	Asthma	Phase I
Kyorin	Ibudilast	NS	Asthma	Marketed

[a]Several other companies have active PDE research programs including SmithKline-Beecham, Celltech, Syntex, Malesci, Glaxo, Zeneca, Schering, and Sterling Winthrop, but detailed information is unavailable.

the T_H1 phenotype secretes interleukin (IL)-2, interferon (IFN)-γ, and tumor necrosis factor (TNF)-β, whereas the T_H2 phenotype secretes IL-4, IL-5, IL-6, and IL-10. Both subsets secrete IL-3 and granulocyte–macrophage colony-stimulating factor (GM-CSF; see Fig. 2). Furthermore, IL-10 released from T_H2 cells can inhibit the ability of T_H1 cells to release IFN-γ and IL-2, whereas the elaboration of IFN-γ from the T_H1 subset suppresses the generation of T_H2-derived cytokines (see Fig. 2). This classification of CD4$^+$ T-cell subsets originally applied to murine T-lymphocyte clones (13,14), but recent evidence is available for a similar, although not absolute, division of T cells in animals and humans in vivo (e.g., 15–20). Of particular relevance is the finding that, in allergic disease, the predominant cytokines detected include IL-4 and IL-5 (with little or no IL-2 or IFN-γ), implying a predominance of the T_H2 subset in these individuals (e.g., 15–17). This contrasts with individuals with delayed hypersensitivity reactions, such as tuberculoid leprosy and Lyme arthritis, who almost exclusively elaborate T_H1 T-cell-derived cytokines (19,20). It is currently unknown what governs the preferential activation of a particular CD4$^+$ T-cell subset, but it is tempting to speculate that factors that directly or indirectly alter the IFN-γ/IL-10 ratio will have a profound influence on this process. It was recently reported that macrophages secrete IL-10 (21,22), which in vivo would theoretically favor the predominance of the T_H2 subset of T cells. If IL-10 is generated by macrophages or other APC following allergen provocation, then this, by inhibiting IFN-γ release from T_H1 T cells, might provide a necessary stimulus for preferential T_H2 T-cell activation.

Antigen processing and presentation initially involve the cleavage of the allergen into small oligopeptides (10- to 20-amino acid residues in length: *processing*), followed by expression of these cleavage products on the surface of the APC in association with an MHC class II molecule: *presentation*. In this form the antigen–MHC class II molecular complex interacts with the T-cell receptor (TCR) expressed on the surface of T lymphocytes. Structurally, the TCR is a heterodimeric molecule composed of an α- and β-polypeptide chain. The genes that encode the $\alpha\beta$-complex can give rise to about 10^{16} receptor variants, which is far more than the total number of T lymphocytes in the body (see Ref. 23). Antigen recognition by T cells also involves the participation of CD4 and CD3 which serve to stabilize the specific immune recognition reactions and to activate T-cells, respectively. Once activated, CD4$^+$ T cells communicate with B-lymphocytes to switch antibody production away from IgM and IgD (which are normally biosynthesized by the cell) to IgE,

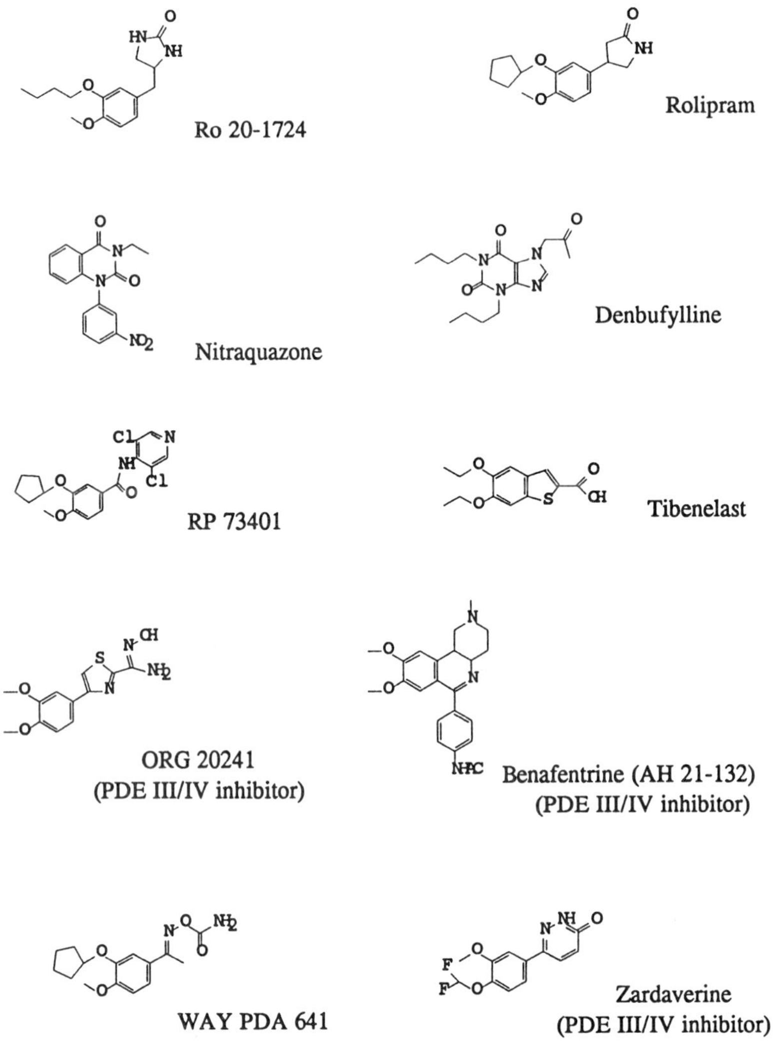

Figure 1   Molecular structure of selected PDE III–IV and PDE IV inhibitors.

IgA, and IgG$_1$. This is brought about by two processes that work in tandem. First, activated CD4$^+$ T cells (and other leukocytes—see below) release a number of cytokines including IL-4 (24) and IL-13 (25,26) which interact with their specific receptors on B cells to induce the transcription of the Cϵ gene through a process of deletional switch recombination (27,28). The mechanism of Cϵ gene transcription is enhanced by IL-6 which can be released from mast cells, basophils, and T$_H$2 T cells (29). Immunoglobulin isotype switching also requires a contact-dependent signal from the T cell which is provided by the CD40 ligand (CD40L) (30,31). This molecule, a 30–39 kDa glycoprotein expressed by activated T lymphocytes, permits the Cϵ mRNA transcripts produced by IL-4 and IL-13 to be translated into functional protein. Immunoglobulin E-bearing mast cells and basophils also express CD40L in response to allergen (32) and, together with their capacity to release IL-4 (33,34), stimulate further IgE synthesis by B lymphocytes. Once produced, the antigen-specific IgE binds to high- and low-affinity IgE Fc-receptors (FcϵRI and FcϵRII, respec-

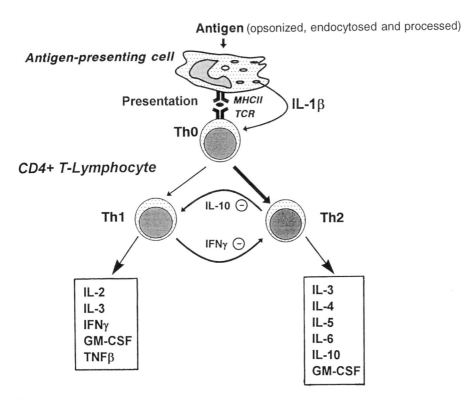

Figure 2   Activation of CD4+ T$_H$2 T lymphocytes by alveolar macrophages in response to allergen. Two functional types of CD4+ T cells have been defined in the mouse, denoted T$_H$1 and T$_H$2, and evidence for a similar classification in humans is available. T$_H$1 and T$_H$2 T cells are derived from putative T$_H$0 T cells but the processes which govern this phenomenon are unknown. Once formed, T$_H$1 and T$_H$2 T cells can inhibit the proliferation of the other through the release of IFN-γ and IL-10, respectively. In addition, these T cells secrete a different profile of cytokines such that T$_H$1 phenotype is better equipped to deal with delayed type hypersensitivity reactions whereas T$_H$2 cells tend to promote immunoglobulin isotype switching and chronic allergic inflammation. See text for further details.

tively) on mast cells, basophils, eosinophils, B cells, and/or macrophages. If the sensitized individual is reexposed to the same allergen, it will be recognized by IgE-bearing cells and effect their activation culminating in an acute allergic response (Fig. 3). This is invariably precipitated by the release of proinflammatory mediators such as histamine, platelet activating factor (PAF), prostaglandins (PG), and leukotrienes (LT).

IgE-INDEPENDENT MECHANISMS AND ALLERGIC INFLAMMATION

Although there is unanimity of opinion that IgE-driven mechanisms are responsible for the immediate short-term exacerbations of many allergic diseases that follow allergen provocation in atopic individuals, the extent to which IgE-mediated mechanisms play a role in late-phase reactions is currently unclear. Indeed, it is likely that IgE represents only one of several, highly complex, components that regulate the chronic ongoing inflammatory

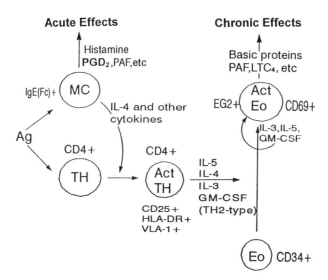

Figure 3 Cartoon outlining a current hypothesis underlying allergen-mediated allergic inflammation (23,36). It is proposed that two pathways operate in tandem culminating in the acute and chronic manifestations of allergen provocation in sensitized individuals. The first involves the activation of granulocytes that express surface-bound Fc receptors for IgE such as mast cells, basophils, and eosinophils with the resultant release of mediators including histamine, prostaglandins, and platelet activating factor. These molecules give rise to the immediate symptoms following allergen exposure and may be responsible for acute exacerbation of allergic symptoms in atopic individuals. In the second pathway, allergen may be presented to CD4+ T_H2 T cells, resulting in their activation and elaboration of a number of cytokines including IL-3, IL-4, IL-5, TNF-α, and GM-CSF. One major action of these so-called chronic proinflammatory mediators is the attraction and activation of eosinophils (CD69+ and EG2+) at sites of allergen entry. Through their ability to release basic proteins and lipid mediators together with the generation of reactive oxygen species, the chronic effects of allergic diseases may, at least in part, be manifest. It is important to note that activation of this second pathway need not invovle the participation of allergen-specific IgE.

responses that characterize many allergic diseases (Fig. 3). There is now overwhelming evidence that activation of macrophages and CD4+ T_H2 T cells in addition to, or instead of, promoting immunoglobulin isotype switching can elicit the release of a plethora of pro-inflammatory cytokines that may induce and perpetuate allergic inflammation. In particular, the elaboration of IL-3, IL-5, GM-CSF, and TNF-α by T cells and macrophages may orchestrate, at least in part, the infiltration and activation of eosinophils, which are implicated in several chronic allergic diseases, including atopic dermatitis (35), asthma (36), and rhinitis (37; see Fig. 3).

Although allergic disorders and atopy are closely related, the disease process can occur (apparently) in the absence of local IgE production or the excessive elaboration of IL-4. Given this finding, IgE-mediated mechanisms appear neither necessary nor sufficient for the development of allergy. Indeed, there are many reports documenting that nonatopic individuals can develop diseases such as allergic asthma, whereas not all atopic subjects become asthmatic. This tempts speculation that these apparently IgE-independent disorders are antigen-driven, cell-mediated phenomena, dependent on the elaboration of proinflammatory cytokines. If this is true, what antigen is responsible for inducing chronic, nonatopic allergy? Various possibilities have been proposed (36), including viral antigens and autoantibodies arising from damaged tissue around the site of inflammation. Inhalation of common allergens, such as house dust mite, can also indirectly activate CD4$^+$ T cells in nonatopic individuals (38).

This chapter will focus primarily on two allergic disorders: atopic dermatitis and allergic asthma which, in the context of PDEs and PDE inhibitors, are the most studied. In both diseases, allergen provocation can evoke an immediate, IgE-driven response, culminating in a variety of acute symptoms, including bronchoconstriction, wheezing, edema, and erythema. This may be followed, hours later, by cell-mediated (predominantly T cells and eosinophils) inflammatory responses involving the release of cytokines, which are believed to ultimately give rise to the more chronic, and in some individuals irreversible, symptoms of these disorders.

GENERAL PROPERTIES AND CLASSIFICATION OF PDE ISOENZYMES

Cyclic nucleotide PDEs (EC 3.1.4.17) were discovered more than 30 years ago (39). These enzymes hydrolyze the phosphodiester bond of purine cyclic nucleotides (cAMP, cGMP) to their corresponding 5′-mononucleotides (5′-AMP, 5′-GMP), which do not activate cyclic nucleotide-dependent protein kinases. Although enzymes have been identified that metabolize cyclic pyrimidines (40), attention has largely focused on those PDEs that hydrolyze cAMP and cGMP, the second-messenger roles of which are well established in cells.

The multiple PDE isoenzymes that have been identified (41–44) differ in their substrate specificity, kinetic properties, responsiveness to endogenous regulators (Ca^{2+}–calmodulin, cGMP) and susceptibility to inhibition by various compounds. Molecular biological studies have demonstrated that many cyclic nucleotide PDEs are separate gene products with multivariant regulatory (Ca^{2+}/calmodulin- or cGMP-binding sites) and other ill-defined domains linked to highly conserved (> 60% amino acid identity) and homologous catalytic sequences (approximately 270 amino acids) that are located near the COOH-terminus of the enzyme. Several attempts to categorize PDE isoenzymes have been made, the most widely adopted system of nomenclature being that proposed by Beavo and Reifsnyder (41) that has been recently updated by Michaeli et al. (42). Seven major families have been proposed (Table 2), although it is likely that there will be additions to these. The families are designated by the Roman numerals I, II, III, IV, V, VI, and VII and correspond to Ca^{2+}–calmodulin-stimulated, cGMP-stimulated, cGMP-inhibited, cAMP-specific, cGMP-specific, photoreceptor- and rolipram-insensitive (cAMP-specific) PDEs, respectively. Members of one family share 20–25% sequence homology with members of another. These families contain two or more related subfamilies (designated with a capital letter) that are derived from similar (70–90% homology), but distinct, genes. Furthermore, several of the subfamilies have multiple members (designated with Arabic numerals) produced by alternative mRNA splicing or different start sites for translation of the protein. For the sake of completeness, a brief description of the seven PDE families identified thus far is presented in the following sections. Readers requiring more detailed information should consult recent reviews of this subject (43,44).

PDE I Isoenzyme Family

The PDE I, or Ca^{2+}–calmodulin-stimulated PDE, is a family of isoenzymes that, as the name implies, is activated by calmodulin, and micromolar concentrations of Ca^{2+}–calmodulin can induce a marked increase in catalytic activity (5- to 20-fold; 45,46). Kinetic

Table 2　Properties and Selective Inhibitors of Cyclic Nucleotide Phosphodiesterase Isoenzymes

PDE family[a]	Subunit size[b] (kDa)	K_m (μM)[b] cAMP	K_m (μM)[b] cGMP	Selective inhibitors	Refs.
I. Ca^{2+}–calmodulin-stimulated	59–75	2–70	2–20	Vinpocetine, trifluoperazine,[c] KS-505a	89
					90
					91
II. cGMP-stimulated	102–105	30–100	10–30	EHNA[d]	92
III. cGMP-inhibited	63–135	0.1–0.5	0.1–0.5	Siguazodan, SK&F 94120	93
				SK&F 95654	94
				Milrinone	95
				Enoximone	96
IV. cAMP-specific	60–83	0.5–2	>50	Rolipram	71
				Ro 20-1724	71
				Nitraquazone	97
				Denbufylline	98
V. cGMP-specific	90–100	>40	1.5	Zaprinast	89
				SK&F 96231	99
VI. Photoreceptor	84–99	>500	17–20	Zaprinast	100
VII. Rolipram-insensitive cAMP-specific	—	0.2	—	None	

[a]Nomenclature based on Beavo and Reifsnyder (41) and Micheali et al. (42).
[b]The K_m values and the subunit sizes are taken from Refs. 41, 96–98. The kinetic heterogeneity within an isoenzyme family is probably related to the tissue, species, isolation procedure, and enzyme purity as well as the existence of multiple subtypes.
[c]Trifluoperazine inhibits PDE I by acting as a calmodulin antagonist.
[d]erythro-9-(2-hydroxy-3-nonyl)-adenine.

analyses have demonstrated that this is due to an increase in V_{max} as well as slight decrease in K_m (45,46). From the functional (kinetic) data, two major forms of the PDE I family appear to exist. Isoforms purified from bovine brain (PDE I_{EI}; 47) and lung (PDE I_{FI}; 46) display substrate selectivity for cGMP (K_m ~3 μM) over cAMP (K_m ~ 40 μM), whereas subtypes identified in mouse testes (PDE I_{DI}; 48) and canine trachealis (49) exhibit similar affinities for both substrates (K_m 1–2 μM). The former group of Ca^{2+}–calmodulin-stimulated PDEs have been referred to as PDE Iα and the latter as PDE Iβ (49).

PDE II Isoenzyme Family

Cyclic GMP-stimulated PDEs display a low affinity for both cAMP (K_m, 30–100 μM) and cGMP (K_m, 10–30 μM) and exhibit positive homotropic cooperativity relative to substrate (50,51). This effect is related to the high-affinity binding of cGMP to an allosteric site (K_d, ~ 0.1 μM). Relatively low concentrations of cGMP (1–5 μM) stimulate cAMP hydrolysis. There is evidence for multiple forms of PDE II, but the structural basis for this is unknown (41).

PDE III Isoenzyme Family

The GMP-inhibited PDE family is characterized by its high-affinity for cAMP (K_m, 0.1–0.5 μM) and cGMP (K_m, 0.1–0.5 μM) (V_{max} greater for cAMP than for cGMP) and competitive inhibition of its cAMP hydrolytic activity by cGMP and certain positive inotropic agents (52). PDE IIIs with similar characteristics have been isolated form a variety of tissues and evidence for multiple molecular forms of PDE III has recently been reported (53,54).

PDE IV Isoenzyme Family

Selective inhibitors of the PDE IV isoenzyme family are receiving considerable attention with regard to their potential anti-inflammatory and immunomodulatory activity. Indeed, it is conceivable that these drugs could exert a steroid-sparing influence in humans. If this is proved, then a number of allergic diseases, including atopic dermatitis and bronchial asthma, may be more effectively managed. Given the importance of PDE IV as a possible target for therapeutic intervention, it is appropriate to describe in greater detail the characteristics and properties of these proteins and how they may be regulated.

The PDE IV isoenzymes are the most rapidly expanding family of PDEs. At the time of writing, four mammalian cDNA homologues (ratPDE 1–4; 55–58) of the *Drosophila melanogaster* "dunce" cAMP PDE (59) had been cloned, establishing a molecular basis for the observed heterogeneity of gene products within this PDE family. These clones are believed to represent transcripts of four different genes and have been reclassified according to the nomenclature proposed by Beavo and Reifsnyder (41). Thus, ratPDE 1, PDE 2, PDE 3, and PDE 4 are now known as PDE IV_C, PDE IV_A, PDE IV_D, and PDE IV_B, respectively. A remarkable finding that has emerged from the molecular cloning of PDE IV isoenzymes, is the presence of mRNA transcripts of different sizes for each of the four variants that are differentially expressed among tissues (55–58,60,61). For example, mRNA transcripts corresponding to members of the PDE IV_A subfamily were identified in rat brain, heart, and testis, but not in liver or kidney. In contrast, the tissue distribution of mRNA transcripts corresponding to the PDE IV_C subfamily were localized to the liver and testis only (61). Similarly, two forms of PDE IV_B mRNA and two forms of PDE IV_D mRNA are coexpressed in rat Sertoli cells (61). Studies conducted by Conti and his colleagues (62) have established that this profound heterogeneity of PDE IV isoenzymes is the result of alternative mRNA splicing and multiple start sites for the transcription of the protein.

Evidence was recently provided for the existence of at least four human genes that encode PDE IV isoenzymes (63–65). Similar to their rat counterparts, there is a restricted localization of mRNA transcripts among tissues (63,64).

A substantial divergence of opinion exists on the size of PDE IV. Sodium dodecyl sulfate–polyacrylamide gel electrophoresis (SDS–PAGE) of an enzyme purified from canine kidney, for example, shows a subunit molecular mass of 82 kDa (66,67), whereas the PDE IV isoenzymes in rat liver (68), rat Sertoli cells (69), and human monocytes (70) have apparent molecular masses of 52, 67, and 88 kDa, respectively. Although limited proteolysis of the native protein could account for these discrepancies, the recent appreciation of marked PDE IV heterogeneity within and among tissues provides an alternative and more convincing explanation. Furthermore, the structure of PDE IV may differ significantly among species.

Confusion is also apparent concerning the quaternary structure of the native protein. For example, Nemoz et al. (71) purified a PDE IV isoenzyme from rat brain cytosol that had a molecular mass of 44 kDa by gel filtration, but of 89 kDa when the protein was electrophoresed on polyacrylamide gels under nondenaturing conditions. Identical results were obtained when rat heart cytosol was used as a source of PDE IV (71). These findings may suggest that the quaternary structure of the native enzyme is either dimeric, composed of two apparently identical subunits, or that an equilibrium exists between the monomeric and dimeric PDE IV variants (71). The former possibility is attractive from the point of view that members of the PDE II, PDE III, PDE V, and PDE VI isoenzyme families all exist as homo- or heterodimers (see Ref. 43). Furthermore, these data tempt speculation that the assembly of PDE monomers into dimers may represent a common feature among all PDEs. Further experiments, however, noted that gel filtration of a crude rat brain supernatant identified a PDE IV activity with a molecular mass of 250 kDa, significantly heavier than that of the purified enzyme (71). It is conceivable that the 44-kDa PDE represents a catalytic subunit that is part of a native enzyme of quaternary structure more complex than a dimer (71).

In contrast, a human monocyte PDE IV cDNA clone that was engineered for overexpression in *Saccharomyces cerevisiae* yields a protein that is significantly different (apparently) from the brain and heart enzyme (70). Gel filtration and SDS–PAGE indicate molecular masses of 320 and 88 kDa, respectively (70). One interpretation of these data is that the monocyte PDE IV exists as a homotetramer in the native state. It is also possible that PDE IV is monomeric, and that the tetramer represents an artifact. Indeed, kinetic analyses of cAMP hydrolysis failed to reveal any evidence of cooperativity among the subunits, which would be expected of a PDE with a tetrameric quaternary structure (70). Recently conducted hydrodynamic studies indicate that the quaternary structure of the human monocyte-cloned PDE IV is probably dimeric (72).

In another study, purification of a PDE IV from canine kidney produced a protein of 60 kDa that did not form higher molecular mass species (dimers or tetramers) by cross-linking with chemical reagents (73). These results indicate that the native PDE IV in this tissue may exist as a monomer.

Rolipram-Binding Site

The observation that [³H]rolipram labels high-affinity sites in rat brain membranes in a saturable and stereoselective manner was first reported in 1987 (74). Although initial attempts failed to establish that purified PDE IV features high-affinity sites for rolipram, a monocyte-derived, recombinant PDE IV$_A$ isoenzyme expressed in yeast, showed significant rolipram binding, indicating that the catalytic site and rolipram-binding site reside on the same gene product (75). Further studies with the expressed enzyme identified a single class of high-affinity ($K_d \sim 2$ nM) noninteracting ($n_H = 1$) sites for rolipram (75). Interestingly, similar studies performed with the recombinant PDE IV$_B$ from human brain, suggest the presence of two noninteracting, high-affinity, rolipram-binding sites ($K_d = 0.4$ and 6 nM) (64).

Evidence that the catalytic and rolipram-binding sites are distinct entities is derived from several experiments. Perhaps the most compelling is the finding that the rank order of potency of several structurally dissimilar PDE inhibitors for inhibiting cAMP hydrolysis does not correlate with their abilities to displace [^{3}H]rolipram (75). Furthermore, the affinity of rolipram for the binding site is approximately 100-fold higher than for the catalytic site (75). These marked discrepancies question the role of the rolipram-binding site in relation to catalytic activity. In particular, does the high-affinity site represent an allosteric domain? The functional role, if any, of this noncatalytic site is still unclear, but raises important questions about the therapeutic implications of selective inhibitors. In particular, can occupation of the rolipram-binding site affect catalytic activity and, if so, is it desirable or undesirable for PDE IV inhibitors to have preferential affinity for the rolipram-binding site, or is it irrelevant? With the remarkable resurgence of interest in cyclic nucleotide PDEs and their regulation, it is likely that the role of the rolipram-binding site will soon be made clear.

Regulation of PDE IV

Until very recently (see later) there was no published evidence for short-term regulation of PDE IV; however, a prolonged elevation of cAMP results in the induction of this protein (60,76–80). Indeed, PDE IV induction represents a common homeostatic mechanism of cyclic nucleotide regulation. Recent studies have shown that incubating U937 cells with albuterol (salbutamol) and rolipram for up to 24 h results in a time-dependent increase in the amount of a rolipram-sensitive PDE activity (77). This phenomenon is dependent on cAMP accumulation, on protein kinase A (PKA) activation, and is slowly reversible after agonist removal (77). Moreover, the induction involves protein and mRNA synthesis, for it is abolished in cells treated with dactinomycin (actinomycin D) and cycloheximide (77). Similar results were obtained when albuterol was used alone (although the induction was not as marked), and after treatment of the cells with prostaglandin E$_2$ and 8-bromo-cAMP (77). These results are consistent with data recently published by Swinnen et al. (61), who reported that increasing the cAMP content of rat Sertoli cells with gonadotropin follicle-stimulating hormone initiates the transcription of two genes that encode PDE IV$_B$ and PDE IV$_D$.

An increase in PDE IV activity has also been reported for several proinflammatory and immunocompetent cells in response to a variety of stimuli (78,79) but, in contrast with rat Sertoli and U937 cells, the increase in activity is manifest rapidly after the application of the stimulus. Indeed, in concanavalin A-stimulated T lymphocytes, in lipopolysaccharide-activated macrophages, and in monocytes treated with IFN-γ and histamine, an increase in PDE IV activity is apparent within 1 h (78–82). The finding that the time courses for increased cAMP PDE activity range from several minutes (83) to many hours (77) suggests that different mechanisms regulate PDE IV and that a rapid increase in cAMP hydrolytic activity is unlikely to involve protein synthesis. If this is true, then what short-term processes could effect a rapid change in PDE IV-catalyzed cAMP hydrolysis? The most obvious mechanism is one involving protein phosphorylation. Indeed, recent preliminary data suggest that, similar to members of the PDE I, PDE III, and PDE V isoenzyme families (see Ref. 43), PDE IV is also subject to a similar regulatory influence (84,84a,84b). In one of those studies, Chan et al. (84) reported that histamine stimulated the phosphorylation of a 61-kDa protein that had the characteristics of an atypical, rolipram-sensitive cAMP PDE (recently identified and partially characterized in monocytes from individuals with atopic dermatitis; see later section on activity in allergic diseases). It was proposed that histamine promoted the phosphorylation and subsequent stimulation of this enzyme by activating protein kinase C (84). Phosphodiesterase IV is also phosphorylated by a cAMP-dependent mechanism (84a,84b). Further details on the regulation of cAMP PDEs, specifically in relation to atopic dermatitis, are provided in the later section on activity in allergic diseases.

PDE V Isoenzyme Family

Until recently (42), cGMP-specific PDE from peripheral tissues, such as lung, vascular and bronchial smooth muscle, and platelets (PDE V_A), was categorized in the same family as the retinal rod (PDE V_B) and retinal cone (PDE V_C) photoreceptor enzymes (41). The latter two isoenzymes are now categorized as PDE VI (42) because of marked differences in primary sequence. The cGMP PDEs have been purified from lung and platelets (85,86). They display substrate selectivity for cGMP (K_m, 4–6 μM), exhibiting little activity on cAMP (85,86). As with PDE II, a high-affinity, noncatalytic cGMP-binding site exists on PDE V, the function of which is uncertain.

PDE VI Isoenzyme Family

Photoreceptor PDEs are located exclusively in retinal rods and cones where they play an important role in visual transduction (87). They display selectivity for cGMP (Km, 17–20 μM), although they are less discriminating than PDE V (K_m of cAMP, 600–2000 μM). As with PDEs II and V, noncatalytic cGMP-binding sites are associated with rod PDE VI (87).

PDE VII Isoenzyme Family

A gene recently isolated from a human glioblastoma cDNA library was expressed in a cAMP PDE-deficient strain of *Saccharomyces cerevisiae* (42). This novel gene, named *HCP-1* (*h*igh-affinity, *c*AMP-specific *p*hosphodiesterase 1), encodes a cAMP PDE (K_m = 0.2 μM) that is insensitive to cGMP and inhibitors of the PDE III (amrinone, milrinone) and PDE IV (rolipram, Ro 20-1724) isoenzyme families. Furthermore, although *HCP-1* shares sequence homology with the catalytic domain of all cyclic nucleotide PDEs, it does not share extensive homology to the *Drosophila* dunce cAMP PDE. Thus, based on these unique characteristics, *HCP-1* appears to represent a member of a previously unrecognized PDE family that Michaeli and co-workers (42) have designated PDE VII.

PDE VIII (?)

A rolipram- and cilostazol-insensitive cyclic purine hydrolytic activity was recently identified in the soluble fraction of rat cerebrum and was termed a PDE VIII isoenzyme (88). Although the properties and characteristics of this novel protein show similarities to PDE VII, its classification as a PDE VIII may be warranted, given that it hydrolyzes cAMP (K_m = 0.11 μM) and cGMP (K_m = 1.8 μM), exhibits a higher V_{max} for the latter substrate, and is inhibited, albeit weakly (IC_{50} ~ 26 μM), by isobutyl methylxanthine (IBMX) (88). Furthermore, cAMP behaves as a potent and competitive inhibitor of cGMP hydrolysis (K_I = 0.12 μM). Gel filtration indicates that this PDE has a molecular mass of 298 kDa (88).

CYCLIC AMP PHOSPHODIESTERASE ACTIVITY IN ALLERGIC DISEASES

In Leukocytes from Atopic Individuals

The cAMP PDE activity is increased in mononuclear leukocytes (MNL) of individuals with atopic disorders, including atopic dermatitis, allergic rhinitis, and asthma (101–103). Similar observations have also been made in MNL from patients with urticaria pigmentosa (104). However, the suggestion that elevated MNL cAMP PDE is a characteristic feature of psoriasis has been questioned (104) and, in the group of patients with urticaria pigmentosa, several subjects exhibited positive skin prick tests (104).

The abnormally elevated cAMP PDE activity is most prominent in blood monocytes (105), but it is also observed, to a lesser extent, in other immunocompetent cells, such as T lymphocytes (106) and neutrophils (103). The influence of atopy on cAMP PDE levels appears to be limited to bone marrow-derived cells, since there is no difference in the cAMP PDE activities in keratinocytes from normal and atopic individuals (107).

Two immunochemically distinct Ro 20-1724-inhibited cAMP PDEs have been reported to exist in monocytes from patients with atopic dermatitis, whereas only one form exists in monocytes from normal subjects (108). The cAMP PDE unique to monocytes from atopic subjects is difficult to categorize in the nomenclature system of Beavo and Reifsnyder (41). It is cytosolic, inhibited by Ro 20-1724 and rolipram (PDE IV inhibitors), and is stimulated by calcium and calmodulin (106,108,109). Interestingly, the atopic monocyte cAMP PDE is more potently inhibited by rolipram and other PDE IV inhibitors than the nonatopic enzyme and displays distinct kinetic characteristics (106). Furthermore, theophylline exhibits an IC_{50} value of 27 μM against this isoenzyme (106), a potency that is approximately tenfold higher than that reported against eosinophil PDE IV (110,111).

Possible Causes for Increased cAMP PDE in MNL from Atopic Individuals

The cause(s) of the elevated cAMP PDE activity in atopic MNL is uncertain. A primary gene defect may be responsible which, if correct, might implicate increased cAMP PDE as an important factor in the etiology of allergic disorders. The apparent, novel properties of the atopic cAMP PDE may point to such a conclusion. Several further pieces of evidence are cited in support of such a hypothesis: Cord blood MNL of children born to atopic parents exhibits elevated cAMP PDE activity, suggesting that the defect may be inheritable (112). However, not all studies have demonstrated elevated MNL cAMP PDE in young children with atopic dermatitis (113). The cAMP PDE activity remains high in individuals with atopic dermatitis whose disease is in complete remission following steroid therapy (114), indicating that the phenomenon is not a consequence of inflammation. The strength of this evidence is, once again, questionable in view of the results from another study showing that prolonged steroid therapy results in restoration of normal cAMP PDE levels (109). Finally, the genetic hypothesis is further supported by the demonstration of increased MNL cAMP PDE in a Basenji greyhound model of asthma and eczema (115). In these dogs, MNL cAMP PDE is elevated in both unsensitized and sensitized dogs (115).

Alternatively, increased cAMP PDE activity may be a consequence of the atopy itself, or of the associated inflammatory processes. Various studies have demonstrated that cAMP PDE can be induced by various agents that increase the intracellular concentration of cAMP (see earlier section on regulation of PDE IV for general details). Similarly, substances released during inflammatory reactions, such as cytokines and mediators, influence cAMP PDE activity in bone marrow-derived cells. For example, histamine increases cAMP PDE activity in normal monocytes to levels seen in cells purified from atopic individuals, possibly by elevating intracellular cAMP (116). A greater elevation of monocyte cAMP PDE is observed when mixed MNL are exposed to histamine, compared with exposure of purified monocytes (116). Hanifin and his colleagues (83) have suggested that, in atopy, unrestrained mediator release can occur in the skin and the mucosal surfaces of the lung and gut in response to neurohumoral and antigenic stimuli. It was further postulated (83) that this can lead to increased MNL cAMP PDE activity that may initiate the clinically observable signs of atopy. Monocyte cAMP PDE activity is also increased following a 1-h exposure of cells to IFN-γ (81,82), an effect enhanced by IL-4 (81). This occurs only in cells from normal subjects, since IFN-γ does not influence the already elevated cAMP PDE activity in monocytes from patients with atopic dermatitis (82).

Possible Consequences of Elevated MNL cAMP PDE Activity in Atopic Individuals

Decreased responsiveness to agents that stimulate cAMP synthesis, such as histamine, PGE$_1$, and β-adrenoceptor agonists, has been observed in MNL from atopic humans and Basenji greyhounds (101,115,117,118). Ro 20-1724 restores the responsiveness to β-adrenoceptor agonists (115), suggesting that accelerated intracellular cAMP hydrolysis is responsible for this defect in atopic MNL. The contribution that alternative down-regulatory processes make to the unresponsiveness of the cAMP cascade in atopy is uncertain. Heterologous down-regulation of adenylyl cyclase responses can be induced by inflammatory cytokines (119,120). Furthermore, agents that stimulate cAMP synthesis can induce tolerance in inflammatory cells by homologous and heterologous down-regulation of adenylyl-cyclase-linked receptors (121,122).

Elevated cAMP PDE activity has been correlated with the increased histamine release (123) and hyper-IgE synthesis (124) that are characteristic of atopic MNL. The suppression of histamine and IgE production from atopic MNL by Ro 20-1724 (123,124) indicates a causal link between accelerated cAMP hydrolysis and these functional defects.

It has been speculated (125) that the increased cAMP PDE in monocytes from atopics results in lowered intracellular cAMP and enhanced PGE$_2$ generation which, in turn, inhibits IFN-γ production from T$_H$1 T cells. Interferon-γ inhibits cytokine release from T$_H$2 cells, and it was proposed that inhibition of its release would disinhibit the generation of IL-4, causing B-lymphocyte antibody class switching and the production of IgE (125,126). High levels of PGE$_2$ are released from atopic monocytes, and a highly significant negative correlation exists between PGE$_2$ and IFN-γ levels in supernatants of atopic MNL in culture (125,126). Furthermore, the increase in IL-4 production, evoked by anti-CD3 by atopic MNL, correlates with elevated cAMP PDE, and a relatively low concentration (1 μM) of Ro 20-1724 inhibits the release of this cytokine, apparently by an action on monocytes (126).

The observations just detailed are intriguing, given that cAMP PDE inhibitors (127), together with other agents that elevate cAMP (128–130), are considered to be much more effective inhibitors of cytokine production from T_H1 cells than from T_H2 cells. The apparently paradoxical findings show that the effects of cAMP on T lymphocytes in a mixed MNL population are difficult to predict from studies on their counterparts in purified populations. Furthermore, cAMP responses in atopic T lymphocytes may differ substantially from those reported in animal or human T-helper subtype clones.

PDE ISOENZYME DISTRIBUTION IN CELLS IMPLICATED IN ALLERGIC DISEASES

The distribution of PDE isoenzymes in cell-types implicated in allergic and inflammatory reactions is presented in Table 3. The predominant isoenzyme family represented in these cells is PDE IV, which is expressed by mast cells, basophils, eosinophils, neutrophils, monocytes, macrophages, T lymphocytes, endothelial and epithelial cells (8–12). PDE III, which has been identified in basophils, murine (but not guinea pig) macrophages, T lymphocytes, platelets and epithelial cells is less widely distributed. The PDE I- (murine mast cells, epithelial cells) and PDE II- (murine macrophages, rat T lymphocytes, platelets, endothelial and epithelial cells) families are also expressed by certain proinflammatory/immunocompetent cells, but their function is unclear at present (8–12).

EFFECT OF PDE INHIBITORS ON CELLS IMPLICATED IN THE PATHOGENESIS OF ALLERGIC DISEASES

To date, the vast majority of information on the effects of PDE inhibitors on cell types implicated in allergic diseases and inflammation derive from studies on cells from normal subjects or animals (see Table 4). Given the evidence indicating that inflammatory and immunocompetent cells from atopic subjects are defective, the relevance of experiments on normal cells to allergic diseases is questionable. In addition, to extrapolate findings obtained using isolated cells to the in vivo or pathological situation must also be viewed with caution. It is likely, for example, that individual immunocompetent/inflammatory cell types that are highly dependent on other leukocytes for their functional responses behave entirely differently in whole blood or mixed leukocyte preparations than when a single population is isolated.

Mast Cells and Basophils

There are no studies reported on the effects of PDE inhibitors on human lung or skin mast cells. Early studies demonstrated that agents that elevated cAMP, including methylxanthines, inhibited mediator release from human lung (149,150). In murine bone marrow-derived mast cells, rolipram inhibits antigen-induced leukotriene (LT)C_4 release (8). Surprisingly, zaprinast, but not rolipram, blocks antigen-induced release of histamine from rat peritoneal mast cells (131), demonstrating the heterogeneity of second-messenger systems involved in regulating mediator release from different populations of mast cells.

Rolipram inhibits antigen- and anti-IgE-induced mediator (histamine, LTC_4) liberation from human basophils (131,132). The inhibitory effect of rolipram on mediator release is potentiated by the PDE III inhibitors, siguazodan and SK&F 95654 (132). Although zaprinast can, surprisingly, increase the cAMP content in these cells it does not inhibit mediator release (132).

Table 3 PDE Isoenzyme Profiles in Proinflammatory–Immunocompetent Cells Implicated in Allergic Disorders

Cell type	Species and source	PDE isoenzymes present	Comments	Refs.
Mast cell	Murine–bone cleaved	I, IV	Enzyme studies not reported.	8
	Rat peritoneal mast cells	V (?)	Zaprinast inhibits antigen-induced histamine release.	131
Basophil	Human peripheral blood	III, IV		132
Eosinophil	Guinea pig peritoneal	IV	Tightly membrane-bound enzyme displaying nonlinear kinetics.	111
				110
	Human peripheral blood		Membrane-bound enzyme displaying nonlinear kinetics.	133
Neutrophil	Human peripheral blood	IV	Membrane-bound enzyme displaying nonlinear kinetics.	134
Monocyte	Human peripheral blood	IV		135, 136
Macrophage	Guinea pig peritoneal macrophage	IV	Membrane-bound enzyme.	137
	Murine peritoneal macrophage	II, III, IV		138
				78
B lymphocyte		Unknown		
T lymphocyte	Rat T cells	II, III, IV		79
	Rat T cells	II, III, IV, V		139
	Human peripheral blood	IV	PDE III exclusively particulate	80
	Human peripheral blood	III, IV	PDE IV cytosolic and particulate	140, 141
	Human T-cell clones	IV, VII (?)	Enzyme with characteristics similar to the recently cloned PDE IV identified in T-cell lines	142
Platelet	Human peripheral blood	II, III, V		93, 94, 143, 144
Endothelial cell	Bovine aorta	II, IV	PDE profile in the microvasculature has not been determined; however, inhibitory effects of rolipram on microvascular leakage suggest presence of PDE IV in endothelial cells of microvascular beds.	145, 146
	Porcine aorta			
Epithelial cell	Fetal bovine aorta	II, IV, V	Epithelium removed.	147
	Bovine trachea	I, II, III, IV, V	Possible contamination with smooth muscle?	148

Table 4 Effects of Phosphodiesterase Inhibitors on Cells Implicated in Allergic or Inflammatory Diseases

Cell type	Functional effect of PDE IV inhibitor[a]	Comments	Ref.
Mast cells	Inhibition of mediator release (M)	PDE V, but not PDE IV, inhibitors suppress mediator release from rat peritoneal mast cells.	8, 131
Basophils	Inhibition of mediator release (H)	PDE III inhibitors enhance the actions of PDE IV inhibitors.	132
T lymphocytes	Inhibition of proliferation (H)	PDE III inhibitors enhance the inhibitory effect of PDE IV inhibitors.	141, 153
	Inhibition of IL-2 expression (H)		153, 155
B lymphocytes	Unknown	Nonspecific PDE inhibitors suppress proliferation and either increase or decrease IgE production.	163
Monocytes	Inhibition of		
	Arachidonic acid breakdown (H)		169
	Phagocytosis (H)		170
	Superoxide generation (H)		170
	TNF-α release (H)	PDE inhibitors only weakly suppress IL-1β release	171, 172, 175
Macrophages	Inhibition of		
	Superoxide generation (GP)		137, 177
	Mediator release (M)		179
	TNF-α release (M)		179
Eosinophils	Inhibition of		
	Superoxide generation (H/GP)		110, 111
	Thromboxane release (GP)		183
	Chemotaxis (GP)		185
	Degranulation (H/GP)	IBMX-induced inhibition of eosinophil derived neurotoxin	184, 203
Neutrophils	Inhibition of		
	Superoxide generation (H)		189
	Chemotaxis (H)		190
	Phagocytosis (H)		170
	Mediator release (H)		191
	Degranulation (H)		203
Endothelial cells	Reduction of permeability of monolayers (P)	PDE III and PDE IV inhibitors reduce permeability of pulmonary artery endothelial cells	198

[a]GP, guinea pig; H, human; M, mouse; P, pig.

T Lymphocytes and B Lymphocytes

The PDE IV inhibitor Ro 20-1724 and the PDE III inhibitor CI-930 suppress phytohemag-glutinin (PHA)-induced blastogenesis of a mixed population of human purified T lympho-cytes (141). Only partial (50–70%) inhibition was observed when these compounds were tested individually, but a combination of the PDE III and PDE IV inhibitors, or the addition of the mixed-type inhibitor, papaverine, elicited a much greater effect (141). By using highly purified preparations of human CD4$^+$ and CD8$^+$ T cells, Giembycz et al. (151) reported that PHA-induced [^{3}H]thymidine incorporation was inhibited by rolipram. Fur-thermore, in the presence of the PDE III inhibitor, SK&F 95654, which was inactive by itself, the inhibitory effect of rolipram was enhanced (151). Similar data are also available for a human T_H2 T-cell clone established from aeroallergen-specific T cells obtained from atopic donors (152). In that study, the selective PDE IV inhibitor WAY PDA-641 and theophylline suppressed the generation of IL-4 induced by anti-CD3 (152). Inhibition of IL-2 generation may be one mechanism by which cAMP PDE inhibitors exert their antiproliferative effects (151,153,154). Indeed, rolipram potently inhibits the generation of IFN-γ and IL-2 in CD4$^+$ and CD8$^+$ T cells stimulated with PHA under conditions in which SK&F 95654 is inactive (151). This conclusion may have to be reinterpreted, however, given that rolipram and CI-930 inhibit concanavalin A-induced murine splenocyte prolif-eration at concentrations below those required to suppress IL-2 generation (155). This suggests that their antiproliferative effects are independent of IL-2 gene transcription (155), a conclusion supported by the finding that in Jurkat cells, neither rolipram nor CI-930 affected steady-state levels of IL-2 mRNA (155). Alternatively, PDE inhibitors may exert their effects by blocking mitogenic signal transduction systems (156,157). Indeed, agents that elevate cAMP inhibit anti-CD3-induced tyrosine phosphorylation of a 100-kDa protein that is implicated in T-cell activation, as well as decreasing IL-2 biosynthesis and IL-2 receptor expression (157). The decrease in IL-2 evoked by cAMP-elevating agents was ascribed to an effect on IL-2 gene transcription and a decrease in the half-time ($t_{1/2}$) for IL-2 mRNA degradation (157). Collectively, these data suggest that PDE inhibitors may have multiple inhibitory effects on T-cell proliferation.

Few studies have compared the actions of PDE inhibitors on T_H1 and T_H2 CD4$^+$ T-lymphocyte functions. The weak, nonselective PDE inhibitor, pentoxifylline, is more effective at inhibiting the release of IL-2 (T_H1 T–cell derived) than IL-4 (T_H2 T–cell-derived) (127) a finding consistent with a wide body of evidence demonstrating that cAMP is more effective in suppressing the release of IL-2 and IFN-γ than of IL-4 and IL-5 (128–130,158,159). Recently, however, Essayen et al. (160,161) reported that the PDE IV inhibitor rolipram, effectively blocked tetanus toxoid (T_H1)- and ragweed (T_H2)-driven proliferation of peripheral blood mononuclear cells, whereas representative inhibitors of the PDE III (siguazodan) and PDE V (zaprinast) isoenzyme families were inactive. Significantly, rolipram was more effective at suppressing the ragweed-driven proliferative response (161). Reverse transcriptase polymerase chain reaction (RT-PCR) revealed that rolipram attenu-ated IL-5 and IFN-γ, but not IL-4, gene transcription following allergen provocation (161). Furthermore, the T_H1-like Jurkat cell line expressed a low level of mRNA for PDE IV$_A$ (human monocyte enzyme; 63), but no detectable message for PDE IV$_B$ (human brain enzyme; 64). In contrast, the ragweed-specific oligoclonal T_H2 cell line expressed mRNA for both PDE IV variants (161). The authors concluded from these data that the ability of rolipram to suppress T_H2 T-cell proliferation may be dictated by the selective expression of PDE IV isoenzymes in the T_H2 cells (161).

The inhibition of T_H2 T–cell-derived cytokines by cAMP PDE inhibitors is observed only in a mixed population of atopic MNL and not in purified T cells. This effect is apparently mediated indirectly by monocytes (see following section on monocytes and macrophages) and demonstrates that the effects of the cAMP PDE inhibitors on isolated inflammatory–immunocompetent cells may be a poor indicator of their actions in whole blood or in vivo.

A cAMP PDE, named JK-21, which shares several notable similarities with PDE VII, has been identified in several T-cell lines, including Jurkat, MOLT-4, HBP-ALL, and HUT-78 (142). In particular, JK-21 is a cAMP-specific enzyme ($K_m = 0.45$ μM) that does not hydrolyze cGMP and that is largely insensitive to milrinone, zaprinast, IBMX, and rolipram (142). JK-21 is not found in the B-cell lines Jijoye, JY, and Namalwa, implying specificity of expression among cells. It is currently unknown if JK-21 is a member of the PDE VII isoenzyme family and, moreover, if it is present in CD4$^+$ or CD8$^+$ T lymphocytes. However, Bloom and Beavo (161a) have identified a PDE VII in the HUT 78 T-lymphocyte cell line, suggesting that this may be so. Given these data, it is tempting to speculate that the recently reported immunomodulatory effects afforded by low-dose theophylline in allergic asthma (162) are attributable to the inhibition of a JK-21/PDE VII-like isoenzyme in T lymphocytes. Implicit in this suggestion is that theophylline is a potent and selective inhibitor of JK-21/PDE VII. This is important to establish, given that the concentration of theophylline achieved therapeutically produces little, if any, inhibition of other known PDE isoenzymes (cf. atopic cAMP PDE).

The effect of PDE inhibitors on B-lymphocyte function is poorly studied. Agents that elevate cAMP either decrease or increase antibody production; the effect may be dependent on the time of drug addition (163). Proliferation of B lymphocytes is inhibited by cAMP (163). Since reduction of proliferation is associated with differentiation, it is of interest that recent studies (164–168) indicate that, paradoxically, cAMP can induce antibody class-switching in B lymphocytes, leading to production of IgG1 and IgE. In spite of this, the only report, to our knowledge, on the effects of PDE inhibitors on antibody production shows that, in MNL from patients with atopic dermatitis, Ro 20-1724 inhibits spontaneous IgE release (124). This inhibition is not observed in monocyte-depleted cells, demonstrating that the effect is indirect (124). Suppression of IL-4 release in atopic MNL by Ro 20-1724 (126) may be responsible for its inhibition of IgE generation. An action of PDE IV inhibitors on T cells may also contribute to the effects of cAMP on antibody production. Interleukin-2 can contribute to the production of IgE in a mixed population of human leukocytes (168). Inhibition of IL-2 release may explain why PGE$_2$ mildly inhibits IgE synthesis in MNL composed of B and T lymphocytes as well as monocytes (168).

Monocytes and Macrophages

PDE inhibitors suppress several functions of monocytes including arachidonic acid breakdown (169), phagocytosis (170), and superoxide formation (170). Inhibitors of PDE IV are particularly effective in suppressing LPS-induced TNF-α release from human monocytes (171–173) through an effect on gene transcription (Souness JE; unpublished observations). Inhibitors of PDE III (CI-390) elicit only a weak inhibitory effect, PDE I inhibitors (vinpocetine) are inactive, whereas the PDE V inhibitor zaprinast is either inactive (173) or augments the LPS-induced release of TNF-α (172). Although some early reports suggested that cAMP posttranscriptionally inhibits IL-1β release (174), the effect of PDE IV inhibition is weak in comparison with the suppression of TNF-α generation (172). The PDE III inhibitor CI-930 and vinpocetine (PDE I inhibitor) exert little influence on monocyte IL-1β generation; consistent with its effect on TNF-α generation, zaprinast augments the LPS response (172). The inhibitory effects of PDE IV inhibitors on LPS-induced TNF-α generation have also been reported in whole blood (175) and in vivo (176).

Inhibition of guinea pig and human macrophage superoxide release is elicited by PDE IV inhibitors (137,177,178). Inhibition of macrophage LTC_4 generation by PDE IV inhibitors has also been observed (179). As in monocytes, LPS-induced TNF-α generation in macrophages is exquisitely sensitive to the inhibitory effects of PDE IV inhibitors, and much lower concentrations are required for suppression of this cytokine than are required for the inhibition of arachidonic acid metabolite production (179). Expression of MHC II is inhibited by agents that elevate cAMP, including PDE inhibitors (180). This may have implications for the presentation of antigen to T cells in atopic disorders.

Eosinophils and Neutrophils

PDE IV inhibitors as well as mixed PDE III and IV inhibitors suppress superoxide anion and H_2O_2 generation from guinea pig and human eosinophils in response to particulate (serum-opsonized zymosan) and several soluble stimuli (110,111,133,181,182). The PDE IV inhibitors also reduce LTB_4-induced thromboxane release (182,183), IgG- and secretory IgA-induced degranulation (184), and hrC5a-, PAF- and FMLP-induced eosinophil chemotaxis (185,186). A preliminary report also suggests that PDE inhibitors may promote apoptosis of eosinophils maintained in culture with IL-5 (187).

Neutrophils have an uncertain role in atopic disorders. Nevertheless, their sensitivity to selective inhibitors has been studied. Thus, PDE IV inhibitors suppress neutrophil degranulation (188), superoxide anion generation (134,189), phagocytosis (170), chemotaxis (190), and mediator production (191).

Other Cell Types

Platelets have been implicated in the pathophysiological mechanisms of asthma (192). Selective inhibitors of the PDE III isoenzyme family reduce platelet aggregation induced by several stimuli (93,94). Zaprinast potentiates nitric oxide-induced aggregation (193) and adhesion (194).

The functions of endothelial cells, which play an important role in regulating plasma fluid and protein leakage out of blood vessels and in cell recruitment into inflamed tissues, are regulated by cAMP. Agents that elevate endothelial cAMP levels, including PDE inhibitors, reduce albumin flux across endothelial monolayers (195–198) and inhibit TNF-α–induced expression of surface adhesion molecules (ELAM-1, VCAM-1, but not ICAM-1) (199).

Little has been reported on the effects of PDE inhibitors in epithelial cells. Bicarbonate secretion in airways epithelium is stimulated by IBMX (200). Interestingly, although information is not available on PDE inhibitors, agents that increase cAMP synthesis as well as cAMP analogues protect bronchial epithelial cells from the cytotoxic effects of endotoxin (201). Such a cytoprotective effect may be of relevance to asthma therapy, since epithelial sloughing is a prominent feature of the disease (202).

ANTI-INFLAMMATORY EFFECTS OF PDE INHIBITORS IN VIVO

Comparatively little is known of the actions of isoenzyme-selective PDE inhibitors on either the acute (IgE-mediated) or chronic (proinflammatory–immunocompetent cell-mediated) consequences of allergen provocation in vivo. The studies that have been performed are restricted to their effects on passive cutaneous anaphylaxis (PCA), cell infiltration into sites of inflammation, and microvascular leakage.

Immunoglobulin E-Mediated Processes

It is currently unknown if PDE inhibitors are able to reduce the levels of IgE in vivo. The only compound that has been assessed in humans, ibudilast, which is an essentially nonselective and relatively poor inhibitor of PDE IV (183), does not affect IgE levels in asthmatic individuals (204). In contrast, PDE IV and PDE V inhibitors exhibit efficacy at reducing PCA reactions in rats, mice, and guinea pigs (205,206). Furthermore, rolipram, but not zaprinast or SK&F 94120, is effective at reducing the infiltration of indium-labeled eosinophils into the skin of guinea pigs following a PCA reaction (207). Collectively, these data imply that PDE IV inhibitors can suppress the degranulation of IgE-bearing leukocytes and, therefore, allergen-induced mediator release. Further support for this proposal derives from studies in sensitized guinea pigs, in which rolipram, administered intravenously, inhibits antigen-induced, but not LTD_4-induced, bronchoconstriction (208). Thus, rolipram preferentially exerts an inhibitory influence at the level of mast cells and basophils, rather than exerting a direct antispasmogenic action at the level of airway smooth muscle. In contrast, the PDE III inhibitor CI-930 inhibited both allergen- and LTD_4-induced broncho-constriction under identical conditions, indicating a direct smooth-muscle effect of this compound (208).

Proinflammatory Cell Infiltration

Several studies have evaluated the effect of PDE IV, PDE III–IV, and PDE V inhibitors on the infiltration of proinflammatory cells into the airways lumen, skin, and eyes of guinea pigs and in rats in responses to platelet-activating factor (PAF), endotoxin, and allergen (209–218). Schudt et al. (216) reported that pretreatment of sensitized guinea pigs with the PDE III/IV inhibitor zardaverine markedly suppressed allergen-induced infiltration of eosinophils, macrophages, and neutrophils into the bronchoalveolar lavage (BAL) fluid, to a level achieved with dexamethasone. Qualitatively identical data have been reported for the PDE III/IV inhibitor benafentrine on PAF-induced (211,213) and allergen-induced (214) pulmonary eosinophil recruitment in guinea pigs after extended (6 days) dosing. Studies conducted more recently with rolipram have provided results that corroborate the data obtained with zardaverine and benafentrine. Thus, intragastric administration of rolipram to conscious guinea pigs selectively attenuated allergen-induced pulmonary eosinophil influx into the BAL fluid and tissue (210). Similarly, the introduction of rolipram directly into the airways of guinea pigs as a micronized dry powder almost completely prevented the appearance of proinflammatory leukocytes into the BAL fluid in response to allergen provocation (12).

Other models of inflammation are also sensitive to type IV-selective PDE inhibitors. For example, allergen-induced lung eosinophilia in Brown Norway rats, an IgE-producing, steroid-sensitive species that exhibits both early- and late-phase reactions (219), is abolished (218) by rolipram and the hybrid PDE III/IV inhibitor, Org 20241 (182). Similarly, in a guinea pig eye model of tissue eosinophilia, rolipram when administered by gavage, significantly inhibited the number of eosinophils that appeared in the conjunctival epithelium in response to histamine, and a combination of LTB_4 and LTD_4 (220). In another study, Griswold et al. (221), reported that oral administration to mice of rolipram inhibited arachidonate-induced inflammatory cell accumulation and activation, as assessed by myeloperoxidase activity in the inflammatory exudate. Rolipram was also active at suppressing neutrophil accumulation into the peritoneum that was evoked by urate crystals and LTB$_4$ (221). Zaprinast was inactive in these functional assays (221).

There are no reports of the effects of selective PDE inhibitors on eosinophil numbers in humans. However, Kawasaki et al. (204) have reported that the nonselective PDE inhibitor, ibudilast (183), does not reduce the circulating eosinophil count in asthmatic subjects.

Recent data suggest that systemic administration of rolipram, but not zaprinast or SK&F 94120, to guinea pigs suppresses the accumulation of indium-labeled eosinophils into the skin in response to zymosan-activated plasma, PAF, and histamine (207). In this model, however, the accumulation of indium-labeled neutrophils, was unaffected by rolipram under identical experimental conditions (207). The reason for this discrepancy is unclear, but it may be because guinea pig neutrophil function is less sensitive to inhibition by rolipram than that of human cells (222), possibly owing to a lower basal adenylyl cyclase activity. Alternatively, rolipram may act preferentially on endothelial cells. It is known that agents that increase cAMP selectively inhibit the expression of vascular cell adhesion molecule (VCAM)-1 but not intracellular adhesion molecule (ICAM)-1 (199). Locally injected rolipram had little effect on eosinophil accumulation (207).

Although proinflammatory mediators, such as PAF, histamine, and LTB$_4$, elicit pulmonary eosinophil recruitment, it has been emphasized that the eosinophil count in the airways' lumen is considerably less than that seen following antigen provocation (223). This observation, together with the finding that selective antagonists of these mediators do not abrogate eosinophil recruitment following antigen challenge, implicate mediators other than PAF, histamine, and LTB$_4$ in eosinophil accumulation in the lung. It is now recognized that several so-called chronic proinflammatory chemokines, including IL-3, IL-5, GM-CSF, RANTES, TNF-α, and macrophage inflammatory protein (MIP)-1α, can elicit the pulmonary accumulation and activation of eosinophils. Indeed, a recent report by Kings et al. (215) documented the ability of IL-3 and GM-CSF, and mouse TNF-α to selectively attract eosinophils into the lungs of guinea pigs. Significantly, pretreatment of the animals with the PDE III–IV inhibitor benafentrine effectively suppressed this response (215). Comparable data are also available for the actions of zardaverine on endotoxin-induced pulmonary neutrophil recruitment in rats (212), which is partly mediated by the release of TNF-α. In that study, zardaverine also inhibited the elaboration of TNF-α into the BAL fluid following endotoxin challenge (212). Collectively, these are important observations, since they imply that selective PDE inhibitors are effective at blocking the deleterious actions of both immediate (PAF, histamine, or LTB$_4$) and chronic (cytokine) mediators of allergic inflammation.

It is currently unclear how PDE inhibitors attenuate leukocyte trafficking, although it is likely that these drugs act on several cell types, thereby suppressing the generation of chemoattractants and, as briefly mentioned earlier, the expression of certain adhesion molecules. It is noteworthy, however, that in parasite-infected mice, rolipram, given continually for 7 days, decreased the number of circulating eosinophils and of those present in the bone marrow and peritoneum (224). Thus, apparently rolipram exerted a glucocorticoid effect, in that it suppressed the development of eosinophil progenitors. Intriguingly, the mechanism of action of rolipram was unrelated to the inhibition of IL-5 release from a T$_H$2 helper clone or from the bone marrow (224).

Microvascular Leakage and Edema

There is now considerable interest in the potential role of the microcirculation in inflammatory reactions. Under normal conditions, the endothelium lining the postcapillary micro-venules is largely impermeable to blood cells and to macromolecules but following a proinflammatory insult, localized arteriolar vasodilatation occurs with a consequent increase in blood flow. This effect is induced by the liberation of proinflammatory mediators such as histamine and tachykinins. An increase in capillary and microvenular pressure then ensues, together with the liberation of other mediators such as PAF and LTD_4 which contract directly the microvenular endothelial cells. Together these effects, by increasing microvenular permeability, permit the loss of plasma-proteins from the vascular compartment. Furthermore, the resulting increase in osmotic pressure due to loss of solute from the circulation leads to marked fluid exudation and to edema.

Only a few studies have documented the effects of isoenzyme-selective PDE inhibitors upon plasma-protein extravasation. Using the hamster cheek pouch Svensjo et al. (225) have reported that PDE IV and PDE III/IV inhibitors attenuated the increase in microvascular permeability evoked by bradykinin. Qualitatively identical results have been reported for the effect of rolipram and denbufylline upon arachidonate-induced rat ear (see Ref. 12) and mouse ear (226) edema, respectively. In anesthetized guinea pigs, intravenous, oral, and intratracheal administration of representative inhibitors of the PDE IV (rolipram) and PDE V (zaprinast) isoenzyme families markedly attenuated PAF-induced microvascular leakage in both small and large airways, and into the BAL fluid (227,228). Rolipram is also effective against allergen-induced microvascular leakage in sensitized guinea pigs (229). The finding that rolipram and zaprinast were active when given directly into the airways indicates an important local action in the lung and highlights that systemic administration is not necessary for these compounds to exert an anti-inflammatory influence. This is an important observation since the administration of PDE inhibitors by the inhaled route is believed to reduce untoward side effects while maintaining efficacy. Drugs that inhibit PDE I (vinpocetine) and PDE III (siguazodan, milrinone) do not inhibit PAF-induced microvascular leakage in guinea pig airways (227,228). This latter finding is curious given that a PDE III isoenzyme has been identified in endothelial cells, and that the selective PDE III inhibitor motapizone blocks the increase in permeability elicited by H_2O_2 in vitro (198). It is likely, however, that this discrepancy is due to a difference in species, the leak-evoking stimulus or in vessel type. In keeping with this latter possibility, Teixeira et al. (207) have reported that rolipram does not inhibit edema formation in guinea pig skin in response to histamine, zymosan-activated plasma, and PAF (cf. guinea pig lung). It is tempting to speculate that the complement of PDE isoenzymes and/or the regulation of endothelial cell contractility by cyclic nucleotides varies significantly between vessels of the pulmonary and systemic vascular beds.

DISCUSSION

Many of the world's major pharmaceutical companies are developing PDE inhibitors for the treatment of allergic diseases, particularly asthma (Table 1; Fig. 1). In the near future, results from clinical studies will reveal whether the initial optimism in the therapeutic potential of this class of compounds was justified. The greatest interest, understandably in view of the information presented in this review, is in the antiallergic and anti-inflammatory potential of PDE IV inhibitors. Indeed, suppression of antigen-driven responses (bronchospasm, mediator release, eosinophilia, and microvascular leakage) point to efficacy in treating the major pathological components of allergic asthma. However, these effects of PDE IV inhibitors have been demonstrated in acute disease animal models, and whether they translate into useful therapy in the chronic human disease remains to be seen.

Little clinical information is available from the few trials on selective PDE III (230),

PDE IV (231), and PDE V inhibitors (232), as well as mixed PDE III/IV inhibitors (233) that have been conducted thus far. Only simple parameters of airways function have been examined, which revealed little concerning the antiallergic or anti-inflammatory actions of these compounds. Ibudilast, the antiasthmatic actions of which may, at least partly, be a consequence of PDE IV inhibition (183), does not affect blood IgE levels or eosinophil numbers in the clinic (204). However, unlike more potent PDE IV inhibitors (210), ibudilast does not suppress eosinophilia in animal models (211). Whether PDE IV inhibitors will, as previously postulated, display a therapeutic profile similar to that of theophylline, but with fewer side effects, again remains to be seen. Indeed, controversy still surrounds the mechanism by which theophylline exerts its antiasthmatic effects, although studies have implicated cAMP PDE inhibition in its mechanism of action (189).

The clinical effects of PDE inhibitors in skin disorders have been investigated in a limited number of studies. An early report suggested that papaverine, a nonselective PDE inhibitor, is effective in decreasing pruritus in patients with atopic dermatitis (234). Caffeine, which also displays weak PDE inhibitory activity, when used as a 30% cream with 0.5% hydrocortisone, is apparently more effective than the steroid alone in treating atopic dermatitis (235). However, the efficacy of these drugs in the treatment of atopic dermatitis has been disputed (236). Although the use of cAMP PDE inhibitors for the treatment of atopic dermatitis has been vigorously championed (237), to our knowledge, no clinical studies have been reported. However, Ro 20-1724 has been tested successfully in psoriatic patients (238).

An explanation for the elevated cAMP PDE activity in MNL of atopic individuals remains elusive. Although evidence exists suggesting that this phenomenon is a consequence of atopy, elevated MNL cAMP PDE is not secondary to tissue inflammation per se, since levels of the enzyme are normal in patients with allergic (type IV) contact dermatitis (101,237). If the genetic defect hypothesis is correct, cAMP PDE elevation may be of major importance in the etiology of allergic diseases. Although the in vivo consequences of the increased cAMP PDE are unclear, provocative in vitro data indicate that the likely accelerated atopic MNL cAMP hydrolysis has a major influence on the elaboration of important allergic mediators and cytokines.

Although confirmatory sequence data are lacking, recent reports suggest the existence of a novel cAMP PDE in atopic MNL. Since this enzyme may be responsible for the abnormal functional responses of atopic MNL, this may have intriguing implications for future therapeutic intervention in allergic diseases. Since the increased monocyte cAMP PDE has been implicated as contributing to allergic disorders, and because oral administration of PDE IV inhibitors is associated with several side effects, targeting this enzyme may be an attractive new approach for the discovery of new antiallergic agents.

Excluding theophylline, whose mechanism of action still remains uncertain, past experience with PDE inhibitors for the treatment of allergic disorders has been disappointing. The cGMP PDE inhibitor, zaprinast, has been tested in the clinic, with unconvincing results (232). In retrospect, it is not surprising that this compound, which arose from the misconceived mast cell stabilizer approach, did not exhibit the anticipated activity in the clinic. Indeed, evidence for the anti-allergic potential of zaprinast was limited solely to its inhibitory effects on rat mast cell mediator release (131) and activity in the rat PCA test (206). The current optimism over the therapeutic potential of PDE IV inhibitors is based on much firmer evidence, including the demonstration of dampening effects on most human cells implicated in allergic disorders, including those from allergic individuals. Thus, the coming months are awaited with great anticipation by the many pharmaceutical companies who have invested in the development of PDE IV inhibitors.

ACKNOWLEDGMENTS

Research performed by M.A.G. is supported by the Medical Research Council (UK), the British Lung Foundation, the National Asthma Campaign (UK), The Purdue-Frederick Company, and Organon Laboratories Ltd. The authors thank Dr. Chris Corrigan, Department of Allergy and Clinical Immunology, Royal Brompton National Heart and Lung Institute, London, for Figure 3.

REFERENCES

1. Fleming DM, Crombie DL. Prevalence of asthma and hay fever in England and Wales. Br Med J 1987; 294:279–283.
2. Sly RM. Increases in death from asthma. Ann Allergy 1984; 53:2–25.
3. Barnes PJ. Asthma deaths: a continuing problem. In: Sheppard M, ed. Advanced Medicine. Vol. 24. London: Bailliere Tindal, 1988:53–61.
4. Keating G, Mitchell EA, Jackson R, Beaglehole R, Rea H. Trends in the sales of drugs for asthma in New Zealand, Australia and the United Kingdom. Br Med J 1983; 289:348–351.
5. Hay IFC, Higenbottam TW. Has the management of asthma improved? Lancet 1987; 2:609–611.
6. Geha RS. Atopic allergy and other hypersensitivity's: understanding the allergic response as a step towards its eradication. Curr Opin Immunol 1993; 5:935–936.
7. Thompson PJ, Stewart GA. Allergens. In: Holgate ST, Church MK, eds. Allergy. London: Raven Press, 1991:1.1–1.14.
8. Torphy TJ, Undem BJ. Phosphodiesterase inhibitors: new opportunities for the treatment of asthma. Thorax 1991; 46:512–523.
9. Giembycz MA, Dent G. Prospects for selective cyclic nucleotide phosphodiesterase inhibitors in the treatment of bronchial asthma. Clin Exp Allergy 1992; 22:337–344.
10. Giembycz MA. Could isoenzyme-selective phosphodiesterase inhibitors render bronchodilator therapy redundant in the treatment of bronchial asthma? Biochem Pharmacol 1992; 43:2041–2051.
11. Giembycz MA, Souness JE. Characteristics and properties of the cyclic AMP-specific phosphodiesterase in eosinophil leukocytes: a potential target for asthma therapy? In: Postma D, Gerritsen J, eds. Bronchitis V. Assen: Van Gorcum & Co, 1994:319–332.
12. Raeburn D, Souness JE, Tomkinson A, Karlsson J-A. Isozyme-selective cyclic nucleotide phosphodiesterase inhibitors: biochemistry, pharmacology and therapeutic potential in asthma. Prog Drug Res 1993; 40:9–31.
13. Mosmann TR, Cherwinski H, Bond MW, Giedlin MA, Coffman RL. Two types of murine helper T-cell clone. I. Definition according to profiles of lymphokine activities and secreted proteins. J Immunol 1986; 136:2348–2357.
14. Cherwinski HM, Schumacher JH, Brown KD, Mosmann TR. Two types of murine helper T-cell clone. III. Further differences in lymphokine synthesis between Th1 and Th2 clones revealed by RNA hybridization, functionally monospecific bioassays, and monoclonal antibodies. J Exp Med 1987; 166:1229–1244.
15. Field EH, Noelle RJ, Rouse T, Goeken J, Waldschmidt T. Evidence for excessive T_H2 CD4$^+$ subset activity in vivo. J Immunol 1993; 151:48–59.
16. Robinson DS, Hamid Q, Jacobson M, Ying S, Durham SR. Evidence for T_H2-type helper cell control of allergic disease in vivo. Springer Sem Immunopathol 1993; 15:17–27.
17. Kay AB, Ying S, Varney V, Gaga M, Durham SR, Moqbel R, Wardlaw AJ, Hamid Q. Messenger RNA expression of the cytokine gene cluster IL-3, IL-4, IL-5 and GM-CSF, in allergen-induced late phase cutaneous reactions in atopic subjects. J Exp Med 1991; 173:775–778.
18. Kapsenberg ML, Wierenga EA, Bos JD, Jansem HM. Functional subsets of allergen-reactive human CD4$^+$ T cells. Immunol Today 1991; 12:393–395.
19. Haanen JB, de Waal Malefyt R, Res PC, Kraakman EM, Ottenhoff TH, de Vries RR, Spits H.

Selection of a human T helper type-1 T-cell subset by mycobacterium. J Exp Med 1991; 174: 583–592.

20. Yssel H, Shanafelt M-C, Soderberg C, Schneider P, Anzola J, Peltz G. *Borrelia burgdorferi* activates a T helper type-1-like T cell subset in Lyme Arthritis. J Exp Med 1991; 174:593–601.

21. Splits H, de Waal Malefyt R. Functional characterization of human IL-10. Int Arch Allergy Immunol 1992; 99:8–15.

22. de Waal Malefyt R, Abrams J, Bennett B, Figdor CG, de Vries JE. Interleukin 10 (IL-10) inhibits cytokine synthesis by human monocytes: an autoregulatory role of IL-10 produced by monocytes. J Exp Med 1991; 174:1209–1212.

23. Corrigan CJ, Kay AB. Lymphocytes, allergy and asthma. In: Holgate ST, Church MK, eds. Allergy. London: Raven Press, 1991:9.1–9.13.

24. Jabara HH, Schneider LC, Shapira SK, Alfieri C, Moody CT, Kieff E, Geha RS, Vercelli D. Induction of germ line and mature Cε transcripts in human B cells stimulated with rIL-4 and EBV. J Immunol 1990; 145:3468–3473.

25. Punnonen J, Aversa G, Cocks BG, McKenzie ANJ, Menon S, Zurawski G, De Wall Malefyt R, De Vries JE. Interleukin-13 induced interleukin-4-independent IgG$_4$ and IgE synthesis and CD23 expression by human B-cells. Proc Natl Acad Sci USA 1993; 90:3730–3734.

26. Minty A, Chalon P, Derocq J-M, Dumont X, Guillemot J-C, Kaghad M, Labit C, Leplatois P, Liauzun P, Miloux B, Minty C, Casellas P, Loison G, Lupker J, Shire D, Ferrara P, Caput D. Interleukin-13 is a new human lymphokine regulating inflammatory and immune responses. Nature 1993; 362:248–250.

27. Vercelli D, Geha RS. Regulation of isotype switching. Curr Opin Immunol 1992; 4:794–797.

28. Vercelli D, Geha RS. Regulation of IgE synthesis: from membrane to gene. Springer Semin Immunopathol 1993; 15:29–36.

29. Schwart LB. Mast cells: function and contents. Curr Opin Immunol 1994; 6:91–97.

30. Fuleihan R, Ramesh N, Geha RS. Role of CD40–CD40-ligand interaction in Ig isotype switching. Curr Opin Immunol 1993; 5:963–967.

31. Armitage RJ, Fanslow WC, Strockbine L, Sato TA, Clifford KN, Macduff BM, Anderson DM, Gimpel SD, Davis-Smith T, Maliszewski CR. Molecular and biological characterization of a murine ligand for CD40. Nature 1992; 357:80–82.

32. Gauchat J-F, Henchoz S, Mazzei G, Aubry J-P, Brunner T, Blasey H, Life P, Talabot D, Flores-Romo L, Thompson J, Kishi K, Butterfield J, Dahinden CA, Bonnefoy J-Y. Induction of human IgE synthesis in B cells by mast cells and basophils. Nature 1993; 365:340–343.

33. Brunner T, Heusser CH, Dahinden CA. Human peripheral blood basophils primed by interleukin-3 (IL-3) produce IL-4 in response to immunoglobulin E-receptor stimulation. J Exp Med 1993; 177:605–611.

34. Bradding P, Feather IH, Howarth PH, Mueller R, Roberts JA, Britten K, Bews JPA, Hunt TC, Okayama Y, Heusser CH, Bullock CR, Church MK, Holgate ST. Interleukin-4 is localized to and released by human mast cells. J Exp Med 1992; 176:1381–1386.

35. Leung DYM. Immunopathology of atopic dermatitis. Springer Semin Immunopathol 1992; 13: 427–440.

36. Corrigan CJ, Kay AB. T Cells and eosinophils in the pathogenesis of asthma. Immunol Today 1992; 13:501–507.

37. Varney VA, Jacobson MR, Sudderick RM, Robinson DS, Irani AMA, Schwartz LB, MacKay IS, Kay AB, Durham SR. Immunohistology of the nasal mucosa following antigen-induced rhinitis. Am Rev Respir Dis 1992; 146:170–176.

38. O'Hehir RE, Bal V, Quint D, Moqbel R, Kay AB, Zanders ED, Lamb JR. An in vitro model of allergen-dependent IgE synthesis by human B-lymphocytes: comparison of the response of an atopic and non-atopic individual to *Dermatophagoides* spp. (house dust mite). Immunology 1989; 66:499–504.

39. Butcher RW, Sutherland EW. Adenosine 3',5'-phosphate in biological materials. J Biol Chem 1962; 237:1244–1250.

40. Newton RP, Sabih SG, Khan JA, Cyclic CMP-specific phosphodiesterase activity. In: Beavo J, Houslay MD, eds. Cyclic Nucleotide Phosphodiesterases: Structure, Regulation and Drug Action. Chichester: John Wiley & Sons, 1990:141–159.

41. Beavo JA, Reifsnyder DH. Primary sequence of cyclic nucleotide phosphodiesterase isozymes and the design of selective inhibitors. Trends Pharmacol Sci 1990; 11:150–155.

42. Michaeli T, Bloom TJ, Martins T, Loughney K, Ferguson K, Riggs M, Rodgers L, Beavo JA, Wigler M. Isolation and characterization of a previously undetected human cyclic AMP phosphodiesterase by complementation of cyclic AMP phosphodiesterase-deficient *Saccharomyces cerevisiae*. J Biol Chem 1993; 268:12925–12932.

43. Giembycz MA, Kelly JJ. Current status of cyclic nucleotide phosphodiesterase isoenzymes. In: Piper PJ, Costello J, eds. Methylxanthines and Phosphodiesterase Inhibitors and the Treatment of Respiratory Disease. London, Parthenon Publishing, 1994:27–80.

44. Beavo JA. Multiple isozymes of cyclic nucleotide phosphodiesterase. Adv Second Messenger Phosphoprotein Res 1987; 22:1–38.

45. Sharma RK, Wang JH. Regulation of cyclic AMP concentration by calmodulin-dependent cyclic nucleotide phosphodiesterase. Biochem Cell Biol 1982; 64:1072–1080.

46. Sharma RK, Wang JH. Purification and characterization of bovine lung calmodulin-dependent cyclic nucleotide phosphodiesterase. An enzyme containing calmodulin as a subunit. J Biol Chem 1986; 261:14160–14166.

47. Sharma RK, Wang TH, Wirch E, Wang JH. Purification and properties of bovine brain calmodulin-dependent cyclic nucleotide phosphodiesterase. J Biol Chem 1980; 255:5916–5923.

48. Rossi P, Giorgi M, Geremia R, Kincaid RL. Testis-specific calmodulin-dependent phosphodiesterase. A distinct high-affinity isozyme immunologically related to brain calmodulin-dependent cyclic GMP phosphodiesterase. J Biol Chem 1988; 263:15521–15527.

49. Torphy TJ, Cieslinski LB. Characterisation and selective inhibition of cyclic nucleotide phosphodiesterase isozymes in canine tracheal smooth muscle. Mol Pharmacol 1990; 37:206–214.

50. Martins TJ, Mumby MC, Beavo JA. Purification and characterization of a cyclic GMP-stimulated cyclic nucleotide phosphodiesterase from bovine tissues. J Biol Chem 1982; 257:1973–1979.

51. Manganiello VC, Tanaka T, Murashima S. Cyclic GMP-stimulated cyclic nucleotide phosphodiesterases. In: Beavo J, Houslay MD, eds. Cyclic Nucleotide Phosphodiesterases: Structure, Regulation and Drug Action. Chichester: John Wiley & Sons, 1990:61–85.

52. Manganiello VC, Smith CJ, Degerman E, Belrage P. Cyclic GMP-inhibited cyclic nucleotide phosphodiesterases. In: Beavo J, Houslay MD, eds. Cyclic Nucleotide Phosphodiesterases: Structure, Regulation and Drug Action. Chichester: John Wiley & Sons, 1990:87–117.

53. Smith CJ, Krall J, Manganiello VC, Movsesian MA. Cytosolic and sarcoplasmic reticulum-associated low K_m, cyclic GMP-inhibited cyclic AMP phosphodiesterase in mammalian myocardium. Biochem Biophys Res Commun 1993; 190:516–521.

54. Masuoka H, Ito M, Sugioka M, Kozeki H, Konishi T, Tanaka T, Nakano T. Two isoforms of cyclic GMP-inhibited cyclic nucleotide phosphodiesterases in human tissues distinguished by their responses to vesnarinone, a new cardiotonic agent. Biochem Biophys Res Commun 1993; 190:412–417.

55. Davies RL, Takaysasu H, Eberwine M, Myres J. Cloning and characterization of mammalian homologs of the *Drosophila* dunce[+] gene. Proc Natl Acad Sci USA 1989; 86:3604–3608.

56. Swinnen JV, Joseph DR, Conti M. Molecular cloning of rat homologs of the *Drosophila melanogaster* dunce cyclic AMP phosphodiesterase: evidence for a family of genes. Proc Natl Acad Sci USA 1989; 86:5325–5329.

57. Colicelli J, Birchmeier C, Michaeli T, O'Neill K, Riggs M, Wigler M. Isolation and characterisation of a mammalian gene encoding a high-affinity cyclic AMP phosphodiesterase. Proc Natl Acad Sci USA 1989; 86:3599–3603.

58. Swinnen JV, Joseph DR, Conti M. The mRNA encoding a high affinity cAMP phosphodiesterase is regulated by hormones and cAMP. Proc Natl Acad Sci USA 1989; 86:8197–8201.

59. Chen CN, Denome S, Davis RL. Molecular analysis of cDNA clones and the corresponding genomic coding sequences of the *Drosophila* dunce$^+$ gene, the structural gene for cAMP phosphodiesterase. Proc Natl Acad Sci USA 1986; 83:9313–9317.

60. Swinnen JV, Tsikalas KE, Conti M. Properties and hormonal regulation of two structurally related cyclic AMP phosphodiesterases from rat Sertoli cells. J Biol Chem 1991; 266:18370–18377.

61. Conti M, Swinnen JV, Tsikalas KE, Jin S-LC. Structure and regulation of the rat high affinity cyclic AMP phosphodiesterase. Adv Second Messenger Protein Phosphorylation Res 1992; 25:87–99.

62. Monaco L, Vicini E, Conti M. Structure of two rat genes coding for a closely related rolipram-sensitive cAMP phosphodiesterase. Multiple mRNA variants originate from alternative splicing and multiple start sites. J Biol Chem 1994; 269:347–357.

63. Livi GP, Kmetz P, McHale M, Cieslinski LB, Sathe GM, Taylor DJ, Davis RL, Torphy TJ, Balcarek JM. Cloning and expression of cDNA for a human low-K_m, rolipram sensitive cyclic AMP phosphodiesterase. Mol Cell Biol 1990; 10:2678–2686.

64. McLaughlin MM, Cieslinski LB, Burman M, Torphy TJ, Livi GP. A low-K_m, rolipram-sensitive, cyclic AMP-specific phosphodiesterase from human brain. Cloning and expression of cDNA, biochemical characterisation of recombinant protein, and tissue distribution of mRNA. J Biol Chem 1993; 268:6470–6476.

65. Obernolte R, Bhakta S, Alvarez R, Bach C, Zuppan P, Mulkins M, Jarnagin K, Shelton ER. The cDNA of a human lymphocyte cyclic AMP phosphodiesterase (PDE IV) reveals a multigene family. Gene 1993; 129:239–247.

66. Epstein PM, Strada SJ, Sarada K, Thompson WJ. Catalytic and kinetic properties of purified high affinity cyclic AMP phosphodiesterase from dog kidney. Arch Biochem Biophys 1982; 218:119–133.

67. Thompson WJ, Epstein PM, Strada SJ. Purification and characterization of a high affinity cyclic adenosine monophosphate phosphodiesterase from dog kidney. Biochemistry 1979; 18:5228–5237.

68. Pyne NJ, Cooper ME, Houslay MD. The insulin- and glucagon-stimulated "dense vesicle" high affinity cyclic AMP phosphodiesterase from rat liver: purification, characterization and inhibitor sensitivity. Biochem J 1987; 242:33–42.

69. Conti M, Swinnen JV. Structure and function of the rolipram-sensitive, low K_m cyclic AMP phosphodiesterase: a family of highly related enzymes. In: Houslay MD, Beavo JA, eds, Molecular Pharmacology of Cell Regulation: Cyclic Nucleotide Phosphodiesterase Structure, Regulation and Drug Action. New York: John Wiley & Sons, 1990:243–266.

70. Torphy TJ, De Wolf WE, Green DW, Livi GP. Biochemical characteristics and cellular regulation of phosphodiesterase IV. Agents Actions 1993; 43(suppl):51–71.

71. Némoz G, Mouequit M, Prigent A-F, Pacheco H. Isolation of similar rolipram-inhibitable cyclic AMP-specific phosphodiesterases from rat brain and heart. Eur J Biochem 1989; 184:511–520.

72. Torphy TJ. Inhibitors of phosphodiesterase isozymes: new therapeutic possibilities for asthma. In: Postma D, Gerritsen J. Eds. Bronchitis V. Assen: Van Gorcum & Co, 1994; 303–317.

73. Thompson WJ, Pratt ML, Strada SJ. Biochemical properties of high affinity cyclic AMP phosphodiesterase. Adv Cyclic Nucleotide Protein Phosphorylation Res 1984; 16:137–148.

74. Schneider HH, Schmiechen R, Brezinski M, Seidler J. Stereospecific binding of the antidepressant rolipram to brain-specific structures. Eur J Pharmacol 1987; 127:105–115.

75. Torphy TJ, Stadel JM, Burman M, Cieslinski LB, McLaughlin MM, White JR, Livi GP. Coexpression of human cyclic AMP-specific phosphodiesterase activity and high-affinity rolipram binding in yeast. J Biol Chem 1992; 267:1798–1804.

76. Schwartz JP, Passoneau JV. Cyclic AMP-mediated induction of the cyclic AMP phosphodiesterase of C-6 glioma cells. Proc Natl Acad Sci USA 1974; 71:3844–3848.

77. Torphy TJ, Zhou H-L, Cieslinski LB. Stimulation of beta-adrenoceptors in a human monocyte cell line (U937) up-regulates cyclic AMP-specific phosphodiesterase activity. J Pharmacol Exp Ther 1992; 263:1195–1205.

78. Okonogi K, Gettys TW, Uhing RJ, Tarry WC, Adams DO, Prpic V. Inhibition of prostaglandin E$_2$-stimulated cyclic AMP accumulation by lipopolysaccharide in murine peritoneal macrophages. J Biol Chem 1991; 266:10305–10312.

79. Valette L, Prigent AF, Nemoz G, Anker G, Macovschi O, Lagarde M. Concanavalin A stimulates the rolipram-sensitive isoforms of cyclic nucleotide phosphodiesterase in rat thymic lymphocytes. Biochem Biophys Res Commun 1990; 160:864–872.

80. Epstein PM, Hachisu R. Cyclic nucleotide phosphodiesterase in normal and leukemic human lymphocytes and lymphoblasts. Adv Cyclic Nucleotide Protein Phosphorylation Res 1984; 16: 303–324.

81. Li S-H, Chan SC, Toshitani A, Leung DYM, Hanifin JM. Synergistic effects of interleukin 4 and interferon-gamma on monocyte phosphodiesterase activity. J Invest Dermatol 1992; 99:65–70.

82. Li S-H, Chan SC, Kramer SM, Hanifin JM. Modulation of leukocyte cyclic AMP phosphodiesterase activity by recombinant interferon-γ: evidence for a differential effect of atopic monocytes. J Interferon Res 1993; 13:197–202.

83. Hanifin JM, Butler JM, Chan SC. Immunopharmacology of the atopic diseases. J Invest Dermatol 1985; 85:161s–164s.

84. Chan SC, Trask DM, Sherman SC, Hanifin JM. Histamine agonist stimulated protein kinase C phosphorylation of a 61K monocyte protein with characteristics of atopic cyclic AMP phosphodiesterase (abstr). J Invest Dermatol 1986; 86:468.

84a. Sette C, Vicini E, Hess M, Conti M. Short term regulation of a rolipram-sensitive, cAMP-specific phosphodiesterase through cAMP-dependent phosphorylation (abstr.). FASEB J 1994; 8:2141.

84b. Luther M, Holmes B, Kassal D, Lenhard J, Hamacher L, Burkhart W, Moyer M, Patel I, Overton L, Hoffman C, Rocque W. Identification and functional characterization of various phosphorylated forms of human recombinant, rolipram-sensitive cAMP-specific type IV phosphodiesterase (abstr.). FASEB J 1994; 8:2141.

85. Francis SH, Thomas MK, Corbin JD. Cyclic GMP-binding cyclic GMP-specific phosphodiesterase from lung. In: Beavo JA, Houslay MD, eds. Cyclic Nucleotide Phosphodiesterases: Structure, Regulation and Drug Action. Chichester: John Wiley & Sons, 1990:117–140.

86. Robichon A. A new cyclic GMP phosphodiesterase isolated from bovine platelets is a substrate for cyclic AMP- and cyclic GMP-dependent protein kinases: evidence for a key role in the process of platelet activation. J Cell Biochem 1991; 47:147–157.

87. Gillespie PG. Phosphodiesterases in visual transduction by rods and cones. In: Beavo JA, Houslay MD, eds. Cyclic Nucleotide Phosphodiesterases: Structure, Regulation and Drug Action. Chichester: John Wiley & Sons 1990:141–159.

88. Mukai J, Asai T, Naka M, Tanaka T. Separation and characterization of a novel isoenzyme of cyclic nucleotide phosphodiesterase from rat cerebrum. Br J Pharmacol 1994; 111:389–390.

89. Souness JE, Brazdil R, Diocee BK, Jordan R. Role of selective cyclic GMP phosphodiesterase inhibition in the myorelaxant actions of M&B 22948, MY-5445, vinpocetine and 1-methyl-3-isobutyl-8-(methylamino)xanthine. Br J Pharmacol 1989; 98:725–734.

90. Levin RM, Weiss B. Binding of trifluoperazine to the calcium dependent activator of cyclic nucleotide phosphodiesterase. Mol Pharmacol 1977; 13:690–697.

91. Nakanishi S, Osawa K, Saito Y, Kawamoto I, Kuroda K, Kase H. KS-505a, a novel inhibitor of bovine brain Ca^{2+} and calmodulin-dependent cyclic-nucleotide phosphodiesterase from *Streptomyces argenteolus*. J Antibiot 1992; 45:341–347.

92. Müller A, Nennstiel P. Selective inhibition of the cyclic GMP-stimulated cyclic nucleotide phosphodiesterase from pig and human myocardium. J Mol Cell Cardiol 1992; 24(suppl 5):S102.

93. Murray KJ, England PJ, Hallam TJ, Maguire J, Moores K, Reeves ML, Simpson AWM, Rink TJ. The effects of siguazodan, a selective phosphodiesterase inhibitor, on human platelet function. Br J Pharmacol 1990; 99:612–616.

94. Murray KJ, Eden RJ, Dolan JS, Grimsditch DC, Stutchbury CA, Patel B, Knowles A, Worby A, Lynham JA, Coates WJ. The effect of SK&F 95654, a novel phosphodiesterase inhibitor, on cardiovascular, respiratory and platelet function. Br J Pharmacol 1992; 107:463–470.

95. Harrison SA, Reifsnyder DH, Gallis B, Cadd GG, Beavo JA. Isolation and characterization of bovine cardiac muscle cyclic GMP-inhibited phosphodiesterase: a receptor for new cardiotonic drugs. Mol Pharmacol 1986; 29:506–514.

96. Kariya T, Dage RC. Tissue distribution and selective inhibition of subtypes of high affinity phosphodiesterase. Biochem Pharmacol 1988; 37:3267–3270.

97. Glaser T, Traber J. TVX 2706—a new phosphodiesterase inhibitor with anti-inflammatory action: biochemical characterization. Agents Actions 1984; 15:341–348.

98. Nicholson CD, Jackman SA, Wilke R. The ability of denbufylline to inhibit cyclic nucleotide phosphodiesterase and its affinity for adenosine receptors and the adenosine re-uptake site. Br J Pharmacol 1989; 97:889–897.

99. Murray KJ. Phosphodiesterase V_A inhibitors. Drugs News Perspect 1993; 6:150–156.

100. Gillespie PG, Beavo JA. Inhibition and stimulation of photoreceptor phosphodiesterase by dipyridamole and M&B 22,948. Mol Pharmacol 1989; 36:773–781.

101. Grewe S, Chan SC, Hanifin JM. Elevated leukocyte cyclic AMP phosphodiesterase in atopic disease. J Allergy Clin Immunol 1982; 70:452–457.

102. Townley RG. Elevated cyclic AMP phosphodiesterase in atopic disease: cause or effect? J Lab Clin Med 1993; 121:15–17.

103. Goldberg BJ, Lad PM, Ghekiere L. Phosphodiesterase activity and superoxide production in normal and asthmatic neutrophils. J Allergy Clin Immunol 1994; 93:166.

104. Holden CA. Atopic dermatitis: a defect of intracellular secondary messenger systems? Clin Exp Allergy 1990; 20:131–136.

105. Holden CA, Chan SC, Hanifin JM. Monocyte localization of elevated cyclic AMP phospho-diesterase activity in atopic dermatitis. J Invest Dermatol 1986; 87:372–376.

106. Chan SC, Hanifin JM. Differential inhibitor effects on cyclic adenosine monophosphate-phosphodiesterase isoforms in atopic and normal leukocytes. J Lab Clin Med 1993; 121:44–51.

107. Wright S, Navsaria H, Leigh IM. Cyclic adenosine monophosphate-phosphodiesterase activity in cultured keratinocytes from patients with atopic eczema. J Dermatol Sci 1991; 2:263–267.

108. Chan SC, Reifsnyder D, Beavo JA, Hanifin MD. Immunochemical characterization of the distinct monocyte cyclic AMP phosphodiesterase from patients with atopic dermatitis. J Allergy Clin Immunol 1993; 91:1179–1188.

109. Holden CA, Yuen C-T, Coulson IH. The effect of in vitro exposure to histamine on mononuclear leukocyte phosphodiesterase activity in atopic dermatitis. Clin Exp Dermatol 1989; 14:186–190.

110. Dent G, Giembycz MA, Rabe KF, Barnes PJ. Inhibition of eosinophil cyclic nucleotide PDE activity and opsonized zymosan-induced respiratory burst by "type IV"-selective PDE inhibi-tors. Br J Pharmacol 1991; 103:1339–1346.

111. Souness JE, Carter CM, Diocee BK, Hassall GA, Wood LJ, Turner NC. Characterization of guinea-pig eosinophil phosphodiesterase activity: assessment of its involvement in regulating superoxide generation. Biochem Pharmacol 1991; 42:937–945.

112. Heskel NS, Chan SC, Thiel ML, Stevens SR, Casperson LS, Hanifin JM. Elevated umbilical cord blood leukocyte cyclic adenosine monophosphate-phosphodiesterase activity in children with atopic parents. J Am Acad Dermatol 1984; 11:422–426.

113. Coulson IH, Duncan SN, Holden CA. Peripheral blood mononuclear leukocyte cyclic adenosine monophosphate specific phosphodiesterase activity in atopic dermatitis. Br J Dermatol 1989; 120:607–612.

114. Holden CA, Yuen C-T. Response of mononuclear leukocyte cyclic adenosine monophosphate-phosphodiesterase activity to treatment with topical fluorinated steroid ointment in atopic dermatitis. J Am Acad Dermatol 1989; 21:69–74.

115. Chan SC, Hanifin JM, Holden CA, Thompson WJ, Hirshman CA. Elevated leukocyte phospho-diesterase as a basis for depressed cyclic adenosine monophosphate responses in the Basenji greyhound dog model of asthma. J Allergy Clin Immunol 1985; 76:148–158.

116. Holden CA, Chan SC, Norris S, Hanifin JM. Histamine-induced elevation of cyclic AMP phosphodiesterase activity in human monocytes. Agents Actions 1987; 22:36–42.

117. Safko MJ, Chan S-C, Cooper KD, Hanifin JM. Heterologous desensitization of leukocytes: a possible mechanism of beta-adrenoceptor blockade in atopic dermatitis. J Allergy Clin Immunol 1981; 68:218–225.

118. Chan SC, Grewe SR, Stevens SR, Hanifin JM. Functional desensitization due to stimulation of cyclic AMP phosphodiesterase in human mononuclear leukocytes. J Cyclic Nucleotide Res 1982; 8:211–224.

119. Beckner SK, Farrar WL. Interleukin 2 modulation of adenylate cyclase: potential role of protein kinase C. J Biol Chem 1986; 261:3043–3047.

120. van Oosterhout AJM, Stamm WB, Vanderschueren RGJRA, Nijkamp FP. Effects of cytokines on β-adrenoceptor function of human peripheral blood mononuclear cells and guinea-pig trachea. Clin Immunol 1992; 90:340–348.

121. Lefkowitz RJ, Hausdorff WP, Caron MG. Role of phosphorylation in desensitization of the β-adrenergic receptor. Trends Pharmacol Sci 1990; 11:190–194.

122. Chuang TT, Sallese M, Ambrosini G, Parruti G, De Blasi A. A high expression of β-adrenergic receptor kinase in human peripheral blood leukocytes. J Biol Chem 1992; 267:6886–6892.

123. Butler JM, Chan SC, Stevens S, Hanifin JM. Increased leukocyte histamine release with elevated cyclic AMP phosphodiesterase activity in atopic dermatitis. J Allergy Clin Immunol 1983; 71:490–497.

124. Cooper KD, Kang K, Chan SC, Hanifin JM. Phosphodiesterase inhibition by Ro 20-1724 reduces hyper-IgE synthesis by atopic dermatitis cells in vitro. J Invest Dermatol 1985; 84: 477–482.

125. Chan SC, Kim J-W, Henderson WR, Hanifin JM. Altered prostaglandin E_2 regulation of cytokine production in atopic dermatitis. J Immunol 1993; 151:3345–3352.

126. Chan SC, Li S-H, Hanifin JM. Increased interleukin-4 production by atopic mononuclear leukocytes correlates with increased cyclic adenosine monophosphate-phosphodiesterase activity and is reversible by phosphodiesterase inhibition. J Invest Dermatol 1993; 100:681–684.

127. Rott O, Cash E, Fleisher B. Phosphodiesterase inhibitor pentoxifylline, a selective suppressor of T-helper type 1- but not type 2-associated lymphokine production, prevents induction of experimental autoimmune encephalomyelitis in Lewis rats. Eur J Immunol 1993; 23:1745–1751.

128. Betz M, Fox BS. Prostaglandin E_2 inhibits production of Th1 lymphokines but not of Th2 lymphokines. J Immunol 1991; 146:108–113.

129. Novak TJ, Rothenberg EV. Cyclic AMP inhibits induction of interleukin 2 but not of interleukin 4 in T cells. Proc Natl Acad Sci USA 1990; 87:9353–9357.

130. Munoz E, Zubiaga AM, Merrow M, Sauter NP, Huber BT. Cholera toxin discriminates between T helper 1 and 2 cell receptor-mediated activation: role of cyclic AMP in T cell proliferation. J Exp Med 1990; 172:95–103.

131. Frossard N, Landry Y, Pauli G, Ruckstuhl M. Effects of cyclic AMP- and cyclic GMP-phosphodiesterase inhibitors on immunological release of histamine and on lung contraction. Br J Pharmacol 1981; 73:933–938.

132. Peachell PT, Undem BJ, Schleimer RP, MacGlashan DW Jr, Lichtenstein LM, Cieslinski LB, Torphy TJ. Preliminary identification and role of phosphodiesterase isozymes in human basophils. J Immunol 1992; 148:2503–2510.

133. Giembycz MA, Dent G, Virdee H, Rabe KF, Evans PM, Barnes PJ. Cyclic nucleotide phosphodiesterases in human eosinophils: functional and biochemical effects of isoenzyme-selective inhibitors. Br J Pharmacol 1994; 112:26P.

134. Wright CD, Kuipers PJ, Kobylarz-Singer D, Devall LJ, Klinkefus BA, Weishaar RE. Differential inhibition of neutrophil functions: role of cyclic AMP-specific, cyclic GMP-insensitive phosphodiesterase. Biochem Pharmacol 1990; 40:699–607.

135. White JR, Torphy TJ, Christensen SB, Lee JA, Mong S. Purification and characterization of the rolipram sensitive, low-K_m phosphodiesterase from human monocytes. FASEB J 1990; 4: A1987.

136. Thompson WJ, Ross CP, Pledger WJ, Strada SJ, Bannewr RL, Hersh EM. Cyclic adenosine $3':5'$-monophosphate phosphodiesterase. Distinct forms in human lymphocytes and monocytes. J Biol Chem 1976; 251:4922–4929.

137. Turner NC, Wood LJ, Burns FM, Gueremy T, Souness JE. The effect of cyclic AMP and cyclic GMP phosphodiesterase inhibitors on the superoxide burst of guinea-pig peritoneal macrophages. Br J Pharmacol 1993; 108:876–883.

138. Kelly JJ, Barnes PJ, Giembycz MA. Evidence for multiple PDE IV-like phosphodiesterases in guinea-pig macrophages. Am Rev Respir Dis 1993; 147:A935.

139. Marcoz P, Prigent AF, Nemoz G. Modulation of rat thymocyte proliferative responses through the inhibition of different cyclic nucleotide phosphodiesterase isoforms by means of selective inhibitors and cGMP-elevating agents. Mol Pharmacol 1993; 44:1027–1035.

140. Robiscek SA Krzanowski JJ, Szentivanyi A, Polson JB. High pressure liquid chromatography of cyclic AMP phosphodiesterase from purified human T-lymphocytes. Biochem Biophys Res Commun 1989; 163:554–560.

141. Robicsek SA, Blanchard DK, Djeu JY, Krzanowski JJ, Szentivanyi A, Polson JB. Multiple high-affinity cyclic AMP phosphodiesterase in human T-lymphocytes. Biochem Pharmacol 1991; 42: 869–877.

142. Ichimura M, Kase H. A new cyclic nucleotide phosphodiesterase isozyme expressed in the T-lymphocyte cell lines. Biochem Biophys Res Commun 1993; 193:985–990.

143. Hidaka H, Teraka T, Itoh H. Selective inhibitors of three forms of cyclic nucleotide phosphodiesterases. Trends Pharmacol Sci 1984; 5:237–239.

144. Hagiwara M, Endo T, Kanayama T, Hidaka H. Effect of 1-(3-chloroanilino)-4-phenylphthalazine (MY 5445), a specific inhibitor of cyclic GMP phosphodiesterase on human platelet aggregation. J Pharmacol Exp Ther 1984; 228:467–471.

145. Souness JE, Diocee BK, Martin W, Moodie SA. Pig aortic endothelial cell cyclic nucleotide phosphodiesterase. Use of phosphodiesterase inhibitors to evaluate their roles in regulating cyclic nucleotide levels in intact cells. Biochem J 1990; 266:127–132.

146. Lugnier C, Schini VB. Characterization of cyclic nucleotide phosphodiesterases from cultured bovine aortic endothelial cells. Biochem Pharmacol 1990; 39:75–84.

147. Kishi Y, Ashikaya T, Numano F. Phosphodiesterases in vascular endothelial cells. Adv Second Messenger Phosphoprotein Res 1992; 25:201–213.

148. Rousseau E, Gagnon J, Lugnier C. Soluble and particulate cycle nucleotide phosphodiesterases characterized from airway epithelial cells. FASEB J 1993; 7:A146.

149. Lichtenstein LM, Margolis S. Histamine release in vitro: inhibition by catecholamines and methylxanthines. Science 1968; 161:902–903.

150. Orange RP, Kaliner MA, Laraia PJ, Austin KF. Immunological release of histamine and slow reacting substance of anaphylaxis from human lung. II. Influence of cellular levels of cyclic AMP. Fed Proc 1971; 30:1725–1729.

151. Giembycz MA, Corrigan CJ, Kay AB, Barnes PJ. Inhibition of CD4 and CD8 T-lymphocytes (T-LC) proliferation and cytokine secretion by isoenzyme-selective phosphodiesterase (PDE) inhibitors: correlation with intracellular cyclic AMP (cAMP) concentrations. J Allergy Clin Immunol 1994; 93:167.

152. Crocker IC, Townley RG, Khan MM. Phosphodiesterase inhibitors modulate cytokine secretion and proliferation. J Allergy Clin Immunol 1994; 93:286.

153. Averill LE, Stein RL, Kammer GM. Control of human T-lymphocyte interleukin-2 production by a cyclic AMP-dependent pathway. Cell Immunol 1988; 115:88–99.

154. Thanhauser A, Reiling N, Bohle A, Toellner K-M, Duchrow M, Scheel D, Schluter C, Ernst M, Flad H-D, Umler AJ. Pentoxifylline: a potent inhibitor of IL-2 and IFNγ biosynthesis and BCG-induced cytotoxicity. Immunology 1993; 80:151–156.

155. Lewis GM, Caccese RG, Heaslip RL, Bansbach CC. Effects of rolipram and CI-930 on IL-2 mRNA transcription in human Jurkat cells. Agents Actions 1993; 39:C89–C92.

156. van Tits LJH, Michel MC, Motulsky HJ, Maisel AS, Brodde O-E. Cyclic AMP counteracts mitogen-induced inositol phosphate generation and increases in intracellular Ca^{2+} concentrations in human lymphocytes. Br J Pharmacol 1991; 103:1288–1294.

157. Anastassiou ED, Paliogianni F, Balow JP, Yamada H, Boumpas DT. Prostaglandin E_2 and other cyclic AMP-elevating agents modulate IL-2 and IL-2R gene expression at multiple levels. J Immunol 1992; 148:2845–2852.

158. Van der Poow-Kraan T, Van Kooten C, Rensink I, Aarden L. Interleukin (IL)-4 production by human T cells: differential regulation of IL-4 vs IL-2 production. Eur J Immunol 1992; 22:1237–1241.

159. Lee HJ, Koyano-Nakagawa N, Naito Y, Nishida J, Arai N, Arai K-I, Yokota T. Cyclic AMP activates the IL-5 promoter synergistically with phorbol ester through the signaling pathway involving protein kinase A in mouse thymoma line EL-4. J Immunol 1993; 151:6135–6142.

160. Essayan DM, Kagey-Sobotka A, Lichtenstein LM, Huang S-K. Modulation of allergen-induced cytokine gene expression and proliferation by phosphodiesterase (PDE) inhibitors in vitro. J Allergy Clin Immunol 1993; 91:454.

161. Essayan DM, Kagey-Sobotka A, Lichtenstein LM, Huang SK. Studies of phosphodiesterase (PDE) isozyme function and expression in human allergic disease. J Allergy Clin Immunol 1994; 93:286.

161a. Bloom TJ, Beavo JA. Identification of type VII PDE in HUT 78 T lymphocyte cells. FASEB J 1994; 8:A372.

162. Ward AJM, McKenniff M, Evans JM, Page CP, Costello JF. Theophylline—an immunomodulatory role in asthma? Am Rev Respir Dis 1993; 147:518–523.

163. Kammer GM. The adenylate cyclase–cyclic AMP–protein kinase A pathway and regulation of the immune response. Immunol Today 1988; 9:222–229.

164. Paul-Eugene N, Kolb JP, Calenda A, Gordon J, Kikutani H, Kishimoto T, Mencia-Huerta JM, Braquet P, Dugas B. Functional interaction between β_2-adrenoceptor agonists and interleukin-4 in the regulation of CD23 expression and release and IgE production in human. Mol Immunol 1993; 30:157–164.

165. Lycke N, Severinson E, Strober W. Cholera toxin acts synergistically with IL-4 to promote IgG_1 switch differentiation. J Immunol 1990; 145:3316–3324.

166. Lycke NY. Cholera toxin promotes B cell isotype switching by two different mechanisms. J Immunol 1993; 150:4810–4821.

167. Roper RL, Conrad DH, Brown DM, Warner CL, Phipps RP. Prostaglandin E_2 promotes IL-4-induced IgE and IgG_1 synthesis. J Immunol 1990; 145:2644–2651.

168. Phipps RP, Roper RL, Stein SH. Regulation of B-cell tolerance and triggering by macrophages and lymphoid dendritic cells. Immunol Rev 1990; 117:135–158.

169. Godfrey RW, Manzi RM, Gennaro DE, Hoffstein ST. Phospholipid and arachidonic acid metabolism in zymosan-stimulated human monocytes: modulation by cyclic AMP. J Chem Physiol 1987; 131:384–392.

170. Bessler H, Gilgal R, Djaldatti M, Zahavi I. Effect of pentoxifylline on the phagocytic activity, cyclic AMP levels and superoxide anion production by monocytes and polymorphonuclear cells. J Leukoc Biol 1986; 40:747–754.

171. Semmler J, Wachtel H, Endres S. The selective type IV phosphodiesterase inhibitor rolipram suppresses tumour necrosis factor-α production by human mononuclear cells. Int J Immunopharmacol 1993; 15:409–413.

172. Molnar-Kimber K, Yonno L, Heaslip RJ, Weichman BM. Modulation of TNFα and IL-1β from endotoxin-stimulated monocytes by selective PDE isozyme inhibitors. Agents Actions 1993; 39:C77–C79.

173. Seldon PS, Barnes PJ, Giembycz MA. Phosphodiesterase IV inhibitors and β-adrenoceptor agonists suppress lipopolysaccharide-induced tumour necrosis factor-α generation by human peripheral blood monocytes. Br J Pharmacol 1994; 112:215P.

174. Knudsen PJ, Dinarello CA, Strom TB. Prostaglandins posttranscriptionally inhibit monocyte expression of interleukin 1 activity by increasing intracellular cyclic adenosine monophosphate. J Immunol 1986; 137:3189–3194.

175. Hartman DA, Ochalski SJ, Carlson RP. The effects of anti-inflammatory and antiallergic drugs on the release of IL-1β and TNF-α in the human whole blood assay. Agents Actions 1933; 39:C70–C72.

176. Ochalski SJ, Hartman DA, Belfast MT, Walter TL, Glaser KB, Carlson RP. Inhibition of endotoxin-induced hypothermia and serum TNF-α levels in CD-1 mice by various pharmacological agents. Agents Actions 1993; 39:C52–C54.

177. Lim LK, Hunt NH, Widemann MJ. Reactive oxygen production, arachidonate metabolism and cyclic AMP in macrophages. Biochim Biophys Acta 1983; 114:549–555.

178. Dent G, Giembycz MA, Rabe KF, Barnes PJ, Magnussen H. Effects of selective phosphodiesterase inhibitors on human alveolar macrophage cyclic nucleotide hydrolysis and respiratory burst. Br J Pharmacol 1993; 111:74P.

179. Schade FU, Schudt C. The specific type III and IV phosphodiesterase inhibitor zardaverine suppresses formation of tumour necrosis factor by macrophages. Eur J Pharmacol 1993; 230: 9–14.

180. Snyder DS, Beller DI, Unanue ER. Prostaglandins modulate macrophage Ia expression. Nature 1982; 299:163–165.

181. Maruo H, Tanimoto Y, Bewtra AK, Townley RG. Effect of phosphodiesterase IV inhibitor (WAY-PDE-641) on PAF-induced superoxide generation from human eosinophils. J Allergy Clin Immunol 1994; 93:257.

182. Nicholson CD, Shahid M, Bruin J, De Boer J, Van Amsterdam RGM, Zaagsma J, Dent G, Giembycz MA, Barnes PJ. Org 20241: a cyclic nucleotide phosphodiesterase inhibitor for asthma. Br J Pharmacol 1992; 107:252P.

183. Souness JE. Villamil ME, Scott LC, Tomkinson A, Giembycz MA, Raeburn D. Possible role of cyclic AMP phosphodiesterase in the actions of ibudilast on eosinophil thromboxane generation and airways smooth muscle tone. Br J Pharmacol 1994; 111:1081–1088.

184. Kita H, Abu-Ghazaleh RI, Gleich GJ, Abraham RT. Regulation of Ig-induced eosinophil degranulation by adenosine 3′,5′-cyclic monophosphate. J Immunol 1991; 146:2712–2718.

185. Cohan VL, Johnson KL, Breslow R, Cheng JB, Showell HJ. PDE IV is the predominant PDE isozyme regulating chemotactic factor-mediated guinea-pig eosinophil functions in vitro. J Allergy Clin Immunol 1992; 89:663.

186. Tanimoto Y, Maruo H, Bewtra AK, Townley RG. Effects of phosphodiesterase IV inhibitor (WAY-PDE-641) on human eosinophil and neutrophil migration in vitro. J Allergy Clin Immunol 1994; 93:257.

187. Ohta K, Sawamoto S, Nakajima M, Nagai A, Tanaka Y, Hirai BSK, Mano K, Miyashita H. Theophylline induces apoptosis in eosinophils surviving with interleukin-5 in vitro. J Allergy Clin Immunol 1994; 93:200.

188. Nourshargh S, Hoult JRS. Inhibition of human neutrophil degranulation by forskolin in the presence of phosphodiesterase inhibitors. Eur J Pharmacol 1986; 122:205–212.

189. Nielson CP, Vestal RE, Sturm RJ, Heaslip R. Effects of selective phosphodiesterase inhibitors on the polymorphonuclear leukocyte respiratory burst. J Allergy Clin Immunol 1990; 86: 801–808.

190. Harvath L, Robbins JD, Russell AA, Seaman KB. Cyclic AMP and human neutrophil chemotaxis. Elevation of cyclic AMP differentially affects chemotactic responsiveness. J Immunol 1991; 146:224–232.

191. Fonteh AN, Winkler JD, Torphy TJ, Heravi J, Undem BJ, Chilton FH. Influence of isoproterenol and phosphodiesterase inhibitors on platelet-activating factor biosynthesis in the human neutrophil. J Immunol 1993; 151:339–350.

192. Page CP. Platelet activating factor. In: Barnes PJ, Rodger IW, Thompson NC, eds. Asthma, Basic Mechanisms and Clinical Management. London: Academic Press, 1988:283–302.

193. Radomski MW, Palmer RMJ, Moncada S. Comparative pharmacology of endothelium-derived relaxing factor, nitric oxide and prostacyclin in platelets. Br J Pharmacol 1987; 92:181–187.

194. Radomski MW, Palmer RMJ, Moncada S. The role of nitric oxide and cyclic GMP in platelet adhesion to vascular endothelium. Biochem Biophys Res Commun 1987; 148:1482–1489.

195. Stelzner TJ, Weil JV, O'Brien RF. Role of cyclic adenosine monophosphate in the induction of endothelial barrier properties. J Cell Physiol 1989; 139:157–166.

196. Casnocha SA, Eskin SG, Hall ER, McIntire LV. Permeability of human endothelial monolayers: effect of vasoactive agonists and cyclic AMP. J Appl Physiol 1989; 67:1997–2005.

197. Minnear FL, DeMichele MA, Moon DG, Rieder CL, Fenton JW. Isoproterenol reduces thrombin-induced pulmonary endothelial permeability in vitro. Am J Physiol 1989; 257:H1613–H1623.

198. Suttorp N, Weber U, Welsch T, Schudt C. Role of phosphodiesterases in the regulation of endothelial permeability in vitro. J Clin Invest 1993; 91:1421–1428.

199. Pober JS, Slowik MR, De Luca LG, Ritchie AJ. Elevated cyclic AMP inhibits endothelial cell synthesis and expression of TNF-induced endothelial leukocyte adhesion molecule-1, and vascular cell adhesion molecule-1, but not intercellular adhesion molecule-1. J Immunol 1993; 150:5114–5123.

200. Smith JJ, Welsh MJ. Cyclic AMP stimulates bicarbonate secretion across normal, but not cystic fibrosis airway epithelia. J Clin Invest 1992; 89:1148–1153.

201. Koyoma S, Rennard SI, Claassen L, Robbins RA. Dibutyryl cyclic AMP, prostaglandin E_2, and antioxidants protect cultured bovine epithelial cells from endotoxin. Am J Physiol 1991; 261: L126–L132.

202. Djukanovic R, Roche WR, Wilson JW, Beasley CRW, Twentyman OP, Howarth PH, Holgate ST. Mucosal inflammation and asthma. Am Rev Respir Dis 1990; 142:434–457.

203. Karlsson J-A, Souness JE, Webber SE, Pollock K, Raeburn D, Palfreyman MN, Ashton MJ. Suppression of mediator release from granulocytes by RP 73401, a novel, selective PDE IV inhibitor. Am Rev Respir Dis 1994; In press.

204. Kawasaki A, Hoshino K, Osaki R, Mizushima Y, Yano S. Effect of ibudilast: a novel anti-asthmatic agent on airway hypersensitivity in bronchial asthma. J Asthma 1992; 29:245–252.

205. Davies GE, Evans DP. Studies with two new phosphodiesterase inhibitors (ICI 58,301 and ICI 63,197) on anaphylaxis in guinea-pigs, mice and rats. Int Arch Allergy Appl Immunol 1973; 45:467–478.

206. Broughton BJ, Chaplen P, Knowles P, Lunt E, Marshall SM, Pain DL, Wooldridge KRH. Antiallergic activity of 2-phenyl-8-azapurin-6-ones. J Med Chem 1975; 18:1117–1122.

207. Teixeira MM, Rossi AG, Williams TJ, Hellewell PG. Effects of phosphodiesterase isoenzyme inhibitors on cutaneous inflammation in the guinea-pig. Br J Pharmacol 1994; 112:332–340.

208. Howell RE, Sickles BD, Woeppel SL. Pulmonary antiallergic and bronchodilator effects of isozyme-selective phosphodiesterase inhibitors in guinea-pigs. J Pharmacol Exp Ther 1993; 264:609–615.

209. Banner KH, Page CP. Effect of the phosphodiesterase (PDE) III/IV inhibitor, zardaverine, administered acutely and chronically on pulmonary cell influx in ovalbumin-sensitised guinea-pigs (abstr.). Br J Pharmacol 1994; 112:253P.

210. Underwood DC, Osborn RR, Novak LB, Matthews JK, Newsholme SJ, Undem BJ, Hand JM, Torphy TJ. Inhibition of antigen-induced bronchoconstriction and eosinophil infiltration in the guinea-pig by the cyclic AMP-specific phosphodiesterase inhibitor, rolipram. J Pharmacol Exp Ther 1993; 266:306–313.

211. Sanjar S, Aoki S, Boubekeur K, Burrows L, Colditz I, Chapman I, Morley J. Inhibition of PAF-induced eosinophil accumulation of pulmonary airways of guinea-pigs by anti-asthma drugs. Jpn J Pharmacol 1989; 51:167–172.

212. Kips JC, Joos GF, Peleman RA, Pauwels RA. The effect of zardaverine, an inhibitor of phosphodiesterase isoenzymes III and IV, on endotoxin-induced airway changes in rats. Clin Exp Allergy 1993; 23:518–523.

213. Sanjar S, Aoki S, Boubekeur K, Chapman ID, Smith D, Kings MA, Morley J. Eosinophil

accumulation in pulmonary airways of guinea-pigs induced by exposure to an aerosol of platelet activating factor: effect of anti-asthma drugs. Br J Pharmacol 1990; 99:267–272.

214. Sanjar S, Aoki S, Kristersson A, Smith D, Morley J. Antigen challenge induced pulmonary airway eosinophil accumulation and airway hyperreactivity in sensitised guinea-pigs: the effect of anti-asthma drugs. Br J Pharmacol 99:679–686.

215. Kings MA, Chapman I, Kristersson A, Sanjar S, Morley J. Human recombinant lymphokines and cytokines induce pulmonary eosinophilia in the guinea-pig which is inhibited by ketotifen and AH 21-132. Int Arch Allergy Appl Immunol 1990; 91:354–361.

216. Schudt C, Winder S, Litze M, Kilian U, Beume R. Zardaverine: a cyclic AMP specific PDE III/IV inhibitor. Agents Actions 1991; 34:161–177.

217. Sturm RJ, Osborne MC, Heaslip RJ. The effect of phosphodiesterase inhibitors on pulmonary inflammatory cell influx in ovalbumin-sensitized guinea-pigs. J Cell Biochem 1990; 14:337.

218. Elwood W, Sun J, Barnes PJ, Giembycz MA, Chung KF. Inhibition of allergen-induced lung eosinophilia by isoenzyme-selective phosphodiesterase inhibitors in Brown Norway rats. Inflam Res 1995; 44:83–86.

219. Eidelman DH, Bellofiori S, Martin JG. Late airway responses to antigen challenge in sensitized inbred rats. Am Rev Respir Dis 1988; 137:1033–1037.

220. Newsholme SJ, Schwartz L. cAMP-specific phosphodiesterase inhibitor, rolipram, reduces eosinophil infiltration evoked by leukotrienes or by histamine in guinea-pig conjunctiva. Inflammation 1993; 17:25–31.

221. Griswold DE, Webb EF, Breton J, White JR, Marshall PJ, Torphy TJ. Effect of selective phosphodiesterase type IV inhibitor, rolipram, on fluid and cellular phases of inflammatory responses. Inflammation 1993; 17:333–344.

222. Boucheron JA, Verghese MW, Irsula O, Stacy L. Species differences in neutrophil superoxide modulation by cyclic nucleotide phosphodiesterase inhibitors. FASEB J 1991; 5:A510.

223. Aoki S, Boubekeur K, Kristersson A, Morley J, Sanjar S. Is allergic airway hyperreactivity of the guinea-pig dependent on eosinophil accumulation in the lung? Br J Pharmacol 1988; 94:365P.

224. DeBrito FB, Ebsworth KE, Lawrence CE. Regulation of eosinophilia by cyclic AMP. Proceedings International Congress on Inflammation. Rome, Italy, 1991.

225. Svensjo E, Andersson KE, Bouskela E, Cyrino FZGA, Lindgren S. Effects of two vasodilatory phosphodiesterase inhibitors on bradykinin induced permeability increase in the hamster. Int J Microcirc Clin Exp 1992; 11:A179.

226. Crummey A, Harper GP, Boyle EA, Mangan FR. Inhibition of arachidonic acid-induced ear oedema as a model for assessing topical anti-inflammatory compounds. Agents Actions 1987; 20:69–76.

227. Ortiz JL, Cortijo J, Valles JM, Bou J, Morcillo EJ. Rolipram inhibits PAF-induced airway microvascular leakage in guinea-pig: a comparison with milrinone and theophylline. Fundam Clin Pharmacol 1992; 6:247–249.

228. Raeburn D, Karlsson J-A. Effects of isoenzyme-selective inhibitors of cyclic nucleotide phosphodiesterase on microvascular leak in guinea-pig airways. J Pharmacol Exp Ther 1993; 267:1147–1152.

229. Raeburn D, Woodman V, Buckley G, Karlsson J-A. Inhibition of PAF-induced microvascular leakage in the guinea-pig in vivo: the effects of rolipram and theophylline. Eur Respir J 1991; 4(suppl 14):590S.

230. Leeman M, Lejeune P, Melot C, Naeije R. Reduction in pulmonary hypertension and in airway resistance by enoximone (MDL 17,043) in decompensated COPD. Chest 1987; 91:662–666.

231. Israel E, Mathur PN, Tachkin D, Drazen JM. LY 168855 prevents bronchospasm in asthma of moderate severity. Chest 1987; 91:71S.

232. Reiser J, Yeang Y, Warner JO. The effect of zaprinast, an orally absorbed mast cell stabilizer, on exercise-induced asthma in children. Br J Dis Chest 1986; 80:157–163.

233. Foster RW, Rakshu K, Carpenter JR, Small RC. Trials of the bronchodilator activity of the

isoenzyme phosphodiesterase inhibitor AH 21-132 in healthy volunteers during a methacholine challenge. Br J Clin Pharmacol 1992; 34:527–534.

234. Baer RL. Papaverine therapy in atopic dermatitis. J Am Acad Dermatol 1985; 13:806–808.
235. Kaplan HJ, Deman L, Rosenberg EW, Feigenbaum S. Topical use of caffeine with hydrocortisone in the treatment of atopic dermatitis. Arch Dermatol 1978; 114:60–62.
236. Rasmussen JE. Advances in nondietary management of children with atopic dermatitis. Pediatr Dermatol 1989; 6:210–215.
237. Hanifin JM. Pharmacophysiology of atopic dermatitis. Clin Rev Allergy 1986; 4:43–65.
238. Sawiski MA, Rusin LJ, Burns TL, Weinstein GD, Voorhees JJ. Ro 20-1724: an agent that significantly improves psoriatic lesions in double-blind clinical trials. J Invest Dermatol 1979; 73:261–263.

23

Ion Channels and Airway Disease

Peter J. Barnes
National Heart and Lung Institute, London, England

INTRODUCTION

The concentration of intracellular ions, such as calcium (Ca^{2+}) and potassium (K^+) ions has a profound influence on cell activity. The intracellular concentrations of these ions are partly determined by their passage through specific ion channels at the cell surface. Ion channels are protein-lined pores in the cell membrane, several of which have now been cloned. Most channels are made up of distinct subunits that are grouped together in the cell membrane. Whether the channel is open or closed depends on different factors for each channel, but may be determined by receptor activation, the polarization of the cell membrane, or the presence of particular ligands that interact directly with the channel. Drugs that open or block these channels have now been discovered (such as highly specific, naturally occurring toxins) or developed through pharmaceutical research, leading to an enormous increase in our understanding of the role of these channels in different cell types. It has also raised the possibility that these drugs may be useful therapeutically.

Airway caliber is largely determined by the tone of airway smooth muscle, and airway smooth-muscle contraction is determined by the intracellular Ca^{2+} concentration ($[Ca^{2+}]_i$). Drugs that block calcium channels, therefore, should be bronchodilator if airway smooth-muscle cells behave in the same manner as vascular smooth-muscle cells, in which calcium antagonists are potent vasodilators. A reduction in intracellular K^+ leads to hyperpolarization of smooth-muscle cells and thus to relaxation, suggesting that drugs that open K^+ channels (KCOs) may also act as bronchodilators.

In addition to airway smooth muscle, many other cells contribute to airway obstruction in asthma and chronic obstructive airway diseases. Release of neurotransmitters from airway nerves and inflammatory mediators from inflammatory cells, such as mast cells, eosinophils, neutrophils, macrophages, and T lymphocytes, may also be determined by

Ca^{2+} and K^+ channels, so that calcium antagonists or KCOs may have additional effects on bronchodilation.

This chapter reviews the possible roles of Ca^{2+} and K^+ channels in airway disease, with particular emphasis on therapeutic potential in the treatment of airway obstruction.

CALCIUM CHANNELS

Several types of calcium channel have now been identified on the basis of drug selectivity, by electrophysiological properties, and from molecular cloning.

Voltage-Operated Channels

Voltage-operated channels (VOCs) or *L-type* channels (for long-lasting) open in response to depolarization of the cell, resulting in influx of Ca^{2+} to increase intracellular Ca^{2+} concentration; these channels are blocked by dihydropyridines (such as nifedipine and nimodipine), by verapamil, and by diltiazem. Several subtypes of L-type channel have now been recognized in different tissues (1). Each consists of five subunits. Voltage-sensitive calcium channels are important in contractile responses of pulmonary vascular smooth muscle, but are less important in the contractile response of airway smooth muscle, or in the activation of inflammatory cells. T-type calcium channels are also opened by depolarization, but are insensitive to dihydropyridines. Electrophysiological studies have revealed the presence of both L- and T-channels in airway smooth muscle, although the L-channels are less sensitive to dihydropyridines than the L-channels in the myocardium (2). N-type channels, which are largely restricted to neurons, are also sensitive to depolarization and are insensitive to dihydropyridines, but are blocked by the toxin ω-conotoxin.

Receptor-Operated Channels

Receptor-operated channels (ROCs) are envisaged as channels that open in response to activation of certain receptors; these receptors are not well defined, but drugs that block ROCs, such as SK&F 96365, have been developed (3). The ROCs may be regulated by signals from intracellular stores and by inositol phosphates, so that Ca^{2+} enters through ROCs to fill intracellular stores (4–6). It has recently been established that a diffusible cytosolic Ca^{2+} influx factor (CIF) may be the second messenger regulating the influx of Ca^{2+} through ROCs to fill depleted intracellular stores (6). The CIF appears to be a phosphate-containing anion that has yet to be characterized in detail.

A rise in intracellular Ca^{2+} concentration is associated with cell activation, but recovery depends on removal of Ca^{2+} by sequestration or by pumping out of the cell in exchange for Na^+. In airway smooth muscle, there is a pump, which exchanges three Na^+ for each Ca^{2+}, that is linked to the activity of Na^+, K^+-ATPase, which maintains the inwardly directed Na^+ gradient by exchanging intracellular Na^+ for extracellular K^+ (7). In airway smooth muscle there is also an active Ca^{2+} channel into intracellular stores that may be stimulated by cAMP (8).

Airway Smooth Muscle

Activation of an airway smooth-muscle cell by a spasmogen results in a rapid rise in $[Ca^{2+}]_i$, from a resting level of about 0.1 to 10–100 nM. Studies with fluorescent markers of $[Ca^{2+}]_i$, such as aequorin and fura-2 in airway smooth-muscle cells show a rapid elevation and return to baseline within 1 min (2). The rise in $[Ca^{2+}]_i$ leads to contraction by activating a series of enzymes. The source of calcium for contraction may derive from extracellular Ca^{2+}, which enters the cell through calcium channels down electrochemical and concentration gradients, or from intracellular stores (Fig. 1).

Both VOCs and ROCs have been differentiated in airway smooth-muscle cells (2,9–11). Depolarization of airway smooth muscle with potassium chloride (KCl) solutions results in a contraction that is due to influx of Ca^{2+} through VOCs. This contractile response is blocked by calcium antagonists, such as verapamil, nifedipine, and diltiazem. The dihydropyridine calcium *agonist* BAY K 8644 augments KCl-induced contractions of airway smooth muscle, by increasing calcium entry (12). Patch-clamp studies of airway smooth-muscle cells indicate that both T- and L-channels are present, although the L-channels are less sensitive to dihydropyridine agonists and antagonists than the classic L-channels in myocardium (2).

Function studies indicate that VDCs mediate contraction caused by depolarization of airway smooth muscle, but the role of VDCs in response to endogenous mediators and neurotransmitters is questionable. Contraction of airway smooth muscle in response to agonists, such as acetylcholine and histamine, is independent of external Ca^{2+} concentration and is not associated with ^{45}Ca-uptake, suggesting that calcium entry is not important for *initiation* of contractile responses. However, entry of Ca^{2+} through ROCs may be important in refilling intracellular stores and in the maintenance of increased tone. Calcium antagonists have only weak effects against contraction of human airway smooth muscle induced by histamine or methacholine, although they are apparently more effective in *reversing* the contraction induced by these agents (13,14). This may indicate that calcium

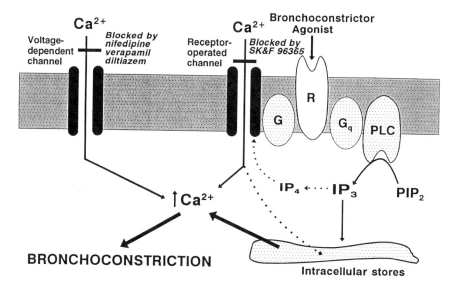

Figure 1 Calcium channels in airway smooth-muscle cells: Calcium ions (Ca^{2+}) may enter the cell by voltage-dependent or receptor-operated calcium channels. The latter are coupled to receptors (R), possibly by G-proteins. Receptors may also stimulate phospholipase C (PLC) through a G-protein (G_q), resulting in an increase in inositol-1,4,5-triphosphate (IP_3), which releases Ca^{2+} from internal calcium stores.

antagonists are not important in the initiation of contraction, but may play a more important role in the maintenance of tone.

Most spasmogens contract airway smooth muscle in the absence of extracellular calcium, suggesting that the source of Ca^{2+} for contraction must be intracellular. By analogy with striated muscle, it is likely that the calcium stores in smooth muscle are the endoplasmic reticulum, and specialized stores of calcium, called *calciosomes*, have been recognized. The molecular mechanisms by which activation of a surface receptor leads to release of intracellular Ca^{2+} and contraction have now been elucidated, and involve the breakdown of a certain pool of membrane phospholipids, phosphoinositides.

Phosphoinositide (PI) hydrolysis is an important mechanism of signal transduction in airway smooth-muscle cells (15,16). Activation of surface receptors (e.g., muscarinic receptors on airway smooth-muscle cells) leads to the activation of the enzyme phospholipase C (PLC or phosphoinositidase) by a coupling guanine nucleotide regulatory protein (G-protein), termed G_q. The PLC activation converts phosphoinositide-4,5-biphosphate (PIP_2) in the cell membrane to two intracellular messengers, myoinositol-1,4,5-triphosphate (IP_3) and 1,2-diacylglycerol (DAG).

Contraction of airway smooth muscle is associated with a fall in PIP_2 and a rise in IP_3 concentrations. IP_3 is broken down by the enzyme 5-phosphatase to IP_2 and then to IP and inositol, which are inactive. Inositol is subsequently reincorporated into the PI pool in the cell membrane. Lithium ions inhibit the conversion of IP back to inositol; thus, if PI hydrolysis is stimulated, IP accumulates and provides a measure of PI turnover in the cell. In airway smooth muscle, muscarinic agonists increase IP accumulation in a concentration-dependent manner, and there is a close relation between occupation of muscarinic receptors and the simulation of PI hydrolysis. Other spasmogens of smooth muscle also stimulate PI hydrolysis in airway smooth muscle. More recently, it has been possible to measure IP_3 directly using a competitive-binding assay. Mass measurements of IP_3 after exposure to a cholinergic agonist, have demonstrated a rapid increase (within seconds) that precedes the development of tension (17,18).

IP_3 is the intracellular messenger that leads to the release of Ca^{2+} from intracellular stores. It binds to specific sites (receptors) on endoplasmic reticulum, which have now been cloned. Binding to these specific sites opens channels that allow the efflux of Ca^{2+} from the stores into the cytoplasm. IP_3 is rapidly degraded in airway smooth muscle, since cholinergic stimulation leads to a transient peak. This may be because the 5-phosphatase that dephosphorylates and inactivates IP_3 is activated by the rise in $[Ca^{2+}]_i$. IP_3 may also be phosphorylated by the enzyme 3-kinase to inositol (1,3,4,5)-tetrakisphosphate (IP_4), which has been proposed as an activator of Ca^{2+} entry to refill intracellular stores by preferential channels. However, in airway smooth muscle there is little rise in concentration of IP_4 after cell activation (19).

Other Cells

A rise in $[Ca^{2+}]_i$ is important in the secretion of inflammatory mediators from inflammatory cells, such as mast cells, neutrophils, and eosinophils. Calcium antagonists, such as nifedipine, however, have no significant inhibitory effect on mediator release from these cells, suggesting that calcium release from intracellular stores may be more important (20). The nature of the calcium channels in inflammatory cells, such as eosinophils, has not been explored in detail. Agonists, such as platelet-activating factor (PAF) cause a transient rise in $[Ca^{2+}]_i$ that is not blocked by dihydropyridines, but is blocked by EDTA, suggesting that a

ROC is involved (21). The ROCs appear to be involved in the activation and secretion of mediators from inflammatory cells, such as mast cells (6,22), and this is an area of intense investigation.

Similarly calcium antagonists have no significant effect on the release of neurotransmitters, since calcium entry into nerve terminals is dependent on N-channels that are not susceptible to calcium antagonists such as dihydropyridines.

Calcium antagonists have little effect on airway microvascular leakage induced by inflammatory mediators and, therefore, are unlikely to have an inhibitory effect on airway edema formation (23). The potent vasodilator action of calcium antagonists theoretically could increase plasma exudation by increasing the delivery of blood to leaky postcapillary venules.

Calcium Antagonists in Asthma

Although calcium antagonists, which block VDCs, have been very effective in cardiovascular disease, their use in asthma has been disappointing (14,24).

Calcium antagonists are only weakly effective in human airways in vivo. They do not cause bronchodilation in either normal or asthmatic subjects, and give only weak protection against histamine-, methacholine-, allergen-, or exercise-induced bronchoconstriction. Even high doses of nifedipine, given by nebulization, have little protective effect against histamine-induced bronchoconstriction in asthmatic patients (25).

Consequently, calcium antagonists are of no value in the clinical management of obstructive airway diseases. However, they may be safely used to treat hypertension and ischemic heart disease in patients with asthma in whom even selective β-adrenergic blockers are contraindicated.

POTASSIUM CHANNELS

Recovery of cells after depolarization depends on the movement of K^+ out of the cell through K^+ channels in the cell membrane. This results in hyperpolarization of the cell, with relaxation of smooth muscle and inhibition of cell activity. Conversely, blockade of K^+ channels with drugs, such as tetraethylammonium (TEA) and 4-aminopyridine (4-AP), results in increased excitability or hyperresponsiveness of cells. Many different types of K^+ channel have now been defined, using selective toxins, patch-clamping techniques, and cloning (26,27).

Differentiation of Potassium Channels

Although more than ten different types of K^+ channel have been described, they may be subdivided into four main classes (Fig. 2).

Voltage-Gated Channels

The voltage-gated channels are the delayed rectifier channels (K_{dr}) that open on depolarization of the membrane and return the cell membrane to its previous polarized state. This is a diverse group of channels, some of which are blocked by α-dendrotoxin: TEA and 4-AP effectively block all K_{dr}.

Calcium-Activated Channels

The Ca^{2+}-activated channels (K_{Ca}) open in response to elevation of intracellular Ca^{2+} concentration. Large-conductance (maxi-K) K^+ channels are found in smooth muscle and

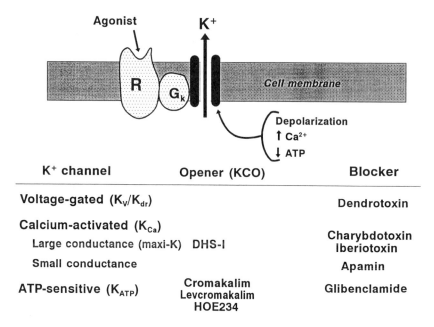

| K⁺ channel | Opener (KCO) | Blocker |

K^+ channel	Opener (KCO)	Blocker
Voltage-gated (K_v/K_{dr})		Dendrotoxin
Calcium-activated (K_{Ca})		
Large conductance (maxi-K)	DHS-I	Charybdotoxin Iberiotoxin
Small conductance		Apamin
ATP-sensitive (K_{ATP})	Cromakalim Levcromakalim HOE234	Glibenclamide

Figure 2 Potassium channel diversity: K^+ channels may be opened by depolarization of the cell membrane, by an increase in intracellular calcium ions, by a fall in ATP, or by receptor (R) activation through a coupling protein (G_k).

neurons and are blocked by the scorpion venoms charybdotoxin and iberiotoxin. Small-conductance channels, some of which are blocked by apamin, are found predominantly in neurons, although they are also found on some types of smooth muscle.

Receptor-Coupled Channels

Receptor-coupled channels are opened by certain receptors through a G-protein, but no specific blockers have been found.

ATP-Sensitive Channels

ATP-sensitive channels (K_{ATP}) are opened by a fall in intracellular ATP concentration. These channels are found in smooth muscle and in the islet cells of the pancreas. They are blocked by sulfonylureas, such as glyburide (glibenclamide), and are opened by drugs, such as cromakalim (BRL 34915), its active enantiomer levcromakalim (BRL 38227), aprikalim (RP 53891), and HOE 245.

Airway Smooth Muscle

Potassium channels play an important role in relaxation of airway smooth muscle (28–30; Fig. 3). β-Agonist-induced bronchodilation is markedly inhibited by charybdotoxin and iberiotoxin (31–33), indicating that opening of a maxi-K channel is involved in the relaxant response. Neither apamin nor glyburide have any inhibitory effect on the relaxation response to β-agonists. A rise in intracellular AMP causes opening of maxi-K channels in airways-smooth muscle (34), but there is also evidence from patch-clamping studies that β-adrenoceptors are directly coupled, by G_s, to maxi-K channels (35,36). This suggests that

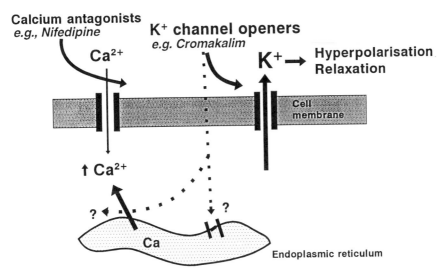

Figure 3   Potassium channels in airway smooth muscle: K^+ channel openers result in an efflux of K^+, with hyperpolarization and relaxation, and may also inhibit the release of calcium from intracellular stores.

it may be possible for airway smooth muscle to relax in response to β-agonists, without an increase in intracellular AMP. Since charybdotoxin appears to have a greater inhibitory effect at low concentrations of β-agonists, and no effect at high concentrations, this suggests that maxi-K channels may be directly opened by β-receptor coupling at low concentrations of agonist, but as concentrations rise there is an increase in AMP that leads to relaxation through other mechanisms.

The KCOs, which open ATP-sensitive K^+ channels, relax animal and human airways in vitro (37–40). Thus, levcromakalim and HOE 234 almost completely relax human airway smooth muscle in vitro. The relaxant effect of KCOs in airway smooth muscle is competitively inhibited by the K_{ATP} blocker glibenclamide. This indicates that the channel involved belongs to the ATP-sensitive K^+ channel class, although the low sensitivity to glyburide distinguishes it from the high-affinity ATP-sensitive K^+ channel typical of pancreatic islets. Glyburide itself has no effect on airway smooth-muscle tone, and may bind to the channel only when it is in the open state. The KCOs appear to act as functional antagonists, as they reverse with equal potency contraction induced by cholinergic agonists, histamine, and neurokinin A (38). This is somewhat surprising, since contraction caused by these spasmogens is mediated by PI hydrolysis and intracellular Ca^{2+} release, rather than by depolarization of the cell, and this is why Ca^{2+} antagonists are not effective. The efficacy of K^+ channel activation in airway smooth muscle may indicate that these drugs have additional effects other than repolarizing or hyperpolarizing cells. It is possible that they may also act on endoplasmic reticulum to pump Ca^{2+} back into intracellular stores, thereby lowering $[Ca^{2+}]_i$.

The KCOs are also effective bronchodilators in vivo, both after intravenous administration and by inhalation, and reach the efficacy of β-agonists (41). Therefore, KCOs may form a new class of bronchodilator for use in asthma.

Neurotransmission

Potassium channels are also involved in the release of neurotransmitters from peripheral nerves, including airway nerves (42). In anesthetized guinea pigs, cromakalim has an inhibitory effect on cholinergic neurotransmission and the release of neuropeptides from sensory nerves in airways (43). The inhibitory effect on neuropeptide release has also been demonstrated in guinea pig airways in vitro (44,45), and it is presumably hyperpolarization of the nerve ending that prevents the release of neurotransmitters. This suggests that KCOs may reduce neurogenic inflammation in the airways, and there is evidence that these drugs have an inhibitory effect on neurogenic airway microvascular leakage and vagus nerve-induced mucous secretion from goblet cells (46,47).

Modulation of neurotransmission is also mediated by opening of maxi-K channels, since charybdotoxin reverses the modulatory effect of many agonists, including opioids, neuropeptide Y, and α-adrenergic agonists, on neuropeptide release from airway sensory nerves (45,48). Similarly, charybdotoxin also blocks the modulatory effect of prejucntional inhibitors of cholinergic nerves in guinea pig and human airways (48). Charybdotoxin increases cholinergic, nerve-induced contraction of airway smooth muscle, by inhibition of the inhibitory effects of acetylcholine on muscarinic M_2-autoreceptors (48).

Other Cells

It is likely that K^+ channels are important in the regulation of inflammatory cell activation and secretion, although the nature of the K^+ channels in inflammatory cells, such as mast cells, eosinophils, T lymphocytes, and macrophages, remains to be defined. The KCOs appear to have little or no inhibitory effects on the release of mediators from inflammatory cells. Thus, cromakalim has no effect on IgE-dependent release of mediators from sensitized human lungs. Similarly, KCOs have no inhibitory effect on airway microvascular leakage (49). In rat basophilic leukemia cells K_{Ca} appear to be involved in degranulation and histamine release (50). A recent study suggests that small-conductance K_{Ca} channels may be involved in the activation of mast cells in the airway, since apamin has an inhibitory effect on allergen-induced constriction of guinea pig airways in vitro, but has no effect on the direct contractile response to histamine (51).

Clinical Studies in Asthma

The potent relaxant effect of KCOs in airway smooth muscle in vitro suggests that these drugs may be useful as novel bronchodilators in asthma (29,52). Orally administered cromakilim has a small inhibitory effect on histamine-induced bronchoconstriction in normal individuals (53), but there is evidence for a small protective effect against the nocturnal fall in lung function in asthmatic patients (54). By contrast, orally administered levcromakalim had no significant bronchodilator effect, nor any protective effect against histamine- or methacholine-induced bronchoconstriction in asthmatic patients (55; Fig. 4). The highest dose of levcromakalim administered has significant adverse effects, with postural hypotension and headaches as a consequence of its vasodilator action. This suggests that this class of drug is not likely to be useful by the oral route, since vasodilator side effects will limit the dose that can be given. One way to overcome this problem may be the use of inhaled preparations, and animal studies indicate that this route of administration is effective (41). However, if the drug is absorbed from the lung into the systemic circulation, there may still be a problem of side effects.

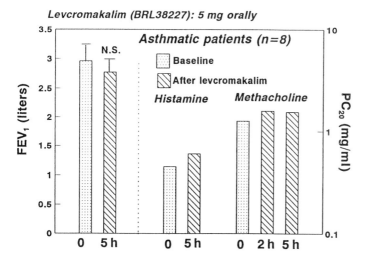

Figure 4 The effect of a K^+ channel opener (levcromakalim) on airway function and histamine and methacholine responsiveness in asthmatic patients. The PC_{20} is the concentration of histamine or methacholine that causes a 20% fall in FEV_1. (Adapted from Ref. 55.)

Whether the additional effects on neurogenic mechanisms may prove useful has yet to be determined. The inhibitory effect of KCOs on neurogenic and cigarette smoke-induced goblet cell secretion (47) suggests that these drugs may have a role in the treatment of mucous hypersecretion in chronic bronchitis.

The KCOs, such as cromakalim and levcromakalim, have cardiovascular side effects that limit their development as antiasthma therapies. In the future, it is possible that KCOs that have a greater selectivity for airway K_{ATP} channels may be developed. The KCO BRL 55834 appears to have less cardiovascular effects than levcromakalim, indicating that such selectivity may be possible (41). The K^+ channel that appears to play a major role in relaxation of airway smooth muscle is the maxi-K channel, suggesting that drugs that selectively open this channel may be more useful than K_{ATP} openers. Extracts from a medicinal herb used in asthma therapy in Ghana appear to have a selective effect on maxi-K channels (56). The most active ingredient is dehydrosoyasaponin I (DHS-I), which reversibly activates maxi-K channels in tracheal smooth-muscle preparations and may form the basis of a new class of bronchodilator therapy. The recent cloning of a maxi-K channel gene, termed *mSlo*, may help in the discovery of such new drugs (57). The recognition that there are a large number of variant *mSlo* cDNAs in mouse indicate that there may be several types of maxi-K channels, indicating that selective openers might be developed in the future.

CHLORIDE CHANNELS

Little is known about chloride channels in the airways. Although several types of Cl^- channel can be distinguished electrophysiologically, these are not well defined, and selective inhibitors and activators are lacking. An inwardly directed calcium-activated Cl^- channel has been described in airway smooth-muscle cells (58), but the functional roles of this channel are not yet clear.

The loop diuretic furosemide was observed to inhibit exercise-induced asthma (59), and subsequently several other indirect challenges (60–62), suggesting that such drugs may have potential as antiasthma compounds (63–65). The protective effect in indirect challenges and the lack of effect against bronchoconstriction induced directly by spasmogens, such as histamine and methacholine, are analogous to the effects of cromolyn sodium and nedocromil sodium. Additionally, inhaled furosemide was also effective in reducing induced cough responses in asthmatic patients (66,67), indicating a possible effect on sensory nerves, as also observed with cromones (68). In addition, furosemide inhibits the IgE-dependent release of mediators from human lung in vitro (69) and the release of mediators from eosinophils (70).

The mechanism of action of furosemide is still uncertain. That bumetanide, a more potent loop diuretic, does not share the same antiasthma effects as furosemide suggests that inhibition of the $Na^+-K^+-Cl^-$ cotransporter is unlikely to account for its antiasthma effects. Furosemide, unlike bumetanide, appears to block Cl^- channels in certain cells (71). Thus, the effects of furosemide may be mimicked by Cl^- channel blockers, 4,4′-diisothiocyano-2,2′-stilbene-disulfanic acid DIDS and NPPB (70). It is of interest that nedocromil sodium also appears to block Cl^- transport in nerves (72). This indicates that cromones may also work through inhibition of certain Cl^- channels. In the future development of more potent and selective inhibitors may help to define these channels more clearly and lead to the development of new antiasthma drugs in the future.

REFERENCES

1. Tsien RW, Tsien RY. Calcium channels, stores, and oscillations. Annu Rev Cell Biol 1990; 6: 715–760.
2. Kotlikoff MI. Calcium currents in isolated canine airway smooth muscle cells. Am J Physiol 1988; 254:C793–C901.
3. Merritt JC, Armstrong WP, Benham CD, et al. SK&F 96365, a novel inhibitor of calcium entry. Biochem J 1990; 271:5–15.
4. Putney JW. Receptor-regulated calcium entry. Pharmacol Ther 1990; 48:427–434.
5. Putney JW, Bird GStJ. The signal for capacitative calcium entry. Cell 1993; 75:199–201.
6. Fasolato C, Innocenti B, Pozzan T. Receptor-attractant Ca^{2+} influx: how many mechanisms for how many channels? Trends Pharmacol Sci 1994; 15:77–83.
7. Bullock CG, Fettes JJF, Kirkpatrick CT. Tracheal smooth muscle—second thoughts on sodium calcium exchange. J Physiol 1981; 318:46–52.
8. Twort CAC, van Breemen C. Human airway smooth muscle in cell culture: control of the intracellular calcium store. Pulm Pharmacol 1989; 2:45–53.
9. Murray RK, Kotlikoff MI. Receptor-activated calcium influx in human airway smooth muscle cells. J Physiol 1991; 435:123–144.
10. Marthan R, Martin C, Amedee T, Mirroneau J. Calcium channel currents in isolated smooth muscle cells from human bronchus. J Appl Physiol 1989; 66:1706–1714.
11. Kotlikoff M. Receptor–effector coupling in smooth muscle. In: Chung KF, Barnes PJ, eds. Pharmacology of the Respiratory Tract. New York: Marcel Dekker, 1993; 27–45.
12. Marthan R, Armour CL, Johnson PRA, Black JL. The calcium channel agonist BAY K8644 enhances the responsiveness of human airway muscle to KCl and histamine, but not to carbachol. Am Rev Respir Dis 1987; 135:185–189.
13. Barnes PJ. Calcium channel blockers in asthma. Thorax 1983; 38:481–485.
14. Löfdahl C-G, Barnes PJ. Calcium channel blockade and asthma—the current position. Eur J Respir Dis 1985; 67:233–237.

15. Grandordy BM, Barnes PJ. Phosphoinositide turnover in airway smooth muscle. Am Rev Respir Dis 1987; 136:S17–S20.

16. Hall I, Chilvers ER. Inositol phosphates and airway smooth muscle. Pulm Pharmacol 1989; 2:113–120.

17. Chilvers ER, Challiss RAJ, Barnes PJ, Nahorski SR. Mass changes of inositol (1,4,5)trisphosphate in trachealis muscle following agonist stimulation. Eur J Pharmacol 1989; 164:587–590.

18. Chilvers ER, Batty IH, Challiss RAJ, Barnes PJ, Nahorski SR. Determination of mass changes in phosphatidyl inositol 4,5-bisphosphate—evidence for agonist-stimulated metabolism of inositol 1,5-trisphosphate in airway smooth muscle. Biochem J 1991; 275:373–379.

19. Chilvers ER, Batty IH, Barnes PJ, Nahorski SR. Formation of inositol polyphosphates in airway smooth muscle after muscarinic receptor stimulation. J Pharmacol Exp Ther 1990; 252:786–791.

20. Krause K-H, Demaurex N, Lew DP. Mechanisms and pharmacology of receptor-mediated Ca^{2+} flux in nonexcitable tissues. In: Chung KF, Barnes PJ, eds. Pharmacology of the Respiratory Tract. New York: Marcel Dekker, 1993; 63–102.

21. Kroegel C, Pleass R, Yukawa T, Chung KF, Westwick J, Barnes PJ. Characterization of platelet-activating factor-induced elevation of cystolic free calcium concentration in eosinophils. FEBS Lett 1989; 243:41–46.

22. Penner R, Neher E. Secretory responses of rat peritoneal mast cells to high intracellular calcium. FEBS Lett 1988; 226:307–313.

23. Boschetto P, Roberts NM, Rogers DF, Barnes PJ. The effect of antiasthma drugs on microvascular leak in guinea pig airways. Am Rev Respir Dis 1989; 139:416–421.

24. Barnes PJ. Clinical studies with calcium antagonists in asthma. Br J Clin Pharmacol 1985; 20:289–298S.

25. Cuss FM, Barnes PJ. The effect of inhaled nifedipine on bronchial reactivity to histamine in man. J Allergy Clin Immunol 1985; 76:718–723.

26. Cook NS. The pharmacology of potassium channels and their therapeutic potential. Trends Pharmacol Sci 1988; 9:21–24.

27. Garcia M, Galvez A, Garcia-Calvo M, King VF, Vazquez J, Kaczorowski GJ. Use of toxins to study potassium channels. J Bioenerg Biomembr 1991; 23:615–646.

28. McCann JD, Welsh MJ. Calcium-activated potassium channels in canine airway smooth muscle. J Physiol (Lond) 1986; 372:113–127.

29. Black JL, Barnes PJ. Potassium channels and airway function: new therapeutic approaches. Thorax 1990; 45:213–218.

30. Kotlikoff MI. Potassium currents in canine airway smooth muscle cells. Am J Physiol 1990; 259:L384–L-395.

31. Jones TR, Charette L, Garcia ML, Kaczorowski GJ. Selective inhibition of relaxation of guinea-pig trachea by charybodotoxin, a potent Ca^{2+}-activated K^+ channel inhibitor. J Pharmacol Exp Ther 1990; 225:697–706.

32. Miura M, Belvisi MG, Stretton CD, Yacoub MH, Barnes PJ. Role of potassium channels in bronchodilator responses in human airways. Am Rev Respir Dis 1992; 146:132–136.

33. Jones TR, Charette L, Garcia ML, Kaczorowski GJ. Interaction of iberiotoxin with β-adrenoceptor agonists and sodium nitroprusside on guinea pig trachea. J Appl Physiol 1993; 74:1879–1884.

34. Kume H, Takai A, Tokuno H, Tomita T. Regulation of Ca^{2+}-dependent K^+-channel activity in tracheal myocytes by phosphorylation. Nature 1989; 341:152–154.

35. Kume H, Graziano MP, Kotlikoff MI. Stimulatory and inhibitory regulation of calcium-activated potassium channels by guanine nucleotide binding proteins. Proc Natl Acad Sci USA 1992; 89:11051–11055.

36. Kume H, Hall IP, Washabau RJ, Taaakagi K, Kotlikoff MI. β-Adrenergic agonists regulate K_{Ca} channels in airway smooth muscle by cAMP-dependent and independent mechanisms. J Clin Invest 1994; 93:371–379.

37. Arch JRS, Buckle DR, Bumstead J, Clarke GD, Taylor JF, Taylor SR. Evaluation of the potassium channel activator cromakalim (BRL 34915) as a bronchodilator in the guinea pig: comparison with nifedipine. Br J Pharmacol 1988; 95:763–770.

38. Black JL, Armour CL, Johnson PRA, Alouan LA, Barnes PJ. The action of a potassium channel activator BRL 38227 (lemakalim) on human airway smooth muscle. Am Rev Respir Dis 1990; 142:1384–1389.

39. Buckle DR, Arch JRS, Bowring NE, et al. Relaxant effects of the potassium channel activators BRL 30227 and pinocidil on guinea-pig and human airway smooth muscle and blockade of their effects by glibenclamide and BRL 31660. Pulm Pharmacol 1993; 6:77–86.

40. Miura M, Belvisi MG, Ward JK, Tadjkarini M, Yacoub MH, Barnes PJ. Bronchodilatory effects of the novel potassium channel opener HOE 234 in human airways in vitro. Br J Clin Pharmacol 1993; 35:318–320.

41. Bowring NE, Arch JRS, Buckle DR, Taylor JF. Comparison of the airways relaxant and hypertensive potencies of the potassium channel activators BRL 55834 and levcromakalin (BRL 38227) in vivo in guinea pigs and rats. Br J Pharmacol 1993; 109:1133–1139.

42. Barnes PJ. Modulation of neurotransmission in airways. Physiol Rev 1992; 72:699–729.

43. Ichinose M, Barnes PJ. A potassium channel activator modulates both noncholinergic and cholinergic neurotransmission in guinea pig airways. J Pharmacol Exp Ther 1990; 252:1207–1212.

44. Burka JF, Berry JL, Foster RW, Small RC, Watt AJ. Effects of cromakalim on neurally-mediated responses of guinea-pig tracheal smooth muscle. Br J Pharmacol 1991; 104:263–269.

45. Stretton CD, Miura M, Belvisi MG, Barnes PJ. Calcium-activated potassium channels mediate prejunctional inhibition of peripheral sensory nerves. Proc Natl Acad Sci USA 1992; 89:1325–1329.

46. Lei Y-H, Barnes PJ, Rogers DF. Inhibition of neurogenic plasma exudation and bronchoconstriction by K^+ channel activator BRL 38227 in guinea pig airways in vivo. Eur J Pharmacol 1993; 239:257–259.

47. Kuo H-P, Rohde JAL, Barnes PJ, Rogers DF. K^+ channel activator inhibition of neurogenic goblet cell secretion in guinea pig trachea. Eur J Pharmacol 1992; 221:385–388.

48. Miura M, Belvisi MG, Stretton CD, Yacoub M, Barnes PJ. The role of K^+ channels in the modulation of cholinergic neural responses in guinea pig and human airways. J Physiol 1992; 455:1–15.

49. Martin CAE, Advenier C. Effects of cromakalim on bradykinin-, histamine- and substance P-induced airway microvascular leakage in the guinea-pig. Eur J Pharmacol 1993; 239:119–126.

50. Labrecque GF, Holowka D, Baird B. Characterization of increased K^+ permeability associated with the stimulation of receptors for immunoglobulin E on rat basophil leukemia cells. J Biol Chem 1991; 266:14912–14917.

51. Yamauchi H, Miura M, Ichinose M, et al. Involvement of aspirin sensitive K^+ channels in antigen-induced spasm of guinea-pig isolated trachea. Br J Pharmacol 1994; 112:958–962.

52. Buckle DR. Prospects for potassium channel activators in the treatment of airways obstruction. Pulm Pharmacol 1993; 6:161–169.

53. Baird A, Hamilton TC, Williams A, et al. Inhibition of histamine-induced bronchoconstriction in healthy volunteers by a potassium channel activator, BRL 34915. Br J Clin Pharmacol 1988; 25:114P.

54. Williams AJ, Lee TH, Cochrane GM, et al. Attenuation of nocturnal asthma by cromakalim. Lancet 1990; 336:334–336.

55. Kidney JC, Fuller RW, Worsdell Y-M, Lavender EA, Chung KF, Barnes PJ. Effect of an oral potassium channel activator BRL 38227 on airway function and responsiveness in asthmatic patients: comparison with oral salbutamol. Thorax 1993; 48:130–134.

56. McManus OB, Harris GH, Giangiacomo KM, et al. An activator of calcium-dependent potassium channels isolated from a medicinal herb. Biochemistry 1993; 32:6128–6133.

57. Butler A, Tsunoda S, McCobb DP, Wei A, Salkoff L. *mSlo*, a complex mouse gene encoding "maxi" calcium-activated potassium channels. Science 1993; 261:221–224.

58. Janssen LJ, Sims SM. Acetylcholine activates non-selective cation and chloride conductances in canine and guinea-pig tracheal smooth muscle cells. J Physiol 1992; 453:197–218.

59. Bianco S, Vaghi A, Robuschi M, Pasargi K, Lian M. Prevention of exercise-induced bronchoconstriction by inhaled frusemide. Lancet 1988; 2:252–255.

60. Bianco S, Pieroni MG, Refini RM, Rottoli L, Siestini P. Protective effect of inhaled furosemide on allergen-induced early and late asthmatic reactions. N Engl J Med 1989; 321:1069–1073.

61. Nichol GM, Alton EWFW, Nix A, Geddes DM, Chung KF, Barnes PJ. Effect of inhaled furosemide on metabisulfite- and methacholine-induced bronchoconstriction and nasal potential difference in asthmatic subjects. Am Rev Respir Dis 1990; 142:576–580.

62. O'Connor BJ, Chung KF, Chen-Wordsell YM, Fuller RW, Barnes PJ. Effect of inhaled furosemide and bumetamide on adenosine 5'-monophosphate and sodium metabisulphite-induced bronchoconstriction. Am Rev Respir Dis 1991; 143:1329–1333.

63. Bianco S, Pieroni MG, Refini RM, Robuschi M, Vaghi A, Sestini P, Inhaled loop diuretics as potential new anti-asthmatic drugs. Eur Respir J 1993; 6:130–134.

64. Chung KF, Barnes PJ. Loop diuretics and asthma. Pulm Pharmacol 1992; 5:1–7.

65. Barnes PJ. Diuretics and asthma. Thorax 1993; 48:195–197.

66. Ventresca GP, Nichol GM, Barnes PJ, Chung KF. Inhaled furosemide inhibits cough induced by low chloride content solutions but not by capsaicin. Am Rev Respir Dis 1990; 142:143–146.

67. Ventresca P, Nichol GM, Barnes PJ, Chung KF. Effect of frusemide on the induction and potentiation of cough induced by $PGF_{2\alpha}$. Br J Clin Pharmacol 1992; 33:514–516.

68. Jackson DM, Norris AA, Eady RP. Nedocromil sodium and sensory nerves in the dog lung. Pulm Pharmacol 1989; 2:179–184.

69. Anderson SD, Wei HE, Temple DM. Inhibition by furosemide of inflammatory mediators from lung fragments (letter). N Engl J Med 1991; 324:131.

70. Perkins RS, Dent G, Chung KF, Barnes PJ. Effects of anion transport inhibitors and extracellular Cl^- concentrations on eosinophil respiratory burst activity. Biochem Pharmacol 1992; 43:2480–2482.

71. Candia OA. Short circuit current related to active transport of chloride in the frog cornea. Biochim Biophys Acta 1973; 298:1011–1014.

72. Jackson DM, Pollard CE, Roberts SM. The effect of nedocromil sodium on the isolated rabbit vagus nerve. Eur J Pharmacol 1992; 221:175–178.

24

Neuropeptides

James N. Baraniuk

Georgetown University, Washington, D.C.

INTRODUCTION

The human respiratory mucosae are complex, dynamic structures designed to protect the nasal, pharyngeal, laryngeal, tracheal, and bronchial airways from injury caused by inhaled factors, microbial colonization, and infection. Sensory, parasympathetic, and sympathetic nerves combine to regulate these protective processes (1–5). These nerves release the classic neurotransmitters and neuropeptides.

Sensory nerves sense the conditions of the mucosal microenvironment. Through synapses with the central nervous system, local parasympathetic ganglia, and local axon response mechanisms, these nerves recruit systemic parasympathetic and sympathetic reflexes, local parasympathetic responses, and local neuropeptide-induced neurogenic inflammation (Fig. 1). Epithelial, vascular, glandular, smooth-muscle, and probably other cell processes are modulated by these integrated neural reflexes (1,2,4–7).

Each population of sensory, parasympathetic, and sympathetic nerves contains a unique combination of classic neurotransmitters (e.g., acetylcholine and norepinephrine) and neuropeptides (Table 1). In a single neuron, depolarization releases the same combination of neurotransmitters from all peripheral (mucosal) and central (CNS) neurosecretory sites (Dale principle; 8,9). Because coreleased peptides and other transmitters may have synergistic, antagonistic, or autoregulatory effects, it may be difficult and misleading to ascribe functions of nerve populations to individual neurotransmitters. Despite these concerns, investigations using exogenous administration of neurotransmitters in vitro and in vivo, and capsaicin to trigger nociceptive sensory nerves, the autoradiographic determination of the receptor distributions for each neurotransmitter, inhibition of neutral endopeptidase, and more recently, the use of specific receptor antagonists, have provided much insight into the functions of each neural system and many of the neurotransmitters.

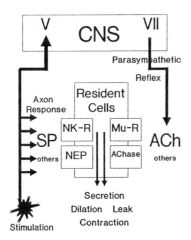

Figure 1 Stimulation of sensory nerve fibers releases SP and other sensory neuropeptides in the periphery that act upon receptors on mucosal resident cells (vessels, glands, epithelium, connective tissue cells) to stimulate acute effects. CNS stimulation by trigeminal fibers recruits parasympathetic neural reflexes that release ACh, VIP, and other peptides that act upon their specific receptors. The actions of neuropeptides and ACh are limited in part by degradation by neutral endopeptidase (NEP) and acetylcholinesterase (AChase), respectively.

These insights predict that neuropeptide antagonists will be of great benefit in treating some respiratory disorders. Their value is foreshadowed by the widespread use of the cholinergic and adrenergic blocking agents that led to the "discovery" of nonadrenergic, noncholinergic (NANC) actions of nerves. Pharmacologically defined NANC actions were once thought to define a new system of nerves; the situation is now known to be much more complex, since the anatomically defined *sensory*, *parasympathetic*, and *sympathetic* neural systems contain heterogenous populations of nerve fibers with often unique combinations of neurotransmitters, and unique functions in tissue-specific locations. Combinations of neuropeptides in nociceptive, parasympathetic, and sympathetic neurons may vary by species, location, and specific nerve function (10).

NOCICEPTIVE SENSORY NERVES

Nasal sensory nerves originate in the trigeminal ganglion and innervate the nose through ethmoidal and posterior nasal nerves (3,6,7). These highly branched neurons innervate vessels, glands, and the epithelium, where they extend between basal cells. Some endings have fine terminal extensions that reach up between epithelial cells to the region of the tight junctions. Nociceptive (pain message) nerves are nonmyelinated bare fibers (type C) that do not have specialized sensory organs. The turbinate, septal, and sinus mucosae do not appear to have other specialized sensory organs, as in the skin or tendons. The olfactory mucosa, which covers the superior portion of the nasal cavity, is innervated by cranial nerve I, which will not be discussed at this time. The nervus terminalis, or cranial nerve XIII also innervates this region (11). In the CNS, trigeminal nociceptive neurons enter the pons through the sensory root, turn caudally in the trigeminal spinal tract to terminate in the pars caudalis of the nucleus of the spinal tract in the lower medulla and upper three cervical segments of the spinal cord (12). Pars caudalis interneurons cross the midline to enter the

Table 1 Neurotransmitters and Additional Peptides

Neurotransmitter peptide	Abbrev.
Trigeminal sensory neurons	
Tachykinins:	
Substance P	SP
Neurokinin A	NKA
Neuropeptide K	
Neurokinin B	NKB
Calcitonin gene-related peptide	CGRP
Gastrin-releasing peptide	GRP
Postganglionic parasympathetic neurons	
Acetylcholine	ACh
Vasoactive intestinal peptide	VIP
Peptide with *histidine* at the NH_2-terminal and *methionine* at the COOH-terminal	PHM
Peptide with *histidine* at the NH_2-terminal and *isoleucine* at the COOH-terminal	PHI
Peptide with *histidine* at the NH_2-terminal and *valine* at the COOH-terminal	PHV
Helodermin	
Postganglionic sympathetic neurons	
Norepinephrine	
Neuropeptide tyrosine (Y)	NPY
Other neuropeptides that may occur in respiratory mucosa	
Galanin	GAL
Atrial natriuretic peptide	ANP
Neurotensin	NT
Enkephalins	ENK
Dynorphin	DYN
Cholecystokinin octapeptide	CCK-8
Pituitary adenylate cyclase-activating peptide	PACAP; PACAP-27
Somatostatin	SOM
Calcitonin	CALC
Endothelin I, II, and III	ET_1, ET_2, ET_3
Proteolytic peptide products from plasma and mucosal proteins	
Bradykinin	BK
Kallidin (lysyl-bradykinin)	Lys-BK
Complement fragments	C3a, C5a

trigeminothalamic tract and terminate in the medial part of the ventral posterior thalamic nucleus (arcuate or semilunar nucleus). Painful and strong thermal stimuli are appreciated at the thalamic level. Tertiary neural relays to the lower third of parietal cortical somesthetic areas provide greater localization of painful stimuli.

The dorsal part of the trigeminal spinal tract includes a small bundle of thermosensitive and nociceptive neurons from the facial, glossopharyngeal, and vagal nerves (12). The glossopharyngeal nerve innervates the posterior third of the tongue, upper pharynx, tonsils, eustachian tube, and middle ear. Glossopharyngeal afferents from the carotid sinus baroreceptors and carotid body chemoceptors assist in the regulation of arterial blood pressure and oxygen tension/ventilatory function, respectively. Vagal afferents with cell bodies in the small superior or nodose vagal ganglia innervate the lower pharynx, epiglottis, larynx (recurrent laryngeal nerve), trachea, main stem and subsegmental bronchi, and esophagus; the vagal auricular branch innervates a portion of the external ear, auditory canal, tympanic membrane, middle ear, and eustachian tube. Central glossopharyngeal and vagal afferents descend in the medullary solitary tract and end in the more caudal part of its nucleus. From these nuclei, interneuronal connections are made with the dorsal motor neurons of the vagus nerve, reticular visceral centers, and subsequently to hypothalamic nuclei. The neurotransmitters of these interneurons are not known. However, substance P (SP) receptors in the ventrolateral medulla regulate ventilatory responses (13), suggesting that tachykinins are candidate neurotransmitters.

Fibers transmitting data for touch from the posterior tongue, pharynx, and larynx may terminate in either the nucleus of the trigeminal spinal tract or the nucleus of the solitary tract. These serve as the afferent limbs of the *gag reflex* (12). The efferent limb of the gag reflex involves activation of the nucleus ambiguus and hypoglossal nucleus and stimulation of the striated muscle of the soft palate, pharynx, larynx, and upper esophagus. The motor division of the accessory nerve innervating these structures could be thought of as a division of the vagal motor nerve, but common convention does not support this contrary view. Connections between the afferent interneurons of the nuclei of the trigeminal spinal tract and the solitary tract with the nucleus ambiguus establish the reflexes for sneezing, coughing, gagging, and vomiting that have critical functions in protecting the integrity and patency of the nasal, pharyngeal, and laryngeal airways. These connections also regulate parasympathetically mediated glandular secretion in the nose (superior salivatory nucleus and facial nerve), and bronchial glandular and smooth-muscle function in trachea and bronchi (dorsal motor nuclei of the vagal nerve). Parasympathetic function is described later.

Two types of nerve fibers mediate nociceptive functions. A_{delta} fibers convey initial sharp pain, which is followed by the delayed transmission of dull, more prolonged pain sensations conveyed by unmyelinated C fibers. The C fibers have bare neural endings that appear to be the most evolutionarily primitive sensory apparatus. These chemosensitive and mechanothermal-sensitive neurons can be stimulated by inflammatory mediators, such as histamine, bradykinin, serotonin, K^+, and H^+ that are released following mucosal injury or mast cell degranulation after allergen exposure (6,14–16). Prostaglandins (PGs) and peptidoleukotrienes (LTs) modulate sensory nerve function by altering the threshold to depolarization, making it easier to stimulate these nerves. Other inhaled agents such as SO_2, O_3, formaldehyde, nicotine, cigarette smoke, and capsaicin can also stimulate these nerves.

Depolarization of the peripheral nociceptive nerve ending generates a wave of depolarization that extends throughout the entire length of the nerve axon and to all the extensively branched rami. The wave of depolarization releases colocalized combinations of neuropeptides from neurosecretory swellings (varicosities) that are found near glands and vessels. The neuropeptides including calcitonin gene-related peptide (CGRP), gastrin-releasing peptide (GRP), the tachykinins substance P (SP) and neurokinin A (NKA), and possibly other, as yet unidentified, neuropeptides (1,3,6,17–19). The varicosities are strung like beads on a string along the extensively branched peripheral sensory nerve. The same combination of neuropeptides is packaged in vesicles in all the varicosities, and released from all the central and peripheral varicosities of a single neuron (Dale principle) (8,9). Sensory neuropeptides act on specific receptors on target cells to initiate and amplify inflammatory responses to mucosal injury. This "axon response" mechanism mediates cutaneous wheal-and-flare reactions (1,2,10) and, in the respiratory tract, initiates and amplifies local mucosal vasodilation, vascular permeability, and glandular exocytosis, and may facilitate vascular wall leukocyte adhesion (19,20). Substance P likely plays a central role in this inflammatory process, since ^{125}I-SP-binding sites are widely distributed (Tables 2 and 3) and SP stimulates many proinflammatory effects in various models in vivo and in vitro (Tables 4 and 5; 21,22). Calcitonin gene-related peptide may be an important long-acting vasodilator and contribute to filling of venous sinusoids (17). Sensory nerve stimulation and central reception of nociceptive nerve impulses in the brain stem and higher centers leads to the appreciation of sensations of itch, burning, and congestion, and the initiation of important central reflexes such as sneeze, cough, and parasympathetic secretory reflexes (7).

Neuropeptide actions are limited by the enzyme neutral endopeptidase (NEP; 23–26). It is thought that all cells bearing peptide receptors also express NEP. Destruction of NEP activity may lead to prolonged, unopposed inflammatory effects of neuropeptides, and may contribute to respiratory hyperresponsiveness that can develop in some inflammatory rhinitic conditions.

PARASYMPATHETIC NERVES

Nociceptive sensory nerve stimulation leads to central recruitment of parasympathetic reflexes. This is possibly the most important function of nociceptive nerves in the human respiratory tract. Parasympathetic efferent connections in the nasal cavity, ethmoid sinuses, and anterior nasopharynx are derived from preganglionic seventh nerve motor fibers from the superior salivary nucleus that synapse in the sphenopalatine ganglion. Vagal efferent fibers originating in the dorsal motor nucleus innervate laryngeal and tracheobronchial parasympathetic ganglia. The brain stem parasympathetic nuclei appear capable of regulating independent nasal, laryngeal, and tracheobronchial efferent responses to irritant stimulation in each respiratory tract location, a response that contrasts with the generalized, all-or-nothing response of the sympathetic nervous system.

Postganglionic fibers innervate glands and some vessels in the nasal, pharyngeal, laryngeal, and tracheobronchial mucosa. Additional glossopharyngeal, vagal, and spinal accessory motor neurons innervate pharyngeal, laryngeal, and upper esophageal striated muscle and participate in the gag reflex that serves to protect the laryngonasal airway and clear obstructions from this critical passage.

Preganglionic parasympathetic nerves release acetylcholine and possibly other neurotransmitters that act on nicotinic receptor–ion channels on postganglionic neurons in airway walls. Postganglionic neurons may act as electrical filters by assessing various stimulatory and inhibitory inputs before being triggered to depolarize. Stimulation of excitatory autoreceptors by substance P or other tachykinins may increase the likelihood of postganglionic cell depolarization (4,5). Stimulation of inhibitory autoreceptors, such as muscarinic M_2, neuropeptide Y (NPY-Yz), γ-aminobutyric acid (GABA$_B$), histamine H_3, α_2- and β_2-adrenergic, and other receptors may decrease postgangionic cell depolarization (Table 6).

Postganglionic parasympathetic secretory neurons release acetylcholine (ACh), vasoactive intestinal peptide (VIP; 27), and other VIP-related peptides (4,5). The cholinergic component of parasympathetic reflexes is a predominant stimulus for mucous secretion in allergic rhinitis and perhaps other respiratory diseases (6,7). Nitric oxide (NO) has been proposed as a postganglionic transmitter, since constitutively expressed nitric oxide synthetase-immunoreactive material has been detected in airway nerves (28), but functional evidence has been mixed (29,30).

Table 2 Radioligand Binding Sites for Various Mediators in Human Nasal Mucosa

	Sensory				Parasympathetic				Sympathetic			Inflammatory		
	SP	NKA	CGRP	GRP	VIP	M_1	M_2	M_3	α	β	NPY	BK	Hist	ET_1
Epithelium	+	0	0	++	+	+	0	+[a]	?	?	0	0	0	0
Serous cells	+	0	0	++	+	+	0	+	?	?	0	0	0	0[b]
Mucous cells	+	0	0	++	+	+	0	+	?	?	0	0	0	0[b]
Vessels														
Resistance (artery, AVA)	+	+	++	0	+	+	0	+	?	?	++	++	+	+
Capacitance (sinusoids)	+	0	±	0	0	+	0	+	?	?	0	++	+	+
Permeable (postcap ven)	+	0	±	0	0	+	0	+	?	?	0	++	+	±

See Table 1 for abbreviations.
?, not reported; 0, not present; ±, weak binding suggesting low density of binding sites; +, binding sites present; ++, dense binding, suggesting high density of binding sites.
[a]M_3 autoradiography results confirmed by in situ hybridization for M_3 receptor mRNA.
[b]Myoepithelial cell-binding sites appear to be present.

Table 3 Radioligand-Binding Sites for Neurotransmitters in Human
Tracheobronchial Mucosa

	Sensory				Parasympathetic					
	SP	NKA	CGRP	GRP	VIP	M_1	M_2	M_3	M_4	M_5
Epithelium	+	?	0	+	+	0	0	+	0	0
Glands	+	?	0	+	+	0	0	+	0	0
Vessels	+	?	+	0	+	0	0	+	0	0
Smooth muscle										
Large a/w	+	+	0	±	+	0	+	+	0	0
Small a/w	+	+	0	?	0	0	+	+	0	0
Alveoli	+	?	+	?	?	+	0	0	0	0

See Table 1 for abbreviations.
?, not reported; 0, not present; ±, weak binding, suggesting low density of binding sites; +, binding
sites present; ++, dense binding, suggesting high density of binding sites.
[a]Muscarinc receptor-binding sites demonstrated by in situ hybridization.

Table 4 Putative Actions of Neurotransmitters

System	Transmitter	Receptor	Actions
Sensory	SP > NKA	NK_1	Arterial dilation, vascular permeability, mucous secretion, leukocyte infiltration
	NKA > SP	NK_2	Bronchoconstriction
	CGRP	CGRP	Arterial dilation
	GRP	GRP	Serous secretion, mucous secretion, tropic factor
Parasympathetic	Acetylcholine	M_1	Glandular secretion
		M_2	Inhibitory autoreceptor
		M_3	Glandular secretion, vasodilation, smooth-muscle contraction
		M_4	?
		M_5	?
	VIP	VIP	Arterial dilation, gland secretion
	Nitric oxide?	Guanylate cyclase	Bronchodilation, vasodilation
Sympathetic	Norepinephrine	α_1, α_2	Vasoconstriction
	Epinephrine[a]	$\beta_2 > \beta_2$	Bronchodilate, vasodilate
	NPY	Y_1	Postsynaptic receptors stimulate vasoconstriction
		Y_2	Presynaptic receptors inhibit neurotransmitter release

[a]Adrenal origin.

Table 5 Major Mucosal Functions That Are Regulated by Neural Pathways

Airflow resistance	
Determined by:	Smooth-muscle contraction
	Acetylcholine (M_3)
	Sensory (NKA, SP)
	Smooth-muscle relaxation
	NO?, VIP?, prostaglandins?
	β_2-Adrenergic stimuli
	Nasal mucosal thickness (sinusoidal filling)

	Vasodilation:	Sensory (SP, CGRP)
		Parasympathetic (acetylcholine, VIP)
	Vasoconstriction:	Sympathetic (norepinephrine, NPY)

Vascular permeability	
Plasma extravasation:	Sensory (SP)
Vasoconstriction:	Sympathetic (noradrenaline, NPY)
Glandular secretion of antimicrobial defense factors, mucins, and other products	
Exocytosis and Expulsion:	Sensory (SP, GRP)
	Parasympathetic (muscarinic M_3, possibly M_1, VIP)
	Sympathetic (α-adrenergic)

At least five muscarinic receptor genes (m1 to m5) have been cloned (31,32). However, since there are partially selective pharmacological ligands for only three receptors (M_1 to M_3; 33), it is not known with certainty which of these receptor subtypes mediates acetylcholine's actions in vivo. In addition, the kinetic binding affinities of cloned receptors expressed in cell lines does not correlate with the apparent pharmacological subtypes of receptors found in vivo and in vitro (34). Initial evidence implicates the M_3 receptor as the preeminent functional subtype on cells in human nasal and bronchial mucosa (33,35). Sensory nerve stimulation and parasympathetic reflexes likely contribute to the pathology of inflammatory conditions, such as allergic rhinitis, vasomotor rhinitis, infectious rhinitis

Table 6 Putative Autoreceptor Functions of Various Mediators on Neural Depolarization

Depolarize neurons	Enhance depolarization	Inhibit depolarization
Thermal stimuli	Prostaglandins	μ-Opioid
Mechanical stimuli	Leukotrienes	β_2-Adrenergic
Capsaicin (ruthenium red-sensitive)	Substance P	α_2-Adrenergic
Bradykinin (B_2) and electrical field		NPY
stimulation (ω-conotoxin-sensitive)		5-HT_3
(voltage-gated Ca^{2+} channel)		$GABA_B$
H^+, K^+		M_2-muscarinic
SO_2, O_3		
Histamine (H_1)		
Serotonin (5-HT)		
PAF		
Peroxides, free radicals, TDI		
Neurotensin, CCK_8, $GABA_A$		
IL-1, IL-8?		

(common cold), chronic bronchitis, asthma, and infectious bronchitis. Anticholinergics and muscarinic mechanisms are discussed in depth elsewhere in this text.

SYMPATHETIC NERVES

Sympathetic reflexes have been poorly studied, yet probably play a crucial role in the normal homeostasis of nasal mucosa and the responses to exercise and other stresses that require a patent nasal and bronchial airway (36,37). Preganglionic sympathetic nerve fibers originate in the intermediolateral cell column of thoracic spinal segments (12). Those destined to regulate respiratory vascular functions in the head synapse with postganglionic cells in the superior cervical ganglion, whereas those regulating thoracic functions synapse predominantly in the superior, middle, and lower cervical ganglia and in the upper five thoracic ganglia. Sympathetic reflexes induce vasoconstriction in respiratory mucosa and may stimulate some glandular secretion in the trachea and bronchi. In the lower respiratory tract, sympathetic neural reflexes do not appear to contribute to bronchodilation. Adrenal release of epinephrine may be of greater significance in bronchospasm.

Sympathetic nerves contain either norepinephrine or norepinephrine plus neuropeptide Y (NPY; 37–39). Both are potent vasoconstrictors. Agonists of α_1- and α_2-adrenergic receptors are popular "nasal decongestants" that effectively reduce mucosal thickness in vivo, whereas β_2-adrenergic agonists are the mainstay of bronchodilator therapy. The adrenergic system is discussed elsewhere in this text.

TACHYKININS

Stimulation of nociceptive sensory nerves leads to the release of the tachykinins SP and neurokinin A (NKA), as well as the release of CGRP and probably GRP.

Substance P and NKA are the products of the preprotachykinin A (or *PPT-I*) gene (19,40,41). The *PPT-I* gene contains seven exons: SP is coded by exon 3 and NKA by exon 6. *PPT-I* generates three distinct mRNAs: α-*PPT-I* lacks exon 6 and codes for SP alone; β-*PPT-I* contains all the exons and codes for both NKA and SP; whereas γ-*PPT-I* mRNA excludes exon 4 and codes for SP, NKA, and neuropeptide-γ. Nerve growth factor and noxious stimuli may up-regulate *PPT-I* transcription, whereas glucocorticoids may down-regulate transcription (41–44). In rats, the δ-*PPT* gene codes for a theoretical, novel tachykinin called NP-δ (45). Neurokinin B is produced from the *PPT-II* gene, but has not yet been described in peripheral mammalian tissue (41).

Three tachykinin receptors, NK_1, NK_2, and NK_3, have been cloned (46–49): SP is the preferred ligand for NK_1 receptors; NKA is the preferred ligand for NK_2 receptors; and NKB binds preferentially to NK_3 receptors. Pharmacological data suggest that there may be additional SP receptors and that there may be additional subtypes of NKA-preferring receptors (50,51). Each of the three receptors stimulates phosphoinositol (PI) metabolism when activated.

Tachykinin receptors belong to the seven-transmembrane region, rhodopsin-like receptor gene superfamily (Fig. 2; 52). These proteins have a glycosylated extracellular NH_2-terminal, seven transmembrane regions, three extracellular loops, three intracellular loops, and an intracellular COOH-tail. The transmembrane regions stack parallel to each other in the membrane. Specific amino acid side chains of the extracellular domains and upper portions of the transmembrane regions form the ligand-binding pocket and determine the specificity and avidity of ligand binding. The third intracellular loop binds to specific

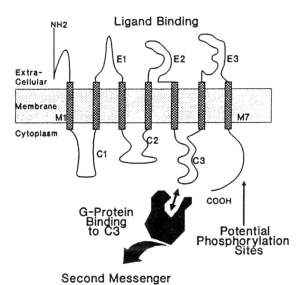

Figure 2 Prototypic G-protein-related receptor showing extracellular amino terminal, three extracellular loops (E1, E2, and E3), seven transmembrane helical regions (M1 to M7), three intracellular loops (C1, C2, and C3), and the intracellular carboxy terminal. Binding of receptor-specific G-proteins is determined by ligand binding with consequent conformational changes of C3, and phosphorylation of the C-terminal region.

G-proteins that are stimulated when the ligand binds the receptor and transduce that signal into the cytoplasm (53). The COOH-tails contain phosphorylation sites that regulate the binding of G-proteins, and thus the activity of the receptor. Phosphorylation of this tail after receptor binding may be one mechanism of receptor tachyphylaxis.

Over 100 structurally and evolutionarily related G-protein–associated receptors have been cloned, including α- and β-adrenergic, dopamine, serotonin, histamine, bradykinin, GRP, NPY, atrial natriuretic peptide (ANP), cholecystokinin (CCK) and IL-8 receptors. The nature of the G-proteins associated with each receptor is under intense scrutiny, but is beyond the scope of this review (54).

The distribution of NK_1-receptors has been suggested by autoradiographic studies of ^{125}I-SP-binding sites. ^{125}I-SP binds to epithelium, vessels, glands, and smooth muscle in the upper and lower respiratory tracts (21,22). This distribution is consistent with the known ability of SP to induce vasodilation, vascular permeability, glandular secretion, and tracheobronchial smooth-muscle contraction in vivo and in vitro (1,2,4,5,21,55). Substance P nasal provocation apparently has minimal effects in normal subjects, but induces albumin secretion and obstructs nasal airflow in allergic rhinitis subjects (56,57). Responses appear to be greater in subjects with established inflammatory syndromes, such as allergic rhinitis or asthma, suggesting that neurogenic inflammatory mechanisms play a role in these diseases or airway hyperresponsiveness. The effects of neutral endopeptidase on tachykinins and neurogenic inflammation are discussed later.

Substance P induces serous and mucous glandular secretion from human nasal mucosal explants in vitro (21). In pig nasal mucosa, SP increases nasal blood flow and the thickness of the mucosa (58). The SP-immunoreactive material can be collected in nasal lavage fluid (59) and bronchoalveolar lavage (BAL) fluid (60) from allergic subjects after allergen challenge, suggesting that SP is released during this process. It is most likely that nociceptive nerves are the source of this SP, although other sources, such as inflammatory cells, have been suggested in the past (61).

The SP-induced vasodilation and plasma extravasation could be due to stimulation of endothelial cell nitric oxide (NO) production (62). SP can stimulate endothelial cell proliferation in vitro (63).

Neurokinin A is probably the dominant tachykinin inducing bronchoconstriction in human airways (51,64), although SP may have activity in some other species (4,5). This action is mediated by NK_2 receptors. Tachykinin-induced bronchoconstriction may play a role in the maturation of neural responses in the developing airway (65).

Capsaicin, the hot spicy essence of chili peppers (66), specifically stimulates and depolarizes nociceptive sensory nerves and induces the sensation of burning pain. Capsaicin has proved invaluable for the investigation of these nerves (1,2,66). It has been used to estimate the magnitude of the axon response in pig nasal mucosa (58) and stimulates an increase in nasal blood flow and mucosal volume. This effect is ablated by ganglionic blocking drugs, indicating that the recruited parasympathetic reflexes mediate most of the vascular reaction induced by capsaicin. When higher doses of capsaicin are combined with ganglionic blockade, then the axon response can be detected as a small increase in superficial blood flow (58). This indicates that, in higher animals, the axon response mechanism exists, but that the major effect of sensory nerve stimulation is recruitment of parasympathetic nerves. The effects of axon responses on glandular secretion are suggested, but have not been definitively shown. Evaluation of the precise role of SP and other neuropeptides in the axon response and in respiratory inflammation will require the use of SP-specific antagonists (64,67–69). The magnitude of tracheobronchial axon responses in humans in vivo continues to be a subject of debate.

In guinea pigs, CP 96345 markedly inhibits substance P-induced decreases in pulmonary resistance (R_L) and blood pressure, but has no effect in allergen-induced bronchial changes, suggesting that substance P has no role in the acute allergen-induced bronchoconstriction (70). FK-888 is also effective against SP- and capsaicin-induced plasma extravasation in vivo and against bronchial smooth-muscle contraction in vitro (71).

Cigarette smoke has been used to stimulate neurogenic inflammation, with plasma extravasation and goblet cell exocytosis, in guinea pig and rat trachea in vivo. These effects are antagonized by the tripeptide SP antagonists FR 113680 and FK 224, implicating SP in cigarette smoke-induced neurogenic inflammation (72). Dry gas hyperpnea in guinea pigs induces bronchoconstriction that can be blocked by NK_1 antagonists, indicating that irritant-induced neurogenic inflammation can lead to bronchoconstriction in vivo (73). Nociceptive sensory neuropeptides appear capable of stimulating bronchoconstriction in vivo, but this neurogenic effect is a minor component of allergen-induced bronchoconstriction (74), in which mast cell-derived mediators are of much greater importance.

Effects of tachykinins and other neuropeptides on immune responses and inflammatory cells have been suggested. The SP antagonist spantide reduced cutaneous inflammation induced by tuberculin (delayed-type hypersensitivity) and benzoic acid-induced contact urticaria, but not inflammation induced by benzalkonium chloride (irritant delayed reaction) or UV_B irradiation (75). Substance P and NKA may modulate human B-lymphocyte maturation (76). These immunological changes are discussed in greater detail elsewhere in this text.

The specificity of the SP binding to NK_1 receptors appears to reside in the positively charged NH_2-terminal region of the peptide and interactions with the second and third extracellular loops of the receptor. Cross-reactivity between tachykinin peptides is likely to be determined by the shared COOH-terminal regions, whereas specificity is determined by the vastly different peptide NH_2-terminal regions. An epitope near the sixth transmembrane region may be critical for SP or NKA binding (77). Interactions with residue 290 of the seventh transmembrane region account for differences in rat and human receptor binding (78).

The molecular actions of tachykinin antagonists (Table 7; 69,79) have been elegantly demonstrated by kinetic-binding studies using chimeric receptors and the nonpeptide anatagonist CP 96345 (77,80). CP 96345 appears to bind to His-197 of the NK_1 receptor, located at the junction of the second-extracytoplasmic loop and the extracellular side of the fifth transmembranous region. This amino acid does not appear to be necessary for SP binding to the receptor, or for the activation of associated G-proteins. Binding of CP 96345 to His-197 and surrounding moieties appears to fill the "well" that is formed between the seven transmembranous loops of the receptor, and prohibits SP "docking" into that well. By blocking access, CP-96345 denies SP the opportunity to interact with its receptor and activate its associated G-protein. These antagonist actions of CP-96345 are probably prototypic of other receptor antagonists (81). However, CP-96345 and its nonantagonistic stereoisomer have calcium channel antagonist properties that may also cause effects in experimental systems. Hence, both stereoisomers should be tested to ensure NK_1 receptor specificity.

Modification of these antagonist compounds is very likely to lead to the development of receptor subtype-specific antagonists, which will be of great use for defining pharmacological events, and which will likely be useful as very specific treatments for neurotransmitter-mediated conditions. The explosion in the number of nonpeptide receptor agonists and antagonists (see Table 7) is in stark contrast to recent opinions that the complexity of the peptide-binding sites could demand unique peptide derivatives that could be difficult and expensive to produce, and be subject to proteolysis. The lipophilicity of the nonpeptide antagonist compounds suggests that they may readily pass through the blood–brain barrier and be active in the CNS. These drugs may unlock many of the mysteries of the human

Table 7 Tachykinin Agonist and Antagonist Drugs

	NK_1	NK_2	NK_3
Agonists	[Sar^9]SP	[βALA^8]NKA(4–10)	Senktide
	GR 73632		
Antagonists	CP 96345	GR 100679	GR 138676
	CP 99994	L-659,877	R487
	FK224	MEN 10,208	
	FK888	MEN 10,207	
	L-668,169	MEN 10,282	
	R454	MEN 10,376	
	R455	R396	
	RP 67580	SR 48968	
	SR 140333		

psyche, the actions of peripheral and central nerves, neurotransmitters, and other inflammatory mediators that bind to the seven-transmembrane-type receptors.

Currently available drugs may have tachykinin antagonist properties, including imipramine (82), dactinomycin (actinomycin-D; 83), lithium (84), and cromolyn sodium (sodium cromoglycate; 85). New classes of tachykinin antagonists are being rapidly discovered, including the indole–anthranilic acid derivatives fiscalin A, B, and C (86), anthrotainin (87), FK224 (88), pyrrolomycin (89), RP 67580 (90), and heterosteroids (91). Potent NK_2-receptor antagonists have also been discovered (64,92), suggesting that receptor antagonists to many other G-protein–related receptors will in time be characterized and available for investigation and therapy.

In addition to interactions with NK_1 receptors and possible cross-reactivity on NK_2 receptors, some of SP's remarkable effects may be mediated by nonspecific biophysical interactions with membranes or membrane components (93). The substance P NH_2 terminal is strongly anionic, whereas its tail is hydrophobic. The NH_2-terminal may interact with membrane phospholipids by binding to cationic phosphate groups through hydrostatic forces, whereas the hydrophobic COOH-terminal tail inserts itself between membrane lipids. This unique interaction may explain some of SP's profuse phenomenology.

These data suggest that SP released from nociceptive sensory nerves may induce vasodilation, vascular permeability, and glandular secretion in respiratory mucosa, but that tachykinin effects may be more prominent during inflammation. Neurokinin A released from the same neurons may be more potent than SP for induction of bronchoconstriction. The most important effects of tachykinins may be their actions on interneurons in the brain stem, spinal cord, and local parasympathetic ganglia that lead to the recruitment of systemic and parasympathetic reflexes and the supratentorial appreciation of pain.

CALCITONIN GENE-RELATED PEPTIDE

Calcitonin gene-related peptide is 37-amino acid residues long, and is produced in two forms: CGRP-I (CGRP-α, A-CGRP), and CGRP-II (CGRP-β, B-CGRP) which differ by three amino acids. Both forms are vasodilators. CGRP is produced by alternative processing from the same genes as calcitonin (94).

Calcitonin gene-related peptide is the predominant gene product in neural tissue, and either or both forms may be produced. It is also produced in tracheobronchial neuroendocrine cells (95). In the fetal human, CGRP is present in trigeminal ganglion cells, either alone or colocalized with SP. The percentage of ganglion cells staining for CGRP or SP reaches adult levels in the immediate preterm period (95). The roles of these neurons during development of the airways are unknown. Recently, CGRP has been reported to be present in rat stomach lamina propria mononuclear cells (96) and in rat tracheal epithelial serous cells (97). It has not been reported in human respiratory epithelial cells other than neuroendocrine cells. The functions of nonneural CGRP is open to speculation.

In the adult human nasal mucosa, CGRP-containing nerve fibers densely innervate arterial vessels, but also innervate venous vessels, some gland acini, and extend into the epithelium (3,17). CGRP appears to be colocalized with SP in tracheobronchial nerves (4,5). The binding sites for ^{125}I-CGRP are concentrated on arterioles in nasal and bronchial mucosa (17,98). These distributions of CGRP nerve fibers and binding sites are consistent with the physiological role of CGRP as a long-acting and potent arterial vasodilator (99,100).

The CGRP receptor genes have not been characterized as yet, but two, or possibly three, receptor subtypes that are linked to G_s and stimulate adenylate cyclase have been suggested by pharmacological studies using the $CGRP_1$-selective agonist CGRP[8-37], the $CGRP_2$-selective agonist [Cys(acetamidomethyl)^{2,7}]-hCGRPα, and amylin, a CGRP-like peptide with about 50% sequence homology to CGRP-α and CGRP-β (101). Studies of CGRP receptor subtypes may prove difficult, since CGRP and CGRP-related peptides may also interact with tachykinin and CCK receptors. Further pharmacological studies and receptor cloning are required to evaluate these possibilities.

Nasal provocation by CGRP has been attempted (102,103). Topically applied CGRP had no effects on protein secretion, although this peptide could have some difficulty gaining entry to the region of its receptors deep in the mucosa, or could be degraded by proteases. CGRP could still play a role in vivo, since it can synergistically interact with other vasomotor agents to increase the blood flow (99,100,104). CGRP agonists may have some usefulness as arterial dilators, whereas its antagonists could act as decongestants of CGRP-induced arterial dilation.

The CGRP-binding sites have not been found on glandular cells (17). In short-term explant cultures of human nasal mucosa, CGRP failed to stimulate release of mucus (17). Although CGRP immunoreactive nerve fibers are present in gland acini, the release of CGRP from nerves in glands probably does not lead to exocytosis, since there are no CGRP-binding sites on those cells. In contrast, CGRP stimulated nasal glandular secretion from guinea pig nasal mucosa (105), indicating that there are significant differences in the responses to peptides in different species, and that conclusions drawn from animal experiments may not be representative or extrapolated to human conditions.

Calcitonin gene-related peptide may play a valuable role as a potent, long-lasting vasodilator in the treatment of congestive heart failure (106–108), cardiac arrhythmias (109,110), Raynaud's disease (111), erectile dysfunction (112,113), and salvage of traumatic tissue flaps with compromised blood supply (114).

GASTRIN-RELEASING PEPTIDE

Gastrin-releasing peptide (GRP) is a 27-amino acid peptide that shares sequence homology with GRP_{10} (GRP[18-27] or neuromedin C), and bombesin (14-amino acid amphibian peptide) (115). Related peptides include porcine neuromedin B (NMB) and NMB_{10}, ranatensin, litorin, and phyllolitorin. Mammalian and amphibian GRP and NMB are derived from genes having three exons, whereas it is thought that amphibian bombesin, ranatensin, and phyllolitorin are derived from genes with only a single exon. Mammalian bombesin, ranatensin, and phyllolitorins have not yet been identified.

The GRP–bombesin peptides share a common aminidated heptapeptide COOH-terminal sequence (WAVGHLM-NH$_2$) that is the active part of the peptide (115–117). Bombesin-immunoreactive peptides are expressed by normal human bronchial epithelial lung neuroendocrine cells (118) and can be detected in bronchoalveolar lavage fluids (119). Bombesin-reactive antiserum recognizes GRP, GRP_{10}, bombesin, and possibly other peptides as well.

The GRP gene transcripts are processed differently in endocrine and neural tissues (120,121), suggesting that mRNA splicing may contribute to the diversity of bombesin-immunoreactive peptides. Three prepro-GRP mRNAs have been identified that code for a NH$_2$-terminal signal peptide, GRP_{27}, and a COOH-terminal extension peptide, CTEP. Each of the three mRNAs codes for a different CTEP. Functions for the signal peptides and CTEPs have not been determined. Gastrin-releasing peptide and related peptides are NEP substrates; some of the "diversity" of peptides detected by high-performance liquid chromatography (HPLC) may represent proteolytic digestion in vivo.

The GRP and NMB receptor subtypes have been cloned from human cell lines: GRP receptors (122,123) preferentially bind GRP, neuromedin C, and bombesin, whereas NMB receptors (124) prefer neuromedin B and bombesin over GRP. The distributions of each receptor subtype in normal respiratory mucosa have not been determined. Since these receptors may play autocrine, tropic roles in small cell carcinoma in vitro (115), it is possible that GRP has tropic properties in respiratory mucosa in vivo.

In human nasal mucosa, GRP nerve fibers are present in the walls of arterial and venous vessels, and around glandular acini (18). Their distribution is very similar to that of CGRP and NKA (3,17,18,21) and suggests, but does not prove, that GRP is colocalized in the same trigeminal sensory neurons. The ^{125}I-GRP-binding sites are localized to the epithelium and submucosal glands of human nasal and tracheal mucosa (see Tables 2 and 3; 18). In vitro, GRP induces both serous and mucous cell exocytosis from human nasal mucosa (18,125). In vivo, bombesin stimulates mucous glycoconjugate and lysozyme secretion from human nasal mucosa, but does not stimulate albumin secretion (126), suggesting an effect on submucosal (and possibly goblet cell) secretion without increases in vascular permeability. The COOH-terminal region is essential for function, since GRP, bombesin, and GRP[20-27] stimulate secretion in human nasal and feline tracheal mucosa in vitro and guinea pig nasal mucosa in vivo, while GRP[1-16], an NH_2-terminal fragment, is inactive (18,117,127). Bombesin is a bronchoconstrictor in guinea pig tracheal smooth muscle in vitro and in vivo (128).

The GRP-containing neuroendocrine cells are rare in normal, nonsmoking humans adults, but are as much as ten times more common in cigarette smokers and in hamsters exposed to cigarette smoke (115,119,129). GRP, NMB, and their receptors are present in small-cell carcinomas and cell lines derived from these tumors, and are proliferation factors for these cells. GRP and related peptides may also stimulate proliferation of nonneoplastic cells in inflammatory conditions, such as asthma and bronchopulmonary dysplasia, suggesting that autocrine release of GRP may play a role in many bronchial disorders.

These varied effects suggest that GRP may be released from trigeminal sensory nerves and bronchial neuroendocrine cells, and may act as a serous and mucous cell secretogue, bronchoconstrictor, and potential growth factor in human respiratory mucosa.

NEUTRAL ENDOPEPTIDASE

The actions of neuropeptides are limited by their degradation by neutral endopeptidase EC 3.4.24.11 (NEP; 23–26), with contributions by other enzymes (angiotensin-converting enzyme, aminopeptidase M, carboxypeptidase N, or others) in some systems (24,130). NEP is active on SP, NKA, CGRP, GRP, bombesin, enkephalins, endothelin, atrial natiuretic peptide (ANP), bradykinin, and many other peptides. Neutral endopeptidase is postulated to be present on all cells that possess peptide receptors (24–26; Fig. 3).

The NEP gene of 24 exons codes for a 749-amino acid–long membrane-bound protein (131,132). Alternative mRNA splicing generates several different-sized mRNAs including one with a deletion of exon 16 that yields a nonfunctional protein (133), and a hypothetical product with a deletion of exons 5 through 18 (134).

The inhibition of NEP enzyme activity with phosphoramidon or thiorphan augments many peptide-induced effects, including epithelial cell ciliary-beat frequency, goblet cell secretion, mucous secretion from ferret and feline tracheas, airway microvascular leak

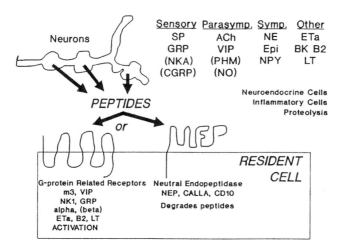

Figure 3 Peptides released from sensory, parasympathetic, or sympathetic neurons, or inflammatory or neuroendocrine cells, may activate resident cell surface receptors or be degraded by neutral endopeptidase (NEP).

induced by tachykinins, bradykinin, depolarization of the vagal nerve, electrical field stimulation, and capsaicin and neutrophil adhesion to the endothelial surface of vessels (19,20,23–26,135). These functional data indicate that NEP activity is present on epithelial, glandular, vascular, and smooth-muscle cells. The distributions of NEP-immunoreactive material and mRNA are consistent with these activities. In situ hybridization of NEP mRNA and immunohistochemistry of NEP-immunoreactive material have revealed NEP in epithelium, glands, and vessels of human nasal mucosa (136,137), as well as tracheo-bronchial smooth-muscle cells (138). These cells are innervated by neuropeptide-containing nerves and possess neuropeptide-binding sites (see Tables 2 and 3). These data are consistent with the hypothesis that NEP is present in all cells that bear neuropeptide receptors, and that NEP plays a role in regulating neuropeptide-mediated responses.

Neutral endopeptidase may have many diverse functions in vivo; jejunal mucosal NEP may digest peptides (139). A limited amount of longitudinal and circular intestinal muscle also expresses NEP mRNA, but vessels in the lamina propria and ganglion cells have been negative. Renal proximal tubule brush border contains abundant NEP that may degrade urinary filtrate peptides so that their amino acids can be absorbed. NEP may also help regulate renal blood flow by actions on atrial natriuretic peptide, renin, bradykinin, or other vasoactive peptides. It may play a role in vascular remodeling in rats exposed to chronic hypoxia (140) and regulate other vascular events through actions on arterial and venous endothelial cells (141). The enzyme may play a regulatory role in the developing human fetal lung, since it is expressed at the growing front of airway epithelium (142).

There has been intense speculation over the role of NEP in neurogenic inflammation (see Fig. 1). Inhibition of neutral endopeptidase potentiates inflammation and bronchial smooth-muscle contraction induced by SP, capsaicin, and vagal nerve stimulation, suggesting that tachykinins or other NEP substrate peptides can cause neurogenic inflammation and that their effects are regulated by NEP (143,144). Decreases in NEP activity may underlie the increased responses of respiratory mucosa to neurogenic inflammation and to some agonists (hyperresponsiveness) found during and after viral and mycoplasmal infections (137,145,146), and after exposure to cigarette smoke (147), ozone (148), and hypochlorous acid (149,150). The release of peptides into areas with reduced NEP activity could lead to enhanced peptide-induced epithelial cell function, glandular secretion, vascular permeability, and smooth-muscle contraction. Cell surface NEP activity may also be modulated by rapid internalization and proteolytic degradation, as occurs in human neutrophils that are activated by phorbol ester or diacylglycerol (151). Although alterations of NEP activity or expression in human diseases have yet to be demonstrated in vivo, inhalation of thiorphan, an NEP inhibitor, permits inhaled NKA to exert a mild bronchoconstrictor effect in nonasthmatic subjects who otherwise do not respond to inhaled NKA (152). This suggests that tonic peptide and NEP activities exist in the normal airway, and that the balance between the two influences can be altered to produce bronchoconstriction in an otherwise normal airway.

Glucocorticoid treatment, on the other hand, increases NEP mRNA and enzymatic activity in a cultured, SV-40-transformed human epithelial cell line (153) and Calu-1 cells (human lung epidermoid carcinoma cell line; 150). This enhancement of NEP expression may explain the beneficial effects of glucocorticoids on neurogenic plasma extravasation in virus-infected rat trachea (135,146). Glucocorticoid treatment also alters the size of NEP mRNA transcripts (153), suggesting complex regulation at the level of mRNA transcription or pretranslational processing. Expression of NEP by lung fibroblasts in culture can be increased by incubation with cytokines, such as IL-1α, tumor necrosis factor (TNF)-α, transforming growth factor (TGF), IL-6, and GM-CSF (154). Cyclic nucleotide and prostaglandin-dependent mechanisms may mediate these effects. These cytokines may play a role in the induction of NEP in perivascular cells of synovial vessels from rheumatoid arthritis and osteoarthritis patients (155). Synovium from normal joints demonstrates no immunohistochemical staining, indicating that some aspect of the disease state can induce NEP immunoreactivity. Induction or suppression of NEP would be expected to alter the responses of cells to other peptides and could represent a very efficient method of autoregulation (156). These studies indicate that glucocorticoids and cytokines can modulate transcription or posttranscription processing (157) of NEP expression and neurogenic inflammation in some cells, models, and diseases. Although these investigations of NEP and its complex regulation continue to direct speculations concerning the significance of neurogenic inflammation in human disease, there is still a need to measure actual NEP activities in vivo in human tissues to clearly define whether NEP or its absence plays any significant pathogenic role in human disease.

VASOACTIVE INTESTINAL PEPTIDE

Vasoactive intestinal peptide (VIP) is colocalized with acetylcholine in parasympathetic neurons in the bronchi and nose (3,4,5,27,158,159). It may also be present in some subsets of sensory nerves (160). The VIP gene complex has been cloned and demonstrates that posttranslational modification of prepro-VIP (161) yields VIP plus PHM (*p*olypeptide with *h*istidine at the NH$_2$-terminal and *m*ethionine at the COOH-terminal). PHM is the human form of PHI (*i*soleucine at the COOH-terminal) which was previously described in porcine neural tissues (162). Other VIP-like peptides have also been described including PHV (*p*eptide with *h*istidine at the NH$_2$-terminal and *V*aline at the COOH-terminal), helodermin, helospectin, pituitary adenylate cyclase-activating peptide (PACAP and PACAP-27), extendin-3, growth hormone-releasing factor, and secretin (4,5). These peptides share sequence homology, may interact with VIP receptors, and have similar vasodilatory, bronchodilatory, and secretomotor effects. Separate VIP-preferring (163,164) and secretin-preferring (165) receptors have been cloned, and it is likely that additional PACAP and extendin-3 receptors will also be discovered. In general, VIP and these related peptides are thought to stimulate adenylate cyclase to increase cAMP levels through receptor-mediated activation of G_s. Vasoactive intestinal peptide is a neutral endopeptidase substrate (166).

Standard autoradiographic receptor localization studies with ^{125}I-VIP have identified VIP-binding sites on nasal epithelium, glands, and vessels (see Tables 2 and 3; 27). In the lung, VIP-binding sites are found on epithelium, submucosal glands, vessels, and smooth muscle of large airways (167). The VIP receptor density appears to decrease as airways become smaller. This may be related to a decrease in the parasympathetic innervation in these smaller bronchi. Some VIP-binding sites are also present on alveolar cells, but their functions and the alveolar source of VIP in vivo are unclear.

Vasoactive intestinal peptide has been touted as a major NANC bronchodilator, that is, a bronchodilating neurotransmitter released after vagal nerve stimulation in the presence of adrenergic and cholinergic blockade, but this contention is controversial (29,30). As will be discussed elsewhere in this text, it is likely that nitric oxide (NO) released from parasympathetic or other nerve populations or stimulated end-organs that express the constitutive NO-synthetase have more potent bronchodilating effects (30).

Both resistance and capacitance vessels in nasal mucosa are dilated by VIP (168). In vitro, VIP stimulates serous cell exocytosis of lactoferrin and mucin-immunoreactive material from human nasal mucosal explants (125). Acetylcholine and VIP did not have additive effects in this system. VIP increases mucous secretion from cat trachea (169) and epithelial cell secretion in dog and ferret trachea (170). In contrast, VIP may inhibit mucous secretion from human bronchial explants (171,172). Anti-VIP antibodies may play a pathological role in some cases of chronic bronchitis (173).

In vivo, VIP may be more active as a vasodilator than as a secretagogue, since atropine blocks essentially all gland secretion, but only partially blocks neurogenically induced blood flow (58,168,174,175). Effective VIP antagonists will be required to determine the relative importance of acetylcholine and VIP in parasympathetically mediated secretion.

Increased immunohistochemical staining of VIP-immunoreactive material has been reported in vasomotor rhinitis (176). Increased glandular secretion and vasodilation may contribute to chronic vascular congestion and hypersecretion. An absence of VIP immunoreactive nerve fibers has been reported in cystic fibrosis (177), which could contribute to a decrease in VIP-induced serous cell secretion and formation of thick, mucoid secretions.

The rate of nerve depolarization may vary the amounts of acetylcholine, VIP, and PHM released from parasympathetic nerves (178). At low rates, ACh is released, whereas at high rates, ACh plus VIP are released. VIP may augment the postsynaptic acetylcholine-induced secretory response in glands (e.g., cat salivary glands; 174), but may also have presynaptic inhibitory effects that act to limit neuropeptide release. This mechanism would conserve the amount of stored peptide, since there are no reuptake mechanisms, and peptides can be resupplied only by axonal transport from the neural cell body. Pharmacological regulation of nasal parasympathetic nerve function by these autoreceptors has not yet been reported in humans. Evaluation of the full range of VIP-related effects will result from the use of peptide and nonpeptide VIP antagonists (79). The VIP agonists may be developed as clinically useful vasodilating agents. They would be of value in asthma only if peptidase-resistant agonists were found that could be effectively inhaled or injected, if their effects were synergistic with β_2-adrenergic agonist bronchodilator drugs, and if hypotension did not limit their effective dose. Treatment of hypertension is an alternative application.

Localization of VIP with SP in human eosinophils (179), and rat basophilic leukemia cells (a model mast cell; 180) is discussed elsewhere in this text.

NEUROPEPTIDE Y

Neuropeptide tyrosine (neuropeptide Y; NPY) is present with norepinephrine in a population of sympathetic neurons (3,37,38,181). This peptide has many of the same actions as norepinephrine (182). The NPY-induced vasoconstriction is slower in onset, but longer in duration, than that of norepinephrine. The walls of arterioles and arteriovenous anastomoses are very densely innervated by NPY nerve fibers (3,37). They intercalate between smooth-muscle cells and individual fibers are also located in venous vessels; a few are present in glandular acini.

In addition to VIP plus acetylcholine fibers, pigs also possess a small population of NPY plus VIP nerve fibers that originate in the sphenopalatine ganglia and innervate glands (39). They may represent a separate population of parasympathetic fibers; their function is unknown. This finding makes it difficult to be dogmatic about the localization of specific neuropeptides in specific neural systems. Furthermore, it indicates that there may be great species-to-species and organ-to-organ variability both in the distributions and functions of autonomic and sensory nerves and their neuropeptides. The functions of colocalized neuropeptides, such as NPY plus VIP, are difficult to predict, since complex synergistic and antagonistic interactions can occur when mixtures of peptides are released (99,100, 102,104,183).

The ^{125}I-NPY-binding sites have been localized by autoradiography on the smooth muscle of arterioles and the arteriolar portion of arteriovenous anastomoses, with less dense representation on the adjacent venous portions (37). There is a strong correlation among the locations of NPY nerve fibers, NPY-binding sites on vessels, and the vasoconstrictor function of this peptide. Exogenous administration of NPY to the human nasal mucosa in vivo reduces nasal airflow resistance and albumin exudation, without stimulating submucosal gland secretion (184), suggesting that NPY agonists may be useful for the treatment of mucosal diseases characterized by vasodilation, vascular permeability, and plasma exudation. Because NPY is a long-acting vasoconstrictor, its agonists may offer advantages over α-agonists for the treatment of chronic vascular congestion. Further study on the mechanisms of NPY's effects, its effects in vivo, and the development of appropriate peptides for therapy are required before NPY agonists replace α-adrenergic agonists.

Subtypes of NPY receptor have been suggested. Postsynaptic Y_1 receptors may be linked to phosphatidylinositol hydrolysis (185,186) and may potentiate the postjunctional effects of norepinephrine (38). Prejunctional Y_2 receptors are coupled to adenylate cyclase inhibition (185). Prejunctional Y_2 receptors on sympathetic nerves may inhibit norepinephrine release and serve to prevent depletion of these neurotransmitters (38). NPY inhibits cholinergic transmission in guinea pig trachea by a direct effect upon NPY receptors on postganglionic cholinergic nerves or other unresolved presynaptic sites (187). An analogous effect on sensory nerves has been suggested for opiates (188). The roles of autoreceptors in nasal mucosal nerves have not been investigated. The diversity and distributions of NPY receptors and their different relative affinities for NPY fragments (38) suggest that it may be possible to selectively design NPY analogue peptides that bind to peripheral vascular NPY receptors and perform as potent, long-acting vasoconstricting agents (189). However, NPY is a substrate for neutral endopeptidase in human nasal mucosa (37) and so NPY peptide and nonpeptide analogues that are relatively resistant to proteolytic degradation may be required for therapeutic use.

SUMMARY

Sensory nerves detect the conditions of inspired air and respond to inhaled noxious agents and mucosal injury. Different forms of insults may generate a wide variety of mediators including H^+, K^+, prostaglandins, leukotrienes, bradykinin, and histamine that may stimulate or modulate nociceptive sensory nerves by acting on specific receptors, ion channels, or other macromolecules in nerves. These mediators may also act directly on vessels to induce vascular permeability and venous sinusoidal filling. Release of sensory neuropeptides, such as SP, NKA, CGRP, GRP, and others, causes the local axon response. The magnitude of the axon response may be subtle in large animals, as demonstrated by the modest increase in superficial blood flow found in the pig (58), and be less potent than the effects found in rodent airways (20).

The most important effects of sensory nerve stimulation in the nose are the recruitment of parasympathetic and other central reflexes, and the induction of the sensation of pain. These lead to sneezing and other avoidance behaviors that attempt to rapidly clear the upper airway of offending agents while protecting the lower airways. Parasympathetic reflexes cause rapid and copious secretion of submucosal gland mucus, and vasodilation which increases nasal airflow resistance (see Tables 4 and 5). Muscarinic M_3, and possibly M_1, receptors most likely mediate glandular secretion. The sensory nerve–parasympathetic reflex arc is of paramount importance in the normal nose and contributes significantly to the pathology of allergic, infectious, and other nonallergic rhinitis. Thus, nociceptive sensory nerves and the recruitment of parasympathetic reflexes are potent proinflammatory mechanisms in the nasal mucosa. Nociceptive sensory nerve stimulation in the tracheobronchial tree may induce bronchospasm, vasodilation, vascular permeability, and glandular secretion, and contribute to the hyperresponsiveness characteristic of asthma and rhinitis. However, in allergen-induced bronchoconstriction, this neural component has only a minor contribution, compared with the overwhelming effects of mast cell mediators (74). The sympathetic nervous system acts to reduce mucosal blood flow, sinusoidal filling, and mucosal thickness, and so induces restoration of nasal airflow and nasal patency. Short-acting norepinephrine and long-acting NPY are potent vasoconstrictors. Loss of sympathetic influences may contribute to some chronic, nonallergic rhinopathies.

Neutral endopeptidase may also act in an anti-inflammatory fashion by degrading neuropeptides and so limiting the duration of their actions in vivo. Destruction or down-regulation of NEP may contribute to the hyperresponsiveness of this mucosa that can occur after infection or exposure to cigarette smoke or other toxic gases. Restoration of NEP activity may be a beneficial effect of glucocorticoid use.

As has been shown, sensory, parasympathetic, and sympathetic nerves play key, coordinated roles in respiratory homeostasis, and in pathological situations. Drugs based on neurotransmitters, such as the α- and β-adrenergic agonists and anticholinergic agents, have been among the most successful medications marketed. Further investigations with neuropeptide analogues, such as substance P antagonists, will reveal more information about the roles of these nerves and their neurotransmitters in health and disease.

ACKNOWLEDGMENTS

Dr. Baraniuk has been awarded the Edward Livingston Trudeau Scholar Award by the American Lung Association, and is a Tobacco Council for Research Scholar.

REFERENCES

1. Lundblad L. Protective reflexes and vascular effects in the nasal mucosa elicited by activation of capsaicin-sensitive substance P-immunoreactive trigeminal neurons. Acta Physiol Scand Suppl 1984; 529:1–42.
2. Hua XY. Tachykinins and calcitonin gene related peptide in relation to peripheral functions of capsaicin-sensitive sensory nerves. Acta Physiol Scand Suppl 1986; 551:1–45.
3. Uddman R, Sundler F. Innervation of the upper airways. Clin Chest Med 1986; 7:201–209.
4. Barnes PJ, Baraniuk JN, Belvisi MG. Neuropeptides in the respiratory tract. Part 1. Am Rev Respir Dis 1991; 144:1187–1198.
5. Barnes PJ, Baraniuk JN, Belvisi MG. Neuropeptides in the respiratory tract. Part 2. Am Rev Respir Dis 1991; 144:1391–1399.
6. Baraniuk JN. Neural control of human nasal secretion. Pulm Pharmacol 1991; 4:20–31.
7. Raphael GR, Baraniuk JN, Kaliner MA. How and why the nose runs. J Allergy Clin Immunol 1991; 87:457–467.
8. Dale HH. Pharmacology and nerve endings. Proc R Soc Med 1935; 68:319–324.
9. Eccles JC. Chemical transmission and Dale's principle. Prog Brain Res 1986; 68:3014–3020.
10. Baraniuk JN, Kowalski M, Kaliner M. Neuropeptides in the skin. In: Bos JB, ed. Skin Immune System (SIS). Baton Rouge, LA: CRC Press, 1990:307–326.
11. Demski LS, Schwanzel-Fukuda M, eds. The terminal nerve (nervus terminalis). Ann NY Acad Sci 1987; 519:1–213.
12. Barr ML. The Human Nervous System. 2nd ed. Hagerstown, MD: Harper & Row, 1974.
13. Chen Z, Hedner J, Hedner T. Local effects of substance P on respiratory regulation in the rat medulla oblongata. J Appl Physiol 1990; 68:693–699.
14. Baraniuk JN, Lundgren JD, Goff J, Gawin AZ, Mizuguchi H, Peden D, Merida M, Shelhamer JH, Kaliner MA. Bradykinin receptor distribution in human nasal mucosa, and analysis of in vitro secretory responses in vitro and in vivo. Am Rev Respir Dis 1990; 141:706–714.
15. Martins MA, Shore SA, Drazen JM. Release of tachykinins by histamine, methacholine, PAF, LTD$_4$, and substance P from guinea pig lungs. Am J Physiol 1991; 261:L449–L455.
16. Raphael GD, Igarashi Y, White MV, Kaliner MA. The pathophysiology of rhinitis. V. Sources of protein in allergen-induced nasal secretions. J Allergy Clin Immunol 1991; 88:33–43.
17. Baraniuk JN, Lundgren JD, Goff J, Mullol M, Castellino S, Merida M, Shelhamer JH, Kaliner MA. Calcitonin gene related peptide (CGRP) in human nasal mucosa. Am J Physiol 1990; 258:L81–L88.
18. Baraniuk JN, Lundgren JD, Goff J, Peden D, Merida M, Shelhamer J, Kaliner MA. Gastrin releasing peptide (GRP) in human nasal mucosa. J Clin Invest 1990; 85:998–1005.
19. Holzer P. Local effector functions of capsaicin-sensitive sensory nerve endings: involvement of tachykinins, calcitonin gene related peptide and other neuropeptides. Neuroscience 1988; 24:739–768.
20. McDonald DM. Neurogenic inflammation in the rat trachea. I. Changes in venules, leukocytes and epithelial cells. J Neurocytol 1988; 17:605–628.
21. Baraniuk JN, Lundgren JD, Okayama M, Goff J, Mullol M, Merida M, Shelhamer JH, Kaliner MA. Substance P and neurokinin A (NKA) in human nasal mucosa. Am J Respir Cell Mol Biol 1991; 4:228–236.
22. Carstairs JR, Barnes PJ. Autoradiographic mapping of substance P receptors in lung. Eur J Pharmacol 1988; 127:295–296.

23. Nadel JA. Decreased neutral endopeptidases: possible role in inflammatory diseases of airways. Lung 1990; 123(suppl):123–127.
24. Nadel JA. Membrane-bound peptidases: endocrine, paracrine, and autocrine effects. Am J Respir Cell Mol Biol 1992; 7:469–470.
25. Borson DB. Roles of neutral endopeptidase in airways. Am J Physiol 1991; 260:L212–L225.
26. Roques BP, Noble F, Dauge V, Fournie-Zaluski MC, Beaumont A. Neutral endopeptidase 24.11: structure, inhibition, and experimental and clinical pharmacology. Pharmacol Rev 1993; 45: 87–146.
27. Baraniuk JN, Okayama M, Lundgren JD, Mullol M, Merida M, Shelhamer JH, Kaliner MA. Vasoactive intestinal peptide (VIP) in human nasal mucosa. J Clin Invest 1990; 86:825–831.
28. Kobzik L, Bredt DS, Lowenstein CJ, Drazen J, Gaston B, Sugarbaker D, Stamler JS. Nitric oxide synthetase in human and rat lung: immunocytochemical and histochemical localization. Am J Respir Cell Mol Biol 1993; 9:371–377.
29. Watson N, MacIagan J, Barnes PJ. Vagal control of guinea pig tracheal smooth muscle—lack of involvement of VIP or nitric oxide. J Appl Physiol 1993; 74:1964–1971.
30. Fisher JT, Anderson JW, Waldron MA. Nonadrenergic noncholinergic neurotransmitter of feline trachealis: VIP or nitric oxide? J Appl Physiol 1993; 74:31–39.
31. Barnes PJ. Muscarinic receptor subtypes: implications for lung disease. Thorax 1989; 44: 161–167.
32. Levine RR, Birdsall NJM, North RA, Holman M, Watanabe A, Iversen LL. Subtypes of muscarinic receptors III. Trends Pharmacol Sci 1991; 9(suppl):1–93.
33. Mak JCW, Barnes PJ. Autoradiographic visualization of muscarinic receptor subtypes in human and guinea pig lung. Am Rev Respir Dis 1990; 141:1559–1568.
34. Dorje F, Wess J, Lambrecht G, Tacke R, Mutschler E, Brann MR. Antagonist binding profiles of five cloned human muscarinic receptor subtypes. J Pharmacol Exp Ther 1991; 256: 727–733.
35. Okayama M, Baraniuk JN, Merida M, Kaliner MA. Autoradiographic localization of muscarinic receptor subtypes in human nasal mucosa. Am J Respir Cell Mol Biol 1993; 8:176–185.
36. Richerson HB, Seebohm PB. Nasal airway response to exercise. J Allergy 1968; 41:269–284.
37. Baraniuk JN, Castellino S, Goff J, et al. Neuropeptide Y (NPY) in human nasal mucosa. Am J Respir Cell Mol Biol 1990; 3:165–173.
38. Potter EK. Neuropeptide Y as an autonomic neurotransmitter. Pharmacol Ther 1988; 37: 251–273.
39. Lacroix JS, Anggard A, Hokfelt T, O'Hare MM, Fahrenkrug J, Lundberg JM. Neuropeptide Y: presence in sympathetic and parasympathetic innervation of the nasal mucosa. Cell Tissue Res 1990; 259:119–128.
40. Nakanishi S. Substance P precursor and kininogen: their structures, gene organizations, and regulation. Physiol Rev 1987; 67:1117–1142.
41. Helke CJ, Drause JE, Mantyh PW, Couture R, Bannon MJ. Diversity in mammalian tachykinin peptidergic neurons: multiple peptides, receptors, and regulatory mechanisms. FASEB J 1990; 4:1606–1615.
42. Lindsay RM, Lockett C, Sternberg J, Winter J. Substance P and calcitonin gene related peptide levels are regulated by nerve growth factor. Neuroscience 1989; 33:53–65.
43. MacLean DB, Bennett B, Morris M, Wheeler FB. Differential regulation of calcitonin gene related peptide an substance P in cultured neonatal rat vagal sensory neurons. Brain Res 1989; 478:349–355.
44. Kageyama R, Sasai Y, Nakanishi S. Molecular cloning of transcription factors that bind to the cAMP responsive region of the SP precursor gene: cDNA of a novel c/EBP-related factor. J Biol Chem 1991; 266:15525–15531.
45. Harmar AJ, Hyde V, Chapman C. Identification and cDNA of delta-preprotachykinin, a fourth splicing variant of the rat substance P precursor. FEBS Lett 1990; 275:22–24.

46. Yokata Y, Sasai S, Tanaka K, Fujiwara T, Tsuchida K, Shigemoto R, Nakanishi S. Molecular characterization of a functional cDNA for rat substance P receptor. J Biol Chem 264:17649–17652.

47. Gerard NP, Eddy RL, Shows TB, Gerard C. The human neurokinin A (substance K) receptor. Molecular cloning of the gene, chromosome localization, and isolation of cDNA from tracheal and gastric tissues. J Biol Chem 1990; 265:20455–20462.

48. Ohkubo H, Nakanishi S. Molecular characterization of the three tachykinin receptors. Ann NY Acad Sci 1991; 632:53–62.

49. Takahashi K, Tanaka A, Hara M, Nakanishi S. The primary structure and gene organization of human substance P and neuromedin K receptors. Eur J Biochem 1992; 204:1025–1033.

50. Petitet F, Saffroy M, Torrens Y, Lavielle S, Chassaing G, Loeuillet D, Glowinski J, Beaujouans JC. Possible existence of a new tachykinin receptor subtype in the guinea pig ileum. Peptides 1992; 13:383–398.

51. Astolfi M, Meini S, Treggiari S, Maggi CA, Manzini S. Characteristics of the NK-2 receptor which mediates the motor response to tachykinins in humans isolated bronchus. Neuropeptides 1993; 24:198–199A.

52. Venter JC, Di Porzio U, Robinson DA, Shreeve SM, Lai J, Kerlavage AR, Fracek SP Jr, Lentes KU, Fraser CM. Evolution of neurotransmitter receptor systems. Prog Neurobiol 1988; 30:105–169.

53. Boyd ND, MacDonald SG, Kage R, Luber-Narod J, Leeman SE. Substance P receptor: biochemical characterization and interactions with G proteins. Ann NY Acad Sci 1991; 632:79–93.

54. Birnbaumer L, Brown AM. G proteins and the mechanisms of action of hormones, neurotransmitters, and autocrine and paracrine regulatory factors. Am Rev Respir Dis 1990; 141:S106–S114.

55. Solway J, Leff AR. Sensory neuropeptides and airway function. J Appl Physiol 1991; 71:2077–2087.

56. Devillier P, Dessanges JF, Rakatosihanaka J, Ghaem A, Boushey HA, Lockhart H. Nasal response to substance P and methacholine in subjects with and without allergic rhinitis. Eur Respir J 1988; 1:356–361.

57. Braunstein G, Fajac I, Lacronique J, Frossard N. Clinical and inflammatory responses to exogenous tachykinins in allergic rhinitis. Am Rev Respir Dis 1991; 144:630–636.

58. Stjarne P, Lacroix JS, Anggard A, Lundberg JM. Compartment analysis of vascular effects of neuropeptides and capsaicin in the pig nasal mucosa. Acta Physiol Scand 1991; 141:335–342.

59. Mosimann BL, White MV, Hohman RJ, Goldrich MS, Kaulbach HC, Kaliner MA. Substance P, calcitonin gene related peptide, and vasoactive intestinal peptide increase in nasal secretions after allergen challenge in atopic patients. J Allergy Clin Immunol 1993; 92:95–104.

60. Nieber K, Baumgartern CR, Rathsack R, Furkert J, Oehme P, Kunkel G. Substance P and β-endorphin-like immunoreactivity in lavage fluids of subjects with and without allergic asthma. J Allergy Clin Immunol 1992; 90:646–652.

61. Payan GP, Levine JD, Goetzl EJ. Modulation of immunity and hypersensitivity by sensory neuropeptides. J Immunol 1984; 132:1601.

62. Busija DW, Chen J. Effects of trigeminal neurotransmitters on piglet pial arterioles. J Dev Physiol 1992; 18:67–72.

63. Ziche M, Morbidelli L, Pacini M, Geppetti P, Alessandri G, Maggi CA. Substance P stimulates neovascularization in vivo and proliferation of cultured endothelial cells. Microvasc Res 1990; 40:264–278.

64. Advenier C, Naline E, Toty L, Bakdach H, Emons-Alt X, Vilain P, Breliere JC, le Fur G. Effects on the isolated human bronchus of SR 48968, a potent and selective nonpeptide antagonist of neurokinin A (NK$_2$) receptors. Am Rev Respir Dis 1992; 146:1177–1181.

65. Tanaka DT, Grunstein MM. Maturation of neuromodulatory effect of substance P in rabbit airways. J Clin Invest 1990; 85:345–350.

66. Holzer P. Capsaicin: cellular targets, mechanisms of action, and selectivity for thin sensory neurons. Pharmacol Rev 1991; 43:143–201.
67. Maggi CA, Patacchini R, Astolfi M, Rovero P, Guilliani S, Giachetti A. NK$_2$-receptor agonists and antagonists. Ann NY Acad Sci 1991; 632:184–190.
68. Regoli D, Nantel F, Tousidgnant C, Jukic D, Rouissy N, Rhaleb E. Neurokinin agonists and antagonists. Ann NY Acad Sci 1991; 632:170–183.
69. Watling KJ. Nonpeptide antagonists herald new era in tachykinin research. Trends Pharmacol Sci 1992; 13:266–269.
70. Sakamoto T, Barnes PJ, Chung KF. Effect of CP-96,345, a non-peptide NK$_1$ receptor antagonist, against substance-, bradykinin-, and allergen-induced airway microvascular leakage and bronchoconstriction in the guinea pig. Eur J Pharmacol 1993; 231:31–38.
71. Murai M, Maeda Y, Hagiwara D, Miyaka H, Ikari N, Matsuo M, Fujii T. Effects of an NK$_1$ receptor antagonist, FK888, on constriction and plasma extravasation induced in guinea pig airway by neurokinins and capsaicin. Eur J Pharmacol 1993; 236:7–13.
72. Morimoto H, Yamishita M, Matsuda A, Miyake H, Fujii T. Effects of FR113680 and FK 224, novel tachykinin receptor antagonists, on cigarette smoke-induced rat tracheal plasma extravasation. Eur J Pharmacol 1992; 224:1–5.
73. Solway J, Koa BM, Jordan JE, Gitter B, Rodger IW, Howbert JJ, Alger LE, Necheles J, Leff AR, Garland A. Tachykinin receptor antagonists inhibit hyperpnea-induced bronchoconstriction in guinea pigs. J Clin Invest 1993; 92:315–323.
74. Didier A, Kowalski ML, Jay J, Kaliner MA. Neurogenic inflammation, vascular permeability, and mast cells. Capsaicin desensitization fails to influence IgE–anti-DNP-induced vascular permeability in rat airways. Am Rev Respir Dis 1990; 141:398–406.
75. Wallengren J. Substance P antagonist inhibits immediate and delayed type cutaneous hypersensitivity reactions. Br J Dermatol 1991; 124:324–328.
76. Laurenzi MA, Persson MA, Dalsgaard CJ, Ringd'en O. Stimulation of human B lymphocyte differentiation by the neuropeptides substance P and neurokinin A. Scand J Immunol 1989; 30:695–701.
77. Gether U, Yokata Y, Emonds-Alt X, Brell'ere JC, Lowe JC III, Snider RM, Nakanishi S, Schwartz TW. Two nonpeptide tachykinin antagonists act through epitopes on corresponding segments of the NK$_1$ and NK$_2$ receptors. Proc Natl Acad Sci USA 1993; 90:6194–6198.
78. Sachais BS, Snider RM, Lowe JA III, Krause JE. Molecular basis for the species selectivity of the substance P antagonist CP 96,345. J Biol Chem 1993; 268:2319–2323.
79. Presti ME, Gardner JD. Receptor antagonists for gastrointestinal peptides. Am J Physiol 1993; 264:G399–G406.
80. Fong TM, Cascieri MA, Yu H, Banasal A, Swain C, Strader CD. Amino–aromatic interaction between histidine 197 of the neurokinin-1 receptor and CP 96345. Nature 1993; 362:350–353.
81. Beinborn M, Lee YM, McBride EW, Quinn SM, Kopin AS. A single amino acid of the cholecystokinin-B/gastrin receptor determines specificity for nonpeptide antagonists. Nature 1993; 362:348–350.
82. Iwashita T, Shimizu T. Imipramine inhibits intrathecal substance P-induced behavior and blocks spinal substance P receptors in mice. Brain Res 1992; 581:59–66.
83. Fujii T, Murai M, Morimoto H, Nishikawa M, Kiyotoh S. Effects of actinomycin-D on airway constriction induced by tachykinins and capsaicin in guinea pigs. Eur J Pharmacol 1991; 194:183–188.
84. Vincent MB. Lithium inhibits substance P and vasoactive intestinal peptide-induced relaxations on isolated porcine ophthalmic artery. Headache 1992; 32:335–337.
85. Crossman DC, Dashwood MR, Taylor GW, Wellings R, Fuller RW. Sodium cromoglycate: evidence of tachykinin antagonist activity in the human skin. J Appl Physiol 1993; 75:167–172.
86. Wong SM, Musza LL, Kydd GC, Kullnig R, Gillum AM, Cooper R. Fiscalins: new substance P inhibitors produced by the fungus *Neosartorya fischeri*. Taxonomy, fermentation, structures, and biological properties. J Antibiot 1993; 46:545–553.

87. Wong SM, Kullnig R, Dedinas J, Appell KC, Kydd GC, Gillum AM, Cooper R, Moore R. Anthrotainin, an inhibitor of substance P binding produced by *Gliocladium catenulatum*. J Antibiot 1993; 46:214–221.

88. Hashimoto M, Hayashi K, Murai M, Fujii T, Nishikawa M, Kiyoto S, Okuhara M, Kohsaka M, Imanaka H. WS9326A, a novel tachykinin antagonist isolated from *Streptomyces violaceus-niger* no. 9326. II. Biological and pharmacological properties of WS9326A and tetrahydro-WS9326A (FK224). J Antiobiot 1992; 45:1064–1070.

89. Masuda K, Suzuki K, Ishida-Okawara A, Mizuno S, Hotta K, Miyadoh S, Hara G, Koyama M. Pyrrolomycin group antibiotics inhibit substance P-induced release of myeloperoxidase from human polymorphonuclear granulocytes. J Antiobiot 1991; 44:533–540.

90. Garret C, Carruette A, Fardin V, Moussaoui S, Peyronel JF, Blanchard JC, Laduron PM. Pharmacological properties of a potent and selective nonpeptide substance P antagonist. Proc Natl Acad Sci USA 1991; 88:10208–10212.

91. Venepalli BR, Aimone LD, Appell KC, et al. Synthesis and substance P receptor binding activity of androstanol[3,2-*b*]pyrimido[1,2-a]benzimidazoles. J Med Chem 1992; 35:374–378.

92. Emonds-Alt X, Golliot F, Pointeau P, Le Fur G, Brelioere JC. Characterization of the binding sites of [^{3}H]SR 48968, a potent nonpeptide radioligand antagonist of the neurokinin-2 receptor. Biochem Biophys Res Commun 1993; 191:1172–1177.

93. Reptke H, Bienert M. Structural requirements for mast cell triggering by substance P-like peptides. Agents Actions 1988; 23:207–210.

94. Steenbergh PH, Hoppener JW, Zandberg Q, Visser A, Lips CJ, Jansz HS. Structure and expression of the human calcitonin/CGRP genes. FEBS Lett 1986; 209:97–103.

95. Springall DR, Collins G, Barer G, Suggett AJ, Bee D, Polak JM. Increased intracellular levels of calcitonin gene related peptide-like immunoreactivity in pulmonary endocrine cells of hypoxic rats. J Pathol 1988; 155:259–267.

96. Jakab G, Webster H deF, Salamon I, Mezey E. Neural and nonneural origin of calcitonin gene related peptide (CGRP) in the gastric mucosa. Neuropeptides 1993; 24:117–122.

97. Baluk P, Nadel JA, McDonald DM. Calcitonin gene related peptide in secretory granules of serous cells in the rat tracheal epithelium. Am J Respir Cell Mol Biol 1993; 8:446–453.

98. Mak JCW, Barnes PJ. Autoradiographic localization of calcitonin gene related peptide (CGRP) binding sites in human and guinea pig lung. Peptides 1988; 9:957–963.

99. Gamse R, Saria A. Potentiation of tachykinin induced plasma protein extravasation by calcitonin gene related peptide. Eur J Pharmacol 1985; 114:61–66.

100. Brain SD, Williams TJ. Inflammatory oedema induced by synergism between calcitonin gene-related peptide (CGRP) and mediators of increased vascular permeability. Br J Pharmacol 1985; 86:855–861.

101. Chin SY, Hall JM, Brain SD, Morton IKM. Do amylin and CGRP interact with similar receptors in the perfused rat isolated kidneys? Neuropeptides 1993; 24:207.

102. Geppetti P, Fusco BM, Marabini S, Maggi CA, Faniullacci M, Sicuteri F. Secretion, pain and sneezing induced by the application of capsaicin to the nasal mucosa in man. Br J Pharmacol 1988; 93:509–514.

103. Guarnaccia S, Baraniuk JN, Bellanti J, Duina M. Calcitonin gene related peptide (CGRP) nasal provocation in humans. Ann Allergy 1993;

104. Brain SD, Williams TJ. Substance P regulates the vasodilator activity of calcitonin gene related peptide. Nature 1988; 335:73–75.

105. Gawin A, Baraniuk JN, Kaliner M. Effects of substance P and calcitonin gene related peptide (CGRP) on guinea pig nasal mucosal secretion in vivo. Acta Otolaryngol (Stockh) 1993; In press.

106. Shekhar YC, Anand IS, Sarma R, Ferrari R, Wahl PL, Poole-Wilson PA. Effects of prolonged infusion of human α-calcitonin gene-related peptide on hemodynamics, renal blood flow and hormone levels in congestive heart failure. Am J Cardiol 1991; 67:732–736.

107. Gennari C, Nami R, Agnusdei D, Fischer JA. Improved cardiac performance with human

calcitonin gene related peptide in patients with congestive heart failure. Cardiovasc Res 1990; 24:239–241.

108. Stevenson RN, Roberts RH, Timmins AD. Calcitonin gene related peptide: a hemodynamic study of a novel vasodilator in patients with severe chronic heart failure. Int J Cardiol 1992; 37:407–414.

109. Zhang JF, Lui J, Lui XZ. Stabilization of cardiac rhythm in subsequently life-threatening ventricular tachycardia and fibrillation by calcitonin gene related peptide. Int J Cardiol 1992; 34:101–103.

110. Zhang JF, Lui J, Lui XZ, Sheng SL, Zhang WJ, Chen YJ. The effect of calcitonin gene related peptide on arrhythmia caused by adenosine diphosphate and desacetyldigilanide-C in rats. Int J Cardiol 1991; 33:43–46.

111. Shawket S, Dickerson C, Hazleman B, Brown MJ. Prolonged effect of CGRP in Raynaud's patients: a double-blind randomized comparison with prostacyclin. Br J Clin Pharmacol 1991; 32:209–213.

112. Djamilian M, Stief CG, Kuczyk M, Jonas U. Follow-up results of a combination of calcitonin gene related peptide and prostaglandin E_1 in the treatment of erectile dysfunction. J Urol 1993; 149:1296–1298.

113. Steif CG, Wetterauer U, Schaebsdau FH, Jonas U. Calcitonin gene related peptide: a possible role in human penile erection and its therapeutic application in impotent patients. J Urol 1991; 146:1010–1014.

114. Jernbeck J, Dalsgaard CJ. Calcitonin gene related peptide treatment of flaps with compromised circulation in humans. Plast Reconstr Surg 1993; 91:236–244.

115. Sunday ME, Kaplan LM, Motoyama E, Chin WW, Spindel ER. Gastrin releasing peptide (mammalian bombesin) gene expression in health and disease. Lab Invest 1988; 59:5–24.

116. Willey JC, Lechner JF, Harris CC. Bombesin and the C-terminal tetradecapeptide of gastrin releasing peptide are growth factors for normal human bronchial epithelial cells. Exp Cell Res 1984; 153:245–248.

117. Lundgren J, Ostrowski N, Baraniuk JN, Shelhamer JH, Kaliner M. Gastrin releasing peptide stimulates glycoconjugate release from feline tracheal explants. Am J Physiol 1990; 258: L68–L74.

118. Tsutsumi Y. Immunohistochemical localization of gastrin releasing peptide in normal and diseased human lung. Ann NY Acad Sci 1988; 547:336–350.

119. Aguayo SM, Kane MA, King TE Jr, Schwartz MI, Grauer L, Miller YE. Increased levels of bombesin-like peptides in the lower respiratory tract of asymptomatic cigarette smokers. J Clin Invest 1989; 84:1105–1113.

120. Spindel ER, Zilberberg MD, Chin WW. Analysis of the gene and multiple messenger ribonucleic acids (mRNAs) encoding human gastrin releasing peptide: alternate RNA splicing occurs in neural and endocrine tissue. Mol Endocrinol 1987; 1:224–230.

121. Spindel ER, Sunday ME, Hofler H. Transient elevation of mRNAs encoding gastrin releasing peptide (GRP), a putative pulmonary growth factor, in human fetal lung. J Clin Invest 1987; 80:1172–1177.

122. Battey JF, Way JM, Corjay MH, Shapira H, Kusano K, Harkins R, Wu JM, Slattery T, Mann E, Feldman RI. Molecular cloning of the bombesin/gastrin releasing peptide receptor from Swiss 3T3 cells. Proc Natl Acad Sci USA 1991; 88:395–399.

123. Corjay MH, Dobrzanski DJ, Way JM, Viallet J, Shapira H, Worland P, Sausville EA, Battey JF. Two distinct bombesin receptor subtypes are expressed and functional in human lung carcinoma cells. J Biol Chem 1991; 266:18771–18779.

124. Wada E, Way J, Shapira H, Kusano K, Lebacqu-Verheyden AM, Coy DH, Jensen RT, Battey J. cDNA cloing, characterization and brain region-specific expression of a neuromedin-B-preferring bombesin receptor. Neuron 1991; 6:421–430.

125. Mullol J, Rieves RD, Lundgren JD, Baraniuk JN, Mérida M, Hausfeld JH, Shelhamer JH,

Kaliner MA. The effects of neuropeptides on mucous glycoprotein secretion from human nasal mucosa in vitro. Neuropeptides 1992; 21:231–238.

126. Baraniuk JN, Silver PB, Lundgren JD, Cole P, Kaliner MA, Barnes PJ. Bombesin stimulates mucous cell and serous cell secretion in human nasal provocation tests. Am J Physiol 1992; 262:L48–L52.

127. Gawin A, Baraniuk JN, Kaliner MA. The effects of gastrin releasing peptide (GRP) and analogues on guinea pig nasal mucosa. Am Rev Respir Dis 1990; 141:A173.

128. Belvisi MG, Stretton CD, Barnes PJ. Bombesin-induced bronchoconstriction in the guinea pig: mode of action. J Pharmacol Exp Ther 1991; 255:36–41.

129. Moody TW. Bombesin-like peptides in the normal and malignant lung. In: Becker KL, Gazdar AF, eds. The Endocrine Lung in Health and Disease. Philadelphia: WB Saunders, 1984:328–336.

130. Desmazes N, Lockhart A, Lacroix A, Dusser DJ. Carboxypeptidase M-like enzyme modulates the noncholinergic bronchoconstrictor response in guinea pig. Am J Respir Cell Mol Biol 1992; 7:477–484.

131. Shipp MA, Richardson NE, Sayre PH, Brown NR, Masteller EL, Clayton LK. Molecular cloning of the common acute lymphoblastic leukemia antigen (CALLA) identifies a type of type II integral membrane protein. Proc Natl Acad Sci USA 1988; 85:4819–4823.

132. D'Adamio L, Shipp MA, Masteller EL, Reinherz EL. Organization of the gene encoding common acute lymphoblastic leukemia antigen (neutral endopeptidase 24.11): multiple mini-exons and separate 5′ untranslated regions. Proc Natl Acad Sci USA 1989; 86:7103–7107.

133. Iijima H, Gerard NP, Squassoni C, Ewig J, Face D, Drazen JM. Exon 16 del: a novel form of human neutral endopeptidase (CALLA). Am J Physiol 1992; 262:L725–L729.

134. Llorens-Cortes C, Giros B, Schwartz JC. A novel potential metallopeptidase derived from the enkephalinase gene by alternate splicing. J Neurochem 1990; 55:2146–2148.

135. Piedemonte G, McDonald DM, Nadel JA. Glucocorticoids inhibit neurogenic plasma extravasation and prevent virus-potentiated extravasation in the rat trachea. J Clin Invest 1990; 86:1409–1415.

136. Baraniuk JN, Ohkubo K, Kwon OJ, Mak J, Rohde J, Durham SR, Barnes PJ. Localization of neutral endopeptidase mRNA in human nasal mucosa. J Appl Physiol 1993; 74:272–279.

137. Ohkubo K, Baraniuk JN, Hohman RJ, Kaulbach HC, Hausfeld JN, Merida M, Kaliner MA. Human nasal mucosal neutral endopeptidase (NEP): location, quantitation and secretion. Am J Respir Cell Mol Biol 1994; In press.

138. Baraniuk JN, Mak J, Letarte M, Davies R, Twort C, Barnes PJ. Neutral endopeptidase mRNA expression. Am Rev Respir Dis 1991; 143:A40.

139. Bunnett NW, Wu V, Sternini C, Klinger J, Shimomaya E, Payan D, Kobayashi R, Walsh JH. Distribution and abundance of neutral endopeptidase (EC 3.4.24.11) in alimentary canal of the rat. Am J Physiol 1993; 264:G497–G508.

140. Winter RJD, Zhoa L, Krausz T, Hughes JMB. Neutral endopeptidase 24.11 inhibition reduces pulmonary vascular remodeling in rats exposed to chronic hypoxia. Am Rev Respir Dis 1991; 144:1342–1346.

141. Llorens-Cortes C, Huang H, Vicart P, Gase JM, Paulin D, Corvol P. Identification and characterization of neutral endopeptidase in endothelial cells from venous or aterial origins. J Biol Chem 1992; 267:140112–14018.

142. Sunday ME, Hua J, Torday JS, Reyes B, Shipp MA. CD10/neutral endopeptidase 24.11 in developing human fetal tissue. J Clin Invest 1992; 90:2517–2525.

143. Umeno E, Nadel JA, Huang HT, McDonald DM. Inhibition of neutral endopeptidase potentiates neurogenic inflammation in the rat trachea. J Appl Physiol 1989; 66:2647–2653.

144. Honda I, Kohrogi H, Yamaguchi T, Ando M, Araki S. Enkephalinase inhibitor potentiates substance P- and capsaicin-induced bronchial smooth muscle contractions in humans. Am Rev Respir Dis 1991; 143:1416–1418.

145. Jacoby DB, Tamaoki J, Borson DB, Nadel JA. Influenza infection increases airway smooth

muscle responsiveness to substance P in ferrets by decreasing enkephalinase. J Appl Physiol 1988; 64:2653–2658.

146. McDonald DM. Infections intensify neurogenic plasma extravasation in the airway mucosa. Am Rev Respir Dis 1992; 146:S40–S44.

147. Dusser DJ, Djoric TD, Borson DB, Nadel JA. Cigarette smoke induces bronchoconstrictor hyperresponsiveness to substance P and inactivates airway neutral endopeptidase in the guinea pig. J Clin Invest 1989; 84:900–906.

148. Yeadon M, Wilkinson D, Payan AN. Ozone induces bronchial hyperreactivity to inhaled substance P by functional inhibition of enkephalinase. Br J Pharmacol 1990; 99:191.

149. Murlas CG, Murphy TP, Lang Z. HOCl causes airway substance P hyperresponsiveness and neutral endopeptidase hypoactivity. Am J Physiol 1990; 258:L361–L368.

150. Lang Z, Murlas CG. Neutral endopeptidase of a human airway epithelial cell line recovers after hypochlorous acid exposure: dexamethasone accelerates this by stimulating neutral endopeptidase mRNA synthesis. Am J Respir Cell Mol Biol 1992; 7:300–306.

151. Erdos EG, Wagner B, Harbury CB, Painter RG, Skidgell RA, Fa XG. Down-regulation and inactivation of neutral endopeptidase 24.11 (enkephalinase) in human neutrophils. J Biol Chem 1989; 263:9456–9461.

152. Cheung D, Bel EH, Den Hartigh J, Dijkman JJ, Sterk PJ. The effect of an inhaled neutral endopeptidase inhibitor, thiorphan, on airway responsiveness to neurokinin A in normal humans in vivo. Am Rev Respir Dis 1992; 145:1275–1280.

153. Borson DB, Gruenert DC. Glucocorticoids induce neutral endopeptidase in transformed human trachea epithelial cells. Am J Physiol 1991; 260:L83–L89.

154. Kondepudi A, Johnson A. Cytokines increase neutral endopeptidase activity in lung fibroblasts. Am J Respir Cell Mol Biol 1993; 8:43–49.

155. Mapp PI, Walsh DA, Kidd BL, Cruwys SC, Polak JM, Blake DR. Localization of the enzyme neutral endopeptidase to the human synovium. J Rheumatol 1992; 19:1838–1844.

156. Stefano GB, Paemen LR, Hughes TK. Autoimmunoregulation: differential modulation of CD10/neutral endopeptidase 24.11 by tumor necrosis factor and neuropeptides. J Neuroimmunol 1992; 41:9–14.

157. Mattox W, Ryner L, Baker BS. Autoregulation and multifunctionality among trans-acting factors that regulate alternative pre-mRNA processing. J Biol Chem 1992; 267:19023–19026.

158. Klaassen ABM, van Megen YJB, Kuipers W, van den Broek P. Autononmic innervation of the nasal mucosa. ORL J Otorhinolaryngol Relat Spec 1988; 50:32–41.

159. Costa M, Furness JB, Gibbons IL, Morris JL, Bornstein JC, Llewellyn-Smith IL, Murphy R. Colocalization of VIP with other neuropeptides and neurotransmitters in the autonomic nervous system. Ann NY Acad Sci 1988; 527:103–109.

160. Hartschuh W, Weihle E, Reinecke M. Peptidergic (neurotensin, VIP, substance P) nerve fibres in the skin. Immunohistochemical evidence of an involvement of neuropeptides in nociception, pruritus, and inflammation. Br J Dermatol 1983; 109(suppl 25):14.

161. Yiangou Y, Requejo F, Polak JM, Bloom SR. Characterization of a novel prepro VIP derived peptide. Biochem Biophys Res Commun 1986; 139:1142.

162. Christiophides ND, Polak JM, Bloom SR. Studies on the distribution of PHI in mammals. Peptides 1984; 5:261.

163. Sreedharan RP, Patel DR, Huang JX, Goetzl EJ. Intestinal peptide receptor. Biochem Biophys Res Commun 1993; 193:546–553.

164. Ishihara T, Shigemoto R, Mori K, Takahashi K, Nagata S. Functional expression and tissue distribution of a novel receptor for vasoactive intestinal polypeptide. Neuron 1992; 8:811–819.

165. Ishihara T, Nakamura S, Kaziro Y, Takahashi T, Takahashi K, Nagata S. Molecular cloning and expression of a cDNA encoding the secretin receptor. EMBO J 1991; 10:1635–1641.

166. Goetzl EJ, Sreedharan SP, Turck CW, Bridenbaugh R, Malfroy B. Preferential cleavage of amino- and carboxy-terminal oligopeptides from vasoactive intestinal polypeptide by human

recombinant enkephalinase (neutral endopeptidase, ED 3.4.24.11). Biochem Biophys Res Commun 1989; 158:850–854.

167. Carstairs JR, Barnes PJ. Visualization of vasoactive intestinal peptide receptors in human and guinea pig lung. J Pharmacol Exp Ther 1986; 239:249–55.

168. Malm L, Sundler F, Uddman R. Effects of vasoactive intestinal peptide (VIP) on resistance and capacitance vessels in nasal mucosa. Acta Otolaryngol (Stockh) 1980; 90:304–308.

169. Shimura S, Sasaki T, Ekeda K, Sasaki K, Takishima T. VIP augments cholinergic-induced glycoconjugate secretion in tracheal submucosal glands. J Appl Physiol 1988; 65:2537–2544.

170. Richardson PS, Webber SE. The control of mucous secretion in the airways by peptidergic mechanisms. Am Rev Respir Dis 1987; 136:S72–S77.

171. Coles SJ, Said SI, Reid LM. Inhibition by vasoactive intestinal peptides of glycoconjugate and lysozyme secretion by human airways in vitro. Am Rev Respir Dis 1981; 124:531–536.

172. Marom Z, Goswami SK. Respiratory mucus hypersecretion (bronchorrea): a case discussion—possible mechanism(s) and treatment. J Allergy Clin Immunol 1981; 87:1050–1055.

173. Eccles R, Wilson H. The autonomic innervation of the nasal blood vessels of the cat. J Physiol 1974; 238:549–560.

174. Lundberg JM, Angaard A, Fahrenkrug J. Complementary role of vasoactive intestinal peptide (VIP) and acetylcholine for cat submandibular gland blood flow and secretion. Acta Physiol Scand 1981; 113:329–336.

175. Larsson O, Duner-Engstrom M, Lundberg JM, Freholm BB, Anggard A. Effects of VIP, PHM and substance P on blood vessels and secretory elements of the human submandibular gland. Regul Pept 1986; 13:319–326.

176. Kurian SS, Blank MA, Sheppard MN. Vasoactive intestinal polypeptide (VIP) in vasomotor rhinitis. Clin Biochem 1983; 11:425–427.

177. Heinz-Erian P, Dey RD, Said SI. Deficient vasoactive intestinal peptide innervation in sweat glands of cystic fibrosis patients. Science 1985; 229:1407–1409.

178. Hokfelt T, Fuxe K, Pernow B. Coexistence of neuronal messengers: a new principle in chemical transmission. Prog Brain Res 1987; 68:1–37.

179. Aliakbari J, Sreedharan SP, Turck CW, Goetzl EJ. Selective localization of vasoactive intestinal polypeptide and substance P in human eosinophils. Biochem Biophys Res Commun 1987; 148:1440–1445.

180. Goetzl EJ, Sreedharan SP, Turck CW. Structurally distinctive vasoactive intestinal polypeptides from rat basophilic leukemia cells. J Biol Chem 1988; 263:9083–9086.

181. Pernow J. Co-release and functional interactions of neuropeptide Y and noradrenaline in peripheral sympathetic vascular control. Acta Physiol Scand 1988; 568(suppl):1–55.

182. Lacroix JS. Adrenergic and non-adrenergic mechanisms in sympathetic vascular control of the nasal mucosa. Acta Physiol Scand Suppl 1989; 581:1–49.

183. Khalil Z, Andrews PV, Helme RD. VIP modulates substance P induced plasma extravasation in vivo. Eur J Pharmacol 1988; 151:281–287.

184. Baraniuk JN, Silver PB, Kaliner MA, Barnes PJ. Neuropeptide Y (NPY) is a vasoconstrictor in human nasal mucosa. J Appl Physiol 1992; 73:1867–1872.

185. Hakanson R, Wahlestadt C. Neuropeptide Y acts via prejunctional (Y_2) and postjunctional (Y_1) receptors. Neuroscience 1987; 22:S679.

186. Hinson J, Rauh C, Coupet J. Neuropeptide Y stimulates inositol phospholipid hydrolysis in rat brain miniprisms. Brain Res 1988; 446:379–382.

187. Stretton CD, Barnes PJ. Modulation of cholinergic neurotransmission in guinea pig trachea by neuropeptide Y. Br J Pharmacol 1990; 93:672–678.

188. Rogers DF, Barnes PJ. Opioid inhibitions of neurally mediated mucus secretion in human bronchi. Lancet 1989; 1:930–932.

189. Wahlenstedt C, Reis DJ. Neuropeptide Y-related peptides and their receptors—are the receptors potential therapeutic drug targets? Annu Rev Pharmacol Toxicol 1993; 33:309–352.

25

Histamine Receptors and Antihistamines

Anoop J. Chauhan and Stephen T. Holgate
University Medicine, University of Southampton, Southampton, England

INTRODUCTION

Major advances have been made in the understanding and treatment of allergic diseases, particularly in the development of effective and specific antihistamine drugs in the past 30 years, despite which they continue to be a leading cause of morbidity.

In this chapter, the clinical role of histamine in relation to allergic diseases is described, followed by discussion of the biochemical and physiological roles of histamine-specific receptors. An appraisal of the role of newer antihistamines, particularly in relation to asthma, rhinitis, and urticaria, is subsequently described.

Histamine, a naturally occurring biogenic amine, was incriminated as a broncho-constrictor substance in asthma in 1911 following the pioneering experiments of Dale and Laidlaw on the airway of sensitized guinea pigs (1). Riley and West subsequently confirmed that histamine in skin was located almost entirely in mast cells, and that a similar cellular store of histamine was present in airways (2). The discovery that immunoglobulin (Ig)E (the reaginic antibody) binds with high affinity to specific mast cell receptors provided the crucial link between antigen sensitization and mediator release from mast cells and basophils. The widespread biological activities of histamine are mediated through activation of specific cell surface receptors, and the use of selective antagonists of the pharmacological action of histamine has led to the classification of histamine receptor subtypes H_1, H_2 (3), and more recently, H_3 (4) receptors. These drugs, therefore, have also served as useful tools to dissect the contribution of histamine in allergic disease, particularly asthma. The receptor-mediated effects of histamine are shown in Table 1.

Table 1 Receptor-Mediated Biological Activities of Histamine in Humans

Target tissue	Effect	Receptor type
Leukocytes		
Lymphocytes	↓ lymphocyte production	H_2
	↓ lymphokine production	
	↓ Ig production	
	Activates suppressor cells	
Basophils	↓ chemotaxis	H_2
	↓ histamine secretion	
	↓ IgE dependent degranulation	
Eosinophils	Activates chemotaxis	H_1/H_2
	Stimulates cAMP	H_2
Neutrophils	Activates chemotaxis	H_2
	↓ lysosome secretion	
Upper Airways	Rhinorrhea (muscarinic reflex)	H_1
	Mucosal edema	
Lower airways		
Bronchiolar smoooth muscle	Contraction/relaxation	H_1
		H_2 (?)
Bronchial epithelium	↑ permeability	H_2
Secretory glands/goblet cells	↑ glycoprotein secretion	H_1/H_2
	Mucus secretion	H_1
	Activation of cough receptors	
General	Probably inhibition of histamine synthesis and secretion	H_3
Adrenal medulla	Adrenalin secretion	H_1
Gastrointestinal		
Oxyntic mucosa	↑ acid and pepsin secretion	H_2
Gastrointestinal smooth muscle	Relaxation/contraction	H_1
Cardiovascular		
Smooth-muscle arteries and veins	Contraction	H_1
Pulmonary artery	Constriction	H_1
	Dilation	H_2
Basilar artery	Constriction	H_1
Carotid artery	Dilation	H_2
Postcapillary venules	Dilation	H_1
Facial cutaneous	Dilation	H_2
Vascular endothelium	↑ Permeability	H_1/H_2
	Prostaglandin-I_2 release	H_1
Cardiac	↑ Sinoatrial activity	H_2
	↑ Force of contraction	
	↑ Atrial and ventricular automaticity	
Nervous system		
Central nervous system	Inhibition of histamine metabolism	H_3
	Neural regulation	$H_1/H_2/H_3$
Peripheral nervous system	Stimulates sensory nerves (pain and itching) flare of triple response	H_1

HISTAMINE RECEPTORS

Clinical Effects of Histamine

Although the actions of histamine are mediated through three distinct receptors defined pharmacologically, the most important effects in allergic diseases are mediated through the H_1 receptor, including pruritus, smooth-muscle contraction, increased vascular permeability, tachycardia, and activation of vagal reflexes. The H_2 receptor-mediated effects include esophageal contraction, gastric acid secretion, and increased lower airways secretion. H_2 receptor antagonists have been developed over the last 15 years, with remarkable therapeutic gains in upper gastrointestinal disease. There are also combined H_1 and H_2 receptor-mediated effects, mainly involving vasoactive-induced symptoms, such as headaches, flushing, tachycardia, and hypotension (5).

In addition to contracting airways smooth muscle, histamine also has a powerful effect on pulmonary vasculature, producing dilation of the precapillary arterioles and increased leakage of the postcapillary venules and fenestrated capillaries (6), a microvascular effect seen in asthma, urticaria, allergic rhinitis, and anaphylaxis. This results in the tissue response accounting for the histamine-induced skin wheal. Histamine also mediates pruritus, probably by stimulation of afferent fibers (pain and itch of the triple response) by its H_1 receptor effects.

In the nasal model, glandular mucous secretion is indirectly mediated by histamine through its H_1 receptor muscarinic vagal reflex, a mechanism supported by the observation that unilateral nasal histamine challenge results in contralateral glandular secretion that is inhibited by atropine (7). The major clinical effects of histamine are summarized in Table 2.

Finally, a new receptor for histamine has been described, designated H_3, that by its presynaptic locations in the central nervous system (CNS) inhibits histamine synthesis and release from neural tissue (8). Although the primary importance of the H_3 receptor may be to turn off histamine secretion, its exact physiological role is currently unknown. Indeed, the ability of the H_2 receptor to inhibit histamine secretion may be mediated by the H_3 receptor, and the presence of both the H_3 and H_2 receptors may down-regulate H_1-mediated effects. This would be a possible explanation for the common observation that, in patients with allergic disease, the severity of a histamine-mediated tissue response varies, even within the same patient, despite exposure to the same total quantity of allergen.

Heterogeneous Activities of Histamine and Histamine Receptors

Although three histamine receptors have been individually defined, growing evidence suggests that the complex and heterogeneous activities of histamine both in vitro and in vivo cannot be explained solely by interaction of the three receptor subtypes. To describe how histamine is capable of diverse cellular functions, its metabolism will be briefly discussed.

Histamine in tissues is synthesized by decarboxylation of histidine by histidine decarboxylase (HDC) and also by aromatic-L-amino acid decarboxylase (DDC) (9). Histamine (together with other mediators) is then released by IgE-specific (10) or nonspecific (11) mechanisms from tissue mast cells and basophils.

Released histamine then binds to at least three different histamine-specific receptors (H_1, H_2, and H_3) and is also capable of activating other receptors, such as the serotonin 1c receptors. Histamine is then catabolized by either diamine oxidase (DAO) or histamine–

Table 2 Clinical Effects and Ligands of Histamine Receptors in Humans

	H_1	H_2	H_3
Locations	Brain, gastrointestinal and bronchial smooth muscle	Brain, stomach, uterine smooth muscle	Brain, bronchial smooth muscle, sensory nerve endings
Functions	↑ Vascular permeability	↑ Gastric acid secretion	? Reduces cholinergic neurotransmission in human airways
	Smooth-muscle contraction	↑ Esophageal motility	? Cerebral vasodilation
	Pruritus	↑ Lower airways mucous secretion	
	Atrioventricular node conduction		
	Airways vagal afferent nerves stimulation		
Typical agonist	N_α-Methylhistamine	4,5-Methylhistamine	$(R)\alpha$-Methylhistamine
Typical antagonist	First-generation: chlorpheniramine, Second-generation: cetirizine	cimetidine, ranitidine	Thioperamide

methyltransferase (HMT), the dominant pathways varying according to species and tissue type (e.g., HMT is the major pathway in mammals, whereas DAO is the main metabolic pathway in invertebrates; (12). Intracellular histamine may induce cellular functions such as activation in T-lymphocyte suppressor cells and platelet aggregation after release and before catabolism by HMT and DAO.

Histamine H_1 Receptors

Selective H_1 Receptor Ligands

Because of the lack of available potent and highly specific ligands for the H_1 receptor, histamine still remains the most potent of agonists. In the development of highly specific H_1 receptor agonists, changes in the configuration of the histamine molecule sacrifices receptor potency for disproportionately minor improvements in selectivity. For example, although N_α-methyl- and N_α,N_α-dimethylhistamine are the next most potent histamine analogues, they are not selective, as higher N_α-alkyl analogues of histamine become less potent. Recent evidence has suggested that the selectivity of H_1 receptor agonists may not be a function of the imidazole ring, as has been commonly understood (13). These authors suggest that modification of histamine at sites a certain distance from the imidazole moiety, results in tissue-selective H_1 agonists. Table 3 shows a subclassification of antihistamines according to their chemical group, and Figure 1 illustrates the structural formulas of selected H_1 receptor antagonists.

Although many potent and highly selective H_1 receptor antagonists have been developed over the past 30 years, classic H_1 antagonists, such as ethylenediamine and pyrilamine (mepyramine), have suffered from an affinity for both CNS and peripheral H_1 receptors, leading to CNS sedation, despite their relative selectivity (14). The use of specific H_1 receptor antagonists in allergic diseases will be discussed later.

Table 3 Subclassification of Antihistamines

Chemical group	Generic name	Trade name	
		United Kingdom	United States
Alkylamine	Chlorpheniramine	Piriton	Chlor-Trimeton, Teldrin, others
	Triprolidine	Pro-Actidil	Actifed (component)
	Acrivastine	Semprex	Semprex-D
Ethanolamine	Clemastine	Tavegil	Tavist
	Diphenhydramine	Benadryl	Benadryl
Phenothiazine	Promethazine	Phenergan	Phenergan, Anergan
Piperazine	Hydroxyzine	Atarax, Ucerax	Visteril
	Cetirizine	Zirtex	Reactine
Piperidine	Cyproheptadine	Periactin	Periactin
	Astemizole	Hismanal	Hismanal
	Ketotifen	Zaditen	Zaditen
	Loratadine	Clarityn	Claritin
	Terfenadine	Triludan	Seldane
Others	Azelastine	Rhinolast nasal spray	Astelin

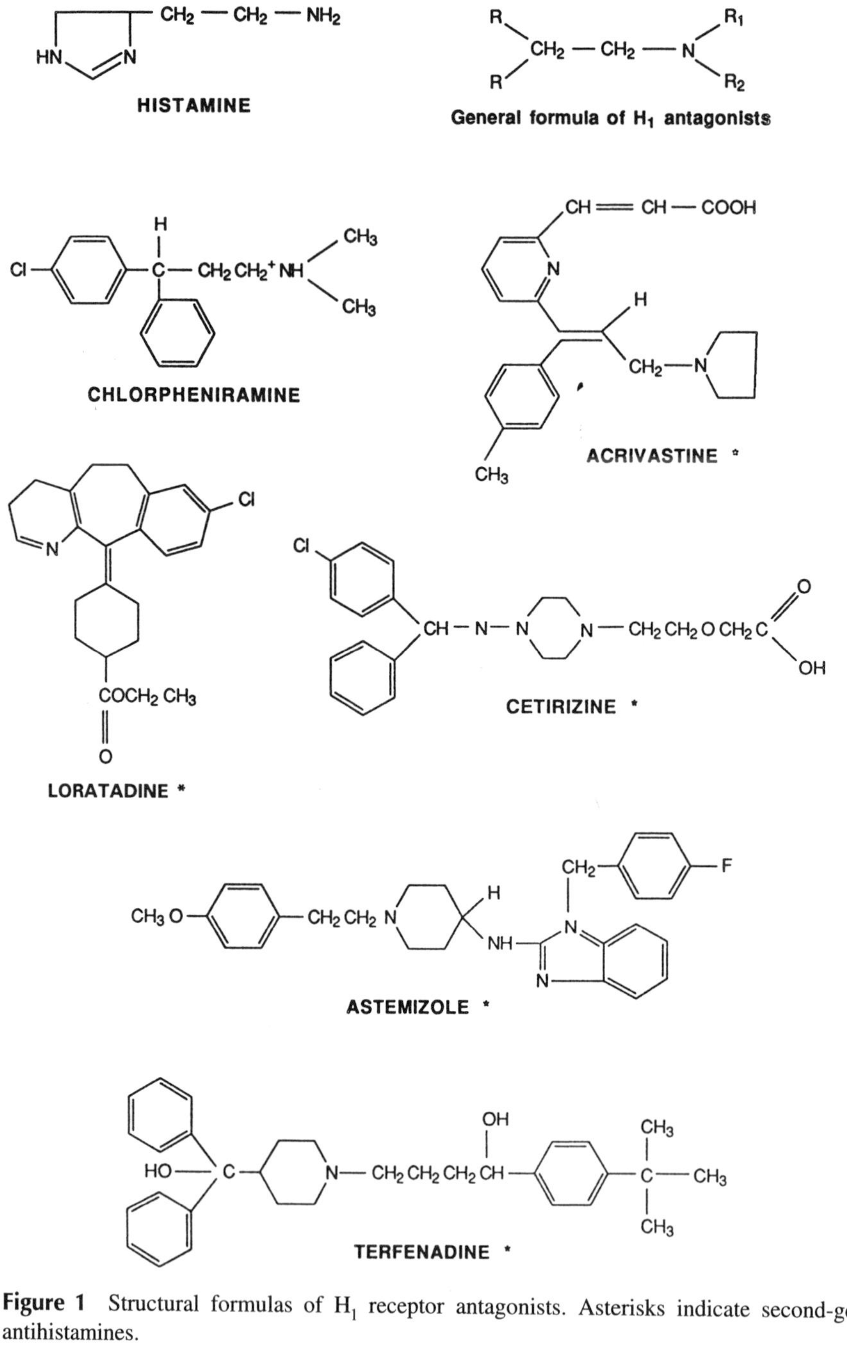

Figure 1 Structural formulas of H_1 receptor antagonists. Asterisks indicate second-generation antihistamines.

Calcium Flux

The histamine H_1 receptor acts by increasing the Ca^{2+} concentration in the cytosol of target cells (15) and, depending on the presence of Ca^{2+}-specific enzyme and substrates, fluxes in Ca^{2+} in the cytosol may account for different responses according to the cell type. There is strong evidence for the Ca^{2+}-mobilizing potency of histamine (16,17); rises in peak cytosolic Ca^{2+} concentrations after 30 s following histamine application have been recorded, followed by sustained elevations of up to threefold basal levels. Also, because this response can be inhibited by pyrilamine and mimicked by histamine derivatives (which are also potent H_1 agonists), the receptors involved can thus be classified as the H_1 receptor subtype.

Furthermore, observations of a biphasic Ca^{2+} response (16) seen in experiments in Ca^{2+}-free media and in the presence of Ca^{2+} entry blockers (e.g., Co^{2+} and Mn^{2+}) suggests there are two distinct pathways for Ca^{2+} mobilization. The peak response may be accounted for by *intracellular* stores and occurs even in the absence of extracellular calcium. The second sustained response can be depressed in the presence of Ca^{2+} entry blockers, thereby providing indirect evidence for an extracellular influx of Ca^{2+}. This is illustrated clinically; in vitro studies of human bronchial muscle show reduced contractions when extracellular Ca^{2+} influx is prevented, however, the muscle is still able to contract in a Ca^{2+}-free medium through its intracellular stores (18). Moreover, a receptor-dependent Ca^{2+} channel (RDC) is likely to account for fluxes in cytosolic Ca^{2+}, as opposed to protein kinase C-related voltage-dependent Ca^{2+} channels (VDC), which have previously been suggested (19), particularly as the VDC-antagonist verapamil does *not* alter basal or post-histamine challenge Ca^{2+} levels (16).

How are the RDCs controlled? There is mounting evidence to support the role of inositol phosphates in the regulation of the extracellular Ca^{2+} influx, possibly by direct activation of Ca^{2+} channels by inositol-1,4,5-triphosphates (IP_3), which has been suggested following the observation of current fluctuations in human T-lymphocyte plasma membranes (20). Further studies on this point have shown that IP_3 probably has to be metabolized to other derivatives for its activity, particularly as IP_3 does not stimulate Ca^{2+} release in purified plasma membranes (21). Another study records the same conclusions (22).

Role of G-Proteins

The H_1 receptor is known to be coupled to phosphatidylinositol hydrolysis pathways, in which the H_1 receptor–specific-induced hydrolysis of phosphatidylinositol (with formation of IP_3 and diacylglycerol; DAG) leads to intracellular Ca^{2+} mobilization and activation of protein kinase C (PKC) (23). Figure 2 summarizes the relationship. However, the exact mechanism of phospholipase C (PLC) activation in relation to H_1 receptor stimulation is as yet unknown. Several studies have suggested the presence of G-proteins (guanine nucleotide-binding regulatory proteins, or GTPs) for this regulatory role. The GTP-binding proteins are a family of molecules that are signal transducers from membrane receptors to intracellular effectors. In smooth muscle a phosphatidylinositol-4,5-biphosphate (PIP_2)-specific phospholipase C has been activated by a stable GTP analogue (24), and in human astrocytes, a stable GTP analogue has stimulated histamine-induced phosphatidylinositol turnover (25). Although the identity of the G-protein(s) coupled to PKC is still unknown, newer G-proteins have recently been identified (16) that show a distribution in the brain resembling that of phospholipase C. The idea of multiple, different G-proteins in phospholipase C regulation has also been suggested. (26)

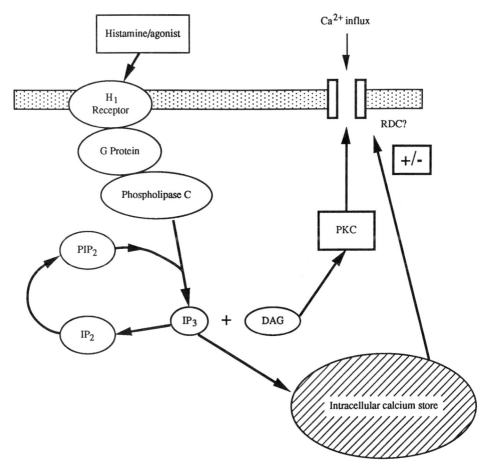

Figure 2 Coupling of inositol hydrolysis pathways to H_1 receptor and Ca^{2+} stores. The H_1 receptor coupled to unidentified G-proteins activates phospholipase C, followed by hydrolysis of PIP_2 to IP_3 and DAG. The RDC channels may then be stimulated in turn by activated PKC. PIP_2, phosphatidylinositol diphosphate; IP_3, inositol-1,4,5-triphosphate; IP_2, inositol biphosphate; DAG, diacylglycerol; PKC, protein kinase C; RDC, receptor-dependent channel.

Signal Transfer and Secondary Messengers

The inositol phosphate metabolism following phospholipase C activation is complex (see Fig. 2). The proposed mechanisms involve hydrolysis of PIP_2 to produce IP_3 and DAG, dephosphorylation of IP_3 to free inositol, followed by rephosphorylation by membrane-bound kinases to produce PIP_2, and the cycle completed (27). There is evidence to suggest that some of the metabolites in this pathway may act as signal transducers or secondary messengers (15,28). Diacylglycerol is also another important contributor to the signal transfer of Ca^{2+}-mobilizing receptors occurring by an increase in affinity of PKC for Ca^{2+}. Exactly how PKC and the inositol phosphates affect the receptor-dependent Ca^{2+} channel is unknown.

The RNA expression of the H_1 receptor from bovine adrenal medulla in *Xenopus laevis* oocytes has recently been established (29), followed by identification of cDNA encoding the bovine histamine H_1 receptor (30). Similar work by sequence homology analysis or polymerase chain reaction (PCR) to clone human H_1 receptor cDNA can similarly be expected in the near future, with exciting results.

Histamine H_2 Receptors

Whereas H_1 receptors are linked to inositol phosphate pathways, H_2 receptors are coupled to adenylate cyclase, resulting in histamine-induced increases in intracellular cAMP (31). Although histamine responses are thus regulated in H_1 receptors by secondary Ca^{2+} pathways, as described, and in H_2 receptors by cAMP pathways, evidence is now emerging of the role of Ca^{2+} fluxes in H_2 receptor responses. The H_2 receptor stimulation increases cAMP and Ca^{2+} levels in gastric parietal cells (32) and in human granulocytic leukocytes (33). In the latter study, histamine-induced mobilization of Ca^{2+} remained unaltered both by reducing the extracellular Ca^{2+} and by the addition of known Ca^{2+} channel blockers (33), and histamine increased the levels of IP_3, suggesting that the H_2 receptor (similarly to the H_1 receptor) is capable of activating the inositol phosphate hydrolysis pathways. Attempts have been made to show a connection between H_2 receptors and the adenylate cyclase system, and although models have been proposed, the exact mechanism is unknown. Recent evidence suggests the presence of two different G-proteins that may activate adenylate cyclase and phospholipase C simultaneously (33). Figure 3 shows a possible model based on this current knowledge.

The cDNA for the H_2 receptor has recently been cloned with the polymerase chain reaction (34). The cloned genes for both H_1 and H_2 receptors encode for seven transmembrane domains (NH_2-terminals for extracellular and COOH-terminals for intracellular), all of which show a high degree of homology with other receptors that couple with G-proteins. Given these rapid developments, cloning of genes for other possible histamine receptor subtypes can be similarly anticipated.

Histamine H_3 Receptors

Since the discovery of the H_3 receptor in 1983 (35), it has become apparent that this presynaptic receptor shows distinct pharmacology and, on available evidence, may have an important role in allergic diseases, as well as being a novel neurotransmitter. Although initially it was considered to be restricted to the CNS, it is now also known to be located at sensory nerve endings and on neurons in several peripheral organs. Specific H_3 receptor ligands have been developed with (R)-α-methylhistamine, a potent and selective histamine H_3 agonist, being a stronger agonist at this receptor than histamine itself, whereas thioperamide is a potent competitive H_3 antagonist.

There is little available information on the molecular characteristics, agonist binding, and signal transfer mechanisms of the presynaptic H_3 receptor. What is known, is that the release of histamine from the neurons is highly dependent on the presence of extracellular Ca^{2+}; H_3 receptor effects diminish as the extracellular Ca^{2+} concentration is raised (36). The H_3 receptor may also be linked to hyperpolarizing K^+ channels (see Chap. 23).

The Role of H_3 Receptors in Allergic Disease

Although well described in the CNS (more recently in humans), insights into possible therapeutic uses of central H_3 receptors remains limited. The recent observation that histaminergic neurons control the process of sleep and wakefulness in mammals shows

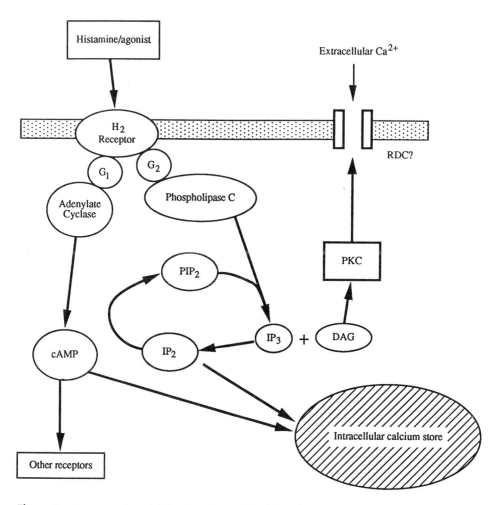

Figure 3 A proposed model for coupling of the histamine H_2 receptor to inositol phosphate pathways and adenylate cyclase, including the effects on Ca^{2+} mobilization, based on current knowledge. cAMP, cyclic adenosine monophosphate; G_1 and G_2, probable two distinct peptides coupling the H_2 receptor to cAMP system and inositol phosphate hydrolysis pathways; PIP_2, phosphatidylinositol diphosphate; IP_3, inositol-1,4,5-triphosphate; IP_2, inositol biphosphate; DAG, diacylglycerol; PKC, protein kinase C; RDC, receptor-dependent channel.

promise, particularly as these processes can be modulated by centrally acting H_3 receptor ligands (37).

The H_3 receptors in peripheral tissues are of more relevance in allergic disease. They have been identified in human lower airways, and are probably not located on smooth muscle. This is supported by the observation that thioperamide or $(R)\alpha$-methylhistamine have no effect (in vitro or in vivo) on airway tone or bronchial responses to histamine or acetylcholine (38). Similar observations have also concluded that cholinergic neurotransmission appears to be subjected to H_3–receptor-mediated inhibition in human airways in vitro (H_3 receptors are present on cholinergic nerves in human airways). Besides inhibition of cholinergic neurotransmission, H_3 receptors also control the nonadrenergic, noncholinergic (NANC) neurotransmission in guinea pig airways. Part of the neurogenic inflammatory process seen in allergic disease involves bronchoconstriction and increased microvascular leakage that are in part H_3-mediated responses, as they can be manipulated by the appropriate H_3 receptor ligands (39). In theory, H_3 receptors might offer potential therapeutic targets for the treatment of asthma.

ANTIHISTAMINES

Introduction

Histamine was first implicated in the pathogenesis of allergic diseases by Dale and Laidlaw, after its structural identification (40). However, not until the 1940s, when it was observed to cause bronchoconstriction when administered intravenously to asthmatic subjects, was it implicated as a mediator of asthma (41). Similar findings prompted a search for drugs capable of antagonizing the effects of histamine safely and effectively, which have resulted in the clinical introduction of numerous antihistamines in the past 50 years and, currently, more than 50 competitive antagonists have been used. Their use, however, has too often been associated with unwanted side effects, either CNS depression, causing sedation or, particularly the older antagonists, have had side effects not attributable to histamine antagonism, such as blockade of muscarinic–cholinergic, serotoninergic, and α-adrenergic receptors. The narrow therapeutic index of the early antihistamines, and introduction of other safer treatments (particularly β_2-adrenergic receptor agonists) had subsequently resulted in their diminished use until a decade ago, when the introduction of newer, second-generation antihistamines justified their reappraisal for use in clinical practice.

First- Versus Second-Generation Antihistamines

The older, first-generation sedating antihistamines have been used in the treatment of allergic diseases since their introduction over 50 years ago, such as phenbenzamine (42), pyrilamine (43), and diphenhydramine (44). Although limited by their unwanted effects, their therapeutic efficacy as antihistamines led to a search for more potent drugs devoid of limiting side effects. Since the 1980s, many potent and specific, yet less-sedating anti-histamines have been developed. These new compounds include terfenadine, astemizole, azelastine, cetirizine, loratadine, and acrivastine. They are relatively lipophobic; hence, they penetrate the CNS poorly, producing less sedation. The CNS side effects have been quantified, and comparisons made between first- and second-generation antihistamines. For example, the time interval from administration of a single dose to the onset of electro-encephalographic (EEG) stage 1 sleep has been used extensively as an objective test of drowsiness. Subjective scores of sedative effect and changes in task performance and alertness have also been used with a variety of timed and scored tests (45). On all similar assessments, the newer antihistamines have generally shown a marked reduction in CNS side effects compared with their predecessors. Table 4 illustrates some differences between the first- and second-generation compounds.

Pharmacokinetically, most antihistamines are well absorbed after oral administration. All of the first-generation and most second-generation antihistamines are metabolized by the hepatic cytochrome P-450 system, and a few subsequently form active metabolites. For example, terfenadine undergoes extensive first-pass metabolism in which 99% of the drug is transformed to two major metabolites, and cetirizine is a metabolite of hydroxyzine by

Table 4 Pharmacological Profile of Nonsedating Second-Generation Antihistamines Compared with Classic First-Generation Antihistamines

Antihistamine	Antihistamine activity[a]	Sedative activity[a]	Anticholinergic activity[a]
Nonsedating			
Terfenadine	+++	0	0
Astemizole	+++	0	0
Loratadine	+++	0/+[b]	0
Cetirizine	+++	0/+[b]	0
Classic			
Chlorpheniramine	+++	+/++[b]	+/++[b]
Diphenhydramine	+++	+++	++
Promethazine	+++	+++	++
Clemastine	+++	++	+/++

[a]0, none; +, mild; ++, moderate; +++, marked;
[b]Dose-dependent.
Source: Ref. 162.

the same hepatic pathway and is now a drug in its own right. Once absorbed, the antihistamines are excreted either by renal (cetirizine and ketotifen) or fecal (astemizole and terfenadine) routes. Their half-lives vary greatly from 1.5 h for acrivastine to 10 days for astemizole. Also, the half-lives of all antihistamines are shorter in children and prolonged in the elderly, compared with healthy middle-aged adults, accounting for the increase in incidence of sedation in the elderly (46). Antihistamines are also excreted in breast milk in a concentration comparable with that in serum.

Central Nervous System Sedation

Sedation is generally considered an adverse effect of antihistamines; however, with some drugs, this effect has been taken advantage of (although usually outside their use for treating allergic disease), notably in the treatment of motion sickness, petit mal seizures, and insomnia. In allergic disease, however, sedation caused either by antihistamines or otherwise can have clinical benefits. In one study of allergic rhinitis (47), phenobarbitone was added as a third choice to the drug-versus-placebo regimen in evaluation of a new antihistamine. Phenobarbitone caused subjectively less sedation, and the symptom scores decreased similarly to those for chlorpheniramine. This was significant, particularly as phenobarbitone is a sedative, and not a known H_1 receptor antagonist. Although the mechanism of CNS sedation is not known, possible explanations, including H_1 and cholinergic receptor blockade in the CNS, have been postulated (48,49). The latter view is supported by the observation that the sedative effects of antihistamines are not mirrored by their peripheral histamine antagonist properties, suggesting effects on other receptor types, or they are less specific for peripheral H_1 receptors when compared with centrally located ones. Perhaps the most important reason for the lack of CNS sedation of the newer antihistamines is their poor penetration into the CNS, owing to their larger molecular size and larger, charged side chains, rendering increased lipophobic properties. The experience of sedation has been reported to be between 10 and 25% by second-generation antihistamine users and is frequently dose-related and may correlate with high concentrations in the lung (50–52). As might be predicted, the new generation antihistamines show a comparatively reduced interaction with alcohol, compared with the older antihistamines, which potentiate the sedative effects of alcohol and tranquilizers (53).

Other Effects of Antihistamines

In addition to the competitive inhibition of the H_1 receptors, some antihistamines have additional effects on other cell types, receptors, and mediators, with specific reference to allergic disease. Of particular importance, however, is the relatively high concentrations of drug required to produce these effects, frequently leading to concern over their relevance in a disease setting.

Prevention of Mediator Release

Antihistamines prevent mast cell and basophil mediator release at low serum concentrations, an effect known from the earliest studies in the 1950s (54). This has been demonstrated in vitro with terfenadine, azatadine, loratadine, azelastine, and astemizole. Of particular importance is the ability of these drugs to inhibit mediator release from mast cells and basophils, unrelated to their ability to antagonize the target tissue effects of histamine at H_1 receptors (49). The proposed explanations for these effects include a direct interaction with the mast cell membrane to stabilize it, or interference with Ca^{2+} mobilization, which as described earlier, is an integral part of the mediator release process.

Anti-Inflammatory Effects

Ketotifen, azelastine, and cetirizine have additional effects on human inflammatory cells. Ketotifen inhibits platelet migration and platelet mediator release (55), and cetirizine is associated with decreased eosinophil chemotaxis and activation at the sites of mast cell activation (56).

Effects of β_2-Adrenergic Receptors

There is evidence to suggest that lymphocyte β_2-adrenergic receptor function and density are reduced in asthmatic subjects treated with β_2-agonist bronchodilators (traditionally attributed to down-regulation of receptors) when compared with untreated asthmatics (57). The resulting subsensitivity to bronchodilation by β_2-agonists has also been documented in asthmatics as well as controls (58). More recently, ketotifen (and corticosteroids)have been reported to prevent the down-regulation of β_2-receptors, leading to bronchial hyperresponsiveness in an animal model (59). Furthermore, specific β_2-adrenergic blockers can prevent this beneficial effect, confirming an action of ketotifen (direct or indirect) on the β_2-adrenergic receptor.

Effects of Other Receptors

Interactions of the first-generation of antihistamines with other receptors have been responsible for many unwanted effects. Cholinergic blockade leads to dry mouth, micturition difficulty, and occasionally, impotence, and α-adrenergic blockade (e.g., promethazine) causes hypotension. Of the newer generation of antihistamines, terfenadine binds only weakly to serotoninergic receptors, and cetirizine, in particular, shows no significant binding with other receptors (60).

Assessing the Efficacy of Antihistamines

There are four main clinical pharmacology models currently in use for assessing the efficacy of antihistamines in patients with allergic disease involving skin, nasal, bronchial, and less commonly, ocular antigen challenge models (61). Patients are challenged "out of season" with histamine or antigen, and following challenge, symptoms and signs are recorded and inflammatory mediators and cells quantified in recovered body fluids. In antigen provocation tests the ability of H_1 receptor antagonists to inhibit mediator release from mast cells and basophils has been studied in the nasal and skin antigen challenge models, as illustrated in Table 5. For histamine, dose–response curves can be constructed and relative efficacy and specificity of the different H_1 antagonists derived.

Although antihistamines penetrate rapidly into body tissues, their relative efficacy and duration of action, which is not predictable by peak serum concentrations or half-life, needs to be measured by clinical effect in the antigen challenge models. For example, in the skin, maximal duration of allergen-provoked wheal suppression (as part of the triple response of erythema, wheal, and flare) occurs several hours after peak serum concentrations are achieved and can persist for hours (62). These discrepancies can be accounted for either by differing sensitivities of antagonists to the H_1 receptor, or by the production of active metabolites and the wide tissue distribution of antihistamines in the body (63). The relation between half-life and wheal suppression for the second-generation antihistamines is illustrated in Table 6. From this information, it can be concluded that it is optimal to administer antihistamines several hours before the expected allergic reaction.

NEW H_2 RECEPTOR ANTAGONISTS IN ALLERGIC DISEASE

The development of more potent second-generation antihistamines, with fewer adverse effects than their predecessors, has led to a reexamination of their role in allergic disease, particularly asthma.

Astemizole

Astemizole, a 2-amino-benzimidazole derivative, has no chemical relation to any other known drug, particularly histamine and, therefore, has no anticholinergic or serotoninergic effects. Hepatic metabolism to two active metabolites is reflected by the delay on histamine-induced skin wheal suppression (64; see Table 6). There is mild drowsiness at

Table 5 Ability of Second-Generation Antihistamines to Inhibit Mediator Release from Mast Cells and Basophils In Vivo and In Vitro[a]

Antihistamine	In vitro	In vivo	
		Skin model	Nasal model
Azelastine	+	0	0
Astemizole	+	−	0
Cetirizine	+	+	−
Ketotifen	+	+	−
Loratadine	+	0	+
Terfenadine	+	0	+

[a]+, inhibition; −, no inhibition; 0, not known.
Source: Ref. 61.

Table 6 Relation of Half-Lives and Wheal Suppression
for Second-Generation Antihistamines

Antihistamine	Serum elimination half-life (h)	Significant wheal suppression (h—dose-dependant)
Azelastin	25	>4
Astemizole	10 d	≥ 2 wk
Cetirizine	7.5	24
Ketotifen	22.1	NA[a]
Loratadine	11	24
Terfenadine	4.5	12–24

[a]NA, data not available.

therapeutic doses, occurring in 5–15% of patients (a figure similar to that seen with placebo). It has no direct bronchodilator effect, but can antagonize histamine-induced bronchoconstriction (65). Astemizole has been tested in several placebo-controlled trials in comparison with the older antihistamines. For trials in allergic disease, the results have been confounded by fluctuations in environmental allergen levels, such as grass pollen. In a study of 63 patients with known grass pollen allergy, astemizole 10 mg versus placebo was compared over a 5-week period (66). A significant reduction in symptoms and in the need for rescue antihistamine treatment was recorded with administration of astemizole. Increases in body weight were also reported, possibly owing to an agonist effect on the satiety center.

Loratadine

Loratadine is structurally related to azatadine and is devoid of anticholinergic effects. After daily oral administration, it is converted to an active metabolite and excreted by the renal route. Loratadine is indicated for relief of symptoms of seasonal (67) and allergic (68) rhinitis and urticaria (69). In a double-blind, placebo-controlled study of 330 patients with seasonal allergic rhinitis, loratadine, 10 mg daily, was compared with clemastine, 1 mg twice daily. The incidence of sedation was comparable with that of placebo for loratadine and was significantly lower than that of clemastine (70). Furthermore, the efficacy of loratadine was similar to clemastine and more efficacious than placebo. A more recent study compared loratadine (10 mg) with astemizole (2 mg/10 kg body weight) in 41 children with seasonal allergic rhinoconjunctivitis (71). Both drugs improved symptoms, with loratadine being slightly superior. Loratadine has also been compared with mequitazine in a double-blind, parallel group, placebo-controlled study of seasonal allergic rhinitis in 69 patients. Both drugs were significantly more effective than placebo in reducing nasal symptoms, and loratadine was significantly more effective than mequitazine after 3 days of treatment (72).

Although there is no known bronchodilator activity in asthmatic airways, loratadine causes rightward displacement of the histamine concentration—FEV_1 response curve (73). A recent study reported a significant (5.5-fold) reduction in bronchial reactivity to inhaled histamine when a single, 10-mg dose of loratadine was given to 11 patients with stable asthma. Withdrawal of loratadine for 6 days yielded an increase in bronchial hyperresponsiveness (74).

Terfenadine

Terfenadine, which is structurally related to butyrophenone neuroleptics and to alkylamine H_1 antihistamines, has no anticholinergic or antiserotoninergic properties (75). After rapid oral absorption, it is converted to two active metabolites before its excretion.

In seasonal allergic rhinitis, a once-daily dose of 120 mg is equipotent to 60 mg twice daily (the recommended adult dosage) (76), although some patients may require up to 240 mg or more to be efficacious (77). This view is supported by the observation in one study that regular doses of terfenadine differ significantly, but not biologically from a fairly high rate of placebo responses (78). However, the use of high doses of both astemizole and terfenadine is associated with the rare risk of precipitating potentially fatal cardiac arrhythmias (especially torsades de point). The risk increases with elevated serum concentrations of the drugs; therefore, high doses in clinical use are not recommended, particularly in those patients who are receiving concomitant imidazole antifungal (e.g., ketoconazole) or macrolide (e.g., erythromycin) treatment, during which hepatic metabolism may be impaired.

In controlled clinical trials, terfenadine has been compared with placebo and sedative (e.g., clemastine) and nonsedative (e.g., astemizole or cetirizine) antihistamines in seasonal and perennial allergic rhinitis and urticaria. Terfenadine has matched short-acting sedative antihistamines in efficacy in the treatment of allergic rhinitis and urticaria, whereas astemizole (10 mg daily) has shown superior control of symptoms, particularly in trials that have lasted several weeks (79); probably because terfenadine has a faster onset of action). Controlled trials in adults (80) and children (78) have shown terfenadine to be effective in seasonal allergic rhinitis, but less satisfactory in perennial allergic rhinitis (81), according to symptom scores and need for rescue antihistamines.

Terfenadine prevents histamine-induced bronchoconstriction in asthmatic airways (82), with large single or prolonged dosing regimens protecting against particularly hyperventilation- and exercise-induced bronchoconstriction (83,84). The use of larger doses can increase the potential of CNS sedation as well as produce ECG abnormalities.

Ketotifen

Ketotifen, with the advantage of oral administration, has a mode of action similar to chromolyn sodium (sodium cromoglycate) and has been introduced for the prophylaxis of asthma. It is a potent mast cell and basophil mediator-release inhibitor (at least in animals) (85), and is extensively metabolized in the liver and excreted by both the renal and fecal routes. It is protective against histamine-induced bronchoconstriction in asthmatic airways (86) both in single doses and when administered long-term, but has no anticholinergic activity in the airways of asthmatic individuals. The incidence of sedation is low and declines during extended periods of treatment, the incidence being 14% after 3 months and 2% after 12 months (87).

Ketotifen has been studied extensively in clinical asthma. In a study of ketotifen versus placebo in 50 adult asthmatics, daytime symptoms improved with ketotifen at 2 mg twice daily, but only in patients whose concomitant medication did not include steroids (88). However, for asthmatics already taking corticosteroids, a small steroid-sparing effect of ketotifen has been demonstrated (89). Ketotifen achieves its maximum effect on symptoms or requirements for other medications only following regular administration. In a 6-month double-blind placebo study of 41 asthmatics, a significant reduction in symptoms and attack frequency was seen with ketotifen. However, the effect began 1 month after the start of treatment and became more pronounced at 6 months (90). Ketotifen has also been used for treatment of seasonal allergic rhinitis in adults, with limited success.

Cetirizine

Cetirizine is modified from its structural relation to the antihistamine hydroxyzine by carboxylation of the alcohol side chain that, although eliminating anticholinergic and antiserotoninergic effects, increases its H_1 receptor potency. Following rapid absorption after oral administration, it is excreted by the renal route, and the dose has to be reduced accordingly in renal disease. Cetirizine has no direct bronchodilator action in asthmatic airways, but it does protect against histamine-induced bronchoconstriction in these airways (91,92). Furthermore, in a recent study of cetirizine, given at 15 mg twice daily, a significant protective effect against an allergen-induced late-allergic bronchoconstriction was observed (93). In view of its relatively recent introduction, its full role in treatment of asthma and other allergic disorders remains to be established. Of special interest is its modulating effect on eosinophil migration and activation in the skin (94).

Azelastine

Azelastine, as a phthalazione derivative, is a histamine H_1 and a weak leukotriene-D_4 (LTD$_4$) receptor antagonist (95). It produces bronchodilation in asthmatic airways (96) and protects against the bronchoconstrictor action of histamine (97). Despite its early promise in animal models, no significant effect has been found on either methacholine- or leukotriene-C_4-induced bronchoconstriction (98). More recently, in a double-blind, placebo-controlled study of ten patients, azelastine significantly inhibited the development of the early asthmatic response, but had no effect on the late response or on the development of methacholine- and prostaglandin-D_2-induced bronchoconstriction. Similarly, in a study of pollen-allergic patients, azelastine, 4 mg twice daily, had no effect on bronchial responsiveness to methacholine (99). There are few comparative studies of azelastine in the treatment of seasonal allergic rhinitis. In a 155-patient, placebo-controlled study, azelastine was compared with chlorpheniramine and placebo, over 4 weeks, and was reported as significantly better than placebo at every weekly assessment (100).

ANTIHISTAMINES IN ASTHMA

Provocation of asthmatic airways with inhaled allergen produces an immediate broncho-constriction, reaching a peak at about 15–20 min, and recovering over 90 min. This early bronchoconstrictor response (EAR) is the result of histamine and other (PGD$_2$ or LTC$_4$) mediator release from activated mast cells, and an underlying responsiveness of the airway smooth muscle and vasculature to these mediators.

The role of the mast cell in the late asthmatic response is not well established, although its activation may occur in conjunction with other cell populations and inflammatory mediators that also possess IgE receptors and can be allergen-activated. In experimental asthma, predosing with antihistamines shifts the bronchoconstrictor dose–response curve with inhaled allergen to the right (101,102). Furthermore, histamine antagonists attenuate the time course response of the early asthmatic response, with greater inhibition seen during the early part of the bronchoconstrictor response, commensurate with histamine release from the mast cells. In 60% of patients with atopic asthma, allergen provocation results in a late-phase airways obstruction at 3–9 h after challenge, which is accompanied by increased

Table 7 Recent Studies Examining the Role of New Generation H_1 Receptor Antagonists in Asthma

Ref.	Study (yr)	Study design[a]	Patient no.	Dose (mg)	Results	Duration (wk)	Statistical significance	Clinical importance
Terfenadine								
111	Taytard (1987)	DB, PC, CO	46	120 bid	Terfenadine better than control	2	Yes	Yes: mild atopic asthma
112	Rafferty (1987)	DB, PC, CO	18	180 tid	Terfenadine better than control	4	Yes	High dosages in atopic asthma[c]
113	Teale (1991)	DB, PC	8	120 single-dose	Terfenadine better than control	One dose	Yes	Minimal
Cetirizine								
114	Kurzeja (1989)	DB, PG	20	10 bid	Cetirizine better than control	NK[b]	Yes	Controls received terfenadine 60 mg bid
115	Bousquet (1990)	DB, PG	80	10, 15 bid	Cetirizine better than control	2	Yes	Minimal
116	Brutman (1990)	DB, PC, PG	57	15 od	Cetirizine better than control	2	Yes	Many dropouts, especially in controls; mild atopic asthma
117	Dijkman (1990)	DB/PG	43	10 bid	Cetirizine better than control	6	Yes	Yes: controls received terfenadine 60 mg bid
Astemizole								
118	Backer (1990)	DB, PC, CO	20	20 od	Astemizole better than control	3	No	Yes: chronic asthma in children
119	Cistero (1992)	DB, PC, CO	12	10, 30 od	Astemizole better than placebo in allergen-induced bronchoconstriction	4	No	Yes: atopic asthma
					Astemizole *no* better than placebo for symptoms		No	

Ketotifen

	Study	Design	n	Dose	Result	Duration (wk)	Sedation	Comments
88	Dyson (1980)	DB, PC, PG	50	1, 2 bid	Ketotifen better than control	4	Yes	Yes: high frequency of drowsiness
89	Lane (1980)	DB, PC, PG	86	1 bid	Ketotifen better than placebo	2	Yes	Yes: steroid sparing
120	Tinkelman (1985)	DB, PC, PG	374	1 bid	Ketotifen better than placebo; no difference in efficacy between ketotifen/theophylline	52	Yes	Yes: high dropout rate owing to treatment failure
121	Rackham (1989)	DB, PC, PG	138	1 bid	Ketotifen better than placebo	7 mo	Yes	Yes: asthmatic children

Loratadine

	Study	Design	n	Dose	Result	Duration (wk)	Sedation	Comments
122	Dirksen (1989)	DB, PC, PG	17	10 od	Loratadine better than placebo	8	No	Yes: chronic asthma
123	Kroll (1993)	Open	25	10 od	Loratadine improved symptoms	6	No	No: uncontrolled study

Azelastine

	Study	Design	n	Dose	Result	Duration (wk)	Sedation	Comments
124	Tinkelman (1990)	DB, PC	221	2, 4, 6, 8 od	Azelastine (6 mg) better than placebo	12	Yes	Yes: drowsiness and dry mouth common
					Azelastine (2, 4 mg) better than placebo		No	
99	Balzano (1992)	DB/PC/CO	12	4 bid	Azelastine no better than placebo	4	No	Yes: Only rhinitis symptoms improved by azelastine

[a]DB, double blind; PC, placebo control; PG, parallel group.

[b]NK, not known.

[c]High dosages now associated with rare risk of cardiac arrhythmia (see text).

Table 8 Review of Published Studies of Antihistamines in Seasonal Allergic Rhinitis

Ref.	Study (yr)	Study design[a]	Patient no.	Drugs studied (doses: mg)[b]	Duration (wk)	Clinical importance
New vs. new antihistamines
134	Loephonte (1984)	DB	134	Mequitazine (5 bid) vs. terfenadine (60 bid)	1	Mequitazine more effective with a more rapid onset of action than terfenadine; sedation similar
72	Skassa-Brocek (1988)	DB, PC, PG	69	Loratadine (10 od) vs. mequitazine (5 bid)	2	Both active drugs equally efficacious and superior to placebo
135	Gervais (1989)	DB	83	Acrivastine (8 tid) vs. terfenadine (60 mg bid)	56	Both drugs efficacious but *no* control group in study
136	Del-Carpio (1989)	DB, PC	317	Loratadine (10 od) vs. terfenadine (60 bid)	2	Both active drugs comparable for symptom relief and superior to placebo; sedation similar to placebo
137	Rijntes (1990)	DB, PC	105	Astemizole (10 od) vs. cetirizine (10 od)	2	No difference between active drugs, superior to placebo; astemizole had longer duration of action
138	Reed (1991)	DB, PC	270	Astemizole (10 od) vs. cetirizine (10 od)	3	No difference between active drugs and placebo for nasal congestion, otherwise superior to placebo
139	Lockley (1993)	SB, PG	160	Cetirizine (10 od) vs. terfenadine (60 bid)	1	No control group; cetirizine led to better patient satisfaction, but otherwise equally efficacious

New vs. old antihistamines

131	Kemp (1985)	DB, PC	397	Terfenadine (60 bid) vs. chlorpheniramine (4 qid)	1	Terfenadine as efficacious as, but not superior to, chlorpheniramine; both drugs superior to placebo
70	Dockhorn (1987)	DB, PC, PG	330	Loratadine (10 od) vs. clemastine (1 bid)	2	Efficacy of both active drugs similar and superior to placebo; clemastine more sedative
132	Wieler (1988)	DB, PC, PG	155	Azelastine (0.5, 1, and 2 od) vs. chlorpheniramine (4 qid)	4	Both drugs superior to placebo; chlorpheniramine better than azelastine for symptoms, but not statistically significant
140	Katelaris (1990)	DB, PG	34	Loratadine (10 od) vs. azatadine (1 bid)	2	Loratadine as efficacious (but less sedative) as azatadine; no control group

New antihistamines vs. nonantihistamines

141	Wood (1986)	DB, PC	74	Astemizole (10 od) vs. beclamethasone (100/nostril bid)	8–9 d	Symptom severity and scores similar for both drugs; "itchy" eyes relieved significantly better by astemizole
142	Backhouse (1986)		99	Terfenadine (60 bid) vs. fluocinolone (50/nostril bid) vs. combined treatment	11	Combined treatment was significantly better than monotherapy for either drug; not controlled or blinded study
127	Meran (1990)	DB, CO, PC	40	Acrivastine (8 tid) vs. pseudoephedrine (60 od) vs. combined	6 d	Combined therapy better than monotherapy or placebo; acrivastine as efficacious as pseudoephedrine.

New antihistamine vs. placebo (selected)

130	Falliers (1991)	DB, PC	419	Cetirizine (5, 10, and 20 od) vs. placebo	1	Cetirizine superior to placebo at all doses, sedation more frequent at 10 and 20 mg doses.
128	Bedard (1992)	DB, PC	185	Loratadine (10 od) vs. placebo	3 d	Symptom relief in 65% of loratadine vs. 48% in placebo; sedation rates similar, loratadine no better than placebo statistically

[a]DB, double-blind; PC, placebo-controlled; PG, parallel group; SB, single-blind.

[b]od, once-daily (every 24-h) administration; bid, twice daily (every 12-h) administration; tid, 3 times daily (every 8-h) administration.

airway responsiveness. The role of histamine in this second phase of bronchoconstriction is not well defined. Factors that are thought to contribute to this response are edema and hypersecretion, particularly in peripheral airways, as opposed to smooth-muscle contraction in the early response.

Although a rise in plasma histamine levels during the late response has been demonstrated, controversy exists about whether this is due to mast cell or basophil activation, or whether it is an in vivo or ex vivo phenomenon occurring during venepuncture. The role of newer antihistamines during both the early and late reactions to antigen have been reviewed recently by Townley, who concluded that the ability of these compounds to inhibit eosinophil, basophil, and neutrophil migration, and platelet-activating factor-induced eosinophil accumulation in skin, at usual therapeutic doses, is a potentially useful tool in dissecting the role of these mediators in the late reaction (LAR) (103).

Hirxheimer pointed out in 1949 that the administration of chlorpheniramine in patients with asthma could produce bronchodilation (104). This led to the evaluation of other older antihistamines, such as clemastine, in asthma, and those studies clearly confirmed their bronchodilator activity. These drugs, however, had anticholinergic, serotoninergic, and α-adrenergic properties and, as a consequence, bronchodilation could not be attributed to histamine blockade alone. However, the observed bronchodilator effect of some of the newer antihistamines has led to the concept of basal histamine airway tone in asthma, which is unrelated to interaction with other receptor types. This follows the observation that, at concentrations achieved at therapeutic doses, the newer antihistamines have little or no effect against cholinergic or adrenergic receptors; hence, the observed bronchodilation is presumed to be a result of basal histamine blockade (105). Furthermore, the bronchodilator activity of antihistamines may last for only 1–2 weeks (106).

The clinical efficacy of the relatively nonselective older antihistamines was difficult to demonstrate following their introduction and, as a consequence, their therapeutic use was discouraged (107), despite enthusiasts (108) vindicating their use for childhood asthma. Furthermore, some investigators have since proposed that they may even be harmful in asthma (109), although the rationale for this has been difficult to understand. However, the advent of the newer antihistamines has led to a reappraisal of their role in asthma, with fresh impetus from a position statement issued by the American Academy of Allergy and Immunology in 1988, which proposed that the newer drugs were safe and could be used in the treatment of asthma (110).

Review of Clinical Studies of Antihistamines in Asthma

Although many studies have been performed examining the effects of second-generation antihistamines in asthma, many of these studies are of limited use because they have studied only mild atopic asthma, usually in patients with coexistent rhinitis. Relatively few have studied chronic asthma (116,122; Table 7). A review of these studies show, in general, a small beneficial effect of the new antihistamines in seasonal asthma. However, many have suffered from flaws in study design, such as a lack of control groups and use of antihistamines at doses now considered to be either ineffective in asthma (114,117), or at high doses that add to the risk of cardiac arrhythmias. Furthermore, other studies have had high dropout rates in placebo groups (116), the reasons for which are not clear, particularly whether they were due to rhinitic or asthmatic symptoms.

Of the studies of chronic perennial asthma, Backer (118) showed that 20 asthmatic children tolerated significantly higher concentrations of histamine challenge when treated

Table 9 Review of Published Studies of Antihistamines in Perennial Allergic Rhinitis

Ref.	Study (yr)	Study design[a]	Patient no.	Drugs studied (doses: mg)	Duration (wk)	Clinical importance
New vs. new antihistamines						
143	Renton (1991)	DB, PC, CO	60	Cetirizine (10 od) vs. terfenadine (120 od)	3	No difference between active drugs, both superior to placebo; adverse events more frequent with cetirizine; terfenadine given once daily
New vs. old antihistamines						
133	Frolund (1990)	DB, PC, PG	155	Loratadine (10 od) vs. clemastine (1 bid)	3	Both active drugs superior to placebo; faster relief of symptoms and less sedation with loratadine
144	Pukander (1990)	DB, PC, CO	29	Mequitazine (5 bid) vs. dexchlorpheniramine (6 bid)	4	Dexchlorpheniramine markedly superior to mequitazine or placebo; mequitazine only slightly superior to placebo
New antihistamines vs. nasal steroids						
145	Bunnag (1992)	DB, PG	69	Astemizole (10 µg od) vs. budesonide (100 µg/nostril bid)	4	Budesonide superior to astemizole for relief of nasal congestion, runny nose and eyes, and patient satisfaction
146	Gastpar (1993)	PG	193	Azelastine (140/nostril bid) vs. budesonide (50/nostril bid)	6	Azelastine comparable with *low*-dose budesonide, but associated with unpleasant taste or smell with nasal spray of azelastine
New antihistamine vs. placebo (selected)						
129	Mansmann (1992)	DB, PC	215	Cetirizine (10 and 20 mg od) vs. placebo	4	Cetirizine more effective than placebo at both doses, but higher dose gave no *additional* benefit.

[a]DB, double-blind; PC, placebo-controlled; PG, parallel group; od, once every 24-h administration; bid, once every 12-h administration; tid, once every 8-h administration.

Table 10 Review of Published Studies of Antihistamines in Chronic Idiopathic Urticaria

Ref.	Study (yr)	Study design[a]	Patient no.	Drugs studied [doses: [mg]]	Duration (wk)	Clinical importance
New vs. new antihistamines						
148	Paul (1989)	DB, PC	40	Terfenadine (30 qid) vs. astemizole (2.5 qid)	8 d	Both active drugs efficacious for pruritus and wheal severity, but no significant differences between them; doses divided too frequently
149	Van Joost (1989)	DB, PC, CO	56	Acrivastine (4 and 8 od) vs. terfenadine (60 od)	10 d	Both active drugs better than placebo, acrivastine as efficacious as terfenadine, despite terfenadine given once daily
150	Kietzmann (1990)	DB	84	Cetirizine (10 od) vs. terfenadine (60 bid)	6 wk	No placebo; cetirizine as efficacious as terfenadine for wheals, but superior for control of erythema
151	Belaich (1990)	DB, PG, PC	187	Loratadine (10 od) vs. terfenadine (60 bid)	28 d	Overall relief of symptoms in 64, 52, and 25% in loratadine, terfenadine, and placebo groups, respectively; high response rate in placebo
152	Alomar (1991)	DB, PG	47	Cetirizine (10 od) vs. astemizole (10 od)	4 wk	Comparable efficacy, but cetirizine had significantly better patient symptom scores and a trend toward wheal reduction; however, it did not reach statistical significance
153	Andri (1993)	DB, PG	30	Cetirizine (10 od) vs. terfenadine (60 bid)	20 d	Cetirizine more effective than terfenadine in controlling urticaria symptoms and in symptom scores

No.	Author (year)	Design	N	Treatment	Duration	Results
154	Fredrikson (1986)	DB, PC, CO	60	Terfenadine (60 bid) vs. clemastine (1 bid)	6 wk	Terfenadine more effective than clemastine and less sedative; both active drugs better than placebo
155	Paul (1986)	DB	45	Terfenadine (60 bid) vs. ranitidine (150 bid) vs. both together (combined)	2 wk	Interesting results; pruritus and wheals improved significantly with dual therapy compared with monotherapy of either drug
156	Grant (1988)	DB, PG, PC	122	Terfenadine (60 bid) vs. chlorpheniramine (4 qid)	6 wk	Pruritus and symptom scores better with active drugs, terfenadine less sedative than chlorpheniramine
157	Boggs (1987)	DB, PG, PC	37	Loratadine (10 od) vs. hydroxyzine (25 qid)	3 wk	Terfenadine as efficacious as hydroxyzine, both more efficacious than placebo.
158	Kalivas (1990)	DB, PG, PC	219	Cetirizine (5–20 od) vs. hydroxyzine (25–75/day) both divided doses	4 wk	Cetirizine as efficacious as hydroxyzine, lower incidence of sedation
159	Sussman (1991)	DB, PG	36	Astemizole (10 mg od) vs. diphenhydramine (25 qid) vs. hydroxyzine (25 qid)	3 mo	Withdrawal rates 58, 18, and 15% for astemizole, diphenhydramine, and hydroxyzine, respectively; greater improvement in wheals and symptoms with astemizole than diphenhydramine and hydroxyzine
160	Monroe (1992)	DB, PG, PC	203	Loratadine (10 bid) vs. hydroxyzine (25 qid)	4 wk	Loratadine and hydroxyzine more effective than placebo, but clinically comparable with each other
New antihistamine vs. placebo (selected)						
161	Honsinger (1990)	DB, PC	51	Astemizole (10 od) vs. placebo	8 wk	75% improvement in symptoms for astemizole, but also significant (20%) improvement in placebo

[a]DB, double-blind; PC, placebo-controlled; PG, parallel group; od, once every 24-h administration; bid, once every 12-h administration; tid, once every 8-h administration.

with astemizole compared with placebo, confirming powerful H_1 blockade. However, there were no differences between the crossover treatment periods in symptoms or in peak expiratory follow. Similarly, in 17 patients with perennial asthma, Dirksen (122) found that the bronchial response to histamine was attenuated by loratadine, but found no differences from placebo in symptom scores, lung function, and use of rescue medication. Taytard's study (111) showed a favorable effect of antihistamines in chronic perennial asthma; patients taking terfenadine, 120 mg twice daily, presented significantly less symptoms, less β_2-agonist use, and had modest improvements in FEV_1. This improvement in pulmonary function was small and probably does not translate into clinical importance. More recently, Cistero (119) found astemizole to be superior to placebo in allergen-induced asthma, except in symptom control and β_2-adrenergic agonist use. Studies of other second-generation antihistamines in asthma therapy are shown in Table 7.

Indications for Antihistamines in Asthma

Despite the recent reevaluation of antihistamines in asthma, the indications for their use in this disease remain unclear. However, given the current evidence, they are unlikely to be clinically beneficial on the basis of H_1 receptor blockade alone. Nevertheless, they provide a useful tool in dissecting the role of histamine in the different forms of asthma.

ANTIHISTAMINES IN ALLERGIC RHINITIS

Histamine has been recognized as an important mediator in allergic rhinitis, and intranasal challenge with histamine reproduces all the typical symptoms of allergic rhinitis. Predosing with antihistamines in patients who are intranasally challenged with antigens to which they are naturally sensitized, effectively prevents the symptoms of sneezing, itching, and rhinorrhea during the immediate reaction to allergen. Terfenadine, loratadine, and cetirizine have been particularly useful (125); both terfenadine and loratadine inhibit histamine release in nasal lavage fluid following challenge; however, similar observations have not been made for ketotifen and cetirizine (126).

Although effective for symptoms of the early reaction after nasal challenge, both older and newer generation antihistamines have demonstrated little or no effect on nasal blockage, which is relieved significantly only when they are administered together with other decongestants (127).

In randomized, prospective, double-blind studies in patients with seasonal (Table 8) or perennial (Table 9) allergic rhinitis, the newer antihistamines have been more effective than placebo (128–130) and comparable in efficacy with the first-generation antihistamines (130–133); however, there is little difference between the newer antihistamines (72,137–139,143). Any minor differences have usually been in incidence of sedation, onset of action, and patient satisfaction (139).

There has been renewed interest in topical application of antihistamines. In a recent study, azelastine nasal spray was comparable with budesonide nasal aerosol in perennial rhinitis, but was associated with a higher incidence of unpleasant taste and smell (146).

ANTIHISTAMINES IN URTICARIA

Histamine mediates all the pathological features of urticaria: vascular permeability, vasodilation, wheals, flares, and pruritus (8). Although other mediators, such as bradykinin and leukotrienes-C_4 and D_4, play a role in vascular permeability and edema, histamine remains the only proved mediator of pruritus; it has been observed that histamine levels from the skin of individuals with urticaria are elevated compared with normal skin, despite normal circulating histamine levels (147).

Antihistamines are useful in relieving pruritus and in reducing the number, duration, and size of wheals. Of the first-generation H_1 antagonists, hydroxyzine is particularly helpful in the treatment of urticaria when compared with the older antihistamines, such as chlorpheniramine, promethazine, cyproheptadine, and diphenhydramine. None of the newer antihistamines provide total, or near total, relief of pruritus and, as a consequence, no clear "pecking order" exists in terms of potency among them (Table 10).

CONCLUDING COMMENTS

The release of histamine from mast cells and basophils undoubtedly contributes to airway obstruction in asthma; the symptoms following nasal allergen challenge; and the local edema, vascular permeability, and pruritus observed in urticaria. However, it is unlikely to play a role as a sole mediator in the clinical expression of the group of allergic diseases described and is more likely to exert its effects in allergic disease in combination with other mediators. Furthermore, following the development of potent, less-sedating antagonists to the effects of the H_1 receptor, it has been evident that these compounds exert other effects pertinent to the pathogenesis of allergic tissue responses, such as actions on the eosinophil. These non–H_1 receptor-mediated effects, could be therapeutically useful and merit further study.

REFERENCES

1. Johansson SGO. Raised levels of a new immunoglobulin class (19ND) in asthma. Lancet 1967; 42:951–953.
2. Tomioka H, Ishizaka K. Mechanism of passive sensitisation. II. Presence of receptors for IgE on monkey mast cells. J Immunol 1971; 107:971–978.
3. Black JW, Duncan WAM, Durant CJ, Ganellin CR, Parsons EM. Definition and antagonism of histamine H_2 receptors. Nature 1972; 236:385–390.
4. Arrang JM, Garbarg M, Lancelot JC, Leconte JM, Pollard H, Robba M, Schunack W, Schwartz JC. Highly potent and selective ligands for histamine H_3-receptors. Nature 1987; 327:117–123.
5. Druce HM, Kaliner MA. Allergic rhinitis. JAMA 1988; 259:260–263.
6. White MV, Slater JE, Kaliner MA. Histamine and asthma. Am Rev Respir Dis 1987; 135:1165–1176.
7. Raphael GD, Meredith SC, Baraniuk JN, Druce HM, Banks SM, Kaliner MA. The pathophysiology of rhinitis II. Assessment of the sources of protein in histamine induced nasal secretion. Am Rev Respir Dis 1989; 139:791–800.
8. Schwartz JC, Arrang JM, Garbarg M, Pollard H, A third histamine receptor subtype: characterisation, localisation and functions of the H_3 receptor. Agents Actions 1990; 30:13–23.
9. Green JP, Prell GP, Khandelwal JK, Blandina P. Aspects of histamine metabolism. Agents Actions 1987; 22:1–15.
10. Ishizaka T. Role of GTP-binding protein in histamine release from mast cells. Clin Immunol Immunopathol 1989; 50:20–29.
11. Morrison DC, Roser JF, Cochrane CG, Hensen PM. Two distinct mechanisms for the initiation of mast cell degranulation. Int Arch Allergy Appl Immunol 1975; 49:172–178.
12. Mitsuhashi M, Payan DG. Functional diversity of histamine and histamine receptors. J Invest Dermatol 1992; 98:85–115.

13. Khan MM, Melmon KL, Marr-Leisy D, Verlander MS, Egli M, Lok S, Goodman M. Congener derivatives and conjugates of histamine: synthesis and tissue receptor selectivity of the derivatives. J Med Chem 1987; 30:2115–2120.

14. Hill SJ, Young JM, Marrian DM. Specific binding of ^{3}H-mepyralline to histamine H_1 receptors in intestinal smooth muscle. Nature 1977; 270:361–363.

15. Abdel Latif AA. Calcium mobilising receptors, polyphosphoinositides and the generation of second messengers. Pharmacol Rev 1986; 38:227–272.

16. Rotrosen D, Gallin JI. Histamine type-1 receptor occupancy increases endothelial cytosolic calcium, reduces F-actin, and promotes albumin diffusion across cultured endothelial monolayers. J Cell Biol 1986; 103:2379–2387.

17. Kotilikoff MI, Murray RK, Reynolds EE. Histamine induced calcium release and phorbol antagonism in cultured airway smooth muscle cells. Am J Physiol 1987; 253:C561–C561.

18. Raeburn D, Roberts JA, Rodger IW, Thompson NC. Agonist-induced contractile responses of human bronchial muscle in vitro: effects of Ca^{2+} removal, La^{3+} and PY108068. Eur J Pharmacol 1986; 121:251–255.

19. Dereimer SA, Strong JA, Albert KA, Greengard P, Kaczmarek LK. Enhancement of calcium current in Aplysia by phorbol ester and protein-kinase C. Nature 1985; 313:313–316.

20. Kuno M, Gardner P. Ion channels activated by inositol-1,4,5,-triphosphate in plasma membrane of human T-lymphocytes. Nature 1987; 326:301–304.

21. Putney JW Jr. Calcium-mobilising receptors. Trends Pharmacol Sci 1987; 8:481–486.

22. Morris AP, Gaucher DV, Irvine RF, Peteren OH. Synergism of inositol triphosphate and tetrakophosphate in activating Ca^{+2} dependent K^+ channels. Nature 1987; 330; 653–655.

23. Hill SJ. Distribution, properties and functional characterisation of three classes of histamine receptor. Pharmacol Rev 1990; 42:45–83.

24. Roth BL. Modulation of phosphatidylinositol-4,5-biphosphate hydrolysis in rat aorta by guanine nucleotides, calcium and magnesium. Life Sci 1987; 41:629–634.

25. Nakahata N, Marin MW, Hughes AR, Heplar JR, Harden TK. H_1-histamine receptors on human astrocytoma cells. Mol Pharmacol 1986; 29:188–195.

26. Pizzi M, D'Agostini F, Da Prada M, Spanos PF. Haefely WE. Dopamine D_2 receptor stimulation decreases the inositol triphosphate level of rat striatal slices. Eur J Pharmacol 1987; 136: 263–264.

27. Haakoma EEJ, Leurs R, Timmerman H. Histamine receptors: subclasses and specific ligands. Pharmacol Ther 1990; 47:73–104.

28. Guillemette G, Bella T, Baukal AJ, Spat A, Catt KJ. Intracellular receptors for inositol-1,4,5-triphosphate in angiotensin II target tissues. J Biol Chem 1987; 262:1010–1015.

29. Sugama K, Yamashita M, Fukui S, Ito S, Wada H. Functional expression of H-histaminergic receptors in Xenopus laevis oocytes injected with bovine medullary mRNA. Jpn J Pharmacol 1991; 55:278–290.

30. Yamashita M, Fukui H, Sugama K, Horio Y, Ito S, Mizuguchi H, Wada H. Expression cloning of a cDNA encoding the bovine histamine H_1 receptor. Proc Natl Acad Sci USA 1991; 88:11515–11519.

31. McNeil JH. Histamine receptors and cyclic AMP. Can J Physiol Pharmacol 1980; 58:1028–1030.

32. Chen CS. Cholecystokinin, carbol, gastrin, histamine and forskolin increase intercellular Ca^{2+} in gastric glands. Am J Physiol 1986; 250:G814–G823.

33. Mitsuhashi M, Mitsuhashi T, Payan DG. Multiple signalling pathways of histamine H_2 receptors. Identification of an H_2 receptor-dependent Ca^{2+} mobilisation pathway in human HL-60 promylocytic leukaemia cells. J Biol Chem 1989; 264:18356–18362.

34. Gantz I, Munzert G, Tashiro T, Schaffer M, Wang L, Delvalle J, Yamada T. Molecular cloning of the human histamine H_2 receptor. Biochem Biophys Res Commun 1991; 178:1386–1392.

35. Arrang JM, Garbarg M, Schwartz JC. Auto-inhibition of brain histamine release by a novel class (H_3) of histamine receptor. Nature 1983; 302:832–837.

36. Arrang JM, Garbarg M, Schwartz JC. Autoinhibition of histamine synthesis mediated by pre-synaptic H_3 receptor. Neuroscience 1987; 23:149–157.

37. Schwartz JC, Arrang JM, Garbarg M, Pollard M, Ruat M. Histaminergic transmission in the mammalian brain. Physiol Rev 1991; 71:1–51.

38. Ichinose M, Stretton CD, Schwartz JC, Barnes PJ. Histamine H_3 receptors inhibit cholinergic neurotransmission in guinea-pig airways. Br J Pharmacol 1989; 97:13–15.

39. Ichinose M, Belvisi MG, Barnes PJ. Histamine H_3 receptors inhibit neurogenic microvascular leakage in airways. J Appl Physiol 1990; 68:21–25.

40. Windaus A, Vogt W. Synthese des Iminazolethylamins. Ber Dtsch Chem Ges 1907; 40:369.

41. Curry J. The action of histamine on the respiratory tract in normal and asthmatic subjects. J Clin Invest 1946; 25:785.

42. Halpern BN. Les antihistaminiques de synthese: essais de clinicotherapie des etats allergiques. Arch Int Pharmacodyn Ther 1942; 68:339–408.

43. Bovet D, Horclois R, Walthert F. Propiétés antihistaminiques de la N-p-methoxybenzyl-N-dimethylaminoethyl-α-amino-pyridine. CR Soc Biol (Paris) 1944; 138:99–100.

44. Lowe ER, Macmillan R, Kaiser ME. The antihistamine properties of Benadryl, β-dimethyl aminoethyl benzhydryl ether hydrochloride. J Pharmacol Exp Ther 1946; 86:229–238.

45. Meltzer EO. Antihistamine and decongestant induced performance decrements. J Occup Med 1990; 32(4):327–334.

46. Simons FER. H_1 receptor antagonists: clinical pharmacology and therapeutics. J Allergy Clin Immunol 1989; 84:845–861.

47. Valentine MD, Norman PS, Lichtenstein LM. Evaluation of an antihistamine in ragweed hay fever. In: McMahon FG, ed. Evaluation of Gastrointestinal, Pulmonary, Anti-inflammatory and Immunological Agents. New York: Futura, 1975; 227–237.

48. Diffley D, Tran VT, Snyder SH. Histamine H_1 receptor labelled in vivo: antidepressant and antihistamine interactions. Eur J Pharmacol 1980; 64:177–181.

49. Rimmer ST, Church MK, The pharmacology and mechanisms of action of histamine H_1-antagonists. Clin Exp Allergy 1990; 20:3–17.

50. Friedman HM. Loratadine: a potent, non-sedating and long acting H_1 antagonist. Am J Rhinol 1986; 1:95–99.

51. Meltzer EO, Storms WW, Pierson WE, et al. Efficacy of azelastine in perennial allergic rhinitis: clinical and rhinomanometric evaluation. J Allergy Clin Immunol 1988; 82:447–455.

52. Simons FER, Simons KJ. H_1 receptor antagonist treatment of chronic rhinitis. J Allergy Clin Immunol 1988; 81:975–980.

53. Cohen AF, Hamilton MJ, Peek AN. The effect of acrivastine (BW825C), diphenhydramine and terfenadine in combination with alcohol on human CNS performance. Eur J Clin Pharmacol 1987; 32:279–288.

54. Arunlakshana O, Schald HO. Histamine release by antihistamines. J Physiol (Lond) 1953; 119:47P–48P.

55. Page CP, Tomiak RHH, Morley J, Saunders R. Susceptibility of platelet dependent broncho-constriction by antihistamine drugs. Am Rev Respir Dis 1984; 129:A24.

56. Van Epps DR, Kutvirt SG, Potter JW. In vitro effects of cetirizine and histamine on human neutrophil function. Ann Allergy 1987; 59:13–19.

57. De Vos C. Pharmacologic modulation of allergic cutaneous inflammation. Proceedings 14th Congress European Academy of Allergol Clinical Immunology, 1989.

58. Holgate ST, Baldwin CJ, Tattersfield AE. beta Adrenergic resistance in normal airways. Lancet 1977; 2:375–377.

59. Koshimo T, Agrawal DK, Townley RG. Effect of ketotifen on the down regulation of beta adrenoreceptors in guinea pig lung and spleen. Am Rev Respir Dis 1988; 137–27.

60. Snyder SH, Snowman AM. Receptor effects of cetirizine? Ann Allergy 1987; 59:4–8.

61. Simons FER. The antiallergic effects of antihistamines (H_1-receptor antagonists). J Allergy Clin Immunol 1992; 90:705–715.

62. Trzeciakowski JD, Mendelsohn N, Levi R. Antihistamines. In: Middleton E, et al., eds. Antihistamines in Allergy; Principles and Practice. St Louis: CV Mosby, 1988:71–38.

63. Simons EF, Simons KJ. Optimum pharmacological management of chronic rhinitis. Drugs 1989; 38:314–331.

64. Bateman D, Chapman P, Rawlings M. Effects of astemizole on histamine induced wheal and flare. Eur J Clin Pharmacol 1986; 31:247.

65. Holgate ST, Emanuel M, Howarth PH. Astemizole and other H_1-antihistamine drug treatment of asthma. J Allergy Clin Immunol 1985; 76:375.

66. Howarth PH, Emanuel M, Holgate ST. Astemizole, a potent histamine H_1-receptor antagonist; effect in allergic rhinoconjunctivitis on antigen and histamine induced skin wheal responses and relationship to serum levels. Br J Clin Pharmacol 1984; 18:108.

67. Horak F, Bruttman G, Pedrali P, et al. A multi-centric study of loratadine, terfenadine and placebo in patients with seasonal allergic rhinitis. Drug Res 1988; 38:124–128.

68. Bruttman G, Chardin D, Germouth J, Horak F, Kunkel G, Wittman G. Evaluation of the efficacy and safety of loratadine in perennial allergic rhinitis. J Allergy Clin Immunol 1989; 83:411–416.

69. Monroe EW, Fox RW, Green AW, et al. Efficacy and safety of loratadine (10 mg od) in the management of idiopathic chronic urticaria. Ann Allergy 1990; 19:138–139.

70. Dockhorn RJ, Bergner A, Connell JT, et al. Safety and efficacy of loratadine (SCH 29851) a new non-sedating antihistamine in seasonal allergic rhinitis. Ann Allergy 1987; 58:407–411.

71. Boner AL, Richelli C, Castellani C, Marchesi E, Andreoli A. Comparison of the effects of loratadine and astemizole in the treatment of children with seasonal allergic rhinoconjunctivitis. Allergy 1992; 47:98–102.

72. Skassa-Brociek W, Bousquet J, Montes F, et al. Double blind controlled study of loratadine, mequitazine and placebo in the symptomatic treatment of seasonal allergic rhinitis. J Allergy Clin Immunol 1988; 81:725–730.

73. Town GI, Holgate ST. Comparison of the effect of loratadine on the airway and skin responses to histamine, methacholine and allergen in asthmatic subjects. J Allergy Clin Immunol 1990; 86:886–893.

74. Grzelewska-Rzymowska I, Gondorowicz K, Cieslenkz G, Rozniecki J, Wojcieshowsha B. [Effect of Loratadine, a sedative H_1 antagonist on histamine induced bronchoconstriction.] Pneumol Allergol Polska 1992; 60:16–21 [in Polish].

75. Cheng H, Woodward J. Antihistaminic effect of terfenadine: a new piperidine-type antihistamine. Drug Rev Res 1982; 2:181–196.

76. Henauer S, Hugonot L, Hugonot S, et al. Multi-centre, double blind comparison of terfenadine once daily versus twice daily in patients with hayfever. J Int Med Res 1987; 15:212–223.

77. Bantx EN, Dozen WK, Nelson HS. A double-blind evaluation of skin test suppression produced by two dose of terfenadine. J Allergy Clin Immunol 1987; 80:99–103.

78. Lockhart JDI, Maneksha G. Children with allergies. Terfenadine suspension plus placebo. Practitioner 1983; 227:1313–1315.

79. Dollery CT, ed. Terfenadine. In: Therapeutic Drugs. Vol. 2. New York: Churchill Livingstone, 1991:T12–T16.

80. Kemp JP, Buckley CE, Gerschwin ME, et al. Multicentre, double-blind placebo controlled trial of terfenadine in season allergic rhinitis and conjunctivitis. Ann Allergy 1985; 54:502–509.

81. Brostoff J, Lockhart JDF. Controlled trial of terfenadine and chlorpheniramine maleate in perennial rhinitis. Postgrad Med J 1982; 58:422–423.

82. Rafferty P, Holgate ST. Terfenadine (Seldane) is a potent and selective H_1 receptor antagonist in asthmatic airways. Am Rev Respir Dis 1987; 135:181–184.

83. Badier M, Beaumont D, Orehek J. Attenuation of hyperventilation induced bronchospasm by terfenadine: a new antihistamine. J Allergy Clin Immunol 1988; 81:437–440.

84. Patel KR. Terfenadine in exercise-induced asthma. Br Med J 1984; 288:1496–1497.

85. Martin UL, Romer D. The pharmacological properties of a new, orally active antianaphylactic compound: ketotifen a benzocylcoheptathiophene. Drug Res 1987; 28:770–782.

86. Mattson D, Poppins H, Nikander-Hurme R. Preventative effect of ketotifen, a new antiallergic agent on histamine induced bronchoconstriction in asthmatics. Clin Allergy 1979; 9:411–416.

87. Maclay WP, Crowder D. Post-marketing surveillance of ketotifen (Zaditen): an interim report. Res Clin Forums 1982; 4:51–57.

88. Dyson AS, Mackay AD. Ketotifen in adult asthma. Br Med J 1980; 280:360–361.

89. Lane DJ. A steroid sparing effect of ketotifen in steroid-dependent asthmatics. Clin Allergy 1980; 10:519–525.

90. Guybout P, Choffel C, Constans P, Fabre C, Robillard M. Efficacy of ketotifen in adult asthmatic patients: a six month double-blind versus placebo study. Respiration 1984; 46(suppl 1):20–21.

91. Brik A, Tashkin DP, Gong H Jr, Dauphinee B, Lee E. Effect of cetirizine, a new antihistamine H_1-antagonist, on airway dynamics and responsiveness to inhaled histamine in mild asthma. J Allergy Clin Immunol 1987; 80:51–56.

92. Wood-Baker R, Holgate ST. The comparative actions and adverse effect profile of single doses of H_1-receptor antihistamines in the airways and skin of subjects with asthma. J Allergy Clin Immunol 1993; 91:1005–1014.

93. Wasserfallen JB, Leuenberger P, Pecoud A. Effect of cetirizine, a new H_1 antihistamine, on the early and late allergic reactions in a bronchial provocation test with allergen. J Allergy Clin Immunol 1993; 91:1189–1197.

94. Fadel R, Herpin-Richard N, Rihoux JP, Henocq E. Inhibitory effect of cetirizine 2HCl on eosinophil migration in vivo. Clin Allergy 1987; 17:373–379.

95. Chand N, Diamantis W, Sofia R. Antagonism of histamine and leukotrienes by azelastine in isolated guinea pig ileum. Agents Actions 1986; 19:164–168.

96. Kemp J, Meltzer E, Orge H. A dose–response study of the bronchodilator action of azelastine in asthma. J Allergy Clin Immunol 1987; 79:893–899.

97. Magnussen H, Alba AS, Bohatiuk G, Saporito L, Lee M. The inhibitory effect of azelastine and ketotifen on histamine-induced bronchoconstriction in asthmatic patients. Chest 1987; 91:855–858.

98. Albazazz M, Patel K. Effect of azelastine in bronchoconstriction induced by histamine and leukotriene C_4 in patients with extrinsic asthma. Thorax 1988; 43:306–311.

99. Bazzano G, Gallo C, Masi C, Cocco G, Ferranti P, Melillo E, Seccia G. Effect of azelastine on the seasonal increase in non-specific bronchial responsiveness to methacholine in pollen allergic patients. A randomised double blind, placebo-controlled, crossover study. Clin Exp Allergy 1992; 22:371–377.

100. Weiler JM, Donnelly A, Campbell BH, et al. Multicentre, double blind, multiple dose, parallel groups efficacy and safety trial of azelastine, chlorpheniramine and placebo in the treatment of spring allergic rhinitis. J Allergy Clin Immunol 1988; 82:810–811.

101. Gong H Jr, Tashkin DP, Dauphinee B, Djahed B, Wu TC. Effects of oral cetirizine, a selective H_1 antagonist, on allergen- and exercise-induced bronchoconstriction in subjects with asthma. J Allergy Clin Immunol 1990; 85:632–641.

102. Rafferty P, Ng WH, Phillips G, Clough J, Church MK, Aurich R, Ollier S, Holgate ST. The inhibitory actions of azelastine hydrochloride on the early and late bronchoconstrictor responses to inhaled allergen in atopic asthma. J Allergy Clin Immunol 1989; 84:649–657.

103. Townley RG. Antiallergic properties of the second generation H_1 antihistamines during the early and late reactions to antigen. J Allergy Clin Immunol 1992; 90:720–725.

104. Hirxheimer H. Antihistamines in bronchial asthma. Br Med J 1949; 2:901–905.

105. White J, Eiser NM. The role of histamine and its receptors in the pathogenesis of asthma. Br J Dis Chest 1983; 77:215–226.

106. Bousquet J, Godard PH, Michel FB. Antihistamines in the treatment of asthma. Eur Respir J 1992; 5:1137–1142.

107. Karlin JM. The use of antihistamines in asthma. Ann Allergy 1972; 30:342–347.

108. Groggins RC, Milner AD, Stokes GM. The bronchodilator effects of chlorpheniramine in childhood asthma. Br J Dis Chest 1979; 73:279–301.

109. Schuller DE. The spectrum of antihistamines adversely affecting the pulmonary function in asthmatic children. J Allergy Clin Immunol 1983; 71:147–150.

110. Sly RM, Kemp JP, Anderson JA, et al. The use of antihistamines in patients with asthma. Position statement of the Committee on Drugs of the American Academic of Allergy and Immunology. J Allergy Clin Immunol 1988; 82:481–482.

111. Taytard A, Beaumont D, Pujet JC, Sapène M, Lewis PJ. Treatment of bronchial asthma with terfenadine: a randomised controlled trial. Br J Clin Pharmacol 1987; 24:743–746.

112. Rafferty P, Jackson L, Smith R, Holgate ST. Terfenadine, a potent histamine H_1 receptor antagonist in the treatment of pollen sensitive asthma. Br J Clin Pharmacol 1990; 30:229–235.

113. Teale C, Morrison JFJ, Pearson SB. Effects of H_1-receptor blockade with terfenadine in nocturnal asthma. Br J Clin Pharmacol 1991; 32:371–373.

114. Kurzesa A, Riedelsheimer B, Hulhoven R, Bernheim H. Cetirizine in pollen associated asthma (letter). Lancet 1989; 1:556.

115. Bousquet J, Emonot A, Germouty J, et al. Double blind multi-centre study of cetirizine in grass pollen induced asthma. Ann Allergy 1990; 65:504–508.

116. Bruttman G, Pedrali P, Arendt C, Rihoiux JD. Protective effect of cetirizine in patients suffering from pollen asthma. Ann Allergy 1990; 64:224–228.

117. Dijkman JH, Hecking PRM, Molkenboer JF, et al. Prophylactic treatment of grass pollen induced asthma with cetirizine. Clin Exp Allergy 1990; 20:483–490.

118. Backer V, Bach-Mortensen N, Becker U, Brink L, Howiz P, Hansen KK, Jensen DW, Laursen EM. Bronchial hyperresponsiveness and exercise induced asthma in children. Allergy 1989; 44:209–213.

119. Cistero A, Abadias M, Lleonart R, La Fuente V, Pinto E, Torrent H, Jane F. Effect of astemizole on allergic asthma. Ann Allergy 1992; 69:123–127.

120. Tinkelman DG, Moss BA, Bukantz SC, et al. A multi-centre trial of the prophylactic effect of ketotifen, theophylline and placebo in atopic asthma. J Allergy Clin Immunol 1985; 76:487–497.

121. Rackham A, Brown CA, Chandra RK, et al. A Canadian multi-centre study with Zadifen (ketotifen) in the treatment of bronchial asthma in children aged 5–17 years. J Allergy Clin Immunol 1989; 84:286–295.

122. Dirksen A, Engel T, Frolund L, Heinig JH, Svendsen UG, Weeke B. Effect of a nonsedative antihistamine (loratadine) in moderate asthma. A double blind, controlled, clinical cross-over trial. Allergy 1989; 44:566–571.

123. Kroll VM, Nothofer B, Werdermann K. [Allergic bronchial asthma treated with loratadine.] Forsch Med 1993; 3:76–78 [in German].

124. Tinkelman DG, Bucholtz GA, Kemp JP, Koepke JW, Repsher LH, Spector SL, Storms WW, Van-As A. Evaluation of the safety and efficacy of multiple doses of azelastine to adult patients with bronchial asthma over time. Am Rev Respir Dis 1990; 141:569–574.

125. Majchel AM, Proud D, Kagey-Sobotka A. Ketotifen reduces sneezing but not histamine release following nasal challenge with antigen. Clin Exp Allergy 1990; 20:701–705.

126. Nacleiro RM, Proud D, Kagey-Sobotka A. The effect of cetirizine on early allergic response. Laryngoscope 1989; 99:596–599.

127. Meran A, Morse J, Gibbs TG. A cross-over comparison of acrivastine, pseudoephedrine and their combination in seasonal allergic rhinitis. Rhinology 1990; 28:33–40.

128. Bedard PM, Del Carpio, Drouin MA, et al. Onset of action of loratadine and placebo and other efficacy variables in patients with seasonal allergic rhinitis. Clin Ther 1992; 10:266–275.

129. Mansmann HC Jr, Actman RA, Berman BA, et al. Efficacy and safety of cetirizine therapy in perennial allergic rhinitis. Ann Allergy 1992; 68:348–353.

130. Falliers CJ, Brandon ML, Buchman E, et al. Double blind comparison of cetirizine and placebo in the treatment of seasonal rhinitis. Ann Allergy 1991; 66:257–262.

131. Kemp JP, Buckley CE, Gershwin MR, et al. Multi-centre, double blind, placebo-controlled trial of terfenadine in seasonal allergic rhinitis and conjunctivitis. Ann Allergy 1984; 54:502–509.

132. Weler JM, Donnelly A, Campbell BH, et al. Multi-centre, double blind, multiple dose, parallel groups efficacy and safety trial of azelastine, chlorpheniramine and placebo in the treatment of spring allergic rhinitis. J Allergy Clin Immunol 1988; 82:801–811.

133. Frolund L, Etholm B, Irlander K, Johannessen TA, Odkuist L, Ohlander B, Weeke B. A multicentre study of loratadine, clemastine and placebo in patients with perennial allergic rhinitis. Allergy 1990; 45:254–261.

134. Leophonte P, Leophonte-Domairon SC, Carre JC, Goyeau E, Vaylwux M. Etude comparative de la mequitazine et de la terfenadine dans les rhinites allergiques. Allerg Immunol 1984; 16: 213–220.

135. Gervais P, Bruttmam G, Pedrali P, Charpin H, Michel FB, Griluat JP. French multicentre double-blind study to evaluate the efficacy and safety of acrivastine as compared with terfenadine in seasonal allergic rhinitis. J Int Med Res 1989; 17(suppl 2):47B–53B.

136. Del Carpio, Kabbash L, Turenng Y, et al. Efficacy and safety of loratadine (10 mg once daily), terfenadine (60 mg twice daily), and placebo in the treatment of allergic rhinitis. J Allergy Clin Immunol 1989; 84:741–746.

137. Rijntes E, Ghys L, Rihoux JP. Astemizole and cetirizine in the treatment of seasonal allergic rhinitis: a comparative, double-blind multi-centre study. J Int Med Res 1990; 18:219–224.

138. Reed CE, Aaronson DW, Bahna SL, et al. Comparison of cetirizine and astemizole treatment of seasonal allergic rhinitis. [abstract]. Ann Allergy 1991; 66:104.

139. Lockley RF, Findley S, Mitchell DQ, Woehler T, Lieberman P, Nicodemus CF. Effect of cetirizine versus terfenadine in seasonal allergic rhinitis. Ann Allergy 1993; 70:311–315.

140. Katelaris C. Comparative effects of loratadine and azelastine in the treatment of seasonal allergic rhinitis. Asian Pac J Allergy Immunol 1990; 103–107.

141. Wood SF. Oral antihistamine or nasal steroid in hay fever: a double blind, double dummy comparative study of once daily oral astemizole vs twice daily nasal beclomethasone dipropionate. Clin Allergy 1986; 16:195–201.

142. Backhouse CL, Finnamore VP, Gosden CN. Treatment of seasonal allergic rhinitis with flunisolide and terfenadine. J Int Med Res 1986; 14:35–41.

143. Renton R, Fidler C, Rodenberg R. Multicentre, crossover study of the efficacy and tolerability of terfenadine 12 mg versus cetirizine 10 mg in perennial allergic rhinitis. Ann Allergy 1991; 67:416–420.

144. Pukander JS, Varma PH, Penttila MA, Peraca ME, Ylitalo P, Kataja MJ. Mequitazine and dexchlorpheniramine in perennial rhinitis. A double-blind cross-over placebo controlled study. Rhinology 1990; 28:249–256.

145. Bunnag C, Jareoncharspi P, Wong FC. A double-blind comparison of nasal budesonide and oral astemizole for the treatment of perennial rhinitis. Allergy 1992; 47:313–317.

146. Gastpar H, Aurich R, Petzold U, et al. Intranasal treatment of perennial allergic rhinitis. Comparison of azelastine nasal spray and budesonide nasal aerosol. Arznemittelforschung 1993; 43:475–479.

147. Shalit M, Schwartz LB, Von Allmen C, et al. Release of histamine and tryptase during continuous and interrupted cutaneous challenge with allergen in humans. J Allergy Clin Immunol 1990; 86:117.

148. Paul E, Bodeker RH. Comparative study of astemizole and terfenadine in the treatment of chronic idiopathic urticaria. A randomised double-blind study of 40 patients. Ann Allergy 1989; 62:318–320.

149. Van Joost T, Blog FB, Westerhof N, et al. A comparison of acrivastine versus terfenadine and placebo in the treatment of chronic idiopathic urticaria. J Int Med Res 1989; 17(suppl 2): 14B–17B.

150. Kietzmann H, Macher E, Rihoux JP, Ghys L. Comparison of cetirizine and terfenadine in the treatment of chronic idiopathic urticaria. Ann Allergy 1990; 65:498–500.

151. Belaich S, Bruttman G, DeGreef H, Lachapelle JM, Paul E, Pedrali P, et al. Comparative effects

of loratadine and terfenadine in the treatment of chronic idiopathic urticaria. Ann Allergy 1990; 64:191–194.

152. Alomar A, De La Caudra, Fernandez J. Cetirizine vs astemizole in the treatment of chronic idiopathic urticaria. J Int Med Res 1990; 18:358–365.
153. Andri L, Senna GE, Betteli C, et al. A comparison of the efficacy of cetirizine and terfenadine. Allergy 1993; 48:258–265.
154. Fredriksson Hersle K, Hjorth N, Mobacken H, et al. Terfenadine in chronic urticaria: a comparison with clemastine and placebo. Cutis 1986; 38:128–130.
155. Paul E, Bodeker RH. Treatment of chronic urticaria with terfenadine and ranitidine—a randomised double-blind study in 45 patients. Eur J Clin Pharmacol 1986; 31:277–280.
156. Grant JA, Bernstein DI, Buckley CI, et al. Double-blind comparison of terfenadine chlorpheniramine and placebo in the treatment of chronic idiopathic urticaria. J Allergy Clin Immunol 1988; 81:574–579.
157. Boggs PB, Ellis CN, Grossman J, et al. Double blind placebo-controlled study of terfenadine and hydroxyzine in patients with chronic idiopathic urticaria. Ann Allergy 1989; 63:616–620.
158. Kalivas J, Breneman D, Tharp M, Bruce S, Bigby M. Urticaria: clinical efficacy of cetirizine in comparison with hydroxyzine and placebo. J Allergy Clin Immunol 1990; 86:1014–1018.
159. Sussman G, Jan Celenicz Z. Controlled trial of H_1 antagonists in the treatment of chronic idiopathic urticaria. Ann Allergy 1991; 67:433–439.
160. Monroe EN, Bernstein DI, Fox RN, et al. Relative efficacy and safety of loratadine, hydroxyzine and placebo in chronic idiopathic urticaria. Arzneimittelforschung 1992; 42:1119–1121.
161. Honsinger RN Jr, Thomsen RJ. Prolonged benefit in the treatment of chronic idiopathic urticaria with aztemizole. Ann Allergy 1990; 65:194–200.
162. Woodward JK. Pharmacology and toxicology of nonclassical antihistamines. Cutis 1988; 42(4A):5.

26

Pharmacological Modulation of Bronchial Challenges: Direct, Indirect, and Antigen

Russell J. Hopp and Robert G. Townley
Creighton University School of Medicine, Omaha, Nebraska

BACKGROUND

Asthma is recognized clinically by reversible airway obstruction and airway hyperrespon-siveness. Airway hyperresponsiveness is essential to the definition of asthma, and an understanding of its mechanism is crucial to the elucidation of the pathogenesis of asthma (1–4). The severity of asthma is correlated with the degree of hyperresponsiveness (1–4). In asthma, airway hyperresponsiveness appears to arise from both genetic and acquired mechanisms, but increased airways responsiveness can be temporarily associated with exposure to environmental stimuli, such as allergens, infection, or ozone (5). A recent study reported (6) that bronchial hyperresponsiveness can exist in healthy subjects (PC_{20} FEV_1 to histamine < 8 mg/ml), without histological evidence for inflammation, which supports a noninflammatory explanations for its presence (6; Fig. 1).

Bronchial challenges, using both physiological (indirect) and pharmacological (direct) methods, have provided an important tool to advance the understanding of airway reactivity and the pathogenesis of bronchial asthma. The purpose of such testing includes diagnosis, occupational screening, research, epidemiology, and evaluation of the efficacy of various pharmacological agents for the treatment of asthma (5–8). Precise inhalation methods are essential for the study of airway hyperresponsiveness, regardless of the purpose of such testing, and detailed reviews of the methodology of measuring airway responsiveness have been published (9,10).

Although the asthmatic individual shows hyperresponsiveness to a wide variety of indirect and direct challenges, it is quite certain that there are important differences in the mechanism whereby these stimuli induced bronchoconstriction. Methacholine or histamine directly induces smooth-muscle constriction; exercise, inhalation of cold, dry air, or inhala-tion of ultrasonically nebulized distilled water (UNDW) appear to do this by more indirect mechanisms, including mast cell mediator release. Furthermore, the response to the direct

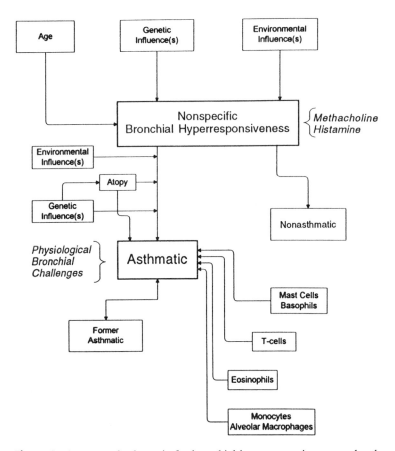

Figure 1 A proposed schematic for bronchial hyperresponsiveness and asthma.

stimuli provides a more sensitive parameter than that of the indirect stimuli. The latter, however, provides a higher degree of specificity. Thus, all current asthmatics respond to methacholine inhalation, whereas only 75–80% will respond to the various indirect stimuli to the point of resulting in a 20% decrease in the 1-s forced expiratory volume (FEV_1) (3,11,12).

The differences between the direct and physiological (indirect) challenges are both qualitative and quantitative. Tests with exercise, inhaled water, or hyperventilation of cold, dry air will not produce a response of 20% fall in the FEV_1 in subjects without asthma, even with the maximum stimulus. In contrast, direct challenges with methacholine or histamine can produce significant airway narrowing in some subjects without asthma.

INDICATIONS FOR TESTING

The primary clinical indication for inhalation challenge with methacholine, histamine, UNDW, or cold air hyperventilation challenge (CAHC) is to identify the presence of bronchial reactivity, an essential component of the asthmatic state (1,7,8,13–18). A negative methacholine challenge test rules out current bronchial asthma and would guide the clinician to consider other causes of bronchial disease, such as tumor, bronchiectasis, or possibly chronic bronchitis.

In the research setting, studies using indirect, direct, or antigen challenge can be used to determine the potential efficacy of a pharmacological agent, either as a potential agent for clinical use or to investigate the pathophysiology of asthma. In this chapter we review the effects of pharmacological agents on bronchial challenge tests. The pertinent methods of bronchial challenge procedures as they relate to performing these tests in the evaluation of pharmacological agents are reviewed. Detailed methods for the different challenge procedures have been published (9,10).

MEASUREMENT OF RESPONSE

The FEV_1 remains as the most important measurement of airway responsiveness and should be included in all pharmacological studies. Its virtues are its simplicity and reproducibility, and its measurement is readily available. It also provides the best differentiation between patients who have asthma and those who do not. Other tests may be used; however, it is important that an FEV_1 is also included for comparison.

Other commonly used tests are airway resistance and conductance (R_{aw} and SG_{aw}), and partial expiratory flow volume curves. These measurements provide sensitive measures of response and avoid the full inspiratory maneuver of the FEV_1, which may have a minimal bronchodilator effect. Therefore, they are useful for measuring responses to a smaller stimulus, or if the challenge agent (procedure) is only minimally effective as a bronchoconstrictor. Changes in these parameters can be obtained even when nonasthmatics are challenged with agents that would not ordinarily produce a PD_{20} FEV_1. They have the disadvantage of being more variable and less reproducible than the FEV_1.

FACTORS INFLUENCING RESPONSE

Factors that can influence the response to bronchial challenge should be avoided, or if unavoidable, taken into consideration in evaluating bronchial challenge results. These include acute viral respiratory infections, bacterial respiratory infections, and pollutants, such as NO_2 and SO_2, that are known to increase reactivity. Seasonal exposure to naturally occurring antigen or recent antigen challenge may increase airway hyperresponsiveness. Similarly, the power of suggestion can also influence airway reactivity.

EXPRESSION OF RESULTS

Each challenge procedure has particular characteristics, with different methods of reporting results. this has been previously reviewed (10). The purpose of using an investigational drug is to determine the effect of that drug on the bronchial responsiveness to a bronchial challenge procedure that has reasonable similarity to that inducing the underlying immediate bronchoconstriction seen in asthma (direct challenges) or that which may occur in the daily life of the asthmatic (antigen, exercise, cold air).

The PD_{20} FEV_1 is the usual method of expressing results of a bronchoprovocation test. Some subjects without asthma, particularly those with allergic rhinitis, may have a positive reaction to histamine or methacholine, as evidenced by attaining an FEV_1 PD_{20}, and then demonstrating a plateau phenomenon (2,3,19,20). In these subjects, further administration of methacholine or histamine will fail to produce progressive airway narrowing. In contrast, patients with asthma, when administered increasing doses of inhaled histamine or methacholine, have a progressive airway narrowing. Woolcock et al. (20) and Townley et al. (2,3,19) have shown that when a FEV_1 PD_{35} is used, one can clearly differentiate individuals with this plateau phenomena versus those with asthma. However, as one goes beyond the FEV_1 PD_{35} a concern for the severity of airway narrowing makes further administration of the bronchoconstrictive agent too uncomfortable or dangerous (19,20).

An important advantage of determining the area under the dose–response curve is that it allows quantitative measurements in subjects who never achieve a 20% fall in FEV_1 (PD_{20} FEV_1) to either histamine or methacholine (2,19,20). The determination of an area under the dose–response curve is not necessary for diagnostic studies, but it is valuable in epidemiological and pharmacological studies.

REPRODUCIBILITY

It is preferable to assess the airway response to mediators at the same time of day as circadian variation in histamine levels has been observed. The 95% confidence limits for the reproducibility of the PC_{20} for methacholine and histamine challenges done on different days with an interval of 1–2 weeks was $\pm$ 1 single twofold concentration (21). This same degree of reproducibility was shown for both the dosimeter and continuous tidal breathing methods (21).

DIRECT BRONCHIAL CHALLENGES

Histamine and Methacholine

Of the pharmacological challenge agents, methacholine and histamine are the most commonly used and have been well standardized. Methacholine is a parasympathomimetic agent that appears to directly stimulate the muscarinic receptors on bronchial smooth muscles, increasing the bronchomotor activity. Methacholine is inhibited by atropine and its analogues (2,5,22). Histamine induces bronchoconstriction, primarily by a direct histamine receptor-mediated bronchoconstrictive effect and partly by reflex vagal stimulation (22).

Methacholine and histamine are both extensively used in research as well as in diagnostic testing, and the methodology of testing has been previously reviewed (10).

Other Pharmacological (Direct) Agents

Bronchial challenges with methacholine or histamine have widespread clinical applications; however, research in asthma includes bronchial provocation testing with various other chemicals. Many of these agents are known to be released during mast cell-dependent events and may partially mimic naturally occurring asthma. These agents are not likely to be widely used, except as tools for the investigation of basic mechanisms in asthma.

The technical aspects, as they related to inhalation challenge tests with these agents, are quite variable when compared with more standardized challenge protocols. It is important for investigators to clearly outline the inhalation technique used to permit a comparison between studies. Dose concentrations and nebulizer outputs should be detailed in published manuscripts.

Prostaglandin-D_2 (PGD_2) is released in significant amounts after immunoglobulin (Ig)E-mediated stimulation of human lung mast cells. Inhaled PGD_2 has an effect on airways that is ten times more potent than that of histamine (23). The PGD_2 activity is mediated through thromboxane receptors in the lung (24). Prostaglandin D_2 had a minimal effect in normal subjects (23), whereas $PGF_{2\alpha}$ showed no effect at various doses in normal subjects (25).

Leukotrienes (LT)C_4, LTD_4, and LTE_4 have potent bronchoconstrictive properties in humans (26). In vitro, LTD_4 is up to 6000 times more potent than histamine or methacholine (27), supporting a direct mode of action. In vivo, the leukotrienes are up to 1000 times more potent than methacholine (28). A metabolite of LTC_4 and LTD_4, LTE_4 is recoverable in increased amounts in urine following allergen challenge in allergic and asthmatic subjects (29). Leukotriene receptors are found in human airways and lung homogenates (30).

Asthmatics respond to neurokinin-A with a bronchospastic response, and the response appears to be partly mediated through a direct mechanism (31).

INDIRECT BRONCHIAL CHALLENGES

As with inhalation studies of methocholine, histamine, and antigen, graded exercise and cold air hyperventilation (CAHC) can also produce bronchoconstriction in susceptible individuals. These tests are used to assess latent asthma, evaluate the severity of known exercise-induced bronchoconstriction, and to evaluate the effects of medications (11,16,17). The specificity approaches 100%; however, the sensitivity varies from 50 to 100%, depending on the criteria for a positive response. Reproducibility is high if performed more than 2 h apart (32). A detailed review of the methods involved with these challenges has been previously published (10).

Exercise

Exercise studies entail free running, treadmill running, and the cycloergometer (33). Free running, though, has many uncontrollable factors that make the test less than optimal (33). As a result, treadmill running and cycle studies in a controlled environment are more popular.

Cold Air Hyperventilation

In those whom exercise testing is contraindicated, cold air hyperventilation may be used to produce similar results; a good correlation exists between the two (18,34,35). Isocapnic hyperventilation is a variation of a cold air challenge, substituting dry, room temperature air for dry subfreezing air (36).

Ultrasonic Nebulized Distilled Water Challenge

Anesthesiologists were first to observe an increase in airway resistance after inhalation of ultrasonicated water. Allegra and Bianco used UNDW as bronchial provocation in 1974 (37). Anderson introduced a dose–response curve and calculated the PD_{20} of UNDW (38).

The test appears to be very specific, but the sensitivity ranges between 30 and 100% (20). The correlation of UNDW challenge to methacholine is variable; there is a better correlation with exercise and CAHC (39).

Hypertonic aerosols with osmolarity up to 1280 have been used as a bronchial challenge.

The bronchoconstriction induced by inhalation of 3.6% normal saline was equal to that induced by UNDW inhalation (40), although the mechanism of the two challenges is not necessarily equivalent (41).

Other Indirect Challenges

Platelet-activating factor (PAF) has been implicated as an active bronchoconstrictive agent in vivo, but not in vitro, suggesting an indirect mechanism of action. A recent study suggested leukotriene release is responsible for the measurable bronchoconstriction induced by PAF inhalation (42).

Adenosine inhalation challenges (adenosine 5'-monophosphate; AMP) have gained limited use, predominantly in the United Kingdom. Adenosine, and its precursor nucleotide AMP, induces bronchial constriction in asthmatics, but not in normal individuals (43). Adenosine likely induced bronchoconstriction through release of mediators from mast cells by A_2-purinoceptor stimulation (44), although additional mechanisms have been suggested (45,46).

The well-recognized clinical observation that β-adrenergic receptor blocking agents can induce bronchoconstriction in asthmatics has resulted in the use of a propranolol-inhalation challenge procedure. Propranolol sensitivity in asthmatics is less than that seen with histamine (47) or methacholine (48). Propranolol-induced bronchoconstriction is thought to be caused indirectly, partially through the release of mast cell mediators (49).

Following the ingestion of aspirin, a percentage of asthmatics will experience bronchospasm, nasal symptoms, and hives. Bronchial challenge can be performed using lysine-aspirin, which elicits bronchoconstriction in aspirin-sensitive, but not in aspirin-nonsensitive asthmatics. The observation that aspirin or lysine-aspirin induces an increase in urinary LTE_4 suggests an indirect mode for aspiring bronchoconstriction (50,51).

Asthmatics, but not normal persons, bronchoconstrict to inhaled bradykinin, kallidin, but not desArg9-bradykinin (52). Bradykinin and kallidin are bradykinin$_2$ receptor agonists, and desArg9-bradykinin is a bradykinin$_1$ receptor agonist. Bradykinin-induced bronchoconstriction probably has an indirect mechanism of action.

Metabisulfite challenges are occasionally performed. The profile of agents that protect against this agent suggest an indirect method of action.

ALLERGEN

Antigen provocation was first described by Lowell and Schiller (53). It is widely used by many investigators as a research tool as it has the advantage of duplicating the early- and late-phase responses of clinical asthma. In addition, the late-phase response is often associated with a significant increase in nonspecific bronchial reactivity. This provides the opportunity to test an investigational agent for its effect on the early- or late-phase change in airway caliber, and its potential benefit in ameliorating the change in bronchial hyperresponsiveness.

There is a good correlation between skin tests and in vitro tests and bronchial provocation. The stronger the skin reaction, the greater the chance of positive bronchial provocation (1,54). A recent report has suggested that an allergen challenge test to determine an early asthmatic response to a particular antigen could be replaced with a skin test and a measure of nonspecific bronchial reactivity (55). Pollens, house dust mites, molds, and animal danders have been used in antigen provocation tests.

PHARMACOLOGICAL MODULATION OF DIRECT CHALLENGES

Overview

A wide variety of pharmacological agents, many currently used in clinical asthma treatment, provide insights into the mechanism of action of the different bronchial challenge procedures. The immediate bronchial responses of all direct challenges are completely or largely inhibited by β-adrenergic receptor agonists. The action of other pharmacological antagonists against direct bronchial challenges will be reviewed.

Methacholine, Histamine, and Other Direct Challenges

Pharmacological antagonism is the only possible method available for inhibiting or attenuating bronchoconstriction caused by methacholine or histamine. All β_2-adrenergic agonists, both short- and long-acting, can block both histamine and methacholine bronchoconstriction (56–58). Atropine and atropine analogues can successfully block methacholine-induced bronchoconstriction through the mechanism of receptor antagonism (2,5,22), whereas muscarinic blockers partially attenuate histamine challenges (22). Oral antihistamines attenuate histamine challenges by competitive antagonism of the H_1 receptor (59). Antihistamines do not have anticholinergic properties against methacholine challenge (59).

In a recent report, inhaled gallopamil (60) attenuated the histamine response in asthmatics, but not the methacholine response, suggesting an involvement of voltage-dependent Ca^{2+} channels in histamine-induced bronchoconstriction. Oxatomide, an inhibitor of the release of allergic mediators, including histamine, has a chemical structure similar to calcium antagonists and interferes with intracellular calcium release and calcium uptake. Oral administration significantly shifted the dose–response to metacholine to the right in nine asthmatic children, using a double-blind, placebo-controlled crossover (DPPCCS) study design (61). This would suggest involvement of intracellular calcium movement in methacholine-induced bronchoconstriction.

Inhaled furosemide does not modify methacholine (62) or histamine (63) bronchial responsiveness.

Bronchoconstriction mediated by inhaled PGD_2 is mediated by thromboxane receptors in the lung. BAY u 3405 a selective thromboxane-A_2 receptor antagonist significantly attenuated PGD_2 challenges in a double-blind, placebo controlled, crossover study of 12 asthmatics (64), with a geometric mean PC_{20} for PGD_2 of 0.0380 ± 2.6 before antagonist and 0.554 ± 5.9. One-half of the subjects did not bronchoconstrict to the top dose of PGD_2 (2 mg/ml) while receiving active drug.

Leukotriene D_4-induced bronchoconstriction is potent, rapid, and relatively long-lasting (65). Its action is not inhibited by lidocaine, inhaled atropine, or cyclooxygenase inhibitors (66,67). An oral leukotriene receptor antagonist zafirlukast (ICI 204,219) provided a marked protective effect (117-fold) against LTD_4-induced bronchospasm (measured using SG_{aw}) in six nonasthmatics, 2 h after drug administration, with a residual effect (ninefold) at 12 h, in a DBPCCS (65). Oral SR 2640, an LTD_4–LTE_4 antagonist attenuated LTD_4-induced bronchoconstriction by 48% (11–137%; 68). Leukotriene receptor antagonists have been used against other bronchial challenges, predominantly indirect, and will subsequently be reviewed.

PHARMACOLOGICAL MODULATION OF INDIRECT CHALLENGES

Overview

The presumed mode of action of all indirect challenges is by mast cell degranulation. The predominate mast cell mediators considered have been histamine, prostaglandins, adenosine, and leukotrienes. Specific receptor antagonists and synthesis inhibitors of these mast cell mediators have been evaluated for their protection against indirect bronchial challenge-induced bronchospasm.

As mentioned for direct challenges, the β_2-adrenergic receptor agonists inhibit the bronchospasm induced by any indirect challenge, and will not be discussed for each challenge, unless of particular interest or study design.

Exercise

Exercise challenge is considered the grandfather of all other "natural" (physiological) bronchial challenges, and the pharmacological approach to exercise-induced asthma (EIA) has been closely duplicated and has been similarly successfully (or unsuccessfully), for cold air, ultrasonic distilled water, isocapnic hyperventilation, and hypertonic saline challenges.

The oral thromboxane receptor antagonist BAY u 3405 has been used to investigate the role of PGD_2 in combined CAHC- and exercise-induced asthma protocol (64). Twelve adult asthmatics performed a 6-min bicycle ergomometer exercise while breathing cold air ($-15°C$). After challenge pulmonary function was monitored for 30 min. In a DPPCCS the agent had no bronchodilator properties and did not block the EIA–CAHC challenge, which suggests PGD_2 does not play a role in indirect challenges using exercise and cold air. Another thromboxane receptor antagonist vapiprost (GR32191) was also ineffective against EIA (69).

Cromolyn sodium and nedocromil sodium both significantly attenuate EIA, although the protection is not complete or universal, and it is clearly dose-dependent (70).

Furosemide, a loop diuretic, significantly attenuates exercise challenge (71). In fact, furosemide has a profile of action that closely mimics cromolyn sodium. Furosemide protection against bronchoconstriction is reduced if subjects are pretreated with indomethacin (72), suggesting an involvement with the bronchodilating PGE_2. However, inhaled furosemide alone has not consistently induced bronchodilation.

Anticholinergic agents are minimally effective against EIA, certainly owing to bronchodilation (73). Similarly, theophylline has bronchodilator properties and is partially effective in EIA in some patients (70).

The antihistamine, terfenadine, at doses higher than standard therapy, has significantly attenuated EIA, providing direct evidence for the action of histamine, released from mast cells, in exercise challenge responsiveness (70). In addition, a leukotriene receptor antagonist, MK 571, attenuated exercise challenges, strongly suggesting a role for these products, presumably released from mast cells (70).

Several calcium channel blockers have shown some benefit in EIA. This suggests a role for calcium movement in the induction of bronchospasm, either at a membrane level (calcium channels) or by the release of stored intracellular calcium. The protection is neither complete, nor universal, but provides further avenues for investigation.

Oxatomide, an inhibitor of the release of allergic mediators, including histamine, has a chemical structure similar to calcium antagonists, and interferes with intracellular calcium release and calcium uptake. In a DPPCCS in nine asthmatic children, the mean maximal percentage fall in FEV_1 improved from 22 to 13.5% ($p < 0.05$) with administration of oxatomide (61).

Hyperventilation of Cold Air or Dry Air

In general, the profile of action of agents used in EIA, when evaluated, have been successful in attenuating bronchospasm caused by CAHC or by dry air (ISH). Inhaled dry air and CAHC are likely more potent stimuli, given a similar amount of minute ventilation between EIA, CAHC, and ISH (70). Isocapnic hyperventilation challenge increases recoverable leukotrienes in bronchoalveolar lavage fluid (74).

Medications with significant, but partial, benefit in EIA may have less protection against CAHC or ISH. These would include cromolyn, nedocromil, terfenadine, calcium antagonists, and furosemide (70). Atropine analogues appear minimally effective in ISH (70).

Acetazolamide, a diuretic, but not an inhibitor of the $Na^+/K^+/2Cl^-$ cotransporter, significantly attenuated CAHC in a DBPCCS (75) and compared favorably to furosemide (75). In another study (76), amiloride, an Na^+ channel blocker, did not protect against ISH, whereas in the same subjects furosemide significantly attenuated ISH. In the study of O'Donnell et al. (75) furosemide actually caused bronchodilation, an observation that is unique to this report.

The 5-lipoxygenase inhibitor zileuton (A-64077) allowed 13 asthmatics to tolerate 47% more ($p < 0.002$) cold air hyperventilation to induce a 20% fall in FEV_1 when compared with placebo (77). The leukotriene receptor antagonist tomelukast (LY171883) attenuated the CAHC by 20%, compared with placebo, in a 2-week oral prechallenge treatment schedule (78). The magnitude of attenuation would suggest a modest leukotriene release by CAHC, or to a meager blockade of the LTD_4 effect by tomelukast.

The oral antihistamine terfenadine attenuates bronchial challenges with CAHC (79).

Distilled Water and Hyperosmolar Saline Challenges

The assumption is that, although similar, the exact mechanism of UNDW- and hyperosmolar saline (HS)-induced bronchoconstriction may not be the same (41). It has been argued the parallel responses for HS challenge and EIA collaborate the theory for "osmolarity" changes in the airway. Similar reasoning would extend to UNDW and EIA. In large part, agents effective in CAHC and ISH, when studied, have been successful in attenuating HS or UNDW challenges. These include cromolyn, nedocromil, furosemide, and terfenadine.

Oral aspirin, but not oral sodium salicylate, significantly attenuated the UNDW bronchial response in a dose-dependent manner (80). Additionally, inhaled lysine-aspirin and indomethacin, but not inhaled sodium salicylate, significantly attenuated UNDW challenges in asthmatics (81). These results suggested a role for prostaglandin synthesis in UNDW-induced bronchoconstriction.

Inhaled furosemide attenuates HS bronchoconstriction (82); and furosemide was significantly effective against UNDW challenge, although the protection was variable, as some asthmatics were equally responsive to UNDW even after furosemide administration (83). Torasemide, although two to four times more effective than furosemide as a diuretic, was less protective than furosemide against UNDW, although the overall protection afforded by inhaled torasemide was significant (83). When inhaled, piretanide, a loop diuretic, was effective in attenuating bronchial responses to UNDW in a dose-dependent fashion in a randomized single-blind, placebo-controlled protocol (84). Piretanide had a marked diuretic effect in this study, which generally has not been seen in various studies using inhaled furosemide, with the exception of a study by O'Donnell et al. (75).

The oral antihistamine terfenadine significantly attenuates the bronchoconstriction induced by nebulized distilled water (79).

Studies using different diuretics in physiological challenges (UNDW, HS, CAHC) suggest that the pharmacokinetics of the agent is a critical component for success. Effectiveness may depend on factors, such as lipid solubility, that would influence the absorption property and contact time with the airway. There has been variable evidence for a bronchodilation after inhaled furosemide, which would raise the possibility that protective prostaglandins are released. The ability to release the bronchodilator PGE_2 may be variable in asthmatics, accounting for a variable response in individual asthmatics, but with an overall protective benefit in a study population.

Atrial natriuretic peptide (ANP) has a bronchodilator action in normal and asthmatic persons when given intravenously. In an interesting study, intravenous ANP, at increasing doses, attenuated UNDW challenge at doses of ANP below the bronchodilator dose (85). ANP reduces bronchial activity to histamine in asthmatics (86).

It has been suggested that hypertonic saline challenge induces bronchoconstriction by neurogenic reflexes. In support of a role for neurogenic reflexes, was a study using ten asthmatics with positive responses to HS who received atropine (0.6 mg intramuscularly), ipratropium bromide (500 μg in 2 ml saline by inhalation), or lidocaine hydrochloride (2 ml by inhalation) in a random fashion (87). Atropine and ipratropium caused small (not significant) improvements in FEV_1, and lidocaine induced a small decrease in FEV_1. Premedication with atropine, ipratropium bromide, and lidocaine afforded a 2.5, 2.0, and 2.6 times improvement in HS responsiveness. The protection was, however, variable among subjects, suggesting individual differences in the importance of vagal and neurogenic mechanisms in HS challenge. Similar variability has been seen in EIA (88) and with UNDW (89).

Other Indirect Challenges

Adenosine (Adenosine 5'-Monophosphate)

Challenges with adenosine or AMP are almost totally blocked using the antihistamines terfenadine or astemizole (90,91). Ipatropium bromide has a singular modest (2.5 times) effect on PC_{20} AMP and an additive benefit with terfenadine (9.5 times) in inhibiting AMP-bronchoconstriction, whereas terfenadine alone afforded a 5.3 times protective effect in this study (92).

Not surprisingly, inhaled furosemide significantly attenuated AMP challenge and shifted the dose–response curve to the right in all 12 subjects evaluated (44). In the same study, inhaled bumetadine, a diuretic with a site of action dissimilar to that of furosemide, when given in a dose equidiuretic to furosemide, also shifted the dose–response curve to the right in 9 of the 12 subjects, and significantly attenuated the AMP response overall, but less than did the furosemide, which was 2.5 times more potent.

Both cromolyn and nedocromil give significant protection against adenosine challenge, with nedocromil having greater protection (93).

Aspirin and Lysine-Aspirin

The observation that aspirin or lysine-aspirin induces an increase in urinary LTE_4 suggests an indirect mode for aspirin bronchoconstriction (50,51). An inhibitor of 5-lipoxygenase (5-LO), zileutin, was evaluated in eight aspirin-sensitive asthmatics. Oral zileutin completely abolished the fall in FEV_1 after the ingestion of aspirin in a DBPCCS design (51). The usefulness of leukotriene receptor antagonists against lysine-aspirin was using oral verlukast (MK-0679). In a DPPCCS 750 mg of verlukast inhibited the bronchoconstriction induced by inhaled lysine-aspirin in eight aspirin-sensitive asthmatics (mean shift 4.4-fold; 94). Collectively, these findings provide evidence for 5-LO products as critical mediators in aspirin-sensitive asthmatics.

Inhaled furosemide significantly attenuated the bronchial response to inhaled lysine-aspirin in six female aspirin-sensitive asthmatics (95). The FEV_1 fell below 20% in all subjects with placebo, and in none of the six after furosemide.

Platelet-Activating Factor

Platelet-activating factor challenges were not inhibited by pretreatment with the oral antihistamine terfenadine (96). Surprisingly, the leukotriene D_4 receptor antagonist zafirlukast (ICI 204,219) attenuated PAF challenges in normals (42). Platelet-activating factor antagonists inhibit the action of inhaled platelet-activating factor (97).

Propranolol

Propranolol challenges are modestly attenuated with cromolyn sodium and nedocromil sodium (98). Cromolyn, however, significantly protects against propranolol (99). In a double-blind, crossover design, inhaled ipratropium bromide at 40 and 160 μg did not block propranolol challenge, whereas, in the same subject, inhaled fenoterol at 800 μg shifted the PC_{20} of propranolol twofold (100). The authors suggest the findings argue against a cholinergic influence on propranolol bronchoconstriction. Intramuscular oxyphenonium bromide (2 mg) was able to shift the dose–response curve to propranolol, suggesting an influence of cholinergic activity in propranolol challenge, in this study intramuscular fenoterol had only a slight effect on propranolol reactivity (48). A very recent study (101) showed that pilocarpine, an agonist of M_2-muscarinic receptors that inhibits acetycholine release, attenuated the response to inhaled propranolol. The authors suggested that β-adrenergic receptor blockers inhibit endogenous catecholamine activity, allowing unopposed muscarinic activity, to which the asthmatic is inherently sensitive.

These conflicting results leave the issue of propranolol-induced responsiveness in asthmatics open to continued study.

Metabisulfite

Both inhaled furosemide (frusemide; 40 mg) and piretanide (24 mg), loop diuretics, significantly attenuated the bronchoconstriction in 12 mild asthmatics (102). Both agents induced a significant diuresis that lasted 24 h. Furosemide was more potent than piretanide, inducing a 3.8-fold shift in the PC_{20} to metabisulfite, compared with a 2.5-fold shift with piretanide, although neither agent protected beyond 90 min after administration of the inducing agent. Amiloride, unlike furosemide, had no effect on metabisulfite (103), nor did bumetanide (63). Inhaled ipratropium bromide modestly attenuated metabisulfite, but was variable among studied subjects (104).

Both cromolyn and nedocromil significantly attenuate metabisulfite challenges, and nedocromil is more potent (105). The prostaglandin PGE_2 significantly (mean 2.5 doubling doses) attenuating metabisulfite challenge, but did not cause a significant increase in FEV_1 (106). The selective H_3-receptor antagonist (R)-α-methylhistamine did not affect metabisulfite responsiveness (107).

Neuropeptides

Oral terfenadine failed to protect against neurokinin A-induced bronchoconstriction (108), and oral astemizole was unable to block substance P-induced bronchoconstriction (109). These results would support the hypothesis that histamine, released from mast cells or basophils, plays no role in neuropeptide-induced bronchoconstriction in asthma. The inhalation of ipratropium bromide induced a small, but significant, shift in the dose–response curve to substance P (109).

Oxitropium bromide did not protect against neurokinin A-induced bronchoconstriction in mild asthmatic subjects (110). Inhaled nedocromil sodium had a significant effect on the FEV_1 response to neurokinin A challenge, with a twofold shift (111).

The specific tachykinin (neurokinin) receptor antagonist FK224 significantly attenuated (eightfold) bradykinin-induced bronchoconstriction in ten asthmatics (112). The pharmacological modulation of bradykinin challenges using terfenadine and flurbiprofen in separate evaluations showed small, but significant, attenuation, suggesting histamine and prostanoids have a modest contribution to bradykinin-induced bronchoconstriction (113).

PHARMACOLOGICAL MODULATION OF ANTIGEN CHALLENGES

Antigen challenge-induced bronchospasm can be demonstrated in both allergic asthmatics and in subjects with allergic rhinitis, strongly supporting the intimate role of mast cells in this process, separate from the condition of being asthmatic. The morbidity and scope of this phenomenon in allergic rhinitis has not been adequately evaluated. For example, given similar degrees of skin titration responsiveness to an antigen, are allergic rhinitis subjects with preexisting bronchial hyperresponsiveness more responsive to inhaled antigen than are allergic rhinitis subjects with minimal or no nonspecific bronchial responsiveness? Which allergic rhinitis subjects have late asthmatic responses to antigen? Do allergic rhinitis subjects react to pharmacological modulation of an antigen challenge—both early and late phases—similarly to asthmatics?

It has long been presumed that the early phase of antigen-induced bronchoconstriction is due to released mast cell mediators, and the use of specific receptor antagonists or production inhibitors would attenuate a portion of the bronchoconstriction. The late phase appears to have a major inflammatory component and, thus, is multifactorial; therefore, only a broad-spectrum approach could attenuate this segment of the antigen challenge. In many ways, the model has been supported by the findings of pharmacological modulation.

The early-phase response to inhaled antigen, when compared with placebo, is significantly attenuated by nonsedating antihistamines (114–117), various oral leukotriene receptor antagonists (118–120), and synthesis inhibitors (121). Prostaglandin synthesis inhibitors have a minimal role in early-phase protection, suggesting a role for prostaglandins or thromboxane (122), whereas platelet-activating factor has minimal to no effect on the early-phase response (123).

Standard β_2-adrenergic agonists (124) and inhaled PGE_2 (125) block early antigen challenges because β-agonists provided pharmacological antagonism to the bronchospastic mediators inducing bronchoconstriction, and PGE_2, although a mild bronchodilator, appears to have an alternative pathway of protection (125). The new long-acting bronchodilators appear to have effects on the late-phase antigen response (126,127). High doses of the standard β_2-adrenergic agonist albuterol attenuates both the early- and late-phase response to antigen challenge (128). This raises the possibility that all β_2-adrenergic agonists, when given at sufficient doses, can attenuate the late-phase responses, either as antibronchospastic or, potentially, as anti-inflammatory agents.

Inhaled furosemide (129), cromolyn sodium (124), and nedocromil sodium (130–132), all attenuate the early-phase and late-phase response after antigen challenge. The mechanism involved in the protection afforded by these three drugs remains an enigma. A recent study has suggested that cromolyn sodium has tachykinin antagonist properties, affecting both substance P and neurokinin B activity (133). In vitro animal studies have recently shown that furosemide may have an inhibitory effect on sensory and cholinergic nerves (134). This line of investigation is pertinent, as cromolyn, nedocromil, and furosemide all have similar profiles against indirect challenges, but not against direct challenges.

Theophylline (135) and atropine analogues (136) provide marginal protection against the early-phase response to allergen. Inhaled corticosteroids attenuate the late-phase antigen response (124).

Other than exercise challenge, allergen bronchial challenge provides clinical correlation with the daily life of an asthmatic. The lessons learned using research studies of allergen challenge pharmacological modulation are beneficial and applicable to clinical practice.

REFERENCES

1. Townley RG, Dennis M, Itkin JM. Comparative action of acetyl-beta-methacholine, histamine and pollen antigens in subjects with hay fever and patients with bronchial asthma. J Allergy 1965; 36:121–137.
2. Townley RG, Bewtra AK, Nair NH, Brodkey FD, Watt GD, Burke KM. Methacholine inhalation challenge studies. J Allergy Clin Immunol 1979; 64:569–574.
3. Reed C, Townley RG. Asthma: classification and pathogenesis. In: Middleton E Jr, Reed CE, Ellis EF, eds. Allergy: Principles and Practice. St Louis: CV Mosby, 1983:811–831.
4. Cockcroft DW, Killian DN, Mellon JJA, Hargreave FE. Bronchial reactivity of inhaled histamine: a method and clinical survey. Clin Allergy 1977; 7:235–243.
5. Boushey HA, Holtzman MJ, Sheller JR, Nadel JA. Bronchial hyperreactivity. Am Rev Respir Dis 1980; 121:389–413.
6. Power C, Sreenan S, Hurson B, Burke C, Poulter LW. Distribution of immunocompetent cells in the bronchial wall of clinically healthy subjects showing bronchial hyperresponsiveness. Thorax 1993; 48:1125–1129.
7. Chai H, Farr RS, Froehlich LA, Mathison DA, McLean JA, Rosenthal RR, Sheffer AL II, Spector SL, Townley RG. Standardization of bronchial inhalation challenge procedures. J Allergy Clin Immunol 1975; 56:322–327.
8. Cropp GJ, Bernstein IL, Boushey HA Jr, Hyde RW, Rosenthal RR, Spector SL, Townley RG. Guidelines for bronchial inhalation challenges with pharmacologic and antigenic agents. ATS News, Spring 1980; Vol 11.
9. Spector SL. Provocative Challenge Procedures: Bronchial, Oral, Nasal, and Exercise. Vol. 1. Boca Raton, FL: CRC Press, 1983.
10. Townley RJ, Hopp RJ. Inhalation methods for the study of airway responsiveness. J Allergy Clin Immunol 1987; 80:111–127.
11. Townley RG, Hopp R, Weiss S, Lang W, McCall M. Mechanisms and management of bronchial asthma. In: Spittell, JA Jr, ed. Clinical Medicine. Philadelphia: Harper & Row, 1986:1–29.

12. Ramsdale EH, Morris MM, Roberts RS, Hargreaves FE. Bronchial responsiveness to metha-choline in chronic bronchitis: relationship to airflow obstruction and cold air responsiveness. Thorax 1984; 39:912–918.

13. Findlay SR, Lichtenstein LM. Basophil releasibility in patients with asthma. Am Rev Respir Dis 1980; 122:53–59.

14. Felarca AB, Itkin I. Studies with the quantitative inhalation challenge technique. I. Curve of dose response to acetyl-beta-methacholine in patients with asthma of known and unknown origin, hayfever subjects and non-atopic volunteers. J Allergy 1966; 37:223–235.

15. Itkin IH. Bronchial hyperreactivity to Mecholyl and histamine in asthma subjects. J Allergy 1967; 40:245–256.

16. Bewtra AK, Townley RG. Bronchoprovocative tests: clinical usefulness and limitations. Arch Intern Med 1984; 144:925–926.

17. Rosenthal RR. Inhalation challenge in asthma. In: Kaplan AP, ed. Allergy. New York: Churchill Livingstone, 1985:Chap. 14.

18. Deal EC, McFadden ER, Ingram RH, Breslin FJ, Jaeger JJ. Airway responsiveness to cold air and hyperpnea in normal subjects and in those with hay fever and asthma. Am Rev Respir Dis 1980; 121:621–628.

19. Townley RG, Ryo UY, Kolotkin BM, Kang B. Bronchial sensitivity to methacholine in current and former asthmatic and allergic rhinitis patients and control subjects. J Allergy Clin Immunol 1975; 56:429–442.

20. Woolcock AJ. Expression of results of airway hyperresponsiveness in airway responsiveness. In: Hargreave FE, Woolcock AJ, eds. Mississauga, Ontario: Astra Pharmaceuticals, 1985: 80–85.

21. Ryan G, Dolovich MB, Roberts RS, Frith PA, Juniper EF, Hargreave FE, Newhouse MT. Standardization of inhalation provocation tests: two techniques of aerosol generation and inhalation compared. Am Rev Respir Dis 1981; 123:195–199.

22. Simonsson BG, Jacobs FM, Nadel JA. Role of the autonomic nervous system and the cough reflex in the increase responsiveness of airways in patients with obstructive airway disease. J Clin Invest 1967; 46:1812–1818.

23. Hardy CC, Robinson C, Tattersfield AE, Holgate ST. The bronchoconstrictor effect of inhaled prostaglandin D_2 in normal and asthmatic men. N Engl J Med 1984; 311:209–213.

24. Featherstone RL, Robinson C, Holgate ST, Church MK. Evidence for thromboxane receptor-mediated contraction of guinea pig and human airways in vitro by prostaglandin (PG) D_2, 9 alpha, 11 beta-PGF_2 and PGF_2-alpha. Naunyn Schmiedebergs Arch Pharmacol 1990; 341: 439–443.

25. Lewis RA, Hardy C, Tattersfield AE. Low and high dose response to prostaglandin F_2 in normal subjects. Clin Sci 1982; 63:7P.

26. Smith LJ, Greenberger PA, Patterson R, Krell RD, Bernstein PR. The effect of inhaled leuko-triene D_4 in humans. Am Rev Respir Dis 1985; 131:368–372.

27. Barnes NC, Piper PJ, Costello JF. Comparative effects of inhaled leukotriene C_4, leukotriene D_4, and histamine in normal human subjects. Thorax 1984; 39:500–504.

28. Weiss JW, Drazen JM, McFadden ER Jr, Weller P, Corey EJ, Lewis RA, Austen KF. Airway constriction in normal humans produced by inhalation of leukotriene D. JAMA 1983; 249:2814–2817.

29. Kumlin M, Dahlen B, Bjorck T, Zetterstrom O, Granstrom L, Dahlen S-E. Urinary excretion of leukotriene E_4 and 11-dehydro-thromboxane B_2 in response to bronchial provocations with allergen, aspirin, leukotriene D_4, and histamine in asthmatics. Am Rev Respir Dis 1992; 146:96–103.

30. Lewis MA, Mong S, Vessella RL, Crooke ST. Identification and characterization of leukotriene D_4 receptors in adult and fetal human lung. Biochem Pharmacol 1985; 34:4311–4317.

31. Barnes PJ, Baraniuk JN, Belvisi MG. Neuropeptides in the respiratory tract. Am Rev Respir Dis 1991; 144:1187–1198.

32. Anderson SD, Schoeffel RE. Standardization of exercise training in the asthmatic patient: a challenge in itself. In: Hargreave FE, Woolcock AJ, eds. Airway Responsiveness: Measurement and Interpretation. Mississauga, Ontario: Astra Pharmaceuticals, 1985:51–59.

33. Godfrey S. Exercise-induced asthma—clinical, physiological, and therapeutic implications. J Allergy Clin Immunol 1975; 56:1–17.

34. Souhrada JF, Kivity S. Exercise testing. In: Spector SL, ed. Provocative Challenge Procedures: Bronchial, Oral, Nasal, and Exercise. Vol. 2. Boca Raton, FL: CRC Press, 1983:75–102.

35. Anderson SD. Issues in exercise-induced asthma. J Allergy Clin Immunol 1985; 76:763–772.

36. Phillips YY, Jaeger JJ, Laube BL, Rosenthal RR. Eucapnic voluntary hyperventilation of compressed gas mixture. A simple system for bronchial challenge by respiratory heat loss. Am Rev Respir Dis 1985; 131:31–35.

37. Allergra L, Bianco S. Non-specific broncho-reactivity obtained with an ultrasonic aerosol of distilled water. Eur J Respir Dis 1980; 106(suppl):41–49.

38. Anderson SD. Bronchial challenge by ultrasonically nebulized aerosol. Clin Rev Allergy 1985; 3:427–439.

39. Bascom B, Bleecker ER. Bronchoconstriction induced by distilled water. Am Rev Respir Dis 1986; 134:248–253.

40. Schoeffel RE, Anderson SD, Altounyan REC. Bronchial hyperreactivity in response to inhalation of ultrasonically nebulized solutions of distilled water and saline. Br Med J 1981; 283:1285–1287.

41. Smith CM, Anderson SD, Black JL. Methacholine responsiveness increases after ultrasonically nebulized water but not after ultrasonically nebulized hypertonic saline in patients with asthma. J Allergy Clin Immunol 1987; 79:85–92.

42. Kidney JC, Ridge SM, Chung KF, Barnes PJ. Inhibition of platelet-activating factor-induced bronchoconstriction by the leukotriene D_4 receptor antagonist ICI 204,219. Am Rev Respir Dis 1993; 147:215–217.

43. Cushley JM, Tattersfield AE, Holgate ST. Adenosine antagonism as an alternative mechanism of action of methylxanthines in asthma. Agents Actions 1983; 13(suppl):109–113.

44. Polosa R, Rajakulasingam K, Prosperini G, Church MK, Hogate ST. Relative potencies and time course of changes in adenosine $5'$-monophosphate airway responsiveness with inhaled furosemide and bumetanide in asthma. J Allergy Clin Immunol 1993; 92:288–297.

45. Polosa R, Phillips GD, Rajakulasingam K, Holgate ST. The effect of inhaled ipratropium bromide alone and in combination with oral terfenadine on bronchoconstriction provoked by AMP and histamine in asthma. J Allergy Clin Immunol 1991; 87:939–947.

46. Polosa R, Rajakulasingam K, Church MK, Holgate ST. Repeated inhalation of bradykinin attenuates AMP-induced bronchoconstriction in asthmatic airways. Eur Respir J 1992; 5: 700–706.

47. Woolcock AJ, Cheung W, Salome C. Relationship between bronchial responsiveness to propranolol and histamine. Am Rev Respir Dis 1986; 133:A177.

48. De Vries K, Gokemeyer JDM, Koeter GH, De Monchy JGR, Van Bork LE, Cauffman HL, Meurs H. Cholinergic and adrenergic mechanisms in bronchial reactivity. In: Morley J, ed. Bronchial Hyperreactivity. London: Academic Press, 1982:107–129.

49. Nosal R, Ondrias K, Pecivova J, et al. Histamine release and membrane fluidisation of mast cells exposed to beta-adrenoceptor blocking drug propranolol. Agents Actions 1988; 23:143–145.

50. Christie PE, Tagari P, Ford-Hutchinson AW, Black C, Markendorf A, Schmitz-Schumann M, Lee TH. Urinary leukotriene E_4 after lysine-aspirin inhalation in asthmatic subjects. Am Rev Respir Dis 1992; 146:1531–1534.

51. Israel E, Fischer AR, Rosenberg MA, Lilly CM, Callery JC, Shapiro J, Cohn J, Rubin P, Drazen JM. The pivotal role of 5-lipoxygenase products in the reaction of aspirin-sensitive asthmatics to aspirin. Am Rev Respir Dis 1993; 148:1447–1451.

52. Polosa R, Cacciola RR, Holgate ST. The response of the airways in asthmatic patients to kinin inhalations define a type-B_2 receptor profile. Ann Ital Med Int 1992; 7:220–225.

53. Lowell FC, Schiller IW. Measurement of change in vital capacity as a means of detecting pulmonary reactions to inhaled aerosolized allergenic extracts in asthmatic subjects. J Allergy 1984; 19:100–107.

54. Bruce CA, Rosenthal RR, Lichtenstein LM, Norman PS. Quantitative inhalation bronchial challenge in ragweed hayfever patients: a comparison with ragweed-allergic asthmatics. J Allergy Clin Immunol 1975; 56:331–337.

55. Cockcroft DW, Murdock KY, Kirby J, Hargreave F. Prediction of airway responsiveness to allergen from skin sensitivity to allergen and airway responsiveness to histamine. Am Rev Respir Dis 1987; 135:264–267.

56. Van Essen-Zandvliet EEM, Kerrebjin KF. The effect of antiasthma drug on bronchial hyper-responsiveness. Immunol Allergy Clin North Am 1990; 10:483–501.

57. Campos Gongora H, Wisnieuwski AFZ, Tattersfield AE. A single dose comparison of inhaled albuterol and two formulations of salmeterol on airway reactivity in asthmatic subjects. Am Rev Respir Dis 1991; 144:626–629.

58. Derom EY, Pauwels RA, Van der Straeten MEF. The effect of inhaled salmeterol on methacholine responsiveness in subjects with asthma up to 12 hours. J Allergy Clin Immunol 1992; 89:811–815.

59. Wood-Baker R, Holgate ST. The comparative actions and adverse effect profile of single doses of H_1-receptor antihistamines in the airways and skin of subjects with asthma. J Allergy Clin Immunol 1993; 91:1005–1014.

60. Ahmed T, Danta I. Modification of histamine- and methacholine-induced bronchoconstriction by calcium antagonist gallopamil in asthmatics. Respiration 1992; 59:332–338.

61. Kishida M, Sasamoto A, Saito S, Iikura Y. Oxatomide modifies methacholine- and exercise-induced bronchoconstriction in asthmatic children. Ann Allergy 1992; 69:455–461.

62. Grubbe RE, Hopp R, Dave NK, Brennan B, Bewtra A, Townley R. Effect of inhaled furosemide on the bronchial response to methacholine and cold-air hyperventilation challenges. J Allergy Clin Immunol 1990; 85:881–884.

63. O'Connor BJ, Chung KF, Chen-Worsdell YM, Fuller RW, Barnes PJ. Effect of inhaled furosemide and bumetanide on adenosine 5'-monophosphate- and sodium metabisulfite-induced bronchoconstriction in asthmatic subjects. Am Rev Respir Dis 1991; 143:1329–1333.

64. Magnussen H, Boerger S, Templin K, Baunack AR. Effects of a thromboxane-receptor antagonist, BAY u 3405, on prostaglandin D_2- and exercise-induced bronchoconstriction. J Allergy Clin Immunol 1992; 89:1119–1126.

65. Smith LJ, Geller S, Ebright L, Glass M, Thyrum PT. Inhibition of leukotriene D_4-induced bronchoconstriction in normal subjects by the oral LTD_4 receptor antagonist ICI 204,219. Am Rev Respir Dis 1990; 141:988–992.

66. Weiss JW, Drazen JM, McFadden ER, et al. Airway constriction in normal humans produced by inhalation of leukotriene D. JAMA 1983; 249:2814–2817.

67. Smith LJ, Kern R, Patterson R, Krell RD, Bernstein PR. Mechanism of leukotriene D_4-induced bronchoconstriction in normal subjects. J Allergy Clin Immunol 1987; 80:338–345.

68. Frolund L, Madsen F, Nielsen J. Reproducibility of leukotriene D_4 inhalation challenge in asthmatics. Effect of a novel leukotriene D_4/E_4-antagonist (SR 2640) on leukotriene D_4-induced bronchoconstriction. Allergy 1991; 46:355–361.

69. Finnerty JP, Twentyman OP, Harris A, Palmer JBD, Holgate ST. Effect of GR32191, a potent thromboxane receptor antagonist, on exercise-induced bronchoconstriction in asthma. Thorax 1991; 46:190–192.

70. Anderson SD. Exercise-induced asthma. In: Middleton E Jr, Reed CE, Ellis EF, Adkinson NF Jr, Yuninger JW, Busse WW, eds. Allergy: Principles and Practice, 4th ed. St. Louis: CV Mosby, 1993:1343–1367.

71. Bianco S, Vaghi A, Robuschi M, et al. Prevention of exercise-induced bronchoconstriction by inhaled furosemide. Lancet 1988; 2:252–255.

72. Pavord ID, Wisniewski A, Tattersfield AE. Inhaled frusemide and exercise induced asthma: evidence of a role for inhibitory prostanoids. Thorax 1992; 47:797–800.

73. Thomson NC, Patel KR, Kerr JW. Sodium cromoglycate and ipratropium bromide in exercise-induced asthma. Thorax 1978; 33:694–699.

74. Pliss LB, Ingenito EP, Ingram RH Jr, Pichurko B. Assessment of bronchoalveolar cell and mediator response to isocapnic hyperpnea in asthma. Am Rev Respir Dis 1990; 142:73–78.

75. O'Donnell WJ, Rosenberg M, Niven RW, Drazen JM, Israel E. Acetazolamide and furosemide attenuate asthma induced by hyperventilation of cold, dry air. Am Rev Respir Dis 1992; 146:1518–1523.

76. Rodwell LT, Anderson SD, du Toit J, Seale JP. Different effects of inhaled amiloride and frusemide on airway responsiveness to dry air challenge in asthmatic subjects. Eur Respir J 1993; 6:855–861.

77. Israel E, Dermarkarian R, Rosenberg M, Sperling R, Taylor G, Rubin P, Drazen JM. The effects of a 5-lipoxygenase inhibitor on asthma induced by cold, dry air. N Engl J Med 1990; 323:1740–1744.

78. Israel E, Juniper EF, Callaghan JT, Mathur PN, Morris MM, Dowell AR, Enas GG, Hargreave FE, Drazen JM. Effect of a leukotriene antagonist, LY171883, in cold air-induced bronchoconstriction in asthmatics. Am Rev Respir Dis 1989; 140:1348–1353.

79. Townley RG, Hopp RJ, Bewtra AK, Nabe M. Effect of terfenadine on pulmonary function, histamine release, and bronchial challenges with nebulized water and cold-air hyperventilation. Ann Allergy 1989; 63:455–460.

80. Bianco S, Robuschi M, Damonte C, Simone P, Vaghi A, Pasargiklian M. Bronchial response to nonsteroidal anti-inflammatory drugs in asthmatic patients. Prog Biochem Pharmacol 1985; 20:132–142.

81. Bianco S, Vaghi A, Pieroni MG, Robuschi M, Refini RM, Sestini P. Protective activity of inhaled nonsteroidal antiinflammatory drugs on bronchial responsiveness to ultrasonically nebulized water. J Allergy Clin Immunol 1992; 90:833–839.

82. Rodwell LT, Anderson SD, du Toit JI, Seale JP. The effect of inhaled frusemide on airway sensitivity to inhaled 4.5% sodium chloride aerosol in asthmatic subjects. Thorax 1993; 48:208–213.

83. Foresi A, Pelucchi A, Mastropasqua B, Cavigioli G, Carlesi RM, Marazzini L. Effect of inhaled furosemide and torasemide on bronchial response to ultrasonically nebulized distilled water in asthmatic subjects. Am Rev Respir Dis 1992; 146:364–368.

84. Bianco S, Robuschi M, Vaghi A, Pieroni MG, Sestini P. Protective effect of inhaled piretanide on the bronchial obstructive response to ultrasonically nebulized H_2O. A dose–response study. Chest 1993; 104:185–188.

85. McAlpine LG, Hulks G, Thomson NC. Effect of atrial natriuretic peptide given by intravenous infusion on bronchoconstriction induced by ultrasonically nebulized distilled water (FOG). Am Rev Respir Dis 1992; 146:912–915.

86. Hulks G, Jardine AG, Connell JMC, Thomson NC. Influence of elevated plasma levels of atrial natriuretic factor on bronchial reactivity in asthma. Am Rev Respir Dis 1991; 143:778–782.

87. Makker HK, Holgate ST. Respiratory pathophysiologic response. The contribution of neurogenic reflexes to hypertonic saline-induced bronchoconstriction in asthma. J Allergy Clin Immunol 1993; 92:82–88.

88. Tullett W, Patel KR, Berkin KE, Kerr JW. Effect of lignocaine, sodium cromoglycate and ipratropium bromide in exercise-induced asthma. Thorax 1982; 37:737–746.

89. Sheppard D, Rizk NW, Boushey HA, Bethel RA. Mechanism of cough and bronchoconstriction induced by distilled water aerosol. Am Rev Respir Dis 1983; 127:691–694.

90. Phillips GD, Rafferty P, Beasley CRW, Holgate ST. The effect of oral terfenadine on the bronchoconstrictor response to inhaled histamine and adenosine 5'-monophosphate in nonatopic asthma. Thorax 1987; 42:939–945.

91. Rafferty P, Beasley CRW, Holgate ST. The contribution of histamine to immediate bronchoconstriction provoked by inhaled allergen and adenosine 5'-monophosphate in atopic asthma. Am Rev Respir Dis 1987; 136:369–373.

92. Polosa R, Phillips GD, Rajakulasingam K, Holgate ST. The effect of inhaled ipratropium bromide alone and in combination with oral terfenadine on bronchoconstriction provoked by adenosine 5'-monophosphate and histamine in asthma. J Allergy Clin Immunol 1991; 87: 939–947.

93. Altounyan REC, Lee TB, Rocchiccioli KMS, Shaw CL. A comparison of the inhibitory effects of nedocromil sodium and sodium cromoglycate on adenosine monophosphate-induced bronchoconstriction in atopic subjects. Eur J Respir Dis 1986; 69(suppl):277–279.

94. Dahlen B, Kumlin M, Margolskee DJ, Larsson C, Blomqvist H, Williams VC, Zetterstrom O, Dahlen SE. The leukotriene-receptor antagonist MK-0679 blocks airway obstruction induced by inhaled lysine-aspirin in aspirin-sensitive asthmatics. Eur Respir J 1993; 6:1018–1026.

95. Vargas FS, Croce M, Teixeira LR, Terra-Filho M, Cukier A, Light RW. Effect of inhaled furosemide on the bronchial response to lysine-aspirin inhalation in asthmatic subjects. Chest 1992; 102:408–411.

96. Hopp RJ, Townley RG, Agrawal DK, Bewtra AK. The effect of terfenadine on the bronchoconstriction, dermal response, and leukopenia induced by platelet-activating factor. Chest 1991; 100:994–998.

97. Adamus WS, Heuer HO, Meade CJ, Schilling JC. Inhibitory effects of a new PAF acether antagonist WEB 2086 on pharmacologic changes induced by PAF inha' tion in human beings. Clin Pharmacol Ther 1990; 47:456–462.

98. Foresi A, Chetta A, Pelucchi A, Cavigioli G, Mastropasqua B, Olivieri D. Effect of inhaled disodium cromoglycate and nedocromil sodium on propranolol-induced bronchoconstriction. Ann Allergy 1993; 70:159–163.

99. Koeter SH, Meurs H, de Monchy JG, de Vries K. Protective effect of disodium cromoglycate on propranolol challenge. Allergy 1982; 37:587–590.

100. Latimer KM, Ruffin RE. The effect of inhaled fenoterol and ipratropium bromide on propranolol induced bronchoconstriction in the asthmatic airways. Clin Exp Pharmacol Physiol 1990; 17:627–635.

101. Okayama M, Shen T, Midorikawa J, Lin J-T, Inoue H, Takishima T, Shirato K. Effect of pilocarpine on propranolol-induced bronchoconstriction in asthma. Am J Respir Crit Care Med 1994; 149:76–80.

102. Yeo CT, O'Connor JB, Chen-Worsdell M, Barnes PJ, Chung KF. Protective effect of loop diuretics, piretanide and frusemide, against sodium metabisulfite-induced bronchoconstriction in asthma. Eur Respir J 1992; 5:1184–1188.

103. Baldwin DR, Grange KL, Pavord I, Knox AJ. The effect of amiloride on the airway response to metabisulphite in asthma: a negative report. Eur Respir J 1992; 5:1189–1192.

104. Bellingan GJ, Dixon CM, Ind PW. Inhibition of inhaled metabisulphite-induced bronchoconstriction by inhaled frusemide and ipratropium bromide. Br J Clin Pharmacol 1992; 34:71–74.

105. Dixon CM, Ind PW. Inhaled sodium metabisulphite induced bronchoconstriction: inhibition by nedocromil sodium and sodium cromoglycate. Br J Clin Pharmacol 1990; 30:371–376.

106. Pavord ID, Wisniewski A, Mathur R, Wahedna I, Knox AJ, Tattersfield AE. Effect of inhaled prostaglandin E_2 on bronchial reactivity to sodium metabisulphite and methacholine in patients with asthma. Thorax 1991; 46:633–637.

107. O'Connor BJ, Lecomte JM, Barnes PJ. Effect of an inhaled histamine H_3-receptor agonist on airway responses to sodium metabisulphite in asthma. Br J Clin Pharmacol 1993; 35:55–57.

108. Crimi N, Oliveri R, Polosa R, Palermo F, Mistretta A. The effect of oral terfenadine on neurokinin-A-induced bronchoconstriction. J Allergy Clin Immunol 1993; 91:1096–1098.

109. Crimi N, Palermo F, Oliveri R, et al. Influence of antihistamine (astemizole) and anticholinergic

drugs (ipratropium bromide) on bronchoconstriction induced by SP. Ann Allergy 1990; 65: 115–120.

110. Joos G, Pauwels R, van der Straeten M. The effect of oxitropium bromide on neurokinin A-induced bronchoconstriction in asthmatic subjects. Pulm Pharmacol 1988; 1:41–45.

111. Crimi N, Palermo F, Oliveri R, Palermo B, Polosa R, Mistretta A. Protection of nedocromil sodium on bronchoconstriction induced by inhaled neurokinin A (NKA) in asthmatic patients. Clin Exp Allergy 1992; 22:75–81.

112. Ichinose M, Nakajima N, Takahashi T, Yamauchi H, Inoue H, Takishima T. Protection against bradykinin-induced bronchoconstriction in asthmatic patients by neurokinin receptor antagonist. Lancet 1992; 340:1248–1251.

113. Polosa R, Phillips GD, Lai CK, Holgate ST. Contribution of histamine and prostanoids to bronchoconstriction provoked by inhaled bradykinin in atopic asthma. Allergy 1990; 45: 174–182.

114. Morgan DJR, Moodley I, Cundell DR, et al. Circulating histamine and neutrophil chemotactic activity during allergen-induced asthma: the effect of inhaled antihistamines and antiallergic compounds. Clin Sci 1985; 69:63–67.

115. Holgate ST, Emanuel MB, Howarth PH. Astemizole and other H_1-antihistaminic drug treatment of asthma. J Allergy Clin Immunol 1985; 76:375–380.

116. Rafferty P, Ng WH, Phillips G. The inhibitory actions of azelastine hydrochloride on the early and late bronchoconstrictor responses to inhaled allergen in atopic asthma. J Allergy Clin Immunol 1989; 84:649–657.

117. Hamid M, Rafferty P, Holgate ST. The inhibitory effect of terfenadine and flurbiprofen on early and late-phase bronchoconstriction following allergen challenge in atopic asthma. Clin Exp Allergy 1990; 20:261–267.

118. Taniguchi U, Tamura G, Honma M, Aizawa T, Maruyama N, Shirato K, Takishima T. The effect of an oral leukotriene antagonis, ONO-1078, on allergen-induced immediate bronchoconstriction in asthmatic subjects. J Allergy Clin Immunol 1993; 92:507–512.

119. Findlay SR, Barden JM, Easley CB, Glass M. Effect of the leukotriene antagonist, ICI 204,219, on antigen-induced bronchoconstriction in subjects with asthma. J Allergy Clin Immunol 1992; 89:1040–1045.

120. Rasmussen JB, Eriksson L-O, Margolskee DJ, Tagari P, Williams VC, Andersson K-E. Leukotriene D_4 receptor blockade inhibits the immediate and late bronchoconstrictor responses to inhaled antigen in patients with asthma. J Allergy Clin Immunol 1992; 90:193–201.

121. Friedman BS, Bel EH, Buntinx A, Tanaka W, Han YH, Shingo S, Spector R, Sterk P. Oral leukotriene inhibitor (MK-886) blocks allergen-induced airway responses. Am Rev Respir Dis 1993; 147:839–844.

122. Kirby JG, Hargreave FE, Crockcroft DW, O'Bryne PM. The effect of indomethicin on allergen-induced asthmatic responses. J Appl Physiol 1989; 66:578–583.

123. Kuitert LM, Hui KP, Uthayarkumar S, Burke W, Newland AC, Uden S, Barnes NC. Effect of the platelet-activating factor antagonist UK-74,505 on the early and late response to allergen. Am Rev Respir Dis 1993; 147:82–86.

124. Cockcroft DW, Murdock KY. Comparative effects of inhaled salbutamol, sodium cromoglyate, and beclomethasone dipropionate on allergen-induced early asthmatic responses, late asthmatic responses, and increased bronchial responsiveness to histamine. J Allergy Clin Immunol 1987; 79:734–740.

125. Pavord ID, Wong CS, Williams J, Tattersfield AE. Effect of inhaled prostaglandin E_2 on allergen-induced asthma. Am Rev Respir Dis 1993; 148:87–90.

126. Taylor IK, O'Shaughnessy KM, Choudry NB, Adachi M, Palmer JB, Fuller RW. A comparative study in atopic subjects with asthma of the effects of salmeterol and salbutamol on allergen-induced bronchoconstriction, increase in airway reactivity, and increase in urinary leukotriene E_4 excretion. J Allergy Clin Immunol 1992; 89:575–583.

127. Pedersen B, Dahl R, Larsen BB, Venge P. The effect of salmeterol on the early- and late-phase reaction to bronchial allergen and postchallenge variation in bronchial reactivity, blood eosinophils, serum eosinophil cationic protein, and serum eosinophil protein X. Allergy 1993; 48:377–382.

128. Twentyman OP, Finnerty JP, Holgate ST. The inhibitory effect of nebulized albuterol on the early and late asthmatic reactions and increase in airway hyperresponsiveness provoked by inhaled allergen in asthma. Am Rev Respir Dis 1991; 144:782–787.

129. Bianco S, Pieroni MG, Refini RM, et al. Protective effect of inhaled furosemide on allergen-induced early and late asthmatic reactions. N Engl J Med 1989; 321:1069–1073.

130. Nair N, Hopp RJ, Townley RG. Effect of nedocromil on antigen-induced bronchoconstriction in asthmatic subjects. Ann Allergy 1989; 62:329–331.

131. Crimi E, Violante B, Pellegrino R, Brusasco V. Effect of multiple doses of nedocromil sodium given after allergen inhalation in asthma. J Allergy Clin Immunol 1993; 92:777–783.

132. Pelikan Z, Knottnerus I. Inhibition of the late asthmatic response by nedocromil sodium administered more than two hours after allergen challenge. J Allergy Clin Immunol 1993; 92:19–28.

133. Crossman DC, Dashwood MR, Taylor GW, Wellings R, Fuller RW. Sodium cromoglycate: evidence of tachykinin antagonist activity in human skin. J Appl Physiol 1993; 75:167–172.

134. Verleden GM, Pype JL, Demedts MG. Furosemide and bumetanide, but not nedocromil sodium, modulate nonadrenergic relaxation in guinea pig trachea in vitro. Am J Respir Crit Care Med 1994; 149:138–144.

135. Cockcroft DW, Murdock KY, Gore BP, O'Bryne PM, Manning P. Theophylline does not inhibit allergen-induced increase in airway responsiveness to methacholine. J Allergy Clin Immunol 1989; 83:913–920.

136. Gross NJ, Boushey HA, Gold WM. Anticholinergic drugs. In: Middleton E, Reed CE, Ellis EF, Adkinson NF, Yunginger JW, Busse WW, eds. Allergy: Principles and Practice. St. Louis: CV Mosby, 1993; 941–962.

27

Mast Cells and Antidegranulating Agents

Frederick L. Pearce
University College London, London, England

INTRODUCTION

The mast cell is widely distributed throughout the human body, but is found in the largest numbers in those areas that come into direct contact with foreign substances from the environment. Thus, the cell predominates in the loose connective tissues of the bronchi, conjunctiva, gut, ear, nose, throat, and skin. As such, it is uniquely placed to participate in a range of allergic and immediate hypersensitivity reactions and has been incriminated in the etiology and pathogenesis of asthma, rhinitis, conjunctivitis, and inflammatory disorders of the gastrointestinal tract and skin. Given the diversity and widespread occurrence of these conditions, it is essential to our understanding of the origins and management of allergic disorders to appreciate that mast cells from different locations may exhibit marked variations in their functional properties.

Much of our knowledge concerning mast cell heterogeneity comes from studies in rodents in which two distinct phenotypes—mucosal mast cells (MMC) and connective tissue mast cells (CTMC)—may be identified (1,2). These cells differ in their morphology, granular contents, sensitivity to regulation by different growth and other factors, and responsivity to various stimuli. Although these differences are profound, there is considerable evidence that the phenotypic characteristics of the populations can change reversibly in response to alterations in the microenvironment (1,2).

In contrast with the rodent, the extent of mast cell heterogeneity in the human has been much less clearly defined. Two subtypes have been identified on the basis of their content of neutral proteases (3): one contains only the enzyme tryptase (MC_T) and the other both tryptase and chymase (MC_{TC}). The MC_{TC} cells predominate in the skin and intestinal submucosa and are also present as a minority of the cells in the lung. The MC_T cells represent the majority of pulmonary mast cells and essentially all of the cells in the mucosa of the gut. A spectrum of human mast cell types seems to exist, as judged by their proteoglycan content. At one extreme, cutaneous mast cells contain heparin, whereas at the other, human intestinal mucosal cells contain only chondroitin sulfate E. Mast cells in the lung appear to represent a transitional population containing both heparin and chondroitin sulfates (for references, see Ref. 2). The skin cell further represents a divergent subpopulation in that, unlike the other human mast cells studied that metabolize arachidonic acid to form both prostaglandin-D_2 (PGD_2) and leukotriene-C_4 (LTC_4), it generates only the prostanoid on immunological stimulation (4). Finally, different human mast cell subtypes may again vary in their responses to secretory and inhibitory stimuli (4,5).

This heterogeneity clearly renders difficult the development and design of mast cell-stabilizing or antidegranulating drugs for clinical use. Moreover, most allergic conditions are now recognized to be complex inflammatory disorders involving a range of effector cells and neural elements. However, the mast cell has long been centrally implicated in the pathology of such conditions, and many hundreds of compounds have been developed in an attempt to modulate the function of this cell. It is not useful to attempt to review the properties of all of these agents. Instead, this chapter concentrates largely on those agents that have been accepted into clinical practice, for one reason or another, and discusses the extent to which their therapeutic activity depends on mast cell stabilization.

CROMOLYN AND NEDOCROMIL

Development

The prototype antiallergic drug, cromolyn sodium (disodium cromoglycate), was first introduced into clinical practice in the United Kingdom for the prophylaxis of bronchial asthma in 1968 (6). The drug was developed from studies on the naturally occurring furanochromone khellin, which was the active constituent of the eastern Mediterranean plant *Ammi visnaga*, known since biblical times for its bronchodilating properties. Several analogues of khellin were produced but, although several were potent bronchodilators, their associated side effects prevented their therapeutic application. To make the molecules water-soluble so that they could be inhaled as an aerosol spray, a series of chromones were prepared bearing a carboxylic acid function at the 2-position of the benzopyran ring system (6). These compounds were then tested directly in humans and, although they were ineffective as bronchodilators, they possessed an entirely novel type of activity. When the agents were inhaled before antigen provocation, they prevented the normal broncho-constriction associated with the challenge. However, the drugs were ineffective when administered after the provocation, in contrast with conventional bronchodilators that could reverse the existing bronchoconstriction (6). Further testing in the same way ultimately led to the development of the bis-chromone, cromolyn sodium, and its subsequent marketing as a novel, prophylactic antiasthmatic agent. Detailed study then showed that cromolyn sodium apparently acted by inhibiting the release of anaphylactic mediators, typified by the autacoid histamine, from tissue mast cells (7,8). As such, the chromone was the first example of an antiasthmatic drug thought to act in this way.

Following the introduction of cromolyn, more than 50 pharmaceutical companies throughout the world attempted to develop similar and more potent compounds. Many of these agents were considerably more active than cromolyn in standard laboratory tests, principally passive cutaneous anaphylaxis in the rat and the inhibition of histamine release from chopped fragments of human lung (9). However, none of these drugs was effective in the management of clinical asthma until the development, some 20 years later, of the pyranoquinoline dicarboxylic acid derivative nedocromil sodium (10). Some of the reasons for this delay are considered in the following.

Effects on Isolated Mast Cells

Cromolyn and nedocromil produce a comparable dose-dependent inhibition of immuno-logical histamine release from rat peritoneal mast cells (Fig. 1). The degree of inhibition produced is related to the strength of the stimulus used to provoke histamine release: the greater the stimulus, the smaller the degree of inhibition achieved with the drugs (5). Both drugs exhibit a sharp tachyphylaxis, and activity is rapidly lost on preincubation with the cells before challenge (see Fig. 1). Cromolyn exhibits cross-tachyphylaxis to nedocromil and a variety of other experimental compounds (for references, see Ref. 11), which is normally taken to indicate that the drugs share a common mode of action, at least in terms of their effects on rat serosal mast cells. The origin of tachyphylaxis in this system is unclear, but it is not dependent on the uptake, metabolism, or other inactivation of the compound, because addition of more drug does not overcome the effect.

Cromolyn and nedocromil show a startling heterogeneity in their effect on mast cells from other laboratory animals (5,11). They exhibit a moderate activity against peritoneal cells from the hamster, but are completely ineffective against these cells from the mouse. Both drugs are also inactive against tissue mast cells from the guinea pig and mucosal mast cells from the rat intestine. The latter finding, compared with the potency of the compounds against rat serosal mast cells, provides a striking example of functional mast cell hetero-geneity within a single species (12).

Cromolyn shows an interesting spectrum of activity against human histaminocytes (Fig. 2). In complete contrast to the rat, the compound is most active against mast cells recovered from the musoca of the gastrointestinal tract, or from the surfaces of the airways by bronchoalveolar lavage (BAL). The drug shows intermediate activity against mast cells from the uterus, lung parenchyma, and intestinal submucosa, but is totally inactive against

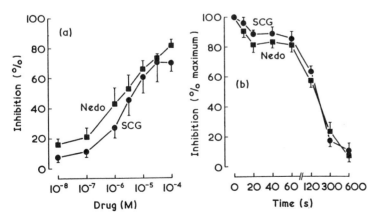

Figure 1   Effect of cromolyn (solid circle, SCG) and nedocromil (solid square, Nedo) on histamine release from rat peritoneal mast cells. Cells were obtained from actively sensitized animals and challenged with allergen from *Nippostrongylus brasiliensis*. (a) Drugs added simultaneously with the secretory stimulus and (b) cells preincubated with the drugs for the indicated times before challenge. Values are means ± SEM for four experiments. (From Ref. 5.)

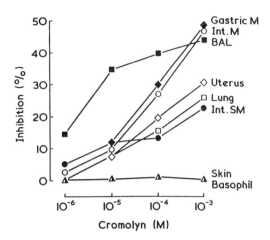

Figure 2 Inhibition by cromolyn of histamine release from human basophils (solid triangles) and mast cells isolated by bronchoalveolar lavage (BAL; solid squares); and by enzymatic dispersion of gastric (solid diamonds) and intestinal (open circles) mucosa; uterus (open diamonds); lung parenchyma (open squares); intestinal submucosa (solid circles); and skin (open triangles). (Data from Refs. 5, 13–17, and unpublished results.)

human cutaneous mast cells and peripheral blood basophils. Nedocromil shows a similar spectrum of activity, but is generally more potent (5,11).

In further contrast to the rat, human mast cells recovered by BAL or from the gastric and intestinal mucosae do not exhibit tachyphylaxis (5,13–17). Instead, the activity against these cells increases on preincubation with cromolyn. This finding is much more in keeping with the clinical usefulness of the drug, which is ideally administered prophylactically before allergen exposure. Moderate tachyphylaxis is, however, observed with the mast cells from the uterus, lung parenchyma, and intestinal submucosa (5,13–17). This may indicate that, in the respiratory tree, the mast cell recoverable from the lumenal surface by BAL, rather than that located in the parenchyma, is the primary target for the action of cromolyn (17). In total, human mast cells thus show a graded decrease in responsivity to cromolyn, and an increasing tachyphylaxis, on passing from the BAL and gastrointestinal mucosal cells, through the lung parenchyma, intestinal muscle and uterine cells, to the skin cells (Fig. 3).

Mechanism of Action

Despite intense effort, the mechanism by which cromolyn and nedocromil inhibit histamine release from mast cells is still poorly understood. This release is a calcium-dependent, secretory process, and a number of workers have suggested that the drug may interfere with calcium mobilization or transport. Initially, it was observed that cromolyn could bind and complex calcium ions, and it was suggested that the drug might thereby block calcium influx into the mast cell (18). This is improbable, however, since the drug is active at micromolar concentrations in the presence of millimolar concentrations of calcium. Moreover, it does not account for the phenomenon of tachyphylaxis. More interestingly, cromolyn blocks calcium-45 uptake following immunological activation of rat mast cells (19) and also prevents the rise in intracellular calcium, as assessed by measurement of quin-2 fluorescence, produced by stimulation of the cell in the presence and absence of the

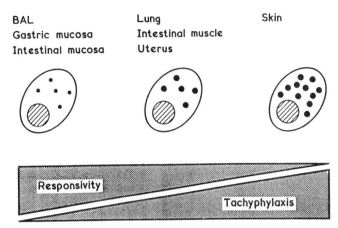

Figure 3 Changing reactivity of human mast cells to cromolyn. Activity decreases and ta-chyphylaxis increases on moving from left to right.

extracellular cation (20,21). This strongly suggests that cromolyn may inhibit histamine release by suppressing both calcium uptake from the external milieu and the release of the cation from sequestered internal stores. The mechanism by which the chromone might block calcium movements has been investigated by Pecht and co-workers. These authors reported (22) that the drug bound in a calcium-dependent manner to the surface of rat basophilic leukemia cells (RBL-2H3) by interaction with a specific protein, the cromolyn-binding protein (CBP). Variants of the cell line lacking the protein did not release histamine on immunological activation, but reactivity was restored by restitution of the CBP with fusogenic carriers, suggesting that it played an essential role in the release process (23). Finally, these workers showed that cross-linking of purified CBP, incorporated into a planar lipid bilayer, permitted a calcium conductance and concluded that the protein constituted the calcium channel itself (24). These experiments appear elegant and persuasive, but it is difficult to assess their significance, as they have not been confirmed by any independent laboratory, and the RBL-2H3 cell, which formed the basis for all of the work, is completely unresponsive to cromolyn.

Other theories on the mode of action of cromolyn have involved the study of protein phosphorylation (25,26). Activation of rat mast cells with immunoglobulin (Ig)E-directed or nonimmunological ligands leads to the rapid phosphorylation of three proteins of relative molecular masses (M_r) 42,000, 59,000, and 68,000, followed by the slower phosphorylation of a protein with an M_r of 78,000. It was suggested that the early rapid phosphorylation was involved in the initiation of secretion, whereas the late phosphorylation of the 78,000-M_r protein was involved in the termination of the response. Most interestingly, treatment of the cells with cromolyn alone also led to the phosphorylation of the 78,000-M_r protein. The time course, tachyphylaxis, and concentration-dependence of this effect paralleled the inhibition of histamine release. As such, cromolyn would appear to activate, in a unique manner, the natural mechanism for the termination of histamine release.

Finally, recent studies have suggested the importance of chloride channels in mast cell activation. Penner and co-workers (27) performed simultaneous patch–clamp and calcium indicator dye (fura-2) measurements in rat peritoneal mast cells. They discovered three ionic mechanisms that were activated following stimulation with compound 48/80 or substance P and that could enhance secretion by maintaining elevated levels of intracellular calcium: (1) a voltage-independent cation channel of about 50-pS conductance, through which divalent cations can permeate according to their thermodynamic driving force; (2) a hyperpolarization-driven calcium influx, activated both by external stimuli and by intracellularly applied inositol triphosphate; and (3) a chloride current of 0.5- to 1-pS single-channel conductance, activated following external stimulation and also induced by internal application of adenosine 3′,5′-cyclic monophosphate (cAMP). This current will clamp the membrane potential of the intact mast cell to negative values, thereby providing the driving force for calcium influx through the first two mechanisms. Immunological activation of RBL-2H3 cells also resulted in the activation of chloride channels, and these were blocked by application of cromolyn to the cytoplasmic side of an inside out membrane patch (28). These studies are of great interest and may provide new insights into the molecular basis of the action of cromolyn and related drugs. (For further information on the role of chloride and other ion channels in allergic diseases see Chapter 23.)

Effects on Other Inflammatory Cells and Neural Mechanisms

Many allergic disorders, such as bronchial asthma, are now recognized to be chronic inflammatory conditions. Late-phase asthmatic reactions, which are thought to accurately reflect the day-to-day manifestations of the disorder, are accompanied by the active migration of granulocytes, such as eosinophils and neutrophils, into the bronchial lumen. These cells may be directly involved in the pathological changes seen in the chronic disease, including mucosal edema, fluid exudation, increased production of mucus, and desquamation of the surface respiratory epithelium. Interestingly, nedocromil and cromolyn are able to suppress the activity of both neutrophils and eosinophils, as assessed by several criteria, including the stimulated expression of complement (C3b) and IgG (Fc) receptors, cytotoxicity toward complement-coated schistosomula of *Schistosoma mansoni*, chemotaxis, and mediator release (11,29–31).

Finally, cromolyn and nedocromil may be clinically active under conditions in which mast cells are not necessarily involved. Thus, the drugs will prevent the bronchoconstriction in asthmatics induced by exercise, cold air, hyperventilation, sulfur dioxide, and aerosols of distilled water (11,32). The mechanisms involved in these responses are of considerable interest and probably involve neural components. Significantly, cromolyn is able to inhibit reflex bronchoconstriction and C-fiber activation in the dog (32), which may explain the effectiveness of the compound in preventing responses induced by nonspecific challenge procedures in humans.

In total, it is clear that cromolyn and nedocromil have important actions other than mast cell stabilization. These properties almost certainly contribute toward their clinical usefulness and, together with the high degree of cellular selectivity of the compounds, help explain the great difficulties experienced in developing similar drugs.

COMPOUNDS AFFECTING INTRACELLULAR LEVELS OF CYCLIC NUCLEOTIDES

Theophylline and Phosphodiesterase Inhibitors

Theophylline and its more water-soluble derivative aminophylline have been mainstays in the treatment of bronchial asthma for more than 50 years. Their therapeutic value stems from a combination of anti-inflammatory and bronchodilator activities, in addition to an ability to increase diaphragmatic contractility (33,34).

Theophylline has several pharmacological actions of which inhibition of cyclic nucleotide phosphodiesterase (PDE) may be the most important. In principle, at least two therapeutically beneficial effects could arise from the inhibition of PDE and the consequent rise in intracellular cAMP or cGMP. First, both cyclic nucleotides can relax airway smooth muscle and cause bronchodilation. Second, elevated levels of cAMP can suppress the activity of inflammatory cells, including mast cells. Accordingly, theophylline inhibits histamine release from all the mast cells so far studied, with the possible exception of the rat intestinal mucosal mast cell (12), and is essentially equiactive against the different human mast cell subpopulations (Fig. 4).

Although it is useful and widely applied in the treatment of asthma, the value of theophylline is limited by its narrow therapeutic index and a wide range of gastrointestinal, central nervous system, and cardiovascular side effects (33,34). There has thus been considerable interest in the development of other PDE inhibitors that circumvent these problems. This approach has been greatly facilitated by the identification of multiple, distinct PDE isozymes that differ in their characteristics and tissue distribution. The general properties of these isozymes are shown in Table 1.

The main regulator of intracellular cAMP levels in both mast cells and basophils appears to be PDE IV (33,35). This isozyme is often referred to as the cAMP-specific PDE because

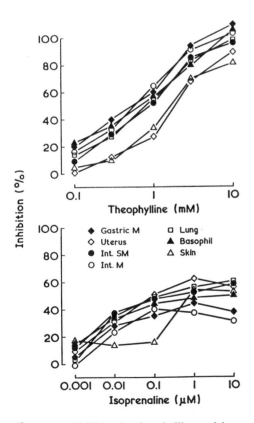

Figure 4 Inhibition by theophylline and isoproterenol (isoprenaline) of histamine release from human basophils (solid triangles); mast cells from the gastric (solid diamonds) and intestinal (open circles) mucosa; uterus (open diamonds); lung parenchyma (open squares); intestinal submucosa (solid circles); and skin (open triangles). (Data from Refs. 5, 13–17, and unpublished results.)

Table 1 Characteristics of Phosphodiesterase
Isozymes

Family	Isozyme	K_m (μM) cAMP	cGMP
I_α	Ca/calmodulin-stimulated	30	3
I_β	Ca/calmodulin-stimulated	1	2
II	cGMP-stimulated	50	50
III	cGMP-inhibited	0.2	0.3
IV	cAMP-specific	2	100
V	cGMP-specific	150	1

Source: Ref. 33.

its affinity for cAMP (K_m = 2 μM) is much greater than for cGMP (K_m = 100 μM). Consistently, rolipram and Ro 20-1724, which are selective inhibitors of PDE IV, block immunological histamine release from human lung mast cells and basophils and from mouse bone marrow-derived mast cells (33,35–37). As expected, neither SK&F 95654 nor zaprinast, inhibitors of PDE III and V, respectively, have any major effect on human lung cells or basophils (33). However, zaprinast is a potent inhibitor of histamine release from rat peritoneal mast cells (36). Whether this reflects a particular distribution of the isozyme in this cell type, or some unrelated activity of the drug, remains to be determined. (For further information on phosphodiesterase inhibitors in allergic diseases, see Chapter 22.)

β-Adrenoceptor Agonists

Although the mechanistic significance was not understood at the time, it is more than half a century since it was first demonstrated that a β-adrenoceptor agonist, epinephrine, could inhibit antigen-induced histamine secretion (38). This finding has since been amply confirmed, and it is clear that conventional agonists, such as isoproterenol (isoprenaline), can inhibit histamine release from all human mast cell phenotypes so far investigated (see Fig. 4). The compound is extremely potent, with an IC_{50} of approximately 1 μM.

Selective β$_2$-adrenoceptor agonists such as albuterol (salbutamol) now provide the mainstay of symptomatic relief in human bronchial asthma and are the most effective bronchodilators currently available (39). Similar to isoproterenol, they are very effective inhibitors of histamine release from human lung mast cells (40,41) and, in fact, are much more potent than cromolyn, with IC_{50} values in the micromolar, compared with the millimolar range. However, unlike cromolyn, they have little effect on the chronic inflammatory changes in the airways that underlie bronchial hyperresponsiveness and the everyday manifestations of asthma (42,43). This has been widely interpreted to mean that mast cell activation is not obligatory for these events (44). However, an alternative explanation is that the duration of action of current β-adrenoceptor agonists is too short to protect against extended exposure to allergens. In this context, recent studies with the newly developed agonist salmeterol are of interest (45). This compound was designed to provide prolonged bronchodilation to control nocturnal symptoms and improve maintenance therapy in asthmatic patients. Salmeterol is considerably more lipophilic than albuterol and has a higher affinity for the β$_2$-adrenoceptor. It appears to have a novel mode of action that involves binding of the lipophilic moiety to a specific exosite domain of the β$_2$-receptor protein to produce continuous stimulation of the active site of the receptor. The prolonged activation of β_2-receptors in the airways results in an extended bronchodilation, reduced vascular permeability, inhibition of inflammatory mediators, stimulation of ciliary function, and modulation of ion and water transport across the bronchial mucosa (45). Also, pretreatment of asthmatic subjects with salmeterol prevents the late asthmatic response and, importantly, attenuates the increase in airway responsiveness following airway challenge (46). These data would indicate that salmeterol has genuine anti-inflammatory properties. (For further information on the role of β-adrenergic agents in allergic diseases see Chapter 21.)

CORTICOSTEROIDS

Glucocorticoids represent the most potent anti-inflammatory agents available for the treatment of asthma. When administered before a bronchial challenge with allergen in a sensitized patient, they block the late-phase asthmatic response and the development of bronchial hyperresponsiveness. Continuous administration also reduces the immediate response to allergen provocation (47). The mechanism of action of these agents is thus of considerable significance. Detailed studies (48) have shown that glucocorticoids inhibit immunological release of histamine from human basophilic leukocytes with an order of potency that very closely parallels that found in vivo (i.e., triamcinolone acetonide > dexamethasone > betamethasone > prednisolone > hydrocortisone). The effect is seen after a 24-h preincubation with nanomolar to micromolar concentrations of glucocorticoid. Dexamethasone and betamethasone also inhibit LTC_4 release from mixed leukocyte preparations (49). Glucocorticoids similarly block mediator release from murine and guinea pig mast cells (50–52) but, surprisingly, have no effect on isolated human mast cells derived from lung parenchyma, intestine, or skin (53). However, topical intranasal glucocorticoids can substantially reduce the number of mast cells in the nasal mucosa (54,55), whereas oral steroids reduce the number of mast cells recovered by BAL of asthmatic subjects (56). Importantly, both the spontaneous and immunological release of histamine from the latter cells is also dramatically attenuated (56; Pearce FL, et al., unpublished work). It is not clear whether these data reflect the much longer time scale of these in vivo studies, or an indirect effect mediated by secondary cells. However, whatever the mechanism, glucocorticoids can clearly have a dramatic effect on human mast cell numbers and reactivity in clinical situations. (For additional information on corticosteroids in allergic disease, see Chapter 28.)

ANTIHISTAMINES

The effects of histamine are mediated through activation of three receptor subtypes, namely, H_1, H_2, and H_3 receptors. The symptoms of immediate-type hypersensitivity reactions are largely produced by stimulation of H_1 receptors and include contraction of bronchial smooth muscle, vasodilation, and increased capillary permeability. These effects may be antagonized by classic antihistamines, such as chlorpheniramine, and the newer, more selective H_1 antagonists, such as astemizole and terfenadine (57). Although these drugs are of proved benefit in allergic rhinitis, conjunctivities, and urticaria, their usefulness in asthma has been considered dubious (57). However, the availability of the newer compounds, which lack the central sedative actions of their predecessors, has made it possible to examine this effect in more detail. When given before allergen challenge, both terfenadine and astemizole attenuate the immediate bronchoconstriction in asthmatic subjects. Regular treatment with these drugs also reduces overall symptoms in mildly asthmatic subjects (57).

In addition to their specific antagonism of cellular histamine receptors, it has long been appreciated that antihistamines have a direct, biphasic action on mast cells (58). At low concentrations they inhibit immunological activation of the cell, whereas at higher concentrations they themselves induce histamine release. Some data for rat peritoneal mast cells are given in Table 2. Terfenadine and astemizole are seen to be the most effective histamine liberators, the phenothiazines, chlorpromazine, promethazine, and trimeprazine, together with ketotifen, show comparable activity, whereas antazoline, cyclizine, diphenhydramine, and triprolidine release histamine only at very high concentrations. Terfenadine and astemizole are also the most potent inhibitors of immunological histamine release (Fig. 5), but these two effects do not appear to be directly related as the ratio ED_{50}/ID_{50} (the concentrations required to produce and inhibit 50% of release, respectively) varies from higher than 100 to 1.0 (see Table 2). Different physicochemical features may then determine these two effects, and identification of these elements may facilitate the development of antihistamines devoid of histamine-releasing activity. The ability of the H_1-antagonists to inhibit release does not appear to correlate with their recorded pA_2 values on the guinea pig ilium, suggesting that the effect is not mediated through H_1 receptors (see Table 2). Instead, the compounds seem to produce their effects by acting directly on the cell membrane, with low concentrations of the drugs becoming intercalated into the lipid bilayer in a way such as to stabilize the structure and high concentrations disrupting the membrane and leading to

Table 2 Effect of Histamine H_1-Antagonists on the Induction and Inhibition of Histamine Release from Rat Peritoneal Mast Cells[a]

Drug	ED_{50} (μM)	ID_{50} (μM)	ED_{50}/ID_{50}	pA_2
Antazoline (ANT)	3,450	80	43.1	7.2
Astemizole (ATZ)	50	20	2.5	9.7
Brompheniramine (BPM)	>10,000	90	>111.1	8.5
Chlorpheniramine (CPM)	>10,000	120	>83.3	8.8
Chlorpromazine (CPZ)	170	20	8.5	8.1
Cyclizine (CYZ)	1200	540	2.2	7.6
Dimethindene (DMD)	>10,000	140	>71.4	10.0
Diphenhydramine (DPM)	2,500	400	6.3	7.6
Ketotifen (KET)	320	320	1.0	8.6
Mepyramine (MPM)/pyrilamine	>10,000	250	>40.0	9.0
Oxatomide (OXT)	>100	40	>2.5	8.4
Promethazine (PMZ)	180	20	9.0	8.9
Temelastine (SK&F 93944; SKF)	>100	>100	—	9.5
Terfenadine (TER)	20	10	2.0	8.2
Tripolidine (TPN)	6,200	120	51.7	9.9
Trimeprazine (TPZ)	160	20	8.0	8.1

[a]Results are recorded as ED_{50} (dose required to produce 50% histamine release during a standard 10-min period of incubation), ID_{50} (dose required to produce 50% inhibition of the histamine release induced by antigen) and pA_2 (literature value for antagonism of the H_1 receptor on the guinea pig ileum). All values are based on at least four experiments.
Source: Ref. 59.

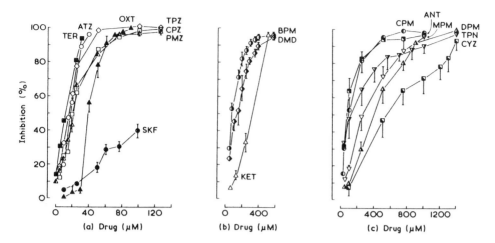

Figure 5 Inhibition of immunological histamine release from rat peritoneal mast cells by various histamine H_1 receptor antagonists. Cells were preincubated with the drugs for 5 min. Values are means ± SEM, $n = 4–7$. Abbreviations used are (a) astemizole (ATZ), chlorpromazine (CPZ), oxatomide (OXT), promethazine (PMZ), temelastine (SK&F 93944; SKF), terfenadine (TER), and trimeprazine (TPZ); (b) brompheniramine (BPM), dimethindene (DMD); and ketotifen (KET); and (c) antazoline (ANT), chlorpheniramine (CPM), cyclizine (CYZ), diphenhydramine (DPM), pyrilamine (mepyramine; MPM), and triprolidine (TPN). (From Ref. 59.)

cell lysis (59). Antihistamines can also inhibit histamine release from human lung parenchymal mast cells and basophilic leukocytes (60), and it seems possible that this may contribute to their clinical usefulness.

CYCLOSPORINE

Cyclosporine is a cyclic undecapeptide of fungal origin that is used as an immunosuppressive agent in the prevention of organ allograft rejection and a variety of inflammatory and autoimmune diseases (61,62). The major intracellular receptor for cyclosporine appears to be cyclophilin, a protein of M_r 17,000, which possesses peptidyl-prolyl *cis–trans*-isomerase activity (62).

Cyclosporine is thought to produce its effects largely by preventing the activation of and production of lymphokines by T lymphocytes (63). These cells have also been implicated in the pathogenesis of human bronchial asthma and, given that the immunosuppressive activity of cyclosporine resembles that of glucocorticoids, it has been suggested that the peptide may be of benefit in patients with severe steroid-dependent asthma (61,64). However, its activity is not confined to the T lymphocyte; it also affects a number of other inflammatory cells. In particular, it inhibits antigen presentation to T lymphocytes by monocytes and macrophages; production of interleukins and superoxide by macrophages; chemotaxis of neutrophils; blood, tissue, and bone marrow eosinophilia; cutaneous late-phase reactions; and bronchoconstriction induced by platelet-activating factor (61). The peptide also suppresses the release of mediators from mast cells and basophils. In particular, cyclosporine prevents the secretion of histamine and LTC_4 from human basophils (65,66), histamine, and PGD_2 from human lung (67,68) and skin (69) mast cells, and histamine from rat peritoneal mast cells (65,68) and RBL-2H3 cells (66). The compound also depletes intestinal mucosal mast cells in the rat, probably by suppressing proliferatory signals from T cells, and inhibits the release of mediators from these cells in vivo (70). The inhibitory effects are very rapid and, hence, presumably do not involve protein synthesis, and studies with a range of cyclosporine analogues indicated that they are probably produced by interaction with cyclophilin (71). In total, the ability of cyclosporine to modulate the activity of histaminocytes and other inflammatory cells may contribute to its therapeutic efficacy.

FUROSEMIDE

Diuretics have been used clinically for several decades for the treatment of hypertension, congestive heart failure, and a range of the conditions characterized by edema and fluid retention. Of these agents, the loop diuretics typified by furosemide (frusemide in Europe) and bumetanide are the most powerful (72). Recent studies, however, have suggested an additional use for these compounds in the management of human bronchial asthma. This derives from the surprising observation of Bianco and colleagues that inhalation of nebulized furosemide almost completely inhibits the airway response to exercise and ultrasonically nebulized water and also blocks the early and late responses to antigen (73–75). Since then, several studies have confirmed the inhibitory effects of furosemide on a range of bronchoconstrictor stimuli, including sodium metabisulfite and adenosine, but have shown that the compound is inactive against agents acting directly on the bronchial smooth muscle, including histamine, methacholine, and $PGF_{2\alpha}$ (76). It may be relevant that this pattern of response is identical with that observed with cromolyn and nedocromil. Also, furosemide blocks the release of histamine and sulfidopeptide leukotrienes from sensitized human lung fragments (77) and the secretion of histamine from isolated rat peritoneal and human lung mast cells (78). The drug exhibits tachyphylaxis in the latter systems, again similar to that observed with cromolyn and nedocromil.

The mechanism by which these effects are produced is unknown, but the diuretic action of the drug is due to prevention of the inward movement of chloride by inhibition of the Na/K/2Cl cotransporter located on the lumenal surface of the thick ascending limb of the kidney nephron (72). Given the potential role of chloride channels in the activation of mast cells (see foregoing), it is tempting to speculate that the drug might act by blocking these channels and preventing the associated movement of calcium. Further study will be required to resolve this possibility, but furosemide may well prove to be a very valuable tool in defining the mechanisms involved in mast cell activation and the mode of action of antiallergic drugs.

ACKNOWLEDGMENTS

Work from the author's laboratory was supported by grants from Fisons PLC and the Wellcome Trust.

REFERENCES

1. Barrett KE, Pearce FL. Heterogeneity of mast cells. Handb Exp Pharmacol 1991; 97:93–117.
2. Barrett KE, Pearce FL. Mast cell heterogeneity. In: Foreman JC, ed. Immunopharmacology of Mast Cells and Basophils. London: Academic Press, 1993; 29–42.

3. Schwartz LB. Mediators of human mast cells and human mast cell subsets. Ann Allergy 1987; 58:226–235.
4. Benyon RC. The human skin mast cell. Clin Exp Allergy 1989; 19:375–387.
5. Pearce FL, Al-Laith M, Bosman L, Brostoff J, Cunniffe TM, Flint KC, Hudspith BN, Jaffar ZH, Johnson NMcI, Kassessinoff TA, Lau HYA, Lee PY, Leung KBP, Liu W, Tainsh KR. Effects of sodium cromoglycate and nedocromil sodium on histamine secretion from mast cells from various locations. Drugs 1989; 37(suppl 1):37–43.
6. Suschitzky JL. Antiasthmatic agents: the discovery of Intal. Chem Br 1985; 21:554–555.
7. Assem ESK, Mongar JL. Inhibition of allergic reactions in man and other species by cromoglycate. Int Arch Allergy 1970; 38:68–77.
8. Cox JSG. Disodium cromoglycate (FPL 670) ("Intal"): a specific inhibitor of reaginic antibody–antigen mechanisms. Nature 1967; 216:1328–1329.
9. Stokes TC, Morley J. Prospects for an oral Intal. Br J Dis Chest 1981; 75:1–14.
10. Cairns H, Orr TSC. The development of a new agent for the treatment of inflammatory/allergic conditions. Int Arch Allergy Appl Immunol 1987; 82:513–517.
11. Foreman JC, Pearce FL. Cromolyn and nedocromil. In: Middleton E, Reed CE, Ellis EF, Adkinson NF, Yunginger JW, Busse WW, eds. Allergy: Principles and Practice. Vol. 1, 4th ed. St. Louis: CV Mosby, 1993:926–940.
12. Pearce FL, Befus AD, Gauldie J, Bienenstock J. Mucosal mast cells. II. Effect of anti-allergic compounds on histamine secretion by isolated intestinal mast cells. J Immunol 1982; 128:2481–2486.
13. Pearce FL, Boulos PB, Lau HYA, Liu WL, Tainsh KR. Functional heterogeneity of human mast cells. Int Arch Allergy Appl Immunol 1991; 94:239–240.
14. Tainsh KR, Lau HYA, Liu, WL, Pearce FL. The human skin mast cell: a comparison with the human lung cell and a novel mast cell type, the uterine mast cell. Agents Actions 1991; 33:16–19.
15. Liu WL, Boulos PB, Lau HYA, Pearce FL. Mast cells from human gastric mucosa: a comparative study with lung and colonic mast cells. Agents Actions 1991; 33:13–15.
16. Liu WL, Bosman L, Boulos PB, Lau HYA, Pearce FL. Mast cells from human colonic mucosa and submucosa/muscle: a comparison with human lung mast cells. Agents Actions 1990; 30:70–73.
17. Leung KBP, Flint KC, Brostoff J, Hudspith BN, Johnson NMcI, Lau HYA, Liu WL, Pearce FL. Effects of sodium cromoglycate and nedocromil sodium on histamine secretion from human lung mast cells. Thorax 1988; 43:756–761.
18. Mazurek N, Geller-Bernstein C, Pecht I. Affinity of calcium ions to the antiallergic drug, dicromoglycate. FEBS Lett 1980; 111:194–196.
19. Foreman JC, Hallett MB, Mongar JL. Site of action of the antiallergic drugs cromoglycate and doxantrazole. Br J Pharmacol 1977; 59:473P–474P.
20. White JR, Ishizaka T, Ishizaka K, Sha'afi R. Direct demonstration of increased intracellular concentration of free calcium as measured by quin-2 in stimulated rat peritoneal mast cell. Proc Natl Acad Sci USA 1984; 81:3978–3982.
21. Tasaka K, Mio M, Okamoto M. Intracellular calcium release induced by histamine releasers and its inhibition by some antiallergic drugs. Ann Allergy 1986; 56:464–469.
22. Mazurek N, Bashkin P, Pecht I. Isolation of a basophilic membrane protein binding the antiallergic drug cromolyn. EMBO J 1982; 1:585–590.
23. Mazurek N, Bashkin P, Loyter A, Pecht I. Restoration of Ca^{2+} influx and degranulation capacity of variant RBL-2H3 cells upon implantation of isolated cromolyn binding protein. Proc Natl Acad Sci USA 1983; 80:6014–6018.
24. Mazurek N, Schindler H, Schürholz TH, Pecht I. The cromolyn binding protein constitutes the Ca^{2+} channel of basophils opening upon immunological stimulus. Proc Natl Acad Sci USA 1984; 81:6841–6845.
25. Sieghart W, Theoharides TC, Douglas WW, Greengard P. Phosphorylation of a single mast cell protein in response to drugs that inhibit secretion. Biochem Pharmacol 1981; 30:2737–2738.
26. Wells E, Mann J. Phosphorylation of a mast cell protein in response to treatment with anti-allergic

compounds. Implications for the mode of action of sodium cromoglycate. Biochem Pharmacol 1983; 32:837–842.

27. Penner R, Mathews G, Neher E. Regulation of calcium influx by second messengers in rat mast cells. Nature 1988; 334:499–504.

28. Romanin C, Reinsprecht M, Pecht I, Schindler H. Immunologically activated chloride channels involved in degranulation of rat mucosal mast cells. EMBO J 1991; 10:3603–3608.

29. Moqbel R, Walsh GM, Macdonald AJ, Kay B. Effect of disodium cromoglycate on activation of human eosinophils and neutrophils following reversed (anti-IgE) anaphylaxis. Clin Allergy 1986; 16:73–83.

30. Moqbel R, Cromwell O, Walsh GM, Wardlaw AJ, Kurlak L, Kay AB. Effects of nedocromil sodium (Tilade) on the activation of human eosinophils and neutrophils and the release of histamine from mast cells. Allergy 1988; 43:268–276.

31. Bruijnzeel PLB, Warringa RAJ, Kok PTM. Inhibition of platelet-activating factor and zymosan-activated serum-induced chemotaxis of human neutrophils by nedocromil sodium, BN 5201 and sodium cromoglycate. Br J Pharmacol 1989; 97:1251–1257.

32. Richards IM, Dixon M, Jackson DM, Vendy K. Alternative modes of action of sodium cromoglycate. Agents Actions 1986; 18:294–300.

33. Torphy TJ, Undem BJ. Phosphodiesterase inhibitors: new opportunities for the treatment of asthma. Thorax 1991; 46:512–523.

34. Aronson JK, Hardman M, Reynolds DJM. Theophylline. Br Med J 1992; 305:1355–1362.

35. Peachell PT, Undem BJ, Schleimer RP, Lichtenstein LM, Torphy TJ. Action of isozyme-selective phosphodiesterase (PDE) inhibitors on human basophils. FASEB J 1990; 4:A639.

36. Frossard N, Landry Y, Pauli G, Ruckstuhl M. Effects of cyclic AMP- and cyclic GMP-phosphodiesterase inhibitors on immunologic release of histamine and on lung contraction. Br J Pharmacol 1981; 73:933–938.

37. Busse WW, Anderson VL. The granulocyte response to the phosphodiesterase inhibitor Ro 20-1724 in asthma. J Allergy Clin Immunol 1981; 67:70–74.

38. Schild HO. Histamine release and anaphylactic shock in isolated lungs of guinea-pigs. Q J Exp Physiol 1936; 26:165–179.

39. Barnes PJ. β-Adrenoceptors on smooth muscle, nerves and inflammatory cells. Life Sci 1993; 52:2101–2109.

40. Peters SP, Schulman ES, Schleimer RP, MacGlashan DW, Newball HH, Lichtenstein LM. Dispersed human lung mast cells: pharmacologic aspects and comparison with human lung fragments. Annu Rev Respir Dis 1982; 126:1034–1038.

41. Church MK, Young KD. The characteristics of inhibition of mediator release from human lung fragments by sodium cromoglycate, salbutamol and chlorpromazine. Br J Pharmacol 1983; 78:671–679.

42. Cockcroft DW, Murdock KY. Comparative effects of inhaled salbutamol, sodium cromoglycate and beclamethasone diproprionate on allergen-induced early asthmatic response, late asthmatic responses, and increased bronchial responsiveness to histamine. J Allergy Clin Immunol 1987; 79:734–740.

43. Kraan J, Koeler GH, Mark TW, Shuter HJ, De Vries K. Changes in bronchial hyperreactivity induced by 4 weeks of treatment with anti-asthmatic drugs in patients with allergic asthma: a comparison between budesonide and terbutaline. J Allergy Clin Immunol 1985; 76:628–631.

44. Kay AB. The mode of action of anti-allergic drugs. Clin Allergy 1987; 17:153–164.

45. Johnson M, Butchers PR, Coleman RA, Nials AT, Strong P, Sumner MJ, Vardey CJ, Whelan CJ. The pharmacology of salmeterol. Life Sci 1993; 52:2131–2143.

46. Twentyman OP, Finnerty JP, Harris A, Palmer J, Holgate ST. Protection against allergen-induced asthma by salmeterol. Lancet 1990; 336:1338–1342.

47. Stempel DA, Szefter SJ. Management of chronic asthma. Ped Clin N Am 1992; 39:1293–1310.

48. Schleimer RP, MacGlashan DW, Gillespie E, Lichtenstein LM. Inhibition of basophil histamine release by anti-inflammatory steroids. J Immunol 1982; 129:1632–1636.

49. Schleimer RP, Davidson DA, Peters SP, Lichtenstein LM. Inhibition of human basophil leuko-triene release by antiinflammatory steroids. Int Arch Allergy Appl Immunol 1985; 77:241–243.
50. Daeron M, Sterk AR, Hirata F, Ishizaka T. Biochemical analysis of glucocorticoid-induced inhibition of IgE-mediated histamine release from mouse mast cells. J Immunol 1982; 129:1212–1218.
51. Marquardt D, Wasserman SI. Modulation of rat serosal mast cell biochemistry by in vivo dexamethasone administration. J Immunol 1983; 131:934–939.
52. Schleimer RP, Undem BJ, Meeker S. Dexamethasone inhibits the antigen-induced contractile activity and release of inflammatory mediators in isolated guinea pig lung tissue. Am Rev Respir Dis 1987; 135:562–566.
53. Cohan VL, Undem BJ, Fox CC, Adkinson NF, Lichtenstein LM, Schleimer RP. Dexamethasone does not inhibit the release of mediators from human mast cells residing in airway, intestine or skin. Am Rev Respir Dis 1989; 140:951–954.
54. Pipkorn U. Budesonide and nasal mucosal histamine content and anti-IgE induced histamine release. Allergy 1982; 37:591–595.
55. Okuda M, Sakaguchi K, Ohtsuka H. Intranasal beclomethasone: mode of action in nasal allergy. Ann Allergy 1983; 50:116–120.
56. Millar AB, Hudspith BN, Lau A, Pearce F, Johnson NMcI. A mechanism for the role of steroids in the treatment of asthma? Thorax 1989; 44:359P.
57. Wood-Baker R, Church MK. Histamine and asthma. Immunol Allergy Clin North Am 1990; 10:329–336.
58. Mota I, Dias da Silva W. The anti-anaphylactic and histamine releasing properties of the antihistamines. The effect on mast cells. Br J Pharmacol 1960; 15:396–404.
59. Lau HYA, Pearce FL. Effects of antihistamines on isolated rat peritoneal mast cells and on model membrane systems. Agents Actions 1990; 29:151–161.
60. Lau HYA, Pearce FL. Effects of antihistamines on isolated human lung mast cells, basophil leucocytes and erythrocytes. Agents Actions 1989; 27:83–85.
61. Calderon E, Lockey RF, Bukantz SC, Coffey RG, Ledford DK. Is there a role for cyclosporine in asthma? J Allergy Clin Immunol 1992; 89:629–636.
62. Sigal NH, Dumont FJ. Cyclosporin A, FK-506, and rapamycin: pharmacologic probes of lymphocyte signal transduction. Annu Rev Immunol 1992; 10:519–560.
63. Kahan BD. Cyclosporine. N Engl J Med 1989; 321:1725–1735.
64. Sczeklik A, Nizankowska E, Dwoski R, Domagala B, Pinis G. Cyclosporin for steroid-dependent asthma. Allergy 1991; 46:312–315.
65. Perdersen C, Permin H, Stahl Skov P, Norn S, Svenson M, Mosbech H, Bendtzen K. Inhibitory effect of cyclosporin A on histamine release from human leukocytes and rat mast cells. Allergy 1985; 40:103–107.
66. Ezeamuzie CI, Assem ESK. Anti-allergic properties of cyclosporin A: inhibition of mediator release from human basophils and rat basophilic leukemia cells (RBL-2H3). Immunopharmacology 1990; 20:31–43.
67. Triggiani M, Cirillo R, Lichtenstein LM, Marone G. Inhibition of histamine and prostaglandin D_2 release from human lung mast cells by ciclosporin [sic] A. Int Arch Allergy Appl Immunol 1989; 88:253–255.
68. Ezeamuzie IC, Assem ESK. Inhibition of histamine release from human lung and rat peritoneal mast cells by cyclosporin A. Agents Actions 1990; 30:110–113.
69. Stellato C, de Paulis A, Ciccarelli A, Cirillo R, Patella V, Casolaro V, Marone G. Anti-inflammatory effect of cyclosporin A on human skin mast cells. J Invest Dermatol 1992; 98:800–804.
70. Cummins AG, Munro GH, Ferguson A. Effect of cyclosporin on rat mucosal mast cells and the associated protease RMCPII. Clin Exp Immunol 1988; 72:136–140.
71. Cirillo R, Triggiani M, Siri L, Ciccarelli A, Pettit GR, Condorelli M, Marone G. Cyclosporin A rapidly inhibits mediator release from human basophils presumably by interacting with cyclophilin. J Immunol 1990; 144:3891–3897.

72. Hendry BM, Ellory JC. Molecular sites for diuretic action. Trends Pharmacol Sci 1988; 9: 416–421.

73. Bianco S, Vaghi A, Robuschi M, Pasargikliian M. Prevention of exercise-induced bronchoconstriction by inhaled frusemide. Lancet 1988; 2:252–255.

74. Robuschi M, Vaghi A, Gambaro G, Spagnotto S, Bianco S. Inhaled frusemide is highly effective in preventing ultrasonically nebulized water bronchoconstriction. Am Rev Respir Dis 1988; 137:412.

75. Bianco S, Pieroni MG, Refini RM, Rottoli L, Sestini P. Protective effect of inhaled frusemide on allergen-induced early and late asthmatic reactions. N Engl J Med 1989; 321:1069–1073.

76. Chung KF, Barnes PJ. Loop diuretics and asthma. Pulm Pharmacol 1992; 5:1–7.

77. Anderson SD, He W, Temple DM. Inhibition by furosemide of inflammatory mediators from lung fragments. N Engl J Med 1991; 324:131.

78. Redrup AC, Pearce FL. Effect of loop diuretics on rat peritoneal and human lung mast cells. Agents Actions 1994; 41:C47–C48.

28

Corticosteroids: Mechanisms of Action and Treatment of Allergic Disease

John H. Toogood and Frederick A. White
University of Western Ontario, London, Ontario, Canada

MECHANISMS

A cascade of different cell types, cytokines, and mediators participate in the process of allergic inflammation (1,2). Among these, T lymphocytes play a central role, because they control immunoglobulin (Ig)E synthesis and are an important source of cytokines necessary to the recruitment, accumulation, and activation of inflammatory cells. The balance between different subsets of T-helper cells determines the type of allergic inflammation expressed clinically; namely, delayed-type hypersensitivity (associated with predominant T_H1 cell activation) or atopic disease (associated with predominant T_H2 cell activation). Furthermore, cytokines, acting by the expression of adhesion molecules on the surface of effector cells (e.g., eosinophils) and target cells (e.g., vascular endothelium), may determine which organ is targeted in a particular allergic response.

Glucocorticoids exert many important effects on this inflammatory process (2). These include inhibition of the secretion of cytokines and proinflammatory mediators; inhibition of leukocyte priming; decreases in vascular permeability; inhibition of the release of arachidonic acid metabolites and platelet-activating factor (PAF); synergistic or permissive effects on cell responsiveness to other hormones, such as catecholamines; and modulation of the whole process by inhibition of synthesis or release of certain inflammatory enzymes, coupled with induction of the synthesis of other enzymes with anti-inflammatory activity. This broad spectrum of anti-inflammatory activities makes the glucocorticoids uniquely valuable therapeutically because it allows them to interfere with the evolution of the pathogenetic process at many different points. This is well illustrated in bronchial asthma, for which the dynamics of the inflammatory process can be differentiated into early and late asthmatic responses and the associated phenomenon of airways hyperresponsiveness (AHR).

Early Asthmatic Response

The early asthmatic response (EAR) to antigen or exercise typically begins about 10 min after the provocation challenge, reaches a maximum within 30 min, resolves spontaneously within 1–3 h, and is fully reversible with a β-adrenergic bronchodilator. Evidence of mediator release from mast cells accompanies the decrease in airflow. Additional chemotactic mediators are also released that contribute to the cellular influx responsible for the late asthmatic response (LAR), which may follow resolution of the EAR (3).

The EAR is not preventable by steroid treatment given immediately before the provocative challenge, but it may be reduced if the drug is administered long enough beforehand to allow its inhibitory intracellular effects to be fully expressed. A 3-h interval was sufficient in sensitized sheep treated with prednisolone (4). In humans, 1–4 weeks of daily treatment with an inhaled steroid (I-S) inhibits the EAR, the degree of protection increasing with the duration of treatment (5).

Late Asthmatic Response

The LAR begins about 3–5 h after spontaneous recovery from the EAR that typically (but not invariably) precedes it, peaks at about 8 h, and resolves within 12. However, it may commence later than 8 h, persist as long as 24 h, and recur repeatedly over several days after a single evocative challenge. Unlike the EAR, the LAR is only partially and transiently reversible with adrenergic treatment—reflecting the inflammatory component that coexists with bronchospasm.

The LAR to allergens, isocyanates, or exercise can be blocked by steroid treatment given systemically or by inhalation, at or before the provocatory challenge, or soon thereafter (3,6,7). This inhibitory effect is probably critically dependent on the capacity of the steroid to prevent the accumulation and activation of neutrophils or eosinophils in the airways.

Airways Hyperresponsiveness

The LAR is strongly associated with AHR; that is, an increase in nonspecific airways responsiveness to inhaled cholinergics, histamine, cold air, and other nonallergic stimuli. The degree of both AHR and the LAR correlate significantly with the clinical severity of chronic asthma. It has been postulated that the two phenomena interact synergistically to amplify the intensity of the bronchial response to antigen exposure. This could explain the susceptibility of patients with allergic asthma to nonantigenic triggering factors, such as exercise or the inhalation of cold air. Furthermore, it could also explain why symptoms persist in some patients long after their removal from exposure to the causative antigen (8).

The LAR and associated increase in AHR can be blocked by pretreatment with steroid given systemically or by inhalation. However, it is possible to demonstrate an increase in AHR in response to antigen challenge, despite blockage of the usual antecedent LAR by steroid pretreatment (9). This suggests that the two phenomena are not directly linked in a chain of causation; possibly different cell populations are involved.

Although the mechanisms of AHR may vary in different patient populations, airways inflammation is involved to an important degree in patients with asthma. This is evidenced by the capacity of steroid treatment to prevent or to reverse the seasonal rise in AHR that occurs in patients sensitized to pollen antigens (10), and its corrective effect on the persisting AHR characteristically found in patients with perennial asthma (11). The beneficial effect of I-S therapy on AHR is dose-dependent and topically mediated, being discernible with doses so low that they are devoid of measurable systemic glucocorticoid activity (11).

The inhibitory action of glucocorticoid drugs on AHR involves a very prompt initial response, presumably owing to a reduction in capillary permeability (12). This is followed by a slower accumulative response that may evolve over weeks, months, or even years (12–14). This may reflect the progressive resolution of airways inflammation.

Neurohumoral Regulation

The synthesis and release of inflammatory and anaphylactic mediators are normally inhibited by β-adrenergic mechanisms and stimulated by α-adrenergic and cholinergic mechanisms. In patients with atopy or asthma, an imbalance in these systems has been observed that is thought to be intrinsic. Additionally, acquired β-adrenergic insufficiency caused by viral infections, or prolonged treatment with β-adrenergic agonist drugs may further perturb this system to augment the local and systemic release of proinflammatory mediators (15–18). These changes may adversely affect the clinical course of patients with chronic asthma and impair the responsiveness of severe asthma to emergency bronchodilator treatment (19,20).

Systemic steroid therapy can prevent or reverse the desensitizing effect of sustained β-adrenergic agonist treatment on cell responsiveness. In doing so, it enhances receptor affinity for the agonist, corrects the down-regulation (15) or functional uncoupling (21) of adrenoreceptors, and activates various protein kinases involved in the β-adrenergic response (21).

These effects on β-adrenoceptors require several hours to evolve. In this manner, they differ from the capacity of glucocorticoid treatment to prolong the action of endogenous catecholamines (but not albuterol or metaproterenol) (22,23), which is manifest in vitro within minutes (24).

INHALED STEROID FOR CHRONIC ASTHMA

Treatment Rationale

Among the I-S drugs currently used to treat asthma, beclomethasone dipropionate (BDP), flunisolide, and triamcinolone acetonide are available for clinical use in the United States, whereas—at the time of writing—fluticasone and budesonide (BUD) are undergoing clinical investigation as new drugs. Budesonide is clinically available in Europe and Canada. Betamethasone valerate is also used in Europe.

The topical anti-inflammatory activity of these drugs reflects their lipophilic properties and high affinity for the glucocorticoid receptor. At low doses their clinical efficacy appears to be entirely due to their topical action in the airways (25). The fraction that is systemically absorbed is therapeutically inert (25). At high doses, the possibility of a contributory systemic effect cannot be excluded.

Pathogenetic Rationale for Inhaled Steroid Therapy

Because airways inflammation is the primary pathogenetic determinant of asthma, and the glucocorticoids are the most potent of the anti-inflammatory agents currently available and the I-S formulations have a more favorable therapeutic index than the oral or parenteral glucocorticoids, I-S therapy is now generally accepted as the preventative treatment of choice for most patients with asthma (26,27).

Clinical Rationale

The I-S drugs have the capacity to reduce the risks and also increase the benefits of asthma treatment.

In terms of reducing risk, I-S can diminish the need for oral bronchodilators, with a corollary reduction in the adverse effects and risk of mortality that complicate theophylline use, and the less serious, but uncomfortable, systemic side effects of oral β-adrenergic agonists (28). The I-S can also reduce or eliminate the excessive dependence on inhaled β-agonists, which is known to be associated with an increased risk of morbidity and mortality (29–33).

In terms of increased benefits, I-S therapy is more effective than "as needed" or regular inhaled β-adrenergic agonist therapy (34–36,47), more effective than cromolyn (37,38), nedocromil (39,40), or ketotifen (41); at least as effective as regular theophylline, and less toxic (42,43); and (provided an adequate dose is given) as effective as prednisone given daily (44,45). Also, I-S is more effective than alternate-day prednisone, if the two regimens are compared at systemically equivalent doses (45).

Also, I-S therapy may ameliorate the progression of asthma to chronic irreversible airflow limitation. Until recently, the evidence that this can be accomplished has been circumstantial and entirely related to oral steroid (O-S) treatment (46), but several controlled prospective studies now suggest that I-S therapy may decelerate the process of progressive airflow limitation (33,48,49).

Inhaled Steroid Versus Oral Steroid

Few published studies have systematically compared the clinical potency and toxicity of O-S and I-S over a wide dosage range in the same patients.

In one such study (a double-blind, crossover comparison of I-S given qid versus graded doses of prednisone given orally once daily on alternate mornings), BUD was significantly more effective when the two regimens were compared at equivalent levels of systemic activity, as measured by their respective effects on the morning cortisol level (45,50).

In a separate study, graded doses of prednisone administered daily as a single morning dose, were compared with BUD inhaled four times daily over a range of doses extending from low and nontoxic to high and potentially toxic levels (41).

Either drug proved equally effective, provided that a large enough dose was administered (Fig. 1). Furthermore, regardless of the dose of I-S used, its systemic glucocorticoid activity was consistently about six times less than that produced by the dose of prednisone required to achieve the same level of asthma control in the same patients (41).

These results favor I-S over either daily or alternate-day O-S for patients who have steroid-dependent asthma. The findings are assumed to apply in principle to the other I-S drugs currently used to treat asthma. However, the margin of the therapeutic advantage of the I-S over prednisone might be less if a different I-S with a topical anti-inflammatory potency lower than that of BUD were used, or if the I-S were administered less frequently than four times a day. Either of these factors may reduce efficacy (see also sections on dosing frequency and formulations).

Substitution of Prednisone with Inhaled Steroid

A reliable estimate of patients' minimum requirements for O-S and I-S requires a dose titration and follow-up period of at least 6 months (51)—preferably longer. We use an 18-month dose titration periods (52). Our schedule, modified for use in clinical practice, is shown in Table 1.

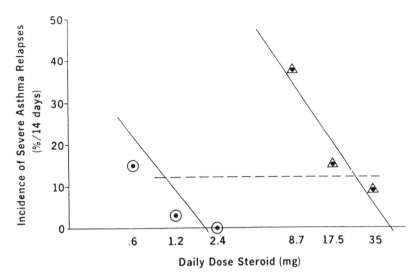

Figure 1   Incidence of disabling asthma relapses during a double-blind crossover comparison of
BUD (⊙) inhaled qid, versus prednisone (△), single AM dose. Every patient took three graduated
doses of each drug, 2 weeks at each dose level. The individual doses varied depending on the patient's
severity of asthma. Doses shown are group means $n = 34$. If a sufficiently large dose is given, either
oral or inhaled steroid may effectively control severe chronic asthma. Potency of BUD to prednisone
= 25:1; $n = 34$. (From Ref. 46.)

The 18% success rate for complete prednisone withdrawal that we were able to achieve
in the aforementioned study (52) indicates that many patients with severe asthma cannot be
optimally controlled on low doses of I-S alone. Such patients are candidates for higher than
conventional doses of I-S (which can be achieved only with a concentrated formulation), or
for combined oral–I-S treatment. The systemic activities of I-S and O-S are additive.
However, provided the doses of each are titrated to minimum effective levels, the overall
effect of such combined treatment can be clinically worthwhile (i.e., major improvements
in asthma control can be achieved with no accompanying increase in the level of systemic
toxicity; 53). In this particular study group, the factors that determined the need for
continuing prednisone use, regular or intermittent—despite the use of BDP doses up to 1.6
mg/day—were the presence of associated nasal polyposis, aspirin intolerance, chronic
bronchitis, a previous need for more than one dose of prednisone per day, and a record of
poor compliance with past treatment (51). The last was the most important single factor (51).

Tests of the morning serum cortisol level or corticotropin (adrenocorticotropic hormone;
ACTH) responsiveness proved unreliable in these patients as predictors of the risk of severe
asthma relapse complicating the attempted prednisone withdrawal (53). Furthermore, the
hypothalamic–pituitary–adrenal (HPA) axis tests have shown no predictive value for the
deaths that have occasionally complicated prednisone withdrawal under the aegis of I-S
treatment (54). Asthma relapse—not adrenocortical insufficiency—is the primary problem
in these patients, and close clinical surveillance is the only reliable way to contain this risk.

Table 1 Schedule for Conversion to Inhaled Steroid Therapy in Asthma Patients Chronically Dependent on Prednisone

Phase	Approximate duration	Treatment
1	2 wk	In severely obstructed patients, precede inhaled steroid with a course of prednisone (e.g., 40–60 mg/d; adult dose) to clear the small airways of mucus. For less severe asthma, omit this step.
2	2 wk	Initiate inhaled steroid at high dosage, (e.g., >1 mg/d; nominal dose). Halve prednisone dosage by converting to alternate mornings.
3	2–4 mo	Reduce prednisone at 2-wk intervals by 10 mg/dose. Terminate prednisone if possible. Continue as high a daily dose of inhaled steroid as is practical.
4	2–4	If patient cannot stay off prednisone, determine minimum requirements. Continue high-dose inhaled steroid.
5	6–12 mo	Reduce inhaled steroid to lowest dose that maintains optimal control. Continue minimum prednisone if required.

Source: Ref. 52.

Intermittent Prednisone

When close clinical surveillance is maintained and, especially, if peak expiratory flow rate (PEFR) is measured daily by the patient, it is often possible to prevent or attenuate severe asthma relapse by intervening with a burst of O-S therapy. This is feasible because the occurrence of such relapses may be heralded days or weeks beforehand by a gradual deterioration in pulmonary function.

Intermittent short bursts of prednisone or prednisolone are effective for this purpose and are generally well tolerated. Either may be used because the two are freely and rapidly interconvertible after absorption (55,56). After 3 weeks of treatment with 20 mg prednisolone twice daily, endogenous cortisol production typically returns to normal within 3 days of abruptly stopping the drug (57). Furthermore, during the 3-day recovery period, the responsiveness of the HPA axis to stress remains prompt, although slightly reduced in magnitude (58).

The O-S-induced growth retardation in children is negligible if prednisone bursts total 3 weeks or less per year, and slight to moderate with more frequent treatment (e.g., 4–12 weeks/year). With longer periods of O-S use, growth is likely to be materially slower than that of matched nonasthmatic controls (59).

If a burst of prednisone is required more than once per year to control severe asthma relapse, this suggests the daily dose of I-S should be increased, with the objective of eliminating the need for intermittent prednisone, if possible.

Determinants of Inhaled Steroid Efficacy

The major determinants of the success of I-S therapy are the dose per day, dosing frequency, drug delivery system, duration of therapy, and patient compliance.

Daily Dose

The benefits and adverse effects of I-S treatment are dose-dependent, the relation being approximately linear on log daily dose (Fig. 2). The frequency distribution of the daily doses currently required by adults attending our asthma clinic is shown in Table 2. About

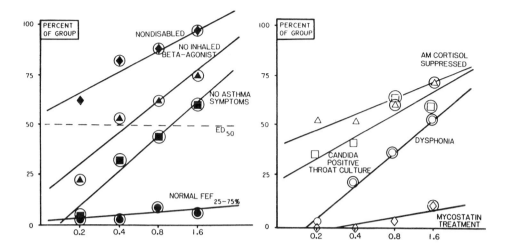

LOG DOSE BECLOMETHASONE (mg/day)

Figure 2 Clinical and systemic responses of 34 prednisone-dependent adult asthmatics to graded dosages of BDP. At each encircled point the mean change from the pre-BDP baseline value was significant ($p < 0.05$ or better). The effective BDP dose for 50% of the group (ED_{50}) may be determined by relating the intercepts of the dashed line with each regression line to the abscissa scale. The antiasthmatic effects, and the systemic and oropharyngeal complications of inhaled BDP are all dose-dependent. The high incidence of adrenal suppression in this group reflects their past systemic steroid therapy plus the effect of combined oral and I-S treatment. Their current prednisone dosage was held stable at an average of 11.0 mg/day while the stepwise BDP increments were added as shown. (From Ref. 61.)

Table 2 Frequency Distribution of Daily Dose Requirements for Inhaled Steroids Among Asthmatic Adults[a]

Nominal dose (mg/day)[b]	% of inhaled steroid users	Puffs per day	
		Dilute	Concentrated[c]
<1.0	55	<20	<5
1.0–2.0	40	20–40	5–10
>2.0	5	>40	>10

[a]Data from a 1989–1990 adudit of the entire adult population receiving ambulatory care for asthma from three specialist physicians in a tertiary health care faculty.

[a]For the Canadian formulations of budesonide or beclomethasone used by these patients, nominal dose = labeled dose.

[b]Concentrated formulations currently marketed: triamcinolone (Azmacort) and flunisolide (Aerobid), and beclomethasone (Becloforte) and budesonide (Pulmicort) (Canada and Europe). See section on comparing I-S formulations on nominal dosage.

Source: Ref. 216.

half these patients require more than 1.0 mg/day (nominal dose) to maintain optimal asthma control. As shown in Table 2, such doses entail an excessively large number of puffs per day unless a concentrated formulation of I-S is used.

For the purposes of an initial therapeutic trial, it is advantageous to begin with a high, rather than a low, dose of I-S because (1) many patients who do not respond to low doses do so with higher doses (60,61); (2) high doses give more accurately predictable results than low doses within a trial period of limited duration, such as 14 days (62); (3) a higher dose is required to normalize pulmonary function than simply to control symptoms (61); and (4) normalization of pulmonary function, insofar as this is feasible in the individual patient, is considered a more efficient goal of long-term asthma treatment than symptomatic treatment alone, since abnormal forced expiratory volume (FEV_1) and airways hyperresponsiveness values are both known to carry prognostic significance for the persistence of childhood asthma into adulthood (63,64). After securing optimal control, down titration of the dose is feasible (65).

Dosing Frequency

The ideal dosing frequency for I-S is a matter of controversy. Once-daily treatment may be as effective as twice-daily (66) and twice-daily treatment may be as effective as four times daily for periods of weeks to months, provided the asthma has been well stabilized (67–69). However, when asthma is unstable, twice-daily dosing is less effective than four times daily (69), and the difference between the regimens can be large enough to be clinically important. For example, in the study illustrated in Figure 3, the therapeutically equivalent dose rose from 0.4 mg/day (with qid treatment) to more than 3 mg/day (with bid treatment) (70). Thus, halving the dose frequency was associated with a shift in the therapeutically equivalent dose from low and nontoxic to high and potentially toxic levels, with a corollary increase in the cost of treatment. For BUD, the greater efficacy of four- versus two-times-daily dosing during long-term treatment has been confirmed by controlled trial in patients with moderate to severe asthma (71), and more recently in patients with milder asthma (72).

In view of the characteristically variable course of chronic asthma, these cost–benefit and risk–benefit considerations suggest it is prudent to recommend four-times-daily dosing as the standard regimen for long-term I-S use, when this is feasible.

Intrapulmonary Delivery

The efficacy of I-S therapy depends ultimately on how much gets into the lung. Under ideal conditions and in well-trained healthy subjects, about 10% of each dose emitted from the metered-dose inhaler (MDI) enters the lung. This figure is lower in patients who have obstructive pulmonary impairment. Furthermore, many asthmatic patients who use the MDI coordinate their inspiratory effort so poorly (73) that it significantly reduces the effectiveness of I-S treatment. Maximizing the efficiency of intrapulmonary drug delivery requires discharge of the aerosol bolus from the MDI early in the inspiratory effort, and a slow inspiration (commencing from FRC, rather than RV) at about 25 L/min, followed by a 5- to 10-s breath-hold (74). As shown in Table 3, coaching the patient in the correct inhalation technique can materially improve drug delivery. Further improvement can be achieved by attaching a "spacer" device to the MDI.

Spacers differ in design (Table 4), but share certain operational principles. They reduce particle velocity and allow more of the propellant to evaporate by increasing the transit distance of the aerosol jet, thereby increasing the proportion of small to large particles in the inspired bolus (75). Only the small particles of I-S are useful, because the larger ones

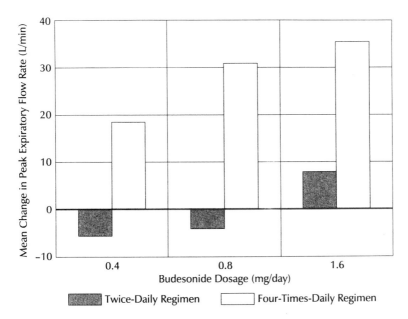

Figure 3 When budesonide was given to the same 34 patients twice daily (dark boxes) or four times daily (light boxes), improvement in peak expiratory flow rate was greater with the four-times-daily regimen. Values shown are 14-day means of the lower of two daily measurements. Thus, dosing frequency has a pronounced effect on the antiasthmatic efficacy of inhaled steroid. In practical terms, the difference observed here implied that a patient taking two puffs four times a day from a 0.05-mg/ puff inhaler would require 17 puffs twice a day from a 0.2-mg/puff inhaler to derive equal benefit. This applied only when the asthma of these patients was unstable; when asthma was well controlled and stable, the two dosing frequencies were equally effective. (Adapted from Ref. 69.)

preferentially deposit in the oropharynx or large airways, where they may cause oro- pharyngeal complications or reflex cough. If it is used properly, a large-volume spacer may double the delivery of the drug to the lung in comparison with what a well-trained patient can achieve by using an MDI alone (73,76). Large-volume spacers appear potentially more efficient than smaller ones (see Table 3). Indeed, if a small spacer is used incorrectly, asthma control may paradoxically deteriorate because of excessive trapping of the drug within the device causing a reduction in intrapulmonary drug delivery (77,78).

Patients often err by expelling more than one puff of drug at a time into the spacer, by allowing more than 1 s to elapse before starting to inspire from the spacer, by inspiring too rapidly (faster than about 25 L/min), or by failing to breath-hold for 10 s at the end of the inspiration. Each of these errors can reduce intrapulmonary drug delivery.

Prescribing a spacer for patients receiving I-S treatment ought not to be restricted to those who obviously use the MDI ineptly, because virtually anyone can benefit in terms of a decrease in oropharyngeal complications or augmented delivery of the I-S to the lung, or both (76). Cost–benefit considerations also favor the use of a spacer (76).

Some published guidelines for asthma management recommend that spacers by used to reduce the systemic effects of I-S to allow larger doses of I-S to be taken with safety (79). Our studies indicate that a spacer may either increase (76) or decrease (78) the systemic effects of an I-S, depending on factors such as the size of the device and how the patient

Table 3 Intrapulmonary Deposition of Radiolabeled Aerosol: MDI Versus MDI Plus Spacer[a]

Clinical diagnosis	MDI without spacer	MDI plus spacer					Spacer's effect on intrapulmonary deposition[b]	Ref.
		Valved, rigid spacer (100 ml)	Unvalved tube spacer (110 ml)	Valved cone spacer (750 ml)	Patient coaching without spacer	Coaching plus spacer (700 ml)		
Normal	10.4	9.85					−5	214
Bronchitis	8.65	9.02					+5	214
Asthma	7.9		11.5				+46	215
				13			+65	215
					11.2		+72	73
COPD	6.5					14.8	+128	73

MDI, metered-dose inhaler; COPD, chronic obstructive pulmonary disease.
[a]Expressed as percentage of dose emitted from valve on pressurized canister of MDI.
[b]Expressed as percentage deposition relative to MDI without spacer.
Source: Ref. 51.

Table 4 Spacers That May Be Used with an MDI

Feature	Valved, rigid (Aerochamber)	Collapsible plastic bag spacer (InspirEase)	Pear-shaped, valved, rigid spacer (Nebuhaler)	Tube spacer (Azmacort)	Pear-shaped valved, rigid spacer (ACE)
Volume (ml)	145	700	750	113	170
Valve assembly	Yes	No	Yes	No	Yes
Flow rate monitor	Yes	Yes	No	No	Yes
Compatible with all MDIs	Yes	Yes	No	No	Yes
Designed for children <4 yr	Yes	No	No	No	No
Coordination needed	No	No	No	Yes	No
Lung deposition achieved (%)[a]	17	15–20	15–20	11	ND
Response ≥ MDI response	Yes	Yes	Yes	ND	ND

MDI, metered-dose inhaler; ND, no data; ACE, Aerosol Cloud Enhancer.

[a]Expressed as percentage of dose emitted from valve of pressurized canister. Using the open-mouth inhalation technique with the MDI alone, about 10% of the emitted dose is delivered to the lung.

Source: Ref. 79.

uses it. When a spacer is observed to reduce the systemic activity of I-S, this may be due to a reduction in intrapulmonary delivery of the drug, with accompanying deterioration in asthma control (77,78).

Another alternative to the conventional MDI (without spacer) is the breath-activated MDI, which releases each dose from the pressurized canister early in inspiration. This device cannot enhance the results achieved in patients who already use, or can be trained to use, their conventional MDI efficiently. However, it may significantly improve intra-pulmonary drug delivery in patients who, despite careful instruction, fail to master the conventional MDI (80).

Duration of Treatment

Three to nine months of I-S treatment may be required to show significant improvement of AHR, depending on the severity of the asthma, and some patients may require more than a year of treatment before the therapeutic response plateaus (13,36). During this time, the use of a clinical surveillance system designed to maximize patient compliance may be critically important for optimizing the final therapeutic response (13). Despite the two- to fourfold, and occasionally as much as tenfold improvement in AHR that may be achieved with prolonged I-S treatment, fully normal values are seldom attained (13,36)—at least with conventional doses of I-S. Thus, symptoms and functional impairment recur in most patients, commonly within a month if the I-S treatment is abruptly withdrawn. Therefore, unless a specific etiologic factor can be identified and removed from the patient's environment, the process that engenders the chronic airways inflammation in asthma appears to be self-perpetuating, and the need for sustained anti-inflammatory treatment is likely to persist indefinitely.

Safety of Inhaled Steroid Therapy

Effects on the HPA Axis

Most of each I-S dose that enters the lung is absorbed in fully bioactive form, as evidenced by its inhibitory effect on HPA axis function. The "safe-dose" cutoff generally adopted by most regulatory authorities specifies the daily dose of I-S above which a statistically significant reduction in the morning serum cortisol level is demonstrable in test groups of approximately 30 patients. This implies a clinically meaningful risk (i.e., acute adrenocortical insufficiency) in the event the patient is subjected to a severe physiological stress.

More sensitive tests of HPA axis function, such as metyrapone responsiveness or measurement of the 24 h urinary free-cortisol output, show unequivocal evidence of systemic activity with low doses of I-S (81,82). However, in the presence of a normal 8 AM serum cortisol level, the clinical importance of these small departures form normal HPA axis function is questionable.

In a few patients treated with high-dose BUD for more than 5 years, we observed a decline in HPA axis function that did not begin until after the cumulative dose exceeded 1 g (83). These patients use doses of BUD averaging 1.6 mg/day, and in most, cotreatment with regular or intermittent prednisone was a contributing factor. Consequently, it is my practice to monitor patients who receive high-dose I-S or combined I-S and O-S therapy by periodically checking their morning serum cortisol level.

Judged by the rarity of published reports, stress-induced addisonian crisis appears to be very rare in patients receiving I-S therapy. Nevertheless, because patients differ markedly in their tolerance of glucocorticoid drugs, it is prudent to routinely administer a preventative glucocorticoid supplement to all patients receiving I-S treatment if they experience major metabolic stress triggered by an acute trauma, infection, or surgery. For this purpose, it is our practice to administer 25 mg oral prednisone (effective after approximately 1 h) or 100 mg of intravenous hydrocortisone (effective immediately). It may be advisable to add 4 mg of intravenous dexamethasone to prolong the effectiveness of the first agent. If the patient's blood pressure drops, the intravenous hydrocortisone is repeated as frequently as needed.

It is less expensive and more expeditious to prescribe steroid prophylaxis routinely for all patients taking an I-S than to perform preliminary tests of HPA axis function in an attempt to identify which ones may be at risk for stress-induced addisonian crisis.

Ocular Complications

The risk of posterior subcapsular cataract (PSC) formation is generally assumed to be much lower with I-S than with systemic steroid therapy. The most rigorously designed assessments of this risk that have been published to date support this assumption (84,85).

In a cross-sectional, slit-lamp survey of 48 asthmatic adults who had had prolonged exposure to unusually high doses of I-S or prednisone, we found the prevalence of PSC correlated significantly with the current daily dose and duration of prednisone use. However, there was no evidence in these patients that I-S either caused PSC, or increased the risk of PSC by acting additively with past or current oral prednisone use or the various nonsteroidal risk factors for cataract also present in some patients (84). A similar survey of 100 asthmatic children treated with high-dose I-S (but no prednisone) for a mean of 2 years found no cases of PSC (85).

Thus, the risk of PSC complicating I-S therapy appears negligible, even if high doses are used for a long time. This does not exclude the possibility that PSC might occur if a particular patient has exceptionally high inherent susceptibility. However, whatever the level of susceptibility, the data indicate that I-S treatment is more likely to reduce than to increase the risk of PSC formation, by virtue of its well-documented ability to reduce or eliminate the need for prednisone. Thus, routine ophthalmological surveillance of I-S-treated patients for cataract is not warranted.

Growth Inhibition

The surveys of the effect of I-S treatment on growth that have now been published relate to the use of low doses only (i.e., < 1 mg/day; nominal dose). Among those published before 1991, only one found evidence of growth inhibition(86), and this might be explained by factors other than the I-S treatment (87). The only study to follow children treated with low-dose BDP through to adulthood found they attained normal height (88). On the other hand, isolated case reports document clinically important stunting occurring in a few children treated with BDP or BUD at various dose levels (89,90). The stunting was clearly related to the drug, rather than to the severity of the asthma, because it reversed after the drug was withdrawn.

More recently, controlled prospective studies clearly show that low-dose BUD or BDP can inhibit growth velocity (44,91–93). For low-dose BUD, the magnitude of the effect has been less than that produced by 2.5 mg/day of prednisone (92). Thus, the effect of low-dose I-S on growth appears clinically unimportant. However, the effect is dose-dependent, and no studies of the effect of high-dose I-S on growth have yet been reported. There is an urgent need for such studies, because an unknown (and possibly, large) number of children currently receive high-dose I-S therapy by nebulization or MDI plus spacer, using concentrated formulations of BDP or BUD in Canada, or triamcinolone acetonide or flunisolide in the United States.

Effects on Bone

The effects of I-S drugs on bone are just beginning to be characterized.

Either BUD or BDP can interfere with laboratory measures of bone formation and resorption (94–97). These effects are dose-related and are greater with BDP than with BUD (97). The magnitude of BUD's effect is significantly less than that of therapeutically equivalent doses of prednisone (98). Similar data are not yet available for the other I-S drugs.

Surveys of bone mineral density in I-S-treated patients show conflicting results (99–103). When reduced density has been observed, the effect of past or current prednisone use or of nonsteroidal factors, such as the postmenopausal state, that also reduce bone density, confound the question of the causal role of the I-S (100–106). The only pediatric study published to date found no evidence of bone depletion among children treated for approximately 2 years with an intermediate dose of BDP (101).

We found, in a cross-sectional survey of bone density among 69 adults who had received long-term I-S and O-S therapy, that doses of I-S higher than 1.2 mg/day were associated with a statistically significant reduction in bone density, whereas lower doses were not; that this effect was consistently less in postmenopausal women treated with estrogen supplements than in men who had had equivalent exposures to I-S and O-S; and that there was evidence of significant bone repair occurring in both men and women during their long-term I-S treatment, presumably consequent to their withdrawal from prednisone after switching to the I-S (107).

Additional studies are needed to elucidate the influence of the choice of I-S drug, dose, and delivery system, and how these may relate to patient age and other risk factors for osteoporosis, in determining the risk of fracture.

Comparing Inhaled Steroid Formulations

Because the regulatory requirements for labeling I-S drugs vary from one formulation to another and from one regulatory jurisdiction to another, as shown in Table 5 (compare columns B vs. C), the "nominal" dosage provides the only common denominator for

Table 5 Comparison of I-S Formulations

Drug (generic)	A Puffs per day to release a nominal dose of 1.0 mg/d	B Nominal dose per puff (mg)	C Labeled dose per puff (mg) USA	Canada
Vanceril or Beclovent (beclomethasone)	20	0.05	0.042	0.05
Azmacort (triamcinolone acetonide)	5	0.20	0.10	0.10
Pulmicort[a] (budesonide)	5	0.20	—	0.20
Aerobid (flunisolide)	4	0.25	0.25	0.25
Becloforte (beclomethasone)	4	0.25	—	0.25

[a]Dry powder formulation.

estimating the relative toxicity of different formulations. Therefore, the daily doses cited here and elsewhere in the text refer to a *nominal* dose (i.e., the amount released at the valve of the pressurized metered-dose inhaler). The number of valve activations required to release a nominal dose of 1.0 mg/day of various inhaled steroid formulations is shown in Table 5, column A.

If the systemic activities of these various agents are assumed to be approximately equivalent milligram for milligram, the figures in column A provide a rough guide for the doses of each drug likely to share equivalent toxicity. However, the figures in column A may not be therapeutically equivalent, because major differences exist among these drugs relative to their topical anti-inflammatory potencies, as determined from their vasoconstrictor activity on human skin, on their in vitro receptor-binding affinities. These differences may reflect clinically discernible differences in antiasthmatic potency, but this assumption has never been validated. If such differences in clinical potency do, in fact, exist, the number of puffs per day shown in column A would need to be adjusted (with corollary changes in the milligram dose per day) to display therapeutically equivalent dosages. These adjustments could alter their relative cost-effectiveness and relative efficiency. *Efficiency* may be defined as the increase in therapeutic efficacy achieved per unit increase in unwanted systemic activity.

In addition to the possible effect of the aforementioned differences in topical anti-inflammatory potency, clinical efficacy (and toxicity) may also be influenced by factors that affect the intrapulmonary delivery of the drug. The latter will vary depending on (1) various characteristics of the aerosol—for example, the percentage of the emitted particles that falls within the "respirable range"; (2) the delivery device used to inhale the drug—for example a conventional MDI used with or without a spacer (and by the design of the spacer), or a breath-activated MDI or a dry powder delivery device; (3) the degree of pulmonary impairment; and most importantly, (4) the individual patient's inhalation technique.

The net effect of this multiplicity of interacting factors will determine the therapeutic efficiency of any particular I-S formulation in any particular patient, and also the efficiency of one relative to another if any pair of I-S drugs are compared.

Given these practical difficulties, and until a generally accepted standard methodology has evolved for making such comparisons, one reasonable approach for the clinical practitioner, faced with a need to choose between different I-S formulations, may be to select any one of them as the drug of choice—based on considerations of cost, convenience, efficiency of drug delivery, and patient preference. Then, using this agent, the factors that have been shown to influence the therapeutic response to I-S may be manipulated to the best advantage of each patient. These are discussed elsewhere in this chapter, and they include the dose per day, dosing frequency, drug delivery system, duration of treatment, and the system used by the physician to encourage long-term patient compliance.

Oral Steroid Preferred

In our view, I-S therapy is the preventative treatment of choice for all but the mildest grades of chronic asthma. This accords with current national and international guidelines for asthma treatment (26,108). Yet, regular prednisone may be preferable to I-S for selected patients in whom adverse social or economic circumstances, poor compliance, or inept use of the MDI compromise the usefulness of I-S treatment. In particular, patients in whom severe labile asthma is combined with a "track record" of social instability and poor compliance with preventative treatment, constitute a high-risk population (109). In such patients, shifting from prednisone to I-S for the preventative arm of their treatment may incur the risk of sudden death caused by asthma, especially if low-dose I-S with unconcentrated formulations is used (109).

Systemic steroid therapy is also required for asthma associated with pulmonary infiltration and eosinophilia (PIE syndrome), the various forms of systemic necrotizing vasculitis that may be accompanied by asthma, and probably for allergic bronchopulmonary aspergillosis (ABPA). In patients with ABPA, I-S treatment may improve the asthma symptoms, without reducing the recurrence rate of the segmental pulmonary consolidations that lead to the widespread lung fibrosis characteristic of end-stage ABPA. Since regular prednisone can prevent these segmental inflammatory lesions, it should probably remain the mainstay of long-term management in this disease.

In ABPA patients who require prednisone doses large enough to carry a risk of significant adverse effects, I-S therapy may be used to facilitate reduction of the prednisone dose to less toxic levels. If an I-S regimen is adopted, it is advisable that the patient be monitored objectively, rather than by symptoms alone, because, in some patients, I-S treatment may be associated with a paradoxical increase in the aspergilli content of the sputum (110). Also, in at least one such patient, disseminated aspergillosis has complicated the use of combined oral and inhaled steroid therapy (110). Spirometry, chest radiographs, sputum cultures, total serum IgE, specific aspergillus IgE or IgG titers, and blood eosinophil counts, provide useful guides to the activity of the disease.

The potential for complications such as those just cited may apply only in patients who have advanced ABPA associated with structural lung defects which may harbor a mycetoma. Some experts consider that the use of I-S to treat ABPA in its earlier and milder stages may, in fact, prevent the syndrome from evolving into its later stages when bronchiectasis, pulmonary fibrosis, and disabling pulmonary insufficiency dominate the clinical picture.

Oral Steroid Regimens

In patients who require regular O-S treatment, alternate-morning, rather than daily dosing, may minimize the risk of some of the adverse systemic effects of prolonged O-S use (111,112). However, it does not diminish the risk of steroid osteoporosis (113,114).

Patients who have difficulty converting from daily prednisone to an alternate-morning regimen because of the lesser efficacy of the latter can usually accomplish this by adding I-S treatment.

STEROIDS FOR ACUTE ASTHMA

Placebo-controlled trials have clearly demonstrated the efficacy of steroid therapy for acute asthma (20,115,116). A ventilatory response may become discernible after 1 h, but it is not prominent until 5–9 h later (117,118). Therefore, it is not possible to demonstrate a significant response to steroid treatment in a clinical trial unless observation continues for more than 6 h after the start of the steroid therapy and concomitant bronchodilator is either withheld (117,119) or maintained at a stable level while the steroid treatment is added to it (20). Failure to attend to these exigencies of trial design has generated controversy about the usefulness of steroids for acute asthma (120,121), whereas the value of prompt and aggressive bronchodilator treatment is generally conceded.

The rationale for treating acute, severe asthma with a systemic steroid rests on the following considerations:

1. It is not possible to accurately predict which patient presenting with severe asthma may suddenly die (122–124).
2. Failure to use steroids early and in adequate dosage has been cited as a frequent correlate of sudden death or near death during severe asthma (125,126).
3. The risks from using steroids in conventional dosage to treat asthma are negligible.
4. Steroids exert an early normalizing effect on the arterial oxygen tension in acute asthma that is not attainable with bronchodilators alone (116,118). Because hypoxemia is an important determinant of the risk of death during asthma, this effect may be clinically valuable.
5. In patients who have become refractory to β-adrenergic agonist drugs owing to down-regulation of adrenoreceptors, steroids may correct this refractory state within a few hours.
6. In some patients with severe acute asthma, iatrogenic adrenocortical insufficiency may contribute to the risk of death (127). Replacement steroid treatment could be critical in such patients.
7. The use of steroids to supplement bronchodilators in the emergency treatment of severe asthma significantly reduces the need for hospital admission (128–130), and also the incidence of asthma relapse soon after hospital discharge (20,131,132) in comparison with what can be achieved with bronchodilators alone.

Oral Versus Parenteral

The oral and intravenous routes of administration differ little relative to the onset of their antiasthmatic effects (55). Prednisolone has approximately equivalent bioavailability by either route, and oral doses achieve peak blood levels in 1 h or less. Either prednisone or prednisolone may be used, because they are rapidly interconvertible, and the peak blood levels achieved are influenced more by the particular patient's metabolic conversion ratio than by which drug was administered (56).

Dosage

A review of the results of several dose-ranging studies, summarized in Figure 4, indicates that an adult dose below 40 mg/day of methylprednisolone may be suboptimal for some patients with acute asthma; that 80–160 mg/day of methylprednisolone is sufficient to achieve optimal results; and that no additional benefit is likely to accrue if larger doses are used. A better result can be achieved in a shorter time by assuring prompt aggressive bronchodilator treatment than by pushing the steroid dose to heroic levels. Furthermore, sudden death may accompany high-dose intravenous prednisolone therapy, presumably as a consequence of arrhythmias triggered by electrolyte shifts (133). Also high-dose systemic steroid treatment for more than 1 week can produce a protracted generalized myopathy (134,135). Fatal varicella-zoster is a rare complication of concern in children.

As a general rule, the intravenous steroid (if used) may be switched after 24–48 h to oral prednisone in divided doses ranging from 50 to 150 mg/day, depending on the severity of the asthma and the patient's tolerance. We generally use 60–80 mg/day of prednisone (0.85–1.5 mg/kg per day) because adverse neuropsychiatric effects are less frequent if the

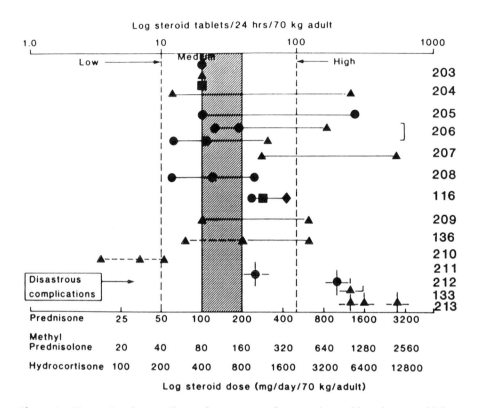

Figure 4   The results of ten studies on the treatment of acute asthma with various steroid drugs and dosages are summarized. To facilitate comparison, all doses have been adjusted to per diem adult dosage. Doses joined by a dashed line showed significant differences in antiasthmatic efficacy ($p <$ 0.05). Doses joined by a solid line were equally effective ($p > 0.05$). The shaded zone demarcates an optimal dose range. Individual studies cited are identifiable by the reference list numbers on the right. The bottom 4 numbers identify reports of serious complications with high-dose systemic steroid treatment. (▲) Methylprednisolone or prednisone; (●) hydrocortisone; (■) dexamethasone; (♦) betamethasone. (From Ref. 46.)

prednisone dose does not exceed 80 mg/day. At this dosage normalization of the airflow may occur within 3 days (136), although patients vary widely in their rate of recovery. Our experience, using 0.85 mg/kg prednisone per day, is that 10–14 days are generally required for improvement in the forced midexpiratory flow ($FEF_{25-75\%}$) to plateau in the adult asthmatics with associated chronic obstructive pulmonary disease (COPD) who constitute most of our hospital admissions. This recovery period will appear shorter if a less sensitive index of the therapeutic response is chosen, such as symptoms alone or PEFR. Serial spirometry provides the most reliable guide for how long the high-dose regimen should continue, because the signs and symptoms of asthma clear well before the pulmonary functional improvement reaches a plateau (137–139).

Tapering

The rate at which the initial high dose of steroid is withdrawn after clinical recovery, remains empiric. It is customary to "taper" the dose gradually because abrupt withdrawal has been reported to be associated with a high rate of relapse and an increased risk of mortality during the 14 days following hospital discharge (139). However, if high-dose I-S is introduced at this point, this may allow the O-S to be stopped abruptly without incurring serious risk (140); assuming the patient's compliance with the I-S treatment can be relied on and providing an adequate system of patient surveillance is in place.

STEROIDS FOR ANAPHYLAXIS

Injectable epinephrine is the drug of choice for anaphylaxis, and maintenance of an effective airway and circulatory system are the primary therapeutic goals. There are no controlled data to support the use of steroids in acute anaphylaxis. Systemic steroids do not suppress the primary phase of anaphylaxis and would not be expected to play a role in its immediate management, because many of their anti-inflammatory effects require hours, days, or weeks to achieve maximal expression (141–143). Nevertheless, steroids continue to be used clinically in the hope of averting late sequelae.

Biphasic anaphylaxis is increasingly being recognized (144,145). Although the second phase may occur despite steroid treatment of the acute phase (144,145), the corticosteroid (CS) may moderate its severity by increasing β-adrenoceptor responsiveness and inhibiting cell activation and mediator release (146,147). In the cutaneous model of the late-phase allergic response, a single dose of prednisolone immediately before antigen challenge may reduce the 6-h lesion diameter by 50% (148).

Therefore, the administration of intravenous hydrocortisone (4–8 mg/kg) or methyl-prednisolone, 2 mg/kg, seems prudent—with repetition every 6 h as needed.

Recurrent Idiopathic Anaphylaxis

In addition to its use for acute anaphylaxis, oral CS may be useful for the prevention of recurrent exacerbations of idiopathic anaphylaxis, urticaria, or angioedema (149–151). Prednisone 60–100 mg is administered each morning for 7–14 days, along with oral albuterol or hydroxyzine. Following this, the patient is converted to alternate-day prednisone, then titrated down by 5 mg every 2–4 weeks as symptoms permit (152). This regimen is reportedly effective in achieving remission rates of 30–50% in patients with recurrent idiopathic anaphylaxis (153). A subset of such patients may require regular administration of preventative CS (152,154), and a small number are CS-resistant (155).

Reactions to Radiocontrast Medium

In patients who give a history of previous anaphylactoid reaction to iodinated radiocontrast medium, CS premedication may reduce the incidence of reaction about sixfold (156–159). If a noninvasive diagnostic procedure cannot be substituted, it is prudent to pretreat any patient with a history of a previous anaphylactic reaction to a radiocontrast medium. Three 50-mg doses of prednisone are recommended at 6-h intervals, with the third dose scheduled 1 h before the procedure (along with diphenhydramine, 50 mg intramuscularly, and ephedrine, 25 mg orally, when not contraindicated) (160). The use of a low-osmolar contrast agent will further reduce the reaction rate if the previous reaction involved a high-osmolar agent. The combination of prophylaxis and a low-osmolar agent has been estimated to reduce the expected recurrence rate from 16–30% to 0.6% (161). Although this pretreatment protocol is highly effective in reducing the frequency and severity of anaphylactoid reactions, it cannot prevent all life-threatening reactions caused by noncardiogenic pulmonary edema (162,163).

STEROIDS FOR OTOLARYNGOLOGICAL DISEASE

Because of their potential for systemic complications, long-term O-S therapy is now reserved for use in patients with severe otolaryngological (OTL) disease, whereas the topically active intranasal steroids (INS) are increasingly used for rhinitis, often as first-line therapy.

Controlled clinical trials have documented the efficacy of INS for seasonal and perennial atopic rhinitis (164–166), nonallergic hyperplastic rhinitis with eosinophilia (NARES syndrome), and nasal polyposis (167–169).

Beclomethasone, budesonide, flunisolide, triamcinolone, and fluticasone are marketed in the United States or Canada as pressurized aerosol suspensions or aqueous sprays for intranasal use. Comparative studies of the different drugs and formulations demonstrate equal efficacy, by and large, although a few suggest BUD may be marginally more effective than BDP (165).

Intranasal Steroid Efficacy Relative to Other Therapies

Most studies comparing INS with intranasal cromolyn in seasonal or perennial allergic rhinitis have demonstrated the INS to be more effective (170,171). Few studies have directly compared INS with antihistamines. Some suggest that INS and long-acting antihistamines may provide equal benefit; others found INS to be more effective (172–174). In practice, these therapies are complementary and may provide the most effective relief if used in combination. There are as yet no studies comparing INS with immunotherapy relative to long-term cost–benefit or efficacy.

Systemic Steroid Use for OTL Disease

In seasonal allergic rhinitis the therapeutic role of O-S is limited to patients who present with severe symptoms and nasal obstruction at the peak of seasonal pollination. Such patients are at risk for developing complicating infective sinusitis, eustachian tube dysfunction, and potentially, sleep apnea (175,176). Intranasal steroids are not effective at this stage because of poor access to the nasal passages. A 1- or 2-week course of prednisone will carry such patients through the peak of the season and allow the INS to be introduced later if needed.

Patients with chronic allergic rhinitis may sometimes be treated with direct injection of steroid into a turbinate or polyp. Although effective for symptomatic relief, this practice should be abandoned because it is occasionally complicated by permanent blindness caused by retinal vessel spasm (177,178).

Use of an INS may be effective in the management of small nasal polyps, both for treatment and for the prevention of recurrence after surgical resection (179–182). However, INS are much less effective than O-S for large polyps that obstruct the airway and prevent successful application of the topical agent. It has been our experience that large polyps and the acute exacerbations of polyps commonly triggered by viral respiratory infection respond promptly and consistently to 3–4 weeks of prednisone, commencing at 40 mg/day (adult dose) (183). The remission can usually be sustained thereafter with an INS.

Intranasal Steroid Use in Other Conditions

There are no published trials of the effectiveness of O-S or INS in the treatment of rhinitis medicamentosa. In our clinical experience, a 2- to 4-week course of prednisone is predictably effective for relieving the symptoms, facilitating abrupt withdrawal from the causative agent, and preventing rebound nasal obstruction, with recurrence of the patient's previous dependence on vasoconstrictor nose sprays. Others report success with INS (165).

The variable response of primary vasomotor rhinitis to O-S or INS reflects the pathogenetic diversity of patients with this nonspecific diagnosis.

Early suggestions of the value of preventative INS therapy for chronic serious otitis media complicating chronic allergy have not been substantiated by subsequent double-blind, controlled studies (185).

Adverse Effects of Intranasal Steroids

The systemic toxicity of all the INS formulations appears to be negligible when they are used in conventional doses. This is evidenced by the results of tests of HPA axis function, the absence of symptoms of hypercortisolism in INS-treated patients, and by the resolution of preexisting signs of hypercortisolism after previous prednisone therapy has been substituted with INS. In children younger than 6 years neither safety nor efficacy data are available.

Routine nasal swabs for candida during long-term treatment with INS are very rarely positive, and there are no reported cases of nasal thrush in immunocompetent patients (although it has been observed in an immunodeficient patient; 186). As with systemic steroids, INS should be avoided or be used with caution in the immunocompromised patient because of the risk of opportunistic infection.

The most common complication of chronic INS use is a small erosion of the nasal septum, the presence of which is usually signaled by epistaxis. The problem is easily resolved by applying petrolatum to the ulcerated area immediately before using the INS. Habitual nose picking may prevent healing, however, and could lead to septal perforation. Perforation has been observed in a few patients treated with INS (187,188); therefore, it is prudent to document whether the nasal septum is intact or not before starting INS therapy.

Nasal biopsy specimens, studied by light and electron microscopy (189,190), have not shown atrophic changes or other evidence of cumulative damage similar to the connective tissue atrophy that the same topically active steroids produce when applied continuously to the skin. The more rapid clearance of the drug from the respiratory tract presumably accounts for this difference.

Animal safety data suggest that the steroids prescribed for inhalation into the nose of lower airways probably do not have carcinogenic or mutagenic potential in humans. Very large doses of these drugs are teratogenic and fetotoxic in rabbits and rats, but BDP inhaled by pregnant mothers with severe asthma did not increase the incidence of congenital malformations in the newborn (191). Some steroids are known to be distributed in human milk and might conceivably suppress growth in nursing infants, but there are no relevant data for the steroids currently prescribed for inhalation use. Because of the absence of data from controlled studies in humans, INS should be used with caution in pregnant or nursing women.

STEROIDAL THERAPY FOR DERMATOSES

Systemic or topical CS are useful in the treatment of allergic dermatoses. Their mechanism of action is incompletely understood, but relates to their anti-inflammatory effects. They are available in a great variety of formulations, the effects and adverse effects of which have been reviewed (192–194). In general, the more potent formulations are indicated for use over thick skin (palms and soles), and low-potency formulations should be used on the thin skin of the face or groin.

Adverse Effects

Prolonged or intensive topical CS therapy may lead to cutaneous or systemic adverse effects, particularly if applied to large areas under occlusion and in infants and children. Iatrogenic Cushing's syndrome occurs rarely. Suppression of normal HPA axis function is more common (195–198).

Localized cutaneous effects include dermal atrophy, striae, hypopigmentation, hypertrichosis, impaired wound healing, and local infection. Contact dermatitis is increasingly reported. Rarely, I-S therapy for rhinitis or asthma may cause similar adverse effects on the perioral skin (199).

Formulations

Corticosteroids stronger than 1% hydrocortisone or 0.5% desonide should be avoided on the face to prevent CS-induced rosacea or perioral dermatitis. Because of the potential for these complications, patients should be monitored closely, and the frequency of application or potency of the drug reduced if possible. The standard frequency of application is controversial; two to three times per day is usually recommended, but once daily may be sufficient for mild to moderate dermatitis (200). The choice of a particular agent varies with the severity and location of the dermatitis and patient preference. It is important to consider the latter to ensure patient compliance. Creams spread more easily than an ointment and are more cosmetically acceptable. However creams require a preservative in the formulation, which may cause allergic sensitization. Ointments are preferred for dry areas and fissured or scaling lesions on the hands or feet. Gels and lotions are convenient for hairy areas, but the alcohol may be drying.

Atopic Dermatitis

Skin hygiene and topical CS therapy are the mainstay of atopic dermatitis therapy. Prolonged systemic CS use should be avoided, but an occasional short course may be needed to control a severe exacerbation and restore responsiveness to topical therapy. For milder exacerbations, 1–2 weeks of treatment with a moderate- to high-potency topical agent (avoid face and body folds) is indicated, switching thereafter to maintenance therapy with a low-potency agent to avoid a CS withdrawal rebound in severity.

Urticaria

In chronic urticaria, systemic CS therapy should be restricted to intermittent short-term use to control disabling exacerbations resistant to other therapy, including combinations of H_1 and H_2 antihistamines. Prolonged O-S treatment should not be given for chronic urticaria unless it is associated with other disorders for which such treatment is indicated (e.g., systemic vasculitis).

Other Dermatoses

High-dose systemic CS is the treatment of choice for acute pemphigus vulgaris or bullous pemphigoid (201,202). It is often used in erythema multiforme, although in the absence of controlled trials, the indications for its use remain empiric and controversial.

Prednisone, 20–40 mg/day for 1 week, is rapidly and consistently effective for acute dermatitis caused by drug allergy or widespread allergic contact dermatitis (e.g., poison ivy). Chronic contact dermatitis is appropriately treated with topical CS, provided a diagnostic allergy assessment and appropriate avoidance procedures have been undertaken.

REFERENCES

1. Boutin Y, Brunet C, Gagnon R, Hebert J. Cytokines involved in allergic reactions. Pract Allergy Immunol 1994; 9:23–26.
2. Schleimer RP. Glucocorticosteroids, their mechanisms of action and use. In: Middleton E, Reed CE, Ellis EF, Adkinson NF, Yunginger JW, Busse WW, eds. Allergy Principles and Practice. St. Louis: Mosby-Year Book, 1993:893–925.
3. Venge P, Dahl R, Hakansson L. Heat-labile neutrophil chemotactic activity in subjects with asthma after allergen: relation to the late asthmatic reaction and effects of asthma medication. J Allergy Clin Immunol 1987; 80:679–688.
4. Delehunt JC, Yeger L, Ahmen T, Abraham WM. Inhibition of antigen-induced bronchoconstriction by methylprednisolone succinate. J Allergy Clin Immunol 1984; 73:479–483.
5. Dahl R, Johansson SA. Importance of duration of treatment with inhaled budesonide on the immediate and late bronchial reaction. Eur J Respir Dis 1982; 63:167–175.
6. Abraham WM, Delehunt JC, Yerger L, Marchette B. Characterization of a late phase pulmonary response after antigen challenge in allergic sheep. Am Rev Respir Dis 1983; 128:839.
7. Mapp C, Boschetto P, Dal Vecchio L, Crescioli S, De Marzo N, Paleari D, Fabbri LM. Protective effect of antiasthma drugs on late asthmatic reactions and increased airway responsiveness induced by toluene diisocyanate in sensitized subjects. Am Rev Respir Dis 1987; 136:1403–1407.
8. Cockcroft DW. Mechanism of perennial allergic asthma. Lancet 1983; 2:253–256.
9. Lanes S, Stevenson JS, Codias E, Hernandez Z, Sielczak MW, Abraham WM. Effects of budesonide on late bronchial responses and the associated airway hyperresponsiveness in allergic sheep. In: Hogg JC, Ellul-Micallef R, Brattsand R, eds. Glucocorticoids, Inflammation and Bronchial Hyperactivity. Amsterdam: Excerpta Medica, 1985:38–50.
10. Ryan G, Latimer KM, Juniper EF, Roberts RS, Hargreave FE. Effect of beclomethasone dipropionate on bronchial responsiveness to histamine in controlled non-steroid-dependent asthma. J Allergy Clin Immunol 1985; 75:25–30.
11. Kraan J, Koeter GHVD, Mark TW, Sluiter HJ, de Vries K. Changes in bronchial hyperreactivity induced by 4 weeks of treatment with antiasthmatic drugs in patients with allergic asthma; a comparison between budesonide and terbutaline. J Allergy Clin Immunol 1985; 76:628–636.
12. Vathenen AS, Knox AJ, Wisniewski A, Tattersfield AE. Time course of change in bronchial reactivity with an inhaled corticosteroid in asthma. Am Rev Respir Dis 1991; 143:1317–1321.
13. Woolcock AJ, Yan K, Salome CM. Effect of therapy on bronchial hyperresponsiveness in the long-term management of asthma. Clin Allergy 1988; 18:165–176.
14. Juniper EF, Kline PA, Vanzieleghem MA, Hargreave FE. Reduction of budesonide after a year of increased use: a randomized controlled trial to evaluate whether improvements in airway responsiveness and clinical asthma are maintained. J Allergy Clin Immunol 1991; 87:483–489.
15. Hui KKP, Connolly ME, Tashkin DP. Reversal of human lymphocyte beta-adrenoceptor desensitization by glucocorticoids. Clin Pharmacol Ther 1982; 32:566–571.
16. Vathenen AS, Knox AJ, Higgins BG, Britton JR, Tattersfield AE. Rebound increase in bronchial responsiveness after treatment with inhaled terbutaline. Lancet 1988; 1:554–558.

17. Busse WW. The precipitation of asthma by upper respiratory infections. Chest 1985; 85: 44S–48S.
18. Busse WW. Decreased granulocyte response to isoproterenol in asthma during upper respiratory infections. Am Rev Respir Dis 1977; 115:783–791.
19. Ellul-Micallef R, Fenech FF. Effect of intravenous prednisolone in asthmatics with diminished adrenergic responsiveness. Lancet 1975; 2:1269–1270.
20. Fanta CH, Tossing TH, McFadden ER Jr. Glucocorticoids in acute asthma. A clinical controlled trial. Am J Med 1983; 74:845–851.
21. Samuelson WM, Davies AO. Hydrocortisone-induced reversal of beta-adrenergic receptor uncoupling. Am Rev Respir Dis 1984; 130:1023–1026.
22. Jeffrey JL, Avner BP. Blockade of uptake 2: the mechanisms of rapid corticosteroid induced potentiation of bronchodilator drugs in tracheal smooth muscle. Proc West Pharmacol Soc 1980; 23:355.
23. Foster PS, Goldie RG, Peterson JW. Effect of steroids on beta-adrenoceptor-mediator relaxation of pig bronchus. Br J Pharmacol 1983; 78:441–445.
24. Geddes BA, Jones TR, Dvorsky RJ, Lefcoe NM. Interactions of glucocorticoids and bronchodilators on isolated guinea pig tracheal and human bronchial smooth muscle. Am Rev Respir Dis 1974; 110:420–427.
25. Toogood JH, Frankish CW, Jennings BH, Baskerville JC, Borga O, Lefcoe NM, Johansson S-A. A study of the mechanism of the antiasthmatic action of inhaled budesonide. J Allergy Clin Immunol 1990; 85:872–880.
26. U.S. Department of Health and Human Services. International consensus report on diagnosis and management of asthma. Publication 92-3091, 1992:1–71.
27. Corticosteroids, Inhalation Local monograph. In Drug Information for the Health Care Professional. U.S. Pharmacopeia. 15th ed. 1995 1:840–846.
28. Sly RM, Committee on Drugs, The American Academy of Allergy and Immunology. Adverse effects and complications of treatment with beta-adrenergic agonist drugs. J Allergy Clin Immunol 1985; 75:443–449.
29. Spitzer WO, Suissa S, Ernst P, et al. The use of β-agonists and the risk of death and near death from asthma. N Engl J Med 1992; 326:501–506.
30. Ernst P, Habbick B, Suissa S, et al. Is the association between inhaled beta-agonist use and life-threatening asthma because of confounding by severity? Am Rev Respir Dis 1993; 148: 75–79.
31. Reisman AE. Asthma induced by adrenergic aerosols. J Allergy 1970; 46:162–177.
32. Sears MR, Lake DC, Yates DM, et al. Regular inhaled beta-agonist treatment in bronchial asthma. Lancet 1990; 336:1391–1396.
33. van Schayck CP, Van Herwarden CLA. Do bronchodilators adversely affect the prognosis of bronchial hyperresponsiveness? Thorax 1993; 48:470–473.
34. Haahtela T, Jarvinen M, Kava T, et al. Comparison of β_2-agonist, terbutaline, with an inhaled corticosteroid, budesonide, in newly detected asthma. N Engl J Med 1991; 325:388–392.
35. Waalkens HJ, Gerritsen J, Koeter GH, Krouwels FH, van Aalderen WMC, Knol K. Budesonide and terbutaline or terbutaline alone in children with mild asthma: effects on bronchial hyperresponsiveness and diurnal variation in peak flow. Thorax 1991; 46:499–503.
36. Juniper EF, Kline PA, Vanzieleghem MA, Ramsdale EH, O'Bryne PM, Hargreave FE. Effect of long-term treatment with an inhaled corticosteroid (budesonide) on airway hyperresponsiveness and clinical asthma in nonsteroid-dependent asthmatics. Am Rev Respir Dis 1990; 142: 832–836.
37. Dawood AG, Hendry AT, Walker SR. The combined use of betamethasone valerate and sodium cromoglycate in the treatment of asthma. Clin Allergy 1977; 7:161–165.
38. Toogood JH, Jennings B, Lefcoe NM. A clinical trial of combined cromolyn/beclomethasone treatment for chronic asthma. J Allergy Clin Immunol 1981; 67:317–324.
39. O'Byrne PM, Cook D. Is nedocromil sodium effective treatment for asthma? Eur Respir J 1993; 6:5–6.

40. Wong CS, Cooper S, Britton JR, Tattersfield AE. Steroid sparing effect of nedocromil sodium in asthmatic patients on high doses of inhaled steroids. Clin Exp Allergy 1993; 23:370–376.

41. Dawson KP, Fergusson DM, Horwood LJ, Mogridge N. Ketotifen in asthma. Aust Paediatr J 1989; 25:89–92.

42. American Academy of Allergy and Immunology Study Group. Comparison of aerosol beclomethasone and oral theophylline as primary treatment of chronic asthma: IV. Conclusions. J Allergy Clin Immunol 1991; 87:202.

43. Tinkelman DG, Reed CE, Nelson HS, Offord KP. Aerosol beclomethasone dipropionate compared with theophylline as primary treatment of chronic, mild to moderately severe asthma in children. Pediatrics 1993; 92:64–77.

44. Toogood JH, Baskerville J, Jennings B, Lefcoe NM, Johansson S-A. Bioequivalent doses of budesonide and prednisone in moderate and severe asthma. J Allergy Clin Immunol 1989; 84:688–700.

45. Toogood JH. Efficiency of inhaled versus oral steroid treatment of chronic asthma. N Engl Reg Allergy Proc 1987; 8:98–103.

46. Toogood JH. Bronchial asthma and glucocorticoids. In: Schleimer RP, Claman HN, Oronsky A, eds. Anti-inflammatory Steroid Action: Basic and Clinical Aspects. San Diego: Academic Press, 1989: 423–468.

47. Laitinen LA, Laitinen A, Haahetela T. A comparative study of the effects of an inhaled corticosteroid, budesonide, and a β_2-agonist, terbutaline, on airway inflammation in newly diagnosed asthma: a randomized, double-blind, parallel-group controlled trial. J Allergy Clin Immunol 1992; 90:32–42.

48. Dompeling E, van Schayck CP, et al. Slowing the deterioration of asthma and chronic obstructive pulmonary disease observed during bronchodilator therapy by adding inhaled corticosteroids. Ann Intern Med 1993; 118:770–778.

49. Haahtela T, Jarvinen M, Kava T, et al. First line treatment of newly detected asthma: an inhaled steroid? One year's follow up after two years treatment. Eur Respir J 1992; 5(suppl 15):13s.

50. Toogood JH, et al. Bioequivalent doses of inhaled vs oral steroids for severe asthma. Chest 1983; 84:349.

51. Toogood JH, Jennings BH, Baskerville JC, Lefcoe NM. Aerosol corticosteroids. In: Weiss EB, Stein M, eds. Bronchial Asthma Mechanisms and Therapeutics, 3rd ed. Boston: Little, Brown & Co, 1993:818–841.

52. Toogood JH, et al. Minimum dose requirements of steroid-dependent asthmatic patients for aerosol beclomethasone and oral prednisone. J Allergy Clin Immunol 1978; 61:355–364.

53. Toogood JH, Jennings B, Baskerville J, Lefcoe NM. Personal observations on the use of inhaled corticosteroid drugs for chronic asthma. Eur J Respir Dis 1984; 65:321–338.

54. Mellis CM, Phelan PD. Asthma deaths in children—a continuing problem. Thorax 1977; 32:29–34.

55. McAllister WAC, Winfield CR, Collins JV. Pharmacokinetics of prednisolone in normal and asthmatic subjects in relation to dose. Eur J Clin Pharmacol 1981; 20:141–145.

56. Wilson CG, Ssendagire R, May CS, Paterson JW. Measurement of plasma prednisolone in man. Br J Clin Pharmacol 1975; 2:321–325.

57. Webb J, Clark TJH. Recovery of plasma corticotrophin and cortisol levels after a three-week course of prednisolone. Thorax 1981; 36:22–24.

58. Streck WG, Lockwood DH. Pituitary adrenal recovery following short-term suppression with corticosteroids. Am J Med 1979; 66:910–914.

59. Chang KC, Miklich DR, Barwise G, Chai H, Miles-Lawrence R. Linear growth of chronic asthmatic children: the effects of the disease and various forms of steroid therapy. Clin Allergy 1982; 12:369–378.

60. Smith MJ, Hodson ME. High-dose beclomethasone inhaler in the treatment of asthma. Lancet 1983; 1:265–269.

61. Toogood JH, et al. A graded dose assessment of the efficacy of beclomethasone dipropionate aerosol for severe chronic asthma. J Allergy Clin Immunol 1977; 59:298–308.

62. Toogood JH, Baskerville J, Errington N, et al. Determinants of the response to beclomethasone aerosol at various dose levels: a multiple regression analysis to identify clinically useful predictors. J Allergy Clin Immunol 1977; 60:367–376.

63. Roorda RJ, Gerritsen J, van Aalderen WMC, et al. Follow-up of asthma from childhood to adulthood: influence of potential childhood risk factors on the outcome of pulmonary function and bronchial responsiveness in adulthood. J Allergy Clin Immunol 1994; 93:575–584.

64. Gerritsen J, Gerard H, Koeter H, et al. Prognosis of asthma fro childhood to adulthood. Am Rev Respir Dis 1989; 140:1325–1330.

65. Agertoft L, Pedersen S. Effects of long-term treatment with an inhaled corticosteroid on growth and pulmonary function in asthmatic children. Respir Med 1994; 88:373–381.

66. Gagnon M, Cote J, Milot J, Turcotte H, Boulet L-P. Comparative safety and efficacy of single or twice daily administration of inhaled beclomethasone in moderate asthma. Chest 1994; 105:1732–1737.

67. Boyd G, Abdallah S, Clark R. Twice or four times daily beclomethasone dipropionate in mild stable asthma? Clin Allergy 1985; 15:383–389.

68. Nyholm E, Frame MH, Cayton RM. Therapeutic advantages of twice-daily over four-times daily inhalation budesonide in the treatment of chronic asthma. Eur J Respir Dis 1984; 65: 339–345.

69. Toogood JH, Baskerville J, Jennings B, Lefcoe NM, Johansson S-A. Influence of dosing frequency and schedule on the response of chronic asthmatics to the aerosol steroid budesonide. J Allergy Clin Immunol 1982; 70:288–298.

70. Toogood JH. Concentrated aerosol formulations in asthma. Lancet 1983; 2:790–791.

71. Malo J-L, Cartier A, Merland N, et al. Four-times-a-day dosing frequency is better than a twice-a-day regimen in subjects requiring a high-dose inhaled steroid, budesonide, to control moderate to severe asthma. Am Rev Respir Dis 1989; 140:624–629.

72. Malo J-L, Trudeau C, Cartier A, et al. Comparison of four-times-a-day dosing with a twice-a-day regimen in subjects requiring 1200 μg or less of budesonide to control mild to moderate asthma. J Allergy Clin Immunol 1994; 93:186.

73. Newman SP, Woodman G, Clarke SW, et al. Effect of Inspir-Ease on the deposition of metered-dose aerosols in the human respiratory tract. Chest 1986; 89:551.

74. Newman SP, Pavia D, Clark SW. How should a pressurized beta-adrenergic bronchodilator be inhaled? Eur J Respir Dis 1981; 62:3–21.

75. Corr D, Dolovich M, McCormack D, et al. Design and characteristics of a portable breath actuated particle size selective medical aerosol inhaler. J Aero Sci 1982; 13:1–7.

76. Toogood JH, Baskerville J, Jennings B, Lefcoe NM, Johansson S-A. Use of spacers to facilitate inhaled corticosteroid treatment of asthma. Am Rev Respir Dis 1984; 129:723–729.

77. Toogood JH. Budesonide in children with asthma. Eur J Clin Pharmacol 1988; 34:113–114.

78. Toogood JH, et al. Assessment of a device for reducing oropharyngeal complications during beclomethasone treatment of asthma. Am Rev Respir Dis 1981; 123:113.

79. Toogood JH. Helping your patients make better use of MDIs and spacers. J Respir Dis 1994; 15:151–166.

80. Newman SP, Weisz AWB, Talaee N, et al. Improvement of drug delivery with a breath-actuated pressurised aerosol for patients with poor inhaler technique. Thorax 1991; 46:712–716.

81. Vaz R, Senior B, Morris M, Binkiewicz A. Adrenal effects of beclomethasone inhalation therapy in asthmatic children. J Pediatr 1982; 100:660–662.

82. Law CM, Marchant JL, Honour JW, Preece MA, Warner JO. Nocturnal adrenal suppression in asthmatic children taking inhaled beclomethasone dipropionate. Lancet 1986; 1:942–944.

83. Toogood JH, Josephson D, Dervish G, Toogood PB. Safety of long term budesonide (BUD) therapy. Clin Invest Med 1989; 12:B5.

84. Toogood JH, Markov AE, Baskerville J, Dyson C. Association of ocular cataracts with inhaled and oral steroid therapy during long-term treatment of asthma. J Allergy Clin Immunol 1993; 91:571–579.

85. Simons FER, Persaud MP, Gilespie CA, Cheang M, Shuckett EP. Absence of posterior subcapsular cataracts in young patients treated with inhaled glucocorticoid. Lancet 1993; 342: 776–778.

86. Littlewood JM, Johnson AW, Edwards PA, Littlewood AE. Growth retardation in asthmatic children treated with inhaled beclomethasone dipropionate. Lancet 1988; 1:115–116.

87. Balfour-Lynn L. Growth retardation in asthmatic children treated with inhaled beclomethasone dipropionate. Lancet 1988; 1:475–476.

88. Balfour-Lynn L. Growth in childhood asthma. Arch Dis Child 1986; 61:1049–1055.

89. Wales JKH, Barnes ND, Swift PGF. Growth retardation in children on steroids for asthma. Lancet 1991; 338:1535.

90. Priftis K, Everard ML, Milner AD. Unexpected side-effects of inhaled steroids: a case report. Eur J Pediatr 1991; 150:449.

91. Wolthers OD, Pederson S. Growth of asthmatic children during treatment with budesonide: a double blind trial. Br Med J 1991; 303:163–165.

92. Wolthers OD, Pedersen S. Controlled study of linear growth in asthmatic children during treatment with inhaled glucocorticosteroids. Pediatrics 1992; 89:839–842.

93. Wolthers OD, Pedersen S. Short term growth during treatment with inhaled fluticasone propionate and beclomethasone diproprionate. Arch Dis Child 1993; 68:673–676.

94. Sorva R, Rurpeinen M, Juntunen-Backman K, Karonen SL, Sorva A. Effects of inhaled budesonide on serum markers of bone metabolism in children with asthma. J Allergy Clin Immunol 1992; 90:808–815.

95. Toogood JH, Jennings B, Hodsman AB, Baskerville J, Fraher LJ. Effects of dose and dosing schedule of inhaled budesonide on bone turnover. J Allergy Clin Immunol 1991; 88:572–580.

96. Ali NJ, Capewell S, Ward MJ. Bone turnover during high dose inhaled corticosteroid therapy. Thorax 1989; 44:900P.

97. Jennings BH, Larsson B, Andersson K-E, et al. A comparison of budesonide and beclomethasone dipropionate in healthy volunteers in the assessment of systemic effects of inhaled glucocorticoids. B. Jennings. Doctoral dissertation, University of Lund, Sweden, 1990; VII:1-VII-14.

98. Hodsman AB, Toogood JH, Jennings B, Fraher LJ, Baskerville JC. Differential effects of inhaled budesnide and oral prednisolone on serum osteocalcin. J Clin Endocr Metab 1991; 72:530–540.

99. Wolff AH, Adelsberg B, Aloia J, Zitt M. Effect of inhaled corticosteroid on bone density in asthmatic patients: a pilot study. Ann Allergy 1991; 67:117–121.

100. Packe GE, Douglas JG, McDonald AF, Robbins SP, Reid DM. Bone density in asthmatic patients taking high dose inhaled beclomethasone dipropionate and intermittent systemic corticosteroids. Thorax 1992; 47:414–417.

101. Konig P, Hillman L, Cervantes C, Levine C, Maloney C, et al. Bone metabolism in children with asthma treated with inhaled beclomethasone dipropionate. J Pediatr 1993; 122:219–226.

102. Ip MSM, Lam KSL, Yam LYC, Kung AWC, Wong PO. Decreased bone mineral density in asthma patients on long term inhaled steroids. Am Rev Respir Dis 1993; 147:A293.

103. Boulet LP, Giguere MC, Milot J, Brown J. Long-term effects of high dose inhaled steroids on bone turnover and density. Am Rev Respir Dis 1993; 147:A293.

104. Reid DM, Nicoll JJ, Smith MA et al. Corticosteroids and bone mass in asthma: comparisons with rheumatoid arthritis and polymyalgia rheumatica. Br Med J 1986; 293:1463–1466.

105. Crompton GK. Corticosteroids and bone mass in asthma. Br Med J 1987; 294:123.

106. Stead RJ, Horsman A, Cooke NJ, Belchetz P. Bone mineral density in women taking inhaled corticosteroids. Thorax 1990; 45:792.

107. Toogood JH, Baskerville J, Markov AE, Hodsman AB, Fraher LJ, Jennings B, Haddad RG, Drost D. Bone mineral density and the risk of fracture in patients receiving long-term inhaled steroid therapy for asthma. J Allergy Clin Immunol 1995; 96:157–166.

108. U.S. Department of Health and Human Services. Guidelines for the diagnosis and management

of asthma. National Asthma Education Program. Expert Panel report. 1991; Publication 91-3042 and 91-3042A, pp 1–135; 1–44.

109. Strunk RC, et al. Physiologic and psychological characteristics associated with deaths due to asthma in childhood. JAMA 1985; 254:1193–1198.

110. Anderson CJ, Craig S, Bardana EF Jr. Allergic bronchopulmonary aspergillosis and bilateral fungal balls terminating in disseminating aspergillosis. J Allergy Clin Immunol 1980; 65: 140–144.

111. Auerback HS, Williams M, Kirkpatrick JA, Colten HR. Alternate-day prednisone reduces morbidity and improves pulmonary function in cystic fibrosis. Lancet 1985; 2:686–688.

112. Huner GG, Allen GL. Daily and alternate day corticosteroid regimens in treatment of giant cell arteritis. Ann Intern Med 1975; 82:613–618.

113. Gluck OS, Murphy WA, Hahn TJ, Hahn B. Bone loss in adults receiving alternate day glucocorticoid therapy. Arthritis Rheum 1981; 24:892–898.

114. Ruegsegger P, Medici TC, Anliker M. Corticosteroid-induced bone loss. A longitudinal study of alternate day therapy in patients with bronchial asthma using quantitative computed tomography. Eur J Clin Pharmacol 1983; 25:615–620.

115. Loren M, Chai H, Leung P, Rohr C, Brenner AM. Corticosteroids in the treatment of acute exacerbations of asthma. Ann Allergy 1980; 45:67–71.

116. Pierson WE, Bierman CW, Kelley VC. A double-blind trial of corticosteroid therapy in status asthmaticus. Pediatrics 1974; 54:282–288.

117. Collins FV, Clark TJH, Brown D, Townsend J. The use of corticosteroids in the treatment of acute asthma. Q J Med 1975; 44:259–273.

118. Ellul-Micallef R, Borthwick RC, Hardy GJR. The effect of oral prednisolone on gas exchange in chronic bronchial asthma. Br J Clin Pharmacol 1980; 9:479–482.

119. Ellul-Micallef R. The acute effects of corticosteroids in bronchial asthma. Eur J Respir Dis 1982; 63(suppl 122):118–122.

120. Stein LM, Cole RP. Early administration of corticosteroids in emergency room treatment of acute asthma. Ann Intern Med 1990; 112:823–827.

121. Luksza AR. A new look at adult asthma. Br J Dis Chest; 1982; 76:11–15.

122. Fletcher HJ, Ibrahim SA, Speight N. Survey of asthma deaths in Northern region, 1970–85. Arch Dis Child 1990; 65:163–167.

123. Macdonald JB, Seaton A, Williams DA. Asthma deaths in Cardiff 1963–74: 90 deaths outside hospital. Br Med J 1976; 1:1493–1495.

124. Wilson JD, Sutherland DC, Thomas AC. Has the change to beta-agonists combined with oral theophylline increased cases of fatal asthma? Lancet 1981; 1:1235–1237.

125. Renato S, Canny GJ, Bohn D, Reisman JJ, Levison H. Severe acute asthma in a pediatric intensive care unit: six years' experience. Pediatrics 1989; 83:1023–1028.

126. Kallenbach JM, Frankel AH, Lapinsky SE, et al. Determinants of near fatality in acute severe asthma. Am J Med 1993; 95:265–272.

127. Speizer FE, Doll R, Heaf P, Strang LB. Investigation into use of drugs preceding death from asthma. Br Med J 1968; 1:339–343.

128. Scarfone RJ, Fuchs SM, Nager AL, Shane SA. Controlled trial of oral prednisone in the emergency department treatment of children with acute asthma. Pediatrics 1993; 92:513–518.

129. Tal A, Levy N, Bearman JE. Methylprednisolone therapy for acute asthma in infants and toddlers: a controlled clinical trial. Pediatrics 1990; 86:350–356.

130. Littenberg B, Gluck EH. A controlled trial of methylprednisolone in the emergency treatment of acute asthma. N Engl J Med 1986; 314:150–152.

131. Fiel SB, Swartz MA, Glanz K, Francis ME. Efficacy of short-term corticosteroid therapy in outpatient treatment of acute bronchial asthma. Am J Med 1983; 75:259–262.

132. Chapman K, Verbeek R, White JG, Rebuck A. Effect of a short course of prednisone in the prevention of early relapse after the emergency room treatment of acute asthma. N Engl J Med 1991; 324:788–794.

133. Bocanegra TS, Castaneda MO, Espinoza LR, et al. Sudden death after methylprednisolone pulse therapy. Ann Intern Med 1981; 95:122.

134. Griffin D, Coursin D, Grossman JE. Acute myopathy during treatment of status asthmaticus with corticosteroids and steroidal muscle relaxants. Chest 1992; 102:510–514.

135. Silk HJ, Perez-Atayde AR. Fatal varicella in steroid-dependent asthma. J Allergy Clin Immunol 1988; 81:47–51.

136. Haskell RJ, Wong BM, Hansen JE. A double-blind, randomized clinical trial of methylprednisolone in status asthmaticus. Arch Intern Med 1983; 143:1324–1327.

137. McFadden ER Jr. The chronicity of acute attacks of asthma mechanical and therapeutic implications. J Allergy Clin Immunol 1975; 56:18–26.

138. Rebuck A, Read J. Assessment and management of severe asthma. Am J Med 1971:51: 788–798.

139. Kelsen SG, Kelsen DP, Fleegler BF, Jones RC, Rodman T. Emergency room assessment and treatment of patients with acute asthma. Am J Med 1978; 64:622–627.

140. O'Driscoll BR, Kalra S, Wilson M, Pickering CAC, Carroll KB, Woodcock AA. Double-blind trial of steroid tapering in acute asthma. Lancet 1993; 341:324–327.

141. Gronneberg R, Strandberg K, Stalenheim G, Zetterstrom O. Effect in man of anti-allergic drugs on the immediate and late phase cutaneous allergic reactions induced by anti-IgE. Allergy 1981; 36:201–208.

142. Burge PS, Efthimiou J, Turner-Warwick M, Nelmes PTJ. Double-blind trials of inhaled beclomethasone dipropionate and fluocortin butyl ester in allergen-induced immediate and late asthmatic reactions. Clin Allergy 1982; 12:523–531.

143. Saavedra-Delgado AM, Mathews KP, Pan PM, Kay DR, Muilenberg ML. Dose-response studies of the suppression of white blood histamine and basophil counts by prednisone. J Allergy Clin Immunol 1980; 66:464–471.

144. Popa VT, Lerner SA. Biphasic systemic anaphylactic reaction: three illustrative cases. Ann Allergy 1984; 53:151–155.

145. Stark BJ, Sullivan TJ. Biphasic and protracted anaphylaxis. J Allergy Clin Immunol 1986; 78:76–83.

146. Davies AO, Lefkowitz RJ. Regulation of β-adrenergic receptors by steroid hormones. Ann Rev Physiol 1984; 46:119–130.

147. Schleimer RP, Davidson DA, Lichtenstein LM, Adkinson NF. Selective inhibition of arachidonic acid metabolite release from human lung tissue by antiinflammatory steroids. J Immunol 1986; 136:3006–3011.

148. Poothullil J, Umemoto L, Dolovich J, Hargreave FE, Day RP. Inhibition by prednisone of late cutaneous allergic responses induced by antiserum to human IgE. J Allergy Clin Immunol 1976; 57:164–167.

149. Sonin L, Grammer LC, Greenberger PA, Patterson R. Idiopathic anaphylaxis. Ann Intern Med 1983; 99:634.

150. Boxer MB, Greenberger PA, Patterson R. The impact of prednisone in life-threatening idiopathic anaphylaxis: reduction in acute episodes and medical costs. Ann Allergy 1989; 62: 201–204.

151. Song Sansan, Yarnold PR, Yango C, Patterson R, Harris KE. Outcome of prophylactic therapy for idiopathic anaphylaxis. Ann Intern Med 1991; 114:133–136.

152. Greenberger PA. Idiopathic anaphylaxis. Immunol Allergy Clin North Am 1992; 23: 571–583.

153. Wong S, Dykewicz MS, Patterson R. Idiopathic anaphylaxis: a clinical summary of 175 patients. Arch Intern Med 1990; 150:1323–1328.

154. Wiggins CA, Dykewicz MS, Patterson R. Corticosteroid-dependent idiopathic anaphylaxis: a report of five cases. J Allergy Clin Immunol 1989; 84:311–315.

155. Patterson R, Wong S, Dykewicz MS, Harris KE. Malignant idiopathic anaphylaxis. J Allergy Clin Immunol 1990; 85:86–88.

156. Greenberger PA, Patterson R, Radin RC. Two pretreatment regimens for high-risk patients receiving radiographic contrast media [abstract]. J Allergy Clin Immunol 1984; 74:164.

157. Greenberger PA, Patterson R, Radin RC. Two pretreatment regimens for high-risk patients receiving radiographic contrast media. J Allergy Clin Immunol 1984; 74:540–543.

158. Greenberger PA, Patterson R, Tapio CM. Prophylaxis against repeated radiocontrast media reactions in 857 cases. Ann Intern Med 1985; 145:2197–2200.

159. Marshall C, Lieberman P. Analysis of 3 pretreatment procedures to prevent anaphylactoid reactions to radiocontrast in previous reactors. J Allergy Clin Immunol 1989; 83:254.

160. Patterson R, DeSwarte RD, Greenberger PA, Grammer LC. Drug allergy and protocols for management of drug allergies NER. Allergy Proc 1986; 7:325–342.

161. Lieberman P, Siegle RL, Treadwell G. Radiocontrast reactions. Clin Rev Allergy 1986; 4: 229–245.

162. Borish L, Matloff SM, Findlay SR. Radiographic contrast media—induced noncardiogenic pulmonary edema: case report and review of the literature. J Allergy Clin Immunol 1984; 74:104–107.

163. Madowitz JS, Schweiger MJ. Severe anaphylactoid reaction to radiographic contrast media. JAMA 1979; 241:2813–2815.

164. Storms W, Bronsky E, Findlay S, et al. Once daily triamcinolone acetonide nasal spray is effective for the treatment of perennial allergic rhinitis. Ann Allergy. 1991; 66:329–334.

165. Siegel SC. Topical intranasal corticosteroid therapy in rhinitis. J Allergy Clin Immunol 1988; 81:984–991.

166. Simons FER, Simons KJ. Pharmacologic treatment of rhinitis. Clin Rev Allergy 1984; 2: 237–253.

167. Brodgen RN, Pinder RM, Sawyer PR, et al. Beclomethasone dipropionate. II. Allergic rhinitis and other conditions. Drugs 1975;10:211.

168. Mygind N, Pedersen CB, Prytz S, et al. Treatment of nasal polyps with intranasal beclomethasone dipropionate aerosol. Clin Allergy 1975;5:159.

169. Pedersen CB, Mygind N, Sorensen H, Prytz S. Long term treatment of nasal polyps with beclomethasone dipropionate aerosol. II. Clinical results. Acta Otolaryngol (Stockh) 1976;82: 256–259.

170. Tandon MK, Strahan EG. Double-blind cross-over trial comparing beclomethasone dipropionate and sodium cromoglycate in perennial allergic rhinitis. Clin Allergy 1980;10:459–462.

171. Brown HM, Engler C, English JR. A comparative trial of flunisolide and sodium cromoglycate nasal sprays in the treatment of seasonal allergic rhinitis. Clin Allergy 1981; 11:169–173.

172. Bjerrum P, Illum P. Treatment of seasonal allergic rhinitis with budesonide and disodium cromoglycate. Allergy 1985;40:65–69.

173. Simons FER, Simons KJ. Pharmacologic treatment of rhinitis. Clin Rev Allergy 1984;2: 237–253.

174. Meltzer EO, Schatz M. Pharmacotherapy of rhinitis—1987 and beyond. Immunol Allergy Clin 1987; 7:57–91.

175. Ackerman MN, Friedman RA, Doyle WJ, et al. Antigen-induced eustachian tube obstruction: an intranasal provocative challenge test. J Allergy Clin Immunol 1984; 73:604–609.

176. Zwillich CW, Pickett C, Hanson FN, Weil JV. Disturbed sleep and prolonged apnea during nasal obstruction in normal men. Am Rev Respir Dis 1981; 124:158–160.

177. Mabry RI. Intraturbinal steroid injection: indications, results and complications. South Med J 1978; 71:789.

178. McCleve D, Goldstein J, Silver S. Corticosteroid injections of the nasal turbinates: past experience and precautions. Otolaryngology 1978; 86:851.

179. Hartwig S, Linden M, Laurent C, Vargo A-K, Lindqvist N. Budesonide nasal spray as prophylactic treatment after polypectomy. J Laryngol Otol 1988; 102:148–151.

180. Chalton R, Mackay I, Wilson R, Cole P. Double blind, placebo controlled trial of betamethasone nasal drops for nasal polyposis. Br Med J 1985; 291:788.

181. Sorensen H, Mygind N, Pedersen CB, Prytz S. Long-term treatment of nasal polyps with beclomethasone dipropionate aerosol. Acta Otolaryngol (Stockh) 1976; 82:260–262.

182. Dingsoer G, Kramer J, Olsholt R, Doederstroem T. Flunisolide nasal spray 0.025% in the prophylactic treatment of nasal polyposis after polypectomy; a randomized double blind parallel placebo controlled study. Rhinology 1985; 23:49–59.

183. Toogood JH. Role of inhaled steroids in the management of chronic rhinitis. Contemp Allergies 1991; 1:4–19.

184. Toogood JH. Some clinical aspects of the pharmacotherapy of rhinitis and asthma. In: Mygind N, Pipkorn U, Dahl R, eds. Rhinitis and Asthma: Similarities and Differences. Copenhagen: Munksgaard, 1990:289–306.

185. Lildholdt T, Kortholm B. Beclomethasone nasal spray in the treatment of middle-ear effusion— a double-blind study. Int J Pediatr Otorhinolaryngol 1982; 4:133.

186. Webb EL. Nasal candidiasis in a patient on long-term topical intranasal corticosteroid therapy. J Allergy Clin Immunol 1993; 91:680–681.

187. Schoelzel EP, Menzel ML. Nasal sprays and perforation of the nasal septum (letter). JAMA 1985; 253:2046.

188. Soderberg-Warner ML. Nasal septal perforation associated with topical corticosteroid therapy. J Pediatr 1984; 105:840–841.

189. Holopainen E, Malmberg H, Binder E. Long-term follow-up of intranasal beclomethasone treatment. A clinical and histologic study. Acta Otolaryngol 1983; 386:270–273.

190. Mygind N, Sorensen H, Pedersen CB. The nasal mucosa during long-term treatment with beclomethasone dipropionate aerosol. Acta Otolaryngol 1978; 85:437–443.

191. Greenberger PA, Patterson R. Beclomethasone dipropionate for severe asthma during pregnancy. Ann Intern Med 1983; 98:478–480.

192. Barber KA. Uses and abuses of topical corticosteroids. Med North Am 1989; 32:5812–5820.

193. Ortonne JP. Clinical potential of topical corticosteroids. Drugs 1988; 36(suppl 5):38–42.

194. Takeda K, Arase S, Takahashi S. Side effects of topical corticosteroids and their prevention. Drugs 1988; 36(suppl 5):15–23.

195. Cook LJ, Freinkel RK, Zugerman C, et al. Iatrogenic hyperadrenocorticism during topical steroid therapy: assessment of systemic effects by metabolic criteria. J Am Acad Dermatol 1982; 6:1054–1060.

196. Himathongkam T, Dasanabhairochana P, Pitchayayothin N, et al. Florid Cushing's syndrome and hirsutism induced by desoximetasone. JAMA 1978; 239:430–431.

197. James VHT, Munro DD, Feiwel M. Pituitary–adrenal function after occlusive topical therapy with betamethasone-17-valerate. Lancet 1967; 2:1059–1061.

198. May P, Stein EJ, Ryter RJ, Hirsh FS, Michel B, Levy RP. Cushing syndrome from percutaneous absorption of triamcinolone cream. Arch Intern Med 1976; 136:612–613.

199. Degreef H, Dooms-Goossens A. The new corticosteroids: are they effective and safe? Dermatol Ther 1993; 11:155–160.

200. Sudilovsky A, Muir JG, Bocobo FC. A comparison of single and multiple applications of halcinonide cream. Int J Dermatol 1981; 20:609–613.

201. Becker BA, Gaspari AA. Pemphigus vulgaris and vegetans. Dermatol Clin 1993; 11:429–451.

202. Korman NJ. Bullous pemphigoid. Dermatol Clin 1993; 11:483–497.

203. Sue MA, Kwong FK, Klaustermeyer WB. A comparison of intravenous hydrocortisone, methylprednisolone, and dexamethasone in acute bronchial asthma. Ann Allergy 1986; 56:406–409.

204. Pedersen BK, Laursen LC, Lervang HH, et al. Methylprednisolone pulse therapy in severe acute asthma. Allergy 1987; 42:154–157.

205. Raimondi AC, Figueroa-Casas JC, Roncoroni AJ. Comparison between high and moderate doses of hydrocortisone in the treatment of status asthmaticus. Chest 1986; 89:832–835.

206. Britton MG, Collins JV, Brown D, Fairhurst NPA, Lambert RG. High-dose corticosteroids in severe acute asthma. Br Med J 1976; 2:73–74.

207. Harfi H, Hanissian AS, Crawford LV. Treatment of status asthmaticus in children with high doses and conventional doses of methylprednisolone. Pediatrics 1978; 61:829–831.

208. McFadden ER, Kiser R, deGroot WJ, Holmes B, Kiker R, Viser G. A controlled study of the effects of single doses of hydrocortisone on the resolution of acute attacks of asthma. Am J Med 1976; 60:52–59.

209. Tanaka RM, Santiago SM, Kuhn GJ, Williams RE, Klaustermeyer WB. Intravenous methyl-prednisolone in adults in status asthmaticus. Comparison of two dosages. Chest 1982; 82: 438–440.

210. Webb JR. Dose response of patients to oral corticosteroid treatment during exacerbations of asthma. Br Med J 1986; 292:1045–1047.

211. Knox AJ, Mascie-Taylor BH, Muers MF. Acute hydrocortisone myopathy in acute severe asthma. Thorax 1986; 41:411–412.

212. Marle WV, Woods KL. Acute hydrocortisone myopathy. Br Med J 1980; 281:271.

213. McDougal BA, Whittier FC, Cross DE. Sudden death after bolus steroid therapy for acute rejection. Transplant Proc 1976; 8:493–496.

214. Dolovich M, Ruffin R, Newhouse MT. Clinical evaluation of a simple demand inhalation device MDI aerosol delivery device. Chest 1983; 84:36–41.

215. Newman SP, Moren F, Pavia D, Little F, Clarke SW. Deposition of pressurized suspension aerosols inhaled through extension devices. Am Rev Respir Dis 1981; 124:317–320.

216. Laity A, Toogood JH, Mazza JA, Moote DW. Profile of ambulatory care for chronic asthma in a tertiary referral clinic. Clin Invest Med 1991; 14(suppl):A6.

Index

Active catalytic subunit, 3
Adenylate cyclase pathway, 3
ADP-ribosylation, 9, 15
Adrenergic receptors, 3, 5, 245, 491–497,
    501–504, 506, 508, 615, 617, 626
  α- and β-adrenergic receptors, 3, 5, 245,
    491, 495, 615
  effect of corticosteroids, 17, 114
  regulation, 18
  role in asthma, 437, 497, 626
  site-directed mutagenesis, 53, 390, 397,
    398, 496
Allergen presentation, 217
Alveolar marcrophage, 274, 510
γ-Aminobutyric acid (GABA) receptor, 2
Anaphylatoxins, 132, 133, 199
Antigen receptor-associated motif (ARAM), 86
Antigen-binding fragment (Fab), 33, 35, 80,
    123, 124, 128
Antihistamines, 246, 345, 609–611, 615–621,
    624, 629–631, 667–669
  in urticaria, 630, 631
Apoptosis, 45, 120, 237
Arthritis, 113, 170, 204, 420, 478
Arylsulfatase, 13
Axon reflex, 336, 344

B-cell activation, 129

B7, CD80, 123, 217
BALT, 165, 292
Bordetella pertussis, 272
Bradykinin, 589–590, 650
Bronchial brushing, 267
Bronchial challenge, 268, 643–646
  direct bronchial challenges, 645
  indications for testing, 630, 640, 697
  pharmacological modulation of indirect
    challenges, 241–243, 249, 650–651
  reproducibility, 641–643
Bronchoalveolar lavage, 267–268, 661–662

Cadherins, 100, 102
Calcitonin gene-related peptide (CGRP), 109,
    292, 335–337
Calcium antagonists, 563, 564, 645, 647
Calcium channels, 563–564, 645–647
  receptor-operated channels, 562
  voltage operated channels, 562
CALLA, 125
cAMP-dependent protein kinase, 3, 48, 247
CD106, 103, 104
CD11b/CD18 (Mac-1), 57, 106
CD15s, 100, 102
CD23, 89, 126, 271, 275, 316, 366–372
CD31, 103, 104, 107
CD54, 103, 104, 100, 113, 184, 271

About the Editors

ROBERT G. TOWNLEY is Chief of the Division of Allergy and Professor in the Departments of Medicine and Medical Microbiology and Immunology at Creighton University School of Medicine, Omaha, Nebraska. A Fellow of the American College of Chest Physicians and the American Academy of Allergy, Asthma and Immunology and a member of the American Federation for Clinical Research and the American Thoracic Society, among other organizations, he is the coeditor of two books on asthma and allergy mechanisms and the author or coauthor of more than 165 professional papers and book chapters and over 250 abstracts. Certified by the American Board of Internal Medicine and the American Board of Allergy and Immunology, Dr. Townley received the M.D. degree (1955) from Creighton University School of Medicine. In 1988 he was awarded the Creighton University School of Medicine Distinguished Research Career Award and he was named among the Best Doctors in America in 1992, 1993, and 1994.

DEVENDRA K. AGRAWAL is Director of Research at the Allergic Disease Center and the Creighton Vascular Center and Associate Professor in the Departments of Internal Medicine and Medical Microbiology and Immunology at Creighton University School of Medicine, Omaha, Nebraska. The author or coeditor of four books and the author or coauthor of over 250 peer-reviewed papers, book chapters, and abstracts, he is a member of the American Academy of Allergy, Asthma and Immunology, the American Society for Pharmacology and Experimental Therapeutics, and the American Thoracic Society, among other organizations. Dr. Agrawal received the Ph.D. degree (1978) in biochemistry from Lucknow University, India, and the Ph.D. degree (1984) in medical sciences from McMaster University, Hamilton, Ontario, Canada.